# Individualized Healthcare Plans for the School Nurse

## Concepts, Framework, Issues, and Applications for School Nursing Practice

**Editors**
Cynthia K. Silkworth, Martha J. Arnold,
Judith F. Harrigan, Donna Shipley Zaiger

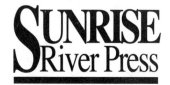

**S**UNRISE
**R**iver **P**ress

The publisher and authors have made a conscientious effort to ensure any recommendations or procedures outlined in this book are proper, accurate, and in accordance with accepted school nursing practices at the time of publication. As is the case with health care in general and school nursing in particular, each specific health issue and each individual question combine to form a unique situation, not easily addressed at a distance nor from the pages of a book designed to provide generic information on a wide range of subjects. While this work provides recognized structures, processes and procedures, the recommendations found in this book are for illustrative purposes only, and are not a substitute for professional on-site assessments and evaluations to determine the appropriate recommendations for each situation. The publisher and authors make no representations or warranties of any kind regarding the materials in this work nor shall they be liable for any damages resulting, in whole or in part, from the use of or reliance upon this material.

## Dedications

To my fellow editors and the authors, for their commitment and expertise that made this book possible. CKS

To my three grandgirls, AlexAnn Koecher, Hannah Koecher and Emma Arnold, who have really taught me how to be a compassionate school nurse and grandma. MJA

To the many school nurses in New York, Colorado, and across the nation who have inspired me to seek answers, develop resources, and continue to progress in my learning. JFH

To the professional nurses who plan and care for the health needs of children and adolescents in the school setting. I appreciate the inspiration and encouragement these school nurses provide which continually enhances my practice. I acknowledge the faithful support of my family that allowed me time to work on this project. DSZ

ISBN-13  978-0-9624814-6-8
ISBN-10  0-9624814-6-7

39966 Grand Avenue
North Branch, MN 55056 USA
(651) 277-1400 or (800) 895-4585
www.schoolnursebooks.com

Library of Congress Cataloging-in-Publication Data

Individualized healthcare plans for the school nurse : concepts, framework,
    issues and applications for school nursing practice / edited by Cynthia K.
    Silkworth ... [et al.].
      p. ; cm.
    Includes bibliographical references and index.
    ISBN-13: 978-0-9624814-6-8
    ISBN-10: 0-9624814-6-7
    1. School nursing.  2. Nursing care plans.
I. Silkworth, Cynthia K.
    [DNLM: 1. School Nursing--methods.  2. Nursing Assessment--Adoles-
  cent.  3. Nursing Assessment--Child.  4. Nursing Care--Adolescent.
    5. Nursing Care--Child.    WY 113 I39 2005]
    LB3405.I53 2005
    371.7'12--dc22

                            2005022199

# Contents

# Editors and Contributors

## Editors

**Cynthia K. Silkworth, R.N., M.P.H, C.S.N.P., F.N.A.S.N.**
Coordinator for School Health Services and School Nurse, White Bear Lake Area Schools, White Bear Lake, Minnesota

**Martha J. Arnold, R.N, B.S.N, P.H.N., F.N.A.S.N.**
Licensed School Nurse, Lifelong Learning Early Childhood Center, St. Francis Public Schools, St. Francis, Minnesota

**Judith F. Harrigan, R.N., M.S.N., F.N.A.S.N.**
Principal Consultant, School Health Services
Colorado Department of Education, Denver, Colorado

**Donna Shipley Zaiger R.N., B.S.N., N.C.S.N., F.N.A.S.N.**
Independent School Health Consultant and Author
School Nurse, Lee's Summit R-7 School District, Lee's Summit, Missouri

## Contributors

**Valerie S. Baldocchi, R.N., M.S.N.**
Graduate Student, Lewis University, Romeoville, Illinois

**Elisabeth Barclay, R.N., B.S.N., M.A., Ed.**
Certified School Nurse, Kinglsey Junior High School and Towanda Elementary School, McLean County Unit District No. 5, Normal, Illinois

**Martha Dewey Bergren, R.N., D.N.S., B.C., N.C.S.N., F.N.A.S.N.**
Clinical Assistant Professor, Coordinator of School Nurse Master Program, Department of Public Health, Mental Health, & Administrative Nursing, University of Illinois, Chicago College of Nursing, Chicago, Illinois

**Sue Boos, R.N., M.S., C.S., A.R.N.P.**
Associate Professor of Nursing, Fort Hays State University, Hays, Kansas

**Patricia Brandstaetter, B.A., M.A.**
Minnesota Other Health Disabilities Specialist, Northeast Service Cooperative, Mt. Iron, Minnesota

**Cheryl R. Brubaker, R.N., M.S.N, A.P.R.N-B.C., F.N.P.**
Special Education Resource Nurse, Albuquerque Public Schools Nursing Services, Albuquerque, New Mexico

**Jayne Chatterton, R.N., B.S.N., C.D.E.**
Diabetes Education Specialist, Children's Hospitals and Clinics, St. Paul, Minnesota

**Constance M. Cotter, R.N., M.N.**
Clinic Nurse Liaison, Wichita Public Schools, Wichita, Kansas

**Katherine J. Cuddy, R.N., B.S.N**
School Nurse, Guilmette School, Lawrence School Department, Lawrence, Massachusetts

**Tambra R. Dahleheimer, R.N., M.S., C.N.P.-Peds, L.S.N.**
Certified Nurse Practitioner, Children's Hospitals and Clinics of Minnesota, St. Paul, Minnesota

**Janice Denehy, R.N., Ph.D.**
Executive Director, *The Journal of School Nursing*
Associate Professor Emeritus, The University of Iowa College of Nursing, Iowa City, Iowa

**Jacalyn P. Dougherty, R.N., Ph.D.**
Instructor, University of Colorado at Denver and Health Sciences Center, Denver, Colorado

**Colleen J. Duffy, R.N., B.S.N.**
School Nurse, Glenview Academy/ The Gramon School, Fairfield, New Jersey

**Barbara Erickson, R.N., L.S.N., C.P.N.P.**
School Nurse for a Federal Setting IV High School, Minneapolis Public School District, Minneapolis, Minnesota

**Charlotte R. Gorun, R.N., B.S.N., C.S.N.**
School Nurse, Paterson Board of Education, Paterson, New Jersey

**Margarita Fernan Granthom, R.N., N.C.S.N.**
School Nurse and District Coordinator, District 504, Sweetwater County School District Number One, Rock Sprints, Wyoming

**Lorali Gray, R.N., B.S.N., M.Ed., N.C.S.N.**
District Nurse, Mount Baker School District, Deming, Washington

**Kella Haren, R.N., B.S.N.**
Licensed School Nurse, Youngstown State University, Youngstown, Ohio

**Anne L. Hedges, R.N., B.S.N., M.S.N., N.C.S.N.**
School Health Administrator, Health Care District of Palm Beach County, West Palm Beach, Florida

**Denise A. Herrman, R.N., B.S.N., M.S., C.P.N.P.**
Licensed School Nurse, Saint Paul Public Schools, St. Paul, Minnesota

**Carolyn F. Holman, R.N., M.S.N., C.S.N., C.F.N.P., F.N.A.S.N.**
Family Nurse Practitioner, Elberta Family Practice, Elberta, Alabama

**Ann Marie Hoxie, R.N., M.S., L.S.N, C.N.P-P.**
Administrator for Student Wellness, Saint Paul Public Schools, St. Paul, Minnesota

**Emelyn L. Hudson, R.N., B.S.N.**
Health Treatment Specialist, Anchorage School District, Health Services, Anchorage, Alaska

**Deborah Kotlas Ilardi, R.N., B.S.N.**
School Nurse, Cicero-North Syracuse High School, North Syracuse Central School District, North Syracuse, New York

**Tara S. Kaup, R.N., M.S.N., L.S.N., C.D.E., A-C.E.**
School Nurse and Diabetes Resource Nurse, Saint Paul Public Schools, St. Paul, Minnesota

**Sarah Kiel, R.N., M.S.N., C.P.N.P.**
Pediatric Nurse Practitioner Coordinator, Pediatric Epilepsy Surgery, Children's Hospital, Birmingham, Alabama

**Lorali Gray, R.N., B.S.N, M.Ed., N.C.S.N.**
District Nurse, Mount Baker School District, Deming, Washington

**Patricia S. Latona, R.N., M.S.N.**
Special Education Nurse, Department of Integrated Instructional Services, Alamogordo Public Schools, Alamogordo, New Mexico

**Brenda Kay Lenz, R.N., Ph.D.**
Assistant Professor, Department of Nursing Science, St. Cloud State University, St. Cloud, Minnesota

**Marilyn Leifgren, Ed.S.**
School Psychologist, White Bear Lake Public Schools, White Bear Lake, Minnesota

**Elaine D. Level, R.N., B.S.N.**
Clinical Healthcare Consultant, Wichita, Kansas

Tona L. Leiker, R.N., M.N., A.R.N.P.-C.N.S., A.P.R.N, B.C.
Chair, Nursing Department, Tabor College, Wichita, Kansas

Janet L. Lowe, R.N., M.A., C.P.N.P.
Licensed School Nurse, Coordinator of Third Party Reimbursement, Saint Paul Public Schools, St. Paul, Minnesota

Terri Lundquist, R.N., L.S.N., M.P.H.
Licensed School Nurse, Saint Paul Public Schools, St. Paul, Minnesota

Maureen Maguire, R.N., M.S.N., P.N.P.
Assistant Professor, Johns Hopkins University School of Nursing, Baltimore, Maryland

Penny J. Makuchal, R.N., Ph.D., N.C.S.N.
School Nurse, Worcester Career and Technology Center, Newark, Maryland School Nurse Consultant for Worcester County Public Schools, Maryland Part-time Nursing Instructor, Salisbury University, Salisbury, Maryland

Nancy Manzo-Mattucci, R.N., M.S.N.
School Nurse, Baltimore County Public Schools, Baltimore, Maryland

Mary Jo Martin, R.N., B.S.N., M.A.Ed.
Licensed School Nurse, Katherine Curren Elementary, Hopkins, Minnesota

Sharon D. Martin, R.N., M.S.N., A.P.R.N., B.C.
Associate Professor of Nursing, Saint Joseph's College, Standish, Maine

Katelyn A. McGowan, B.S.N. Candidate
Boston College, William F. Connell School of Nursing, Boston, Massachusetts

Jean Mientus, R.N., B.S.N.
Certified School Nurse, Carlow College, Pittsburgh, Pennsylvania

Lindsey W. Minchella, R.N., M.S.N., N.C.S.N.
School Nurse, Consultant for Special Education, Greater Lafayette Area Special Services, Lafayette School Corporation, Lafayette, Indiana

Carole Ellerbe Moore, R.N., B.S.N., N.C.S.N.
School Nurse, Grace School, Houston, Texas

Nancy W. Mosca, R.N., Ph.D.
Professor of Nursing, Coordinator of School Nurse Program, Youngstown State University, Youngstown, Ohio
Marcia S. Mullen, R.N., M.S.
School Nurse, Windham School Department, Windham, Maine

Mary E. Newell, R.N., M.S.N.
Nurse Facilitator, Kent School District, Kent, Washington

Andrea D. Posey, R.N., M.S.N.
Director, Cardiovascular Services Unit, Alaska Regional Hospital, Anchorage, Alaska

Susan Poulton, R.N., C.S., M.S.N.
Health Services Director, Iowa City Community School District, Iowa City, Iowa

Annette L. Perschke, R.N., B.S.N., C.R.R.N., C.N.R.N.
Clinical Nurse I, Johns Hopkins Hospital Children's Center, Baltimore, Maryland Clinical Faculty, Johns Hopkins University School of Nursing, Baltimore, Maryland

Clara J. Richardson, R.N., B.C., M.S.N.
Clinical Assistant Professor, Purdue University School of Nursing, West Lafayette, Indiana

Sally Zentner Schoessler, R.N., B.S.N., S.N.T., M.S.Ed.
School Nurse Teacher, Sherman Elementary School, Rush-Henriette Central School District, Henrietta, New York

Lacy E. Scott, R.N., B.S.N.
Child Find Nurse, Aurora Public Schools, Aurora, Colorado

Jeanne Sedgwick, R.N., M.S., L.S.N., N.C.S.N.
District Special Education Resource for Other Health Disabilities and Traumatic Brain Injury, Saint Paul Public Schools, St. Paul, Minnesota

Mariann Smith, R.N., B.S.N., M.N.
Retired School Nurse and Medical Education Liaison Nurse, Wichita Public Schools, Wichita, Kansas

Linda L. Solum, R.N., M.A., P.H.N., L.S.N.
Health Services Coordinator, ISD 197, West St. Paul/ Mendota Heights/ Eagan School District, Minnesota

Katherine M. Sommer, R.N., M.S., C.N.P-P., L.S.N.
Licensed School Nurse, South Washington County Schools, Cottage Grove, Minnesota

MaryAnn Tapper Strawhacker, R.N., B.S.N., M.P.H.
Special Education Nurse Consultant, Heartland Area Education Agency, Johnston, Iowa

Mary A. Swanson, R.N., B.S.N., M.S.
Licensed School Nurse, Robbinsdale Area Schools, Robbinsdale, Minnesota Adjunct Faculty, University of Minnesota School of Nursing, Minneapolis, Minnesota

Gail Synoground, R.N., A.R.N.P., Ed.D., F.N.A.S.N, retired
Professor emeritus, retired, Intercollegiate College of Nursing, Washington State University, Spokane, Washington

Heidi M. Toth, R.N., M.S., C.I.C.
School Nurse, Freehold Township Schools, Freehold, New Jersey Adjunct Professor, Monmouth University, West Long Beach, New Jersey

Roxanne Truen, R.N., M.S.N., P.N.P.
Licensed School Nurse, Dowling Urban Environmental Learning Center, Minneapolis Public Schools, Minneapolis, Minnesota

Judith A. Vessey, R.N., Ph.D., M.B.A., P.N.P., F.A.A.N
Lelia Holden Carroll Professor of Nursing, Boston College, William F. Connell School of Nursing, Boston, Massachusetts

Jeanette H. Williams, R.N., M.H.S.
Diagnostic Nurse, Special School District, St. Louis County, Missouri

Sharon Yearous, R.N., M.S.N, A.R.N.P., C.P.N.P., N.C.S.N.
Pediatric Nurse Practitioner and Nursing Department Faculty, Joint appointment with Mercy Medical Center/Xavier High School/Mount Mercy College in Cedar Rapids, Iowa

Julie Young-Burns, R.N., M.S.N., C.P.N.P., L.S.N.
Mental and Chemical Health Lead, Safe Schools/Healthy Students Initiative, Positive School Climate Team, Minneapolis Public Schools, Minneapolis, Minnesota

## Reviewers

Margaret Lunney, R.N., Ph.D.
Professor and Graduate Programs Coordinator, College of Staten Island, City University of New York, Department of Nursing, Staten Island, New York.

Nadine C. Schwab, B.S.N, M.P.H., N.C.S.N, F.N.A.S.N.
Supervisor of Health Services, Westport Public Schools, Westport, Connecticut,

## Chapter One

# Individualized Healthcare Plans

### Denise A. Herrmann

## Introduction

The year 2002 marked the 100th anniversary of school nursing in America. In 1902, Lillian Wald, founder of the Henry Street Settlement, assigned Lina Rogers to be the first school nurse in New York City. Lina Rogers' task was to make a difference in the school absentee rate in 1 month. Her success was astonishing, and thus began the specialty practice of school nursing. Throughout the following years, school nurses and the practice of school nursing evolved to meet the changing needs of students, families, communities, and society.

The National Association of School Nurses (NASN) has defined school nursing as a specialized practice of professional nursing that advances the well-being, academic success, and lifelong achievement of students. To that end, school nurses facilitate positive student responses to normal development; promote health and safety; intervene in actual and potential health problems; provide case management services; and actively collaborate with others to build student and family capacity for adaptation, self-management, self-advocacy, and learning (NASN, 1999).

Individualized healthcare plans (IHPs) are a tool that school nurses use to facilitate the well-being and the academic success of all learners. The purpose of this book is to help school nurses develop IHPs that meet the needs of students and clearly document school nursing practice.

## Why Should School Nurses Use IHPs?

The nursing process emerged in the 1970s as the scientific approach to the identification and solution of problems in nursing practice. As the cornerstone of nursing practice, the nursing process provides a systematic, yet dynamic, method for the delivery and evaluation of nursing care. As such, the nursing process forms the foundation of the scope and standards of professional school nursing practice (NASN & American Nurses Association [ANA], 2001). The nursing process includes assessment, diagnosis, outcome identification, planning, implementation, and evaluation. The nursing process takes the guesswork out of providing care, relying on a scientific knowledge base to make decisions about the delivery of nursing care (Denehy, 2004). It is applicable to all areas of nursing practice, including school nursing. Utilization of the nursing process in schools results in the development of IHPs for students who have health-related issues.

When students at school need ongoing nursing management, a documented plan of care is essential (Hootman, 1996a). An IHP documents the information from the assessment phase, a nursing diagnosis, the student goals and outcomes to be achieved, the nursing interventions to be utilized, and ways in which the plan's effectiveness will be measured.

Documentation promotes sound planning, coordination, continuity, and evaluation of care (Schwab, Panettieri, & Bergren, 1998). A review of the literature outlines the many purposes of care planning and IHP development for students. Carpenito (1997) stated that care plans have two professional purposes—administrative and clinical. These categories can be applied to IHPs as follows.

Administrative purposes of IHPs:
- To define the focus of nursing, validating the nurse's position in the school
- To facilitate the management of health conditions to optimize learning
- To differentiate the accountability of the school nurse from others in the school (i.e., paraprofessionals, teachers)
- To provide criteria for reviewing and evaluating care-quality assurance
- To provide data for statistical reports, research, third-party reimbursement, and legal evidence
- To create a safer process for delegation of nursing care in the school setting

Clinical purposes of IHPs:
- To clarify and consolidate health information that is meaningful for students, families, and staff
- To establish the priority set of nursing diagnoses for a student
- To provide a method of communication to direct the nursing care needed by a particular student
- To build the foundation for documentation
- To ensure consistency and continuity of care as students move within and outside of school districts
- To direct specific interventions for the student, family, and other school staff to implement
- To provide a means to review and evaluate nursing goals and outcome criteria

## IHPs: Prioritizing Your Student Population

School nurses often have high to unreasonable student ratios, and in some cases school nurses may be in a particular school only 1 day a week. School nurses can feel overwhelmed by the volume of students, the health needs of students, or both. Every student who has special healthcare needs will require an IHP. Nurses working in the school setting may need to set limits as to which of a student's multiple health issues they can manage within the constraints of the assigned student population (Hootman, 1996b).

School nurses should prioritize students and their needs. Begin by first identifying those students whose health needs overwhelmingly affect their daily functioning or impact their education or educational environment. Consider the following in setting priorities:

- Students who may be medically fragile with multiple health needs
- Students who require extended nursing care or multiple contacts with the nurse/delegatee during the school day
- Students who must have health needs addressed as part of the individualized education program (IEP) or 504 process
- Students with health needs that are addressed on a daily basis

School nurses are also encouraged to consult with other school nurses within the school district, community, or state. Remember that an IHP does not have to address every health issue of the student. Later in this chapter, prioritization of health needs of individual students will be addressed.

## Components of the IHP

The IHP provides a format for assessment (summarizing key information); nursing diagnosis (synthesizing a problem statement); developing goals, interventions, and outcomes to meet the health needs of students; and evaluation.

## Assessment

The assessment provides the foundation for development of an IHP. An accurate assessment is needed for a meaningful IHP. This is the phase where the school nurse collects data that describe the student's health status, risks, concerns, and strengths. There are five main areas to include in the assessment: (1) health history, (2) current health status/management, (3) self-care skills/needs, (4) psychosocial status, and (5) health issues related to learning.

Most nurses utilize a combination of several methods to complete a comprehensive assessment. These include:

- Interview of student and/or family
- Review of past medical, nursing, and educational records, such as hospital or outpatient reports, IHPs, emergency care plans (ECPs), IEPs, and 504 plans
- Review of current medical records
- Consultation with other community providers, physician and primary healthcare providers, hospital staff, home care agency, or counseling services
- Physical assessment/measures of pertinent body systems (i.e., sensory functioning, vision and hearing)

- Interview of other school staff who interact with student
- Observation of student in the classroom

## Nursing Diagnosis

Individual pieces of data by themselves have no meaning. It is the method of organizing the data about a particular student and drawing a conclusion that separates professional school nurses from paraprofessionals, teachers, and other school staff. Nursing diagnoses define what school nurses distinctly identify and contribute as autonomous practitioners in the school setting, rather than as subordinates to another professional (Hootman, 1996a).

The nursing diagnosis gives direction to outcome identification, the selection of nursing interventions, and the evaluation of the interventions implemented (Denehy, 2004). There are three types of nursing diagnoses: actual, risk, and wellness (NANDA International, 2003, p. 263). Each nursing diagnosis has its own definition and may also have defining characteristics, related factors, or risk factors. In deciding upon the most appropriate nursing diagnosis, the school nurse uses clinical judgment to compare the information from the assessment to the definition, defining characteristics, and related/risk factors associated with a specific diagnosis.

NANDA developed definitions and a diagnostic classification system to uniformly and precisely identify the health issues for which nurses are accountable. NANDA defines a nursing diagnosis as "a clinical judgment about an individual, family or a community response to actual and potential health problems or life process. A nursing diagnosis provides the basis for selection of nursing interventions to achieve outcomes for which the nurse is accountable" (NANDA, 2003, p. 263). In 2001, the NASN declared in a position paper that it would support the use of NANDA diagnosis in the school health setting.

## Prioritizing Nursing Diagnoses

The number of nursing diagnoses that may be appropriate for any given student can inundate nurses. Just as school nurses must determine for which students an IHP will be developed, they must determine which health issues can be managed within the limitations of the school environment. When school nurses determine the priority of nursing diagnoses, they then can best direct the resources toward goal achievement. Carpenito (1997) described priority diagnoses as those nursing diagnoses that, if not managed now, will deter progress to the achievement of outcomes or will negatively affect the client's functional status.

School nurses must be realistic and knowledgeable of resources available when prioritizing nursing diagnoses. Resources including the time required and skill of the school nurse and any delegatees must be considered. In setting priorities, school nurses should focus first on the health issues that affect safety (physical and environmental needs that are potentially life-threatening). The next priority would be those diagnoses that affect the student's ability to learn and succeed in the educational setting. Finally, overall consider-

## Goals

Once the nursing diagnoses have been determined and prioritized, goals are developed. A goal is a hoped-for outcome, a statement of what is desired. It should be realistic in terms of student potential and the nurse's abilities. Goals should be worded in a clear and concise manner that can be understood by all team members. Often it is appropriate for the student and/or family to help in the planning of goals. Goals can be short-term or long-term, but in either case they must be measurable. Student goals should describe a measurable behavior of the student that is evident after nursing interventions have been completed. Measurable behaviors include resolution of a problem or evidence of progress toward an improved health status or continued maintenance of good functioning.

Bulechek and McCloskey (1985) define outcomes as the guideposts to the selection of nursing interventions. There should exist readily identifiable and logical links between the diagnosis and plan of care. The activities prescribed should assist or enable the client to meet the identified expected outcome. During evaluation, student goals are used to determine the success or appropriateness of the IHP. If goals are not achieved or progress is not evident, the school nurse should revise the IHP.

## Nursing Interventions

A nursing diagnosis requires that the nurse prescribe the definitive treatment for the situation. A nursing intervention is defined as any treatment, based upon clinical judgment and knowledge, that a nurse performs to enhance patient/client outcomes (Dochterman & Bulechek, 2004). The Nursing Interventions Classification (NIC) provides a standardized language for what nurses do and lists specific activities that nurses can select in implementing the intervention (Denehy, 2004, p. 14). The NIC defines five types of nursing interventions: direct care, indirect care, community interventions, nurse-initiated treatments, and physician-initiated treatments. The school nurse uses clinical judgment in selecting the nursing intervention(s) that will achieve the desired goal.

In the school setting it is important to remember that appropriate interventions may vary across settings, and that some interventions may be delegated to other staff. Additionally, some interventions may be shared with other school staff without necessitating delegation. An example of this is shown in **Figure 1.**

## Expected Student Outcomes

An outcome is what the student is expected to do, experience, or learn. To be measurable, it is paired with a modifier that is the *when, where, and how.* The essential characteristics of outcome criteria are that they must be

- long-term or short-term,
- in measurable behaviors,
- specific in content and time, and
- realistic and achievable.

Measurable verbs are verbs that describe the exact action or behavior of the client that the nurse can validate by seeing or hearing it or less frequently, by touch, taste, or smell. For example, instead of stating, "The student will *experience* less depression," it is better to state, "The student will *report* less depression." School nurses should not choose outcomes that cannot be achieved utilizing the interventions that were selected, in the time frame chosen, or in the context of the school setting.

The use of student outcome language closely mirrors the use of student learning objectives, which educators are familiar with and use when developing an IEP. This similarity can promote understanding and collaboration as school nurses work with the educational team to meet the health needs of students.

School nurses may also find the Nursing Outcomes Classification (NOC) system, which was developed in 1991 after the development of NIC, to be helpful in completing the nursing process. The NOC provides a standardized, concrete method to measure outcomes. A nursing outcome is defined as an individual, family, or community state, behavior, or perception that is measured along a continuum in response to a nursing intervention(s) (Moorhead, Johnson, & Maas, 2004). An outcome has five components:

---

**Figure 1**

| Nursing Diagnosis | Goals | Nursing Interventions | Expected Outcomes |
|---|---|---|---|
| Alteration in communication due to tracheostomy | Student has increased independent communication skills. | In-service training and encouraging staff to utilize methods that promote effective communication<br><br>Staff should stand in front of student, use eye contact and good volume. | Student will increase communication by one verbal or nonverbal cue weekly. |

---

label, definition, code number, indicators, and scales. The third edition of *Nursing Outcomes Classification (NOC)* has added a new outcome designed for school nurses. It is defined as "physical, cognitive/emotion and social status of school-aged children that contribute to school attendance, participation in school activities, and ability to learn" (Moorhead et al., pp. 522-523). Increasingly, it will be important to measure student outcomes that can be linked to student achievement, student attendance, student readiness, and/or student success, all of which can help demonstrate the importance of the role of school nursing.

For the purposes of this book, the chapter authors were directed to use NANDA classification and nursing diagnoses. The NIC is a system of standardized language for nursing interventions. The NOC is a standardized language of nurse-sensitive outcomes. Although the authors were not instructed to specifically use NIC and NOC for the IHPs listed, readers are encouraged to move toward using a systematic standardized nursing language as a mechanism for providing meaningful IHPs (Pavelka, McCarthy, & Denehy, 1999). The use of NANDA, NIC, and NOC by school nurses will promote quality nursing care for our clients, validate school nursing effects on our clients, and promote research endeavors (NASN, 2001).

Figure 1 provides a template for an IHP with abbreviated definitions and explanations.

## Evaluation

An IHP is the written plan of care for a student with health needs in the school setting. The IHP is not a one-time event but is dynamic through the process of evaluation. The evaluation process includes (a) reviewing the desired student goals and outcomes, (b) collecting data to determine the outcomes, (c) comparing the actual outcomes to the desired outcomes, (d) documenting the outcomes on the IHP, (e) relating the appropriateness and effectiveness of the selected interventions to the outcome, and (f) reviewing and modifying the plan of care as necessary (Denehy & Poulton, 1999).

Evaluation allows the school nurse to make judgments about the student's progress toward identified goals. Some questions that should be considered by the school nurse include the following: Is the outcome still appropriate? Does any intervention need to be added or changed to continue progress toward the goal? Is the timeline still appropriate? Can goal achievement be related to the nursing interventions given? Are there any barriers to meeting and achieving student outcomes? Were there unexpected beneficial student out-

comes? Are the nursing diagnoses still pertinent for the student's health condition?

Usually it is not necessary to rewrite the IHP. Revising the plan, making additions or deletions as appropriate, and documenting changes by dating and initialing changes to the IHP may be all that is needed. You may need to write an additional progress note to document your assessment, or subjective or objective data, which was collected or observed and prompted the revision.

IHP evaluations should be completed when any significant change occurs in the student's health status or physician-prescribed medication or treatment. If the student has a relatively stable health status, the school nurse may wish to consider establishing a periodic review so the evaluation is not forgotten.

## Summary

The role of the nurse in the school setting is to assess the health needs of children and to coordinate with staff, families, healthcare providers, and community agencies to provide a comprehensive school health program that facilitates the maximum educational opportunity for students. School nurses are stepping to the forefront of pediatric healthcare, health promotion, and education by developing and adopting standardized language and tools that measure the quality and outcomes of school nursing services (Stock, Larter, Kieckehefer, Thronson & Maire, 2002). The IHP can assist school nurses in many areas (NASN, 2003):

Professional school nurses utilize IHPs to communicate nursing care needs to administrators, staff, students, and parents.

The IHP will create a safer process for delegation of nursing care, supporting the continuity of care.

Planning and delivering care based on standardized IHPs and the use of standardized nursing language will help advance professional school nurses by affording evidence-based practice.

The position of the NASN on IHPs is very clear: "It is the position of the National Association of School Nurses that students whose health needs affect their daily functioning have an IHP. It is also the position of NASN that the professional school nurse should be responsible for the writing of the IHP in collaboration with the student, family, and healthcare providers and for seeing that the IHP is implemented, with periodic evaluation for evidence of desired student outcomes" (NASN, 2003, p.2).

# References

Bulechek, G., & McCloskey, J. (1985). *Nursing interventions: Treatments for potential nursing diagnoses.* Philadelphia: Saunders.

Carpenito, L. J. (1997). *Nursing diagnosis application to clinical practice* (7th ed). Philadelphia: Lippincott.

Denehy, J. (2004). *Using nursing languages in school nursing practice.* Scarborough, ME: National Association of School Nurses.

Denehy, J., & Poulton, S. (1999). The use of standardized language in individualized healthcare plans. *Journal of School Nursing, 15*(1), 38–45.

Dochterman, J., & Bulechek, G. (2004). *Nursing Interventions Classification (NIC)* (4th ed.). St. Louis, MO: Mosby.

Hootman, J. (1996a). *Nursing diagnosis: Application in the school setting.* Scarborough, ME: National Association of School Nurses.

Hootman, J. (1996b). *Quality nursing interventions in the school setting: Procedures, models, and guidelines.* Scarborough, ME: National Association of School Nurses.

Moorhead, S., Johnson, M., & Maas, M. (2004). *Nursing Outcomes Classification (NOC)* (3rd ed.). St. Louis, MO: Mosby.

National Association of School Nurses (NASN). (1999). Definition of school nursing. *Journal of School Nursing, 15*(3), 5.

National Association of School Nurses. (2001). *Position statement. Nursing classification systems: North American Nursing Diagnosis Association, Nursing Interventions Classifications (NIC), and Nursing Outcomes Classifications (NOC).* Scarborough, ME: Author.

National Association of School Nurses. (2003). *Position Statement: Individualized healthcare plan.* Scarborough, ME: Author.

National Association of School Nurses & American Nurses Association. (2001). *Scope and standards of professional school nursing practice.* Washington, DC: American Nurses Publishing.

North American Nursing Diagnosis Association. (2003). *NANDA nursing diagnoses: Definitions and classification, 2003-2004.* Philadelphia: NANDA International.

Pavelka, L., McCarthy, A. M., & Denehy, J. (1999). Nursing interventions used in school nursing practice. *Journal of School Nursing, 15*(1), 29–37.

Schwab, N. C., Panettieri, M. J., & Bergren, M. D. (1998). *Guidelines for school nursing documentation: Standards, issues, and models.* Scarborough, ME: National Association of School Nurses.

Stock, J. L., Larter, N., Kieckehefer, G. M., Thronson, G., & Maire, J. (2002). Measuring outcomes of school nursing services. *Journal of School Nursing, 18*(6), 353–359.

# Bibliography

Bednarz, P. (1998). The Omaha system: A model for describing school nurse case management. *Journal of School Nursing, 14*(3), 24–30.

Carpenito, L. J. (1995). *Nursing care plans & documentation* (2nd ed.). Philadelphia: Lippincott.

Carpenito, L. J. (2004). *Nursing diagnosis application to clinical practice* (10th ed.). Philadelphia: Lippincott.

Cavendish, R., Lunney, M., Luise, B. K., & Richardson, K. (2001). The Nursing Outcomes Classification: Its relevance to school nursing. *Journal of School Nursing, 17*(4), 189–197.

Denehy, J. (2000). Measuring the outcomes of school nursing practice: Showing that school nurses do make a difference. *Journal of School Nursing, 16*(1), 2–3.

Harvey, G. (2001). *Reframing school nursing services in the language of educational outcomes.* Gilmantown, NH: School Nurse Perspectives.

Hootman, J. (1996). Nursing diagnosis—a language of nursing; a language for powerful communication. *Journal of School Nursing, 12*(4), 19–23.

Hootman, J. (2004). *Quality nursing interventions in the school setting: Procedures, models, and guidelines.* Scarborough, ME: National Association of School Nurses.

Johnson, M., Bulechek, G., Maas, M., McCloskey Dochterman, J., & Moorhead, S. (2000). *Nursing diagnosis, interventions, and outcomes: NANDA, NIC, and NOC linkages.* St. Louis, MO: Mosby.

Lunney, M. (1996). The significance of nursing classification systems to school nursing. *Journal of School Nursing, 12*(2), 35–37.

Lunney, M., Cavendish, R., Luise, B. K., & Richardson, K. (1997). Relevance of NANDA and health promotion diagnoses to school nursing. *Journal of School Nursing, 13*(5), 16–22.

Proctor, S., Lordi, S., & Zaiger, D. (1993). *School nursing practice: Roles and standards.* Scarborough, ME: National Association of School Nurses.

Schwab, N. C., & Gelfman, M. H. B. (2001). *Legal issues in school health services.* North Branch, MN: Sunrise River Press.

## Chapter Two

# The Unique Qualities and the Similarities of IHPs and Other Educational, Health, and Home Care Agency Plans

Denise A. Herrmann

## Introduction

An individualized healthcare plan (IHP), emergency care plan (ECP), individualized education program (IEP), and Section 504 plan are all used within an educational setting as a process to document preparation and planning for student success. Often a student may require a combination of two or more of these plans. Distinct differences exist between the plans, yet some of the components, assessments, goals, or student outcomes may overlap. It is important for the nurse to understand these similarities and differences.

Both the IHP and ECP are specifically developed to manage health issues and are part of the nursing process, whereas the IEP and Section 504 plan are developed to deal with learning and/or educational issues, which may or may not include a related health issue. The IHP and ECP are nurse-initiated planning processes; teachers, parents, and/or administrators initiate IEP and Section 504 plans. Although students and families can and are encouraged to be involved in the development of an IHP or ECP, the IEP and Section 504 plan require parent participation. In fact, each has a "due process" component to ensure that the rights of students and parents are not violated.

## The IHP and ECP

Professional nursing standards set the expectation of developing IHPs and/or ECPs in order to deliver quality nursing care. Rarely does a state statute require these plans. In contrast, federal legislation—the Individuals With Disabilities Education Act (IDEA) and Section 504 of the Rehabilitation Act of 1973—and subsequent state laws and rules mandate the use of IEP and 504 plans with qualifying students.

Finally, the components of an IHP and ECP have been developed through professional guidelines and nursing research. To produce an effective IHP and ECP, all components should be included but are not necessarily required by a state or federal statute. There is some flexibility for professional nursing judgment. However, the IEP and, to a lesser extent, the 504 plan have specific components that must be addressed, with exceptions authorized by statute or rule.

There are also specific differences between an IHP and an ECP.

The IHP is developed using the nursing process to address the health needs of students. The ECP also comes out of the nursing process but is developed to deal with a specific potential medical emergency such as hypoglycemia, anaphylaxis, or status epilepticus. Students with special healthcare needs may have both an ECP and an IHP, but the ECP should never be considered as a substitute for a full IHP, which addresses the entire needs of the student (National Association of School Nurses [NASN], 1998). The IHP should be developed first, and within that IHP, the development of an ECP would be listed as a specific nursing intervention.

The ECP is a well-defined step-by-step process that proceeds in a logical order and provides specific directions about what to do in a particular emergency situation. It is usually written in language that can be understood by persons with limited nursing/medical knowledge. The plan includes specific information about the child's medical condition, current and emergency medications, and appropriate emergency intervention(s). Not having an ECP could potentially jeopardize the safety of a student in the school setting if a medical emergency occurred as a result of a known health condition. The ECP must be shared with or given to all appropriate building staff and usually involves specific training to ensure a prepared response by staff members. Practice or rehearsal may also be needed. The goal is to ensure maintenance of the student's health and safety in any anticipated life-threatening emergency.

An IHP may or may not be shared with building staff, depending upon the student's condition and his or her involvement in the plan.

### The IEP and Section 504 Plan

An IEP is written as part of the special education process after it has been determined that the student is eligible and will need special academic or related services to attain academic goals. A Section 504 plan is written when a student requires accommodations in instruction or environment to attain academic goals due to a documented medical condition.

When it has been determined that the student has specific health issues, the IHP can often be incorporated into or added to the IEP or Section 504 plan. In some circumstances, student goals and outcomes from an IHP may be attached to a specific IEP academic goal. In other cases, it is simply adopted as an addendum to the IEP. In the case of a Section 504 plan, the IHP may be the foundation upon which the 504 plan is developed. ~~In many situations the development of an IHP may eliminate the need for a Section 504 plan.~~ Because the implementation of the Section 504 process varies by state, school nurses must know the specifics of the district and state where they work. Chapters seven, eight, and nine in this book deal more specifically with the special education process and 504 mandate.

## Emergency Evacuation Plan

An emergency evacuation plan (EEP) is written for a student who has a health condition that requires special considerations for environmental emergencies, such as fire, tornado, earthquake, hurricane, or bomb scare. It is similar to an ECP in that it is a well-defined, step-by-step process that proceeds in a logical order dependent upon the previous action in response to an event that can only be anticipated.

School nurses and educational staff develop an EEP with knowledge about the student's health condition, physical layout of the school building, school district policies and procedures, and the community's emergency response system. Often this plan is developed in consultation with community agencies such as fire or police departments. Like an ECP, an EEP should not substitute for an IHP and is usually listed as a specific nursing intervention. An EEP must be shared with or given to all appropriate school staff and community response agencies.

## An IHP for Students Who Are Accompanied to School by a Nurse From a Home Care Agency

As students with increasingly complex health needs enter schools, they often are accompanied by a nurse or paraprofessional from an outside agency, such as a home care agency. This situation raises many issues and questions, such as, How are nursing roles differentiated? What type of healthcare plan is needed and who is responsible? There are also many legal and potential ethical questions that are beyond the scope of this book. For the purposes of this book, we will examine roles and responsibilities as they pertain to healthcare planning in the school setting.

## Role of the School Nurse

The school nurse is responsible for health services to all students enrolled in the school. ~~Because the school nurse will not be providing direct care to the student, the IHP will reflect case management or care coordination activities.~~ The school nurse, in the role of case manager, provides oversight of care and services and serves as the point of contact for communication among the student, family, school staff, and healthcare provider (NASN, 2002). The following are some general guidelines:

1. The school nurse meets with the home care case manager and staff who will accompany student to school prior to starting school.

2. The school nurse helps to determine where and when student's medical needs will be met in the school setting.

3. The school nurse orients agency staff to the health office, use of phone, OSHA guidelines for schools, and emergency supplies or procedures.

4. The school nurse obtains the nursing care plan from the home care agency initially and periodically when renewals/reviews are completed. This care plan is part of the pupil health record and may be part of the IHP.

5. The school nurse obtains necessary release of information needed between the home care agency and school, ensuring student confidentiality.

6. The school nurse is not usually responsible for primary/direct nursing care to the student but in the event of an emergency may provide nursing support.

7. The school nurse should develop an ECP and/or EEP if appropriate.

8. The school nurse facilitates storage of needed equipment such as oxygen, suctioning machine, humidity, or IV pole.

9. The school nurse is a member of the IEP team and provides health information needed for special education planning.

10. The school nurse facilitates communication between primary care provider, home care agency, school staff, and parents.

11. The school nurse instructs agency staff to keep confidential any incidental information learned about other students.

12. The school nurse collaborates with classroom staff and the home care agency to provide information to classmates and/or parents, if appropriate.

## Role of the Home Care Agency

The role of the agency staff is to attend to the medical needs of the individual student, provide direct nursing care, and work cooperatively with school staff for the benefit of the student. Following are some general guidelines for home care agency staff:

1. Provide name, address, and telephone number of agency and case manager. Also provide name/title of those attending school with the student.

2. Have case manager meet initially with school nurse to provide care plan, and at each review thereafter. Keep school nurse informed of any changes in health status or procedures performed during the school day.

3. Work with school nurse and classroom staff to decide when and where nursing procedures will be performed to avoid classroom disruption.

4. Indicate the distance the home care staff should be from the student, such as on call outside the classroom or within the classroom.

5. Clearly describe behaviors/conditions of the student that require medical attention.

6. Agency staff is responsible to assist only the student accompanied by the home care agency nurse. Usually school district insurance does not cover agency involvement with other students or staff.
7. Maintain confidential any information derived from parent or home situation. When agency staff believe it is in the child's interest that information be shared, parental written permission will be obtained.
8. Collaborate with school nurse and classroom staff to provide information or in-service to classmates/parents, if appropriate.
9. May attend IEP meetings or educational conferences by invitation of parent, following due process procedures.

10. Does not act as conduit of communication between parent and school about educational concerns, but instead encourages the parent to communicate directly with school staff, so as to avoid misunderstandings.
11. Provide orientation to school nurse and staff regarding agency structure as well as roles and responsibility of agency staff.

The components in the IHP for the student who comes to school with home care nursing remain the same: nursing diagnosis, goals, interventions, and outcomes. The following chart is a small example of such an IHP.

| Nursing Diagnosis | Goals | Nursing Interventions | Expected Outcomes |
|---|---|---|---|
| Disuse syndrome related to congenital myopathy/immobility | Student will maintain health status while achieving educational goals. | Direct care provided by home care nurse<br><br>Multidisciplinary team conference to identify health needs, roles and responsibilities of school staff and home care nurse<br><br>Develop emergency care plan in collaboration with home care nurse and parent.<br><br>Develop emergency evacuation plan and implement drill of plan.<br><br>Provide orientation to home care nurse regarding school space for care and privacy, phone access, equipment storage | Student will maintain present level of physical functioning.<br><br>Student will experience continuity of care to meet his or her needs.<br><br>Student will experience safety, physical and environmental, in the school setting.<br><br>Student will evacuate the building quickly and safely, with assistance from home care nurse and school staff, during emergency evacuations and drills. |

# References

National Association of School Nurses. (1998). *Position Statement: Emergency care plans for students with special health care needs.* Scarborough, ME: Author.

National Association of School Nurses. (2002). *Position Statement: Case management of children with special health care needs.* Scarborough, ME: Author.

# Bibliography

Allen, B. S., Ball, J., & Helfer, B. (1998). Preventing and managing childhood emergencies in school. *Journal of School Nursing,* 14(1), 20–24.

American Academy of Pediatrics Committee on School Health. (2001). Guidelines for urgent care in schools. *Pediatrics,* 107(2), 435–436.

EMSC Task Force on CSHCN. (1997). Coordinating care for children with special health care needs. *Annals of Emergency Medicine,* 30(3), 274–280.

Schwab, N. C., & Gelfman, M. H. B. (2001). *Legal issues in school health services.* North Branch, MN: Sunrise River Press.

University of Colorado Health Sciences Center, School of Nursing. (1996). *Safe at school: Planning for children with special health care needs.* Lawrence, KS: Learner Managed Designs.

Valluzzi, J. L., Brown, S. E., & Dailey, B. D. (1997). Protecting the rights of children with special health care needs through the development of individualized emergency response plans. *Infants and Young Children,* 10(2), 66–80.

## Chapter Three

# Delegation of School Nursing Activities

### Denise A. Herrmann

## Overview

Today, school nurses are often faced with decisions as to how to provide needed healthcare services within the constraints of the school system. Financial and human resources are limited, but student health needs are increasing. Therefore, many school nurses need to delegate some of the intervention activities to unlicensed assistive personnel. This chapter discusses the standards, concepts, and guidelines for delegation decision making. It is always the responsibility of school nurses to consult and follow the rules and regulations established in the Nurse Practice Act in their state.

## Standards and Regulations

School nursing, like all nursing practice, is governed by professional and regulatory agencies. Professional agencies set the standards of practice and determine the scope of practice for nurses. According to the American Nurses Association (ANA, 1991), standards are authoritative statements by which the nursing profession

- describes the responsibilities for which its practitioners are accountable,
- provides direction for professional nursing practice,
- defines the nursing profession's accountability to the public, and
- defines the client outcome for which nurses are responsible.

Regulatory agencies determine the minimum level of preparation for licensure, enforce the agreed-upon scope of practice language of the state Nurse Practice Act, and enforce the laws in order to protect the public. In fact, the state Nurse Practice Act is one of the most crucial elements that the school nurse must understand when delegating intervention activities. The Nurse Practice Act, regulations, and declaratory statements of the state of practice usually take precedence over all other professional guidelines.

## Definition and Concepts

*Delegation* is the transfer of responsibility for the performance of a task from one person to another, with the former retaining accountability for the outcome (ANA, 1994). Delegation presumes that the delegator has greater

knowledge, experience, and judgment and that the delegated task is only a subcomponent of the total student care process. In delegating, the school nurse uses professional judgment to decide what nursing care may be delegated and to whom.

The National Council of State Boards of Nursing (NCSBN, 1995) established the premises that constitute the basis for the delegation decision-making process. Included are the following:

- A licensed nurse must have ultimate responsibility and accountability for the management and provision of nursing care.
- A licensed nurse must be actively involved in and be accountable for all managerial decisions, policymaking, and practices related to the delegation of nursing care.
- Unlicensed assistive personnel are equipped to assist, not replace, the nurse.
- The practice-pervasive nursing functions of assessment, evaluation, and nursing judgment must not be delegated.
- The unlicensed assistive personnel cannot redelegate a task delegated to an unlicensed person.

When school nurses are deciding to delegate an intervention activity, they must remember that they retain the accountability for the student outcome. Many administrators and parents want to decide which nursing tasks school nurses can and cannot delegate and even to whom to delegate. Although non-nurses may suggest which nursing acts may be delegated, it is the school nurse who ultimately decides the appropriateness of the delegation. This delegation is to a selected person for a specific task to a specific child in a specific situation. Once the task has been delegated, the unlicensed person cannot redelegate that task.

## Deciding to Delegate

The American Nurses Association Code of Ethics (1985) states the nurse exercises informed judgment and uses individual competency and qualifications as criteria in seeking consultation, accepting responsibilities, and delegating nursing activities. It continues: Inasmuch as the nurse is accountable for the quality of nursing care rendered to clients, nurses are accountable for the delegation of nursing care activities to other health workers. Therefore, the nurse must assess individual competency in assigning selected components of nursing care to other nursing service personnel. The nurse should not delegate to any member of the nursing team a function for which that person is not prepared or qualified. Employer policies or directives do not relieve the nurse of accountability for making judgment about the delegation of nursing care activities (ANA, 1985).

When deciding to delegate, school nurses must consider professional standards and meet the obligations of the state Nurse Practice Act. To help nurses make appropriate delegation decisions, the Five Rights of Delegation (NCSBN, 1995) can be utilized. These are explained as follows:

### The Right Task

This refers to determination of the task, procedure, or function that is to be delegated. Is the procedure reasonably routine with a reasonably predictable outcome?

### The Right Person

This refers to staff availability. Who is available to do the nursing task, at the required time? Are enough trained staff available?

### The Right Direction

This involves assessment of the potential delegate's competency. What kind of training has this unlicensed assistive person had? Is the person able to understand the limitations of this delegation? Is this person reliable? Will this person seek appropriate help? Will this person complete the appropriate documentation?

### The Right Supervision

This means consideration of the level of supervision available and determination of the level and method of supervision required ensuring safe performance. How much initial and ongoing supervision does this procedure for this specific student require? How will the school nurse document and ensure that adequate training and supervision have occurred? By what method and how frequently does the school nurse need to assess for the student's safety and appropriate outcome?

### The Right Circumstances

This refers to assessment of client needs, including age and vulnerability. Is this child particularly vulnerable on account of age, developmental level, cognitive abilities, gender, or special health need?

### Steps to Safe Delegation

The National Association of State School Nurse Consultants (1995) identified nine steps to safe delegation of nursing care. They are as follows:

1. The registered nurse (RN) validates the necessary physician orders, parent/guardian authorization, and any other legal documentation necessary for implementing the nursing care.

2. The RN conducts an initial nursing assessment of the student's healthcare needs.

3. Consistent with the state's Nurse Practice Act and the school nurse's assessment, the nurse determines what level of care is required.

4. Consistent with the state board of nursing regulations, the RN determines the amount of training required for the unlicensed assistive person. If the individual has not completed standardized training, the RN must ensure that the person obtains such training in addition to receiving child-specific training.

5. Prior to delegation, the nurse must have evaluated the competence of the individual to safely perform the task.

6. The RN provides a written plan of care to be followed by the unlicensed staff member.

7. The RN indicates, within the written care plan, when RN notification, reassessment, and intervention are warranted, on account of a change in the student's condition, the performance of the procedure, or other circumstances.

8. The RN determines the amount and type of RN supervision necessary.

9. The RN determines the frequency and type of student health reassessment necessary for ongoing safety and efficacy.

10. The RN trains unlicensed assistive personnel to document the delegated care according to the standards and requirements of the state's board of nursing and agency procedures.

11. The RN documents activities appropriate to each of the nursing actions listed above.

## Supervision

Inherent in the decision to delegate is the obligation to provide supervision to unlicensed assistive personnel. The American Nurses Association, which sets the standards of professional nursing, defines supervision as the active process of directing, guiding and influencing the outcome of an individual performance of an activity (ANA, 1994). Supervision is generally categorized as on-site (the nurse is physically present or immediately available while the activity is being performed) or off-site (the nurse has the ability to provide direction through various means of written and verbal communications).

What is a reasonable level of supervision of unlicensed assistive personnel in the school setting? Little has been written or researched about this component of nursing delegation. Haas (1990) stated the following:

*A specific amount of time will depend upon the abilities, training and type and number of delegated nursing care tasks. However, a best practice would be to have on-site direct supervision of health aides by professional nurses for 50% or better of the health aide's work time. This means that the nurse is observing the care given by the health aide and training the health aide. Some time will be spent carrying out other professional activities with students and staff as well. A minimum level of supervision would be an overlap of 20% of the health aide and professional work time at each school site. Of course, paraprofessionals should have access to professional nurses 100% of the time by phone should problems develop with particular students. If the nurse is present on-site for less than 20% of the health aide work hours, it is not likely that the nurse can adequately monitor the performance of the health aide, delegate, and train for additional tasks, or monitor students' responses to treatment (Haas, 1990).*

## Rights and Responsibilities

As delegator, the school nurse has the responsibility to make a proper act of delegation by giving clear, specific directions to a person who can perform safely and competently. The burden of determining the competency of the person who will perform the tasks and ongoing evaluation rests with the nurse. The delegator is accountable for the act delegated and may incur liability if found to be negligent in the process of delegating and supervising.

The delegatee has the responsibility of carrying out the delegated act or function correctly and is accountable for accepting the delegation and for his or her own actions in carrying out the act.

Based on a review of the literature, the following is a list of rights and responsibilities that could be used with unlicensed assistive personnel as a guideline that would ensure quality and safety while meeting the needs of children with special healthcare needs.

- The right not to assume responsibility for a nursing task or acknowledge delegation from anyone other than an RN. Depending upon the state, this may constitute practicing nursing without a license
- The right to training education, support, supervision, and monitoring on a regular basis for any delegated task
- The right to ask for support, counseling, and teaching from the school nurse
- The right to refuse delegation if you cannot competently perform task
- The right to expect a written plan of care including emergency information
- The right to expect a health delegation policy at your district level
- The responsibility to maintain health data as confidential
- The responsibility to support the student's healthcare plan as developed by the licensed school nurse
- The responsibility when performing a task to make sure it is done correctly, at the right time, and to report any concerns to the professional nurse
- The responsibility not to transfer the performance of a nursing task from one student to another student without specific delegation for each student from the school nurse
- The responsibility not to redelegate any task to another unlicensed assistive person

## IHP and Delegation Documentation

The individualized healthcare plan (IHP) provides an effective vehicle for the documentation of nursing delegation. When describing the interventions needed to meet the student's goals and objectives, the school nurse can identify those activities that will be delegated on the IHP. The following is an excellent example by Denehy and Poulton.

---

**A sample IHP for a child with spina bifida**

Delegation (NIC 7650)
- Teach association to do catheterization procedure at the beginning of the school year.
- Review procedure with associate every 2 months.
- Teach associate the signs and symptoms of urinary tract infections.

(Denehy & Poulton, 1999)

---

This documentation should not be confused with the documentation of the training and supervision of an unlicensed assistive person. Documentation of training should include dates and times of training, a summary of training techniques employed, evaluation of the person's readiness, and appropriate signatures (Panettieri & Schwab, 1996). Documentation of supervision must be completed each time it is performed, as well as methods of supervision, a statement about the person's performance, and any necessary remedial measures (Panettieri & Schwab 1996). In many situations, the use of a checklist or flow sheet is appropriate.

## Summary

It is the role and responsibility of the school nurse to develop IHPs to meet the health needs of students. School nurses often must rely on the help and cooperation of others in the school setting to help meet those needs. Appropriately, the nurse can choose to delegate intervention activities. The school nurse must know how delegation is addressed in the state Nurse Practice Act, understand the professional and ethical standards related to nursing, and utilize a sound decision-making process for delegation decisions (NASN, 2004). The documentation of these delegated activities can easily be incorporated into the IHP. When delegation is documented, the quality of nursing care and the safety of the student are ensured.

---

# References

American Nurses Association. (1985). *Code for nurses with interpretive statements.* Washington, DC: Author.

American Nurses Association. (1991). *Standards of clinical nursing practice.* Washington, DC: American Nurses Publishing.

American Nurses Association. (1994). *Registered professional nurses & unlicensed assistive personnel.* Washington, DC: American Nurses Publishing.

Denehy, J., & Poulton, S. (1999). The use of standardized language in individualized healthcare plans. *Journal of School Nursing,* 15(1), 38–45.

Haas, M. (1990). Standards of practice: Delegation of care and supervision of health aides. In: *Healthy children healthy schools.* Minneapolis, MN: Minnesota Department of Health.

National Association of School Nurses. (2004). *Issue Brief: Delegation of care in the school setting.* Scarborough, ME: Author.

National Association of State School Nurse Consultants. (1995). Position Paper: Delegation of school health services to unlicensed assistive personnel. *Journal of School Nursing,* 11(2), 17–19.

National Council of State Boards of Nursing (NCSBN). (1995). *Delegation: Concepts and the decision making process.* Chicago: Author.

Panettieri, M. J., & Schwab, N. (1996). Delegation and supervision in school settings. *Journal of School Nursing,* 12(2), 11–18.

# Bibliography

American Federation of Teachers. (1998). *The medically fragile child in the school setting: A resource guide for the educational team* (2nd ed.). Washington, DC: Author.

American Nurses Association. (1997). *Registered nurse utilization of unlicensed assistive personnel.* Washington, DC: American Nurses Publishing.

Cronenwett, L. R. (1995). The use of unlicensed assistive personnel: When to support, oppose or be neutral. *Journal of Nursing Administration,* 25(6), 11–12.

Essex N., Schifani, J., & Bowman, S. (1994). Handle with care your school's tough new challenge: Educating medically fragile children. *American School Board Journal,* 181, 50–53.

Irvine, D., Sidani, S., & Hall, L. (1998). Linking outcomes to nurses' roles in health care. *Nursing Economics,* 16(2), 58–64.

Josten, L., Smoot, C., & Beckley, S. (1995). Delegation to assistive personnel by school nurses. *Journal of School Nursing,* 11(2), 8–16.

Luckenbill, D. (1996). *The school nurse's role in delegation of care: Guidelines and compendium.* Scarborough, ME: National Association of School Nurses.

Minnesota Nurses Association. (1997). *Position Paper: Delegation and supervision of nursing activities.* St. Paul, MN: Author.

National Association of School Nurses. (2002). *Position Statement: Delegation.* Scarborough, ME: Author.

National Association of School Nurses. (2002). *Position Statement: Using assistive personnel in school health services programs.* Scarborough, ME: Author.

National Association of School Nurses, American Nurses Association (NASN, ANA). (2001). *Scope and standards of professional school nursing practice.* Washington, DC: American Nurses Publishing.

National Association of State School Nurse Consultants. (2000). NASSNC *Position Statement: Delegation of school health services.* Kent, OH: Author.

National Education Association. (1998). *Providing safe health care: The role of educational support personnel.* Washington, DC: Author.

Palfry, J. S., Haynie, M., Porter, S., Bierle, T., Cooperman, P., & Lowcock, J. (1992). Project School Care: Integrating children assisted by medical technology into educational settings. *Journal of School Health,* 62(2), 50–54.

Panettieri, M. J., & Schwab, N. (1996). Delegation and supervision in school settings: Standards, issues, and guidelines for practice (part 2). *Journal of School Nursing,* 12(2), 19–27.

Proctor, S., Lordi, S., & Zaiger, D. (1993). *School nursing practice: Roles and standards.* Scarborough, ME: National Association of School Nurses.

Schwab, N. C., & Gelfman, M. H. B. (2001). *Legal issues in school health services.* North Branch, MN: Sunrise River Press.

Schwab, N., & Haas, M. (1995). Delegation and supervision in school settings. *Journal of School Nursing,* 11(1), 26–34.

Todaro, A. W., Failla, S., & Caldwell, T. H. (1993). A model for training community-based providers for children with special health care needs. *Journal of School Health,* 63(6), 262–265.

## Chapter Four

# Evidence-Based Practice in School Nursing

### Judith A. Vessey and Katelyn A. McGowan

## Introduction

Consider this scenario: Michael, an 8-year-old student who is new to the town and school district, comes to your office once again. This is the fourth such visit to the health room since school began 3 weeks ago, and he also has missed several days of school. Although he is not in acute distress, Michael is coughing and has a clear watery nasal discharge. Michael complains that his throat "feels tight and itchy" and he can't sleep at night due to his cough, although he denies that he ever wheezes. Michael goes on to say that he gets sick like this "a lot." Michael's pertinent medical history is positive only for ragweed allergy, for which he takes an over-the-counter antihistamine. His concerned mother initially consulted 2 weeks ago with the family's former doctor, who prescribed over the phone a cough suppressant and antibiotic for bronchitis. Because Michael's condition has not improved, a second phone call to the doctor resulted in a change to a new, more potent antibiotic. You think that Michael may have asthma. What do you do:

1. Go along with the current treatment recommendations but encourage the mother to find a new doctor in the area?
2. Suggest to the mother that she take her child to the emergency department of the local children's hospital?
3. Educate the mother as to the signs and symptoms of asthma and partner with her to get Michael the care he needs?

Depending on your education and experience, you might have chosen either of the first two options. Neither, however, is clinically efficacious and cost-appropriate. The problem with the first option is that a faulty diagnosis has led to a faulty treatment plan. When the wrong care is given, it is always costly. Expensive antibiotics have been unnecessarily prescribed, and a correct diagnosis is further delayed as Michael's mother tries to locate an appropriate provider. For Michael, the result is a prolonged illness, increased absenteeism, and, possibly, worsening academic performance.

With the second option, a correct diagnosis is likely to be forthcoming from an astute pediatric resident in the children's hospital emergency department. But such care is expensive and not designed to promote care continuity. Although Michael will quickly recover from this episode, he is likely to experience another expensive exacerbation in the not-too-distant future.

If, however, you are a savvy nurse who keeps up with emerging research findings that influence school health, you would recognize that Michael has signs and symptoms consistent with a diagnosis of cough-variant asthma. You know that the absence of wheezing does not negate an asthma diagnosis. His symptoms further suggest that the appropriate severity classification would be "moderate persistent asthma" (National Heart, Lung, & Blood Institute, 2002), which requires a comprehensive treatment plan. A rescue medication such as albuterol, followed by a regimen of inhaled low-dose corticosteroids and a long-acting beta2-agonist, accompanied by environmental modifications, is in order (Kieckhefer & Ratcliffe, 2004). Michael needs to be seen by a pediatric primary care provider with expertise in asthma management. You choose to educate his mother about asthma, help her locate and schedule an emergent appointment with a primary care provider in the community, and offer to help her institute a comprehensive treatment plan in collaboration with Michael's new primary care provider.

As a school nurse, what type of care would you like to be the hallmark of your practice? True professionals assertively use all available evidence to guide their clinical practice. Unfortunately, too much of what school nurses do continues to be based on tradition, intuition, or authority. It often seems easier to "go along" with a prescribed regimen than to become knowledgeable about students' health needs, question dubious care, or actively advocate for students and their families. But in today's healthcare arena, nurses are being held to a higher standard of care. By adopting evidence-based practice (EBP), school nurses can ensure that students receive the best possible care available to them.

## Background

### Definition

*Evidence-based practice* refers to the conscientious, explicit, and judicious use of the best current evidence in making decisions about the care of individuals (Sackett, 1997; Sackett, Straus, Richardson, Rosenberg, & Haynes, 2000). A health professional's clinical expertise is integrated with a synthesis of knowledge from research findings, retrospective chart reviews, quality improvement studies, and other clinical data, and from student and family values and preferences (Romyn et al., 2003). Collectively, this information is systematically used in guiding individualized care decisions (Jennings & Loan, 2001). EBP allows for the best possible healthcare to be given using the resources available (Colyer & Kamath, 1999).

## History

In the 1970s, the need to use evidence to guide practice was promulgated by the British physician-epidemiologist Archibald Lemon Cochrane. Becoming interested in the need to use evidence in making treatment decisions, he advised physicians to pay attention to empirically based evidence shown to be effective and the public to pay only for such care (Melnyk, 2003). Shortly after his death, the Cochrane Center and the Cochrane Collaboration were founded in 1992 and 1993, respectively. Their central purpose is to develop, maintain, and update systematic reviews of healthcare interventions for professionals and the public to inform the dialog among providers and patients when making care decisions.

This ideal was coined "evidence-based medicine" (EBM) by Dr Sackett at McMaster University School of Medicine in Canada in the early 1990s. EBM further gained credence when the Evidence-Based Medicine Working Group of the American Medical Association underscored the importance of using research findings to guide clinical practice. In 1989, the Agency for Health Care Policy and Research (AHCPR) (now the Agency for Healthcare Research and Quality [AHRQ]) was formed and funded by the U.S. Congress with a mission to compile and evaluate relevant evidence so that providers and patients could make informed healthcare decisions about selected conditions. It was not until the mid-1990s, however, that healthcare reform initiatives highlighted the problems of spiraling healthcare costs in the absence of concomitant improvement in healthcare outcomes. The term "evidence-based practice" later emerged from the broader healthcare community. The efforts of the Cochrane Collaboration, the AHRQ, and other professional groups sustained the momentum for the EBM and EBP movement.

As EBP was embraced, clinical guidelines emerged. Clinical guidelines provide healthcare personnel with principles and optimal methods of addressing specific aspects of patient care (Hewitt-Taylor, 2003). They combine findings from theory, scientific principles, research studies, case reports, and expert opinions (McNaughton, Klardie, & Meyers, 2004). Although guidelines were first developed by the AHCPR, professional healthcare organizations in medicine, nursing, and allied health assumed the responsibility for constructing clinical guidelines specific to their practice.

To assist all healthcare professionals in obtaining available objective, detailed information needed to provide quality evidence-based patient care, the National Guideline Clearinghouse was created in 1999 by the AHRQ in partnership with the American Medical Association and the American Association of Health Plans (now America's Health Insurance Plans). Today this public resource serves as a comprehensive database of evidence-based clinical practice guidelines and related materials (Vessey, 2004).

EBP represents a profound paradigm shift in the way health professionals practice. Emphasis is placed on comprehensive and systematic reviews of relevant research findings and other objective evidence rather than on authority, opinion, or tradition (Jennings & Loan, 2001). Some groups attacked EBP as "cookbook medicine," seeing it as a tool designed to control healthcare practices, limit practitioners' autonomy, and facilitate healthcare rationing (Tod, Palfreyman, & Burke, 2004). Others saw it as a healthcare delivery fad, destined to fade away in a few years. But despite these early criticisms, research has consistently demonstrated that using evidence to determine best practices is not only cost-effective but clinically efficacious (Young, 2003).

## Significance

Although medicine spearheaded EBP, the idea was not new to nursing. Historically, nurses have systematically collected and used information to improve nursing care. Initially, this was done through the nursing process; later, formalized models for research utilization were incorporated into nursing practice (Windle, 2003). The need to include not only objective data from clinical research but knowledge from other sources, including clinical expertise, helped expand this paradigm, providing a more inclusive framework from which to provide care.

EBP is important to school nurses for several reasons. First and foremost, students deserve the best care that school nurses can provide. Moreover, in today's educational arena, school nurses need to demonstrate that what they do, and how they do it, helps keep students healthy and available for learning. Various constituencies, including school board members, community leaders, legislators, and parents, are demanding better accountability from all school staff as measured by students' academic performance, school safety, and fiscal responsibility (Vessey, in press). Embracing EBP helps school nurses demonstrate that their practice is accountable, clinically efficacious, and cost-effective (Denehy, 2003; Hootman, 2002).

## Components of Evidence-Based Practice

### Sources of Evidence

EBP requires that a series of thematic studies be critiqued for their veracity and pragmatic utility for clinical application and then synthesized into a single conceptual area (Vessey, in press). Evidence used in EBP is not limited to findings from randomized clinical trials. Although empirical research findings are foundational to EBP, quality nursing care cannot be based on scientific findings alone (Stetler et al., 1998). Only when research findings are incorporated with other existing data, clinician expertise, and client values and preferences can students' health needs be best addressed.

## Research Findings

Evidence from the research literature comes from several sources. Findings from experimental studies such as randomized clinical trials are generally considered to be the highest and most appropriate form of research evidence (Hewitt-Taylor, 2003) (see **Box 1**). Experimental research uses highly structured investigative approaches that rely on the statistical analyses of empirical (numerical) data to test the effect of a new procedure or intervention. Initially, hunches and ideas are refined into measurable hypotheses and then tested using the scientific method. Characteristics of experimental research are threefold. First, the investigator does something to, or for, a group of participants, a process referred to as manipulation. Second, the experimenter uses a control group and (at least one) experimental group, and one group of subjects does not receive the intervention and the other does. This allows the investigator to evaluate the effectiveness of the intervention by measuring the differences in outcomes between the groups receiving and not receiving the intervention. Third, the experimenter assigns participants to intervention or control groups randomly, or without systematic bias. There are many different research designs that can be used for conducting intervention research; they vary in their rigor according to the attention they give to each of the three fundamental characteristics—manipulation, control, and randomization. Randomized clinical trials, the gold standard of experimental research, seek to increase the confidence with which interventions can be applied across the population and thus hold the preeminent spot in the evidence hierarchy.

**Box 1. Quality Hierarchy for Evaluating Existing Evidence**

1. Meta-analyses of experimental research, with emphasis on randomized clinical trials

2. Well-designed individual experimental or quasi experimental studies

3. Well-designed individual nonexperimental (e.g., descriptive, correlational, qualitative, case study) research

4. Systematically obtained prospective or retrospective quality improvement data

5. Expert committee reports and consensus statements

6. Opinions of nationally known authorities based on clinical expertise, legal opinions, regulatory statutes

7. Nonsystematic clinical information

Results from nonexperimental research studies also are useful in EBP. Nonexperimental research differs from experimental research primarily in the investigator's level of involvement in manipulating the data. In nonexperimental research, the researcher collects and interprets data about the natural state of affairs. The researcher does not introduce or seek to measure an intervention (Polit, Beck, & Hungler, 2001) and has little control over a study's variables.

Nonexperimental quantitative research (e.g., surveys, questionnaires) is by far the most common type that has been conducted by school nurses. There are several reasons for this. First, there is sufficient data to analyze. Second, there are a number of variables that researchers may be interested in but cannot be manipulated—youths' ages, genders, socioeconomic status, and the like. Third, it is difficult and sometimes unethical to conduct intervention studies (Vessey, in press). Two common types of nonexperimental research are descriptive and correlational. Descriptive research systematically describes or portrays aspects of individuals, groups, or situations and the frequency with which they occur. No attempt is made to explain or predict how the circumstances may change in the future (Fain, 2004). In correlational research, interrelationships of interest are examined between and among identified variables (Fain). Information from both these types of research is helpful in explaining phenomena but can never be used to explain cause-and-effect of relationships among the variables.

Qualitative studies, another form of nonexperimental research, are designed to inform clinicians about the meaning and context of health and illness situations (Vessey, in press). These studies are important to informing nursing practice. Knowledge is generated by using methods of inquiry, such as in-depth unstructured interviews or serial observations. Such techniques emphasize the meaning of the experience for the individual. Narrative (nonnumeric) data are then subjectively interpreted using a set of rules for the specific qualitative methods used.

Although the findings from individual studies are the building blocks for EBP, identifying all the specific studies in a given area is not always easy. Because knowledge expands so rapidly, identifying systematic reviews that have been conducted on topics of interest helps ensure that the majority of evidence is identified (Melnyk, 2003). Systematic reviews are conducted by experts who organize a group of related studies around a single clinical question so that conclusions can be readily drawn by clinicians (Melnyk & Fineout-Overholt, 2002). One type of systematic review is the meta-analysis. Meta-analyses use quantitative methodologies to summarize data from randomized controlled trials and other experimental research. The summary statistic that is produced provides a precise measure of the strength of an intervention. Other types of systematic reviews are review articles, sometimes referred to as metasyntheses. These will include findings from nonexperimental as well as experimental studies.

Both experimental and nonexperimental research studies have a role in EBP. What is important is the quality of the study and what it contributes to clinical practice, not solely the methods employed.

## Other Existing Data

Data from standardized quality improvement programs are useful in determining EBP. Specific outcomes can be benchmarked to "best school health practices" as determined by research evidence (Igoe, 2000). Benchmarking is a structured approach for continuously identifying, measuring, and improving a school nurse's performance. It requires a measurement mechanism so that the performance "gaps" can be identified and rectified (Vessey, in press). Recent position statements, policies, protocols, and clinical guidelines that are released from the National Association of School Nurses (NASN), state and federal agencies, and other professional groups also may be used as evidence. Regardless of the source, the quality of the evidence it contains should be critiqued before it is used.

School nurses have considerable untapped data in their records. One detriment to using such data is that it historically has not been collected or recorded in a systematic fashion. Without a common and consistent classification system, it is impossible to monitor the effectiveness of interventions and use this information to improve the quality of care. The efforts of the North American Nursing Diagnosis Association (NANDA), the Nursing Interventions Classification (NIC), and the Nursing Outcomes Classification (NOC) are all contributing to the development of a standardized nomenclature that will address this need (Denehy & Poulton, 1999).

## Clinician Expertise

Although the emphasis in many discussions on EBP is on the inclusion of research findings, of equal importance is a clinician's expertise. A clinical expert nurse considers not only a condition's pathophysiology but how it interfaces with the complex biopsychosocial and developmental needs of students. This holistic approach allows for the identification of issues not identified in clinical trials. For example, is a treatment protocol too costly for a family to implement, or are its side effects too onerous for therapeutic adherence to be maintained? It is important to remember, however, that clinical expertise is rarely value-free, but reflects a clinician's training and personal health beliefs. For example, clinicians who have a strong belief in the scientific process and randomized clinical trials often discount complementary and alternative therapies that have not been tested in such a fashion.

Decision-making capabilities of school nurses are a function of education, experience, inquisitiveness, and drive. Whereas novice school nurses will likely more strictly adhere to clinical guidelines and structured care plans, more experienced nurses will interpret and alter them in light of individual situations and emerging priorities (Benner, 1984).

## Client and Family Values and Preferences

EBP requires that students and their families be included as full partners in clinical decision making. Through such partnerships, more efficacious care is provided. Core nursing values related to health and illness, personal autonomy, social justice, and professional accountability also will be upheld (Mitchell, 1997; Romyn et al., 2003)

Although finding information describing a phenomenon from the researcher's or provider's view is relatively easy, little information regarding consumer preferences is known (Foster, 2004). This is unfortunate; regardless of the quality of the research evidence and skill of the provider, if the client and family do not see the value of proposed diagnostic and treatment regimens, nonadherence and "treatment failures" are likely. Social and economic circumstances, cultural background, and spiritual beliefs all influence the values of students and their families.

## Identifying and Accessing Evidence

The first step in using evidence is to read evidence-based clinical articles from nursing and related disciplines that are germane to your practice. School nurses can keep abreast of new knowledge, such as new anticonvulsants, interventions for pregnant teens, or reducing latex allergy risks in the school setting. Subscribing to the Journal of School Nursing and a peer-reviewed journal specific to an area of interest—such as adolescence or youths with learning differences—helps school nurses develop a specific area of expertise important to their constituency. Although lay articles and media coverage often present "evidence" in their coverage, these reports are not refereed and there is little attempt to control bias. Using such information without further validating its veracity is problematic.

Becoming Internet savvy helps school nurses identify available evidence. Position statements, policies, protocols, and guidelines that are released from the NASN, state and federal agencies, and other professional groups are also available on the World Wide Web. Such information is particularly helpful as scientific findings are translated in light of clinical pragmatics and policy considerations.

Identifying and accessing specific research and review articles is best done by searching online databases (Montgomery, 2002). Those most commonly used by school nurses are PubMed, CINAHL, PsychINFO, ERIC, and the International Council of Nurses Research Network; many others may be appropriate for a narrow or specialized topic, such as SPORTDiscus for exercise-related topics. Appropriate literature also may be identified through Web-based scanning subscriptions. In most databases, research and conceptually driven articles are included. After identifying potential sources in a database, each reference can be screened for its relevance to the area of interest. By reading the title and abstract and scanning for key words, you can separate useful citations from those that are not.

A second type of database is equally useful in identifying evidence. Such databases have already compiled and synthesized data on a specific topic. For example, some clinical guidelines that support EBP in school settings are posted with the National Guideline Clearinghouse and can be found at www.guidelines.gov. This site compiles the latest evidence from a variety of international professional health and medical organizations and federal agencies. Integrated reviews from the Cochrane Collaboration can be found at www.cochrane.org. A list of the Cochrane reviews that would be of interest to school nurses may be found in **Box 2**. Systematic reviews of specific interest to nursing are published in Sigma Theta Tau International's *Online Journal of Knowledge Synthesis for Nursing* (OJKSN) at www.nursingsociety.org. A list of topics of interest is found in **Box 3**.

In addition to using computerized databases, there are other ways of identifying evidence. Searching the World Wide Web may help locate studies published in electronic journals or other studies that are in progress or have been recently completed but not yet published. Other search methods include searching conference proceedings and citation-index searching, which identifies articles that cite a key reference. Finally, hand searching requires reviewing those specific journals that likely publish articles related to your area of study (Conn et al., 2003; Gennaro, Hodnett, & Kearney, 2001).

Regardless of how the citation was found, literature can be most readily retrieved from university libraries, interlibrary loan, document delivery services, or sometimes directly from the Web. Some databases, such as PubMed, are open access, but many require a subscription, including CINAHL, the Cochrane Reviews, and OJKSN. Generally, universities with schools of nursing subscribe to these databases. School nurses who precept nursing students should consider requesting an academic appointment with library privileges so that they may access this information. An option for members of Sigma Theta Tau (the International Honor Society for Nurses) is to subscribe to the Online Literature Review, a unique, Web-based service that is completely customized to an individual's needs and interests. **Table 1** presents more detailed information on databases.

Finally, your school librarian can assist you in accessing online databases, identifying relevant literature, and obtaining articles. In fact, the librarian is likely to identify twice as many sources as a novice researcher. But if searching is new to you, don't despair. Your searching skills will improve with practice.

## Critiquing the Evidence

Hopefully, a systematic review that addresses the question at hand is available. After identifying potentially useful systematic reviews, the reader needs to "appraise it for validity, strength of the findings, and applicability" (Melnyk, 2003, p. 148). Questions to ask when evaluating the literature may be found in **Box 4**. If a systematic review is not available, all sources of evidence need to be critiqued individually prior to their inclusion, because the quality of evidentiary sources varies dramatically. The scope of critiquing research is too broad to cover in this chapter. **Box 5** lists texts specific for this purpose. Suffice it to say, to effectively critique objective research evidence, nurses need to know research terminology, understand the research process, and evaluate the appropriateness of study findings for their setting.

## Using Evidence in Practice

After the body knowledge is synthesized, the evidence can then be used in practice. This requires that protocols be derived, personnel educated, protocols implemented, and an evaluation of its success be conducted. Textbooks such as this one help in this process. The nursing care plans in this textbook are composed of a series of nursing standards for which the relevant evidence is provided. Each of these standards and supporting evidence serves as the underpinnings for the prescribed actions. Use of standardized nursing care plans also provides a framework for monitoring quality and documentation activities of nursing care and its outcomes (Long, 2003).

EBP is not static. Evidence needs to be updated in all practice documents in a timely fashion. All school health policies, procedures, and standardized care plans need to be continually reviewed; the schedule is determined in accordance with how rapidly knowledge is emerging in a given area or whenever a major report or consensus statement is released by a professional organization (e.g., Juvenile Diabetes Heart Association, Cystic Fibrosis Foundation) or federal group (e.g., National Institutes of Health, Centers for Disease Control) (Vessey, in press). For example, immunization protocols should be reviewed at least once a year, whereas asthma care plans might be reviewed every 2 years and athletic participation policies reviewed less frequently.

Cross-referencing key evidence helps ensure that all updates are made simultaneously. Immunization information, for example, needs to be updated on immunization policies and procedures and also on all condition-specific care plans (e.g., HIV, epilepsy) where immunization protocols are addressed. It is extremely important that all documents contain the latest revision date (so the currency of the information is known) and the list of references from which the evidence was drawn (so the reader can evaluate the quality of the work).

Finally, EBP cannot be done in isolation. All members of the healthcare team need to adopt the EBP approach to client care; if they do not, therapeutic gains are negated when colleagues working with the same student are basing their interventions on the familiar rather than on what has been tested. For school nurses, this frequently means including parents, health aides, administrators, teachers, and coaches on the team. The steps for engaging in EBP are outlined in **Box 6**.

## Barriers to Adopting EBP

Although the need for and appeal of EBP is self-evident, adopting EBP standards has met with resistance in the nursing community. Some of these concerns have merit, others are fallacious. A major criticism of EBP is that the quality and quantity of evidence are insufficient. Unfortunately, this is a valid concern. The majority of healthcare practices are not evidence-based. For example, it is estimated that no more than 20% of all medical practice is supported by evidence (Kongstvedt, 2001), and considerably less research has been done to identify "best practices" in nursing.

Another concern is the quality of evidence available from nursing studies (Hutchinson & Johnston, 2004; Jennings & McClure, 2004). There are few well-conducted clinical trials specific to school nursing practice. In some areas, such as psychosocial issues and mental health interventions, evidence of well-conducted intervention studies is particularly lacking (Short, Kitchiner, & Curran, 2004). Again, this is a valid concern that needs to be addressed by researchers interested in school health and professional organizations.

Personal factors are a major barrier to advancing EBP. Many nurses are often unaware of the scope of nursing research published in interdisciplinary journals or those of other disciplines (Moore, 2003). Other school nurses are uncomfortable or lack skill in evaluating and synthesizing available evidence across domains and applying it to their clinical decision making (Hutchinson & Johnston, 2004). For some, it is easier to be "told what to do" than to have to interpret and use new knowledge. In part, this is a reflection of an education that did not include formal academic research training. Over two-thirds of nurses, for example, think that the statistics in research articles are not understandable (Funk, et al., 1991). However, understanding the "rules of evidence" and using evidence appropriately are an expectation of professional nursing practice. For nurses who lack these skills, self-study, continuing education programs, and/or formal academic training are recommended.

Finally, school nurses may see EBP as too time-consuming (Young, 2003), although this may be used as an excuse for inadequate knowledge or lack of interest. But consider this: Is it more time-consuming and cost efficient to repeatedly call emergency services for a child whose diabetes is out of control because the family (a) does not understand diabetes management, (b) cannot pay for insulin and supplies, (c) cannot provide healthy food choices, (d) appears too unstructured to institute care, or (e) all of these, than to work with the family in finding some common ground that will promote behavior change?

## Summary

Everyone reading this chapter has different levels of clinical expertise and interest in research. All school nurses have the personal responsibility to proactively advance EBP in whatever way is appropriate for their background. The care plans that are presented in this text were developed using the best research evidence available. As you read them and use them in your clinical practice, consider what professional expertise you can add to help improve the care you provide to students and families.

## References

Benner, P. (1984). *From novice to expert: Excellence and power in clinical nursing practice.* Menlo Park, CA: Addison-Wesley.

Colyer, H., & Kamath, P. (1999). Evidence based practice: A philosophical and political analysis; some matters for consideration by professional practitioners. *Journal of Advanced Nursing, 29,* 188–193.

Conn, V. S., Isaramalai, S., Rath, S., Jantarakupt, P., Wadhawan, R., & Dash, Y. (2003). Beyond MEDLINE for literature searches. *Journal of Nursing Scholarship, 35*(2), 177–182.

Denehy, J. (2003). Developing a program of research in school nursing. *Journal of School Nursing, 19*(3), 125–126.

Denehy, J., & Poulton, S. (1999). The use of standardized language in individualized healthcare plans. *Journal of School Nursing, 15*(1), 38–45.

Fain, J. A. (2004). *Reading, understanding, and applying nursing research* (2nd ed). Philadelphia: Davis.

Foster, R.L. (2004). Partnering with children and families for evidence-based practice. *Journal for Specialists in Pediatric Nursing, 9*(1), 3–4.

Funk, S. G., Champagne, M. T., Wiese, R. A., & Tornquist, E. M. (1991). Barriers to using research findings in practice: The clinician's perspective. *Applied Nursing Research, 4*(2), 90–95.

Gennaro, S., Hodnett, E., & Kearney, M. (2001). Making evidence-based practice a reality in your institution: Evaluating the evidence and using the evidence to change clinical practice. *American Journal of Maternal Child Nursing, 26*(5), 236–245.

Hewitt-Taylor, J. (2003). Developing and using clinical guidelines. *Nursing Standard, 18*(5), 41–44.

Hootman, J. (2002). The importance of research to school nurses and school nursing practice. *Journal of School Nursing, 18*(1), 18–24.

Hutchinson, A.M., & Johnston, L. (2004). Bridging the divide: A survey of nurses' opinions regarding barriers to, and facilitators of, research utilization in practice setting. *Journal of Clinical Nursing, 13*(3), 304–315.

Igoe, J. B. (2000). School nursing today: A search for new cheese. *Journal of School Nursing, 16*(5), 9–15.

Jennings, B. M., & Loan, L.A. (2001). Misconceptions among nurses about evidence-based practice. *Journal of Nursing Scholarship, 33*(2), 122–127.

Jennings, B. M., & McClure, M. L. (2004). Strategies to advance health care quality. *Nursing Outlook, 52*(1), 17–22.

Kieckhefer, G., & Ratcliffe, M. (2004). Asthma. In P. Jackson & J. A. Vessey (Eds.), *Primary care of the child with chronic conditions* (4th ed., pp. 174–197). Philadelphia: Mosby.

Kongstvedt, P. R. (2001). *Essentials of managed health care* (4th ed.). Gaithersburg, MD: Aspen Publications.

Long, L. E. (2003). Imbedding quality improvement into all aspects of nursing practice. *International Journal of Nursing Practice, 9*(5), 280–284.

McNaughton, M. A., Klardie, K., & Meyers, W. (2004). Integrating the principles of evidence-based practice: Testing and diagnosis. *Journal of the American Academy of Nurse Practitioners, 16*(1), 2–7.

Melnyk, B. M. (2003). Evidence-based practice. Finding and appraising systematic reviews of clinical interventions: Critical skills for evidence-based practice. *Pediatric Nursing, 29*(2), 125, 147–149.

Melnyk, B. M., & Fineout-Overholt, E. (2002). Key steps in implementing evidence-based practice: Asking compelling, searchable, questions and searching for the best evidence. *Pediatric Nursing, 28*(3), 262–263, 266.

Mitchell, G. (1997). Research issues. Questioning evidence-based practice for nursing. *Nursing Science Quarterly, 10*(4), 154–155.

Montgomery, K. S. (2002). Scientific inquiry. Utilization of research via the Internet. *Journal for Specialists in Pediatric Nursing, 7*(2), 86–88.

Moore, M. L. (2003). Preterm birth. *Journal of Gynecology and Neonatal Nursing, 32*(5), 636–637.

National Heart, Lung, & Blood Institute. (2002). *National Asthma Education and Prevention Program Expert Panel report 2: Guidelines for the diagnosis and management of asthma—Update on selected topics 2002.* National asthma education program expert panel report II. Publication No. 97-4051A. U.S. Department of Health and Human Services.

Polit, D.F., Beck, C.T., & Hungler, B.P. (2001). *Essentials of nursing research: Methods, appraisal and utilization* (5th ed.). Philadelphia: Lippincott Williams & Wilkins.

Romyn, D. M., Allen, M. N., Boschma, G., Duncan, S. M., Edgecombe, N., Jensen, L. A., et al. (2003). The notion of evidence in evidence-based practice by the Nursing Philosophy Work Group. *Journal of Professional Nursing, 19*(4), 184–188.

Sackett, D. L. (1997). …so little time, and … *Evidence Based Medicine, 2*(2), 39–40.

Sackett, D. L., Straus, S. E., Richardson, W. S., Rosenburg, W., & Haynes, R. B. (2000). *Evidence based medicine: How to practice and teach EBM.* London: Churchill Livingstone.

Short, N. P., Kitchiner, N. J., & Curran, J. (2004). Unreliable evidence. *Journal of Psychiatric and Mental Health Nursing, 11,*106–111.

Stetler, C. B., Brunell, M., Giuliano, K. K., Morsi, D., Prince, L., & Newell-Stokes, V. (1998). Evidence-based practice and the role of nursing leadership. *Journal of Nursing Administration, 28*(7/8), 45–53.

Tod, A., Palfreyman, S., & Burke, L. (2004). Evidence-based practice is a time of opportunity for nursing. *British Journal of Nursing, 13*(4), 211–216.

Vessey, J. A. (in press). School nurse's role as a researcher. In J. Selekman (Ed.), *National Association of School Nurses' comprehensive textbook of school nursing.* Philadelphia, PA: W.B. Saunders.

Vessey, J. A. (2004). The guiding light: www.guidelines.gov. *NASN Newsletter, 19*(4), 15.

Windle, P. E. (2003). Understanding evidence-based practice. *Journal of PeriAnesthesia Nursing, 18*(5), 360–362.

Young, K. M. (2003). Where's the evidence? Evidence-based practice is not a reality for most nurses. *American Journal of Nursing, 103*(10), 11.

---

**Box 2. Selected Topics Relevant to School Health in *Cochrane Database of Systematic Reviews***

- Alarm interventions for nocturnal enuresis in children (Glazener, Evans, & Peto)
- Antibiotics for acute otitis media in children (Glasziou, Del Mar, & Sanders)
- Antibiotics for persistent nasal discharge (rhinosinusitis) in children (Morris & Leach)
- Community interventions for preventing smoking in young people (Sowden, Arblaster, & Stead)
- Community-based interventions for the prevention of burns and scalds in children (Turner, Spinks, & McClure)
- Complex behavioural and educational interventions for nocturnal enuresis in children (Glazener, Evans, & Peto)
- Educational interventions for children with asthma (Wolf, Gueavara, & Grum et al.)
- Exercise to improve self esteem in children and young people (Ekeland, Heian, & Hagen)
- Family therapy for asthma in children (Panton & Barley)
- Growth monitoring in children (Panpanich & Garner)
- Interventions aimed at improving immunization rates (Szilagyi, Vann, & Bordley et al.)
- Interventions for educating children who attended the emergency room for asthma (Haby, Waters, & Robertson)
- Interventions for preventing eating disorders in children and adolescents (Pratt & Woolfenden)
- Interventions for treating head lice (Dodd)
- Interventions for treating obesity in children (Summerbell, Ashton, Campbell, Edmunds, Kelly, & Waters)
- Primary prevention for alcohol misuse in young people (Foxcroft, Ireland, & Lister-Sharp)
- School-based programmes for preventing smoking (Thomas)

---

**Box 3. Selected Titles Relevant to School Health in Sigma Theta Tau International's** *Online Journal of Knowledge Synthesis for Nursing*

- A Comparison of the Effectiveness of Accuracy of Children's Self-Reported Adherence to Treatment (Burkhart, Dunbar-Jacob, & Rohay)
- Adolescent Sexual Decision-Making: An Integrative Review (Hulton)
- Affiliative Preferences, Self-Change, and Adolescent Condom Use (Baldwin & Tigges)
- American and Icelandic Parents' Perceptions of the Health Status of their Young Children with Chronic Asthma (Kolbrun, Svavarsdóttir, & Rayens)
- Children's Perception of TV and Health Behaviors Effects (Kennedy, Strzempko, & Danford)
- Children's Exposure to Community Violence (Tener, Goodwin, & Veenema)
- Increasing Perception of Self Worth in Preadolescent Diagnosed with ADHD (Frame, Kelly, & Bayley)

- Maternal Role Attainment in Adolescent Mothers: Foundations and Implications (Sartore)
- Parental Uncertainty and Posttraumatic Stress in Serious Childhood Illness (Judge & Santacroce)
- Pharmacologic Treatment of Otitis Media with Effusion in Children: Integrative and Meta-Analysis (Witmer, Wells, & Seymour)
- Promotion of Safety Helmets for Children Bicyclists: 2002 Update (Coffman)
- Revisiting the Parenting Profile - Assessment to Screen for Child Abuse (Anderson)
- Using Technology to Promote Self-Efficacy for Healthy Eating in Adolescents (Long & Stevens)
- Youth Access to Tobacco in Two Communities (Teall & Clark Graham)

**Box 4. Critical Appraisal Questions for Systematic Reviews of Clinical Interventions/Treatments**

1. Are the results of the review valid?
   - Are the studies contained in the review randomized controlled trials?
   - Does the review include a detailed description of the search strategy to find all relevant studies?
   - Does the review describe how validity of the individual studies was assessed (e.g., methodological quality, including the use of random assignment to study groups and complete follow-up of the subjects)?
   - Were the results consistent throughout the studies?
   - Were individual student data or aggregate data used in the analysis?

2. What were the results?
   - How large were the treatment effects?
   - How precise is the estimate of treatment effects?

3. Will the results assist me in caring for my patients?
   - Are my patients similar to the ones included in the review?
   - Is it feasible to implement the finding in my practice setting?
   - Were all clinically important outcomes considered, including risks and benefits of the treatment?
   - What is my clinical assessment of the patient, and are there any contraindications or circumstances that would inhibit me from implementing the treatment?
   - What are my patient and family's preferences and values about the treatment that is being considered?

From "Evidence-Based Practice. Finding and Appraising Systematic Reviews of Clinical Interventions: Critical Skills for Evidence-Based Practice," by B. M. Melnyk, 2003, *Pediatric Nursing, 29,* p. 148. Copyright 2003 by The Journal of Pediatric Nursing. Adapted with permission.

**Box 5. Useful References for Learning About Research Critique and Evidence-based Practice**

- Burns, N., & Grove, S. K. (2002). *A study guide for understanding nursing research* (3rd ed.). Philadelphia: Saunders.
- Burns, N., & Grove, S. K. (2002). *Understanding nursing research* (3rd ed.). Philadelphia: Saunders.
- Fain, J. A. (2004). *Reading, understanding, and applying nursing research* (2nd ed). Philadelphia: Davis.
- Friedland, D. J., Go, A. S., Davoren, J. B., Shlipak, M. G, Bent, S. W., Subak, L. L., et al. (1998). *Evidence-based medicine: A framework for clinical practice.* Stamford, CT: Appleton & Lange.
- Girden, E. R. (2001). *Evaluating research articles from start to finish* (2nd ed.). Thousand Oaks, CA: Sage.

- Melnyk, B. M., & Fineout-Overholt, E. (2005). *Evidence-based practice in nursing and healthcare: A guide to best practice.* Philadelphia: Lippincott Williams & Wilkins.
- Polit, D. F., & Hungler, B. P. (2005). *Essentials of nursing research: Methods, appraisal and utilization* (6th ed.). Philadelphia: Lippincott Williams & Wilkins.
- Riegelman, R.K. (2000). *Studying a study and testing a test: How to read the medical evidence* (4th ed.). Philadelphia: Lippincott, Williams & Wilkins.

**Box 6. Steps to Using Evidence**

1. Identify an area of concern/answerable question.
2. Identify and collect relevant evidence.
3. Organize the evidence.
4. Systematically evaluate the evidence: examine the veracity of the studies and its clinical relevance and applicability for school nursing.
5. Format the evidence in a way that is convincing and accurate.
6. If the evidence is sufficient, design practice applications: policies, protocols, or guidelines for clinical care. (If evidence is insufficient, consider implementing a research study.)

7. Identify expected outcomes after implementation, and design evaluation tool.
8. Provide in-service education for all stakeholders.
9. Monitor clinician adherence.
10. Evaluate the project's effectiveness; use Continuous Quality Improvement (CQI) mechanism if appropriate.
11. Document the project's success (or failure).
12. Disseminate the results of the project to local constituencies and interested professionals.

From National Association of School Nurses' Comprehensive Textbook of School Nursing, edited by J. Selekman, (in press). Philadelphia: W. B. Saunders. Adapted with permission.

## Table 1. Databases Useful in Conducting Evidence-Based Practice

| Databases | Contents | Address | Cues | Cost |
|---|---|---|---|---|
| PubMed | Electronic database<br><br>Large assortment of medical research<br><br>Abstracts and citations available | www.pubmed.gov | Some citations that have not yet been indexed and reviewed<br><br>New citations for the latest information<br><br>"Due to the size of the database, it can be quite challenging to narrow a search" (Fain, 2004) | Free<br><br>No full-text searching |
| CINAHL (Cumulative Index to Nursing and Allied Health Literature) | Electronic bibliographic database<br><br>Covers many healthcare topics<br><br>Nursing journals, books, and specific sections of books<br><br>Updated monthly | www.cinahl.com | | Print online journals, $16<br><br>Faxed article, $20 |
| ERIC | Electronic bibliographic database<br><br>Largest source of education information<br><br>Monthly updates<br><br>Worldwide | www.edrs.com | | Electronic document, $6.50 per document<br><br>Paper copy, $8 per 25-page increments<br><br>Microfiche, $2.48 per document, plus standard shipping |
| International Council of Nurses (ICN) | Guidelines and regulations on different topics that are important to nursing profession<br><br>"Quick Facts" incorporate current issues nurses are faced with | www.icn.ch | | Full membership, $235 |

## Chapter Five

# Integrating NANDA, NIC, and NOC into Individualized Healthcare Plans

Susan Poulton and Janice Denehy

## Introduction

Nursing leaders have come to recognize the importance of standardized nursing languages to advance the profession of nursing. This awareness has developed for a number of reasons. First, nurses realized that even though their practices were the same or similar in many situations, the words they used to describe their activities differed considerably from nurse to nurse, from region to region, and from one specialty to another. This lack of consistency hindered communication among nurses in their attempts to share information about nursing practice and created confusion when communicating with other health professionals, clients, and families.

Second, as nurses began to use electronic health records, it became evident that use of a standardized nursing language or terminology is essential to meet the requirements of these electronic systems. As more nurses use the electronic health record, this common terminology can be useful to aggregate data and develop large databases for determining what interventions are effective and how nurses use their time. Such standardized information is also important for reimbursement of services that nurses perform.

Even though nursing care is a major component of healthcare, there has been little documentation of what nurses do; therefore, their contribution to healthcare and school health has been largely invisible. Standardized nursing languages provide nurses with a tool to clearly describe their role in promoting health in a systematic manner to other healthcare providers and the public.

Finally, developing a knowledge base for nursing practice is critical to the profession. In order to do research on nursing practice, there needs to be some consensus on how nurses describe their practice. The development of standardized nursing languages is an important step toward meeting these challenges faced by the profession and toward developing a body of knowledge about nursing practice needed to provide evidence-based practice.

Today's school nurses are challenged to meet the needs of a wide array of students of all ages enrolled in a variety of school settings. Many of these students need only periodic episodic care for minor illnesses or injuries, but others require continued monitoring or treatment for serious chronic illnesses or disabilities so they can remain in the classroom. In addition, many students are at risk for health problems due to poverty, abuse, unprotected sexual activity, unsafe environments, poor nutrition, and unhealthy lifestyles.

School nurses provide holistic care for large numbers of students, often in more than one school building. They also serve families, school staff members, and the community at large. The National Association of School Nurses (NASN) has defined school nursing as "a specialized practice of professional nursing that advances the well being, academic success, and life-long achievement of students. To that end, school nurses facilitate positive student responses to normal development; promote health and safety; intervene with actual and potential health problems; provide case management services; and actively collaborate with others to build student and family capacity for adaptation, self management, self advocacy, and learning" (NASN, 1999).

There are high expectations for school nurses. At a time when the need for their services is growing, budgetary shortfalls threaten to reduce their numbers and dilute the positive effect that school nurses have on the school community. Under such conditions, school nurses would benefit from a way to systematically describe what they do that is easily communicated to parents and educators, as well as to administrators and others who make decisions on how to allocate precious resources. Standardized nursing languages are a tool that will not only assist school nurses in accomplishing this goal, but also have the potential for assisting school nurses in measuring the effectiveness of their interventions, data that will be essential to validate their contribution to the health and academic outcomes of students. This chapter discusses the classification of nursing diagnoses developed by the North American Nursing Diagnosis Association (NANDA) International, the Nursing Interventions Classification (NIC), and the Nursing Outcomes Classification (NOC) and illustrates how school nurses can integrate these standardized nursing languages into individualized healthcare plans (IHPs).

## Overview of Standardized Languages

What are standardized nursing languages, and how can they be used in school nursing practice? Standardized languages encompass a group of carefully developed classifications that describe the phenomena that comprise the major components of the nursing process—nursing diagnoses, nursing interventions, and nursing outcomes. A number of standardized languages have been developed in nursing over the last 30 years. In 1973, NANDA International began the development of a classification of nursing diagnoses, which is now widely used and accepted in the nursing profession (NANDA, 2003). Karen Martin (Martin & Schect, 1992) developed the Omaha System of diagnoses and interventions that were used by nurses in community and home care settings as early as the 1980s. In 1987, the Iowa Intervention Project team began its work on the NIC in response to the need for a common nomenclature to describe interventions nurses do on behalf of clients. Finally, in 1992, work began on the NOC, giving nurses a tool to evaluate the outcomes of the care they delivered.

Standardized nursing languages have the power to assist school nurses to clearly communicate what they do and to articulate their contributions to the health of the children they serve. The use of these languages in IHPs is helpful in communicating with other health professionals and the education team. An IHP includes a nursing diagnosis, an outcome goal, nursing interventions designed to reach the identified outcome goal, and a method to determine if the goal has been met within a certain time frame. The use of NANDA nursing diagnoses, NIC nursing interventions, and NOC nursing outcomes assists school nurses in using in a common language to describe the problem identified (nursing diagnosis), the outcome goals for treating the problem exhibited by the student, what they plan to do (nursing interventions) to meet the student's outcome goals, and how they will determine if the outcome goals have been met (outcomes of nursing care). These classifications are an excellent fit with the components of an IHP and can be easily integrated into existing forms.

These classifications provide standardized terminology to describe the nursing diagnoses, nursing interventions, and nursing outcomes. In addition, the classifications have defined these phenomena and operationalized each diagnosis, intervention, and outcome. For example, the NANDA nursing diagnosis Risk for Suicide is defined as "At risk for self-inflicted, life-threatening injury" (NANDA, 2003, p. 183). This diagnosis includes seven clusters of risk factors: (1) behavioral, (2) verbal, (3) situational, (4) psychological, (5) demographic, (6) physical, and (7) social. Each of these clusters includes specific risk factors related to the diagnosis.

The NIC intervention *Suicide Prevention*, defined as "Reducing the risk for self-inflicted harm with the intent to end life" (Dochterman & Bulechek, 2004, p. 678), is an appropriate intervention to implement with individuals having the nursing diagnosis Risk for Suicide. The intervention *Suicide Prevention* lists 45 activities the nurse might carry out to implement this intervention. Examples of activities in this intervention include "Determine if patient has available means to follow through with suicide plan," "Use direct, nonjudgmental approach in discussing suicide," and "Refer patient to mental healthcare provider

for evaluation and treatment of suicidal ideation and behavior, as needed" (pp. 678–679). This intervention provides information to the nurse about what specific activities might be selected to implement this intervention and provides a certain amount of standardization of care, as well as common terminology for this care. However, because the nurse may use only some of the activities listed, may revise activities as appropriate, or can create new activities as needed, it allows for the individualization of nursing care.

Finally, the NOC outcome *Suicide Self-Restraint*, defined as "Personal actions to refrain from gestures and attempts at killing self" (Moorhead, Johnson, & Maas, 2004, p. 527), includes 20 indicators to measure the ability of a person at risk for suicide in restraining from this act. For instance, the indicators "Expresses sense of hope," "Refrains from giving away possessions," and "Uses available mental health services" (pp. 527–528) are evaluated on a 5-point scale from "never demonstrated" to "consistently demonstrated." From these examples, it is evident that these classifications not only offer a standardized language that is easy to use, but also provide valuable information about what these diagnoses, interventions, and outcomes include and how they can be used to provide comprehensive nursing care.

A number of authors have written about standardized languages and their importance for school nurses (Hootman, 1996; Lunney, 1996; Pavelka, McCarthy, & Denehy, 1999; Denehy & Poulton, 1999; Cavendish, Lunney, Luise, & Richardson, 1999; Denehy, 2000; Cavendish, Lunney, Luise, & Richardson, 2001; Fahrenkrug, 2003). In addition, NASN has a position statement, "Nursing Classification Systems: North American Nursing Diagnosis Association (NANDA), Nursing Interventions Classification (NIC), Nursing Outcomes Classification (NOC)," which concludes, "The use of NANDA, NIC, and NOC by school nurses will promote quality nursing care for our clients, validate school nursing effects on our clients and promote research endeavors" (NASN, 2001). NASN supports and encourages the use of NANDA, NIC, and NOC by school nurses in their daily practice and documentation as well as the inclusion of these languages in school health software and school nurse education programs. NASN has published a manual that describes NANDA, NIC, and NOC in greater depth with numerous examples of how standardized languages can be used in school nursing practice (Denehy, 2004).

## Individualized Healthcare Plans

School nurses are well acquainted with IHPs and their value in school nursing practice. A well-written IHP uses the nursing process to delineate the care to be provided for a student with special health needs. The IHP gives a brief history and assessment of the student's current health status, followed by the care to be delivered to the child in the school setting. An IHP includes a nursing diagnosis based on data collected during the assessment phase of the nursing process. The use of a NANDA nursing diagnosis label provides a standardized name for the presenting problem. The nursing diagnosis is followed by specific outcome goals that articulate the desired behavior that the child or family will exhibit after the treatment plan has been implemented. Nursing interventions are selected during the planning stage based on the desired outcome goal. Interventions provide a method to meet the stated goal. Nursing interventions selected from the NIC give a common name for the nursing action selected as well as provide a list of possible activities from which to choose to implement the intervention. Finally, a method to measure the effectiveness of the nursing intervention(s) in reaching the desired goal is given along with the frequency or time parameters for this measurement. Outcomes from the NOC provide a concrete way to evaluate the effectiveness of care in achieving the desired outcome goal. The NOC provides a list of indicators that can be used to measure each outcome on a 5-point scale. The outcome scales can be used to determine baseline behavior and then evaluate behavior at regular time intervals during the school year to determine progress in meeting the specified goal.

In addition to describing the plan of care, IHPs provide information about delegation that specifies who is responsible for the delivery of care—the nurse, health aide, or designated other person. This information may be useful in determining staffing needs in each school. Having a clearly worded IHP helps all involved staff members better understand the unique health needs of a student and improves communication among the people working with the student and family to achieve the outcome goals. Clearly articulating each component of care provides a road map and gives direction to those involved in the delivery of care. A number of publications describe how standardized languages can be incorporated into IHPs and provide sample IHPs for school nurses (Denehy & Poulton, 1999; Poulton & Denehy, 1999; Cavendish, 2001; Cavendish, 2003; Strawhacker & Wellendorf, 2004). These samples give school nurses concrete examples of how to update their IHPs using standardized languages, NANDA, NIC, and NOC.

## NANDA Nursing Diagnoses

NANDA International began its pioneering work in 1973. The work of this association has set the stage for the use of standardized language in the profession of nursing. The NANDA nursing diagnoses have gained widespread acceptance and use in nursing practice and nursing education. The 2003-2004 NANDA classification contains 167 nursing diagnoses. Nursing diagnosis is defined as "A clinical judgment about individual, family, or community responses to actual and potential health problems/life processes. A nursing diagnosis provides the basis for selection of nursing interventions to achieve outcomes for which the nurse is accountable" (NANDA, 2003, p. 263). Nursing diagnoses have a label or name, a definition, relat-

ed factors that describe conditions antecedent to or associated with the diagnosis, and defining characteristics, which are observable signs and symptoms that are manifestations of the diagnosis.

There are three types of nursing diagnoses. The first type is an *actual* diagnosis, which "describes human responses to health conditions/life processes that exist in an individual, family, or community. It is supported by defining characteristics (manifestations, signs and symptoms) that cluster in patterns of related cues or inferences" (NANDA, 2003, p. 263) (e.g., *Constipation, Dysfunctional Family Processes: Alcoholism*, and *Ineffective Community Coping*). Actual nursing diagnoses are frequently used in the school setting with individual children experiencing healthcare concerns.

The second type is a risk diagnosis, which "describes human responses to health conditions/life processes that may develop in a vulnerable individual, family, or community. It is supported by risk factors that contribute to increased vulnerability" (NANDA, 2003, p. 263) (e.g., *Risk for Injury* and *Risk for Impaired Parenting*). (Note: Risk diagnoses were previously referred to as potential diagnoses.) Risk diagnoses are also commonly used in the school setting not only for individuals at risk for health problems, but for aggregates or groups in the school community.

The third type of nursing diagnosis is a *wellness* diagnosis, which "describes human responses to levels of wellness in an individual, family, or community that have a readiness for enhancement" (NANDA, 2003, p. 263) (e.g., *Readiness for Enhanced Spiritual Wellbeing* and *Readiness for Enhanced Family Processes*). At this time there are few wellness diagnoses in the classification.

The NANDA nursing diagnoses classification has developed over the years as practicing nurses have suggested revisions and created new diagnoses related to their practice area and submitted them for review by the NANDA Diagnosis Review Committee for consideration into the classification. The 2003-2004 edition of the NANDA classification has added 12 diagnoses, 11 of which are health promotion/wellness diagnoses, such as *Readiness for Enhanced Nutrition* and *Readiness for Enhanced Self-Concept*. An additional three diagnoses were revised based on feedback from nurses interested in updating existing diagnoses to reflect current practice. School nurses have an opportunity to add nursing diagnoses to the NANDA classification by suggesting or creating new diagnoses that reflect the unique needs identified in the school population. Examples of new nursing diagnoses appropriate for school nursing identified by the author (J.D.) are *Risk for Unintended Pregnancy*, which would be an appropriate diagnosis for sexually active adolescents, and *Risk for Substance Use*, a concern in many high school populations today. Submission guidelines for new nursing diagnoses are outlined in the NANDA classification (NANDA, 2003, pp. 255–260).

The nursing diagnoses in the NANDA classification have been organized into a taxonomy. NANDA's Taxonomy Committee is currently developing a new organizing structure, Taxonomy II, which is similar to Marjorie Gordon's (1998) Functional Health Patterns. The new taxonomic structure is organized into 13 domains from the Functional Health Patterns (**Table 1**). Each domain is then organized into classes that arrange the diagnoses in each domain into smaller groups. Each domain and class have been defined. For example, in the domain Elimination, defined as "Secretion and excretion of waste products from the body" (NANDA, 2003, p. 229), there are four classes: Urinary System, Gastrointestinal System, Integumentary System, and Pulmonary System. The relevant nursing diagnoses are then listed under each class. In the class Gastrointestinal System, defined as "Excretion and expulsion of waste products from the bowel" (p. 229), five nursing diagnoses are listed: *Bowel Incontinence, Diarrhea, Constipation, Risk for Constipation,* and *Perceived Constipation.*

**Table 1. Domains in the NANDA Classification**

| | |
|---|---|
| 1. Health Promotion | 8. Sexuality |
| 2. Nutrition | 9. Coping/Stress Tolerance |
| 3. Elimination | 10. Life Principles |
| 4. Activity/Rest | 11. Safety/Protection |
| 5. Perception/Cognition | 12. Comfort |
| 6. Self-perception | 13. Growth/Development |
| 7. Role Relationships | (NANDA, 2003, pp. 228-237) |

The NANDA taxonomy is designed to organize the 167 diagnoses in the classification and will facilitate retrieval of nursing diagnoses for the practicing nurse. It also shows areas in which additional diagnoses need to be developed. Work continues on this new taxonomic structure and on codes for computerization of nursing diagnoses.

### NANDA Nursing Diagnoses in IHPs

In the IHP, the nursing diagnosis describes the identified problem area that will be addressed in the school setting. Nursing diagnoses are identified by the school nurse using clinical judgment and are based on the assessment data gathered about the student from information obtained from the student, family, school staff, and other healthcare providers. The nurse may identify one or more nursing diagnoses for a particular student. Each diagnosis will lead to specific student outcome goals and appropriate nursing interventions selected to achieve those goals. The use of NANDA nursing diagnoses provides a common language to describe the student's actual or potential problem areas. The written nursing diagnosis includes the diagnostic label (name), related factors, and defining characteristics. For example, the nursing diagnosis *Constipation related to immobility* (related factor), *characterized by hard, infrequent stool* (defining characteristics) is often seen in students with cerebral palsy.

## The Nursing Interventions Classification

The NIC is a comprehensive, standardized language describing treatments that nurses perform in all settings and in all specialties (Dochterman & Bulechek, 2004). It was developed by a research team formed in 1987 at the University of Iowa College of Nursing. The team included nurses representing a wide range of clinical specialties and practice settings. The NIC is based on existing research and clinical practice. The structure of NIC is easy to use with terminology that is familiar and clinically useful to practicing nurses. It has been implemented in numerous clinical and educational settings, including tertiary care and long-term care settings as well as ambulatory settings and schools. The NIC has been recognized by the American Nurses Association as one data set that will meet the guidelines for information system vendors. It is also included in the Methathesaurus of the National Library of Medicine's Unified Medical Language System, has been added to the Cumulative Index to Nursing & Allied Health Literature (CINAHL), and is listed by the Joint Commission on Accreditation of Healthcare Organizations as one classification that can be used to meet the standard on uniform data. It is currently being used in practice, education, and computer information systems.

The NIC includes 514 interventions that are grouped into a taxonomy to facilitate access by the practicing nurse. A nursing intervention is defined as "Any treatment, based upon clinical judgment and knowledge, that a nurse performs to enhance patient/client outcomes" (Dochterman & Bulechek, 2004, p. xxiii). Each nursing intervention has a name or label, a definition, a set of activities that a nurse might do to carry out the intervention, and a short list of background readings.

The NIC describes five types of nursing interventions. The first type is direct care interventions. "A direct care intervention is a treatment performed through interaction with the patient(s)" (p. xxiii). Direct care interventions are those that involve actual nurse to patient or client contact, both physiological and psychosocial treatments. Common direct care interventions for school nurses would include *Asthma Management, Wound Care, Anxiety Reduction,* and *Active Listening.* The second type of nursing intervention is indirect care interventions. "An indirect care intervention is a treatment performed away from the patient but on behalf of a patient or group of patients" (p. xxiii). Examples frequently used by school nurses are *Documentation, Delegation, Referral,* and *Multidisciplinary Care Conference.* The third type of nursing interventions is community health interventions. "A community (public health) intervention is targeted to promote and preserve the health of populations" (p. xxiii). School nurses often implement interventions to groups in the school community to promote health or prevent disease or injury. Other interventions in this group include strategies that address the social and political climate that may contribute to health risks. Examples of community health interventions are *Health Education, Teaching: Sexuality, Bioterrorism Preparedness,* and *Environmental Management: Safety.*

The final two types of nursing interventions are related to who has initiated the intervention. The first is nurse-initiated treatments. "A nurse-initiated treatment is an intervention initiated by the nurse in response to a nursing diagnosis. It is an autonomous action based on scientific rationale that is executed to benefit the client in a predicted way related to the nursing diagnosis and projected outcomes. These actions would include those treatments initiated by advanced nurse practitioners" (p. xxiii). Examples of nurse-initiated treatments are *Latex Precautions, Health Screening, Exercise Promotion,* and *Wound Care.* Because of the autonomous nature of school nursing practice, most of the interventions implemented by nurses in the school setting are nurse-initiated treatments. The final type of nursing interventions is physician-initiated treatments. "A physician-initiated treatment is an intervention initiated by a physician in response to a medical diagnosis but is carried out by a nurse in response to a 'doctor's order.' Nurses may also carry out treatments initiated by other providers, such as pharmacists, respiratory therapists, or physician assistants" (p. xxiii). In some states, advanced nurse practitioners may also initiate these treatments. School nurses require a physician's order for interventions such as *Medication Administration: Oral, Oxygen Therapy,* and *Tube Care: Gastrointestinal.*

The NIC contains interventions that reflect the wide scope of school nursing practice (Pavelka, McCarthy, & Denehy, 1999). It includes interventions for illness management (e.g., *Seizure Management*), disease prevention (e.g., *Immunization/Vaccination Administration*), and health promotion (e.g., *Health Education*). There are also interventions for individuals (e.g., *Nutrition Management*) and for families (e.g., *Family Integrity Promotion*) as well as for aggregates and communities (e.g., *Health Education* and *Environmental Management: Safety*). In IHPs, the NIC label and definition are to be used as stated in the NIC. However, the activities listed under each NIC label are only suggestions. Any of these suggested activities can be selected if needed for the individual student, some may need to be revised to reflect the needs for the particular student in the school setting, or additional activities may be created as appropriate.

The interventions in the NIC also have a taxonomy, consisting of seven domains (**Table 2**) and 30 classes (Dochterman & Bulechek, 2004, p. v). Each domain and class have been defined to assist users. Each of the 514 nursing interventions has been placed in an appropriate class, facilitating organization and retrieval of the interventions. For example, the Safety domain, defined as "Care that supports protection against harm" (p. 122), has two classes, Crisis Management and Risk Management. The Risk Management class, defined as "Interventions to initiate risk reduction activities and continue monitoring risks over time" (p. 122), lists 42 related interventions,

including *Infection Control, Sports Injury Prevention: Youth,* and *Seizure Management.*

**Table 2. Domains in the Nursing Interventions Classification (NIC)**

| | |
|---|---|
| 1. Physiological: Basic | 5. Family |
| 2. Physiological: Complex | 6. Health System |
| 3. Behavioral | 7. Community |
| 4. Safety | (NIC, 2004, pp. 112–125.) |

A coding system has been developed to identify each NIC nursing intervention, based on the domain, class, and specific nursing intervention. This coding system will facilitate the use of NIC interventions in the computerized health record and for reimbursement for school nursing services. The coding system and its use are described in greater depth in the fourth edition of *Nursing Interventions Classification.*

## NIC Interventions in IHPs

In the IHP, the NIC intervention describes the nursing care to be delivered. Each nursing intervention lists specific activities that can be used to implement the intervention. These activities are to be individualized to the student and carried out by the school nurse or other designated person. The intervention is selected to achieve the desired outcome goal stated on the IHP. Interventions implemented in the school setting and listed on the IHP include both direct and indirect care. The interventions may be specific prescribed orders (e.g., *Medication Administration* and *Urinary Catherization: Intermittent*), nursing care and ongoing monitoring of health status (e.g., *Asthma Management* and *Vital Signs Monitoring*), delegating and teaching of nonlicensed personnel, supervision of these staff members (e.g., *Delegation* and *Staff Supervision*), as well as follow-up and ongoing communication with parents, the education team, and healthcare providers (e.g., *Multidisciplinary Care Conference* and *Telephone Follow-up*). It is important to include both direct care (e.g., *Tube Care: Gastrointestinal*) and indirect care (e.g., *Delegation* and *Multidisciplinary Care Conference*) interventions in the IHP. Also included with the intervention and specific activities is the title or name of the person delegated to carry out the activity in the school setting. Remember that delegation includes consideration of the student's health status, the person's willingness to complete the task, the competency level and scope of practice, training and supervision of that person, and safety of the student/potential for harm.

The listed activities in the NIC are suggestions that fit with the particular intervention. If appropriate, these activities might be chosen or individualized to meet student needs. Additional activities should be included if necessary to meet the needs of the student. The authors of the NIC recommend six factors to consider when choosing a nursing intervention (Dochterman & Bulechek, 2004).

---

These same factors can be applied to the process of choosing interventions to include in the IHP. First, consider what is the desired student outcome and which interventions can be implemented to help the student reach the stated outcome goal. Second, consider the nursing diagnoses and what interventions will change the related factors, treat the signs and symptoms, or minimize the risk factors identified. Third, think about the research base of the interventions and choose those for which there is evidence of their effectiveness. Fourth, consider what is pertinent to the student's health status and the feasibility of actually completing the intervention. Fifth, choose interventions that will be acceptable to the student and parents, as well as to the staff involved in the care of the child. Sixth and finally, consider the capability and competence of the staff carrying out the intervention. After consideration of each of these factors, the school nurse can determine what interventions are needed to meet the student outcomes goals to optimize the student's health and academic achievement.

The Iowa Intervention Project team conducted a research project to determine the core interventions for nursing specialties. Core interventions are a "central set of interventions that define the nature of the specialty" (Dochterman & Bulechek, 2004, p. 905). There were 62 core interventions listed for the specialty of school nursing (p. 929). Examination of the interventions on this list will assist school nurses in locating some of the most commonly used nursing interventions in school nursing practice.

School nurses bring a vast knowledge and experience base to their practice. They often know what interventions need to be initiated for students with special healthcare needs. In this case, it is just a matter of using a classification system to put the interventions on paper, using the standardized language provided by the classification. With repeated use, patterns will develop and many of the same intervention labels will be used for groups of students with similar health concerns. Use of the NIC system also may expand the care delivered as school nurses find new activities that may be helpful for the particular student. Once school nurses begin to use the NIC, they will see the benefits of using a standardized system and find it user-friendly and very relevant for use in IHPs.

## The Nursing Outcomes Classification

The NOC was also developed by a research team at the University of Iowa College of Nursing who realized there was a need to evaluate the effectiveness of nursing interventions in a systematic way. This classification consists of 330 nursing outcomes, defined as "An individual, family or community state, behavior, or perception that is measured along a continuum in response to a nursing intervention(s)" (Moorhead, Johnson & Maas, 2004, p. xix). "Outcomes … define a patient status at a particular point in time and may indicate improvement or deterioration of the state compared with a previous assessment" (p. 25). The procedures used by the Iowa Outcomes Project research team to develop the NOC were similar to those

used by the NIC team. The NOC is recognized by the American Nurses Association (ANA), is included in the Metathesaurus in the National Library of Medicine's Unified Medical Language System, is included in CINAHL, and meets the standards of the ANA's Nursing Information and Data Set Evaluation Center.

In the NOC system, each outcome has a neutral label or name and a definition, followed by a list of indicators that describe client behavior or patient status. NOC outcomes are stated in neutral terms. The reason for this is that client status may move in the desired direction, but it may remain unchanged or deteriorate. Therefore, a neutral outcome label is necessary to accurately characterize the actual behavior, whatever the direction. It is important to note that NOC outcomes differ from desired patient outcomes or goals in that outcome goals are stated as the desired end results or behavior and are not neutral in nature. A desired outcome goal might be Pain Reduction, indicating a positive movement in controlling pain. The appropriate NOC outcome to determine if this outcome goal has been achieved would be Pain Level, defined as "Severity of observed or reported pain" (Moorhead, Johnson & Maas, 2004, p. 421). The neutral outcome, *Pain Level*, can determine the level of pain. The result may indicate that the pain is reduced, remains the same, or has in fact gotten worse after intervention. Examples of indicators in this outcome are "Reported pain," "Facial expressions of pain," and "Muscle tension" (p. 421).

Each NOC outcome includes a 5-point scale to rate indicators. Lower scores (1 and 2 indicate minimal performance, and higher scores (4 and 5) indicate that clients are progressing well on that particular indicator. For example, the outcome Pain Level uses the following 5-point scale to measure the related indicators: (1) severe, (2) substantial, (3) moderate, (4) slight, and (5) none. The outcome *Risk Control: Sexually Transmitted Diseases* (STD), uses the 5-point scale (1) never demonstrated, (2) rarely demonstrated, (3) sometimes demonstrated, (4) often demonstrated, and (5) consistently demonstrated, to measure the indicators such as "Acknowledges individual risk for STD," "Uses methods to control STD transmission," and "Inquires of partner's STD status before sexual activity" (Moorhead, Johnson & Maas, 2004, p. 471). The scales can be used to determine baseline status prior to intervention and to compare with client status at different points after interventions have been implemented. By making this comparison, the school nurse can determine the effectiveness of the intervention in reaching the desired outcome goal and modify it accordingly. The third edition of *Nursing Outcomes Classification* has 13 different scales to measure outcomes that are appropriate to the nature of the indicators for a specific outcome.

When using NOC outcomes, one must use the NOC label and definition as written. Outcomes can be customized, however, by choosing indicators that are relevant to the specific child's goals, by modifying indicators to reflect the needs of children in a school setting, or by developing additional indicators as needed.

Like NANDA and NIC, the NOC system has a taxonomy to organize the 330 outcomes and to facilitate retrieval by the practicing nurse. The NOC taxonomy consists of seven domains (**Table 3**). The seven domains contain 31 classes. For example, the domain Functional Health, defined as "Outcomes that describe capacity for and performance of basic tasks of life" (Moorhead, Johnson & Maas, 2004, p. 103), contains the following classes: Energy Maintenance, Growth and Development, Mobility, and Self-Care. Each class groups related outcomes. The class Growth and Development contains 21 outcomes related to an individual's physical, emotional, and social maturation.

**Table 3. Domains in the Nursing Outcomes Classification (NOC)**

| | |
|---|---|
| 1. Functional Health | 5. Perceived Health |
| 2. Physiological Health | 6. Family Health |
| 3. Psychosocial Health | 7. Community Health |
| 4. Health Knowledge and Behavior | (NIC, 2004, pp. 112–125.) |

The NOC outcomes have been coded with a unique 6-digit number reflecting the domain, class, and specific nursing outcome. In addition, each indicator, scale, and scale value can be added to the code to facilitate the computerization and analysis of outcome data. The coding system and its use are described in greater depth in the third edition of *Nursing Outcomes Classification*.

## NOC Outcomes in IHPs

The use of the NOC system in the IHP assists the school nurse in evaluating the effectiveness of nursing interventions in meeting the desired outcome goal. The IHP is reviewed at least yearly or when there is any change in the student's health status. Basically, when evaluating the IHP, the nurse must decide if the stated goal has been achieved or if movement is being made in that direction. "The evaluation process includes: (a) reviewing the desired student outcome, (b) collecting data to determine the outcome, (c) comparing the actual outcome to the desired student outcome, (d) documenting the outcome on the IHP, (e) relating the appropriateness and effectiveness of the selected interventions to the outcome, and (f) reviewing and modifying the plan of care as necessary. The use of NOC outcomes provides a quantitative measure of student progress that is easy for all healthcare providers to use and understand" (Denehy & Poulton, 1999, p. 44).

To review, when writing the actual IHP, the school nurse determines the nursing diagnosis based on assessment data; from this diagnosis the school nurse in collaboration with the multidisciplinary team determines the desired outcome goals for the student; the nursing interventions are selected to meet the outcome goals identified; and finally, the outcomes or effectiveness of the nursing interventions are measured to determine the progress made toward meeting student outcome goals.

The NOC outcome label indicates the area of concern to be monitored. There is a list of indicators for each NOC outcome. These indicators can be tailored to the individual student needs. The outcome statement is *neutral*. When it is time to complete the evaluation of the IHP, the NOC outcomes can be used to determine if the outcomes have been achieved. The NOC scales can be included in the written IHP (see Sample IHP) and used before interventions have been implemented to gather baseline data, as well as after interventions to determine the outcomes of care. By including the NOC scales in the IHP, members of the team can see how student outcomes will be measured and can observe student progress toward reaching the outcome goals established in the IHP.

The Nursing Outcomes Project team has also compiled a list of core outcomes used by different nursing specialties. The core nursing outcomes for school nursing are listed in NOC (Moorhead, Johnson & Maas, 2004, p. 693) and represent outcomes identified as those most frequently used in school nursing practice. This list provides a helpful introduction for school nurses integrating NOC outcomes in IHPs.

## NANDA, NIC, and NOC Linkages

A linkage is defined as "a relationship or association between a nursing diagnosis and a nursing intervention that causes them to occur together in order to obtain an outcome or the resolution of a patient's problem" (Dochterman & Bulechek, 2004, p. 783) or "an association or relationship that exists between a patient problem (nursing diagnosis) and a desired outcome (resolution or improvement of the problem)" (Moorhead, Johnson & Maas, 2004, p. 579). Linkages among the NANDA diagnoses, the NIC interventions, and the NOC outcomes are included in the appendixes of the NIC and NOC books, as well as in a separate book (Johnson, et al., 2001) and computer software package (Johnson, Dochterman, & Moorhead, 2004). These linkages facilitate the selection of NIC nursing interventions and NOC nursing outcomes appropriate for the NANDA nursing diagnosis and outcome goal stated in a child's IHP. The linkages give school nurses structure and assistance in locating relevant interventions and outcomes as they learn to use the nursing classifications.

In *Nursing Interventions Classification*, fourth edition, each NANDA nursing diagnosis is listed, and then suggested nursing interventions for problem resolution are listed. For example, for the nursing diagnosis, *Risk for Aspiration*, 16 NIC interventions are listed. Three priority interventions, the most likely and obvious interventions, are highlighted for this diagnosis—*Aspiration Precautions, Teaching: Infant Safety*, and *Vomiting Management*. For the nursing diagnosis Fear, of the 15 suggested interventions listed, *Anxiety Reduction, Coping Enhancement*, and *Security Enhancement* are highlighted as priority interventions. In addition to the 15 suggested interventions, 25 additional optional interventions are listed. These priority, suggested, and optional interventions give the school nurse a wide range of choices in selecting an appropriate nursing intervention for the nursing diagnosis Fear.

In the *Nursing Outcomes Classification*, third edition, each NANDA nursing diagnosis is listed and followed by a list of suggested outcomes. To follow up on the same example, the nursing diagnosis *Risk for Aspiration* is followed by a list of 17 suggested outcomes. No priority outcomes are highlighted in the NOC linkages. An appropriate outcome for this diagnosis might be *Respiratory Status: Ventilation*, although there are others listed that could be appropriate in different cases. For the nursing diagnosis Fear, three suggested outcomes are listed, and six additional associated outcomes are given. An appropriate suggested outcome might be Fear Level: Child.

The book *Nursing Diagnoses, Outcomes, and Interventions: NANDA, NOC, and NIC Linkages* puts all the linkage information in one source devoted to showing the relationship among the classifications in nursing practice (Johnson et al., 2001). The linkages can also be obtained on CD-ROM from the Center for Nursing Classification and Clinical Effectiveness. This guide provides a quick reference for those planning care using the nursing process and standardized languages in any setting. There are many examples of how NANDA/NIC/NOC linkages are appropriate to school nursing practice (**Table 4**). The use of these linkages is particularly relevant to the development of IHPs, because they cover the major components listed in these documents, as well as a method to measure movement toward the desired outcome goal.

## Summary

School nurses know that it is important to document the delivery of special healthcare services to students. An IHP formalizes the nursing care to be given. To make the IHP a useful document, it is important to write the IHP in a consistent manner that can be easily communicated to other members of the healthcare team and members of the education team. By using standardized nursing language in IHPs, school nurses will be doing just that—documenting the provision of special health services to individual students consistently in a form that is easily communicated to others involved in the care of the student.

The use of a standardized nursing language also provides data on the care provided and the outcomes of that care. This information can then be entered into computerized information systems for data collection and research. By computerizing the data included in IHPs, school nurses have the potential to develop large databases that will help identify common problems, the effectiveness of various nursing interventions, and their success in achieving the desired outcomes. This information can be used to show the contribution of school nurses to the health of children with special needs and lead to the provision of evidence-based care in the school setting. This data also will provide the impetus for research on interventions that school nurses use and how school nurses use their time. In addition, it can be used to examine the linkages between interventions and outcomes—which interventions are

**Table 4. Examples of NANDA, NIC, and NOC Linkages**

| NANDA Nursing Diagnosis | NIC Nursing Intervention | NOC Nursing Outcome |
|---|---|---|
| Ineffective Breathing Pattern | Asthma Management | Asthma Self-Management |
| Social Isolation | Socialization Enhancement | Social Involvement |
| Risk for Injury | Environmental Management: Safety | Safety Status: Physical Injury |
| Ineffective Family Coping | Coping Enhancement | Family Coping |
| Risk for Infection | Teaching: Sexuality | Risk Control: STD |
| Imbalanced Nutrition: More than Body Requirements | Weight Management | Nutritional Status: Body Mass |
| Situational Low Self-Esteem | Self-Esteem Enhancement | Self-Esteem |
| Risk for Other-Directed Violence | Anger Control Assistance | Impulse Control |

most effective in reaching the desired outcome. Coupled with student demographic and educational data, this data allows school nurses to track the academic progress of children with special healthcare needs. This data has the potential to show the value of school nurses in the school setting in promoting optimal health and maximizing learning in children with special healthcare needs. Such data may help make the case for additional nurses or personnel to assist nurses in their work with students. In this age of budget cuts and the replacement of nurses with nonlicensed personnel, it is essential that school nurses document what nursing interventions are necessary and effective in meeting the special healthcare needs of children. This process is assisted through the use of standardized languages.

We live in an era in which healthcare educational costs are a major concern, and reducing these costs by cutting personnel or services is common. Difficult decisions about prioritizing limited educational funding often mean trimming or cutting existing programs and services. Particularly challenging to school nurses is articulating their contribution to the educational mission of the schools in terms educators can understand and appreciate. A new outcome in NOC, Student Health Status (Moorhead et al., 2004, pp. 522-523), lists indicators for educational as well as health outcomes. Some of the educational indicators include school attendance, readiness to learn, academic performance at grade level or better, and participation in curricular school activities. Use of standardized language clearly identifies and defines components of care, as well as providing a mechanism to evaluate the effectiveness of this care. Not only is it important that the activities of today's school nurses be visible, but also nurses need to show in a concrete way that what they do—their nursing interventions—make a difference in the health and educational outcomes of students. The use of standardized nursing languages has the potential to assist school nurses in showing that what school nurses do does make a difference.

---

**Table 5. Example of an IHP Using Standardized Nursing Languages**

*Scenario:* Up-to-date immunization is required for school entry and throughout the childhood years to protect students and the community from common communicable diseases. School nurses are often responsible for keeping records on student immunization status and recommending when immunizations need to be updated according to school policy. The following is a care plan related to immunization compliance using standardized nursing languages.

**Nursing Care Plan:**

| Nursing Diagnosis | Goals | Nursing Interventions | Expected Outcomes |
|---|---|---|---|
| *Risk for Infection* | Immunizations of students will be up to date. | *Immunization/Vaccination Management* | *Immunization Behavior* |

**Intervention: *Immunization/Vaccination Management***

*Activities:*
- Inform families which immunizations are required by law for entering preschool, kindergarten, junior high, high school, and college.
- Follow the American Academy of Pediatrics (AAP), American Academy of Family Physicians, and U.S. Public Health Service (USPHS) guidelines for immunization administration.
- Audit school immunization records for completeness on a yearly basis.
- Notify individual/family when immunizations are not up-to-date.
- Identify providers who participate in federal "Vaccine for Children" program to provide free vaccines.
- Advocate for programs and policies that provide free or affordable immunizations to all populations.
- Support national registry to track immunization status.

| Never Demonstrated 1 | Rarely Demonstrated 2 | Sometimes Demonstrated 3 | Often Demonstrated 4 | Consistently Demonstrated 5 |
|---|---|---|---|---|

**Outcome: *Immunization Behavior***

*Indicators:*
- Acknowledges disease risk without immunization
- Obtains immunizations recommended for age by the AAP or USPHS
- Identifies community resources for immunization

# References

Cavendish, R. (2001). The use of standardized language to describe abdominal pain. *Journal of School Nursing,* 17(4), 266–273.

Cavendish, R. (2003). A Lyme disease case study and individualized healthcare plan. *Journal of School Nursing,* 19(2), 81–88.

Cavendish, R., Lunney, M., Luise, B. K., & Richardson, K. (1999) National survey to identify the nursing interventions used in school settings. *Journal of School Nursing,* 15(2), 12–19.

Cavendish, R., Lunney, M., Luise, B. K., & Richardson, K. (2001). The nursing outcomes classification: Its relevance to school nursing. *Journal of School Nursing,* 17(4), 189–197.

Center for Nursing Classification & Clinical Effectiveness: The University of Iowa College of Nursing. http://www.nursing.uiowa.edu/centers/cncce/

Denehy, J. (2000). Measuring the outcomes of school nursing practice: Showing that school nurses do make a difference: *Journal of School Nursing,* 16(1), 2–3.

Denehy, J. (2004). Using nursing languages in school nursing practice. *Nursing classification systems: North American Nursing Diagnosis Association* (NANDA). Nursing Interventions Classification (NIC), Nursing Outcomes Classification (NOC). Scarborough, ME: National Association of School Nurses.

Denehy, J. & Poulton, S. (1999). The use of standardized language in individualized healthcare plans. *Journal of School Nursing,* 15(1), 38–45.

Dochterman, J., & Bulechek, G.M. (2004). *Nursing Interventions Classification* (NIC) (4th ed.). St. Louis, MO: Mosby.

Fahrenkrug, M.A. (2003). Development of a nursing data set for school nursing. *Journal of School Nursing,* 19(4), 238–248.

Gordon, M. (1998). *Manual of nursing diagnosis.* St. Louis, MO: Mosby.

Hootman, J. (1996). Nursing diagnosis—A language of nursing; a language for powerful communication. *Journal of School Nursing,* 12(4), 19–23.

Johnson, M., Bulechek, G., McCloskey Dochterman, J., Maas, M., & Moorhead, S. (2001). *Nursing diagnoses, outcomes, and interventions: NANDA, NOC, and NIC Linkages.* St. Louis, MO: Mosby.

Johnson, M., Dochterman J., & Moorhead S. (2004). *Nursing diagnoses, outcomes, and interventions: NANDA, NOC, and NIC Linkages, Nursing Interventions Classification 4e, Nursing Outcomes Classification 3e package.* St. Louis, MO: Mosby. [AU: Reference OK as added? This is the package]

Lunney, M. (1996). The significance of nursing classification systems to school nursing. *Journal of School Nursing,* 12(2), 35–37.

Martin, K. S., & Scheet, N. J. (1992). *The Omaha System: Applications for community health nursing.* Philadelphia: Saunders.

Moorhead, S., Johnson, M., & Maas, M. (2004). *Nursing Outcomes Classification (NOC)* (3rd ed.). St. Louis, MO: Mosby.

NANDA International (NANDA). (2003). *NANDA nursing diagnoses: Definitions and classification 2003-2004.* Philadelphia: Author.

National Association of School Nurses (NASN). (1999). Definition of school nursing. *Journal of School Nursing,* 15(3), 5. Available online at: http://www.nasn.org

National Association of School Nurses (NASN). (2001). *Position statement: Nursing classification systems: North American Nursing Diagnosis Association (NANDA), Nursing Interventions Classification (NIC), and Nursing Outcomes Classification (NOC).* Available online at: http://www.nasn.org/positions/nanda.htm

Pavelka, L., McCarthy, A. M., & Denehy, J. (1999). Nursing interventions used by school nurses. *Journal of School Nursing,* 15(1): 27–31.

Poulton, S., & Denehy, J. (1999). Standardized languages in nursing: Integrating NANDA, NIC, and NOC into IHPs. In M. J. Arnold & C. K. Silkworth (Eds.), *The School Nurse's Source Book of Individualized Healthcare Plan—Volume II* (pp. 25–40). North Branch, MN: Sunrise River Press.

Strawhacker, M., & Wellendorf, J. (2004). Caring for children with cystic fibrosis: A collaborative clinical and school approach. *Journal of School Nursing,* 20(1), 5–15.

# Individualized Healthcare Plan

Student name: _____  Birth date: _____  Effective dates: _____

School: _____  Physician: _____  School nurse: _____

| Assessment Data: | Nursing diagnosis: | Student Goals | Interventions (Person responsible listed in parentheses) | Outcomes |
|---|---|---|---|---|
| 12-year old diagnosed asthma at age 9. Carries Proventil inhaler at all times. Independent in identifying symptoms and need for treatment. M.D. order normal PE program | *Ineffective breathing pattern* (NANDA, 2003, p. 25) as characterized by shortness of breath. Coughing, and/or wheezing related to asthma. | 1. _____ will demonstrate appropriate use of inhaler at the beginning of school year. <br><br> 2. _____ will initiate treatment when symptoms appear throughout the school year. <br><br> 3. _____ will keep record of peak flow meter readings if required throughout the school year. <br><br> 4. _____ will keep record of use of inhaler for health office throughout the school year. <br><br> 5. _____ will avoid having an emergency asthma attack during this school year. | *Asthma Management* (NIC) <br><br> **Activities:** <br> • Review use of inhaler with _____ at the beginning of the school year. (Nurse) <br><br> • At the beginning of the school year, review with teacher and other appropriate staff, the signs and symptoms of asthma exacerbation and when _____ should use his inhaler. (Nurse) <br><br> • Every two months, obtain student's record of inhaler use for documentation in health file. Report increased use of inhaler to parents/physician. (Nurse) <br><br> *Emergency plan:* <br> See STUDENT ASTHMA EMERGENCY PROTOCOL: (in classroom, locker room, and nurse's office) | *Asthma Self-Management* (NOC) <br><br> **Indicators:** <br> Recognizes onset of asthma <br> Never Rarely Sometimes Often Consistently <br> 1 2 3 4 5 <br><br> Initiates action to manage personal triggers <br> Never Rarely Sometimes Often Consistently <br> 1 2 3 4 5 <br><br> Self-manages exacerbations <br> Never Rarely Sometimes Often Consistently <br> 1 2 3 4 5 <br><br> Reports asthma controlled <br> Never Rarely Sometimes Often Consistently <br> 1 2 3 4 5 |

**I have read and approve of the above plan for school health care:**

Parent signature _____  Date reviewed by the educational team _____

Nurse signature _____  Physician signature (optional) _____

*Chapter Six*

# HIPAA, FERPA, and the Privacy of Student Health Information in Individual Healthcare Plans

Martha Dewey Bergren

## Introduction

School nurses are serving increasing numbers of medically fragile children and students with chronic illness. Individualized healthcare plans (IHPs) for these students require collecting, analyzing, and summarizing a large amount of individual and family health information. Much of that information is highly sensitive and may include third-party records from the student's primary care provider, specialists, geneticists, treatment facilities, and acute care settings. In fact, the amount and complexity of the health and medical information collected on a substantial percentage of students rival that of many hospitalized patients. The detail and the breadth of the student's health history are essential for creating an appropriate education plan and an adequate plan for care that includes interventions, delegating care, and skilled procedures and protects the student's safety. With that responsibility and as the caretaker of the record, the school nurse must ensure that the data collected and the information shared are maintained with the privacy and security afforded to sensitive health records.

## Privacy

Although school personnel are ethically bound to maintain the privacy of student health information, there are federal and state laws that govern the handling of personally identifiable information in schools. The publicity generated by the Health Insurance Portability and Accountability Act (HIPAA) educated average consumers on their privacy rights in regard to personally identifiable health information (Bergren, 2001a; 2001d).

HIPAA was passed in 1996 with the intent of streamlining the burden of the healthcare reimbursement system. To decrease delays and the burden of manual handling of paper claims, uniform electronic processes were developed for reimbursement and other healthcare transactions. Congress recognized the threat to the health privacy of citizens if a mandate for patient electronic databases and transactions was not accompanied by a strict requirement for privacy and security. As a result, HIPAA confers new rights to privacy, providing all persons with access to their own health record and restricting access to their identifiable health information by others. Any agency that engages in a HIPAA transaction (e.g., electronic reimbursement) is subject to a comprehensive array of privacy and security requirements designed to provide reasonable protection of personally identifiable health information (Bergren, 2004a). Penalties for violating HIPAA protections, whether deliberate or accidental, are significant.

HIPAA specifically exempts education records from the Privacy Rule. The rationale for the exemption is that a federal privacy law since 1974, the Family Educational Rights and Privacy Act (FERPA), already protects education records. Education records include all records, files, and other materials that contain information directly related to a student and are maintained by an educational institution or agency or by a person acting for that agency or institution (FERPA, 1974 ). Therefore, all health records created and maintained by a school nurse are education records (Rooker, 2004; Schwab & Pohlman, 2004). According to FERPA (1974), personally identifiable information about students may be shared only internally among educators and staff or with persons who contract with the school to provide a service and who have a "legitimate educational interest" in the student. To share identifiable student information externally, outside the school district, an authorization to release or exchange information must be obtained.

FERPA governs the privacy of educational records in schools that accept federal funds, affecting all public schools and a large majority of private schools. HIPAA governs the privacy practices in private schools that do not accept any federal funding and do engage in HIPAA transactions, such as electronic reimbursement for healthcare (Bergren, 2004a). Private schools that accept no federal funds and do not engage in HIPAA transactions are not covered by either of the federal privacy laws (Bergren, 2004a).

School-based health clinics managed by independent outside agencies, even if housed on school property, are entities covered by HIPAA and must meet HIPAA privacy standards. Public health departments that conduct health department activities on school property, such as giving flu shots and immunizations, generate records that are health department records and covered by HIPAA (Schwab & Pohlman, 2004). If that same health department is contracted by the school district to provide vision and hearing screening, the health department staff creates education records covered by FERPA (Schwab & Pohlman,

2004). Identifying which privacy law applies is not determined by which agency employs the creator of the record, but the by the purpose of the record. Records created for health department purposes are HIPAA records. Records created for the school are education records.

## State Laws

HIPAA and FERPA provide the minimum standards of privacy and confidentiality afforded health and education records. Many states have laws more restrictive than the federal regulations. School nurses should investigate state school record codes and state health record regulations to ensure that personally identifiable information is handled appropriately. The National Association of State Boards of Education has established a State Level School Health Policies Web page that alerts school officials to any state regulations that exceed FERPA privacy standards. The Alan Guttmacher Institute provides a Web page that is updated monthly with state-by-state analysis detailing the sexual and reproductive health and rights of minors. Both of these links are found in the Resources section of this chapter.

## Confidentiality

Professionals, nurses, educators, social workers, psychologists, and others in both private and public education settings are bound by the standards of practice of their professional group, which includes an ethical responsibility for protecting confidential client information. Confidentiality standards for school nurses are explicit in both the American Nurses Association (ANA) Code for Nurses (ANA, 2003) and the School Nursing Standards of Practice (National Association of School Nurses [NASN] & ANA, 2001). When students or parents reveal personal information about themselves or their minor child to a professional, there is an expectation that that information will not be disclosed.

## Personally Identifiable Health Information

HIPAA and FERPA cover records that contain personally identifiable information. Elements in education records that identify a student are: name, address, date of birth; school entry or dates of treatment; telephone and fax numbers; e-mail addresses; Social Security number; medical record or health plan number, account numbers, medical device identifiers and serial numbers; full-face photographic images (Schwab et al., 2005); IP (Internet protocol) addresses, Web addresses, and other unique numbers, characteristics, or codes that render information identifiable (U.S. Department of Health and Human Services [USDHHS], 2000). Both HIPAA and FERPA exempt directory information from privacy regulations when not associated with other education or health information. However, individuals or parents of a minor child can opt out of sharing directory data.

## Identifying Cases

Many parents contact the school nurse if their child has a health condition that requires intervention and monitoring at school. However, often a student's diagnosis is revealed through the routine collection of the annual health or emergency card or on state-mandated physical examination reports. Most schools send such forms to the student's home in the registration packet prior to the start of school. The forms are returned to school and pass though many hands before finally reaching the school health office (Bergren, 2004b; Schwab et al., 2005). Health information that is requested from parents by the school should be returned in a preaddressed sealed envelope and delivered intact to the school nurse (Bergren, 2004b; Schwab et al., 2005). In addition, emergency contact information that is copied and maintained in the main office and other sites throughout the school building should be collected on a form separate from the annual health update (Bergren, 2004b).

Many school nurses discover that a student with serious health conditions has been in school for many months and they have not been notified (Bergren, 2004c). Often other school staff or officials were notified, but they assumed that the parents had notified the school nurse or they did not understand the necessity for the school nurse to be aware of the problems and provide a plan for the student's healthcare and safety. Sharing health information with the school nurse is within the legitimate educational interests of the student and protects the district from liability should an adverse event occur at school. School districts should establish a policy that when parents or a student alerts a teacher or other school district employee to a student health condition, the staff member should offer to notify the school nurse or request that the parent notify the school nurse.

Students, parents, or concerned staff members who present themselves to the health office should be invited to volunteer the reason for the visit in a location that maintains their privacy. Some school health offices are too small for a discussion of sensitive health issues, and those involved need to move to another area. Office practices can be implemented to enhance privacy, such as creating natural barriers with furniture, asking new arrivals to wait in a marked area if the staff is greeting another student, or posting signs that encourage visitors to ask to speak to the nurse confidentially (Bergren, 1999; Bergren, 2004b).

## Data Collection

Once students are identified as having a health condition necessitating an IHP, a health history is undertaken. Parents and students are interviewed and/or asked to fill out comprehensive health history forms. Physicians, nurse practitioners, and other providers are consulted regarding the student's health status and functional limitations. Records are often requested from their primary care providers, acute care settings, and specialists. Each method of data collection presents privacy and confidentiality issues.

Parents and students must be interviewed in an area that provides reasonable privacy, ideally a private room. Depending on the nature of the health problem, arrangements may be made for supervision of minor children and other waiting facilities provided for extended family members or friends during the interview. Parents should be invited to provide additional information by phone following the interview. If forms or information requests are sent home to the family, the school nurse should provide a preaddressed sealable envelope for the return of the data.

Information regarding a treatment ordered by a physician or nurse practitioner that is provided by a school nurse is exempt from the HIPAA Privacy Rule (Campanelli, 2004). However, a HIPAA-compliant release or exchange of information authorization is required to obtain health records or exchange background information regarding a student's IHP with physicians, nurse practitioners, and other providers, agencies, hospitals, and clinics. A HIPAA-covered provider who releases such information without a properly signed release is subject to a significant financial penalty. A HIPAA-compliant form contains the following elements (Bergren, 2004a; USDHHS, 2000):

- A specific and meaningful description of information requested
- Name of person or class of persons to whom information will be disclosed
- Expiration date
- Statement that the authorization may be revoked at any time
- Instructions on how to revoke authorization
- Statement that once information is disclosed, it may no longer be subject to HIPAA protections
- Signature and date
- Description of the signer's authority to act for the minor student (Bergren, 2003)

The HIPAA-covered provider has a responsibility to ensure that the school district's handling of the information is secure and appropriate. Once any information, including third-party health records, is placed into a student's file, it becomes subject to FERPA privacy provisions. Many HIPAA-covered entities send personally identifiable health information in sealed envelopes that inform the recipient that creating copies of the information is prohibited and the information may not be shared or forwarded to any party not on the signed release form. If the recipient does not agree to these restrictions, the information must be returned unopened. School district policy should allow direct access to third-party records only by those listed on the authorization form, and copying of third-party records should be barred (Schwab et al., 2005). Persons contributing to an IHP should use the original record, and the record should not be taken to the staff member's home. Although FERPA allows any information that is part of the education record to be forwarded to a school to which a student plans to transfer, districts are encouraged to create a policy that prohibits transferring third-party records (Schwab et al., 2005).

If information is faxed to a school, the provider has a responsibility to investigate whether the school has a secure fax machine and has procedures for delivering the information to the health office without violating the confidentiality and privacy rights of the student and the family. Fax machines used for identifiable student information should be located outside of public areas (Schwab et al., 2005; Bergren, 2001c). It is recommended that one individual trained in HIPAA/FERPA regulations be accountable for removing all incoming faxes from the machine, ensuring that all pages were received, and placing the faxes in an envelope addressed to a specific person (Schwab et al., 2005; Bergren, 2001c). Many districts opt to install a fax machine in the school health office to decrease the possibility of breaching a student's health information privacy.

## Individual Healthcare Plans

Once the information is collected from parents, the student, and third parties, IHPs are developed in collaboration with the student, family, and healthcare providers (NASN, 2003). For a student with highly complex health conditions, review of the final draft of the IHP by the primary provider may be necessary. Although HIPAA allows healthcare providers to share information regarding treatment with other providers, FERPA has no such exemption, and the school nurse must verify that a current exchange-of-information form is on file before sharing the IHP, part of an education record, with any external person or agency.

To keep health conditions private, the care plan must take into consideration the location of treatments or care the plan dictates. The IHP must specify that the procedures or care delineated be conducted in an area that ensures the student's privacy. The parent and student should be aware of any privacy risks inherent in the plan. The limitations of the physical environment in ensuring privacy need to be addressed within the school district (American Diabetes Association, 2003). Examples of inadequate privacy are the lack of screening or closed doors for self-catheterization, announcing a student name for medication administration, or not providing a private space for blood glucose testing.

Together with the parent, the school nurse should determine who has a legitimate educational interest in the child within the school and who would require a copy of or part of the IHP to provide educational accommodations, healthcare, and a safe environment for the student. Whereas care should be taken to avoid sharing information inappropriately, every effort should be made to identify all pertinent school district personnel relative to the child's education, health, and safety. Parents sign the IHP, which includes the list of individuals who will receive all or part of the care plan.

### Disseminating the IHP

Historically, school nurses have been asked to provide staff and administrators with lists that identify all students with health conditions. Such lists violate the restriction of sharing personally identifiable student information with only those who have a legitimate educational interest in the child (a violation of FERPA), and are not congruent with the standards of nursing practice (Bergren, 2004b; Schwab & Gelfman, 2001; Schwab, Panettieri & Bergren, 1998; Taliaferro, 2003). Anecdotes abound about health condition lists that were viewed by students, classroom visitors, and parent volunteers after being posted on bulletin boards or left on desks. Students who require staff assistance for a health problem are not adequately served by a health conditions list that merely identifies a name and a diagnosis and does not inform the staff of the monitoring or actions required (Bergren, 2004b). Staff members who provide care or monitor a student with a condition that interferes with health and education must be given a written IHP or part of an IHP that pertains to their role. If a student's condition does not interfere with learning or health, and does not require a staff response or monitoring delineated in an IHP, there is no need to share the information with school personnel (Bergren, 2004b).

The school district must identify policy and procedures for the internal dissemination of the IHP. The school nurse has a responsibility to provide the information to each district employee identified in the care plan, along with guidelines on protecting the student's personally identifiable information, whether in the classroom, on the school bus, or on the athletic field. Anyone privy to the care plan and the treatment environment should receive FERPA privacy training. All district employees should have annual FERPA privacy training and should understand their responsibilities in maintaining and securing student information as well as in not sharing the information beyond those identified as having a legitimate educational interest in the student (Bergren 2001a; Bergren, 2004c).

Ideally, the school nurse meets with each staff member to review the care plan and reinforce the need to maintain the student's privacy. The needs of some students are so complex that a meeting with appropriate school personnel is necessary to review the plans and to answer questions. However, for less serious or common health needs, the school nurse may elect to send the care plan or portions of it in sealed envelopes to appropriate individuals and encourage them to follow up if they have any questions. Individuals in either group may sign a statement that they:

- Understand their role in the student's health and safety
- Must protect the privacy of the student's personally identifiable health information
- Maintain the IHP and any personally identifiable information in a private and secure manner
- Understand that identifiable student information may be shared in the event of an emergency. FERPA exempts privacy protections in emergency situation.

## Safeguarding the IHP

The National Task Force on Confidential Student Health Information (2000; Schwab et al., 2005) recommends that all health information collected and managed by the school nurse be stored in the school health office and not in the cumulative education file in the main office. Cumulative education files are accessed by a wide range of personnel who may not have a legitimate educational interest in the health needs of a student. Through the IHP, the school nurse will ensure that staff will have the information needed to provide a safe environment and be responsive to students' health needs.

The IHP will be distributed to staff and administrators in a wide variety of settings throughout the school district. Care plans or documents guiding the staff will be found in classrooms, on busses, in the gym, on the playground, and in individual offices. Ideally, IHPs should be stored in locked file cabinets (Cheung, Clements, & Pechman, 1997; Schwab et al., 2005; Schwab & Gelfman, 2001). However, immediate access is needed for certain health conditions, and situations may necessitate that IHPs be carried during outside activities, on field trips, and to athletic events in other districts. Every precaution should be taken to prevent the reading or viewing of IHPs by anyone other than the person responsible for the student's care and safety, while at the same time making the information accessible when needed. Opaque envelopes should be used to carry the information within the building or school grounds. In a classroom, IHPs that need to be accessed frequently can be stored in a sleeve or pocket inside a lockable cabinet. Students in wheelchairs may have sealed envelopes with plans in a pocket on the chair.

## Electronic IHPs

When a school district uses electronic student education records, additional precautions must be taken. If the IHP is part of the electronic record, access to records must be limited to those who have both a legitimate educational interest in the student and are included in the IHP distribution list. A teacher or librarian may have a legitimate educational interest in a student but may not necessarily be included on the list of school personnel who have a role in performing the care or the monitoring specified in the IHP. Access to the IHP and student health information should be protected by a password, and the record should be partitioned from the remainder of the student's education record according to password permissions (Bergren, 2001a; 2001d). In other words, the record is programmed to allow only certain individuals access to the IHP based on their password. If the software used by the school district does not allow partitioning, it is not appropriate to put the care plan and other health information within the electronic education record.

HIPAA, FERPA, and the Privacy of Student Health Information

**40**    *Chapter Six: HIPAA, FERPA, and the Privacy of Student Health Information*

The school nurse should also investigate the district's policy regarding sending identifiable information over the school's electronic network. It may not be prudent to send the IHP to individual teachers or staff by email if the system or the network is not secure. Encryption is recommended for sending any identifiable information by electronic mail. Many school districts have opted to bar electronic transfer of sensitive information by e-mail (Bergren, 2001a; 2001b).

## Summary

The complexity of many students' health conditions and the volume of health information created and collected in schools have increased scrutiny of how districts protect student and family FERPA privacy rights. The advent of HIPAA has brought about changes in how districts acquire and manage information needed for IHPs from third-party providers and agencies. School nurses must take both federal privacy laws and state laws into consideration when collecting, preparing, and disseminating IHPs. Students and families should be confident that when care is needed during the school day, their personally identifiable information will be treated with the respect and consideration afforded them by law. School districts need to examine their practices and create new policies and procedures that allow school nurses and staff members to fulfill their legal and ethical responsibilities.

## References

American Diabetes Association. (2003). Care of children with diabetes in the school and daycare setting. Helping the child with diabetes succeed. Diabetes Care, 26(Suppl. I), S131–S135.

American Nurses Association. (2003). *Code for nurses with interpretive statements.* Washington, DC: Author.

Bergren, M. D. (1999). Legal issues: Office management practices. *Journal of School Nursing,* 15(3), 40–41.

Bergren, M. D. (2001a). Electronic records and technology. In N. C. Schwab & M. H.B. Gelfman (Eds.), *Legal issues in school health services: A resource for school nurses, administrators and attorneys.* North Branch, MN: Sunrise River Press.

Bergren, M. D. (2001b). The facts about email. *Journal of School Nursing,* 17, 210–212.

Bergren, M. D. (2001c). The facts about faxing. *Journal of School Nursing,* 17, 274–275.

Bergren, M. D. (2001d). HIPAA hoopla? The privacy and security of identifiable health information. *Journal of School Nursing,* 17, 336–340.

Bergren, M. D. (2003). National conference on HIPAA privacy rule, *NASNewsletter,* 18(4), 20–22.

Bergren, M. D. (2004a). HIPAA—FERPA revisited. *Journal of School Nursing,* 20, 107–112.

Bergren, M. D. (2004b). Privacy questions from practicing school nurses: Answers from an expert. *Journal of School Nursing,* 20, 296–301.

Bergren, M. D. (2004c, February 19). *Testimony of Martha Dewey Bergren, DNS, RN on HIPAA and FERPA in Schools, Representing National Association of School Nurses.* Washington, DC: National Committee on Vital Health Statistics Subcommittee on Privacy and Confidentiality. Retrieved March 19, 2004, from http://www.va.gov/virtconf.htm

Campanelli, R. (2004, July 23). Letter from Richard Campanelli, Director of the Office of Civil Rights, from the Department of Health and Human Services in response to the August 20, 2003 letter from the National Association of School Nurses (NASN), National Association of State School Nurse Consultants (NASSNC) and the National Assembly on School-Based Health Care (NASBHC). Retrieved February 6, 2005, from the NASN Web site: http://www.nasn.org/membersonly/hipcampltr.pdf

Cheung, O., Clements, B. & Pechman, E. (1997). *Protecting the privacy of student records: Guidelines for educational agencies.* NCES. http://nces.ed.gov/pubsearch/pubsinfo.asp?pubid=97527

Family Educational Rights and Privacy Act, 20 U.S.C. § 1232g; Regulations at 34 C.F.R. pt. 99 (1974).

National Association of School Nurses. (2003). *Position statement: Individualized healthcare plan.* Scarborough, ME: Author. Retrieved November 21, 2004, from http://www.nasn.org/positions/careplans.htm

National Association of School Nurses, American Nurses Association (NASN, ANA). (2001). *Scope and standards of professional school nursing practice.* Washington, DC: American Nurses Publishing.

National Task Force on Confidential Student Health Information. (2000). *Guidelines for protecting confidential student health information.* Kent, OH: American School Health Association.

Rooker, L. (2004, February 24). FERPA online library: Letter of disclosure of education records. Washington, DC: Family Compliance Office, U.S. Department of Education. Retrieved January 17, 2004, from http://www.ed.gov/policy/gen/guid/fpco/ferpa/library/alhippaa.html

Schwab, N. C. & Gelfman, M. H. B. (2001). Confidentiality: Principles and practice issues. In N. C. Schwab & M. H. B. Gelfman (Eds.), *Legal issues in school health services: A resource for school nurses, administrators and attorneys. North Branch,* MN: Sunrise River Press.

Schwab, N. C., Panettieri, M. J., & Bergren, M. D. (1998). *Guidelines for school nursing documentation: Standards, issues, and models.* Scarborough, ME: National Association of School Nurses.

Schwab, N., & Pohlman, K. J. (2004). Records: The Achilles heel of school nurses. Answers to some bothersome questions. *Journal of School Nursing, 20,* 236–241.

Schwab, N. C., Rubin, M., Maire, J. A., Gelfman, M. H. B, Bergren, M. D., Mazyck, D., et al. (2005). *The Second National Task Force on Confidential Student Health Information. Protecting and sharing student health information: Guidelines for developing school district policies and procedures.* Kent, OH: American School Health Association.

Taliaferro, V. (2003, October). HIPAA and schools. *School Health Alert Newsletter, (Special Supplement),* 1–4. Retrieved February 6, 2005, from http://www.school-nurse.com/med_info/hipa_and_school.html

U. S. Department of Health and Human Services. (2000, December 20). *Administrative simplification regulation text.* Washington, DC: Author. Retrieved April 2, 2001, from http://aspe.os.dhhs.gov/admnsimp/final/PvcTxt01.htm

## Bibliography

AHIMA. (1996). *Practice brief: Facsimile transmission of health information.* Chicago IL: American Health Information Management Association. Retrieved January 22, 2005 from http://library.ahima.org/xpedio/groups/public/documents/ahima/pub_bok2_000116.html

American Medical Informatics Association. (1998). *Guidelines to the clinical use of electronic mail with patients.* Philadelphia, PA: Hanley & Belfus. Retrieved February 6, 2005, from http://www.amia.org/pubs/other/email_guidelines.html

Bergren, M. D. (1999). Criteria for software evaluation: Legal issues. *Journal of School Nursing, 1(2),* 32–33.

Bollinger, D. M. (2003, February). Protecting and using computer evidence, *Inquiry and Analysis,* 1–4.

Centers for Disease Control, USDHHS. (2003, April). HIPAA Privacy Rule and public health: Guidance from CDC and the U.S. Department of Health and Human Services. *MMWR, 52*(Suppl), 1–20. Retrieved June 4, 2003, from www.cdc.gov/mmwr/preview/mmwrhtml/m2e411a1.htmhttp:///

Hunt, V. (2003). Meeting clarifies HIPAA restrictions, NATA News, 10, 12.

InFocus. (2003, January 13). *The other health privacy law: What FERPA requires for schools.* Washington, DC: The Center for Health and Health Care in Schools, The George Washington University School of Public Health and Health Services. Retrieved April 24, 2004 from http://www.healthinschools.org/focus/2003/no1.htm

Levin, M. & Lalley, P. (2003, January). What to do if the HIPAA beast is at your door. *Inquiry and Analysis,* 1–4.

Levin, M. & Lalley, P. (2003, December). Is the HIPAA beast coming to your school district? *Inquiry and Analysis,* 1–4.

Lumpkin, J. R. (2004, March 5). Letter to The Honorable Tommy G. Thompson, Secretary, U.S. Department of Health and Human Services, from the National Committee on Vital and Health Statistics. Retrieved March 19, 2004, from http://www.ncvhs.hhs.gov/040305l2.htm

National Association of School Nurses. (2004). *Issue brief: Privacy standards for student health records.* Scarborough, ME: Author. http://www.nasn.org/briefs/2004briefprivacy.htm

National Center for Education Statistics. (2003). *Weaving a secure web around education: A guide to technology standards and security.* U.S. Department of Education. National Center for Education Statistics. Washington, DC. [Publication No. NCES 2003-381]. http://nces.ed.gov/pubs2003/2003381.pdf

National Forum on Education Statistics. (2004). *Forum guide to protecting the privacy of student Information: State and local education agencies,* NCES 2004–330. Washington, DC: National Center for Education Statistics.

Office of Civil Rights. (2003) *HIPAA: Frequently asked questions.* Office of Civil Rights, U.S. Department of Health and Human Services. Retrieved November 22, 2003, from http://www.hhs.gov/ocr/hipaa/

Vessey, J. (2002). An evaluation of commercial school health software for use in multisite research studies. *Journal of School Nursing, 18,* 95–100.

Zaiger, D. S. (2000). National Task Force on Confidential Student Health Information offers guidelines. *NASN Newsletter, 16*(2), 1–11.

## Resources

Alan Guttmacher Institute
http://www.agi-usa.org/statecenter/index.html
State Center section of Web site offers directory of state-to-state legislation on minors' rights.

*Journal of School Nursing (JOSN)*
http://www.nasn.org/josn/journal.htm
Contains timely articles on school health records, legislation, and legal issues. The members-only Web site provides archives of JOSN articles from 2000 to the present. Nonmembers may view articles using pay-per-view.

National Association of State Boards of Education
http://www.nasbe.org/HealthySchools/States/State_Policy.html
Presents information on State Level School Health Policies. Directory of state legislation that affects healthcare, health education, and educational records, including privacy requirements that exceed Family Educational Rights and Privacy Act (FERPA).

National Association of School Nurses
http://www.nasn.org
Members-only section of Web site contains HIPAA–FERPA resources.

National Association of State School Nurse Consultants
http://lserver.aea14.k12.ia.us/swp/tadkins/nassnc/nassnc.html
State school nurse consultants can guide school nurses on the state laws that impact education records and health information in schools.

National Center for Education Statistics (NCES)
Forum Unified Education Technology Suite
http://nces.ed.gov/pubs2005/tech_suite/
A compilation of NCES resources on guidelines on education records and technology in schools.

National Center for Vital Health Statistics
http://www.ncvhs.hhs.gov/
Contains testimony and correspondence regarding health privacy in schools.

National School Board Association Council of School Attorneys
www.nsba.org/cosa

U.S. Department of Education
http://www.ed.gov/
Offers full text of FERPA and technical guidance.

U.S. Department of Health and Human Services
Administrative Simplification Privacy and Security
http://aspe.hhs.gov/admnsimp/bannerps.htm
Offers full text of HIPAA and technical guidance.

Workgroup for Electronic Data Interchange
12020 Sunrise Valley Drive
Suite 100
Reston, VA 20191
703-391-2743
Offers for $50 a video of presentation by R. Campanelli et al., at the National Conference on the Health Insurance Portability and Accountability Act (HIPAA) Privacy Rule, Chicago, March 2003.

## Chapter Seven

# Using Individualized Healthcare Plans in the Special Education Process

### Janet L. Lowe

## Introduction

"Special Education means specially designed instruction, at no cost to the parents, to meet the unique needs of a child with a disability" (Individuals with Disabilities Education Act [IDEA], 2004, 34 CFR 300.26 ).

There has been a continual increase in recent years in the number of students with chronic health conditions who are also eligible for and receiving special education services. For some school nurses, working with special education students is a full-time practice. For others, it may be a portion of the myriad responsibilities they have as part of their school nursing practice.

The range of health conditions among special education students has also increased. Some special education students do not have health-related conditions that impact their ability to learn. Other students have conditions that vary widely from mild health conditions to severe, multiple health conditions that have a profound and direct impact on their ability to learn. The school nurse plays a critical role in the special education process, especially when the health and/or physical needs of the student, if left unattended, would prevent or restrict the student from full participation in his or her educational program.

An individualized healthcare plan (IHP) is a valuable tool that can assist school nurses to accomplish their role in the special education process. IHPs can be integrated into the individualized education program (IEP), ensuring that the health needs of the student are addressed and saving the school nurse time.

This chapter provides a description of how the IHP can be used and integrated into the special education process. This chapter also provides background information on special education and gives school nurses guidelines for their role in the special education process.

## Background

The Education for All Handicapped Children Act was enacted in 1975 to protect children with disabilities. This law has been amended many times under the IDEA. The main provisions of this law mandate that children with disabilities are entitled to more than reading, writing, and arithmetic and that schools must also provide other supports and related services as necessary in order for the child to benefit from their education. This law mandates that:

- Education is to be individualized according to the individual needs of the child and an IEP must be developed, reviewed, and revised for each child with a disability. (IDEA, 2004, 34 CFR 300.128). The school nurse is often involved in the development of the IEP process.
- Children must be educated in the least restrictive environment. This means that to the maximum extent appropriate, children with disabilities, including children in public or private institutions or other care facilities, are educated with children who are not disabled. This also means that children with disabilities should not be placed in separate classrooms or removed from regular educational classrooms unless the nature or the severity of the disability is such that education in regular classes cannot be achieved.(IDEA, 2004, 34 CFR 300.550). This means that the school nurse will provide nursing services to children in a variety of educational settings.
- Children with disabilities, and their parents, are afforded procedural safeguards to ensure that the requirements of the laws are met (IDEA, 2004, 34 CFR 300.129). The school nurse must be knowledgeable regarding the special education process to ensure compliance with the laws.
- Special education and related services must be provided in accordance with a *free appropriate public education* (FAPE) (IDEA, 2004, 34 CFR 300.13). This means that special education and related services, including nursing services, must be provided at no cost to the family. It does not mean, however, that school districts cannot bill and be reimbursed for IEP health-related services that are provided to children. The Medicare Catastrophic Coverage Act of 1988 ensured that school districts can bill Medical Assistance for IEP health-related services. Districts cannot bill private insurance exclusively if it would increase a family's insurance rates, cap out their thresholds, and result in a cost to families, because these services must be provided according to FAPE.

## Child Find and Referral and Evaluation Procedures

By federal law, states must have in effect Child Find procedures and policies so that children with disabilities are identified, located, and evaluated (IDEA, 2004, 34 CFR 300.125). School districts are involved in ways to reach out to families with children with special needs in order to help them connect with services and support. School nurses are often involved in identifying children with special needs and assisting parents for further evaluation.

School districts must also have in place a process for referral, evaluation, and determining eligibility for special education (IDEA, 2004, 34 CFR 300.530). The exact process and procedure are individualized by each school district. School nurses should become familiar with their school district's special education policies and procedures.

## IEP Teams

There are multidisciplinary teams, or committees, that manage special education referrals. These teams are identified by different names in school districts, such as special education teams, IEP teams, child study committees, or school support teams. These committees are composed of a multidisciplinary team that must consist of (IDEA, 2004, 34 CFR 300.344):

- Parents of the child. The school district needs to take steps to ensure that one or both of the parents of a child with a disability are present at each IEP meeting or are afforded the opportunity to participate (IDEA, 2004, 34 CFR 300.345). If a parent is not able to come, the school district should keep records of attempts made to contact the parent(s). Also, the school district must ensure that parents understand the proceedings at the meetings, including arranging for an interpreter for parents with deafness or whose native language is other than English.
- At least one regular education teacher of the child
- At least one special education teacher
- A school district representative who is qualified to provide, or supervise the provision of, specially designed instruction to meet the unique needs of children with disabilities; is knowledgeable about the general curriculum; and is knowledgeable about the availability of resources
- An individual who can interpret the instructional implications of evaluation results
- Other individuals who have knowledge or special expertise regarding the child, including related services personnel as appropriate, such as a school nurse, occupational therapist, physical therapist, and speech therapist.
- When appropriate, the student. Attempts should be made to invite the student if the student is 14 or younger and the student's presence is appropriate.

Children in special education are protected under the law, and it is the responsibility of the school district and this interdisciplinary team to follow federal and state laws and determine if a student who is having difficulty learning is eligible for special education and, if eligible, to outline the current level of performance, special education needs, goals, and objectives, and any services and related services that are necessary for the student to benefit from his or her educational program.

The role of the school nurse on this committee is critical. The school nurse brings a unique and valuable perspective on how each child's health may, or does, impact his or her ability to learn. The input of the school nurse in this process may assist the IEP team in determining eligibility for special education. Some of the categories of special education require a review of health history and documentation of a medical diagnosis. The school nurse should make it a priority to participate on the IEP team.

Learners who are having difficulty in school are referred to this committee, which determines special education eligibility. Parents, teachers, or others who are concerned and involved with the student can make referrals. This initial evaluation must include the consent of the parent or guardian. Consent means that the parent has been fully informed of all information relevant to the activity for which consent is sought, in his or her native language, or other mode of communication (such as signing). Consent means that the parent agrees in writing and understands that the consent is voluntary and can be revoked at any time and that revocation is not retroactive (IDEA, 2004, 34 CFR 300.500).

After a referral, the IEP team reviews the needs and concerns of the child and may, if needed, conduct an evaluation, or assessment, for special education services.

## Evaluation

The student is evaluated, or assessed, in all areas related to the suspected disability, including, if appropriate, health, vision, hearing, social and emotional status, general intelligence, academic performance, communicative status, and motor abilities. The evaluation needs to be comprehensive to be able to identify all of the student's special education and related services needs, whether or not commonly linked to the disability category in which the student has been classified (IDEA, 2004, 34 CFR 300.541). Evaluations must be performed in accordance with recognized nursing standards. *Providing an evaluation for special education by the school nurse means providing an assessment of the student's health.*

An evaluation/health assessment is recommended by the school nurse when:

- Medications or healthcare procedures are necessary at school
- A student has a physical or mental health condition (past or present) that may be impacting learning

- A student has a sensory deficit (i.e., fluctuating hearing loss) that requires ongoing monitoring and/or case management by the school nurse
- The school nurse provides medication management (for medications given at home or school)
- A student requires an individual health plan (IHP) and/or emergency care plan
- A student has a complex health/medical history
- Physician or other healthcare provider documentation is required for a category of special education eligibility (i.e., Other Health Impairment, Physical Impairment, Traumatic Brain Injury)
- The school nurse is involved in care coordination and/or case management for a student who has physical and/or mental health conditions
- A health history review is required for a category of special education eligibility. A health history review is also recommended for other special education eligibility categories whenever there are known or suspected health concerns that may impact learning.

A notice must be sent to the parent, or guardian, describing any evaluation procedures the school district proposes to conduct. This notice must include information about the area(s) to be assessed, personnel who will assess the student, including name and title, and the plan for the assessment. The areas to be assessed must be completed by qualified, trained, and knowledgeable personnel. *Qualified* means that a person has recognized certification, licensing, registration, or other requirements that apply to the area in which he or she is providing special education, or related services (IDEA, 2004, 34 CFR 300.23). The school nurse is a qualified individual to complete a health assessment/evaluation. Listed below is an example of language that the school nurse may use when completing this notice to the parent/guardian.

*The school nurse will complete a health assessment/evaluation to determine the learner's health needs that are relative to academic performance and will include: a review of health history, a review and interpretation of medical records, hearing and vision assessment, vital signs and physical inspection (if applicable), a review of school health records, parent or guardian interview, classroom observation, review of attendance patterns.*

Once the parent or guardian has signed this notice, there are strict regulations, according to law, regarding timelines for completion of the reports or assessments. To be compliant with the law, the school nurse must adhere to the guidelines for completing an evaluation/health assessment.

## Evaluation/Health Assessment

The purpose of the evaluation/health assessment is to identify how health problems, or conditions, impact the student's ability to learn and participate in his or her educational program.

Every school district must ensure that evaluations/assessments are administered in accordance with recognized professional standards. Providing a health assessment is part of the Standards of Professional School Nursing Practice (National Association of School Nurses, 2000).

### Standard I. Assessment

The school nurse collects client data.
Measurement criteria:
1. Data collection involves the student, family, school, staff, community, and other providers, as necessary.
2. The priority of data collection is determined by the nursing diagnosis and the client's immediate condition and/or needs.
3. Pertinent individual and aggregate data are collected, using appropriate assessment techniques, and reviewed in light of relevant supporting information.
4. Relevant data are documented in a retrievable form.
5. The data collection process is systematic, organized, and ongoing.

### Standard II Diagnosis

The school nurse analyzes the assessment data in determining nursing diagnoses.
Measurement criteria:
1. Nursing diagnoses are derived from the evaluation of assessment data.
2. Nursing diagnoses are validated with the student, family, school staff, community, and other providers, when appropriate.

Sources of information that the school nurse may use to perform an evaluation/health assessment include:
- Teacher interviews, student interviews, parent interviews (parent concerns)
- Observation of student in education setting
- Performance of nursing physical examination, or physical inspection (otoscopic examination, peak flow readings, blood glucose monitoring, auscultation, etc.)
- Medical records, pupil health records, early childhood screening, and other health history information.
- Review of medication and treatment regimens
- Review of previous special education health assessments

## Evaluation/Health Assessment Components

The following components provide a structure for the school nurse to use while completing an evaluation/health assessment (Burns, Barber, Brady, & Dunn, 1996; Wong & Hess, 2000; Licensed School Nurse Assessment of Health/Physical Status form, School Nurse Organization of Minnesota [SNOM], 2004). Appendix A
  I.   Health History
  II.  Current Health Status
  III. Daily Living
  IV.  Transition Health Issues

V. Health Care
VI. School Setting
VII. Physical Measures/Nursing Observations
VIII. Evaluation Report and Individual Education Plan (IEP) Information

If the student has an IHP, the school nurse may already have much of the information accessible for a special education evaluation/health assessment. Reevaluation is completed at least once every 3 years (IDEA, 2004, 34 CFR 300.536). For a reevaluation, the school nurse can review existing evaluation data of the child, including past evaluations, or health assessments completed, classroom observations, and observations by teachers and related service providers. After reviewing existing data and updating information from the child's parents, the school nurse should identify any additional data needed for the evaluation/health assessment.

## Evaluation Report

The school nurse uses the information from the evaluation/health assessment to assist the multidisciplinary team to write an evaluation report. The report summarizes all assessments completed and determines, along with the parent, if the student meets the eligibility for a disability in special education. The evaluation report must include:

-Whether the child is eligible for special education and related services, or continues to be eligible for special education
  • The licensed school nurse identifies health needs and nursing services that are necessary during the school day to maintain health status and allow the student to benefit from, or be able to participate in, the special education program.
  • For students with complex health needs, the licensed school nurse may refer to the IHP, which describes necessary nursing interventions and emergency care plans required during the school day.
-Modifications needed
  • Describe any special adaptations, or supports, that eliminate health-related barriers to learning, such as preferential seating and use of elevator.
-Parent/guardian concerns
-A summary of all evaluation results and interpretation of the evaluation
  • The school nurse describes the student's general physical status, vision and hearing status, and current health conditions, and their implications on the student's ability to learn and the impact they have in the student's academic environment (e.g., classroom, field trips, job site). The school nurse should not use medical jargon and instead use terminology that everyone on the IEP team can understand.
-Present levels of performance in the areas evaluated and educational needs of the student

Examples of information to include on the evaluation report are listed below. Consult with the case manager as to how she or he would like this information submitted.

*Example:* Student with attention deficit hyperactivity disorder (ADHD). Sally has a history of being in good general health. Her vision and hearing status is within normal limits. She was diagnosed 2 years ago as having ADHD. When she is not taking medication, she exhibits symptoms of distractibility and impulsivity. She is currently taking medication at 8 a.m. and 12 noon daily. With this medication regimen, the teachers have noted increased attending to task and less impulsive behaviors; however, she continues to have problems with work completion. Sally will need adaptations in her classroom, including a reduced workload in her assignments, and well-defined coping skills to continue dealing with the impulsive behaviors. Sally will need nursing services as a related service for daily administration of medication and for medication monitoring and management.

-Documentation of whether the student has a disability. The IEP team makes a determination about whether a student has a disability and is eligible for special education.

Listed below are categories of eligibility for special education. Each category has specific criteria that the student must meet to be eligible to receive special education services.

A child with a disability means a child with any of the following (IDEA, 2004, 34 CFR 300.7):
1. Mental impairments
2. Hearing impairments, including deafness
3. Vision impairments, including blindness
4. Speech or language impairments
5. Deafness and blindness
6. Emotional disturbances
7. Autism
8. Traumatic brain injury
9. Orthopedic impairments
10. Other health impairments
    a. Other health impairments is defined as a chronic or acute health condition that is adversely affecting a student's educational performance. A child with other health impairments may be having limited strength, vitality, or alertness, including a heightened alertness to environmental stimuli, that result in limited alertness in the educational environment.
11. Specific learning disability
12. Developmental delays (ages 3 to 9)
13. Multiple disabilities

It is the school nurse's responsibility to *become familiar with the criteria* for those areas of eligibility that may involve health-related issues. School nurses need to check their state statutes and rules regarding these categories.

Many categories of eligibility, such as emotional disturbances, other health impairments, physical impairments, and traumatic brain injury, will need documentation of a medical diagnosis. The school nurse can assume this responsibility to *assist the IEP team in obtaining the medical diagnosis and other medical documentation and to interpret the information received.*

## Related Services

Related services refers to transportation and such developmental, corrective, and other supportive services as are required to *assist a student with a disability to benefit from special education* (IDEA, 2004, 34 CFR 300.24). *School nursing services* are clearly defined as a related service in the Individuals with Disabilities Education Improvement Act of 2004.

Other related services include speech-language pathology and audiology services, interpreting services, psychological services, physical and occupational therapy, recreation, including therapeutic recreation, social work services, counseling services, including rehabilitative counseling, orientation and mobility services, and medical services for diagnosis and evaluation.

A student must be eligible for special education before he or she can receive *school nursing service* as a related service. It is the school nurse's responsibility to assist the IEP team to determine if nursing services as a related service is a necessary service for the student to benefit from his or her special education program. It is considered necessary if the student cannot attain his or her IEP goals, or participate in the educational program, without the supportive service. Related services must be documented on the IEP and must be provided at no cost to the family.

## IEPs and Individual Family Service Plan

An IEP is a written statement for each child with a disability that is developed, reviewed, and revised at least annually for a student in accordance with federal and state laws. An Individualized Family Service Plan (IFSP) is a written statement for providing services for toddlers and infants with disabilities, and their families, through interagency agreements. Procedural and program requirements for the IEP also apply to the educational components of the IFSP. The IEP must include (IDEA, 2004, 34 CFR 300.347):
- A statement of the child's present levels of educational performance, or for preschool children, how the disability affects the child's participation in appropriate activities
- A statement of annual goals, including short-term instructional objectives
- A statement of specific special education and related services provided
- An explanation of the extent of a disabled child not participating with nondisabled children
- A statement of modifications needed for assessments
- Projected dates for initiation of services and the anticipated duration of the services
- A statement of how the child's progress toward goals will be measured and how the child's parents will be regularly informed (through periodic report cards, or at least as often as parents are informed of the progress of their nondisabled children)
- A statement of transition service needs of the student

### Components of the IEP/IFSP Documentation for School Nursing
*Statement of Related Service Needed*

The IEP/IFSP should include a general statement regarding the supportive and related services needed. Listed below are some examples of general statements describing why nursing as a related service is necessary for the student.
- Student with ADHD

  Nursing service is a necessary related service for medication administration and management to control neurobehavioral status to allow the student to benefit from his or her special education program.
- Student with learning disability and asthma

  Nursing service is a necessary related service for nebulization treatments to maintain respiratory status and attendance patterns to allow the student to benefit from his or her special education program.
- Student with a gastrostomy tube feeding

  Nursing service is a necessary related service for gastrostomy tube feeding to maintain nutritional status and attendance patterns to allow the student to benefit from his or her special education program.
- Student with seizures

  Nursing service is a necessary related service for medication administration and management to maintain neurologic status and attendance patterns to allow the student to benefit from his or her special education program.

### Documentation of Direct and Indirect Nursing Service

Direct and indirect nursing service time should be documented on the IEP. Examples of direct nursing service include:
- Administration of medications
- Administration of nebulization treatments
- Administration of a gastrostomy feeding
- Teaching a student a health-related procedure

Examples of indirect nursing service include:
- Nursing management activities, such as communication with teachers, parents, other disciplines (occupational or physical therapy)
- Writing of IHPs and emergency plans
- Teaching educational staff

## Goals and Objectives

Annual goals and short-term objectives in an IEP are related to the following (IDEA, 2004, 34 CFR 300.347):

1. Meeting the child's needs that result from the child's disability to enable the child to be involved in and progress in the general curriculum, or for preschool children, as appropriate, to participate in appropriate activities; and
2. Meeting each of the child's other education needs that result from the child's disability.

Usually, educational goals and objectives are not needed for a nursing service, unless the student is learning a procedure, or behavior, related to an educational need resulting from the health issue that is impacting the student in school. Listed below is an example of what the school nurses may use if they are required to write educational goals and objectives. Use of the Expected Student Outcomes in the IHP examples will assist in writing student-based objectives.

### Example

Present level of performance area:

John has severe persistent asthma and requires daily nebulization treatments at school to maintain respiratory status. With consistent daily treatments his attendance patterns have been good. He has missed only 2 days of school in 3 months due to illness. He is interested in learning more about his asthma and is ready to learn the tasks of the procedure to do the nebulization treatments.

Pupil-based special education need:

John needs to learn a healthcare procedure that assists him in staying healthy to maintain optimal attendance patterns. John also needs to learn more about managing his asthma.

### Annual goal:

Increase from being dependent on someone else for the nebulization treatment and management of his asthma to being independent in self-care of the nebulization treatment and more knowledgeable regarding management of his asthma.

### Objectives:

1. John will demonstrate proper administration techniques of the nebulization procedure during 90% of the attempts by the end of the school year as documented by the school nurse.
2. John will be able to describe his triggers and symptoms in three out of four tries by the end of the school year as documented by the school nurse.
3. John will be able to initiate and follow his prescribed asthma action plan in three out of four attempts by the end of the school year as documented by the school nurse.

4. John will be able to list motivators and barriers to compliance with the asthma action plan in three out of four attempts by the end of the school year as documented by the school nurse.
5. John will have minimal disruptions in his education program due to asthma and have a good school attendance pattern (absent fewer than 10 days per school year) as documented by the teacher on the attendance card.

## Periodic/Annual Reviews and Reevaluations

IEPs must be reviewed periodically, at least annually, to determine if the annual goals are being achieved. (IDEA, 2004, 34 CFR 300.43). The school nurse's responsibility is to provide an update of the student's health status and health needs. If there are changes in the IEP regarding services needed, services provided, or direct or indirect health services time, they need to be documented in the IEP.

Reevaluations must be completed at least every 3 years, or upon the child's or teacher's request of an evaluation (IDEA, 2004, 34 CFR 300.536).

## Transition Services

The IEP for each student, beginning no later than age 14, and at a younger age if determined appropriate by the IEP team, must include a statement of the needed transition services (IDEA, 2004, 34 CFR 300.347).

Transition services are a coordinated set of activities for a student with a disability that is designed within an outcome-oriented process that promotes movement from school to postschool activities, including postsecondary education, vocational training, integrated employment, continuing and adult education, adult services, independent living, or community participation (IDEA, 2004, 34 CFR 300.29).

The coordinated set of activities must be based on the individual student needs and include instruction, community experiences, development of employment and postschool objectives, and, if appropriate, the acquisition of daily living skills and functional vocational evaluation. Transition services may be specially designed instruction, or related services, if they are required to assist a student with a disability to benefit from special education.

## Evaluation/Health Assessment

When completing the health assessment for a student who is in need of transition services, the school nurse must consider that the student is transitioning from school into postsecondary activities that may include job sites, independent living, and community involvement. The school nurse must assess the health-related needs and the student's level of independence in these new environments. In addition to the health assessment, the school nurse should assess the student's independence and level of healthcare skills. Listed below are examples of healthcare skills (SNOM, 2004). Can the student do the following?:

- Describe his or her chronic illness or disability
- Understand the implication of chronic illness or disability on daily life
- Describe the needs and accommodations for work or for school
- Identify the healthcare provider and insurance coverage
- State the health need at school, or to teacher
- Know what medication he or she is taking and for what, or carry information in wallet
- Be responsible for taking own medication
- Be responsible for carrying out own treatments
- Call for medical appointments and keep a calendar of medical and dental appointments
- Access transportation for medical and dental appointments
- Obtain sex education materials, birth control and family planning information as needed
- Get a prescription filled, if needed

The school nurse should summarize the results of the health assessment and assessment of the healthcare skills in the evaluation report. The summary should include the student's current level of health and independence and any health-related services, or teaching, needed during transitioning.

The IEP must include a statement of the needed transition services, including any special education or related services needed. If the IEP team determines that transition services are not needed in any of the areas, the IEP must include a statement and rationale to that effect.

## Summary of School Nurse's Role in the Special Education Process

The school nurse does the following:
1. Participates in the special education committee
2. Provides initial health assessments/evaluation and 3-year health assessments/reevaluations for students with health needs that may impact learning
3. Assists the IEP team to determine eligibility for special education, particularly regarding the criteria that relates to health, and is knowledgeable about the criteria for eligibility for categories of special education that are health-related
4. Interprets medical/health information and how health conditions are affecting the student in his or her academic environment and assists the evaluation team in completion of the evaluation report
5. Assists the evaluation team to determine if school health services/nursing services as a related service are needed on the IEP for the student to benefit from his or her special education program
6. Participates in the development of the IEP as appropriate
7. Provides further information to the IEP team regarding a student's IHP, including emergency care plans as required.

8. Participates in progress reports as appropriate when there are goals and objectives for students who have health needs that impact learning.
9. Provides updated health information whenever the IEP is reviewed or revised, at least annually

## Conclusion

The number of children and adolescents with chronic health conditions continues to increase. Newacheck and Taylor (1992) found that 31% of 17,110 children under 18 years of age were affected by chronic health conditions, and over two thirds of these children required medications. Many of these students will be eligible for special education. Lowe and Miller (1996) found that the majority of school nurses spend more than 2 hours a day in providing case management activities for children with chronic health problems.

Students who are in special education have an even higher incidence of chronic health conditions. Palfrey, Singer, Walker, and Butler (1986) found that 47.8% of special education students are reported to have at least one health condition and 17.8% were reported to have more than one. All students who are in special education are required to have an IEP, and a large number of these students will require healthcare services that are outlined in IHPs and emergency plans.

IHPs must be integrated into the IEP process (Denehy & Poulton, 1999). This integration, and documentation of services provided, will be beneficial to school nurses, school districts, and students for several reasons:

First, school districts are being financially strained to provide healthcare services to students. To receive reimbursement for these services, the services must be documented and outlined on the IEP and the IHP. Third-party payers, upon parental consent, may request documentation of these services.

Second, school districts may use the amount of time and service documented on IHPs and IEPs as indicators for the numbers of nursing personnel needed and the distribution of nursing services in a school district. By having this documentation, school nurses may be able to increase the number of nurses in a school district and the amount of time assigned to a school.

Third, knowledge of how to integrate IHPs into the IEP process will update school nursing practice to meet mandated state and federal laws and standards of practice. With ensuing litigation in the United States, school nurses are prudent to be knowledgeable of the special education mandates and their role in this process.

Finally, and most important, the integration of the IHP into the IEP process will ensure that children and adolescents receive the necessary healthcare services that will contribute to their educational success.

# References

Burns, C., Barber, N., Brady, M., & Dunn, A. (1996). *Pediatric primary care: A handbook for nurse practitioners.* Philadelphia: Saunders.

Denehy, J., & Poulton, S. (1999). The use of standardized language in individualized healthcare plans. *Journal of School Nursing, 15,* 38-45.

Individuals with Disabilities Education Act (IDEA), 20 U.S.C. et seq., 64 Fed. Reg. 12,418, Last updated 02-18-2004, 34 C.F.R. § 300 et seq. Retrieved May 27, 2004, from Government Printing Office Electronic Code of Federal Regulations (e-CFR) http://ecfr.gpoaccess.gov/cgi/t/text/text-idx?c=ecfr;sid=5f3d60b8ae9e2aea6ea3339965871e37;rgn=div5;view=text;node=34:2.1.1.1.1;idno=34;cc=ecfrhttp://ecfr.gpoaccess.gov/cgi/t/text-

Individuals with Disabilities Education Improvement Act of 2004, December, 2004. Public Law 108-446, 118 Stat.2647. Title 1, Section 602, (26). Retrieved January 27, 2005, from http://edworkforce.house.gov/issues/108th/education/idea/conferencereport/IDEA%20Part%20A.pdf

Lowe, J., & Miller, W. (1998). Health services provided by school nurses for students with chronic health problems. *Journal of School Nursing, 14,* 4–16.

National Association of School Nurses (2000). *Standards of professional school nursing practice.* Scarbough:, ME: Author.

Newacheck, P. G., & Taylor, W. R. (1992). Childhood chronic illness: prevalence, severity, and impact. *American Journal of Public Health, 82,* 364–371.

Palfrey, J. S., Singer, J. D., Walker, D. K., & Butler, J. A. (1986). Health and special education: A study of new developments for handicapped children in five metropolitan communities. *Public Health Reports, 101,* 379–388.

School Nurse Organization of Minnesota (SNOM). Special education. Retrieved August 10, 2004, from http://www.minnesotaschoolnurses.org/spec.html

Wong, D., & Hess, C. (2000). *Wong and Whaley's clinical manual of pediatric nursing* (5th ed.). St. Louis, MO: Mosby.

# Bibliography

National Association of School Nurses. (2001). *Cedar Rapids Community School District vs, Garret F., Impact of on school nursing services* [Issue brief]. Scarborough, ME: Author.

National Association of School Nurses. (2001). *Inclusion* [Issue brief]. Scarborough, ME: Author.

National Association of School Nurses. (Adopted 2001). *Position Statement: Medical services vs. health services in the school setting.* Scarborough, ME: Author.

National Association of School Nurses. (Revised 2002). *Position statement: Case management of children with special health care needs.* Scarborough, ME: Author.

National Association of School Nurses. (2002). *Individuals with Disabilities Act (IDEA). School nurses and the* [Issue brief]. Scarborough, ME: Author.

National Association of School Nurses. (Revised 2002). *Position statement: The school nurse and specialized health care services.* Scarborough, ME: Author.

National Association of School Nurses. (2003). *Position statement: Individualized health care plans.* Scarborough, ME: Author.

Praeger S., Zickler, C., & Mosca, N. W. (2002). *Care of students with special needs in schools: Application of professional school nursing practice standards* [Manual]. Scarborough, ME: National Association of School Nurses.

Using Individualized Healthcare Plans in the Special Education Process

# Licensed School Nurse Assessment of Health/Physical Status

The following components are designed to be a guide that may be utilized in the process of completing an LSN assessment.

Student _____ ☐ M ☐ F DOB: _____

School _____ ID# _____ Grade _____

Parent/Guardian _____ Phone (H) _____

Address: _____ Phone (W) _____

_____ Cell/Pager _____

## I. Health History
☐ Diabetes    ☐ Asthma    ☐ Genetic/Inherited diseases    ☐ Learning Disability
☐ Thyroid    ☐ Mental Illness    ☐ ADHD    ☐ Other _____

Comments: _____

Pregnancy/Labor/Delivery/Neonatal history (gestational age, complications, tobacco, alcohol, or chemical use)

_____

_____

Developmental history (age at which milestones reached)
____ Talked    ____ Walked    ____ Toilet trained    ____ Any concerns _____

Growth history (pattern of growth, any concerns) _____

Childhood illnesses/injuries/lead exposure

_____

Hospitalization/surgeries _____

_____

Chronic health conditions _____

_____

## II. Current Health Status
Medical diagnoses/health conditions _____

_____

Treatments _____

Medications _____

Alternative therapies _____

Immunization status _____

Allergies _____

Vision _____

Hearing _____

## II. Current Health Status – *continued*
Review of systems (any concerns in the following areas)

General Appearance _____

Head _____

Eyes, ears, nose, throat _____

Respiratory _____

Cardiovascular _____

Gastrointestinal _____

Genitourinary _____

Musculoskeletal _____

Neurological _____

Endocrine _____

Skin _____

Mental Health _____

Social/emotional _____

Behavior _____

Cultural _____

Family _____

Chemical use _____

Other _____

## III. Daily Living
Sleep patterns:   Bedtime at _____   Awakens at _____

Problems with sleep _____

Nutritional (limitations/allergies) _____

Feeding _____

Elimination/toileting _____

Menses (onset, frequency, duration, pain) _____

_____

Self care skills _____

Activity/Mobility/Limitations _____

## IV. Transition Health Issues (age 14 and up)
See Transition Addendum, page 57 of this document

## V. Health Care
Health care providers:

| Name | Specialty | Clinic/Location | Phone |
|------|-----------|-----------------|-------|
|      |           |                 |       |
|      |           |                 |       |
|      |           |                 |       |
|      |           |                 |       |

Outside agencies (nursing, equipment, etc.) _____

Health Insurance coverage:  ☐ Yes  ☐ No

Describe insurance/need: _____

## VI. School Setting
Attendance _____

Adaptive equipment or supplies needed in school _____

_____

Medications/treatments needed in school _____

_____

Health problem that can result in an emergency _____

Health problem that could interfere with learning _____

Individual Health Plan (IMP)/Emergency Health Plan (ESP) needed _____

## III. Physical Measures/Nursing Observation (may include the following)
Peak flow meter readings _____

Blood glucose monitoring _____

Vital signs: temp, pulse, BPI, respiration _____

Vision & Hearing screening _____

Physical exam: **may** include general appearance, eyes, ears, nose, mouth, throat, lungs, heart, abdomen, musculoskeletal, neurological, integume

This section is optional. Use this space to record any portion of a physical exam that you do, i.e.: otoscopic exams, auscultation of lungs, inspection of the throat

## VIII. Evaluation Report and Individual Education Plan (IEP) information

The evaluation report is a collective summary of all of the evaluations completed. The evaluation report must include a summary of the information obtained in the Licensed School Nurse Assessment of Health/Physical Status and written in language that is clear to parents and non-health professionals.

The evaluation report includes:
• General health status
• Parent/guardian concerns
• Vision/hearing status
• Past and current health conditions affecting the student in the education environment and the education needs related to the health condition. (Make the link between health and education)
• Nursing service or other accommodation needed in the educational environment

Nursing services grid for the IEP:

| Instruction or Service Provided | Location | | Anticipation Frequency | Total Minutes per Week | | Service | |
|---|---|---|---|---|---|---|---|
| | General Education | Special Education | | Indirect | Direct | Start Date | Anticipation Duration |
| Nursing | | | | | | | |

IEP Adaptations:

Individual Health Plan (IHP)/Emergency Health Plan (EHP) developed ☐ Yes ☐ No

Consent obtained for 3rd party billing ☐ Yes ☐ No

Sources of information utilized:

_____ teacher/classroom staff interviews _____ observation of student

_____ student interview _____ review of medical records

_____ nursing physical exam _____ review of pupil health record

_____ parent interview _____ other

Assessment completed by: _____ Date:_____

# Transition Addendum (for students age 14 and older)

When completing a transition Health Assessment, consider that the student will move from traditional school to community-based activities. Consider skills and accommodations needed for the student to participate in the five areas of transitions:

- Jobs annd jobs training
- Commmunity participation
- Recreation and leisure
- Home living
- Post-secondary education/training

**Transition Health Issues**

Can the student:

- Describe their disability/chronic health condition: _____   _____

_____

- Describe how to manage their disability/chronic health condition in various settings: _____

_____

- Identify health care providers and insurance coverage: _____

_____

- Make medical appointments, record them on a calendar, and arrange transportation: _____

_____

- Be responsible for:

    -taking medications, refilling prescriptions: _____

    -carrying out treatments, ordering supplies: _____

    -limiting risky behaviors including smoking, drinking and driving, unprotected sex: _____

    -carrying identifications: _____

    -caring for menstrual needs and keep a record of periods: _____

- Be responsible for:

    -hygeine: _____

    -nutrition: _____

    -exercise: _____

    -preventative health and dental care: _____

- Understand physical changes during puberty and obtain information as needed:

_____

Completed by: _____ Date: _____

*Chapter Eight*

# Special Education: Other Health Impairment (OHI)

Patricia Brandstaetter, Marilyn Leifgren, and Cynthia K. Silkworth

## Introduction

Schools across the country are serving students with an extraordinary range of chronic and acute health conditions. These conditions may be congenital or acquired. Students with these conditions may have associated characteristics or symptoms ranging from mild to severe. Some of the health conditions may be stable and some progressive. Some of the conditions have symptoms that may vary in intensity from day to day. Medications, treatments, therapies, frequent medical appointments, and repeated hospitalizations can impact the student's ability to learn and function in school. Even a relatively mild health condition may significantly impact academic, behavioral, social, and emotional functioning.

There is no "model" standard for determining who will be eligible for special education and related services based on a medically diagnosed health condition or syndrome. A health condition alone is not sufficient to qualify a student for special education services under any disability category. When a student has a health condition (or even multiple health conditions) that can be managed well medically and the student is making good academic progress and can successfully participate in school and classroom activities, the student may not need any special education services. However, when a health condition adversely affects the student's educational performance, the student may need special education and related services.

Establishment of a link between the health condition and the adverse effect on the student's education performance is critical to determining eligibility for special education services under the category "other health impairment" (OHI). Each eligibility determination must be made on the basis of the needs of the particular student. This requires school special education teams to collaborate in planning and implementing a comprehensive assessment that takes into consideration all aspects of a student's school life— cognitive abilities, academic performance, school attendance, illness and treatment effects, health-related procedures or treatments needed during the school day, physical strength and endurance, alertness, and behavioral, social, and emotional functioning—and determining how the health condition is impacting each of them.

## Students With OHI

Because of advances in medical technology, there are an increasing number of children being diagnosed and surviving for longer periods of time with multiple and complex medical problems, childhood diseases, and chronic health conditions. In addition, there are increasing numbers of children identified and diagnosed with attention deficit hyperactivity disorder. As an increased number of students come to school with a broad variety of medical diagnoses, there appears to be more and more confusion regarding how to make decisions and allocate resources about meeting their health needs and providing a safe environment for learning. School teams struggle to evaluate and determine whether students need specially designed instruction and related services and whether some of these students are eligible for accommodations due to the health condition. Students may have a health diagnosis that is medically managed and require no service, and some may need accommodations to allow them to be successful in school. Schools need to consider a continuum of services for students with health conditions.

The following flow chart was developed to visualize the array of services that may be available to a student who comes to school with a medical diagnosis. After the student has been diagnosed with a medical condition and treatment has been prescribed by a physician, it is the responsibility of the educational community, through a comprehensive evaluation, to determine if the medical diagnosis is linked to the learning and functioning problems at school. It is best practice to consider the medical evaluation and diagnosis as part of the educational evaluation. Only children whose conditions have severe impact on learning may be found eligible for special educational services. There are other options for assistance and support within the school setting that are shown within the flow chart. Children may require no service or support, an individualized healthcare plan (IHP), an emergency care plan, a 504 plan consisting of accommodations to the school settings, or an individualized education program (IEP).

**A licensed physician has diagnosed a medical condition.**

- Parent shares information about a health condition with school staff.
- School nurse comments health condition in the health record.
- School nurse may develop an individualized Health Plan (IHP) or Emergency Cary Plan (ECP)
- Nurse or parent informs the teachers and staff about the health condition.
- School staff may or may not note educational elicit or presenting problems.

Potential Outcomes and Levels of Support within Educational Setting

**No support needed**

Child and family manage condition without accommodation or support in the educational setting. Child maintains academic progress.

Example:
Child has medical diagnosis by a licensed physician of ADHD and is taking medications at home.

Child broke a leg in an accident. Family and child are managing medical needs. Child will remain out of regular PE until leg heals and may use school elevator. No support is needed from the school at this time.

Child has diagnosed allergies to certain pollens, dust, and other substances. Family and child manage medical needs by using prescribed medications when symptoms increase. No support is needed from the school at this time

**When Supports May be Needed in the Educational Setting**

Parent and/or nurse presents to school staff, re: academics and functional concerns and teacher makes accommodations within the classroom. Child is successful.

Or

Develop 504 Plan

Intervention strategies implemented and student is successful

Or

Student is presented to Child Study Team after 2 prior Documented interventions (PDI) have been completed.

Student is not successful.

**504 Evaluation Considered**
Follow district 504 procedure within the general education setting.

**Special Education Evaluation Considered**
- Medical diagnosis is written and signed by the licensed physician.
- Evaluation for Special Education is completed.

| Eligible | Not Eligible | Not Eligible | Eligible |
|---|---|---|---|

504 Plan

If student is not eligible, consider 504 Evaluation

IEP

IEP Team determines service based on students needs

From *Other health disabilities manual,* by Minnesota Department of Health (in press). St. Paul, MN: Author. Reprinted with permission.

Special Education: Other Health Impairment (OHI)

# Definition of OHI

## Federal Definition

According to the Individuals with Disabilities Educational Act (IDEA) of 1975, *other health impairment* means having limited strength, vitality, or alertness, including a heightened alertness to environmental stimuli, which results in limited alertness in the educational environment, that

- is due to chronic or acute health problems such as asthma, attention deficit disorder or attention deficit hyperactivity disorder, diabetes, epilepsy, a heart condition, hemophilia, lead poisoning, leukemia, nephritis, rheumatic fever, and sickle cell anemia; and
- adversely affect a child's educational performance.

## State Definition

Based on the IDEA, federal definitions of various special educational categories are outlined in rule and each state uses this guideline to develop its own definition and eligibility criteria in 13 specific disability areas. It is crucial to define the students who meet eligibility within each criteria to ensure that appropriately trained and licensed staff and allocated resources are available to meet the needs of each disability category.

### Example: Minnesota State Criteria (Minnesota Rule 3525.1335) (1998)

*Definition:* "Other health disability" means having limited strength, endurance, vitality, or alertness, including a heightened or diminished alertness to environmental stimuli, in the educational environment. These limitations are due to a broad range of medically diagnosed chronic or acute health conditions that adversely affect a pupil's educational performance.

*Criteria:* The team shall determine that a pupil is eligible and in need of special education instruction and services if the pupil meets the criteria in A and B.

A. There is:
1. written and signed documentation of a licensed physician of a medically diagnosed chronic or acute health condition; or
2. in the case of a diagnosis of attention deficit disorder or attention deficit hyperactivity disorder (ADD or ADHD), there is written and signed documentation of a medical diagnosis by a physician. The diagnosis of ADD/ADHD must include documentation that *DSM-IV* criteria in items A to E have been met. *DSM-IV* criteria documentation must be provided by either a licensed physician or a mental health or medical professional licensed to diagnose the condition.
3. For initial evaluation, all documentation must be dated within the previous 12 months.

B. In comparison with peers, the health condition adversely affects the pupil's ability to complete educational tasks within routine timelines as documented by three or more of the following.
1. excessive absenteeism linked to the health condition, for example, hospitalizations, medical treatments, surgeries, or illnesses;
2. specialized healthcare procedures that are necessary during the school day;
3. medications that adversely affect learning and functioning in terms of comprehension, memory, attention, or fatigue;
4. limited physical strength resulting in decreased capacity to perform school activities;
5. limited endurance resulting in decreased stamina and decreased ability to maintain performance;
6. heightened or diminished alertness resulting in impaired abilities, for example, prioritizing environmental stimuli; maintaining focus; or sustaining effort or accuracy;
7. impaired ability to manage and organize materials and complete classroom assignments within routine timelines; or
8. impaired ability to follow directions or initiate and complete a task.

*Evaluation:* The health condition results in a pattern of unsatisfactory educational progress as determined by a comprehensive evaluation documenting the required components in criteria, items A and B. The eligibility findings must be supported by current or existing data from items A to E.

A. an individually administered, nationally normed standardized evaluation of the pupil's academic performance;
B. documentation, systematic interviews conducted by a licensed special education teacher with classroom teachers and the pupil's parent or guardian;
C. one or more documented systematic observations in the classroom or other learning environment by a licensed special education teacher;
D. a review of the pupil's health history, including verification of a medical diagnosis of a health condition; and
E. records review.

The evaluation findings may include data from the following: an individually administered, nationally normed test of intellectual ability; an interview with the pupil; information from the school nurse or other individuals knowledgeable about the health condition of the pupil; standardized, nationally normed behavior rating scales; gross and fine motor and sensory motor measures; communication measures; functional skills checklists; and environmental, sociocultural, and ethnic information reviews

## Educational Practices

Due to the fact that each chronic or acute health condition may manifest itself with a variety of learning, functioning, and medical/health needs within the school setting, it is crucial to complete a comprehensive educational evaluation. Each evaluation should consider all areas of concern: cognitive abilities, academic performance, school attendance, communication skills, functional skills, behavioral/social/emotional functioning, physical/health-related needs during the school day, physical strength and endurance, alertness, and illness and treatment effects.

Each person on the educational team brings specific knowledge and skills to the table to develop and implement a plan that provides for accommodations and modifications to the school setting to minimize the impact the health condition has on learning and functioning. The team, at a minimum, needs to include the student's parent(s)/guardian(s), classroom teachers, special education teacher, school psychologist, school nurse, and school administrator or designee. Frequently it is beneficial to include staff from the medical community to share results and protocols and respond to educators' questions. Because there are so many medical conditions and staff are not able to have in-depth knowledge about all conditions, it may also be beneficial to include community agencies at planning meetings. Often agencies are pleased to be considered as part of the team and are able to bring resources and training information to assist the school team to have a broader understanding of how the condition can affect learning and functioning.

It is important for the educational team to identify chronic or acute health conditions that may demonstrate disability within the OHI category:

- Teams must become familiar with the typical presenting problems of students with chronic or acute health conditions.
- Teams must be aware of safety concerns of this at-risk population.
- Teams must be aware of how each health condition impacts learning so strategies may be determined to reduce the impact the health condition has on learning.
- Teams must gather information from appropriate medical and educational staff to evaluate and make decisions about services so the child is learning in a safe environment with educators who understand how the medical condition manifests itself and what services (emergency or specialized health care) are needed.
- Teams must demonstrate a link between the health condition and the student's educational difficulties.

Following are examples of a *link between the health condition and educational difficulties*:

- The health condition, which requires a student to have absences from school for specialized treatments, interferes with the student's ability to maintain satisfactory academic progress due to decreased instructional opportunities in comparison to peers.
- The student's level of distractibility interferes with his or her ability to start, remain on task, and complete classroom work at a level comparable to his or her peers.
- The student's health condition, causing limited endurance, results in the student's inability to compete written assignments and requires intermittent rest time during the school day.

Following are examples of *educational difficulties that do not link to the health condition:*

- The student's lack of academic progress is attributable to motivational concerns not directly linked to the health condition.
- The student's lack of academic progress is attributable to behavioral issues, not directly linked to the health condition.

Because a student with a health disability may have difficulty with maintaining effort due to the health condition, alternative accommodations/modifications and strategies need to be designed to improve success and provide alternative plans to accommodate for inconsistent and inefficient learning and functioning.

Students with health disabilities may benefit from:

- accommodations in teaching strategies and curriculum, such as compensation for work completion, curriculum modifications and adaptations;
- accommodations for organization and independent work skills, such as daily planners, note takers, modified assignments or tests;
- adjustments of the school environment or schedule due to health condition, such as rest needed following a seizure, limitation for physical activity, periodic breaks for endurance, part-time schedule, homebound instruction, building modifications for access, additional time allotted for passing between classes;
- accommodations utilizing behavioral management techniques, such as self-monitoring tools, peer tutors, reinforcement programs, medication compliance;
- development of self-advocacy skills and independence related to their health condition and self-care;
- accommodations in areas of gross and/or fine motor skills, such as ambulation, writing, self-care, daily living skills; and/or
- accommodations for major safety considerations, such as special transportation, emergency plan, additional supervision and health monitoring.

## Issues in OHI

Medical diagnoses are not exclusive to the OHI category. Utilizing federal and many state definitions and typical categories of chronic or acute health conditions, we become aware of the fact that medical diagnoses are found in all special education categories. For example, children with mental health diagnoses (bipolar disorder, depression, anxiety, oppositional defiant disorder) may demonstrate disability within the emotional and behavioral disorders (EBD) category. Children with diagnoses of certain syndromes (Down syndrome, fragile X) may demonstrate disability within the developmental cognitive disability (DCD) category (in some states labeled mentally impaired). There are also diagnoses that affect vision, hearing, movement, and learning that may demonstrate disability as visually impaired, hearing impaired, physically impaired, and specific learning disability (SLD). One of the greatest challenges for special education teams is to determine that the criteria for eligibility for OHI are met, based on linking the presenting problems to the health condition and not just "dumping" the student in OHI because he or she has a medical diagnosis, doesn't meet eligibility criteria in other categories, and needs some assistance with academics.

There continue to be misconceptions about which students to identify as eligible within this special educational category. Some believe that a child who comes to school with a medical diagnosis of any kind requires services as OHI. Others consider this category when a child is not eligible in other categories, but happens to have a medical diagnosis and needs academic assistance. Still others consider this category to be a "kinder" label for students with mental health conditions. For example, a parent or community agency may insist that a school team label a child as having OHI, instead of EBD, if a child demonstrates clinical depression, anxiety, or bipolar disorder, or has ADHD with other coexisting mental health conditions. Often these disorders do not demonstrate disability as a chronic or acute health condition, but rather as an emotional or behavioral disorder.

It is crucial to collaborate with the medical community to provide a safe and healthy learning setting. It is also important to recognize that the medical and educational community play different, but complementary, roles in addressing the needs of students within the school setting. The physician diagnoses the medical condition. The physician prescribes medical treatment, consisting of medication, special healthcare procedures, therapy by other healthcare providers (such as physical therapy or counseling), health monitoring, and other interventions. The physician may discuss educational issues based on parent concerns and medical evaluation. However, the physician cannot decide whether a student meets the criteria for OHI, or any other special education category, and determine whether the student needs special education services. Information from the physician and other healthcare providers needs to be considered by the educational team as they determine the student's abilities and needs within the educational setting.

As the number of children needing assistance in schools appears to increase and the cost to serve them has increased, many states have tightened their special education criteria and require a student to demonstrate a greater degree of disability with learning and functioning to be considered eligible for specially designed instruction and related services under IDEA. Within school districts, as funding decreases, many support services, such as nursing, social work, and family services, are not readily available and teachers and teams struggle to determine how to best meet the needs of this growing population of students. In addition, most states have no teaching license specific to OHI. This means that any teacher with a special education license may serve this growing number of students with broad and diverse educational needs and health conditions.

Some students may require accommodations to their educational program to access learning and be successful in school. There is not targeted additional funding to provide 504 services, and in many schools there is limited training for the general education staff in regard to their role and responsibility for this group of students. The 504 programs are sometimes poorly implemented, and in general education no one seems to be accountable for providing accommodations to meet the needs of these students. This may lead to an increase in referrals by parents and educators for special education assessments to address the needs of students with health conditions. It is important to recognize the educational impact that many chronic or acute health conditions may have on learning. The medical community continues to make progress in identifying medical conditions and interventions that can improve a student's health status and well-being. The educational community must continue to gain knowledge in regard to how these medical conditions may affect learning and functioning and how specific educational interventions may assist a student with a health condition to minimize the impact on the student's academic progress and functioning in the school and community.

## When is ADHD Considered OHI?

ADHD refers to a disorder of behavioral control and self-regulation characterized by developmentally inappropriate extremes of inattentiveness, hyperactivity, and impulsivity. The diagnostic criteria for ADHD in the *Diagnostic and Statistical Manual of Mental Disorders (DSM–IV–TR)*, (American Psychiatric Association, 2000) should be standard practice in diagnostic evaluations by physicians and appropriately licensed mental health professionals. Documentation of the *DSM–IV–TR* diagnosis of ADHD is an essential component for consideration of the special education criteria of OHI.

Students with ADHD present an unpredictable variety and intensity of success in school across age ranges and environments. Across the spectrum, some students with ADHD may be independent high achievers, even gifted students with no need for accommodations or support. Some students may demonstrate the need for minimal accommodations that can be achieved in the regular education classroom, or they may qualify through assessment for a 504 plan. Other ADHD students, experiencing significant educational difficulties, require evaluation to determine the degree and severity of the impact of the ADHD symptoms upon school performance to qualify for OHI. Still others may have coexisting conditions, which significantly impact their educational performance, social adjustments, and behaviors.

A medical diagnosis of ADHD does not ensure accommodations, specialized instruction, or related service. Each student must have a comprehensive educational evaluation to determine eligibility for any special education category or services. Child study teams need to maintain a holistic perspective on a child being evaluated for special education services. In situations where the evaluation process identifies multiple issues, teams must weigh the information to determine the appropriate eligibility category and services. This requires careful analysis of the presenting educational problems. For OHI, teams need to establish and document a link between ADHD and its adverse effect on the student's educational performance, based on evaluation data.

## Assessment Components for ADHD in the School Setting

DuPaul and Stoner (2004) suggest a system to evaluate ADHD in schools. The following stages have been modified to include additional school components.

*Parent and/or teacher concerns of inattention, impulsivity and/or hyperactivity*

Stage I. Screening and prereferral interventions
- Teacher or parent report of ADHD symptoms and academic progress
- Review of school health records
- Prereferral interventions
- Informal observations
- If prereferral interventions are successful, further assessment may not be indicated.

Stage II. Comprehensive special education evaluation—addressing multiple issues
- Modification of prereferral interventions
- Parent and teacher interviews
- Review of school records and health history
- Parent and teacher rating scales
- Observations of classroom behavior
- Academic performance data
- Physician's diagnosis of ADHD

Stage III. Interpretation of results
- Number of ADHD symptoms
- Deviance from age and gender norms
- Age at onset and chronicity
- Pervasiveness across situations
- Established link between ADHD and its adverse effect on educational performance
- Eligibility criteria met for special education category OHI
- Other state disability criteria areas ruled out as primary

Stage IV. Development of IEP, based on:
- Severity of ADHD symptoms and impact of educational performance
- Functional analysis of behavior
- Presence of associated disorders
- Response to prior interventions and treatment
- Community-based and medical resources

### Quantitative Measures and Evaluation Procedures

Questionnaires should be selected in consideration of their reliability, validity, standardization, and age range. They provide one measure of data and should be considered in context of all other sources of information. Goldstein and Goldstein (1998) present a model for the evaluation of school functioning. Additional current questionnaires have been included in the following model.

### A Model for Gathering Data: ADHD Concerns

Attention, impulsivity, and hyperactivity are often inferred as explanations for student's misbehavior, noncompliance, and poor academic performance. These difficulties could be caused by multiple other factors, including mental and physical health issues, motivational issues, environmental and family issues, cultural and linguistic factors, cognitive or learning impairments, as well as the co-occurrence of other disorders with ADHD. Therefore data collection should provide information for differential diagnosis. This includes: a careful social and developmental history, rating scales of both school and home behaviors, observation and functional analysis of a student's presenting problem(s), test results, and an integration of data focusing on differential diagnosis.

### Social and Developmental History

A developmental, health, and social history should be obtained from parents in a direct interview process. Intensity, frequency, and persistence of symptoms are crucial factors. Important questions to have in mind while taking the history are: When, where, how much, and with whom do these behaviors occur? How serious are they? Are they taking a toll on this child's development? Barkley (1998) and Sattler (1998) provide samples of several clinical interview forms to assist in gathering pertinent data.

### Assessment Measures: Suggested Rating Scales

Rating scales are only one part of an evaluation of ADHD. Rating scales should be evaluated on their validity, reliability, and stability. Examiners must keep in mind that the ratings are the informant's subjective opinion about the observed behavior. Although the scales give the appearance of objectivity by quantifying the opinions, the bias of individuals and situational differences are key factors influencing the scales. Rating scales should not be used normatively with cultural or ethnic groups whose behavioral expectations differ markedly from those of the general culture in which norms were derived.

Comprehensive assessment measures:
- Behavior Assessment System for Children (BASC-2). Teacher, parent, and student self-report.
- Auchenbach's Child Behavior Checklist. Caregiver, teacher, and youth self-report.

Specific measures of ADHD symptoms:
- Conners' Rating Scales-Revised (CRS-R)
- ADD-H Comprehensive Teacher Rating Scale (ACTeRS)
- ADHD Symptom Checklist-4 (ADHD-SC4)
- Attention Deficit Disorders Evaluation Scale (ADDES-3)
- Childhood Attention Problems Questionnaire (CAP)
- Academic Performance Rating Scale
- Brown Attention Deficit Disorder Scales (Brown ADD Scales)

Teacher and/or parent report questionnaires (qualitative measures):
- Teacher Observation Checklist
- School Situation Questionnaire
- Home Situations Questionnaire
- Social Skills Assessment
- Adolescent School Situation Questionnaire

## Observational Data

Behavioral observation of a student can be one of the most accurate and valid of all the suggested assessment measures. It provides comparison to others in the same setting, links assessment and intervention, helps clarify discrepancies between informants, and aids in evaluation of treatment. Observers should have training in performing valid observations. Direct classroom observation can also provide the practitioner with insight into many factors that may elicit problem behavior. Antecedent and consequent events can be observed. Single or multiple target behaviors to be observed should be operationally defined. The observer may wish to determine the frequency of a particular behavior during the rating period, the duration of the behavior, or simply whether the behavior occurs during a given interval.

## Observation Considerations

It is recommended that observations last at least 20 minutes.

*When (and how many)*
- During typical class routine
- Consideration given to "troublesomeness" of the situation; for example, structured vs. unstructured, low interest vs. high interest
- More than one observation allows some judgment of interobservation reliability

*Where*
- Classrooms

- Other school settings where behaviors are observable
- Home environment when indicated

*What*
- Identify and define (operationally) target behaviors
- Typical targets when assessing students with attentional problems: (time on task, inappropriate overactivity, compliance issues, negative interactions with adults and peers, behavioral products such as work completion, impulsivity, restlessness)
- Selection of comparison student(s)

*How*
- Unobtrusive, to reduce reactivity from student
- Time sampling
- Formal vs. informal systems
- Duration of sampling period: segments of observing lasting from 4 to 60 seconds recommended, with shorter periods for recording after each segment
- Reported as percentage of time or activity: for example, time on task presented as percentage of total observation time

A number of assessment systems, such as the BASC-2, include observational components. Barkley (1998) developed an ADHD behavior coding system in which the student is observed during the performance of independent academic work in an isolated setting. Behaviors observed include being off-task, fidgeting, vocalizing, playing with objects, and being out of seat. The important point is to choose the observational method that will best gather data of the target behavior of concern.

## Functional Analysis of Student Behavior

A functional analysis of the student's behavior may fine-tune the anecdotal information that has been collected and provides a measurement of the student's problem behaviors, or an indication of the preexisting level of behavior. A functional analysis is accomplished by using the observation of the target behavior and its antecedents and consequences. This information may be useful in identifying and developing an intervention plan.

## School and Clinical Evaluation

A comprehensive evaluation by both the school and medical community is an important component of a thorough evaluation. The evaluation may include intellectual and achievement testing, social/emotional evaluation, adaptive behavior, visual-motor integration, vigilance and sustained attention, and other evaluation procedures deemed necessary to provide a diagnosis.

## Determination of Primary Disability Other Than OHI

The child study team may determine that a student meets the criteria of another special education category as their primary area of disability, such as:

- SLD: coexisting learning disability, information processing concerns
- DCD: IQ below 70, adaptive skills below 15th percentile
- EBD: existing emotional or behavioral disorders, aggressive behaviors, acting-out behaviors

*Example 1:* A student is diagnosed as having oppositional defiant disorder and ADHD. The evaluation information identifies presenting problems as defiance of authority, refusal to comply with directions from adults, threatened aggression toward peers, refusal to complete assignments, and frequent use of inappropriate language. The presenting problems indicate that the student should be considered for eligibility in the EBD category.

*Example 2:* A student is diagnosed as having ADHD. The student is evaluated and has a full-scale IQ of 67. The adaptive skills are all below the 15th percentile. Behaviors of concern are noted as inability to remain focused on a task, assistance needed with self-care tasks, lack of organizational skills, and inability to work independently for more than 3 to 5 minutes. Evaluation indicates that the student is 2 years behind peers in all academic subjects. The evaluation data indicate the student should be considered for eligibility in the DCD category.

*Example 3:* A student is diagnosed as having ADHD. Evaluation indicates that the student has failed to make sufficient academic progress given extensive individualized interventions. Evaluation also indicates a significant discrepancy between the student's intellectual functioning and academic achievement. The student shows information processing deficits. The evaluation data indicate that the student should be considered for the SLD category.

*Example 4:* A student is diagnosed as having ADHD. The evaluation information clearly identifies presenting problems as inability to remain focused on a task, poor organizational skills, consistent out-of-seat behavior, and some difficulty with peer relations. The presenting problems indicate that the student should be considered for eligibility in the OHI category.

## Role of the School Nurse

As a member of the special education team, the school nurse has an important role in evaluation and planning for students with physical and/or mental health conditions that may impact learning. This is especially true when a student's health condition(s) appears to be adversely affecting the student's educational performance. The school nurse can assist the special education team in the following ways:

**Evaluate the sensory and physical/health status** of students for initial evaluation and reevaluation for special education. This includes:

Sensory status
- Auditory: hearing assessment
- Visual: vision assessment
- Tactile and other senses, if appropriate

Physical/health status
- Health history, including review of health records
- Current health status, including current diagnoses and health management plans, growth pattern, nutritional pattern, sleep pattern
- Student's knowledge about his or her health condition(s)
- Student's self-care abilities related to his or her health condition(s)
- Social/emotional status, including peer relationships, relationships with parents, teachers, coaches
- Activity tolerance
- Healthcare access and providers
- School attendance pattern

*Develop IHPs* for students, including relevant nursing diagnoses, student goals, interventions, student outcome criteria

*Develop ECPs* for students who have known health conditions that may result in a medical emergency at school. An ECP includes specific steps and procedures to follow if a specific medical emergency occurs.

*Assist in development of Emergency Evacuation Plans* for students who have a health condition that requires special considerations for environmental emergencies and school building evacuation.

*Assist in obtaining written documentation of health condition(s)* from parents, physicians, and other health care providers.

*Assist in interpreting medical information to the members of the multidisciplinary team,* including the current and potential impact on ability to learn or function in the educational environment.

*Determine the student's healthcare needs and the necessary health-related services* that are needed during the school day to maintain the student's current health status and that will allow the student to benefit from and participate in their educational program.

*Assist the multidisciplinary team to complete the Evaluation Report.*

*Assist the multidisciplinary team to determine eligibility criteria for special education,* particularly regarding the criteria that relates to health.

*Assist in the development of IEP and Individual Interagency Intervention Plan,* including appropriate student health-related goals and objectives, specific accommodations and adaptations needed, and related services needed.

*Provide and develop a system for the provision of health-related services* that are necessary for students to participate in their educational program, including how the procedures are performed and how they are documented. For example:
- Specific healthcare procedures, such as gastrostomy tube feeding, tracheostomy care, bronchial drainage, administration of oxygen, urinary catheterization, ostomy care, blood glucose monitoring
- Administration of medications

*Delegate, train, and supervise unlicensed assistive personnel in providing health-related services* (based on professional school nursing judgment and standards and as defined in individual state nurse practice acts).

*Assist in obtaining resources for inclusion of students with health conditions in the classroom and school setting,* including space and privacy for specialized healthcare procedures, special supplies, or equipment.

*Provide educational opportunities* that help students learn more about their condition, develop self-care skills, and become more independent.

*Assist with providing in-service programs for teachers and staff* regarding educational accommodations and management of students with health conditions in the classroom.

*Develop liaisons and collaborate* with parents, healthcare providers, and others who work with students with health conditions, especially in the communication of information and planning for transitions.

### Which Students Need to Have an IHP?

Not every student who qualifies for special education services, under the category OHI or any other disability category, requires an IHP. Selected students with chronic health conditions that require daily or regular nursing care, students who have multiple healthcare needs that require health services during the school day, or students whose healthcare needs are to be met through an IEP may require an IHP.

## References

American Psychiatric Association. (2000). *Diagnostic and statistical manual of mental disorders (DSM-IV-TR).* Washington, DC: Author.

Barkley, R. A. (1998). *Attention deficit hyperactivity disorder: Handbook for diagnosis and treatment.* New York: Guilford Press.

DuPaul, G., & Stoner, G. (2004). *ADHD in schools: Assessment and intervention strategies.* New York: Guilford Press.

Individual with Disabilities Education Act (IDEA) (1975), 20 U.S.C. 1400 et seq., as amended and incorporating the Education of All Handicapped Children Act (EHA), 1975, P.L. 94-142, and subsequent amendments: Regulations at 34 CFR, 300.7c.*(special education and related services for students).*

Goldstein, S., & Goldstein, M. (1998). *Managing attention deficit hyperactivity disorder in children: A guide for practitioners.* New York: John Wiley.

Minnesota Department of Education (in press). *Other health disabilities manual.* Roseville, MN: Author.

Minnesota Rules, 3525.1335 *Other health disabilities.* (1998).

Sattler, J. M. (1998). *Clinical and forensic interviewing of children and families: Guidelines for mental health, education, pediatric and child maltreatment fields.* San Diego, CA: Jerome M. Sattler.

## Bibliography

Allen, P. J., & Vessey, J. A. (2004). *Child with a chronic condition* (4th ed.). St. Louis, MO: Mosby.

American Academy of Pediatrics (AAP). (2000). Clinical practice guideline: Treatment of the school-aged child with attention deficit/hyperactivity disorder. *Pediatrics,* 105(5), 1158–1170.

American Academy of Pediatrics (AAP). (2004). ADHD: *A complete and authoritative guide.* New York: Author.

Auchenbach, T. M. (2000, 2001). *Auchenbach system of empirically based assessment.* Burlington, VT: Research Center for Children, Youth & Families.

Barkley, R. A. (2000). *Taking charge of ADHD.* New York: Guilford Press.

Batshaw, M. (2002). *Children with disabilities* (5th ed.). Baltimore, MD: Paul H. Brooks.

Blazer, B. (1999). Developing 504 classroom accommodation plans: Parent-student-teacher approach. *Teaching Exceptional Children,* 32, 28–33.

Brown, R. (Ed.). (1999). Cognitive aspects of chronic illness in children. New York: Guilford Press.

Brown, T. E. (1996). Brown Attention-Deficit Disorder Scales. San Antonio, TX: Psychological Corporation.

Connors, C. K. (1997). *Connors' Rating Scales Revised* (CRS-R). North Tonawanda, NY: Multi-Health Systems.

DuPaul, G. J., Rapport, M., & Perriello, L. M. (1991). Teacher ratings of academic performance: The development of the Academic Performance Rating Scale. School Psychology Review, 20, 284–300.

Edelbrock, C. S. (1998). Childhood Attention Problems Questionnaire (CAP). Worchester, MA: University of Massachusetts Medical Center.

Gadow, K. D., & Sprafkin, J. (2002). Child Symptom Inventory-4. CSI-4 Screening Manual. CSI-4 Norms Manual (ADHD-SC4). Stony Brook, NY: Checkmate Plus.

Gregg, S. ( 2001). ADHD and IDEA: A guide to health and mental health professionals. ADHD Report, 9(6),53–60.

Hill, J. L. (1999). Meeting the needs of students with special physical and health care needs. Upper Saddle River, NY: Prentice-Hall.

Kline, F. M., Silver, L. B., & Russell, S. C. (2001). The educator's guide to medical issues in the classroom. Baltimore, MD: Paul H. Brooks.

McCarney, S. B. (2004). Attention Deficit Disorders Evaluation Scale (ADDES-3). Columbia, MO: Hawthorne Educational Services.

Office of Special Education and Rehabilitation Services (OSERS). (1999). Children with attention deficit/hyperactivity disorder—Topic brief. Retrieved July 30, 2004, from http://www.ed.gov/policy/speced/leg/idea/brief6.

Reynolds, C. R., & Kamphaus, R. W. (2004). Behavior Assessment System for Children—BASC-2. Circle Pines, MN: AGS Publishing.

Ullmann, R. K., Sleator, E. K., & Sprague, R. L. (1991). ADD-H Comprehensive Teacher Rating Scale (ACTeRS). Champaign, IL: MetricTech.

## Resources

Attention Deficit Disorder Association
1788 Second Street
Suite 200
Highland Park, IL 60035
847-432-2332
847-432-5874 (fax)
http://www.add.org

Children and Adults With Attention
    Deficit/Hyperactivity Disorder (CHADD)
8181 Professional Place
Landover, MD 20785
1-800-233-4050
301-306-7090 (fax)
national@chadd.org
http://www.chadd.org

Council for Exceptional Children
1110 North Blebe Road
Suite 300
Arlington, VA 22201
1-888-232-7733
703-264-9494 (fax)
service@sped.org
http://www.cec.sped.org

Minnesota Department of Education
1500 Highway 36 West
Roseville, MN 55113-4266
651-582-8200
www.education.state.mn.us

National Information Center for Children and Youth
    with Disabilities (NICHCY)
PO Box 1492
Washington, DC 20013
1-800-695-0285
202-884-8441 (fax)
E-mail: nichcy@aed.org
http://www.nichcy.org

Northeast Service Cooperative
5525 Emerald Avenue
Mountain Iron, MN 55768
218-741-0750
www.nesc.k12.mn.us

Office of Special Education and Rehabilitation Services
    (OSERS)
U.S. Department of Education
400 Maryland Avenue, SW
Washington, DC 20013
202-205-5465
http://www.ed.gov/offices/OSERS

Parent Advocacy Coalition for Educational Rights
    (PACER)
8161 Normandale Boulevard
Minneapolis, MN 55437
952-838-9000
952-838-0199 (fax)
pacer@pacer.org
http://pacer.org

## Chapter Nine

# Using Individualized Healthcare Plans with 504 Plans and Accommodations

Jeanne M. Sedgwick

## What Is Section 504?

Historically, the main interpretation and enforcement of Section 504 of the Rehabilitation Act of 1973 has revolved around employment issues for individuals with disabilities. In 1990, the Americans with Disabilities Act (ADA) expanded on the concepts and protections introduced by Section 504 by providing comprehensive federal civil rights protection for people with disabilities. In recent years, more emphasis has been given to the enforcement of Section 504 in the area of education of individuals with disabilities. This statute prohibits discrimination against individuals with disabilities, including students, by public school districts receiving federal financial assistance. The U.S. Office for Civil Rights (OCR) enforces the provisions of Section 504. Unlike the Individuals with Disabilities Education Act (IDEA), Section 504 does not have state or federal funding provided to assist districts in complying with its implementation . All costs are the obligation of the local school district. (Beta, 2001; Department of Education, 1992). Unlike IDEA, Section 504 is a law of access, not of benefit. Section 504 is an existing federal law, and complying with it is not an option.

Section 504 protects the rights of persons with disabilities. It prohibits agencies or organizations that receive federal funds from discrimination against otherwise qualified individuals solely on the basis of disability. The Section 504 regulations require that students with disabilities, regardless of the nature or severity of the disabilities, be provided with a free appropriate public education (FAPE).

Under Section 504, individuals are determined to have a disability if they have a physical or mental impairment which substantially limits one or more major life activities (walking, seeing, hearing, speaking, breathing, *learning*, working, caring for oneself, performing manual tasks).

A physical or mental impairment qualifying for Section 504 protection may include any disability, long-term illness, or various disorder that "substantially" reduces or lessens a student's ability to access learning in the educational setting because of a learning-, behavior-, or health-related condition. Note that only physical and mental impairments are included; thus environmental, cultural, and economic disadvantages are not in themselves covered under 504 (appendix A to Part 104, #3).

For example, this can mean that a school-aged child who has attention deficit hyperactivity disorder (ADHD) or some other disability and does not qualify for special education services may still be entitled to accommodations or other services in regular education under Section 504. The student has a disability. The disability limits the major life activity of learning. The student must have an accommodation plan under Section 504 if he or she is substantially limited by the disability within the educational setting. The eligible student must have a need for day-to-day, systematic, comprehensive accommodations in order to have an equal opportunity to learn.

All individuals identified as disabled under IDEA are protected under Section 504 requirements. However, all individuals who are identified as disabled under Section 504 are not necessarily disabled under IDEA (see Appendix 1).

School districts are required annually to take appropriate steps to identify and locate every qualified individual who has a disability, even if that individual does not qualify for special education services. If a student is determined to be eligible for consideration of a 504 Plan, the team must outline current levels of performance and what services and/or accommodations are necessary for the student to have an equal opportunity to benefit from his or her educational program. Section 504 is a law of access. These steps must be taken even though the student is not eligible to be covered by the IDEA special education provisions and procedures. The evaluation and accommodation plan must be developed by the building 504 team, not the special education team (Beta, 2001; Department of Education, 1992) (see Appendix 2).

Implementation of Section 504 provisions from state to state has varied on account of the ambiguity in the language and intent of Section 504 (Beta, 2001). Wristen (1997, p. 1) stated, "The best thing about Section 504 is that it is very broad and non-specific—the worst thing about Section 504 is that it is very broad and non-specific." Section 504 does not list specific diseases, conditions, or disorders that qualify as impairments because of the difficulty of ensuring the comprehensiveness of such a list and because a diagnosis alone does not qualify a student for 504 protection. Some examples of *potential* 504 qualifying conditions are diabetes, epilepsy, hemophilia, paralysis, obesity, spina bifida, severe allergies, impaired vision or hearing, heart disease, ADHD, dyslexia, chronic asthma, Tourette syndrome, digestive disorders, cardiovascular disorders, depression, conduct disorder, oppositional defiant disorder, HIV/AIDS, behavior disorders, drug or alcohol addiction (only if student is not currently using drugs or alcohol), learning disabilities, and temporary disabilities (e.g., fractured writing arm, fractured leg).

The rationale for the school nurse to be involved in this process lies within the very definition of eligibility for consideration for 504: the student must have a physical or mental impairment that substantially limits a major life activity. The school nurse's assessment skills are an essential part of that evaluation to help determine the impact of the student's disability on his or her education (substantial limitation). As the medical expert on the team, the school nurse can answer essential questions as to how the student's health condition has an impact upon the student's ability to learn. The school nurse can be involved with identifying eligible students, serving as a liaison between the school and the specialized healthcare teams, and, in some cases, the school nurse's services may involve direct nursing care, interventions in specific types of primary prevention, and case management (Beta, 2001).

## Steps in the 504 FAPE Process

Following is a list of the steps involved in implementing a 504 plan.

1. Referral
   a. Referrals are received from parents, individual teachers, learners, community agencies, or others concerned about the student's educational needs.
   b. However, while anyone can make a referral, the OCR has stated in a staff memorandum (OCR memorandum, April 29, 1993) that "the school district must also have reason to believe that the child is in need of services under Section 504 due to a disability" (Durheim, 2003).

2. Evaluation
   a. Presenting problem(s) and previous interventions are considered and reviewed by the school team. The school team is composed of those persons knowledgeable about the student, the student's school history, the student's individual needs, interpreting the evaluation data, and the placement options.
   b. The summary includes all current information and recommendations for additional evaluation. No *formalized* testing is required for 504 evaluation (Durheim, 2003).
   c. The school notifies the parent(s) of the school's reason and intent to conduct an evaluation.

   d. Section 504 requires that a school district evaluate each identified student with a disability before making an initial placement or any subsequent, significant change in her or his placement.
   e. The 504 law itself does not require parent consent, but the OCR has interpreted Section 504 to require parental consent before the initial evaluation. If a district suspects or believes a student needs special instruction or related services and parental consent is withheld, districts may use due process hearing procedures to override the parent's denial of consent for initial evaluation (OCR, 2001).
   f. In cases in which it is determined that additional evaluation is to be done by the 504 team, the school plans a 504 team meeting and identifies all staff and parent(s) who should be included in the meeting. The 504 team conducting this evaluation consists of the student's teachers and other persons knowledgeable about the student's needs, the meaning of the data, and the placement options.
   g. This evaluation may include:
      • Family history, medical, psychological, social/emotional, and other relevant data
      • Results of assessments/evaluations (no formalized testing is required)
      • Observations
      • Discipline reports
      • Attendance records
      • Grades
      • The student's unmet needs
      • Needed services and/or accommodation(s)
      • Possible staff in-service

3. Eligibility determination
   a. The 504 team will make the final decision of eligibility and inform the student's parents or guardians.
   b. To be eligible the student must be unable to perform, or be significantly limited in the ability to perform, an activity compared to an average person in the general population. It is not a diagnosis or label that determines whether a person is protected by Section 504, but rather the effect of an impairment on that student's life activities (Smith, 2002).

4. Accommodation plan development
   a. Each student's needs are determined individually based on the nature of the disabling condition and what that student needs in order to have an equal opportunity to compete when compared to the nondisabled.

b. Necessary accommodations and/or services are planned and implemented. They are intended to "level the playing field" so that the students with disabilities have an equal opportunity to be successful.

c. A medical professional cannot order educational accommodations.

d. Best practice dictates a written accommodation plan. The plan is developed by a multidisciplinary team knowledgeable about the student, and it is reviewed periodically (OCR, 2001).

e. Examples of possible accommodations are listed in Appendix 2: 504 Accommodation Plan Sample Form.

5. Periodic reevaluation
   a. An annual review is strongly recommended, but not required.
   b. The law does require a review every 3 years.
   c. Students must be reevaluated whenever there is going to be a significant change in placement.
   d. The frequency of reevaluation and the designation of a case manager (not required, but recommended) can be stated in the 504 plan. This helps to ensure compliance and accountability.

First priority must be given to providing this program in the regular education classroom, with a written plan for related aids, services, and accommodations (Durheim, 2003). In 1992, the U.S. Department of Education issued a clarification paper stating that special education and related services as defined under IDEA are required by Section 504 if the child's education cannot be achieved satisfactorily in the regular education classroom with modifications (Department of Education, 1992). If it is determined that a student needs other related services under 504, those services are provided without special education funding. The funding is provided out of the general education budget.

Section 504 requires that districts designate an employee to be responsible for ensuring district compliance with Section 504 and provide a grievance procedure for parents, students, and employees. It also requires that the parent have an opportunity to participate and be represented by counsel. Section 504 requires periodic review. The details of due process are left to the discretion of the school district. The OCR investigates Section 504 complaints (OCR, 2001).

## What to Include in 504 Plans

Appendix 3 includes samples of 504 plans. Although there are many variations of 504 plans, each 504 plan should address these basic elements:

- Description of the nature of the concern
- Description of the basis for the determination of disability
- Description of how the disability affects a major life activity
- Description of supplementary aids, services, and accommodations that are necessary
- Review/reassessment date
- Participants' names and titles
- Case manager

Individualized healthcare plans (IHPs) are one method that may be used to provide health-related accommodations to students. Some districts that choose to use the IHP to provide the health-related accommodations to students may use the 504 plan if classroom accommodations are needed. Both 504 plans and IHPs can help to ensure that modifications and accommodations are made in the regular education program (Sedgwick, 1995).

## References

Beta, C. L. (2001). Use of 540 plans for children and youth with disabilities: Nursing applications. *Pediatric Nursing, 27*(4), 347–352.

Department of Education. (1992). A clarification of state and local responsibility under federal law to address the needs of children with attention deficit disorder. *Office of Special Education and Rehabilitation Services News,* Winter: 7–29.

Durheim, M. (2003). A parent's guide to Section 504. Aug, 36–41. http://www.chadd.org

Office for Civil Rights. (2001). *Protecting students with disabilities: Frequently asked questions about Section 504 and the education of children with disabilities.* Retrieved January 10, 2004, from www.ed.gov/ocr

Sedgwick, J. M. (1995). *Implementation of Section 504 guidelines in the school setting for children diagnosed with attentional disorders.* Mankato, MN: Minnesota State University, Mankato.

Smith, T. E. C. (2002). Section 504: What teachers need to know. *Intervention in School and Clinic, 37*(5), 259–266.

Wristen, E. L. (1997). *Educational accommodations under Section 504 of the Rehabilitation Act of 1973,* (White Paper). Reynoldsburg, OH: Special Education Ohio.

## Bibliography

Moses, M., Gilchrest, C., Schwab, N. C. (2005). Section 504 of the rehabilitation act: Determining eligibility and implications for school districts. *Journal of School Nursing*, 21(1), 48–59.

## Resources

DisabilityInfo.gov
http://www.disabilitydirect.gov
Provides access to resources, services, and information available throughout the federal government

National Information Clearinghouse on Children and Youth and Disabilities
http://www.nichcy.org
Information and referral center that provides information on disability and disability-related issues for families, educators, and other professionals

Office for Civil Rights
U.S. Department of Education
Washington, DC 20202-1100
800-421-3481
ocr@ed.gov
http://www.ed.gov/ocr (Enter "Section 504" under Search; go to "Protecting students with disabilities" and then to "Frequently asked questions about Section 504 and the Education of Children with Disabilities.")

Pacer Center
8168 Normandale Boulevard
Minneapolis, MN 55437
952-838-9000
952-838-0190 (TTY)
pacer@pacer.org
http://www.pacer.org
Parents helping parents of children with disabilities

Rehabilitation Act of 1973, Pub.L. No. 93-112, Section 504
http://www.ed.gov/policy/rights/reg/ocr/edlite-34cfr104.html
http://www4.law.cornell.edu/cfr (Click on "Code of federal regulations"; enter 34 in title box and 104 in section box; 104.31-104.39 apply to education.)

Using Individual Healthcare Plans with 504 Plans and Accommodations

## Appendix I. Special Services for Students

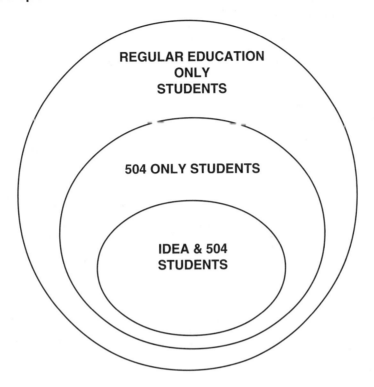

**IDEA/504 STUDENTS**

Are qualified under one or more of thirteen (13) IDEA disabling conditions. Specially designed individual education programs are planned for each student by IEP teams.

**SECTION 504 STUDENTS ONLY**

Substantial mental or physical impairments that limit one or more of the student's major life activities, special accommodations to the student's program are required. A 504 accommodation plan is designed for each student according to individual need. Examples of potential 504 handicapping conditions not typically covered under IDEA are:

- communicable diseases – HIV, tuberculosis
- medical conditions - asthma, allergies, diabetes, heart disease
- temporary medical conditions due to illness or accident
- Attention Deficit Disorder (ADD, ADHD)
- behavior difficulties
- drug/alcohol addiction
- other conditions

NOTE: IDEA refers to students in special education.

## Appendix II. IDEA/504 Flow Chart

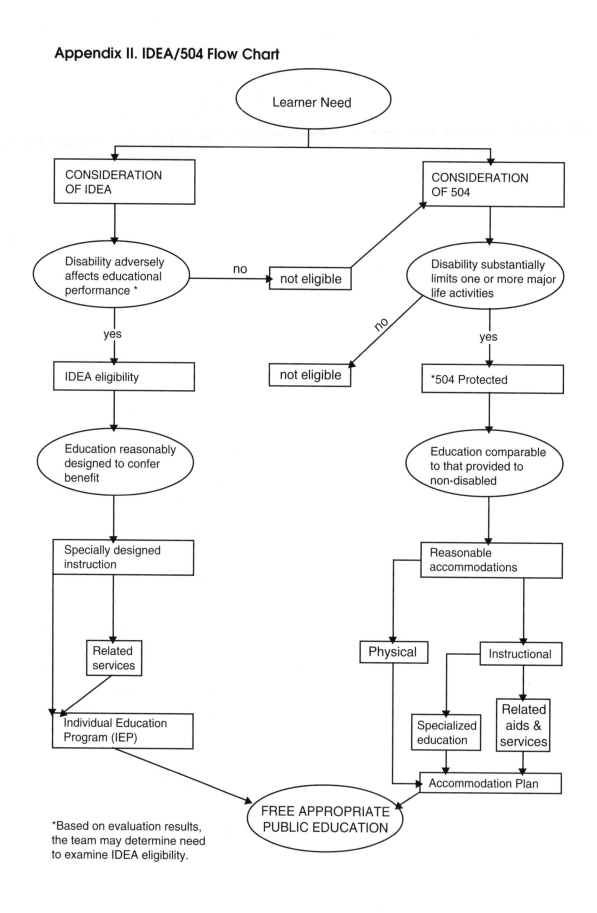

*Based on evaluation results, the team may determine need to examine IDEA eligibility.

## Appendix III. Sample Section 504 Plans

---

**REGULAR EDUCATION PLAN
SECTION 504**

---

Student_____     School_____

Date of Birth_____     Grade_____


1.  Describe the nature of the concern: _____
    _____
    _____


2.  Describe the basis for the determination of disability:_____
    _____
    _____


3.  Describe how the disability affects a major life activity:_____
    _____
    _____


4.  Describe the services and/or accommodations that are necessary:_____
    _____
    _____
    _____
    _____


Review/Reassessment date:_____


Signatures


_____     _____
                                      Title


_____     _____
                                      Title


_____     _____
                                      Title


_____     _____
                                      Title


Cc   Cumulative File

---

---

**STUDENT ACCOMMODATION PLAN**
**SECTION 504**

---

Student _____     School _____
Date of Birth_____     Grade _____

PART I:     JUSTIFICATION FOR SERVICES

1.  Is the student disabled under Section 504?

    (  ) Yes          (  ) No

    (  ) The student has a physical or mental impairment which substantially limits
    one or more of his/hers major life activities.

    (  )     caring for one's self          (  )     hearing
    (  )     performing  manual tasks        (  )     speaking
    (  )     walking                          (  )     working
    (  )     seeing                           (  )     learning
    (  )     breathing                        (  )     other

    How does the disability affect a major life activity? _____
    _____
    _____

OR

    (  ) Has a record of such a disability?_____
    _____
    _____

OR

    (  ) Is regarded (perceived) as having such a disability?_____
    _____
    _____

2.  Briefly document the basis for determining the disability:
    _____
    _____
    _____
    _____

PART II:     STUDENT ACCOMMODATIONS

Accommodation 1:     _____
                     _____
        Objective    _____
                     _____
        Objective    _____
                     _____
Accommodation 2:     _____
                     _____
        Objective    _____
                     _____
        Objective    _____
                     _____
Accommodation 3      _____
                     _____
        Objective    _____
                     _____
        Objective    _____
                     _____
                     _____

DURATION OF ACCOMMODATION(s)  From_____        To_____


Review/Reassessment date: _____

**Participants**

Name                      Title                     Date

_____      _____      _____

_____      _____      _____

_____      _____      _____


cc:     Student's cumulative file

## 504 ACCOMMODATION PLAN
## SAMPLE FORM

NAME _____ DATE _____

STUDENT ID# _____ DATE OF BIRTH _____ CA _____

SCHOOL_____ TEACHER_____ GRADE _____

1. Describe the manner of the concern:_____
   _____

2. Describe the basis of the determination of handicap (if any):_____
   _____

3. Describe how the handicap affects a major life activity:_____
   _____
   _____

4. The Child Study Team/Intervention Assistance Team has reviewed the files of the above named student and concludes that he/she meets the classification as a qualified handicapped individual under Section 504 of the Rehabilitation Act of 1973. In accordance with the Section 504 guidelines, the school has agreed to make reasonable accommodations and address the student's individual needs by:

PHYSICAL ARRANGEMENT OF ROOM:
_____ seating student near the teacher
_____ seating student near a positive role model
_____ standing near the student when giving directions or presenting lessons
_____ avoiding distracting stimuli (air conditioner, high-traffic areas, etc.)
_____ increasing the distance between the desks
_____ additional accommodations_____

LESSON PRESENTATION:
_____ pairing students to check work       _____providing written outline
_____ writing key points on the board      _____allowing student to tape record lessons
_____ providing peer tutoring              _____having student review key points
_____ visual aides                         _____orally teaching through multi-sensory modes
_____ providing peer note taker            _____modes using computer assisted instruction
_____ making sure directions are
_____ including a variety of activities during each lesson
_____ breaking longer presentations into shorter segments
_____ additional accommodations_____

ASSIGNMENTS/WORKSHEETS:
_____ giving extra time to complete tasks  _____using self monitoring devices
_____ simplifying complex directions       _____reducing homework assignments
_____ handing worksheets out one at a time _____not grading handwriting
_____ reducing the reading level of the assignments
_____ requiring fewer correct responses to achieve grade

_____allowing student to tape record assignments/homework
_____providing a structured routine in written form
_____providing study skills training/learning strategies
_____giving frequent short quizzes and avoiding long tests
_____shortening assignments; breaking work into smaller segments
_____allowing typewritten or computer printed assignments
_____additional accommodations_____

## TEST TAKING:

_____allowing open book exams          _____allowing extra time for exams
_____giving exam orally               _____reading test item to student
_____giving take-home tests
_____using more objective items (fewer essay responses)
_____allowing student to give test answers on tape recorder
_____giving frequent short quizzes, not long exams
_____additional accommodations_____

## ORGANIZATION:

_____providing peer assistance with organizational skills
_____assigning volunteer homework buddy
_____allowing student to have an extra set of books at home
_____sending daily/weekly progress reports home
_____developing a reward system for in-school work and homework completion
_____providing student with a homework assignment notebook
_____additional accommodations_____

## BEHAVIORS:

_____praising specific behaviors          _____allowing legitimate movement
_____using self-monitoring strategies    _____contracting with the student
_____giving extra privileges and rewards _____increasing the immediacy of rewards
_____implementing time-out procedures    _____keeping classroom rules simple and clear
_____making "prudent use" of negative consequences
_____allowing for short breaks between assignments
_____cueing student to stay on task (nonverbal signal)
_____marking student's correct answers, not his or her mistakes
_____implementing a classroom behavior management system
_____allowing student time out of seat to run errands, etc.
_____ignoring inappropriate behaviors not drastically outside classroom limits
_____additional accommodations_____

## SPECIAL CONSIDERATIONS:

_____suggesting parenting program(s)       _____alerting bus driver
_____monitoring student closely on field trip _____suggesting agency involvement
_____providing group/individual counseling _____in-servicing teacher(s) on student's
_____providing social skills group experiences          handicap
_____developing intervention strategies for transitional periods (e.g., cafeteria, physical
          education, etc.)

## MEDICATION:

Physician_____Phone_____
Medication(s)_____Schedule_____
_____Schedule_____
Monitoring of medication(s)_____daily_____weekly_____as needed basis
Administered by_____Title_____

COMMENTS:_____

_____

_____

_____

**Participants**

Name                          Title                         Date

_____          _____          _____

_____          _____          _____

_____          _____          _____

_____          _____          _____

Case Manager's Name _____

## Chapter Ten

# Third-Party Reimbursement for Healthcare Services Provided in Schools

Janet L. Lowe and Ann Marie Hoxie

## Introduction

Individualized healthcare plans (IHPs) describe the plan of care that is necessary documentation for third-party reimbursement. Many school districts are developing third-party reimbursement programs in order to fund necessary healthcare services that children need in our schools. This chapter provides the school nurse with guidelines to initiate a third-party reimbursement program.

The goal in providing healthcare services in a school setting is to eliminate or reduce the health-related barriers to learning and assist children to be ready to learn. Many factors impact the increase in the delivery of healthcare services in schools, including:

- An increase in special-needs children with complex health problems
- Thirty percent of the children have at least one chronic health condition. The number of children with asthma is increasing, and treatment regimens have changed for many health conditions (for example, diabetes requires closer monitoring and more injections to maintain stable blood sugar levels)
- Lack of health insurance coverage
- An increase in the required number of immunizations for school attendance
- An increase in immigration and the need for tuberculosis screening
- An increase in children without legal documentation, which results in barriers to health and dental care
- Cultural, language, and transportation barriers that result in problems navigating a very complex healthcare system
- Poverty and the complex variables associated with poverty often delay treatment of health conditions, which impacts attendance, time on task, and readiness to learn
- Health disparities for children of color
- Working families with very limited time for clinic appointments
- Legislation related to physical and mental healthcare for school-aged children

Providing healthcare services and developing IHPs are essential for the educational success of children. However, educational systems are increasingly challenged to fund the healthcare services to meet the health-related needs of students. Therefore, school leaders are compelled to seek other sources of funding for healthcare services, such as third-party reimbursement, grants, and state aid.

## Needs Assessment to Determine Feasibility for a Third-Party Reimbursement Program

A school district can conduct a needs assessment of the population to determine the level of need for healthcare service delivery within the school system. Several indicators need to be considered:

- Percentage of students without healthcare coverage
- Number of students who qualify for free and reduced meals
- Lost schools days related to health issues
- Access to healthcare and barriers such as transportation, interpreters, cultural factors
- Percentage of students in noncompliance with state immunization law
- Percentage of students without preventative healthcare
- Acute health conditions that result in lost school days and could be treated efficiently at school, such as skin infections, ear infections
- Chronic health conditions that result in lost school days, such as asthma, which could benefit from case management and health education

A feasibility study of the district resources and capacity to provide services should be undertaken. This should include:

- Administrative leadership and Board of Education support
- Funding resources, including grants
- Estimates of third-party reimbursement
- Ability to obtain contracts with third-party payers
- Parent and community interest and support of school-based services

## Resources Essential to Third-Party Reimbursement Program Development

Essential resources include the Technical Assistance Guide on Medicaid and School Health 1997 (Centers for Medicare and Medicaid Services [CMS], 2002) (hereafter be referred to as the Guide) and individual state Medicaid program guidelines for technical assistance.

### State Medicaid Plan

The state plan means a comprehensive written commitment by the Medicaid agency submitted under section 1902 (a) of the Social Security Act, to administer or supervise the administration of a Medicaid program in accordance with federal requirements (Title XIX, Social Security Act (Act), 2004, 42 C.F.R.400.203). The state Medicaid plan describes the populations covered and the amount, duration, and scope of services covered by the state Medicaid program.

Title XIX of the Social Security Act, hereafter referred to as the Act, defines the basic services that states are required to provide to eligible individuals. Mandatory services include:

- physician services,
- family planning services and supplies,
- rural health clinic services,
- federally qualified health center services, and
- early and periodic screening, diagnostic, and treatment services for individuals under age 21.

In addition to the mandatory services, states may elect to include in their state plan optional services, for example, prescription drugs. There is no benefit category in Medicaid statute entitled "school health services" or "early intervention services"; therefore, to be reimbursed by Medicaid for health services provided in schools, the services must be those included in the Medicaid statute (section 1905a of the Social Security Act) and included in the state Medicaid plan or be available under Early and Periodic Screening, Diagnostic, and Treatment (EPSDT) services.

### Healthcare Services Reimbursable in Schools

The Guide (CMS, 2002) describes the Medicaid service categories that could typically be provided by schools. The Guide suggests that this list is not all-inclusive and school providers should consult with their state Medicaid agency to identify any additional state requirements.

- Physicians' services and medical and surgical services of a dentist (Act, 2004, 42 C.F.R. 440.50)
- Medical or other remedial care provided by licensed practitioners (Act, 2004, 42 C.F.R. 440.60)
- Clinic services (Act, 2004, 42 C.F.R. 440.90)
- Dental services (Act, 2004, 42 C.F.R. 440.100)
- Physical, occupational, speech therapy (Act, 2004, 42 C.F.R. 440.110)
- Diagnostic services (Act, 2004, 42 C.F.R. 440.130a)
- Preventive services (Act, 2004, 42 C.F.R. 440.130c)

Rehabilitative services (Act, 2004, 42 C.F.R. 440.130d)
- Transportation services (Act, 2004, 42 C.F.R. 440.170a)
- Nurse practitioner services (Act, 2004, 42 C.F.R. 440.166)
- Private duty nursing services (Act, 2004, 42 C.F.R. 440.80)
- Personal care services (Act, 2004, 42 C.F.R. 440.167)
- Family planning services (Act, 2004, 42 C.F.R. 441.20)

### Medical Services Under the Individuals with Disabilities Act (IDEA)

The Guide (CMS, 2004, p. 14) explains that the Medicare Catastrophic Coverage Act of 1988 (Pub.L. No. 100-360) is an amendment to the Social Security Act to allow for Medicaid payment for medical services provided to children under the Individuals With Disabilities Act (IDEA), formerly known as the Education of the Handicapped Act. This amendment was enacted to ensure that Medicaid would cover health-related services provided under IDEA.

The 1997 Reauthorization of IDEA (IDEA, 2004, 34 C.F.R. 300.142) strengthened the expectation that schools work closely with the state Medicaid agency. Since that time, many school districts have developed third-party reimbursement programs for health-related services provided to students with individualized education program (IEP) plans. State Medicaid agencies provide technical assistance to school districts and should be consulted in regard to state specific requirements and IEP health-related services covered in the state plan.

IDEA (IDEA, 2004, 34 C.F.R. 300.24) describes related services as transportation, and such developmental, corrective, and other supportive services as are required to assist a child with a disability to benefit from special education and includes:

- Audiology
- Counseling
- Early identification and assessment
- Medical services
- Occupational therapy
- Orientation and mobility services
- Parent counseling and training
- Physical therapy
- Psychological services
- Recreation
- Rehabilitative counseling
- School health services
- School social work services
- Speech-language pathology services
- Transportation (such as special or adapted buses, lifts, and ramps)

School health services are defined as services provided by a qualified school nurse or other qualified person. Medical services are those services provided by a licensed physician to determine a child's medically related disability that results in the child's need for special education and related services.

States may differ in coverage of IEP health-related services. It is necessary to consult with the state Medicaid agency regarding covered services.

## Early and Periodic Screening, Diagnostic, and Treatment Services

Children under the age of 21 are entitled to the mandatory Medicaid benefit known as Early and Periodic Screening, Diagnostic, and Treatment (EPSDT) services. The Guide (CMS, 2002) states "EPSDT is Medicaid's comprehensive and preventive children's health care program geared toward early assessment of children's healthcare needs through periodic examinations. The goal is to assure that health problems are diagnosed and treated as early as possible, before the problems become complex and treatment more costly."

State Medicaid agencies cannot require prior authorization for EPSDT screens (either periodic or interperiodic screens).

Schools may determine that it is beneficial to provide EPSDT services in certain populations in order to address healthcare disparities and gaps in healthcare services. The identification and early treatment of health problems promotes school success by remediation of conditions that interfere with learning and by increasing school attendance and time on task.

Required screening components are:
1. Screening services
   - Comprehensive health and developmental history, including assessment of physical and mental health development
   - Comprehensive physical examination
   - Immunizations according to the Advisory Committee on Immunization Practices (ACIP)
   - Laboratory tests including blood lead
   - Health education and anticipatory guidance
2. Vision services
3. Dental services
4. Hearing services
5. Other necessary healthcare, diagnostic services, and treatment services to correct and ameliorate defects and physical and mental conditions identified during screening services

Interperiodic screening, outside of the state's established periodicity schedule, must be made available to EPSDT participants when an illness or condition is suspected that was not present during the regular scheduled periodic screening. In order to bill for interperiodic screens, all five elements of the required periodic screening are not necessary.

## Immunization Services

Immunizations administered to Medicaid-eligible children and youth are covered services (Act, 2004, 42 C.F.R. 441.56). Consult the state Medicaid agency to determine providers eligible for reimbursement for immunization services. The federal Vaccines for Children program provides vaccines for low-income children, and the state Medicaid agency can provide specifics about enrollment in the program.

Tuberculosis skin tests are covered Medicaid service and can be provided in schools. Contact the state Medicaid agency and collaborate with the local health department to provide these services.

Healthcare services provided by a nurse practitioner are covered if the services are a covered Medicaid service (consult the state Medicaid plan) and within the scope of practice for an advanced practice registered nurse as defined in the state Nurse Practice act. Federal law (Act, 2004, 42 C.F.R. 441.22) requires that:
- State Medicaid plans provide that nurse practitioner services are provided to the medically needy
- State Medicaid plans specify whether those services are provided to the medically needy
- Services furnished by the nurse practitioner be reimbursed by the state Medicaid agency through an independent provider agreement between the state and the nurse practitioner or be paid through the employing provider.

## Third-Party Reimbursement Requirements

### Free Care Rule

The Guide (CMS, 2004) indicates that Medicaid funds may not be used to pay for services that are available without charge to everyone in the community. If only Medicaid recipients are billed for the service, the care is considered free and Medicaid will not reimburse for this service. If the school plans to bill Medicaid students for healthcare services, then the school must also bill all third-party payers, including private insurance, and must bill the uninsured. A sliding fee schedule must be established to bill uninsured students.

The Guide (CMS, 2004) indicates that there are two exceptions to the free care rule:
1. Services provided under IDEA (IEP health-related services). Schools may bill Medicaid for IEP health-related services provided to children/students in special education even though these services are provided free to non-Medicaid-eligible children.
2. Services provided under Maternal and Child Health (MHC) Services Title V Block Grant. MCH grants provide financial assistance to states for the provision of health services to mothers, children, and adolescents to reduce infant mortality, prevent disease, and improve access to healthcare.

The "free care principle" has been disputed between the Oklahoma Health Care Authority and the Centers of Medicare and Medicaid Services through the U.S. Department of Health and Human Services Departmental Appeals Board. Medicare and Medicaid disallowed

$1,902,390 federal financial participation (FFP) claimed by Oklahoma under title XIX of the Social Security Act (Act) for the cost of school-based health services known as EPSDT services provided. The claims were disallowed on the grounds that Oklahoma did not seek reimbursement for the cost of EPSDT services for students who were not Medicaid-eligible. The U.S. Department of Health and Human Services Departmental Appeals Board reversed this disallowance in full, mainly on the basis that there is no statutory regulation in the Act indicating the free care principle, and that requiring the schools to bill the non-Medicaid students is a barrier to the provision of the EPSDT services (U.S. Department of Health and Human Services, 2004).

### Third-Party Liability

Schools must meet the federal and state Medicaid requirements for third-party liability. Third party refers to any individual, entity, or program that is or may be liable to pay all or part of the expenditures for medical assistance furnished under a State Plan (Act, 2004, 42 C.F.R. 433.136). If a child/student has Medicaid and another insurance policy, the school must first bill the private insurance (Act, 2004, 42 C.F.R. 433.138). If a denial of payment from the private insurance is received, then the school can submit a claim to Medicaid.

IDEA requires schools to provide children with a free and appropriate public education. Schools cannot require parents to file an insurance claim if the claim could realistically result in a financial loss to the parents of a child with a disability.

Schools should consult the state Medicaid agency for state specific requirements.

### Establishing Rates

The school district must establish usual and customary rates for healthcare services by determining costs.

To determine allocable costs that can be used by schools, review Circular A-87 and Circular A-21 from the Office of Management and Budget. Circular A-87 establishes principles and costs for state and local governments, and Circular A-21 establishes principles and costs for educational institutions (OMB, 2004).

1. To determine hourly cost of school nurse services: Average school nurse salary = total cost of nursing salaries + fringe benefits divided by the number of full-time nurse equivalents
2. Add administrative cost (consult school business administration)
3. Add No. 1 and No. 2 and divide by the number of school days
4. Divide by the number of hours in a school day = the hourly cost
5. Divide the units/hour into the hourly cost = unit cost

To determine the cost of a specific service:

1. Determine the average time (minutes) needed to provide the healthcare service
2. Muliply the service time (minutes) by the hourly cost (in minutes) of provider
3. Add overhead costs (i.e., supplies, equipment, administrative and clerical support, facility expenses, telephone). Refer to OMB Circulars to determine allocable costs.
4. Result = cost of service

Example of determining cost of specific nursing service: it is important that they first determine the average time for a specific service so

1. Determine Average time for a specific nursing service = for example 70 minutes for nursing assessment
2. Hourly cost of school nurse service as determined by the above instructions = $50
3. Overhead cost = $6.95

Determine rate per minute:
$50 / 60 minutes = $ 0.833 / minute

Determine cost of assessment:
$0.833 x 70 minutes        = $58.31

Determine total cost:
Cost of assessment        = $58.31
Overhead cost             =   6.95
Cost of service           = $65.28

An example of a Charge Ticket is shown in **Table 1**.

### Health Insurance Portability and Accountability Act of 1996 (HIPAA)

HIPAA was enacted in 1996 to protect the security and privacy of health data and to address the administrative simplification of billing transactions. HIPAA has established national standards for electronic healthcare transactions and national identifiers for providers, health plans, and employers. For more information, see the CMS Web site (http://cms.hhs.gov/hipaa/).

HIPAA excludes individually identifiable health information in education records that are covered by the Family Educational Rights and Privacy Act (FERPA) 20 U.S.C. 1232g (HIPAA, 45 C.F.R. 160.103, 2004).

Even though HIPAA excludes records covered by FERPA, it is necessary for the school nurse to become familiar with the main components of HIPAA because the entire medical community must adhere to HIPAA regulations. There are three components within HIPAA:

1. Privacy (implementation date, April 14, 2004)
2. Security (implementation date, April 20, 2005)
3. Electronic Data Interchange (implementation date, October 16, 2003)

*Transactions:* A transaction is the transmission of information between two parties to carry out *financial or administrative activities related to health care.* The transaction rule was effective on October 16, 2003. Many providers obtained extensions into 2004. School districts that submit claims electronically must comply with HIPAA transactions. The transaction rule does not apply to claims submitted on paper (form CMS-1500). (HIPAA, 2004, 45 C.F.R. 160.103, 45C.F.R.162.900).

*Code sets for diagnosis and procedures:* When completing transactions, code sets as defined in HIPAA must be used. Examples of acceptable code sets to be used during transactions are the *International Classification of Diseases, 9th revision, Clinical Modification (ICD-9-CM), Current Procedural Terminology, Fourth Edition* (CPT-4), and the Health Care Financing Administration Common Procedure Coding System (HCPCS).

*Unique identifiers:* Each provider must be identified by a unique provider identification known as EIN, the Standard Unique Employer Identifier. For school districts, the EIN (employer identification number) will be the district federal tax ID number, and this number must be used when submitting claims (HIPAA, 2004, 45 C.F.R.162.610).

School nurses interact with the medical community and will need to have HIPAA-compliant release-of-information forms in order to access records from many clinics.

*HIPAA-Compliant Release-of-Information Forms* (HIPAA, 2004, 45 C.F.R. 164.508) must include:
- A description of the information to be disclosed
- Specific person disclosing and receiving information
- Plain language
- Expiration date, or an expiration event (i.e., end of the school year)
- Right to revoke permission in writing
- Purpose of each request
- Signature and date
- The ability or inability to condition treatment, payment, enrollment, or eligibility for benefits by stating either:
  a. The school district may not condition treatment on whether the authorization is signed, or
  b. The consequences of not signing the release. The school district may not be able to provide the treatment without your authorization and further information from your physician.
- An explanation of the potential for the information to be subject to redisclosure by recipient and no longer protected by the HIPAA privacy rule
- Copy to the individual. The individual must be given a copy of the signed authorization.

## HIPAA vs. FERPA
- Records created by school districts (including health records) are educational records and are covered by FERPA, not HIPAA Privacy Rules
- When school districts electronically transmit healthcare service records for billing, the school must comply with HIPAA Transaction Rules
- Schools are not subject to HIPAA privacy and therefore do not have "Protected Health Information"

*However:*
- Schools do collect and maintain health information that is subject to FERPA privacy and to HIPAA transaction rules

## Trading Partner Agreement
HIPAA compliance requires a Trading Partner Agreement (TPA) (HIPAA, 2004, 45 C.F.R. 160.103), which is an agreement related to the exchange of information in electronic transactions, whether the agreement is distinct or part of a larger agreement between each party to the agreement. A school district may have a TPA in place when the provider is contracting with a third party for billing.

## Enrollment With State Medicaid Agency and Contracts With Insurance Companies
The State Medicaid Agency provides assistance with provider enrollment, contracting with payers, claim completion, and state-specific regulations. The school district will need to enroll with the state Medicaid agency to obtain a provider number. Many state Medicaid agencies are contracting with individual managed care organizations to coordinate benefits for Medicaid recipients. Therefore, the school district will need to contract individually with other third-party payers to obtain provider numbers.

The provider agreement/contract outlines a statement of terms for participation, which may include but is not limited to:
- Definition of terms
- Administrative requirements: licensure and credentialing, liability insurance, hold harmless and indemnification, quality assurance review
- Scope of services
- Access to records for audit
- Billing and compensation
- Terms and termination
- HIPAA compliance requirements, including trading partner agreement
- Collection, use, and dissemination of records

## Use of Billing Agencies
Depending on the amount of healthcare services billed, the district will need to determine whether or not to contract with a billing agent to process the claims, or to process the claims internally. Many variables affect the decision, including the percentage of students who are eligible for Medicaid, the number and types of healthcare services that will be billed, and the number of providers on staff. If a contract is desired, a district may need to develop a request for proposal and work with their contract/legal department.

A school district may also elect to use a billing agent for some healthcare services and bill other portions of the healthcare services internally.

When a school district completes a contract with a billing agent, the payment to the billing agent should be per claim rather than based on a percentage of the revenue.

## Enrollment in Clinical Laboratory Improvement Amendments (CLIA)

If a school district intends to seek reimbursement for laboratory tests, a CLIA certificate will be necessary. Providers must have a certificate of waiver if they perform only tests that are designated as waived tests or a registration certificate if they perform nonwaived testing.

### Background

The CLIA program began in 1992 following publication of final regulations by the Department of Health and Human Services (Section 353 of the Public Health Services Act, 42 U.S.C. 263a, as revised by the CLIA).

The CLIA law promotes quality and reliability of medical tests performed throughout the nation by clinical laboratories as well as other healthcare providers. All clinical laboratories must be properly certified to receive Medicaid payments (for more information, see www.cms.hhs.gov.clia).

By the CLIA law, waived tests are those tests that are determined by Communicable Disease Control (CDC) or Food and Drug Association (FDA) to be so simple that there is little risk of error. Some testing methods for glucose and cholesterol are waived along with pregnancy tests, fecal occult blood tests, some urine tests, some hemoglobin tests, and others. Currently, 40 tests have been approved for certificate of waiver (COW) status (see the CLIA Web site at http://www.fda.gov/cdrh/clia).

*Certificate of Waiver:* The COW is issued to a laboratory to perform only waived tests.

*Certificate for Provider-Performed Microscopy Procedures:* This certificate is issued to a laboratory in which a physician, midlevel practitioner, or dentist performs no tests other than the microscopy procedures. This certificate permits the laboratory to also perform waived tests.

*Certificate of Registration:* This certificate is issued to a laboratory that enables the entity to conduct moderate or high-complexity laboratory testing, or both, until the entity is determined by survey to be in compliance with the CLIA regulations.

*Certificate of Compliance:* This certificate is issued to a laboratory after an inspection that finds the laboratory to be in compliance with all applicable CLIA requirements.

*Certificate of Accreditation:* This is a certificate that is issued to a laboratory on the basis of the laboratory's accreditation by an accreditation organization approved by HCFA.

## Reimbursement Requirements

When completing claims for reimbursement for healthcare services, providers are required to enter procedure/service codes identifying covered services and diagnosis. Providers must use applicable diagnostic and procedure codes from the most current manuals:

- *International Classification of Diseases, 10th Revision, Clinical Modification 2005* (ICD-9-CM) (AMA, 2004).
- *Current Procedural Terminology* (CPT), (AMA, 2004).

The invoice for the healthcare service is submitted on paper form (CMS-1500) or in an electronic HIPAA-compliant format. Contact state Medicaid agency for training.

All electronic transactions must follow HIPAA guidelines.

HIPAA Standard Transactions (HIPAA, 2004, 45 C.F.R. 160.103):
- Health claim (CMS-1500) and equivalent encounter information (837)
- Enrollment and disenrollment in a health plan (834)
- Eligibility for a health plan (270)
- Eligibility response (271)
- Healthcare payment and remittance advice (835)
- Health plan premium payments
- Health claim status inquiry (276)
- Claim status response (277)
- Referral certification and authorization (278)
- Coordination of benefits

When setting up a third-party reimbursement program, contact the district financial department to determine budget codes for depositing the payment for services and for assistance in setting up an accounting system to post payments. Payment information from all third-party payers will be sent on the remittance advice (835). Review payment remittance, reconcile claims for errors, or make changes as needed and resubmit claims. If a claim is denied, there will be an explanation of this denial on the remittance. To enhance revenue it is important that someone is assigned to review the remittances and denials. Payment can often be received for a denial if a mistake is corrected or further information is supplied.

## Medically Necessary Service

A claim must be for a medically necessary service that is consistent with the diagnosis/health condition of the child. Medical necessity refers to the appropriateness of medical care and treatment for certain medical conditions. Individual states define what medical necessity means for the purposes of covering services under their Medicaid programs. The record must include documentation of assessment of student needs and identification of medical necessity. This information may be included in an assessment or evaluation.

## Qualified Service Provider

The services billed must be within the provider's scope of practice and/or licensure/certification. Schools should maintain these records on site for audit purposes.

## Healthcare Provider Authorization

Some healthcare services require medical orders/authorization from the healthcare provider. The healthcare provider medical order/authorization must be in place at the time service is billed and kept on file.

## Consent to Bill

Informed Consent must adhere to all applicable requirements for consent, including FERPA, HIPAA, and individual state Data Privacy requirements. The consent should follow the FERPA and HIPAA Compliant Release of Information requirements and also should include components authorizing:

- the provision of the service,
- permission to bill Medicaid or other insurance companies for services, and
- authorization to release records for audits and quality assurance reviews.

## Plan of Care

A plan of care must be developed. The plan of care may be included in the IEP document or an IHP or other case management plan of care in order to meet this requirement.

## Health Service Record

In order to receive payment for a healthcare service, documentation is necessary and includes:

1. Date of service
2. Duration (time) of service spent with the student
3. Service description. Standard nomenclature for service description should be used, for example, CPT (AMA, 2004) codes or Nursing Interventions Classification (NIC) (McCloskey & Bulechek, 2000).
4. Progress notes, including response to treatment and changes in treatment or diagnosis
5. Signature and title of the provider

School nurses have the systems in place to provide the documentation necessary for reimbursement. IHPs will support the school nurse in the third-party reimbursement process.

## Audit

Each occurrence of healthcare service must be documented in the record. If these services have been paid and are audited and documentation cannot be produced, then the claims are subject to monetary recovery.

## Retain records

Retain records according to state-specific data practices and record retention requirements.

---

### Audit Checklist

✓ Signed consent for service and for billing
✓ Student health need documented
✓ Healthcare service provided
✓ Healthcare provider order, if applicable
✓ Date of service
✓ Time spent providing service
✓ Service description: response, results, progress
✓ Service provider name, title, and signature, and current licensure documentation

---

## Conclusion

Providing necessary healthcare services and developing IHPs are essential for the educational success and safety of children. As educational systems are increasingly financially challenged, school leaders are compelled to seek other sources of funding. Third-party reimbursement for healthcare services that are necessary and are already being provided is a financial entitlement that school systems need to access.

## References

American Medical Association (AMA). (2004). *Current procedural terminology* (CPT), Chicago: American Medical Association Press.

American Medical Association (AMA). (2004) *International classification of diseases, 2004, 9th revision, clinical modification (6th ed.),* Chicago: American Medical Association Press.

Centers for Medicare and Medicaid Services (CMS): U.S. Department of Health and Human Services (Last modified June 04, 2002). *Technical assistance guide on Medicaid and school health* 1997. Retrieved August 10, 2004, from http://www.cms.hhs.gov/medicaid/schools/scbintro.asp

Family Educational Rights and Privacy Act (FERPA) 20 U.S.C. 1232g, 34 C.F.R.99 et seq. Retrieved September 21, 2004, from Government Printing Office Electronic Code of Federal Regulations (e-CFR) http://ecfr.gpoaccess.gov/cgi/t/text/text-idx?c=ecfr&sid=f5aa3bb942e444878beb15319a3278d3&tpl=/ecfrbrowse/Title34/34cfr99_main_02.tpl

Health Insurance Portability and Accountability Act of 1996 (HIPAA), 42 U.S.C. § 1302(a), 42 U.S.C. § 1320d-11320d-8, and Pub. L. No. 104-191, § 264,110

---

Stat. 2033-22034. Source: 65 Fed. Reg. 882709, December 28, 2000. Source: 65 Fed. Reg. 50367, August 17, 2000. 45 C.F.R. § 160, 162, and 164. Retrieved September 15, 2004, from Government Printing Office Electronic Code of Federal Regulations (e-CFR): http://ecfr.gpoaccess.gov/cgi/t/text/text-idx?sid=1f5fa2603851085905e2c1a3df54b24d&c=ecfr&tpl=/ecfrbrowse/Title45/45cfrv1_02.tpl

Individuals with Disability Education Act (IDEA), 20 U.S.C. et seq., 64 Fed. Reg. 12418, Last Updated February 18, 2004, 34 C.F.R. 300 et seq. Retrieved May 27, 2004, from Government Printing Office Electronic Code of Federal Regulations (e-CFR): http://ecfr.gpoaccess.gov/cgi/t/text/text-idx?c=ecfr;sid=5f3d60b8ae9e2aea6ea3339965871e37;rgn=div5;view=text;node=34:2.1.1.1.1;idno=34;cc=ecfrhttp://ecfr.gpoaccess.gov/cgi/t/text-

McCloskey, J., & Bulechek, G. (2000). *Nursing interventions classification* (NIC) (3rd ed.). St. Louis, MO: Mosby.

Office of Management and Budget (OMB), Executive Office of the President of the United States, *Circulars A-87, and Circular A-21*, revised May 10, 2004, retrieved August 31, 2004, from http://www.whitehouse.gov/omb/ciruclars/

Public Health Services Act of 1992, 42 U.S.C. § 353, 263a. Retrieved May 15, 2004, from the Centers for Medicare and Medicaid: http://www.fda.gov/cdrh/clia

Title XIX of the Social Security Act (Act) of 1965, § 1102 and 1871, 42 U.S.C. 1302 and1395hh and 44 U.S.C. Chapter 35. 42 C.F.R. § 400-429, 430-499. Retrieved August 31, 2004, from Government Printing Office Electronic Code of Federal Regulations (e-CFR), Last Updated August 27, 2004: http://ecfr.gpoaccess.gov/cgi/t/text/text-idx?&c=ecfr&tpl=/ecfrbrowse/Title42/42tab_02.tpl

U.S. Department of Health and Human Services (HHS), Departmental Appeal Board, Subject: Oklahoma Health Care Authority, No. A-03-79, Decision No. 1924, June 14, 2004, Retrieved August 31, 2004, from http:www.hhs.gov/dab/decisions/dab1924.htm

# Bibliography

American Academy of Pediatrics. (Adopted 2001). Position Statement: *The role of the school nurse in providing school health services.* Elk Grove Village, IL: Author.

National Association of School Nurses. (Revised 2002). *Position Statement: Case management of children with special health care needs.* Scarborough, ME: Author.

National Association of School Nurses. (2001). *Cedar Rapids Community School District vs. Garret F., Impact of on school nursing services* [Issue brief]. Scarborough, ME: Author.

National Association of School Nurses. (2002). *School nurses and the Individuals with Disabilities Act (IDEA)* [Issue brief]. Scarborough, ME: Author.

National Association of School Nurses. (Adopted 2001). *Position Statement: Medical services vs. health services in the school setting.* Scarborough, ME: Author.

National Association of School Nurses. (Revised 2002). *Position Statement: The school nurse and specialized health care services.* Scarborough, ME: Author.

National Association of School Nurses. (2002). *State children's health insurance program* [Issue brief]. Scarborough, ME: Author.

Praeger, S., Zickler, C., & Mosca, N. W. (2002). *Care of students with special needs in schools: Application of professional school nursing practice standards* [Manual]. Scarborough, ME: National Association of School Nurses.

# Charge Ticket

**Patient Info.**    CIF#_____

| | |
|---|---|
| Last Name _____ | First name _____ |
| DOB _____   Gender ___ M ___ F | School _____ |

**Insurance Info.**

Insurance Co. _____

Policy Holder _____    DOB(Policy Holder)_____

Insurance ID or PMI # _____    Group # _____

Social Security # _____

## Evaluation/Management Codes

| X | New | X | Est | Patient | V20.2 | ICD-9 | ICD-9 | Code | |
|---|---|---|---|---|---|---|---|---|---|
| | 99381 | | 99391 | C&TC,1 | | | | | AV- Pt. refused |
| | 99382 | | 99392 | C&TC,1-4 | | | | | ST-Referral |
| | 99383 | | 99393 | C&TC,5-11 | | | | | S2-Under tx. |
| | 99384 | | 99394 | C&TC,12-17 | | | | | NO- No referral |
| | 99385 | | 99395 | C&TC,18-39 | | | | | |

| X | New | X | Est | Patient | | | | | |
|---|---|---|---|---|---|---|---|---|---|
| | 99201 | | 99211 | Level I Off. Visit(use 25 modifier if billed with CTC) | | | | | |
| | 99202 | | 99212 | Level II Office Visit | | | | | |
| | 99203 | | 99213 | Level III Office Visit | | | | | |
| | 99204 | | 99214 | Level IV Office Visit | | | | | |
| | 99205 | | 99215 | Level V Office Visit | | | | | |
| | | | | 25E/M Modifier- office visit with separate procedure | | | | | |
| | | | | 59 Modifier on the procedure | | | | | |

### Time As A Key Factor

| New | Established |
|---|---|
| 99201:10min | |
| 99202:20min. | 99212:10min. |
| 99203:30min. | 99213 15 min. |
| 99204:45min. | 99214:25min. |
| 99205:60min. | 99215:40min. |

| Code | Procedure |
|---|---|
| S0302 | C&TC reimbursement** |
| 96110 | Developmental Testing(e.g. MPSI, DDST) |
| 69210 | Ear Lavage |
| 99173 | Vision |
| T1015 | Nsg. Assess. - Old code X5546 |
| T1015 | Nsg. Treatment - Old code X5548 |
| T1015 | Medication Management - Old code X5549 |
| T1015 | Health Promotion and Counseling, individual - Old code X5547 |
| S9446 | Health Promotion and Counseling, group, may be reported on the same day as T1015 |
| 99401 | Preventive med counseling 15 min. |
| 99402 | Preventive med counseling 30 min. |
| 99403 | Preventive med counseling 45 min |
| 99404 | Preventive med counsel 60 min. |
| 99411 | Preventive counseling (group - 30 min.) |
| 99412 | Preventive counseling (group - 60 min.) |
| 92551 | Screening, puretone |
| 92552 | Puretone Threshold |
| 92567 | Tympanometry |
| **Lab** | |
| 85018 | Hemoglobin- (as needed and required for menstruating adolescent) |
| 82962 | Glucometer Testing |
| 83655 | Lead(4-6 yrs. If never tested) |
| 87430 | Strep screen |
| 87081 | Strep culture |
| 81000 | Urinalysis(dipstick)optional 4-6 yrs. Required between 12-20 yrs. |

| Immunizations/Mantoux | | Asthma Codes | |
|---|---|---|---|
| 90700 | Dtap *V06.2* | 94010 | Spirometry |
| 90707 | MMR *V06.4* | 94760 | Pulse Oximetry |
| 90713 | IPV *VO4.0* | 94640 | Inhalation tx.(neb or MDI) |
| 90716 | Varicella *V05.4* | 94664 | Demonst. and/or eval. of Pt. Utilization of neb, or MDI |
| 90718 | Td (Adult) V06.5 | | |
| 90721 | DtaP/Hib Conjugate | 99078 | |
| 90645 | Hib, HbOC Congugate *V03.81* | | NP educ. services in a group setting |
| 90647 | Hib, PRP-OMP Conj *V03.81* . | 97535 | Self care/home management training, one to one contact by provider (15 min.) Parent asthma session |
| 90748 | Hib, PrRP-T Conjugate *V03.81* | | |
| 90744 | Hep B, ped/adolescent *V05.3* | | |
| 90746 | Hep B, adult dosage *V05.3* | | |
| 90748 | HepB-Hib *V05.3 and V03.81* | S9441 | Asthma Education, non-physician provider, per session(Medica) |
| 86580 | Tb Intraderm (as needed) | | |
| 90741 | Admin one unit | | |
| 90742 | Admin each additional | | |

**Provider Name** _____     **Date of Service** _____

**Time As A Key Factor**: time spent in counseling is more than 50% of the visit in face to face contact with the patient/parents. NP has to document the amt. of time spent in this discussion period and what was discussed.

*Chapter Eleven*

# Crisis in Schools – Responding to Students' Needs

### Judith F. Harrigan

## Overview

Crises or emergency situations can occur inside or outside of school. Schools have always planned for large-scale emergencies, but the traditional list was largely related to fire, weather, and transportation. The list has expanded greatly since shootings in schools and the events of September 11, 2001. Regardless of whether the crisis is a man-made or a natural disaster, the range of severity of injuries, or the number of persons involved, school personnel must be prepared to:

- keep children, school staff, and school visitors as safe as possible;
- respond in a timely and coordinated fashion to deliver appropriate first-aid services;
- assist in community disaster response efforts; and
- implement corrective measures as necessary to prevent a recurrence of the emergency, if it was related to the school.

The following chapter provides school nurses and other school personnel with information and considerations for dealing with crises or emergency situations in the school setting. The material in this chapter focuses on situations affecting the entire school population, as opposed to more routine emergencies.

## Description of the Issue

Generally, emergency situations fall into the following categories:

- Accidents, such as falls, fires in school buildings, vehicular incidents, equipment-related events, hazardous materials incidents, or building collapse, which cause injuries, including lacerations, amputations, head and neck injuries, burns, chemical or electrical burns, broken bones, tendon or ligament injuries, mental trauma, etc.
- Substance abuse or misuse, such as, alcohol or other drug intoxication, overdose, or poisoning.
- Violence, such as fist or knife fights, gunshot wounds, assaults, attempted suicides, kidnapping,

homicides, or rapes, which may cause physical and/or mental injuries.
- Natural or other disasters, such as wildfire, explosion, bleacher collapse, bus/vehicular accidents, or storm (flood, hurricane, or tornado.)
- First-response situations, such as attack, which could include chemical or biological weapons

## Violence at School

Public schools continue to be among the safest places in our communities. Even so, each day, serious offenses, including violent crimes and weapon and drug-related offenses, are committed by and against schoolchildren. These offenses endanger the welfare of children and teachers and disrupt the educational process (Colorado Attorney General, 2002).

- Nationally, about 8% of high school students are threatened or injured with a weapon while on school property each year.
- Approximately 30% of students report involvement in bullying at school, either as a bully, one who is bullied, or both.
- Each year about 12% of elementary and secondary school teachers are threatened by students.
- One half of boys and one quarter of girls report being physically assaulted by someone at school (Children's Safety Network, 2001).

Colorado's Attorney General has asked that school staff "keep a watchful eye and ... intervene decisively at the first sign of trouble. It is essential for school officials to be vigilant and to pursue all lawful means to maintain school safety and to keep guns and other weapons, drugs, and alcohol off of school grounds to protect the health or safety of the student or of other individuals" (Colorado Attorney General, 2002).

School nurses have expertise and opportunity to collaborate with school and community members to implement programs to maintain this vigilance, to proactively change behaviors and lead to the creation of a positive, healthy, and safe school environment.

---

The material in this chapter was adapted, with permission, from "Emergency Situations in the School Setting: Guidelines for School Nurses," 2005, Denver, CO: Colorado Department of Education.

## Schools and First Responses to Large-Scale Emergencies

Emergencies or large-scale disasters occurring at or near schools create panic and chaos. Children are disproportionately affected by situations involving health and safety issues. Their smaller size and immature physiology make them more vulnerable than adults, and their medical treatment needs and protocols are unique. Children who are very young or disabled may not be able to walk or follow directions, hampering their ability to get to safety or to respond to instructions calmly. Children of all ages would be at risk of emotional stress from witnessing injuries and deaths and being separated from parents (American Academy of Pediatrics, 2000).

Schools and school nurses must be prepared to respond: to evacuate children and staff, get them to a safe place, notify parents, reunite children with their families, provide or arrange care for children whose parents are incapacitated or cannot reach them, and render first aid. Schools need to consider the unique needs of the children in their schools in such areas as prevention, communication, community preparedness, countermeasures, therapeutics, and emergency response (American Academy of Pediatrics, 2003).

## Schools and First Response to Terrorism

Schools and school nurses have a particular role in responding to a possible terrorist attack. Children are more vulnerable than adults to chemical or biological attacks (American Academy of Pediatrics, 2003). School nurses have immediate access to large populations of children. They are in positions to monitor unusual symptoms or signs, recognize patterns of symptom presentation, act to protect against spread of communicable diseases, and provide immediate treatment and decontamination for members of the school community (National Association of School Nurses, 2002).

## Emergency Planning

Most states have laws and regulations that relate to emergency planning in schools. Generally, these mandates require each school district to adopt and implement a safe school plan. An interdisciplinary team approach is generally recommended with participation from school advisory councils, parents, teachers, administrators, students, students, and the community at large. The team is entrusted with the task of developing a plan that will address situations that could present emergencies, including gang-related activities, disruptive students, use of weapons and/or controlled substances on school property or at school-sanctioned events, bullying, and so on. The plan should include at least:

- a conduct and discipline code,
- safe school reporting requirements,
- agreements with state agencies,
- a crisis management policy,
- a safety and security policy,
- information-sharing agreements,
- an open school policy,
- an employee screening policy, and
- an immunity policy (Colorado Attorney General, 2002).

The school nurse must be prepared to act consistently with the emergency plans of both the individual district and her assigned school building(s). The school nurse may be designated to review and update the school plan and provide emergency training for school staff, either individually or as part of a larger team. If there is no school plan, the school nurse may be the designated person to create policies, procedures, and training to address the emergency needs of her own school.

## Release of Information

The Family Educational Rights and Privacy Act (FERPA) governs release of information from a student's health record. Under provisions of FERPA, a school may not disclose personally identifiable information about a student from any education records, including health records, without the prior written consent of the student's parent or, in the case of students who are 18 or older, the consent of the student. However, FERPA specifies situations and conditions under which a school may disclose information from a student's education records without consent.

One such exception has specific relevance to accessing and sharing information for threat assessment inquiries:

- Health and Safety Emergencies: FERPA provides that schools may disclose information from a student's education records in situations in which there is an immediate need to share that information in order to protect the health or safety of the student or others. Under this exception, schools must define the term "health or safety emergency" narrowly and are permitted to disclose information from education records only to those individuals who need the information in order to protect the student and others.
- Law Enforcement Unit Records: FERPA regulations draw a distinction between records created by a school law enforcement unit for law enforcement purposes and professionals, such as a forensic psychologist, a clinical psychologist, school psychologist, guidance counselor, teacher, coach, and school nurse, who may be able to contribute to the threat assessment process.

## Threat Assessment

A "threat assessment" may be conducted in relation to an individual student or groups of students and is designed to answer two questions: (1) Can we know violence is being planned at school, and if the answer is yes, (2) how can we prevent it from occurring?"

The process appraises behaviors, rather than explicit threats, in order "to help school and law enforcement officials to respond responsibly, prudently, and effectively to threats and other behaviors that raise concern about potential violence" (Fein et al, 2002).

The threat assessment team may be composed of law enforcement officials, school personnel, and individuals who know the student(s) of concern in the threat assessment inquiry.

If the student of concern is being provided services under the Individuals with Disabilities Education Act (IDEA), a representative from the team that developed or manages that student's individualized education plan (IEP) also should be brought onto the threat assessment team as an ad hoc member for the inquiry regarding this particular student (IDEA, 2004).

State laws generally provide that schools and other agencies working with juveniles can share necessary information with the appropriate people under certain circumstances. These laws usually encourage "open communication among appropriate agencies, including criminal justice agencies, assessment centers for children, school districts, and schools, in order to assist disruptive children and to maintain safe schools" and require boards of education to develop written agreements with law enforcement officials, the juvenile justice system, and social services, as allowed under state and federal law, to keep each school environment safe.

## Safe Schools

Other laws that may also have a bearing on safe schools include:

- Administering Restraints: defines the parameters of public school personnel to administer restraints when deemed necessary to ensure the safety of the student and the school community in an emergency situation
- Bullying: any written or verbal expression, or physical act or gesture, or pattern thereof, that is intended to cause distress upon one or more students in the school, on school grounds, in school vehicles, at a designated school bus stop, or at school activities or sanctioned events
- Criminal Acts Related to Schools: various criminal acts that carry specific penalties when occurring on or near school property or school transportation, including carrying or bringing a deadly weapon onto/into school property; making a false report of a bomb, or bringing poisonous materials onto a school bus; carrying a loaded firearm, explosive, or incendiary device on a school bus; and sales of prohibited drugs within 1,000 feet of a school perimeter, in school building, or on school buses
- Searches: specific and random searches on school grounds, including student locker searches
- Safe and Drug Free Schools Acts: address how a district will handle abuse of illegal substances in school or in a way that affects school performance

## Nursing Considerations
### Broad Parameters of the School Nurse

According to the National Association of School Nurses, school nurses bring many skills and roles to emergency preparedness:

- Surveillance and pattern recognition
- Ability to assess potential emergency risks
- Ability to assess the adequacy of emergency trainings and practice activities
- Front-line position when an emergency occurs and involvement in the response to all serious adverse events that threaten the health, safety, or well-being of a school and its community
- Often the first and perhaps the only healthcare professional to assess, treat, and refer a sick child to other healthcare facilities
- Possession of detailed knowledge of the needs of children with special healthcare needs and the ability to plan for these students' needs in emergency situations
- Ability to assist in the short-term and long-term recovery phase after a traumatic event has occurred (National Association of School Nurses, 2002)

### Role of the School Nurse in School Discipline/School Violence

School nurses have been trained to assess situations from an objective perspective and to implement appropriate interventions. Because of these professional skills, school nurses:

- can assess the student and family functioning and ability to cope with changing life stresses;
- have the opportunity to identify mental health issues or developmentally inappropriate behaviors in students;
- are in a unique position to recognize the early warning signs that may lead to violence or the signs that identify a victim of violence;
- have the benefit and knowledge of effective treatment and medical issues related to behavioral concerns and can help determine whether the student's disability or health condition caused or contributed to the behavior (Gelfman, 2002);
- will be knowledgeable about behavioral implications of medications used by the student; and
- are prepared to deal with the physical and emotional results of violence and to contribute to positive youth development and academic success though education and counseling, identification and referral for services, and monitoring follow-up with treatment programs (National Association of School Nurses, 2000).

## Role of the School Nurse in Emergency Planning

Prevention of injuries and emergency situations is a major priority for school nurses. The best way to prevent an emergency is to create an environment where the situation is less likely to arise and procedures to follow if a situation occurs that will lessen the impact or potential for harm. School nurses are qualified to be primary contributors in the development of school emergency plans.

## What Should Be in an Emergency Plan

Crisis response occurs during the emergency, in its immediate aftermath, and during the follow-up of the situation. In each phase, schools must deal with issues surrounding communication, direction and coordination, and health and safety. An emergency plan should cover as many contingencies as possible, both in terms of cause of the emergency and potential impact. There are many questions to consider regardless of whether the emergency is small or large-scale. It is clear from the following partial list of questions that the school nurse's role in providing healthcare and maintaining health supplies and health records for students and staff make her highly valuable in emergency planning.

- Are roles and responsibilities of individual staff members clearly spelled out?
- Do these roles cover as many eventualities as possible?
- How will staff, including substitute staff, be oriented to the plans?
- Is there provision for training and practicing these plans?
- Is there provision for exchanging information with local law enforcement and fire departments on school floor plans, health office layout, utility hookup locations, exits, etc?
- Are there clear plans for communication contingencies?
- Who will be in charge, and what are the lines of reporting back?
- How will staff currently certified to provide first aid be identified?
- Who will keep track of students, and how will that be done?
- How will parents be notified?
- How will safety be ensured?
- How will hygiene needs be met?
- What about food and water?
- How will bodily fluids be handled?
- Are there plans to access necessary records? Medical supplies? Medications currently prescribed for students? Emergency medications (e.g., EPI pen, insulin)? Other supplies?
- Have needs specified in all individual health plans been served?
- Will medications be available?
- Will health procedures be able to be provided?
- Are plans and protocols appropriate to the ages of the students? For example, if the school has an early childhood program on the premises, are there extra diapers?
- Does the plan cover the recovery period as well as the response period?

## Keeping Students Safe

An emergency plan must ensure, insofar as possible, protection and security of students and personnel from threats or acts of violence or terrorism and large-scale environmental hazards. In a large-scale threat, school officials and the school nurse have several general possibilities for interventions:

- schoolwide lockdown of the building with the students in the building;
- evacuation of the students from the school building (conditions outside the building are safer than inside);
- reverse evacuation of students into the school building (when that is the safest alternative);
- sheltering, usually for use in severe weather emergencies (could be in or out of school building);
- shelter in place (for use in external gas or chemical release); or
- Stop, Drop and Hold (for use in earthquake or other imminent danger to building or immediate surroundings) (Kentucky Center for School Safety, 2001).

There should be a clear written set of protocols for each element of the possible interventions listed above. The plan should define what community or school official is empowered to make the final decision for each particular intervention to be used in a particular situation. The procedures should be practiced several times a year if possible, just as fire drills are practiced.

## What to Do in an Emergency

- Stay calm and call 911 immediately.
- Stabilize the immediate situation; make sure all students are safe.
- Keep students in the safest place given the situation; do not allow students to move about the building. See **Table 1** for universal emergency procedures.
- If close to an area that is contaminated by dangerous or unhealthy substances, remove students to another classroom or area of the school.
- In the case of a chemical threat, do not move students to the basement of the building. (Vapors tend to get trapped in basements.)
- In the case of a nuclear radiation exposure, students and teachers should consider moving to the basement or lower-level rooms.
- In all cases, the school nurse should establish and maintain some type of communication system with the designated emergency leader before making a major decision independently.

- Designate a person to shut down the heating, ventilation and air conditioning (HVAC) in event of a biologic or chemical incident.

## Keeping Track of Everyone

Keeping track of everyone and everything is critical in an emergency. The emergency plan should:

- identify "reunion areas" where students, staff, parents, and caregivers should meet in the event of an emergency;
- cover transportation issues, such as adequately providing clear bus routes and an adequate fleet of buses for transporting students to reunion areas or other necessary locations, with these instruction clearly stated to all appropriate personnel;
- establish a clear procedure for releasing students to caregivers and set up accountability system for verifying names (such as copies of the day's attendance records, including a list of students who have left during the school day);
- ensure that emergency files are in order for each child and are kept in a central location, which can be accessed in an emergency (the files should contain current emergency contact and authorization information, immunization and medical records, phone number of child's doctor, medication administration forms and emergency care plans for students with special needs); and
- ensure that first-aid kits are stocked with up-to-date supplies and are available in central locations, in high-risk areas, and for extracurricular activities.

## What Information Should Be Collected Before An Emergency?

Prior to an emergency ever occurring, the school nurse should have collected several types of information. (See Tables 2 & 3.)

- Student Emergency Information Card. An emergency information card should be on file for every student and staff member in the building. The card should include the name of the student and contact information for parents and for an emergency contact person. Ideally, the card should have a photograph of the student. Pertinent health information should be included, such as allergies. One copy of the card should be kept in the school building and a back-up copy should be housed at an outside site, such as the school administration building or the police station.
- List of Emergency Phone Numbers. A list of key emergency phone numbers should be posted by all of the phones in the school building. A set of directions to the school should also be posted with the emergency numbers. Numbers to poison control, fire, police, hospital, department of social services, and local health department, as well as other important numbers, should be included on the list.
- Building Emergency Information. If possible, an instruction sheet that details steps for a school building lockdown, utility shutdown, or evacuation should be posted within every classroom and in the nurse's office.

## Assigning/Delegating Duties Clearly

The school nurse should ensure that staff responsibilities regarding healthcare in case of an emergency are clearly defined in writing. For example, there should be written policies and procedures outlining duties, including:

- specific health delegations;
- rendering healthcare, including standard protocols for common emergency problems and a process for how those orders reach the appropriate staff;
- rendering healthcare and medications to students with special health needs;
- accessing emergency medical services (EMS) from all locations (such as playgrounds, athletic fields, field trips, extracurricular activities);
- notifying the responsible school authority;
- contacting the healthcare providers (physical, dental, and mental health) designated to act as consultants to the school for health- and safety-related questions;
- transportation of an injured or ill student;
- calling on municipal services and effectively using volunteer support;
- notifying parents; and
- supervising uninjured children.

## Training School Staff for Emergencies

The school nurse serves multiple roles in training. The nurse can:

- act as census taker to see who is certified and for what;
- implement or oversee in-house training;
- provide resources for those staff or students who will be certified in various forms of emergency response. There should be at least one individual, other than the nurse, trained in CPR, universal precautions, and first aid, in each building.

## Communicating With Other Responders

Without communication there is potential for chaos. The emergency plan should include:

- a mechanism for gathering and disseminating factual information to parents about the crisis;
- a phone tree of all staff members, including janitors, cooks, bus drivers, and other support staff;
- regular communication between school personnel and local EMS, both during the emergency and in interim periods, regarding the emergency plan, services available, children with special needs, and other important information about the school;
- sufficient modes of communication during emergencies (operable walkie-talkies, cell phones and batteries, multiple phone lines, paper and pencil);
- two-way communication to the school office available from as many rooms in the school as possible;

- updated emergency numbers posted by all telephones, with all employees familiar with emergency numbers;
- defined policy and system for responding to media inquiries. (Response should be fast, reliable, and consistent, with a designated person responsible for communications with the press.); and,
- a procedure for debriefing.

## Following Up

Development of a plan identifying appropriate follow-up after emergency incidents involving individual students is essential. Communication between the school nurse, the teacher(s), the parent/guardian, and the child's primary care provider assists in maintaining awareness of student progress, identifies any new or additional care needs, and reinforces any restrictions or limitations that may have been placed on the child's activities at school.

If an accident or emergency occurs, it is critical that proper documentation be done at the scene. The person who witnessed the event will be responsible for completing an official accident or incident report after the event, but the school nurse may be responsible to see that this gets done. An incident report should include the following information:

- Name, address, telephone number, and date of birth of injured person(s)
- Parent/guardian or contact person's name, address, and telephone number
- Date, time, and place of injury/illness
- Objective description of what occurred at the time of incident/injury
- A list of witnesses
- Type of treatment given at the school
- Record of transport
- Name, address, and telephone number of the receiving hospital or physician
- Additional treatment given at hospital or by the primary care physician
- Record of parents/guardian notification
- Name of person filling out the report
- Development of a plan identifying appropriate follow-up after large-scale emergency incidents is also essential. The contingencies range from habitability of the school facility to counseling staff and students.

## Debriefing Plan Checklist

- Does the plan allow for support and counseling for students and staff?
- Does the plan consider that regular instruction may need to be suspended while the disaster is discussed?
- Does the plan include a decision-making process that is inclusive and responsive?
- Does the plan carefully consider collaborative planning necessary for the first day back at school?

- Does the plan consider alternative sites for conducting school in the event that a disaster destroys school buildings or renders them temporarily unusable?
- Does the plan designate safe rooms or locations for staff and students to receive help before, during, and after school?
- Does the plan allow students to get assistance from additional support staff and outside professionals?
- Does the plan make additional resources available to teachers who will be dealing with students in need of extra attention?
- Does the plan have adequate provisions to address the needs of ALL students, including physically challenged students and students with limited English proficiency?

## Who is on the Team?

During a crisis situation, the school nurse is part of a dedicated team of school staff, working both to help prevent incidents that could result in life- or health-threatening situations and to deal with emergencies in real time and during the aftermath. The nurse interfaces with colleagues by:

- ensuring that the school staff is adequately trained in the emergency plans
- ensuring that the staff is adequately trained to provide first aid and supportive care in an emergency
- ensuring that health information is secured and only released when appropriate

Guidance counselors and social workers will meet with individuals and/or small groups to help students cope with the stressful event and/or grieving process. They may guide students through the initial shock and conduct informal assessments, contacting parents and school administration, when they feel private counseling or long-term treatment is necessary. The school nurse should be included in these discussions.

Building-level administrators are responsible for their buildings and will often be the designated lead on all or some of the pieces of the school emergency plan. They will usually direct first-response relief efforts by trained building personnel and local officials. They cooperate and provide necessary assistance to trained emergency personnel once they arrive on the scene. As soon as practical, they report appropriate details to the central office and building staff.

Teachers and/or other staff members may be the first on the scene, in which case they take whatever immediate steps are necessary to protect life and report to the principal as soon as possible. Teachers inform students of the basic facts surrounding the incident and share concerns with the class. They may be delegated to perform certain health duties. Teachers refer students needing assistance to the appropriate support system. Teachers observe students in the time following the crisis for behaviors that might be related to the incident. They report observations to the principal, school nurse, guidance personnel, and social workers, as appropriate.

District school administrators direct and authorize news releases and/or reports to necessary agencies and report to their school boards in a timely fashion. With assistance from appropriate building level administrators, they will oversee all legal matters surrounding a crisis (Maine School Health Manual, 2002).

Remember, it is not sufficient to write the plan. All school employees should be trained on the emergency plan. A written copy should be available in key locations at all times, and all staff need to know where those locations are. The plan should be periodically reviewed and updated. Staff must be trained in implementation of the plan, with some provision for retraining and orientation.

# References

American Academy of Pediatrics. (March 2000). Chemical-biological terrorism and its impact on children: A subject review (RE9959) *Pediatrics, 105*(3), 662–670. Retrieved January 15, 2005 from http://www.aap.org/policy/re9959.html

American Academy of Pediatrics. (2003). Children, terrorism and disasters toolkit. Retrieved January 15, 2005 from www.aap.org/terrorism

Children's Safety Network. (2001). National Injury and Violence Prevention Resource Center. Available at: http://www.childrenssafetynetwork.org/resources.asp.

Colorado Attorney General. (August 2002). Colorado school violence prevention and student discipline manual. Denver, CO. State of Colorado. Retrieved January 15, 2005 from http://www.ago.state.co.us/cssm/cssm2004.pdf

Fein R, Vossekuil, B., Pollack, W., Borum, R., Modzeleski, W., & Reddy, M. (2002).Threat assessment in schools: A guide to managing threatening situations and to creating safe school climates. National Threat Assessment Center, Secret Service, US Departments of Treasury and Education. Retrieved January 15, 2005 from http://www.secretservice.gov/ntac/ssi_guide.pdf

Gelfman, M. H. B. (2002). Does the school nurse have a role to play in school discipline? *Journal of School Nursing,* 18(1), pp. 48–53.

Kentucky Center for School Safety. (2001). Emergency management guide. Retrieved January 15, 2005 from http://www.kysafeschools.org/pdfs&docs/emg.doc

National Association of School Nurses. (2002). *Position statement: School nurse role in bioterrorism emergency preparedness.* http://www.nasn.org/positions/bioterrorism.htm

Maine Department of Education. (2001). School health manual. Retrieved January 12, 2005 from http://www.state.me.us/education/sh/.

U.S. Department of Education. (2004). Individuals with Disabilities Education Act. 34 CFR 99.31(a) (10).

# Bibliography

Bernado, L. M., & Anderson, L. (1998). Preparing a response to emergency problems. Scarborough, ME: National Association of School Nurse.

Bobo, N., Hallenbeck, P., & Robinson, J. (2003). Recommended minimal emergency equipment and resources for schools: National consensus group report. *Journal of School Nursing 19*(3), 150-156.

The Center for Health and Health Care in Schools. (2002). *Bioterrorism.* Retrieved from www.schoolhealth.org/bioterrorism.htm

Doyle, J., & Loyacono, T. R. (2002). *Disaster preparedness guidelines for school nurses.* Scarborough, ME: National Association of School Nurses.

Illinois Emergency Medical Services for Children. (2003). Emergency care resource manual for the nurse in the school setting. Retrieved from http://www.luhs.org/depts/emsc/Schl_Man.pdf

Indiana State Department of Education. (1998) *Guidelines for emergency care of injuries and illnesses occurring at school.* Indianapolis: Office of Student Services.

Massachusetts Department of Public Health. (1995). *The comprehensive school health manual.* Boston, MA: Bureau of Family and Community Health, School Health Unit.

Nansel, T. R., Overpeck, M., Pilla, R. S., Ruan, W. J., Simons-Morton, B., Scheidt, P. (2001). Bullying behaviors among US youth. *JAMA,* 285(16), 2094–2100.

Ohio Department of Public Safety. (2001). *Emergency guidelines.* Columbus, OH: Division of Emergency Medical Services, Emergency Medical Services for Children Program. Retrieved from www.state.oh.us/odps/division/ems/ems_local/emsc/EMSForChildren.htm

Texas Department of State Health Services. (2001). The Texas guide to school health programs. Retrieved from http://www.tdh.state.tx.us/schoolhealth/program_guide_toc.htm

University of the State of New York. (1993). *Emergency procedures in the school setting.* Albany, NY: The State Education Department, School Health Education and Services.

Virginia Department of Health (1999). *Virginia school health guidelines* (2nd ed.). http://www.vahealth.org/school-health/onlinepubs.htm#vshguidelines

# Resources

Kentucky Center for Safe Schools. (2001). School-centered emergency management guide (http://www.kysafeschools.org/pdfs&docs/emg.doc) Web site contains a current research-based, customizable school-centered emergency management guide being used across Kentucky. The template, developed by the Kentucky Community Crisis Response Board, in collaboration with the KCSS, the Kentucky Department of Education and the Kentucky State Police, provides a research-based foundation for the protocol and emergency management procedures necessary in the event of any crisis. Developed through a grant from the Federal Safe and Drug-Free Schools Program, it has a separate training component. Of note is the School Biological/Chemical Terrorist Response Plan, which provides guidelines on responding to various threats within the schools

National Education Association. (n.d.) *Crisis communication guide and toolkit.* (http://www2.nea.org/crisis/) Assessment guide and checklist to help determine how your school or district crisis plan measure up.

National Institute of Justice. (2002). Conflict resolution for school personnel: An interactive school safety training tool (http://www.ojp.usdoj.gov/nij/pubs-sum/194198.htm). This interactive CD–ROM (NCJ 194198) from NIJ contains five modules (anger, threats, attacks with weapons, suicide, and weapons on campus) that are intended to aid school personnel in their responses to such potentially violent situations. The modules, which can be viewed in any order, are broken down into 12 didactic tutorials (e.g., de-escalating student conflicts, assessing a suicide threat, suspected gunshots) and 14 interactive scenarios (e.g., fight in library, Internet hit list, gun in cafeteria).

St. Louis University, School of Public Health. (2001). The Mass Casualty Disaster Plan Checklist Template (http://www.bioterrorism.slu.edu/bt/quick/disaster-plan.pdf). Adapted from a hospital disaster checklist prepared by the Center for the Study of Bioterrorism and Emerging Infections. A very complete disaster checklist.

UCLA Center for Mental Health in Schools. (2004). School crisis resource packets (http://smhp.psych.ucla.edu/pdfdocs/crisis/crisis.pdf). These toolkits offer a brief set of resources for self-tutorials or providing an in-service session. They include key talking points for a short training session, a brief overview of the topic, fact sheets, tools, and a sampling of other related information and resources for conflict resolution programs, crisis assistance, and reducing barriers to learning.

U.S. Centers for Disease Control and U.S. Department of Education. (n.d.) Resource list (http://www.phppo.cdc.gov/PHTN/schools/resource.asp). Multiple resources to help schools prepare for possible terrorism.

U.S. Department of Education. (n.d.) Early warning, timely response: A guide to safe schools (http://www.ed.gov/about/offices/list/osers/osep/gtss.html?exp=0). This report tells what to look for and what to do to prevent violence, when to intervene and get help for troubled students, and how to respond when violent situations occur. This includes an action-planning checklist for school personnel.

**Table 1**

## Universal Emergency Procedures

**A. Evacuation** (for use when conditions outside are safer than inside)
When announcement is made or alarm sounded:
- Take the closest and safest way out as posted (use secondary route if primary route is blocked or hazardous)
- Take roll book for student accounting
- Assist those needing special assistance
- Do not stop for student/staff belongings
- Go to designated Assembly Area
- Check for injuries
- Take attendance; report according to Student Accounting and Release procedures
- Wait for further instructions

**B. Reverse evacuation** (for use when conditions inside are safer than outside)
When announcement is made:
- Move students and staff inside as quickly as possible
- Assist those needing special assistance
- Report to classroom
- Check for injuries
- Take attendance; report according to Student Accounting and Release procedures
- Wait for further instructions.

**B. Severe weather safe area** (for use in severe weather emergencies)
When announcement is made or alarm sounded:
- Take the closest, safest route to shelter in designated safe areas (use secondary route if primary route is blocked or dangerous)
- Occupants of portable classrooms shall move to the main building to designated safe areas
- Take roll book for student accounting
- Take attendance; report according to Student Accounting and Release procedures
- Assist those needing special assistance
- Do not stop for student/staff belongings
- Close all doors
- Remain in safe area until the "all clear" is given
- Wait for further instructions

**C. Shelter in place** (for use in external gas or chemical release)
When announcement is made:
- Students are to be cleared from the halls immediately and to report to nearest available classroom or other designated location
- Assist those needing special assistance
- Close and tape all windows and doors and seal the gap between bottom of the door and the floor (external gas/chemical release)
- Take attendance; report according to Student Accounting and Release procedures
- Do not allow anyone to leave the classroom
- Stay away from all doors and windows
- Wait for further instructions

**E. Lockdown** (for use to protect building occupants from potential dangers in the building)
When announcement is made:
- Students are to be cleared from the halls immediately and to report to nearest available classroom
- Assist those needing special assistance
- Close and lock all windows and doors and do not leave for any reason
- Cover all room and door windows
- Stay away from all doors and windows and move students to interior walls and drop
- Shut off lights
- BE QUIET!
- Wait for further instructions

**F. Drop, Cover and Hold** (for use in earthquake or other imminent danger to building or immediate surroundings)
When command "Drop" is made:
- DROP to the floor, take cover under a nearby desk or table, and face away from the windows
- COVER your eyes by leaning your face against your arms
- HOLD on to the table or desk legs, and maintain present location/position
- Assist those needing special assistance
- Wait for further instructions

From *Emergency management guide* (p. 80), 2003, (http://www.kysafeschools.org/clear/issues/EMG.html), Richmond, KY: Kentucky Center for School Safety. Copyright 2003 by Kentucky Center for School Safety. Reprinted with permission.

**Table 2**

## Minimal Essential Emergency Equipment and Resources for Schools without a School Nurse Present

| | |
|---|---|
| Accessible keys to locked supplies | One-way resuscitation mask |
| Accessible list of phone resources | Phone |
| Biohazard waste bags | Posters with CPR/Heimlich instructions |
| Blunt scissors | Refrigerator or cooler |
| Clock with a second hand | Resealable plastic bags |
| CPR staff on-site when students are on premises | Schoolwide plan for emergencies |
| Disposable blankets | Soap |
| Emergency cards on all staff | Source of oral glucose (i.e. frosting) |
| Emergency cards on all students | Splints |
| Established relationship with local EMS personnel | Staff that have received basic first aid training |
| Ice (not cold packs) | Variety of bandages and dressings |
| Non-latex gloves | |

From Recommended Minimal Emergency Equipment and Resources for Schools by N. Bobo, P. Hallenbeck, & J. Johnson, 2003, Journal of School Nursing 19 (3) p. 154. Copyright 2003 by the *Journal of School Nursing*. Reprinted with permission.

**Table 3**

## Additional Minimal Essential Equipment and Resources for Schools with a School Nurse

| | |
|---|---|
| C-spine immobilizer | Penlight |
| Glucose monitoring device | Self-inflating resuscitation device in two sizes (500 ml and 1 L) with appropriate-sized masks to meet needs of population being served |
| Medications: All should be in accordance with state laws, pharmacy, and nurse practice acts | |
|     Albuterol | Sharps container |
|     Epinephrine pen | Stethoscope |
|     Oxygen | Suction equipment (does not have to be electric, i.e., turkey baster) |
| Nebulizer | |

From Recommended Minimal Emergency Equipment and Resources for Schools by N. Bobo, P. Hallenbeck, & J. Johnson, 2003, *Journal of School Nursing* 19 (3) p. 154. Copyright 2003 by the Journal of School Nursing. Reprinted with permission.

## Chapter Twelve

# Wellness Promotion in the School Setting

### Deborah Kotlas Ilardi

*"Life involves many possibilities and potentials: physical, emotional, mental, spiritual, relationships and choices. They are constantly interacting. Knowing our own strengths and weaknesses helps us understand our own power."*

*– Lynn Keegan, PhD, RN*

## Introduction

So much emphasis has been given to publicizing the concept of wellness today that its importance has been simplified into a generational colloquialism. Using the concept of wellness in advertising to promote sales of everything from exercise equipment to presumably healthy foods, we have confused consumers of all ages. No longer do wellness, healthy, or "good for you" mean the same things they did a decade ago. To complicate the issue, wellness has been equated with disease prevention. Are these concepts the same thing? Perhaps they are not. In this chapter, we will explore how school health and wellness promotion are related.

Nursing care is so much more than just caring for people when they are ill. For the registered professional school nurse, guiding students in the philosophy of wellness is a welcome challenge and one worth serious consideration. Why, then, does a search of information online about wellness turn up mostly information on diseases? The need to return to basics seems obvious. If you keep yourself fit, healthy, and relaxed, you are better prepared emotionally and physically to tackle the stresses of everyday life. We all need to take care of ourselves. This means relaxing, eating a healthy diet, exercising, having fun, involving ourselves in absorbing activities, taking breaks, being with family and friends, and maintaining a balance between work and play. Research shows that children laugh about 150 times a day, whereas adults laugh only six times. In addition to improving respiration, lowering blood pressure, and tuning up heart muscles, laughter boosts the immune system, making people healthier and protecting them from illness and disease (Powell, 2000).

Information regarding a student's academic performance, social skills, support networks, capabilities in performing daily living skills, and stamina for handling the demands of the school day needs to be assessed and acted on to best help children cope with the limitations that may be encountered in school while helping them maintain independence (Allen & Vessey, 2004). Students requiring school program modifications due to chronic health conditions will have their own level of wellness that differs from that of the average child.

Consideration of cultural diversity cannot be overlooked. For school nurses seeking to address the needs of foreign-born students, it is essential to remember that race, ethnicity, and citizenship status are important variables to consider when assessing a student's health, educational needs, and adaptation. (Arnold & Silkworth, 1999). This is true for immigrants as well as adopted students.

## National Health Studies

The Centers for Disease Control and Prevention (CDC) monitors the nation's health. Within the framework for the U.S. Department of Health and Human Services, in March 2004, the CDC reported statistical data from the National Health Interview Survey for children under 18 years of age, classified by sex, age, race, family structure, parent's education, family income, poverty status, health insurance coverage, place of residence, region, and current health status. Selected highlights from this report in the category of days of school lost due to illness or injury include the following:

- About one quarter of school-aged children in the United States missed no school in the past 12 months due to illness or injury.
- Over one third of non-Hispanic black children and Hispanic children missed no school in the past 12 months due to illness or injury.
- Children in the lowest income families were more likely than children in the highest income families to have missed no school in the past 12 months due to illness or injury.
- Six percent of children missed 11 days or more in the past 12 months due to illness or injury.
- Children in families with the lowest income were more than twice as likely as children in the families with the highest income to have absences of 11 days or more.

- Children in single-mother families were more than twice as likely to have been absent from school for 11 days or more in the past 12 months due to illness or injury, compared with children in single-father families.
- Children with Medicaid coverage were more than twice as likely as children with private health insurance to have missed 11 days of school in the past 12 months due to illness or injury (Dey, Schiller, & Tai, 2004).

This information sheds light on the whole child, which is key to providing best practice in nursing assessment and planning of individualized care. None of the contributing aspects of health promotion discussed in this chapter can be viewed in isolation of any of these factors or without regard to family structure.

## Key Issues

The American Academy of Pediatrics (AAP) recommends and supports the continued strong partnership among school nurses, other school health professionals, and pediatricians. These partners should work together closely to promote the health of children and youth (AAP, 2001). America's children and youth face many compelling health, educational, developmental, and social challenges that may affect their lives and their futures. The behaviors that contribute to the greatest morbidity and mortality in adulthood are usually established during youth. These behaviors—substance use, dietary patterns, and physical inactivity—contribute to the chronic health problems of cardiovascular diseases, cancer, and diabetes. They also contribute to social and educational problems, including school dropout, unemployment, and crime (National Association of School Nurses [NASN], 2004).

The NASN position statement "Coordinated School Health Education" supports the framework of the wellness model. The major health problems facing those living in the United States today are largely preventable and attributed to behaviors that include poor eating habits, physical inactivity, substance abuse, intentional or unintentional injury, and sexual behaviors that result in infection or unintentional pregnancy (NASN, 2004).

## Sleep

Until the 1950s, most people thought of sleep as a passive, dormant part of our daily lives. We now know that our brains are very active during sleep. Moreover, sleep affects our daily functioning and our physical and mental

health in many ways that we are just beginning to understand. Research shows that during deep sleep, growth hormone is released in children and in young adults as well (National Institute of Neurological Disorders and Stroke, 2004). Reading the research on the importance of sleep on our state of wellness will support the conclusions you may have already arrived at in your own life. When you get enough sleep, whatever "enough" means for you, the mind feels clear, the emotions are in check, and the ideas flow freely. Stress can be better handled. Ideas seem to come easily for creative thinking and problem solving.

### Nutrition and Hydration

The role of the U.S. Department of Agriculture's Food and Nutrition Service (FNS) is to establish policy, develop and distribute materials, develop partnerships with other federal agencies and national organizations, and promote these messages through the national media. The FNS designed "Team Nutrition" as a curriculum for just that purpose.

Teachers tell the FNS that they want to promote peak performance by teaching students to eat well. They want to help themselves and their students to enjoy the beauty and joy of good food and good health (USDA Food and Nutrition Services, 2004). School nurses also want to be part of the team that promotes nutrition and hydration as wellness components that support general health. The most important thing one can do to prevent excess exposure or lessen the effects of neurotoxins is to eat a varied, nutritionally sound diet (American Dietetic Association, 2004). Not only can nurses provide education on a one-to-one basis with the students they see, but they can also play a pivotal role in the choices made for school breakfast and lunch programs, foods placed in vending machines, and beverages available for purchase during the school day. Support from agencies like the American Dietetic Association helps provide additional framework. Successful weight management promotes overall health and requires a lifelong commitment to healthful lifestyle behaviors emphasizing sustainable and enjoyable eating practices and daily physical activity (American Dietetic Association).

Staying hydrated seems virtually impossible inside most of our schools as they are structured today. Water is the most necessary nutrient of them all, so necessary that people cannot survive for more than a few days without it. More than half the weight of your body is water: If you weigh 60 pounds, fewer than 25 of those pounds are bones and squishy insides, and the remaining pounds are made up of water (Kidshealth, 2004). Of the many compounds necessary for life, none rivals water in importance. Yet during the school day, during lessons in class, students are discouraged from getting out of their seats to get a drink in rooms that have sinks and fountains. They are prevented from carrying drinks in classes without these facilities. Common complaints from school staff include observations that if they drink too much, they will then disrupt their learning again to use the restroom. The school nurse is the ideal person to help these well-meaning adults to rethink their position. If the brain and body are properly hydrated, the learning process improves. That works for students, and it works for staff also.

## Physical Activity

Exercise needs to be as regular a daily activity as breathing. For good health, children need at least 60 minutes of moderate to vigorous physical activity most days of the week, but ideally every day. School nurses can actively support the continuation of regular, organized physical education classes for all students. Adaptive physical education for those with special needs and altered physical education for those with temporary limitations are crucial to a healthy today and a healthier tomorrow. This total can include a variety of activities, such as participating in sports, dance, or martial arts classes; biking; running; swimming; walking; and even active chores like raking leaves, vacuuming, and dusting. In addition, for healthy muscles and bones, kids should participate in strengthening exercises twice a week. These activities include push-ups, pull-ups, gymnastics, or playing on a jungle gym or other playground equipment. Kids can accumulate their 60 minutes in shorter chunks, such as 30 minutes of walking, 10 minutes of bike riding, and 20 minutes of active play such as tag or jumping rope. Physical education teachers may be more familiar with this data than school nurses, but it is often not discussed outside their own department circles. School nurses can partner with them to spread the word. Knowledge is only one part of the plan for change. Every adult should try to model active behavior. Make every attempt to incorporate as much movement as possible. Encourage appropriate use of the playgrounds. Share ideas on how to use the open grassy fields that surround many elementary schools. Bring back the old games where everyone participated (tag, kickball, races). Put fun back into exercise. All of America will benefit.

## Environmental Health at School

Children are required by law to be at school. From the morning bus ride and breakfast program for pre-kindergarten through 12th grade classes, indoors and out, to closing each day with after-school activities, children may spend more than 40 hours per week at school. Schools are children's workplaces. Few standards have been set to protect children. Schools can and should be role models of environmentally responsible behavior for children, for personnel, and for their communities (Healthy Schools Network, 2000). An appreciation of the importance of environmental factors has become an essential component in treating disease and in educating people to avoid illness. The air we breathe, the water we drink, the noise we hear, the products we use, the way we live—all these factors combine to make an environment that can preserve our health or damage it (Sustainable Buildings Industry Council, 2001).

Day-lighting is the controlled admission of natural light into a space through windows, skylights, or roof monitors. A high-performance school should use as much natural daylight as possible (especially in classrooms) while avoiding excessive heat loss, heat gain, and glare. We now know that daylight is the highest-quality source for visual tasks, because it enhances the color and appearance of objects. Studies clearly indicate that day-lighting can enhance student performance. Views from windows also provide a connection with the natural world and promote healthy vision by allowing frequent changes in focal distance (Sustainable Buildings Industry Council, 2001).

Even the physical surroundings have been studied to the extent that we can document their positive influence on wellness. By participating in building level and district level committees that address change in the physical environment, the school nurse promotes future wellness.

## Who Will Take the Leadership?

Consider yourself a school resource for information on healthy eating, physical activity, and obesity prevention. Your visibility and stability as a stakeholder for wellness will position health services for future funding opportunities. Target the population or community setting that is the current focus of your efforts. Use the Surgeon General's call to action (**Table 1**) as a blueprint for communication and action in five settings: families and communities, schools, worksites, healthcare, and media (Bonam, 2002).

**Table 1. Making Healthy Choices Easy Choices: The Surgeon General's Call To Action**

| Communication goals: | Action steps: |
|---|---|
| 1. Change the perception of overweight/obesity at all ages; focus on health, not appearance. | 1. Ensure daily, quality physical education in all grades to prepare children/youth for active lives. |
| 2. Educate all expectant parents about the benefits of breast-feeding, including promotion of healthy weight for children and mothers. | 2. Reduce TV time and other sedentary pastimes. |
| 3. Provide culturally appropriate education in schools and communities about healthy eating and physical activity; emphasize the consumer's role. | 3. Build physical activity into daily routine and playtime for children and families; adults aim for 30 minutes, children aim for 60 minutes. |
| 4. Educate healthcare professionals about the prevention and treatment of overweight and obesity. | 4. Create more opportunities for physical activity at work sites. Encourage employers to make facilities and opportunities available. |
|  | 5. Make community facilities available and accessible to everyone, including the elderly. |
|  | 6. Promote healthier food choices, including reasonably sized portions and at least five servings of fruit and vegetables daily in homes, schools, and work sites. Ensure that schools provide healthful foods and beverages on campus and at school events. |
|  | 7. Create reimbursement mechanisms for prevention and treatment of overweight and obesity. |

From *The Surgeon General's Call to Action to Prevent and Decrease Overweight and Obesity* (December 2001), Washington, DC: United States Department of Health & Human Services. Copyright 2001 by US Dept of Health & Human Services.

## School Nurse as Advocate for Wellness

Many American children are growing up in warm, loving families and living in stable, supportive communities. For them, life is as it should be—a positive, nurturing experience. But many other children, at every age, among all races and income groups, and in communities nationwide, are in need of an advocate, someone to speak up on their behalf. These are young people growing up in families whose lives are unsettled. Their parents are unable or unwilling to provide the information and guidance needed to enable the children to dream of bright futures with hope (American School Health Association [ASHA], 2000).

The challenges facing young people today arise from a variety of cultural, economic, and political and health problems. These complex problems do not disappear when the child enters school but may actually become magnified when large numbers of youth are brought together. America's schools are struggling to help children learn without adequate resources to address many of the problems brought to them. Consequently, schools and communities must work together to address the barriers that impede children's ability to reach their potential. It has long been recognized that health and learning are interactively linked. Children cannot learn when they are not well or when health concerns interrupt their ability to concentrate. Over one third of the objectives outlined in the Healthy People 2000 initiative related to the health needs of children and youth (ASHA, 2000).

**Table 2. Student Support Services: Coordinated School Health**

Health is not just the absence of disease; it is complete physical, mental, and social well-being. A school that effectively addresses students' health will improve their ability to learn. A healthy school includes eight components that reflect the best supports possible for youth in schools and communities today:

- Healthy school climate/culture
- Family and community involvement
- Counseling, psychological, and social services
- Health promotion for faculty and staff

- School health services
- School nutrition services
- Physical education
- Skills-based health education

These components have been proven to make a difference in the academic achievement of kids in schools and their health behaviors and outcomes. Each component makes a unique contribution while complementing the others, ultimately creating a whole that is more than the sum of its parts.

From *Concepts to Action* (2004) Albany, NY: New York State Education Department. Copyright 2004 by the NYS Education Department. Adapted with permission.

## Accommodation Modification for Chronic Health Problems

Sometimes, even when students have their basic needs in balance, their chronic health problem(s) prevent them from doing their best work ... from academic success. Take the following example:

*A 17-year-old girl with spina bifida feels embarrassed getting to class late when an examination is in progress, even though arriving late on a normal class day doesn't seem to faze her. You uncover this because she comes to your office, instead of going to class, and says she needs to catheterize herself, even though she has done it less than 2 hours before. Something is up and you know it. You uncover the facts as they relate to her classroom examination while you are in the lavatory with her. What can be done?*

In instances like these, the school nurse is the ideal individual to raise the issue of 504 modification. The solution may lie in arranging an alternate testing site, early release from a previous class, or even extended time for the minutes lost in the hallway traversing in a wheelchair. The school nurse's knowledge of the student, understanding of her health needs, and sensitivity to her emotional fragility make the nurse the ideal person to raise this issue. The school nurse used the nursing process, but the problem is an academic one created by healthcare issues.

## Conclusion

Refocusing the attention of administrators and educators on the basic tenets of good health will take many more generations of persistence. Since the primary mission of schools is to impart and teach skills, schools have enormous potential for helping students develop the knowledge and skills needed to be healthy, achieve academic success, and become productive adults (NASN, 2004).

School nurses and the profession of school nursing are constantly in a state of flux. With the constant changes that we face, we need to stop and assess what the major issues of the day are, how they affect our roles and priorities, and how we can address them effectively (Dychkowski, 2002). According to the Surgeon General's Making Healthy Choices Easy Choices Call to Action, successful efforts must focus not only on individual behavioral change, but also on group influences, institutional and community influences, and public policy. Individual behavioral changes can occur only in a supportive environment with accessible and affordable healthy food choices and opportunities for regular physical activity (NYS Community Health Partnership, 2002). The basic recommendations for creating an individual overall program for staying healthy stress two concepts intrinsic to good health: balance and moderation.

The NASN position statement "Coordinated School Health Education" provides guidance for school nurses to make use of their professional education and skills to assist their schools and local communities in the development, implementation, and evaluation of a coordinated school health program. When we can achieve that goal, wellness promotion will be applauded as a professional nursing service, vital to the development of healthy students who are academically successful.

# References

Allen, P. J., & Vessey, J. A. (2004). *Primary care of the child with a chronic condition* (4th ed., pp. 71–87). St. Louis, MO: Mosby.

American Academy of Pediatrics, Committee on School Health. (2001, November). The role of the school nurse in providing school health services. *Pediatrics,* 108(5), 1231–1232. Retrieved April 20, 2004 from http://www.nasn/org posted from http://aappolicy.aap-publications.org/cgi/reprint/pediatrics;108/5/1231.pdf

American Dietetic Association. (2004, March). *Position Statement: Weight management.* Retrieved March 2004 from http://www.eatright.org/Public/GovernmentAffairs/92_ada r0802.cfm

American School Health Association. (2000, August 3). ASHA Advocacy Kit. From a presentation at the Alliance Conference, Ithaca, NY.

Arnold M. J., & Silkworth, C. K. (1999). *The school nurse's source book of individualized healthcare plans: Issues and applications in school nursing practice.* North Branch, MN: Sunrise River Press.

Bonam, S. (2002) Making Healthy Choices Easy Choices. FOCUS: Community Health. NYS Department of Health . Retrieved March 2005 from http://www.hanys.org/newsletters/focus/upload/Spring-2002.pdf

Concepts To Action. New York State Education Department. (2004) Retrieved March 30, 2005, from http://www.emsc.nysed.gov/sss/CHAPS-SSS/SSS-CSHP-Concepts%20to%20Action.doc

Dey, A. N., Schiller, J. S., & Tai DA. (2004). Summary health statistics for U.S. children: National Health Interview Survey, 2002. National Center for Health Statistics. *Vital Health Stat,* 10(221).

Dychkowski, L. (2002). The practice of school nursing in the twenty-first century. School Nurse News, 19(3), 1–22.

Healthy Schools Network, Inc. (2000). *Environmental health at school: Fact sheet.* Albany, NY: Author.

National Association of School Nurses. (2004, March). *Position Statement: Coordinated school health education.* Retrieved April 25, 2004 from http://www.nasn.org/positions/coorded.htm

National Institute of Neurological Disorders & Stroke. *Brain basics: Understanding sleep.* Retrieved March 2004, from http://www.ninds.nih.gov/health_and_medical/pubs/understanding_sleep_brain_basics_html

New York State Community Health Partnership, Office of Disease Prevention and Health Promotion. (Spring 2002). *Nutrition, physical activity and obesity: Making healthy choices easy choices.* Retrieved March 20, 2005, from www.hanys.org/newsletters/focus/focus.cfm

Powell T. (2000). *Stress free living.* New York: DK Publishing.

Sustainable Buildings Industry Council (2001). *High performance school buildings: Resource and strategy guide.* Retrieved April 1, 2005, from http://www.sbicouncil.org/highperformanceschoolbuildings.htm

USDA Food and Nutrition Services. (2004, March). *Team nutrition.* Retrieved from http://www.fns.usda.gov/tn/Educators/index.htm

Why drinking water is the way to go. (February 2004). *Kidshealth.* Retrieved from http://www.kidsheath.org

# Bibliography

Marx, E., & Wooley, S.F. (Eds.). (1998). *Health is academic: A guide to coordinated school health programs.* New York: Teachers College Press.

# Resources

## Web sites

CDC Division of Nutrition and Physical Activity
http://www.cdc.gov/nccdph/dnpa

Children's Defense Fund
http://www.childrensdefense.org/

Cornell Nutrition Works
http://www.nutritionworks.cornell.edu

Food, Nutrition and Consumer Services
http://www.fns.usda.gov/fncs/

Healthfinder
http://www.healthfinder.gov

Healthy People 2010
http://www.healthypeople.gov

National Association of School Nurses
http://www.nasn.org

National Cancer Institute
"Eat 5 A Day For Better Health"
http://www.5aday.gov/

National Center for Bicycling and Walking
http://www.bikefed.org

Office of Disease Prevention and Health Promotion
http://odphp.osophs.dhhs.gov

The Surgeon General's Call To Action to Prevent and
    Decrease Overweight and Obesity
http://www.surgeongeneral.gov/topics/obesity

## Agencies and Organizations

American Dietetic Association
120 South Riverside Plaza
Suite 2000
Chicago, IL 60606-6995
1-800-877-1600
or
1120 Connecticut Avenue, NW
Suite 480
Washington, DC 20036
202-775-8277
ADA's Public Relations Team:
1-800-877-1600, ext. 4802, 4769, 4894, or 4822
http://www.eatright.org

Children's Defense Fund
Leave No Child Behind
25 E Street, NW
Washington, DC 20001
202-628-8787
cdfinfo@childrensdefense.gov

Environmental Protection Agency
1200 Pennsylvania Ave, NW
Washington, DC 20460
202-272-016
 http://www.epa.gov

Healthy Kids Network, American Cancer Society
260-471-3911
305-594-4363
1-800-444-1410
305-592-514 (fax)

Healthy Schools Network, Inc.
773 Madison Avenue
Albany, NY 12208
518-462-0632
http://www.healthyschools.org

National Institute of Neurological
    Disorders & Stroke
BRAIN
PO Box 5801
Bethesda, MD 20824
1-800-352-9424
www.nids.nih.gov

Office of Disease Prevention and Health Promotion
Healthy People 2010
Office of Public Health & Science
Office of the Secretary
200 Independence Avenue, SW
Room 738G
Washington, DC 20201
hp2010@osophs.dhhs.gov
1-800-367-4725
202-205-9478 (fax)

USDA's Team Nutrition
3101 Park Center Drive
Room 632
Alexandria, VA 22302
703-305-1624
703-305-2549 (fax)
http://www.fns.usda.gov/tn/

# Chapter Thirteen

# Chronic Health Conditions: Indicators of Need

Brenda Kay Lenz

## Introduction

Chronic health conditions can have tremendous impact on children and their families. Chronic health conditions disrupt the normal child developmental pattern and result in multiple burdens to the family. These burdens may include hospitalizations, school absences, surgery, medications, medical treatments, managing chronic pain, and activity restrictions due to the illness or fatigue. In turn, the burdens may produce for the family and/or child anxiety, loss of control, coping difficulties, role and responsibility changes, fear, grief, and impaired socialization and, for the child, developmental lags.

The exact number of children with a chronic condition is unknown, but the National Health Interview Survey on Child Health conducted in 1988 estimated 31% of children less than 18 years of age had one or more chronic conditions, not including mental health conditions (Newacheck, McManus, & Fox, 1991). Estimates of children with chronic conditions depend on the definition and method used to identify them (Allen & Vessey, 2004). Jackson and Vessey (2000) defined chronic illness or condition as one that is long term and is either not curable or has residual characteristics that limit activities of daily living and require adaptation or some special assistance. Chronic disease is the foremost set of healthcare problems in the United States today, as one in five Americans report a chronic condition (Kinne, Patrick, & Doyle, 2004). The increase in prevalence of chronic illness stems from improvements in infectious disease control, advances in medical technology, pharmacotherapeutics, improved diagnosis and case finding, and increased birth and injury survival rates (Allen & Vessey). The overall incidence of childhood chronic conditions has not changed in the past 20 years, but improved life expectancy has increased the prevalence of chronic conditions. New categories of childhood chronic conditions are emerging, including extreme prematurity and the increased prevalence in type 2 diabetes resulting from the dramatic rise in childhood obesity (Allen & Vessey). Examples of childhood chronic conditions include diabetes mellitus, cystic fibrosis, cerebral palsy, asthma, inflammatory bowel syndrome, bleeding disorders, cancer, cystic fibrosis, Down syndrome, epilepsy, HIV/AIDS, arthritis, sickle cell disease, neural tube defects, and mental health concerns.

Children with chronic conditions have unique needs compared with adults. Chronic conditions in children are frequently not stable, and children may experience acute exacerbations and remissions that are superimposed on their growth and development (Allen & Vessey, 2004). Nurses must consider the developmental needs for children living with a chronic condition. Developmental needs include cognitive, fine and gross motor, social, personal, communication, and emotional. Variables that contribute to severity of developmental alterations include the natural history of the condition, personal characteristics of the child, and the larger social network (Jackson & Vessey, 2000).

Children's understanding of and response to chronic illness are influenced by their age at the onset of the disorder as well as growth and development throughout the course of the illness (James, Ashwill, & Droske, 2002). As children mature, their view of illness evolves (Leifer & Hartston, 2004). According to these authors, preschoolers experience illness as magical, whereas young school-aged children have concrete and rigid ideas and show little comprehension of the illness, although they can list symptoms. Older school-aged children show greater understanding of the cause of the illness, and adolescents understand abstract principles and concepts involved in illness.

The adolescence period is crucial in regard to adaptation to chronic conditions. Adolescents are already under stress due to developmental changes related to identity, independence, and role changes (Lubkin & Larsen, 2002). Woodgate (1998) conducted an exploratory, qualitative study with teens to elicit detailed descriptions of adolescents' chronic illness experiences. "It's hard" was found as an overall theme regarding the difficulties and hardships that come from having a chronic illness for these adolescents. Most adolescents in the Woodgate study felt that life was not easy because of their chronic illness. Additional themes include the experience required additional energy or extra effort; it meant that the adolescents experienced limitations or restrictions; they experienced distress, suffering, or pain; and in addition to worry about school, friends, and family, these adolescents worried about their health and consequences that come with having a chronic illness.

Children with chronic conditions are twice as likely as other children to have emotional or behavioral problems (Allen & Vessey, 2004). Regardless of the stage of growth and development, concerns related to emotional maladjustment in the areas of self-esteem, self-reliance, and autonomy are prevalent among children (James et al, 2002). They are at significant risk for behavioral difficulties, role performance changes such as the sick or impaired role, and poor resolution of developmental tasks including regression (Lubken & Larsen, 2002). Some children will experience altered body awareness and body image resulting from the physical changes related to the illness or treatment. School absences are a concern for some children. Socialization may be limited as a result of frequent hospitalization as well as side effects of treatment. Altered communication or lack of communication may occur as related to psychological and emotional needs. The condition may contribute to developmental lags compared to unaffected peers, although chronic conditions do not necessarily connote the presence of developmental disturbances (Jackson & Vessey, 2000.

Unlike adults with chronic conditions, children depend on adults for care and it is critical for nurses to keep in mind the context of the family and caregivers. Family health, ethnicity, culture, socioeconomic status, education, and source of health insurance all affect the child's access to services, use of services, and adherence to treatment plans (Allen & Vessey, 2004). Clawson (1996), analyzed the concept of family adaptation to a child with a chronic illness. The author described that initially, upon diagnosis, the family system often reacts with shock and disbelief. Attributes of family adaptation to chronic illness include accepting the child's condition and giving meaning to the condition as a coping strategy. Another adaptive task is to manage the child's condition on a day-to-day basis. Additional tasks described by Clawson include meeting the child's developmental needs, coping with ongoing stress and periodic crisis, assisting family members to manage their feelings, educating others about the condition, and establishing a support system. Chronic illness can strain sibling relationships and take a toll on economic resources of the family (Leifer & Hartston, 2004)

Some families are more able to adapt than others (Diamond, 1994). Studies have shown that some families reorganize and actually become stronger in response to a situational crisis. These families are considered resilient. Traits of a resilient family include balancing the illness with other family needs, attributing positive meaning to the experience, engaging in effective coping efforts, maintaining flexibility, communicating effectively, and collaborating with professionals (James et al., 2002). Unfortunately, some families with a child with disabilities may view the child as a source of stress and maladaptation (Olsen et al.,1999).

Socioeconomic status and ethnicity play important roles in incidence and severity of the conditions (Allen & Vessey, 2004). Poor children have a significantly higher incidence rate and severity level of disability. Additionally, the child's disability has a major impact on the family's finances. Costs for families include increased healthcare expenditures, such as special diets, pharmaceuticals, treatments, cosmetics or clothes to hide or accommodate effects of disease or treatment, counseling and mental health services, respite services, transportation expenses; also there may be a decreased ability of parents to work as a result of the child's needs and babysitting costs for siblings while the child receives treatment.

A final critical issue for nurses is the medical management plan for the treatment of the chronic condition. Adherence by children to the medical management of the condition is related to the beliefs the children and their families hold about the condition. Those children who are more likely to be compromised are those who perceive their illness as more negative and restricting their function (Jackson & Vessey, 2000). Moreover, poor medical management creates a downward spiral that results in more chronic illness symptoms, increased school absences, and further psychosocial adjustment issues. For example, Sherman and Hendeles (2000) reported that many patients with poorly controlled asthma are actually poorly compliant. Children who take their treatments as prescribed have an opportunity to live more normal lives.

Behavioral problems may be related to adherence to the treatment plan. For example, the parents, out of fear for the child's future well-being, may focus their attention on strict compliance to the treatment regimen. This attention may lead to a power struggle between parent and child, as developmentally the child strives for independence or autonomy from parental supervision. In contrast, permissive parents may allow the child to take care of the treatment on his or her own. This permissiveness does not take in account the child's developmental needs for guidance, consistency, and structure.

School nurses are in pivotal positions to help children with chronic conditions and their families to succeed. Working with these children requires knowledge of the condition, the medical treatment plan, potential complications, and side effects of treatment. Nurses hold this knowledge. However, nurses need to recognize the psychosocial and developmental problems associated with chronic conditions and provide nursing interventions specifically for these problems.

Primary psychosocial nursing interventions include care for the child through counseling and ongoing support, health promotion, and, lastly, anticipatory guidance through periods of developmental transition. Secondary nursing intervention may include teaching related to knowledge deficits. However, a knowledge deficit may not be the primary reason for psychosocial issues, and health education should not be substituted for primary psychosocial nursing interventions. If health education is needed, it should be an ongoing process, must be adapted to the child's developmental level, and must be adapted to the family's knowledge base (Diamond, 1994). Lastly, parental support may be necessary to reinforce normal family life and consistent discipline.

School nurses must advocate for the child and the family in the school environment. School nurses have the unique role of facilitating school accommodations and fostering psychosocial support throughout the school setting. Children thrive in schools that support their needs. As described by Lowe and Miller (1998), school nursing services are an essential component to the health and well-being of children and youth with chronic health problems.

## Management

The goal for any child with chronic illness is to achieve and maintain the highest level of health and function possible (James et al., 2002). This includes the child's physical, psychosocial, and emotional health. The attempt is to maintain a normal pattern of living, or normalization, for the child and the family.

"The school nurse has an important leadership role in the provision of school health services for children with chronic conditions" (Allen & Vessey, 2004, p. 81). The most common and familiar nursing role is assessment of student needs, development of an individualized healthcare plan (IHP) to address the needs, either direct nursing service or delegation and supervision of nursing care, and evaluation of care. This includes nursing care of acute, chronic, episodic, and emergency needs.

The second role is one of case or care coordinator. The school nurse is in an ideal position to serve in the role of coordinator of care with the primary care provider, specialists, and local public health and social service agencies (Allen & Vessey, 2004). The nurse has the opportunity to see the child daily and can identify changes in health status, the effectiveness of prescribed treatments and medications, the effectiveness of the individualized education plan (IEP) and assistive technologic devices in meeting the educational goals for the child, and potential problems and changes in the child's condition.

Last, the school nurse, with formal education in pediatrics, child growth and development, mental health, family health, and health promotion, has a unique knowledge base in which to foster the psychosocial adjustment of children with chronic conditions. Nurses need to take an active and leadership role in the promotion of psychosocial and emotional health for children with chronic conditions.

# Individualized Healthcare Plan

### Assessment

Nurses must gather data from many sources, including observations, interviews, physical examinations, and interactions with the child and family. Current health information regarding the child and the chronic illness is essential. References for the section include the fifth edition of *Chronic Illness Impact and Interventions* (Lubken & Larsen, 2002) and the article "Assessment of Stressors in Families With a Child Who Has a Chronic Condition" (Burke, Kauffmann, Harrison, & Wiskin, 1999).

Following are listed the areas for assessment.

*Social isolation*
- Assess for student's feelings; may include marginality or exclusion, alienation, isolation, loneliness, and aloneness (*Example:* Student with brain tumor needs to wear baseball cap due to loss of hair in school where caps are against policy. He feels ridiculed and singled out.)
- Observation assessment by teachers, nurse, or family yields declining quality and number of friends
- Attendance changes that include missed school due to hospitalizations or absences

*Medical Treatment Nonadherence*
- Assess knowledge level, beliefs, and attitudes of student and family.
- Assess for student and family's perception of illness threat.
- Assess student's feelings, which may include hostility, depression, emotional distress, anxiety. (*Example:* Adolescent with cystitic fibrosis refuses to eat additional calories and family provides additional calories through nasogastric tube feeding at night.
- Assess for social support, cultural factors, language barriers, motivation, and personal control. (*Example:* Immigrant student with tuberculosis doesn't understand the need for or the cost of taking antibiotics for 6 months).
- Assess family economic factors related to cost of medical management, including insurance and copay costs, government programs, transportation costs, employment of parents, and out-of-pocket money for sibling babysitting, supplies, and special expenditures above what insurance will pay.

*Body Image*
- Assessment includes observation and interview of student. Assess student's experience and meaning of change, perception of experience, knowledge of illness and effects.

- Learn how much value is placed on appearance to determine impact. (*Example:* Young adolescent who values thin appearance avoids insulin injections in order to lose weight.)
- Assess for self-esteem and support systems.
- Use standardized screening tool if necessary.

### Self-reliance and Autonomy
- Identify student strengths.
- Identify self-care skills student uses.
- Identify self-care skills student doesn't use but would be able to if given the autonomy to do so by provider, family, or others.
- Identify fears or anxiety issues related to chronic illness that prevents autonomy.

### Family Processes
- Assess for impact on family life stage
- Assess family for distribution of tasks/responsibility among family members.
- Assess for stress associated with providing care. Stress is associated with intensity of care, type of care, caregiver obligations, and support from family for care.
- Assess for burden or strain of care or the infringement of the caregiving role upon the individual's space.
- Assess for exhaustion or burnout.
- Assess for neglect, abuse, and excessive caregiving. (*Example:* Mother is present every day at school to ensure proper care of son with cerebral palsy while teenage daughter suffers from lack of parental supervision and seeks attention from older men.)
- Assess financial impact of caregiving and direct costs for care of child.
- Assess sibling issues.
- Assess for social support and relationships that support family including extended family, community, friends, and parents with similar children.

### Coping
- Assess past coping mechanisms used by student during stress and illness crisis.
- Assess effectiveness of coping mechanisms used by student and consequences of use.
- Assess for ineffective or inappropriate coping mechanisms used by student. (*Example:* Student uses anger and lashes out at caregivers when blood glucose needs to be checked.)
- Assess changes in coping mechanisms used over course of chronic illness.

### Self-esteem
- Assess for signs of depression, mood disorders; may need to use depression screening tool.
- Assess for motivation. (*Example:* "I don't feel like taking care of myself.")
- Assess for feelings related to self. (*Example:* "I hate myself.")
- Assess for feelings related to self-efficacy or the ability to care for self.
- Assess for thoughts about suicide and suicide plan.

### Role Performance
- Assess student for the ability to carry out medical regimen.
- Assess student ability to plan ahead related to illness needs and symptoms, modify his or her environment, and plan activities when symptom-free.
- Assess student's ability to manage and prevent crisis. (*Example:* Has student experienced hypoglycemic episode and can she identify early symptoms?)
- Assess student's ability to adjust to changes in the course of the disease.
- Assess student's ability to adjust schedule to cope with managements of health regimens.
- Assess student's ability to hide illness, manage symptoms, and find ways to be treated as normal.

## Nursing Diagnoses (N.D.) (NANDA 2003)

**N.D. 1** Delayed growth and development (00111) related to chronic condition or disability

**N.D. 2** Disturbed body image (00118) related to actual or perceived differences, feelings of being different, inability to participate in specific activities.

**N.D. 3** Interrupted family processes (00060) related to situational crisis (child with chronic condition)

**N.D. 4** Impaired social interaction (00052) related to frequent hospitalizations, frequent school absences, and the inability to initiate or maintain social relationships

**N.D. 5** Ineffective role performance (00055) or impaired role (sick role) performance related to chronic illness or disability (includes risk for school role failure)

**N.D. 6** Low self-esteem (00120) related to effects of chronic condition

**N.D. 7** Impaired adjustment (00070) or ineffective coping (00069) related to chronic condition

**N.D. 8** Self-care deficit (00109; 00108; 00102; 00110), inappropriate dependence, low self-reliance related to chronic condition

## Student Goals

The student will attain maximum expected growth and development. (N.D. 1)

The student will express feelings and concerns and/or will cope with actual or perceived changes caused by illness. (N.D. 2)

The student will have needs met pertaining to family unit and/or will exhibit positive adaptation to child's condition. (N.D. 3)

The student will experience positive interpersonal relationships. (N.D. 4)

The student will exhibit positive adaptation to chronic condition. (N.D. 5)

The student will exhibit improved self-esteem and self-concept. (N.D. 6)

The student will cope with limitations positively. (N.D. 7)

The student will engage in self-care activities; will achieve sense of competence and mastery. (N.D. 8)

The student will experience reduction in fear and anxiety. (N.D 3, 5, 6, 7, 8)

The student will demonstrate understanding of chronic condition. (N.D. 1–8)

## Nursing Interventions

Planning and implementation of nursing care are based on several factors. First, the child's condition must be considered, because each illness will include specific implications. Second, the child's growth and development must be considered. Last, the needs, coping mechanisms, and available resources of the child and family are considered as influencing factors. Nursing care includes assisting the child and family to accept, understand, and incorporate the illness into each stage of growth and development.

*School-wide interventions:*
- Create an empathetic school community by sharing implications of chronic conditions through education of school staff and peers. (N.D. 1–8)
- Balance confidentiality (as requested by family and child) with meeting school health and safety needs. (N.D. 1–8)
- Monitor the results of interventions and document. (N.D. 1–8)

*Individualized Healthcare Plan (IHP):*
- Initiate an IHP and coordinate care for child between teacher, school support services (school social worker, counselors, and psychologist), auxiliary staff (cafeteria, playground), family, and community services and primary provider as appropriate. (N.D. 1–8)
- IHP accommodations related to school performance and attendance should be made on an individualized basis. (N.D. 4, 5)

*Interventions for medical management:*
- Monitor adherence and response to the medical management plan. Evaluate the child's response to the plan. (N.D. 1–8)
- Share information with the health care provider or primary physician while complying with confidentiality and privacy guidelines (HIPAA). (N.D. 1–8)

*Interventions for the family:*
- Be available to child and family. Communicate honestly with child and parents. Build an ongoing trusting relationship with family and child. Return phone calls promptly. (N.D. 1–8)
- Assist family to identify support systems. This may include community camps, extended family, respite, and other community services or programs. (N.D. 3)
- Help family understand chronic condition, therapies, and implications. Reinforce information given by others. Clarify misconceptions. Provide accurate information. (N.D. 1–8)

- Provide anticipatory guidance to family and child related to impending developmental needs (*Example:* the transition from high school to college and the needs of the young adult with inflammatory bowel syndrome). (N.D. 1)
- Support families to find meaning in the condition. (N.D. 3)

### Community-based interventions:
- Advocate for community services for children's mental health needs, family and sibling needs, and respite care at the local, state, and national level. (N.D. 1–8)

### Student interventions:
- Facilitate a school-based support group for children with a chronic condition. Findings from research suggest that children may lack essential information about their illness and have misunderstandings about themselves and their family and friends regarding their illness (Berg, Tichacek, & Theodorakis, 2004). Groups allow children to share the emotional impact of the illness. Studies have found that asthma education programs to students resulted in an increase in students' self-management behaviors (Gregory, 2000). (N.D. 2-7)
- If unable to provide support group, introduce child to others who have adjusted well to this or similar condition. (N.D. 2, 4, 5, 6, 7)
- Facilitate adult-child mentoring. Encourage local adults with similar needs or experiences to support students (Example: adult athlete with asthma talks about asthma with student athlete). (N.D. 4–7)
- Encourage students to acknowledge experiences and feelings through active listening and supportive comments. (N.D. 2–7)
- Develop and facilitate social-skills and/or coping training programs. Network with teachers and school support services (school counselor, school social worker, and school psychologist) to provide program (Example: the use of theater performers to model appropriate responses to social cues). (N.D. 4–7)
- Provide one-on-one counseling. Counseling can assist child to give meaning to condition and to release negative emotions. Counseling can identify positive coping behaviors, extinguish negative behaviors, and set realistic goals. Nurses have the skills and knowledge to provide health counseling. Counseling is supportive and allows children to find their own answer from within themselves rather than being told what to do by authority figures. (N.D. 2, 4–7)
- Monitor and assess students with chronic conditions for maladaptive behaviors, ineffective coping mechanisms, and signs of depression as described in assessment section. (N.D. 1–8)
- Refer students with maladaptive behaviors, early signs of depression, or ineffective coping mechanisms to a professional community-based mental health provider who specializes in chronic conditions. Community-based counseling may be necessary or even supportive to the child's adaptation to the illness. (N.D. 1–8)

- Encourage normal life events. Maximize involvement of the child in school activities. Plan and support the child's attendance on field trips. Advocate and support the child's attendance in extracurricular activities. (Example: Work with family of cystic fibrosis child to pack pulmonary equipment for field trip and ensure that nurse attending field trip is trained regarding the use of the equipment.) (N.D. 2, 4, 5, 6, 7)
- Encourage adequate rest, nutrition, physical activity, and activities of daily living. (N.D. 1)
- Teach self-care on an individual basis to children with chronic conditions. Encourage child to assist in own care as age and capabilities permit. Refer to occupational therapist or physical therapist for equipment adaptation needs. (N.D. 8)
- Conduct classroom education related to hygiene and nutrition. By supporting a healthy school, nurses can assist children with chronic illnesses to develop their full potential. (Example: Good hand washing decreases the infection rate and keeps students with suppressed immune systems [leukemia] in school versus the hospital.) (N.D. 4, 5)
- Ensure safety. Provide for environmental safety needs. Clarify school policy on infection control and environmental hazards (Example: chemistry class and asthma triggers, or animal visitation and asthma triggers). (N.D. 4, 5)
- Help child understand chronic condition, therapies, and implications through health education. Reinforce information given by others. Clarify misconceptions. Provide accurate information. (N.D. 1–8)

### Interventions directed at the school nurse:
- Attend continuing nursing education programs to increase nursing knowledge base regarding chronic conditions and family care. (N.D. 1–8)
- Develop and practice counseling skills. Attend continuing education programs to increase counseling (not teaching) skills. (N.D. 1–8)

## Expected Student Outcomes

The student will:
- Experience minimal disturbance of normal growth and development as evidenced by minimal delays. (N.D. 1)
- Experience minimal disturbance of normal growth and development as evidenced by ability to interact in age-appropriate manner socially, physically, cognitively, to the degree allowed by the disability or illness. (N.D. 1–8)
- Exhibit minimal body image disturbance and will adapt to physical changes caused by illness or disability as evidenced by acceptance of change or loss and ability to adjust to changes. (N.D. 2, 7–8)
- (In conjunction with family) experience normal patterns of functioning as evidenced by maintaining family routines, and meeting family needs. The student and family will experience normal patterns of functioning as evidenced by expressing feelings or coping effectively and using support systems. (N.D. 3–5)
- Develop positive relationships with peers. (N.D. 4–7)
- Develop positive role performance as evidenced by positive comments or behaviors. (N.D. 5)
- Develop positive self-esteem or self-regard as evidenced by positive comments or behaviors. (N.D. 6)
- Display effective coping mechanisms as evidenced by open communication, use of supportive services and resources, acceptance or adaptation to illness. (N.D. 7)
- Succeed in school as evidenced by attendance, grades, and other school achievements. (N.D. 4–7)
- Develop healthy interdependence as evidenced by appropriate self-care. (N.D. 8)

# References

Allen, P. J., & Vessey, J. A. (2004). *Primary care of the child with a chronic condition* (4th ed). St. Louis, MO: Mosby.

Burke, S. O., Kauffmann, E., Harrison, M., & Wiskin, N. (1999). Assessment of stressors in families with a child who has a chronic condition. *American Journal of Maternal Child Nursing 24*(2), 98–106.

Clawson, J. A. (1996). A child with chronic illness and the process of family adaptation. *Journal of Pediatric Nursing 11*(1), 52–61.

Diamond, J. (1994). Family-centered care for children with chronic illness. *Journal of Pediatric Health Care 8, 196–197.*

Gregory, E.K. (2000). Empowering students on medication for asthma to be active participants in their care: an exploratory study. *Journal of School Nursing 16*(1), 20-27.

Jackson, P. L., & Vessey, J. A. (2000). *Primary are of the child with a chronic condition* (3rd ed). St. Louis, MO: Mosby.

James, S. R., Ashwill, J. W., & Droske, S. C. (2002). *Nursing Care of Children Principles and Practice* (2nd ed). Philadelphia: Saunders.

Kinne, S., Patrick, D. L., & Doyle, D. L. (2004). Prevalence of secondary conditions among people with disabilities. *American Journal of Public Health. 94*(3), 443–445.

Leifer, G., & Hartston, H. (2004). *Growth and Development Across the Lifespan: A Health Promotion Focus*. St. Louis, MO: Saunders.

Lowe, J., & Miller, W. (1998). Students with chronic health problems. *Journal of School Nursing, 14*(5). 4–16.

Lubkin, I. ., & Larsen, P. D. (2002). *Chronic Illness: Impact and Interventions*. (5th ed). Sudbury, MA: Jones and Bartlett.

Newacheck, P. W., McManus, M. A., & Fox, H. B. (1991). Prevalence and impact of chronic illness among children. *American Journal of Diseases of Children, 145,* 1367–1373.

NANDA International (2003). *Nursing diagnoses: Definitions & Classification 2003-2004*. Philadelphia: Author.

Olsen, S. F., Marshall, E. S., Mandleco, B. L., Allred, K. W., Dyches, T. T., & Sansom, N. (1999). Support, communication, and hardiness in families with children with disabilities. *Journal of Family Nursing 5*(3), 275–291.

Sherman, J., & Hendeles, L. (2000). Practical pharmacology for pediatric asthma. *Pediatric Annals 29* 768–773.

Berg, J., Tichachek, M., & Theodorakis, R. (2004). Evaluation of an educational program for adolescents with asthma. *Journal of School Nursing 20*(1), 29-35.

Woodgate, R. L. (1998). Adolescents' perspectives of chronic illness: "It's hard." *Journal of Pediatric Nursing 13*(4), 210–223.

## Bibliography

Arnold, M. J., & Silkworth, C. K. (Eds.). (1999). *The school nurse's source book of individualized healthcare plans, Vol II.* North Branch, MN: Sunrise River Press.

*Journal of School Nursing.* Official journal of the National Association of School Nurses; presents projects, research articles, and information relevant for practicing professional school nurses. Available from National Association of School Nurses, 810 East 10th Street, Lawrence, KS 66044.

National Association of School Nurses. (Revised 2002). *Case management of children with special health care needs* (Position Statement). Scarborough, ME: Author.

National Association of School Nurses. (2001). *Cedar Rapids Community School District vs. Garret F., Impact of on school nursing services* (Issues Brief). Scarborough, ME: Author.

National Association of School Nurses. (Revised 2002). *Specialized health care services, The school nurse and* (Position Statement). Scarborough, ME: Author.

Praeger, S., Zickler, C., & Mosca, N. W. (2002). *Care of students with special needs in schools: Application of professional school nursing practice standards* [Manual]. Scarborough, ME: National Association of School Nurses.

Schwab, N., & Gelfman, M. (2001). Legal issues in school health services. (Ed.). North Branch, MN: Sunrise River Press.

Wong, D. L., Hockenberry, M.J., Wilson, D., Winkelstein, M. L., & Kline, N. E. (2003). Behavioral health problems of adolescents. In *Nursing care of infants and children* (7th ed, pp. 884–895). St. Louis, MO: Mosby.

## Resources

Many community resources are available to help children and families succeed. The nurse, as a liaison between the school and the family, can assist the family by providing referrals to current resources.

Local resources include county health and human services agencies. Frequently, these agencies have compiled a listing of local community resources, and this list is available to school nurses simply by calling and inquiring. Community resources include respite care providers, crisis nurseries, domestic abuse shelters, food shelves, used clothing and household furnishing sites, toy-lending libraries, and other public assistance services.

Another resource may be the area's regional hospital. Frequently, regional hospitals (as opposed to local/rural hospitals) have staff that specialize in chronic illness and provide classes and support groups for various chronic illnesses, and families may be willing to drive to obtain that support (example: inflammatory bowel syndrome monthly support group).

Many chronic illnesses and disabilities have national and/or state organizations dedicated to supporting children and their families. A partial list of examples, along with mailing addresses and phone numbers, is included below. Another quick method for identifying resources is to use a search engine to check the Web. The Web page for these organizations will have the most current information, including workshops, support groups, and available print material. If you are unfamiliar with searching the Web, check with the community or school library for assistance. Many libraries and schools, even in rural areas, have access to the Web and search engines.

## Cancer

American Cancer Society
1599 Clifton Road, NE
Atlanta, GA 30329
1-800-ACS-2345
http://www.cancer.org

Corporate Angel Network
Westchester County Airport
1 Loop Road
West Plains, NY 10604
914-328-1313
http://www.corpangelnetwork.org

National Childhood Cancer Foundation
440 East Huntington Drive
PO Box 60012
Arcadia, CA 91066
1-800-458-NCCF
http://www.curesearch.org

## Diabetes

American Diabetes Association
1701 North Beauregard
Alexandria, VA 22311
1-800-DIABETES
http://www.diabetes.org
International Diabetes Center
3800 Park Nicollet Boulevard
Minneapolis, MN 55416
1-888-825-6315
http://www.parknicollet.com/diabetes/

## Gastrointestinal Disorders

American Celiac Society/Dietary Support Coalition
59 Crystal Avenue
West Orange, NJ 07052
973-325-8837

Celiac-Sprue Association USA
PO Box 31700
Omaha, NE 68131
402-558-0600
http://www.csaceliacs.org

Crohn's and Colitis Foundation of America
386 Park Avenue South
17th Floor
New York, NY 10016
1-800-932-2423
http://www.ccfa.org

## Mental Retardation

American Association of Mental Retardation
444 North Capitol Street, NW
Suite 846
Washington, DC 20001
1-800-424-3688
http://www.aamr.org

National Down Syndrome Society
666 Broadway
8th Floor
New York, NY 10012
1-800-221-4602
http://www.ndss.org

## Musculoskeletal Disorders

Arthritis Foundation
PO Box 7669
Atlanta, GA. 30357
1-800-282-7800
http://www.arthritis.org

Muscular Dystrophy Association of American, Inc.
3300 E Sunrise Drive
Tucson, AZ 86718
1-800-572-1717
http://www.mdausa.org

Osteogenesis Imperfecta Foundation, Inc
804 West Diamond Avenue
Suite 210
Gaithersburg, MD 20878
1-800-981-2663
http://www.oif.org

Neurologic Disorders
Epilepsy Foundation
4351 Garden City Drive
Landover, MD 20785
1-800-EFA-1000
http://www.epilepsyfoundation.org

Spina Bifida Association
4590 MacArthur Blvd, NW
Suite 250
Washington, DC 20007
1-800-621-3141
http://www.sbma.org

United Cerebral Palsy
1660 L Street, NW
Suite 700
Washington, DC 20036
1-800-872-5827
http://www.ucp.org

## Respiratory Disorders

American Lung Association
1740 Broadway
New York, NY 10019
1-800-LUNG-USA
http://www.lungusa.org

Asthma and Allergy Foundation of America
1233 20th Street, NW
Suite 402
Washington, DC 20036
1-800-7-ASTHMA
http://www.aafa.org

Terminal Illness
Children's Hospice International
901 North Pitt Street
Suite 230
Alexandria, VA 22314
1-800-242-4453
http://www.chionline.org

Make-A-Wish Foundation of America
3550 North Central Avenue
Suite 300
Phoenix, AZ 85012
1-800-722-WISH
http://www.wish.org

## Other Disorders

National Organization for Rare Disorders (NORD)
55 Kenosia Avenue
PO Box 1968
Danbury, CT 06813
203-744-0100
1-800-999-6673
http://www.rarediseases.org

*Chapter Fourteen*

# Psychosocial Aspects of School-Aged Children With Disabilities and Chronic Health Conditions

Terri J. Lundquist

## Introduction

Medical advancements in the past decade have made it possible for infants and children to survive life-threatening events and health conditions. Some of these children continue to have chronic health problems and disabilities related to these events. Therapeutic interventions are needed to support the child in the activities of daily living. As these children enter the school system, they require continued support to enable them to function in the school setting. School nurses have been called to the challenge of providing care and expertise to students with a variety of health problems. These health problems can last for several months or years. When these children enter or re-enter the school system, they are required to adjust to new routines and situations that can further challenge their ability to function successfully. Simple self-care skills such as toileting, feeding, and dressing may be major challenges. Whereas the physical limitations and problems are plain to see, these children also deal with emotional and psychological adjustments that may not be so obvious. Yet, their impact is enormous. These children will need psychosocial support to function productively. Feelings of low self-esteem, inadequacy, and depression often develop secondarily to the multiple struggles to adapt. A recent survey conducted in 1998 by Minnesota's Children with Special Health Needs Program showed that 13% of these students reported suicide attempts and 22% to 32% (depending on grade or gender) felt discouraged or hopeless. Children with disabilities are three times more likely to suffer psychological stressors that can lead to truancy, learning disabilities and impaired self-esteem (Parent Fact Sheet, 2003). Although chronic illness and disability are stressors, research has indicated that a child's psychosocial health is dependent upon his or her own and the family's functional status and family risk indicators such as low income, maternal depression, and single parenthood. (Witt, Riley, & Coiro, 2003). The school nurse is a community expert for such children. It is the school nurse's role to recognize actual and potential problems of students. Managing a child's chronic health condition requires a coordinated effort between school, home, and community resources. The school nurse can serve as a case manager and community liaison for students. This coordi-nation is reflected in the interdisciplinary school meetings and the development of individualized health care plans and emergency plans. These plans allow the student to attend school and have full access to their education equal to their peers. The school nurse coordinates and supports the interventions needed to allow for successful school experiences by keeping the lines of communication between family, school, and community providers open, providing adaptations and developing a dynamic nurse-student relationship to continuously meet the ever-changing needs of the student.

## Psychosocial Concerns

### Delayed Mastery of Basic Skills

All children go through stages of development as they grow. Students with a chronic disability or illness face challenges in meeting their developmental goals. There are many theorists who have explored the cognitive, emotional, and physical developmental stages of a person's life. One theorist, Erik Erikson, has divided the human life cycle into eight stages (**Table 1**). Each of these stages describes a tension between successful completion and failure of basic developmental tasks. These stages address the process of learning and skill development.

The second through fourth stages are particularly significant for school-aged children. The second stage, Autonomy versus Shame, examines the developmental tasks of toddlers. Toddlers are learning to walk, talk, and do things for themselves. When these tasks are successfully met, and the parent offers positive praise, the child experiences confidence in his ability. This gives the child the energy and focus to move on to the next developmental stage. If a parent is overprotective and attempts to do these tasks for the child, the child begins to doubt his or her ability and may develop shameful feelings regarding his or her behavior. For a child with chronic disabilities, there is greater difficulty in accomplishing these basic tasks. Parents of children with chronic disabilities can become overprotective out of fear and guilt. This overprotection can further complicate the struggle for independence. As these children move into the next stage of initiative versus guilt, the foundation for learning is laid. In this stage, the child has more control over his motor skills,

**Table 1. Erikson's Developmental Stages in School-Aged Children**

| Stage | Resolved | Unresolved |
|---|---|---|
| Autonomy vs. Shame and Doubt | Child feels confident in abilities | Child doubts self and develops feelings of shame |
| Initiative vs. Guilt | Child experiences an increase in personal power | Child develops feelings of guilt and inadequacy |
| Industry vs. Inferiority | Child develops skill mastery and independence | Child feels isolated and becomes dependent on others |
| Identity vs. Role Confusion | Child has feelings of self worth, develops core values and has a stable identity | Child experiences confusion and has an undeveloped and chaotic self-image |

enjoys personal power, and is exposed to more peer-based social interactions. If the child's disability interferes with his or her motor behavior, feelings of inferiority continue from the previous stage. There are complicated feelings of failure and guilt. If the parent continues to overprotect the child, the child begins to believe independence is wrong. It is this independence that propels a child into exploring new territories, and its absence hinders learning.

If all the stages have been successfully completed by the time the child enters school, the child then enters the latency stage, also known as Industry versus Inferiority. Developing new tasks and building upon previously learned skills continue the learning process for the child. However, when a child with disabilities enters the school having struggled through the previous stages with limited mastery, the chance for school success can be greatly diminished. School-aged children are attempting to master basic skills that are essential to successful social and physical development. These skills include reading social cues, dealing with conflict, and mastering fine and gross motor development. These everyday experiences are more difficult and challenging for children with disabilities. They may not be able to understand social cues and lack significant control over their body and, hence, become frustrated more easily. As they struggle to fit in, their peers are moving ahead at a quicker pace. The mastery of these skills affects peer relationships and the ability to recognize societal expectations.

When a child masters a skill, there is inclusion in the peer group. If a student fails to master that skill, there is likely to be isolation. These physical limitations are not just defined by the lack of skills. Susceptibility to infections and the higher risk for trauma and accidents result in increased absenteeism. Absenteeism secondary to the student's disability and functional impairments creates further separation from the peer group. The lack of relational support makes it difficult for the student to become aware of cues and signals that are the dynamics of positive

social interactions. Attempts to decipher social cues and codes are met with frustration, teasing, and alienation by peers. This lack of success in social relationships extends to the mastery of self-care skills and learning. These students view themselves as powerless to achieve and likely to fail. Broatch (2003) reports that disabled students feel they are "slow, lazy and dumb. Rather than developing a sense of pride in their accomplishments...[they] may end up in a quagmire of frustration and shame."

The social skills necessary to adapt to real-world activities are greatly diminished by repeated reminders of failed attempts. These students find it hard to navigate their way through social situations that can lead to further isolation. Friends are a source of support, role modeling, and socializing. They give feedback on acceptable and unacceptable behaviors. Children with disabilities also have difficulty understanding social cues despite interactions with their peer group. Without this feedback, disabled students continue with their self-blaming behavior and feelings of low self-esteem (Richfield, 2002). Learning becomes more difficult and frustrating with the student losing interest in school. Since successful employment depends upon skill mastery and the ability to have positive social interactions, these students' futures are at risk.

Adolescence addresses the conflict between identity and role confusion. It is in this stage of development that the child's previous stages are integrated to form the adult identity. Failure to achieve success in any previous stage can make this integration difficult. There are four components to this adolescent stage: foreclosure, moratorium, confusion, and achievement (Langley, 2000). Foreclosure occurs in the early stage of adolescence. The child has fixed ideas and opinions and does not consider alternatives. Moratorium is a crisis period. The adolescent starts to explore alternatives and develop doubts in previously held ideas. Confusion is not a crisis period, but the adolescent is still struggling with decisions regarding values and personal ideology. This struggle leads to chaotic, erratic, and unpredictable behavior by the adolescent who is trying to integrate different ideologies into a new identity. Finally, the adolescent reaches the stage of achievement. This is a stable integration of ideas and personal identity.

Adolescents with chronic disabilities may not have had the opportunity to fully integrate past stages and conflicts. This can increase the turmoil of adolescence and further delay the completion of this stage. An adolescent may become fixed at the foreclosure stage and believe that no alternatives exist for managing their health conditions. Or the adolescent can enter the moratorium and confusion stages without a sense of independence and competency. These feelings of insecurity can add to the tumult and confusion already present in this stage.

## Functional Limitations

It is no surprise that developmental delays impact the student's functioning at home, in school, and in the community. Functional limitation is defined as "a physical or mental impairment that substantially limits a major life activity, such as hearing, seeing, speaking, breathing, performing manual tasks, walking, caring for oneself or working" (Disability Support Services, 2004).

Hogan, in his research, divided functional status into four areas. They are mobility, self-care, communication, and learning ability. Communication and learning ability directly relate to school expectations and subsequent success. The lack of coherent and fluent communication hinders learning and the development of social relationships. Communication allows a child to express wants and needs. When communication is difficult, needs may not always be met. The child becomes more frustrated, angry, and defeated. This further complicates the student's self-esteem and feelings of inferiority. Lack of mobility can also add to feelings of inferiority. Self-care activities such as feeding, dressing, and washing become difficult, if not impossible. When these children need to rely on other people or adaptive equipment to manage activities of daily living, successful completion of Erikson's second stage is threatened. They remain dependent on their parents and caregivers at a time crucial to the development of self-esteem and feelings of empowerment. It is estimated that students with only one moderate to severe limitation accounted for more than 2 million students.

## Family Issues

Disability and chronic illness affect the family as well. Families endure economic upheaval, altered roles, and loss of perceived family health and stability. In a study by Witt et al., 2003, "found that parent-, child-, and family-related factors were more strongly associated with the children's adjustment [to their disability] than the disease or disability [itself]." Parents, from fear, worry or guilt, may develop a tendency to become overprotective or take over basic skills that the student needs to do.

Many insurance companies require a *spend-down* whereby families must pay out of pocket before coverage starts. State and federally funded programs, such as medical assistance, have increasingly strict income guidelines that limit the type of support services available. Often, one parent stays home to care for the child, giving up a family's second income. This can be due to the family's inability to find suitable day care, a parental desire to stay with the child, or the loss of respite care, requiring the parent to leave work and care for the child periodically.

Typically, it is the mother who stays home with the child, but fathers also take over that role if the mother's employment or insurance is a better choice. The child's disability can consume much time and energy of the caregiver, leaving little for the role of spouse, community volunteer, or parent to other children.

Parents and siblings need to re-define their expectations of health and its impact in day-to-day functioning. Parents may cite a child's disability as cause for another sibling to forfeit community sports, traveling teams, costly camps, and vacations. The entire family can become *disabled* by this chronic health problem. Sibling resentments may develop. Esdaile and Greenwood (2003) note that many studies have "reported that mothers of children with disabilities are particularly vulnerable to parenting stress, which may place them at …psychological risk." If the parents are highly stressed, their ability to cope with the demands of care may be diminished. This can lead to ineffective coping and disturbed family systems. This can further affect the child's ability to successfully reach developmental milestones.

## School Nurse's Role

The school nurse is in an ideal position to serve as case manager for the student. In the National Association of School Nurses' brief (2002) on the role of the school nurse, the roles of providing healthcare, leadership, and liaisons within the community are especially pertinent to the care of disabled children.

The role of providing direct care includes the functions of case management and development of the individualized health and emergency care plans. Case management begins when the nurse assumes a pivotal role in coordinating team members in the care of the student. Because school nurses typically do not work evenings, weekends, or vacations, the case manager works in tandem with community providers to ensure continuity of care. The lines of communication should always be kept open. The case manager is aware of community supports and refers the family to these when appropriate. Examples of these supports are support groups, durable medical equipment providers, camps, and advocacy organizations.

Individualized healthcare plans have two dimensions for those with chronic health concerns. The plan has the historical profile that does not vary through the years and a dynamic profile that changes with present-day circumstances. These can include a change in family roles, new developmental stages, or a change in the functional ability of the student. Though the disability may be chronic, its effects are anything but static. The nurse takes a leadership position when this information is shared with the school staff. The school nurse must be careful to respect the confidentiality of the client while focusing on the functional limitations and adaptations required by the student to have equal access to their education. Emergency plans that highlight specific concerns may be shared with parental permission, but the nurse must focus on standard procedures and safeguards and not the child's diagnosis.

Finally, the nurse serves as a liaison when attending special education meetings and networking with community contacts to ensure that the child's disability is not addressed in a vacuum. The nurse supports the family by serving as an advocate for them during the special education process, integrating the child's adaptive needs within the classroom milieu. The nurse collaborates with the healthcare providers, advocacy organizations, and social services to coordinate the child's care outside of the school experience.

## Summary

The school nurse role is multifaceted, especially with the coordination and delivery of care to students with disabilities. An effective approach recognizes the family, community, and student's resources. The school nurse works with these resources to minimize and eliminate potential psychological and functional disturbances. Collaboration is a key element in this role to make sure the channels of communication are kept open. The nurse models problem-solving skills to the child, family, and school staff, empowering them to proactively address needs as they arise. The goal for the school nurse is to maximize the student's ability and provide access to everyday school experiences.

## References

Broatch, L. (2003). Learning disabilities and psychological problems—An overview. Retrieved December 4, 2004 from Schwab Learning: A Parent's Guide to Helping Kids with Disabilities web site: http://www.SchwabLearning.org/articles.asp?r=746&f=search

Disability Support Services (2004). Retrieved February 18, 2005, from the University of North Dakota Disability Support Services Web site: http://www.und.edu/dept/dss/Accessing%20Services.htm

Esdaile, S.A., & Greenwood, K.M. (2003). A Comparison of mother's and father's experience of parenting stress and attributions for parent child interaction outcomes. *Occupational Therapy International, 2*, 115-126.

Hogan, D., Msall, M., Rogers, M., & Avery, R. (1997). Improved disability population estimates of functional limitation among American children aged 5-17. *Maternal and Child Health Journal, 1*, 203–216.

Hogan, D., Rogers, M., & Msall, M. (2000). Functional limitations and key indicators of well-being in children with disability. *Archives of Pediatric Adolescent Medicine, 154*, 1042–1048.

Langley, T. (2000). Erik Erikson's eight stages of psychosocial development. Retrieved August 10, 2004 from Henderson State University web site: http://www.hsu.edu

Minnesota Children with Special Health Needs. (2001, August) *Mental health disparities in children and youth with chronic illness and disabilities* (Issue brief No. 3). St. Paul, MN: Minnesota Department of Health.

National Association of School Nurses. (Revised 2002). *Position Statement: Case management of children with special health care needs.* Scarborough, ME: Author.

Parent fact sheet on chronic illness (2003). Retrieved February 18, 2005, from The Children's Hospital at Westmead web site: http://www.chw.edu.au/parents/factsheets/chronic_illness.htm

Richfield, S. (2002). Strategies to bolster self-esteem. Retrieved February 18, 2005 from childrensdisabilities.info/parenting/self-esteem.html

Witt, W., Riley, A., & Coiro, M. (2003). Childhood functional status, family stressors, and psychological adjustment among school-aged children with disabilities in the United States. *Archives of Pediatric Adolescent Medicine, 157*, 687–695.

# Bibliography

Adams, R., Gordon, C., & Spangler, A. (1999). Maternal stress in caring for children with feeding disabilities: Implications for health care providers. *Journal of the American Dietetic Association, 99,* 962–966.

Adelman, H., & Taylor, L. (1997-2000). *Nursing assessment of school age youth.* Promoting Mental Health in Schools in the Midst of School Reform. *Journal of School Health, 70,* 171-178.

Bergren, M. D. (2002). Child and adolescent mental health Web resources. The *Journal of School Nursing,* 18(4), 226–228.

DeSocio, J., Hootman, J. (2004). Children's mental health and school success. *The Journal of School Nursing,* 20(4), 189–196.

Lightfoot, J., Wright, S., & Sloper, P. (1998). Supporting pupils in mainstream school with an illness or disability: Young people's views. *Child: Care, Health and Development, 25,* 297–283.

Msall, M., Avery, R., Tremont, M., Lima, J., Rogers, M., & Hogan, D. (2003). Functional disability and school activity limitations in 41,300 school-age children: Relationship to medical impairments. *Pediatrics, 111,* 548–553.

Pain, H. (1999). Coping with a child with disabilities from the parent's perspective: The function of information. *Child: Care, Health and Development, 25,* 299–312.

Palermo, T., Childs, G., Burgess, E., Kaugars, A., Comer, D., & Kelleher, K. (2002). Functional limitations of school aged children seen in primary care. *Child: Care, Health and Development, 28,* 379–389.

Psychosocial Screening (Home Study Module No. 3). Scarborough, ME: National Association of School Nurses.

Weil, C., Wade, S., Bauman, L., Lynn, H., Mitchell, H., & Lavigne, J. (1999). The relationship between psychosocial factors and asthma morbidity in inner-city children with asthma. *Pediatrics, 104,* 1274–1280.

Wildman, B., Kinsman, A., & Smucker, W. (2000). Use of child reports of daily functioning to facilitate identification of psychosocial problems in children. *Archives of Family Medicine, 9,* 612–616.

Williams, P., Williams, A., Graff, C., Hanson, S., Stanton, A., Hafeman, C., et al. (2002). Interrelationships among variables affecting well siblings and mothers in families of children with a chronic illness or disability. *Journal of Behavioral Medicine, 25,* 411–424.

## Chapter Fifteen

# Medically Fragile and Complex Chronically Ill Children in the School Setting

Brenda Kay Lenz

## Introduction

Technological advances in healthcare in the past 50 years have significantly changed the experience of chronic illness in childhood. Children with chronic illnesses are living longer, and an increasing number of children are living with illnesses previously considered to be fatal (James, Ashwill, & Droske, 2002). Chronic illness may include children born with very low-birth-weight or prenatal development disorders, children who experienced traumatic brain injury, or children diagnosed with terminal disease such as cancer and muscular dystrophy. Severity varies among chronic illnesses and includes conditions that require adaptation or special assistance in order for the child to survive and/or function.

In Massachusetts, prevalence rates for children with technology dependence who required daily nursing assistance has been reported as 1 in every 1,000 children from 3 months to 18 years of age, according to Palfrey et al. (1994). These children were reported to have one or more of the following: tracheostomy, respirator, oxygen, suctioning, gastrostomy, jejunal or nasogastric feedings, ostomies, urethral catheterization, ureteral diversion, intravenous access, or dialysis. Furthermore, Palfrey et al. estimated that 101,800 children are assisted by medical technology nationwide.

The goal for any child with a chronic illness is to achieve and maintain the highest level of health and function possible, emotionally, psychosocially, and physically. Nationally, these beliefs have been translated into federal education/health policy. In 1975, the Education for All Handicapped Children Act (EHA) PL94-142 guaranteed access to education in the least restrictive environment for each child with a disability or chronic condition (Schwab & Gelfman, 2001). In 1986, PL 99-457 expanded PL 94-142 to include identification of, and provision of services to, children with disabilities from birth to age 5. The EHA was renamed the Individuals with Disabilities Education Act in 1990 (PL 101-476) and is currently referred to as IDEA. IDEA requires that a free appropriate public education be offered to all children regardless of the nature or severity of their disabilities.

These federal legislative mandates have shaped school health services for children. Since school health services are defined as related services under IDEA, school districts may not deny such services solely based on routine staffing of the school health office. The school district is required to provide additional nursing services and staffing if the individualized education plan (IEP) determines that these services are what the student requires in order to benefit from the IEP or in order for the student to be placed in the least restrictive environment.

School nurses play a pivotal role in the provision of school health services for children with chronic illness. Examples include a child with spina bifida who requires intermittent catheterization every few hours, a child with a chronic and frequent seizure disorder requiring rectal valium, and a child with severe cerebral palsy who requires continuous humidified oxygen and periodic sterile tracheostomy suctioning.

Through the individualized health plan (IHP), the school nurse plans and implements nursing care for these children. Nursing goals include maintaining the highest level of health and function possible, promoting educational goals for the child, and supporting the family by fostering a good relationship and appropriate communication.

### Pathophysiology

A chronic illness or condition is one that is usually long-term and ongoing. Chronic illnesses are defined as interfering with daily functioning for more than 3 months in a year and may cause hospitalizations for more than 1 month in a year. Complex chronic illnesses requiring adaptation or special assistance in order for the child to function in activities of daily living can have a tremendous impact on the child, family, school, and society. Some chronically ill children are terminally ill and have diagnoses such as cancer or muscular dystrophy. Not all children who are chronically ill require special education services.

#### Acquired Chronic Conditions

Common acquired chronic conditions requiring adaptation or special assistance include cancers such as brain tumors and renal cancers; blood cancers such as leukemia; chronic renal failure; traumatic brain injuries; and severe asthma.

## Perinatal and Birth Factors

These can include very low-birth-weight babies or infants born with respiratory alterations, including bronchopulmonary dysplasia and respiratory distress syndrome, cerebral palsy, congenital heart disease, hydrocephalus, and neural tube defects.

## Hereditary-genetic Conditions

Hereditary-genetic conditions include the following examples: cri du chat syndrome; trisomy 18 or Down syndrome; cystic fibrosis; muscular dystrophy; inborn errors of metabolism such as phenylketonuria; sickle cell anemia; hemophilia; and inherited immunodeficiencies.

## Injuries and Infections

Injuries include unintentional injuries, such as motor vehicle crashes, near drowning, head trauma, spinal cord injuries, cardiopulmonary arrest, and burns. Infections include congenital viral infections, osteomyelitis, meningitis, viral encephalitis, and AIDS.

## Management

Chronically ill children receive care based on their particular condition and required adaptation or special assistance that is needed to manage their care at school.

Interventions may include:

- Nutritional management: oral stimulation and feedings, tube feedings, nutritional supplements
- Activity and rest management: oxygen, nebulizers and aerosol therapy, chest percussion, tracheostomy care, suctioning, respiratory and cardiac monitors, BiPAP or CPAP machines, oxygen saturation (Sao2) monitoring, range of motion, frequent repositioning, providing periods of rest and play, and positioning to avoid skin breakdown and promote physical comfort
- Elimination management: diapering, maintaining intake and output records, catheterization, ostomy and colostomy care, administration of laxative and/or fiber
- Cognitive management: educational needs, stimulation, seizure monitoring, seizure medications
- Psychosocial management (includes student's role, coping, self-perception, self-concept): facilitating coping efforts, assisting with the development and maintenance of peer relationships, maintaining social integration, attributing positive meaning to experience, balancing illness with other needs, supporting the family and caregiver roles.

# Indivdidualized Healthcare Plan

## Assessment

### History

- What are the diagnoses (may be multiple), and when they were made?
- What is the history related to the diagnoses? Or etiology?
- What is the prognosis?
- Which bodily systems are involved in the diagnoses? What are the degree and pattern of physical disabilities related to diagnosis? Has there been any change in the disabilities? What was the amount of change, and why was there a change?
- Have there been recent hospitalizations and/or surgery? When? What? How does this affect current care?
- Are there existing growth and developmental delays? What are they?
- What healthcare providers are involved in management, including waivered services, case management, home care, and nursing?
- What technologies, equipment, and medication have been needed to manage health needs in the past?
- What coping strategies and support systems have been used in the past?
- What is the family's role in caregiving and management of the child's needs at home? What are the family's goals for the child?

### Current Status and Management

- Current medical management plan: technologies, equipment, response in an emergency
- Current medications and side effects
- Assessment of bodily systems, including:
  1. Gross and fine motor development, muscle tone, reflexes, mobility needs
  2. Self-care and abilities
  3. Nutrition, including feeding method, additional supplements, additional hydration needs
  4. Respiratory/cardiac
  5. Elimination: toileting, catheterization, or diapering needs
  6. Neurologic/seizures

7. Activity tolerance and rest needs
8. Skin and skin breakdown concerns
9. Communication
10. Sensory: vision, hearing, taste, touch
11. Mental functioning
- How is care provided in the home—family, nurse, personal care attendant, or other? Is a home care agency involved? Are there waivered services? Who provides case management?
- How does the family pay for this care? Will the school be able to bill the insurance carrier for services rendered while at school?
- What equipment is necessary to care for the student? Who will provide the equipment at school? How will the equipment get to school? Can equipment be shared, or does the school need separate equipment?
- What are the transportation needs of the student to/from school? Will the student be safe on the bus alone, or is staff needed to ride along with the student?
- What are the lifting needs: weight of student, does student participate in transfers, number of adults needed to transfer student, equipment needs for transfer to prevent lifting injuries?

*Self-care*
- Student's understanding of medical/health management
- Student's ability to participate in medical/health management and what, if any, can be managed on student's own
- Family or healthcare provider's understanding of needs
- Activities tolerated (dependent on treatments and condition)
- Mobility needs (independent and dependent functioning)
- Nutrition needs
- Toileting needs
- Skin care needs

*Psychosocial Status*
- Age and developmental level
- Student's perception and feelings of condition(s) and technologies
- Student's perception of what friends, students, and family members think and feel about him (her) and his (her) condition
- Student's support systems: family, friends, home care, respite care, other
- Outside activities: school-related, sports, church, community
- Mental health concerns
- Family and caregiver concerns

*Academic Issues*
- Academic or cumulative school records, patterns of academic performance
- Teacher's perception of student's performance and classroom needs
- Comparison of student's performance to peer norms
- School attendance pattern
- Transportation needs: to and from school, field trips
- Need for special education, transportation, classroom adaptations, occupational or physical therapy, vocational guidance
- Amount and type of school health services needed to support the student during school day
- Amount and type of any additional educational support needed during day
- Equipment necessary to care for the child in the school setting. Who will provide the equipment, and how will it get to school? Will a durable supply company need to be contacted and the school billed?
- School environment: privacy and space for needed healthcare activities, storage area for supplies
- Educational needs of teachers and school staff related to student health needs

## Nursing Considerations

Nursing considerations are based on the National Association of School Nurses (NASN) Position Statement "Case Management of Children With Special Health Care Needs" (2002).

Case management is inherent to the role of the school nurse and involves nursing interventions designed to ensure the health and educational success of the child at school. The nurse has the knowledge, experiences, and authority to be the case manager for chronically ill children (NASN, 2002).

A case management team is essential for ensuring care. The school nurse must assume a leadership position as case manager, but team members include school administration, teachers, other school services members as described in the IEP, and the family.

### Determination of the Level of Staffing

On the basis of the student's IEP and IHP, a determination must be made as to the level of nursing care the student will need. Questions to address include:

1. Can the school nurse, in addition to her or his other obligations, provide the necessary nursing care at the frequency and amount the student requires?
2. If the school nurse cannot provide the care, to whom will the school nurse delegate? A paraprofessional or nurse's aide? Or are skilled nursing services from an LPN or an RN required?

Delegation of nursing care by the school nurse (RN) to either an LPN or an assistant typically falls under the Nurse Practice Act and the nurse licensing board in the state in which the school nurse practices. School nurses are encouraged to contact the Board of Nursing in their state if they have questions regarding delegation and supervision of nursing care.

Delegation of nursing care requires training the person delegated to, and periodic follow-up supervision of the delegated cares. Documentation of the training and supervision is recommended for liability reasons.

### Reimbursement of Costs

If hiring additional nursing staff to provide care for the student, the school district will need to determine if the student's health insurance or Medical Assistance can be billed for reimbursement of costs. In some states, school districts are able to, with parents' written permission, bill Medical Assistance for nursing care provided during school. Typically, only "skilled nursing care" performed by an RN is billable. Skilled nursing care is defined as care that only an RN is able to perform. Examples include sterile suctioning, sterile dressing changes, and nasogastric tube insertion. Examples not included are administration of oral medications, nebulizer treatments, and pummeling.

### Hiring Options

There are three options for hiring:

1. The school could hire and employ a licensed nurse (RN or LPN) to work directly with the student.
2. The school could contract with a home care agency to provide needed services, including direct nursing care to the student and case management.
3. The school could contract with the home care agency to provide a nurse for direct cares, but have the school nurse provide case management for the student and supervision of the home care nurse. This option would be less expensive than option 2.

The following points should be considered when deciding who to hire:

- If the student is frequently absent, what will the school-employed nurse do during the time the student is not in school? Will the district find the nurse alternative assignments, and will the nurse agree to these assignments? It may be impossible to find a nurse who is willing to go without pay for extended periods of time while the child is absent or hospitalized.
- School districts frequently have two pay scales, one for professionals such as teachers, and another for paraprofessionals or support staff. On what pay scale will the licensed nurse be paid? Will the district be able to find a nurse to work at a pay level given to support staff?
- If a school-employed nurse is hired and he or she is sick, who will cover the student's care during the absence?
- If a school-employed nurse cannot be hired for an extended period, who will cover the cares during this period? Or if the school-employed nurse resigns his or her position, what will the district do until another nurse is hired?
- Will the nurse provide educational services in addition to the nursing care as directed by the IEP and the licensed teacher? The nurse's contract and job description should reflect all duties assigned to the position.

### Substitutes and School Nurse Availability

- The school nurse will need to train and supervise staff and any substitutes caring for the student. Training and supervision should be documented in the student's chart. Arrangements will need to be made for staff absents.
- Unless the school district contracted with a home health agency to provide nursing care and case management, the school nurse is legally responsible for any nursing care provided to the student as described by the Nurse

Practice Act and the licensing board for each state. In practice, this means that staff should have access to the school nurse at all times. The school nurse may need to carry a pager or cell phone.

*Working With the Physician*

- Physician orders for any medications, medical treatments, and healthcare procedures to be done at school need to be obtained. This may include physical or occupational therapy, chest percussion, oxygen levels, amount and timing of feedings, medications, when and what type of suctioning, and others.
- If the school is able to bill the insurance carrier or Medical Assistance, the physician will need to sign a Report of Professional Worker (RPW) every 2 months to continue care. The school nurse, as the case manager, writes the RPW and procures the required signature. See the discussion that follows.

## Payment of Nursing Services

- Arrange for payment of the nursing care. Frequently, skilled nursing services can be billed to Medical Assistance or another insurance carrier. See individual state regulations, Supreme Court rulings, and healthcare policy about billing options and requirements.
- Insurance providers require detailed records of care completed and periodic reports (usually bimonthly) to the physician for his or her signature. These reports are sometimes referred to as the Report of Professional Worker. Care delegated to a paraprofessional cannot be billed, but the licensed nurse's time to train and supervise the paraprofessional can be.

## Preparing the School Site

- Include the family in preparations. Collaboration between the parents, healthcare providers, and school personnel is a crucial linkage that guides the school entry or reentry process. The family is familiar with the student's needs, physician treatment plan, and home nursing services (Kliebenstein & Broome, 2000).
- Arrange for a secure place to store any needed equipment and medication. This should be close to allow for easy access, but out of the reach of other students.
- Make arrangements for any needed equipment. This may include oxygen, humidifiers, nebulizers, and other equipment. Options: parents provide equipment, school bills provider for additional equipment and orders through a durable service goods company, school provides equipment and equipment remains at school.
- Plan on the unexpected. The student's condition may deteriorate, and he or she may need more nursing care. What if the oxygen doesn't get delivered or the humidifier quits working?
- Develop an emergency plan, and train those involved in working with the student. The emergency plan should include fire drills and evacuation methods.
- Provide a private place for healthcare procedures that is away from the rest of the students, especially if the student receives rectal medications, diapering, catheterizations, or experiences periods of dyspnea, etc.
- Provide education to teachers, administrators, bus drivers, and other school staff as necessary.
- Provide education to the classroom and other children as necessary.

## DNR/DNI Orders: A Special Concern

Many people derive their concept of cardiopulmonary resuscitation (CPR) from what they see in the media. In general, people often overestimate the effectiveness of CPR and rarely appreciate that CPR is a harsh and traumatic procedure and that survival rates for severely chronically ill patients are extremely low (Burkhardt & Nathaniel, 2002).

The general practice in nursing care facilities such as nursing homes and hospitals regarding CPR is that it must be initiated unless it would be clearly futile to do so, or the practitioner has specific instructions not to do so. The legal definition of do not resuscitate (DNR) or do not intubate (DNI) is not to initiate CPR in the event of pulmonary or cardiac arrest. DNR/DNI orders should be documented and signed by a physician (Burkhardt & Nathaniel, 2002).

DNR/DNI orders for children are rare and typically reserved for children in which death is inevitable, such as a terminal condition. DNR/DNI decisions require open communication among the patient, the family, and the physician. This can be a traumatic decision for families and always indicates the seriousness of the child's condition and the child's prognosis and his or her future quality of life.

Considering whether to initiate DNR/DNI orders with a student requires attention to professional, ethical, legal, and institutional considerations. Ethical principles utilized to justify decisions regarding resuscitation include autonomy, self-determination, nonmalfeasance, and respect for persons (Burkhardt & Nathaniel, 2002). The following points are important.

- Before a school or district establishes a policy on DNR orders, or responds to any specific DNR orders, it is imperative that it closely review state statutes to determine how the state interprets constitutional rights and protections (Schwab & Gelfman, 2001; NASN, 2000).

- Districts usually have implemented a Do Not Honor DNR/DNI Policy for several reasons. Staff and the school board may be concerned about the trauma associated with allowing a student in their care to die during a school day. Also, only the school nurse has the medical knowledge to assess the student's health status and make a determination to not intervene as ordered by the physician. When the nurse is out of the building, this will fall to the educational staff, who are not able to access or provide medical treatment as ordered by a physician. They can, however, administer CPR.

- When a child with a DNR/DNI order enters the school, the nurse should review the district's DNR/DNI policy. The school nurse plays a key role in the district's DNR/DNI policy as well as in working with the family and meeting the family's needs and the needs of the student.

## Options concerning DNR/DNI

**Option 1:** The district does not honor DNR/DNI orders. If a life-threatening emergency happens, school staff, including the school nurse, should provide CPR until the paramedics arrive. The paramedics may honor the DNR/DNI order if the family has made these arrangements beforehand.

### Points to think about:

The school nurse may be vulnerable to legal action in this situation because he or she has not followed a direct physician order, especially if the child is rescued and his or her condition has deteriorated severely. The school nurse should consult legal counsel.

The school nurse may want to encourage the family to file a copy of the DNR/DNI order with the paramedics prior to an emergency. The school nurse might also want to provide a copy of the order to the paramedics when they arrive.

**Option 2:** The district honors DNR/DNI orders. If a life-threatening emergency happens, school staff would not provide CPR. Paramedics would be called to transport the child to the hospital. Staff would make the student comfortable until paramedics arrive, but would not administer CPR.

### Points to think about:

How will the school nurse delegate care in this situation? Only a registered nurse is legally able to make assessments and a decision about medical treatment or nontreatment. If the school nurse is unavailable, who will assess the health status of the child and make the decision not to provide CPR? If the school nurse is already delegating care for the child to a registered nurse, this point is mute. How will the school nurse delegate this if the nurse is an LPN? Or a paraprofessional?

**Option 3:** The district doesn't honor DNR orders but has made an exception in the case of this child. The district, after hearing from the physician and family, decides that providing CPR to this child would severely injure the child and cause substantial harm and so have allowed the IHP to include no CPR.

### Points to think about:

These would be the same as noted in Option 2 above.

# References

Burkhardt, M., & Nathaniel, A. (2002). *Ethics and issues in contemporary nursing* (2nd ed.). Albany, NY: Delmar.

James, S.R., Ashwill, J.W., & Droske, S.C. (2002). *Nursing care of children: Principles and practice* (2nd ed.). Philadelphia: Saunders.

Kliebenstein, M., & Broome, M. (2000). School re-entry for the child with chronic illness: Parent and school personnel perceptions. *Pediatric Nursing 26*(6), 579–584.

National Association of School Nurses (2000). Position statement on do not resuscitate. Scarborough, ME: Author.

National Association of School Nurses (2002). Position statement on case management of children with special health care needs. Scarborough, ME: Author.

Palfrey J. S. , Haynie M., Porter S., et al. (1994). Prevalence of medical technology assistance among children in Massachusetts in 1987 and 1990. *Public Health Reports 109*(?), 226–233

Schwab, N. C., & Gelfman, M. H. B. (Eds.). (2001). Legal issues in school health services: *A resource for school administrators, school attorneys, and school nurses.* North Branch, MN: Sunrise River Press.

# Resources

Parents and children with a complex chronic illness have significant needs. This can include financial needs, housing and transportation assistance, medical care and supplies, respite care, health education and health promotion for the child and for family members, and emotional support.

The nurse is a liaison for the family and the school. In this capacity, the nurse can help support the family. Assisting the family may include referrals to various resources such as general and disease-specific support organizations (for example, the American Cancer Society, Make-A-Wish Foundation, National Down Syndrome Society, Muscular Dystrophy Association of America, Epilepsy Foundation, United Cerebral Palsy, and Children's Hospice International). Many of these support organizations sponsor Web sites that can be found by using an Internet search engine.

Local resources include county health and human service agencies, local chapters of national support organizations, community-based hospitals and support programs, waivered service providers, respite care providers, and community volunteers.

## Chapter Sixteen

# Immigrant and Refugee Students: Legal, Health, and Cultural Considerations

### Ann Marie Hoxie

## Introduction

When assessing immigrant and refugee students in order to develop individualized healthcare plans (IHPs), the school nurse takes into consideration cultural issues as well as legal and health issues in order to provide quality, comprehensive, and culturally competent care.

Schools across the United States are changing due to the growth of immigrant and refugee populations as a result of worldwide demographic shifts. As the population grows more diverse, schools face new opportunities and new demands to participate in the promotion of healthy immigrant communities (DeSantis, 1997). School nurses are challenged to provide effective cross-cultural interactions that will benefit students and their families.

The United States accepts approximately 75,000 refugees each year from diverse regions of the world (Center for Applied Linguistics, 1996). The number of refugees admitted each year is established by the President. Over the past two decades more than 2 million refugees have resettled in the United States, predominantly from Southeast Asia as a result of the Vietnam War. Currently refugees are being resettled in the United States from countries in the former Soviet Union, the former Yugoslavia (Bosnia-Herzegovina), Somalia, Iraq, Ethiopia, Sudan, Afghanistan, Cuba, and Haiti. At times, a large group of refugees may settle in one community, presenting particular challenges to educational, health, and social services (Ackerman, 1997). In addition, secondary migration may contribute to the growth of a specific community within a certain geographical area.

According to the 2002 Yearbook of Immigration Statistics, the number of immigrants admitted to the United States that year for lawful permanent residence was 1,063,732. This number includes 384,427 individuals who obtained immigrant visas through the U.S. Department of State and became lawful permanent residents. The remaining were legal immigrants (including former undocumented immigrants, refugees, and asylees) who had their status adjusted following an average of 3 to 4 years of living in the United States.

Immigration and migration are fueled by economic and political forces that make leaving home and country either a necessity or more desirable than staying. People from all over the world still choose to come to the United States, just as they always have. Bringing energy and enthusiasm, they come to join family members, to find a better life, to escape persecution, and to find employment. Chaney and Hernandez (1998) report one of every five people under age 18 in the United States is an immigrant or has parents who are immigrants. Nearly 1 million new arrivals enter this country each year as refugees, immigrants, and foreign-born adopted children and as undocumented immigrants.

For school health staff seeking to address the needs of foreign-born students, it is essential to remember that race, ethnicity, and citizenship status are important variables to consider when assessing student health, educational needs, and adaptation. It is helpful to understand the different categories under which people qualify as immigrants and refugees, potential health conditions, and the medical examinations, which are either required or voluntary.

## Legal Status

Legal status can add to the understanding of the student's background and present health status and may determine what services are available to the student and family. The manner in which a person enters this country determines his or her status. The U.S. Citizenship and Immigration Services (USCIS), formerly known as The U.S. Department of Immigration and Naturalization Service (INS), provides the following definitions:

**Alien** — A person who is not a citizen or national of the United States.

**Asylee** — A foreign-born resident who is not a U.S. citizen and who cannot return to his or her country of origin or last residence because of persecution or the well-founded fear of persecution because of race, religion, nationality, membership in a particular social group, or political opinion, as determined by the USCIS. An asylee receives this status after entering the United States.

**Parolee** — An alien who has been given permission to enter the United States under emergency conditions or when that alien's entry is considered to be in the public interest.

**Refugee** — A foreign-born resident who is not a U.S. citizen and who cannot return to his or her country of origin or last residence because of persecution or the well-founded fear of persecution because of race, religion, nationality, membership in a particular social group, or political opinion, as determined by the USCIS. A refugee receives this status prior to entering the United States.

**Immigrant** — An individual who chooses to make a new home in this country and has a passport from his or her home country and a visa issued by the United States. Immigrants may petition the government to become permanent residents.

**Nondocumented immigrant** — An individual who enters or lives in the United States without official authorization, by entering without inspection, overstaying his or her visa, or violating the terms of his or her visa.

Note: refugees differ from immigrants due to a fear of persecution because of religious or political beliefs or ethnicity. Refugees enter the United States under the Refugee Act and are therefore not subject to the immigration quotas that dictate the entrance of immigrants.

Since immigrants chose to come to the United States, they have had time to prepare emotionally and to thoughtfully plan their new lives. Often they have waited for a lengthy period of time to receive approval for immigration. Most often they have family to provide support and assistance during their resettlement. Immigration law requires that they be able to support themselves. On the other hand, refugees generally do not have marketable job skills, rarely speak English, and may have experienced trauma, disruptions, and deprivations that result in physical and emotional problems. In addition, circumstances have given them no choice but to resettle (Pickwell, 1996).

### Medicolegal Issues

The health status of individuals will be strongly influenced by their background. Many refugees have had poor quality healthcare in their country of origin and in refugee camps. Crowded conditions, poor sanitation, and traumatic experiences all affect current health. Children will have had little or no preventive healthcare or dental care. Immigrants may have had better access to healthcare in their home country but may be without healthcare coverage in the United States.

Undocumented immigrants may be reluctant to seek healthcare due to concerns about their legal status and lack of healthcare coverage. Children of undocumented immigrants often do not have access to preventive care, including prenatal care, dental care, health supervision, or immunizations. According to the American Academy of Pediatrics (1997), family members often have different immigration statuses, which further complicates access to care, because the entire family may be fearful of investigation and therefore delay seeking care.

Eligibility for medical services is determined by legal status and varies from state to state. The Welfare Reform Act of 1996 directs states to determine eligibility for Medicaid, Temporary Assistance to Needy Families

(TANF), the Supplemental Food Program for Women, Infants, and Children (WIC), and Medicaid for pregnant women and children.

In addition, any noncitizen may be subject to deportation as a result of being accused of a serious crime. This can lead to fear and misunderstanding among refugees and immigrants. Families may not seek help for family or emotional issues, fearing accusations of child abuse or concern for other legal repercussions.

## Immigrant and Refugee Medical Examinations

Refugees and/or immigrants may have completed three different medical examinations (Refugee Health Coordinator Network, 1994). The examinations differ significantly in scope and purpose. Criteria for these examinations are found in the Immigration and Nationality Act and amended by the Immigration Act of 1990.

### Overseas Visa Medical Examination

Both refugees and immigrants are required to pass this examination within the year prior to arrival in the United States. The purpose of this examination is to identify medical conditions that would by law prohibit the individual from entering the United States. The examination is not meant to provide healthcare to the person, but rather is structured as an exclusionary process in order to protect the U.S. population and to exclude individuals with conditions that would present a financial burden to the United States. *This examination is mandatory for all immigrants and refugees.* The State Department arranges for refugee examinations, but all other immigrants pay for their own examination. The Overseas Visa Medical Examination is performed under the oversight of the U.S. Centers for Disease Control and Prevention, Center for Prevention Services, Division of Quarantine. The International Organization for Migration conducts the overseas examinations in Southeast Asia and the former Soviet Union under a contract with the U.S. State Department. In other countries, "panel physicians" appointed by U.S. embassies and consulates perform the examination. The quality of the examination varies according to site, the panel physician, and the length of time the overseas examination process has been in place in a given location. The visa medical examination can be completed up to a year prior to departure; therefore, the possibility exists that a person may develop a health condition after the examination but before entrance into the United States. Exclusionary conditions are as follows:

- Communicable diseases of public health significance: infectious tuberculosis, HIV infection, Hansen's disease (leprosy), certain sexually transmitted diseases
- Current or past physical or mental disorder with associated harmful behavior
- Substance abuse or dependence

• Other physical or emotional disorders

Refugees and immigrants pass through a U.S. Public Health Service Quarantine Station at the port of entry into the United States. Individuals are visually inspected for observable conditions and may be denied entrance at that time.

## 2. Domestic Refugee Health Assessment

State refugee health programs manage the Domestic Health Assessment program, and as a result, variations exist in the design and implementation of the services. Questions may be directed to the state refugee health coordinator. This examination is focused on eliminating health-related barriers to successful refugee resettlement. *Immigrants do not participate in this process, and, although highly encouraged, refugees are not required to undergo this examination.* The examination is meant to provide protection for the U.S. population by identifying and treating infectious diseases. This assessment also focuses on the individual's health and, in addition to the comprehensive examination, is meant to assist the individual in securing necessary healthcare and services. Refugees are eligible for Medicaid coverage during their first months of residency in the United States, and Medicaid covers the cost of this examination. The components of this examination generally include evaluation of:

• Immunization status
• Tuberculosis infection and disease
• Hepatitis B infection
• Intestinal parasite infections
• Sexually transmitted disease
• Other health problems, including pregnancy testing, dental abnormalities, vision, and hearing screening
• Referral and follow-up of identified conditions
• Linkage with primary healthcare resources

Refugees are assisted by resettlement agencies, often referred to as sponsors, which are an important source of information and assistance during the refugee's first months in the United States. An agency representative meets the family at the airport, arranges for housing, and prepares a resettlement plan that includes initial contact with governmental services and employment agencies. Resettlement agencies may be religious-based organizations, private organizations, state agencies, or ethnic organizations. Resettlement workers aided by relatives, friends, and volunteers help refugees become established (Center for Applied Linguistics, 1996). Immigrants have no such formalized system of support but rely on family, friends, and ethnic organizations to provide assistance.

## 3. Adjustment of Status Medical Examination

The purpose of this examination is to determine if health conditions exist that require care and intervention prior to the individual being granted legal permanent resident status. *The examination is required for individuals applying for permanent resident status.* Applicants pay for this examination themselves; it is not covered by health insurance. The components of this examination include:

• Physical examination
• Immunizations
• Evaluation of tuberculosis disease and infection
• Serology for syphilis
• Serology for HIV antibody

### Immunizations

Immunization status is a priority for new students entering a school. The American Academy of Pediatrics in the *1997 Red Book: Report of the Committee on Infectious Diseases* outlines clinical guidelines for immunizations. Foreign-born students are at risk for vaccine-preventable diseases because of exposure to disease and the immunization practices unique to their native countries. Some immigrant families do not have immunization records with them and will not be able to retrieve them from the home country. Often vaccine records are incomplete when applied to state school immunization laws. Records that document immunizations, which meet the recommended vaccine schedule of state school immunization laws, are acceptable. Some students may believe they are current because of immunizations (such as yellow fever or cholera) received just prior to departure from the country of origin and may not be familiar with the immunizations required for school in the United States. Some countries give measles vaccine but not the combined MMR (measles, mumps, rubella) required in U.S. schools. Handwritten records, foreign language records, and records that report dates in an unfamiliar manner (i.e., day/month/year) can further complicate interpretation of immunization records. Required vaccines as indicated for age should be administered prior to school entrance.

### Tuberculosis

Tuberculosis (TB) is the most important public health problem of refugees, particularly those from Southeast Asia and other developing countries, such as many African nations, where TB is endemic. Refugees and immigrants have accounted for a substantial and increasing proportion of new cases of TB within the United States in the past decade. The Centers for Disease Control and Prevention (1990) report that during the first 5 years of resettlement, a significant risk exists for development of TB disease. Persons with clinically active TB must begin treatment in the country of origin but may resettle once they are no longer contagious. Tuberculosis treatment must continue in the United States. Screening for TB and appropriate preventive therapy are an important priority in order to protect the U.S population, particularly during the first 5 years of residence in the United States. Therefore, tuberculin skin testing is recommended for all refugees regardless of previous BCG (bacille Calmette-Guérin) vaccinations (American Academy of Pediatrics, 1997). School nurses should collect and record the results of tuberculin skin testing, assist students in obtaining follow-up care, and monitor the results. It is also important to recognize that significant stigma is attached to tuberculosis infection and disease among refugee and immigrant populations.

## Other Health Concerns

Hepatitis B is prevalent in many areas of the world, which results in relatively high rates among refugee populations. Individuals should be tested to detect carriers, and those who are nonimmune should be immunized. Malnutrition and iron deficiency anemia are common. Many refugees have dental caries. Ackerman (1997) reports that intestinal parasites are endemic in tropical areas and occur in up to 40% of refugees. Intestinal parasites can result in malnutrition, anemia, chronic diarrhea, and growth retardation or failure to thrive. Other concerns include sexually transmitted diseases, malaria, and leprosy. Although refugee and immigrant children may have been exposed to infectious diseases, most will be free of contagious conditions (American Academy of Pediatrics, 1997).

Many refugees and some immigrants have experienced significant emotional trauma and torture and/or have witnessed extreme violence. As a result, posttraumatic stress disorder, anxiety, withdrawal, somatic complaints, and depression can be common among individuals of all ages. These conditions occur at higher rates among refugee populations, although significant variations are noted among groups (Ackerman, 1997; American Academy of Pediatrics, 1997; Gavagan and Brodyaga, 1998). Guarnaccia and Lopez (1998) suggest that the family can buffer stresses that affect children and can be a protective factor against the development of emotional disorders.

Posttraumatic stress disorder is characterized by persistent reexperience of the event through intrusive recollections, dreams, and reliving the experience. The person has persistent avoidance of thoughts associated with the event, avoids anything that triggers memories, feels detached from others, and has diminished interest in activities. Posttraumatic stress disorder can cause sleep disruptions, irritability and hypervigilance, concentration difficulties, exaggerated startle responses, and physiologic reactivity (American Psychiatric Association, 1994; James, 1997). Children who suffer from posttraumatic stress disorder can be retraumatized by health procedures (Kathleen McCullough, BSN, oral communication, February 23, 1999).

## Health Issues in Internationally Adopted Children

Each year, U.S. families adopt approximately 10,000 foreign-born children. International adoptions have been primarily from Asian countries (Korea, Philippines, India) and Central and South America. In recent years, however, increasing numbers of adoptions are occurring from Eastern Europe and the Caribbean. Internationally adopted children are required to have an overseas visa medical examination in the country of origin in order to receive an immigrant visa. This examination is for the purposes discussed earlier and is not a comprehensive evaluation (Gavagan & Brodyaga, 1998; American Academy of Pediatrics, 1997). Health problems exhibited by these children are a reflection of the circumstances they have experienced and therefore vary widely. Albers, Johnson, Hostetter, Iverson, and Miller (1997) report that many internationally adopted children have been institutionalized, some for long periods of time, and many have experienced abandonment and deprivation. At least half of the children arrive in the United States with at least one health problem that requires treatment. The health reports that accompany the children vary in the amount of detail and documentation of healthcare, and at times significant discrepancies exist in the preadoptive evaluations and subsequent assessments done in the United States. Health concerns for these children include growth and developmental delays; undiagnosed infectious diseases, including chronic hepatitis B, tuberculosis, and intestinal parasites; and incomplete immunization status (American Academy of Pediatrics, 1997; Albers et al., 1997; Hostetter et al., 1991).

The American Academy of Pediatrics recommends in the *1997 Red Book: Report of the Committee on Infectious Diseases* that all international adoptees, after arrival in the United States, undergo a medical examination that focuses on:

- Vision and hearing assessments
- Developmental testing
- Nutritional assessment
- Physical examination, including complete blood cell count, identification of infectious diseases, and identification of congenital anomalies

## Adjustment Issues for Children and Youth

New immigrants and refugees can be expected to experience culture shock as they discover the profound differences between their practices and beliefs and the values and behaviors of those among whom they now live (Lynch & Hanson, 1998). Adjustments, adaptations, and efforts to understand and navigate the educational, health, and social service systems all demand a great deal of energy and can lead to misunderstanding, frustration, and despair. However, the growth of healthy immigrant communities depends on recognition by mainstream society of the strengths of immigrants and refugees—dignity, resiliency, survivorship skills, and ability to adapt to change—as well as the willingness of society to support the adaptation process (DeSantis, 1997).

The stress of adapting to a new culture and the losses of the familiar homes, routines, languages, and cultures can cause difficulties for children in adapting to new schools and communities. Adjustment problems, school failure, and deviant behaviors that occur as immigrant and refugee children and youth struggle to assimilate put them at risk for mental health problems. The initial phase of adjustment is often characterized by silence due to inability to communicate and/or awareness of different cultural expectations. Children may appear withdrawn yet be actively observing and listening. Reacting to pressures to assimilate into the new culture may cause children to pretend they are not connected to their past, to their culture, and, at times, to their families. Other children may feel and behave one way at home and another at school. Parent-child relationships are altered as the children learn English and adopt American cultural behaviors more quickly than the older generation. In addition, immigrant and refugee children find few support systems within the school and community. Language barriers contribute to difficulties in accessing and benefiting from available services. Efforts are needed to develop multilingual and multicultural programs that meet the mental health needs of immigrant and refugee youth (Guarnaccia & Lopez, 1998; Igoa, 1995; James, 1997).

Healthy adjustment occurs through acculturation as the individual changes, accepts, and participates in mainstream culture without abandoning traditional cultural beliefs and values. When parents are supported and assisted in the parental role, children feel safer. Children also benefit when helped to appreciate and value both cultures—to make sense of both worlds. Schools can provide significant assistance by promoting the value of diversity within the student body, working against prejudice, and developing ways to assist parents to understand and navigate the educational system (DeSantis, 1997; Guarnaccia & Lopez, 1998, James, 1997).

## Cultural Considerations

Culture is how we are raised to understand and live life. Lipson, Dibble, and Minarik (1996) state that culture can be viewed as a framework for how we live. Culture mediates—it affects and influences our perceptions, defines our choices, and affects our interactions with other people.

Nowhere is the impact of culture more powerful than in health, as it affects both the students' health beliefs and behaviors and the school nurse's health beliefs and behaviors. Culture affects perceptions about illness, health, and disability. In addition to determining the student's immigration status and the resultant health and legal issues, it is also crucial for the school nurse to include an assessment of cultural beliefs, practices, and meanings when developing an IHP. The challenge to school nurses when assessing and planning for the needs of immigrant and refugee students is to provide care that conforms to each student's values, beliefs, and practices.

## Transcultural Nursing

School nurses working with students whose cultural background differs from that of the nurse are called upon to develop crosscultural expertise. Transcultural nursing authors and theorists provide a body of research to assist nurses (Andrews & Boyle, 1999; Lipson et al.,1996; Giger & Dacidhizar, 1995; Leininger,1991). Founder and leader of transcultural nursing, Madeline Leininger, was the first to note, in the 1950s, cultural differences between patients and nurses. Her theory of culture care diversity and universality provides the structure on which the transcultural nursing specialty is based. Leininger's Sunrise Model (1991), which depicts this theory, is based on the concept of cultural care. This theory is focused on care which is culturally congruent, that is, care which is meaningful and beneficial to the person involved. Taking into consideration the many influences and factors that may be present, she describes three modalities of nursing decisions and actions that demonstrate how to deliver culturally congruent care:

1. **Culture care preservation and/or maintenance.** The nurse and student agree to use cultural care such as folk medicine or healing rituals known to be helpful and not harmful. The cultural ways are preserved.
2. **Culture care accommodation and/or negotiation.** The nurse accommodates the cultural patterns or habits of the student into the plan of care. For example, extended families are encouraged to participate in decision making.
3. **Culture care repatterning or restructuring.** Together, the nurse and student design different patterns for the health and well-being of the student. With respect for the student's cultural beliefs, the school nurse helps the student to understand and benefit from the American healthcare system, develop self-care skills, or practice preventive health measures (Cooper, 1996; Leininger, 1991; Lynch, & Hanson, 1998).

## Cultural Assessment

Cultural assessment skills are learned. An assessment of student and family values, beliefs, and health practices can be conducted separately using one of the cultural assessment tools that are available (Andrews & Boyle, 1999; Lipson, Dibble, & Minarik; 1996; Giger & Dacidhizar, 1995; Leininger, 1991) or by incorporating a cultural perspective into the usual health history. Use open-ended statements or questions, such as, "Tell me about the problem," "What do you think is causing this,?" "What does your mother say is happening to you,?" "What does your family do at home for this problem?" (Cooper, 1996; Giger & Dacidhizar, 1995). Expect to discover differences in health beliefs and practices when working with a culturally diverse population.

Leininger (1991) reminds us that the plan is for the patient. If there are elements of the family's actions or choices that the school nurse assesses as harmful in light of current professional practice, use problem solving to reach a solution, involve cultural liaisons or mediators, or help the family to restructure their understanding. Continue to evaluate and reassess.

It is important and helpful to learn those beliefs, practices, and unique health problems and needs that are specific to each cultural group. Because this process can take a long time, it is often necessary to attempt to apply what is learned from one group to another while avoiding stereotypes. Certainly the competence and skills developed in assessing a student or several students of a particular culture can enhance the nurse's abilities when assessing a student from another culture.

## Cross-cultural Competence: A Journey for School Nurses

Developing competency in interactions with students and families from other cultures is a journey—a process of acquiring understanding and skills. The skills and abilities to provide culturally competent care are important now and will become increasingly important in the 21st century. Begin the journey with an acknowledgment of the profound effect culture has on health and health outcomes for all people (Center for Cross-Cultural Health, 1997). Examine the effects your own culture has on your beliefs and practices. How are you affected by the way you were brought up, the nursing education you received, the work situations you have experienced, the professional standards that guide your practice? How and why have you changed your values and behaviors from those of your family of origin? Examine how your own cultural beliefs influence your attitudes, behaviors, and expectations.

Next, seek to learn and understand the cultural beliefs and values of students and their families that influence their attitudes, beliefs, and behaviors. If you do not speak the language of the student or family, use an interpreter. Find a cultural liaison or mediator to teach you about the culture. Look for similarities and differences between cultures. Avoid stereotypes, remembering that individuals within a culture vary significantly. Each family modifies the culture of the larger group in ways that are unique. Families will adhere to the old ways that have meaning and adopt new beliefs that work for them. Culture is fluid and is influenced and changed by experiences and environment (Andrews & Boyle, 1999; Randall-Davis, 1989; Refugee Health Program, 1996; Southwest Communication Resources, 1996).

Move toward an acceptance of other cultural perspectives by adapting your thinking to respect and value the students' or families' beliefs and practices. Believe that students have a right to their values, beliefs, and practices. Integrate the family's beliefs with your beliefs and be will-

ing to tolerate ambiguity. Ask questions and find answers, portray a desire to learn, remain nonjudgmental, and keep your sense of humor. Involve the student and family in making decisions about their care. Be sure to consider financial issues and access-to-care issues. Don't expect to do it alone; find resources in your school and community and build partnerships within the immigrant community and the community at large. You will be developing effective cross-cultural communication and understandings, which will increase your skills. You will learn to be effective in assessing students and in planning, implementing, and evaluating the plan of care and health outcomes (Andrews & Boyle, 1999; Center for Cross-Cultural Health, 1997; Refugee Health Program, 1996). Do not expect to complete this journey; it will continue throughout your years of professional practice.

## Assessing Family Patterns

Family characteristics and behaviors can be observed across a continuum (Lynch & Hanson, 1998). Understanding of this can be helpful in working with families when the cultural background of the nurse differs from that of the student. Examples of cultural continua illustrate differences in behavior not only across cultures but also between specific families within cultural groups. There is no right or wrong to these behaviors. However, failure to understand such differences in approaches can cause misunderstanding, conflicts, wasted time and effort, and poor outcomes for the student (Lynch & Hanson, 1998).

Differing perspectives on beliefs and values are not fixed positions. Age, education, friends, economic situations, life experiences, and other variables can affect an individual's beliefs and thus position on the continuum. Also, family members may be at different points. This framework can be used to assess a student or family response to a new situation, to an expectation from school, to a medical or educational diagnosis, to a treatment plan, or to a medication regimen. The seven value sets listed can be used for evaluation and interpretation of individual perspectives, not only those of the student and family members but also those of the school nurse.

The first continuum addresses extended families versus small, independent unit families. Extended families often rely on family members for assistance but may expect help or agreement in return. By contrast, the small unit family may be more independent in decision making but have less access to family support resources. Some families value individuality and foster self-esteem. Other families value the family whole over the individual—the person's worth is determined by his or her contribution to the family.

Nurturing may vary from one family to another. Some families keep children close to them physically, for example, whereas others encourage early independence and value the abilities to calm and entertain oneself.

Time is a variable, which can have significantly different levels of importance among people and can cause significant conflicts. For many, the clock and calendar dictate the day's activities and schedule. For others, it may be more important to respond to the immediate needs of friends and family, as things come up, than to meet a schedule.

For some, the wisdom of the elders and the rituals and traditions of the ancestors are basic to life. In contrast, for many Americans, the emphasis is on the future, on technology, on what is new and better. American children are often taught early about "mine," about ownership and property rights. At the other end of this continuum is the child who grows up in a culture where things are shared by a wide group of family and community members.

The sixth value set contrasts rights and responsibilities. Families define gender roles, responsibilities for childcare, and decision-making power in varying ways. Some families value traditional, established gender roles, whereas others place value on equal rights and responsibilities for each parent.

The final continuum is harmony/control. Some families seek harmony in their environment. Their lives may be centered on this principle and structured spiritually to attain harmony. For others, often those of mainstream U.S. culture, a common belief is that things can be controlled, fixed, changed, and acted upon (Lynch & Hanson, 1998).

## Assessing Students With Special Needs

The challenges of being culturally competent become even more apparent when working with children with special healthcare, developmental, or educational needs. Families with children with special health or developmental needs face many challenges; families of ethnically or culturally diverse backgrounds experience even greater obstacles (Southwest Communication Resources, 1996). The family's perceptions of their child's needs vary greatly among cultures, and it is necessary for school nurses to recognize and assess cultural influences on a family's response to illness, disability, or developmental delays in order to respond appropriately, make effective plans of care, intervene, and evaluate.

The possible responses of parents from diverse cultures to a child with illness or a disability are infinite. Some of these possibilities are described in this paragraph. Family members may seek advice from an elder, seek help from a cultural or spiritual healer, or use native medicines or healing practices in addition to or in place of Western medicine. Family and extended family are very important in many cultures, and decisions may not be made before consulting the extended family or the elders. Often the extended family is very involved in raising the children, with multiple caregivers present in the child's life. Some cultures teach that respect is shown by avoiding eye contact, by not asking questions. Providers can misinterpret these behaviors to mean lack of understanding, agreement, or interest on the part of the family. Because some immigrants and refugees may be cautious of government services and of signing papers that they do not understand based on past experiences in their country of origin, they may refuse services for their child.

Spirituality may be very important. Families may have a strong belief in the possibility of miracles. Some Asian cultures believe that a child's illness or disability is the result of a wrongdoing by an ancestor. Many cultures explain illness or disability as a punishment or a curse, and the community may seek an explanation by attempting to discover what wrong was committed and who is to blame. Others believe that the cause or cure is within the individual. For some cultures, admitting a problem publicly causes humiliation and shame. Touching a child's head is a comforting or friendly gesture to many Americans but is disrespectful in some Asian cultures. Families may feel that a disability was meant to be and that surgical intervention, medication, or therapies are not appropriate. Some believe that surgical procedures, even minor operations such as insertion of tympanostomy tubes for chronic middle ear effusions, may release the child's spirit and that the spirit may never return. Other family issues, such as adjusting to American culture, financial insecurity, and/or feelings of anger or depression, may take precedence over the child's need (Andrews & Boyle, 1999; Lynch & Hanson, 1998; Randall-Davis, 1989; Southwest Communication Resources, 1996).

Perceptions, beliefs, and practices such as these can cause confusion, disbelief, dismay, frustration, and anger in Western healthcare providers and education staff. To be effective, one must embark on the cultural journey described earlier and continually try to understand the meaning of the situation for the student and family.

## Considerations Related to the Nursing Process

Assessment of students from diverse cultural backgrounds requires the school nurse to strive to develop cultural competence and transcultural nursing skills. It is essential to integrate a cultural history into the nursing assessment. It is also essential to recognize that not only will students come from many cultures and subcultures, but they may also be at any point along a continuum of the acculturation process from new arrival to second or third generation. An understanding of culture will be important in assessing all children (Margaret Andrews, PhD, RN, e-mail, March 1, 1999).

When determining nursing diagnoses to define the student's health concern and direct the IHP, the school nurse must be aware of the effect that cultural biases and the perspective of Western medicine may have on his or her selection of nursing diagnoses (Andrews & Boyle, 1999; Geissler, 1991; Giger & Dacidhizar, 1995; Leininger, 1991). It is necessary to guard against describing a condition as impaired or altered when the behavior may be considered normal within a cultural group. An understanding of culture will guide the nurse in making assessments. The culturally competent school nurse determines with the student and the family what the student expects and needs. By clarifying perceptions of the problem and then checking the accuracy of nursing diagnoses with the student and/or family, appropriate nursing diagnoses and plans of care can be achieved. It is essential to develop, together with the student and family, a plan of care that is appropriate and meaningful and that will be effective. The school nurse negotiates differences, individualizes the plan to fit the family patterns, and, when appropriate, incorporates cultural care that is not harmful to the student. Finally, culturally competent care requires the school nurse to frequently evaluate and reassess the IHP.

## Access to Healthcare Issues

In recent years attention has begun to focus on disparities in healthcare and health outcomes for minority populations. Two factors that limit access to care for immigrant and refugee populations and contribute to disparities in health outcomes are health coverage and language barriers. Health insurance coverage provides access to quality care—care that meets standards—and care that is delivered preventively or early in a disease course. However, immigrants and refugees are less likely to be insured than the general population. In 1997, 43% of children and 12% of elders who were noncitizens lacked healthcare coverage, compared with 14% of nonimmigrant children and 1% of nonimmigrant elders (James, 1997). Important determinants of coverage include income, time in the United States, and residency status. Many low-income occupations that employ immigrants do not provide healthcare coverage. Immigrants and refugees face competing needs, such as housing and food. In addition, recent changes in government health programs have limited the eligibility of some refugees and immigrants for these programs. Many of the uninsured are children for whom the lack of health insurance results in delayed and fragmented care (Carrasquillo, Carrasquillo, & Shea, 2000).

Language is often a barrier to obtaining quality care. Title VI of the Civil Rights Act of 1964 prohibits discrimination on the basis of race, color, or national origin in any program receiving federal assistance. Title VI has repeatedly been interpreted to mean that trained and qualified interpreters must be provided in healthcare and other settings. In March 2001, the U.S. Department of Health and Human Services, Office of Minority Health, published the National Standards for Culturally and Linguistically Appropriate Services in Health Care (CLAS Standards). The standards were developed to address the need to provide appropriate services to all patients and to contribute to the elimination of health disparities in minority populations.

## Recommendations for Interventions in Working With Immigrant and Refugee Students

- Determine status of student: refugee, immigrant, nondocumented immigrant.
- Be aware of the health needs of refugee or immigrant populations entering school.
- Assess immunization status.
- Assist student and family to complete immunization series/boosters.
- Screen hearing and vision initially to identify barriers to learning.
- Determine if the refugee health examination has been completed; obtain results.
- Use interpreters and cultural mediators and develop comfortable working relationships.
- Develop a knowledge base about students' culture, background, experiences, cultural view of medical practices, culture-specific diseases.
- Add cultural history to data collection.
- Network with other school support staff, including English as a Second Language teachers, to address educational needs and language needs/barrier.
- Monitor for infectious disease signs/symptoms.
- Monitor nutritional status.
- Monitor for signs/symptoms of depression, grief, posttraumatic stress syndrome.
- Assist students to appreciate, understand, and accept both the culture of their family and American culture.
- Collaborate with local public health to:
  ☐ provide culturally appropriate care
  ☐ follow tuberculosis concerns
  ☐ obtain refugee screening results
  ☐ provide translated health education materials
  ☐ identify healthcare resources
- Develop referral resources for:
  ☐ health
  ☐ medical
  ☐ social services
  ☐ cultural liaisons
  ☐ mutual assistance organizations
- Assist student/family in locating and accessing healthcare resources.
- Display posters, pamphlets, magazines, pictures, and artifacts from the cultures of the students in the school.
- Obtain health education videos in the home languages of the students
- Learn to recognize how one's own culture influences beliefs, behaviors, practices.

- Acknowledge and respect cultural differences, develop appreciation for diverse cultural health beliefs and practices.
- Recognize that within cultures there is a continuum of beliefs and practices; each student is an individual within a culture.
- Explain to student's family that they do not have to answer questions if they are uncomfortable; explain why you are asking questions.
- Ask who is the decision maker regarding health and education within the family.
- Listen to student/family concerns, beliefs, perceptions.
- Ask about student and family perception of illness and response to illness.
- Ask if there are cultural or religious practices that influence health or sickness. Use simple explanations; repeat as necessary, take time.
- Demonstrate skills; monitor student return demonstration of self-care practices.
- Problem solve with student, family, educational staff, and healthcare provider.
- Negotiate mutually acceptable solutions to health-related problems with students and families.
- Become knowledgeable about the healthcare system: eligibility, application process, benefits.

- Explain and assist family to utilize U.S. healthcare system and understand the need for appointments, medication regimens.
- Accept that frustration does occur, be patient, collaborate, problem solve, work with cultural liaisons.
- Support the hiring of multilingual and culturally diverse school staff.
- Work with others to build healthy communities that support all of the population.
- Participate in ethnic celebrations within the community.

Adapted from material in Downing, 1997; Lynch, Hanson, 1998; Randall-Davis, 1989; Southwest Communication Resources,1996.

In school settings, a sibling or another student may be asked to interpret. This arrangement poses concerns for confidentiality, misinterpretation, and role confusion. Lynch and Hanson (1998) explain how role reversal of the child (as the one who imparts information and answers for the family) can cause disruptions in family dynamics and puts significant burdens on the child. In addition, parents may not wish to discuss some issues while their child is interpreting, because they may be embarrassed, reluctant for the child to share in decision making, and/or concerned about the loss of their authority as the parent.

## Use of Interpreters

☐ Determine which language the student and/or family/guardian will use to best express themselves (some individuals speak several languages, or speak English socially but are not able to discuss in depth using English).

☐ Use interpreters who are proficient in the language, including specific dialect, who can communicate, understand, and make your message clear to the student and/or parent/guardian, and who understand the educational and health issues.

☐ Prior to the interview, discuss with the interpreter the purpose of the interaction, including any specific terms that will be used or any forms that will need to be completed.

☐ Consider the interpreter a member of the school team by establishing a working relationship.

☐ Plan adequate time for the interview; interpreting takes more time.

☐ If other school staff need to obtain similar information from the family, schedule a joint interview and share an outline prior to meeting.

☐ Look directly at and speak to the student or parent/guardian, not the interpreter.

☐ Convey concern for and interest in the student and or family/guardian and the information they have to share.

☐ Speak in short sentences and ask one question at a time.

☐ Pause and wait for the interpreter to interpret.

☐ Use simple terms; be cautious of medical or educational terminology.

☐ Use words to express your meaning; gestures can be misinterpreted.

☐ Speak normally, not too loudly and not too fast.

☐ If you are giving instructions, do so in a step-by-step, logical sequence; pictures or other visual aids are helpful.

☐ Say only what you want the student or parent to hear.

☐ Encourage the interpreter to ask you for clarification; check accuracy.

☐ Expect the interpreter to translate directly without adding to or changing the message and to remain impartial.

☐ Listen closely to the student or parent/guardian for clues to their concerns, emotional response, and understanding.

☐ Realize that you may need to repeat or reword your message.

# References

Ackerman L. (1997). Health problems of refugees. *Journal of the American Board of Family Practice, 10,* 337–348.

Albers, L., Johnson, D., Hostetter, M., Iverson, S., & Miller, L. (1997). Health of children adopted from the former Soviet Union and eastern Europe. *Journal of the American Medical Association, 278,* 922–924.

American Academy of Pediatrics, Committee on Community Health Services. (1997). Healthcare for children of immigrant families. Pediatrics, 100, 153–156.

American Academy of Pediatrics (1997). *1997 Red Book: Report of the Committee on Infectious Diseases.* Elk Grove, IL: Author.

American Psychiatric Association (1994). *Diagnostic and statistical manual of mental disorders* (4th ed.). Washington, DC: Author.

Andrews, M. & Boyle, J. (1999). *Transcultural concepts in nursing* (3rd ed). Philadelphia: Lippincott, Williams & Wilkins.

Carrasquillo, O., Carrasquillo, A,. Shea, S. (2000). Health insurance coverage of immigrants living in the United States: Differences by citizenship status and county of origin. *American Journal of Public Health, 90,* 917–923.

Center for Applied Linguistics. (1996). *Welcome to the United States: A guidebook for refugees.* Washington, DC: Refugee Service Center, Author.

The Center for Cross-Cultural Health. (1997). *Caring across cultures: The providers guide to cross-cultural health care.* Minneapolis, MN: Author.

Centers for Disease Control and Prevention. (1990). *Tuberculosis Statistics in the United States, 1988.* Atlanta, GA: Author.

Chaney, E., Hernandez, D. (1998). *The health and well-being of children in immigrant families.* Committee on the Health and Adjustment of Immigrant Children and Families, Board on Children, Youth, and Families, National Research Council, Institute of Medicine. Washington, DC: National Academy Press.

Cooper T. (1996). Culturally appropriate care: optional or imperative. *Advances in Practicing Nursing Quarterly, 2,* 1–6.

DeSantis, L. (1997). Building healthy communities with immigrants and refugees. *Journal of Transcultural Nursing, 9,* 20–30.

Downing, B. (1997). *Guidelines for working with medical interpreters. Caring across cultures.* Minneapolis, MN: Center for Cross-Cultural Health.

Gavagan, T., & Brodyaga , L. (1998). Medical care for immigrants and refugees. *American Family Physician, 57,* 1061–1068.

Geissler, E. (1991). Nursing diagnoses of culturally diverse patients. *International Nursing Review, 35,* 150–151.

Giger, J., & Dacidhizar, R. (1995). *Transcultural nursing: Assessment and intervention.* St. Louis, MO: Mosby-Yearbook.

Guarnaccia, P., & Lopez, S. (1998). The mental health and adjustment of immigrant and refugee children. *Child and Adolescent Psychiatric Clinics of North America, 7,* 537–553.

Hostetter, M., Iverson, S., Thomas, W., Mckenzie, D., Dole, K., & Johnson, D. (1991). Medical evaluation of internationally adopted children. *New England Journal of Medicine, 325,* 479–485.

Igoa, C. (1995). *The Inner World of the Immigrant Child.* New York: St. Martin's Press

Leininger, M. (1991). *Culture care diversity and universality: A theory of nursing.* New York: National League for Nursing Press.

James, D. (1997). Coping with a new society: The unique psychosocial problems of immigrant youth. *Journal of School Health, 67,* 98–102.

Lipson, J., Dibble, S., & Minarik, P. (1996). *Culture and nursing care.* San Francisco, CA: University of California, San Francisco, Nursing Press.

Lynch, E., & Hanson, M. (1998). Developing cross-cultural competence: *A guide for working with young children and their families.* Baltimore, MD: Paul H. Brookes Publishing.

McCullough, K. (1999). Minneapolis, MN: The Center for Cross-Cultural Health.

Pickwell, S. (1996). Providing health care to refugees. *Advances in Practicing Nursing Quarterly, 2,* 39–44.

Randall-Davis, E. (1989). *Strategies for working with culturally diverse communities and clients.* Bethesda, MD: Association for the Care of Children's Health.

Refugee Health Coordinator Network, Office of Refugee Resettlement. (1994). *Issues in refugee health: The overseas medical examination and domestic health examination.* Washington, DC: U.S. Department of Health and Human Services.

Refugee Health Program. (1996). *Six steps toward cultural competence: How to meet the health care needs of immigrants and refugees.* Minneapolis, MN: Minnesota Department of Health.

Southwest Communication Resources. (1996). *Family perspectives: Cultural/ ethnic issues affecting children with special health care needs. Educational fact packets for health and human service providers.* Bernalillo, NM: Author.

# Bibliography

American Academy of Nursing. (1992). AAN Expert Panel Report: Culturally competent health care. *Nursing Outlook, 40,* 277–283.

Binkin, N., Zuber, P., Wells, C., Tipple, M., & Castro, K. (1996). Overseas screening for tuberculosis in immigrants refugees to the United States: current status. *Clinical Infectious Diseases, 23,* 1226–1232.

Cookson, S., et al. (1998) Immigrant and refugee health. *Emerging Infectious Diseases, 4*(3):427–428.

Fadiman, A. (1997). *The spirit catches you and you fall down: A Hmong child, her American doctors, and the collision of two cultures.* New York: Farrar, Straus, and Giroux.

Ingstad, B., Whyte, S. (1995). *Disability and culture.* Berkeley, CA: University of California Press.

Jackson, LE. (1993). Understanding, eliciting, and negotiating client multicultural health beliefs. *Nurse Practitioner, 18,* 30–43.

James, D. (1997). Coping with a new society: the unique psychosocial problems of immigrant youth. *Journal of School Health 67*(3), 98-102.

Kavanagh, K., Kennedy, P. (1992). *Promoting cultural diversity: Strategies for health care professionals.* Newbury Park, CA: SAGE.

Kleinman, A. (1980). Patients and healers in the context of culture. Berkeley, CA: University of California Press.

Kosarchyn, C. (1993) School nurses' perceptions of the health needs of Hispanic elementary school children. *Journal of School Nursing, 9*(1), 37–43.

Leininger, M. (1990). Issues, questions, and concerns related to the nursing diagnosis cultural movement from a transcultural nursing perspective. *Journal of Transcultural Nursing, 2*(1), 23–31.

Leininger, M. (1997). Future trends in transcultural nursing in the 21st century. *International Nursing Review, 44*(1), 19–23.

Pipher, M. (2002). *The middle of everywhere: Helping refugees enter the American community.* Orlando, FL: Harcourt.

Roessler, G. (1990). Transcultural nursing certification. *Journal of Transcultural Nursing, 1,* 59.

Sack, W. (1998). Multiple forms of stress in refugee and immigrant children. *Child and Adolescent Psychiatric Clinics of North America, 7*(1), 153–167.

Suro, R. (1998). *Strangers among us: How Latino immigration is transforming America.* New York: Albert A. Knopf.

Urrutia-Rojas, X., & Aday, L. (1991). A framework for community assessment: Designing and conducting a survey in a Hispanic immigrant and refugee community. *Public Health Nursing, 8*(1), 20–26.

Vincent, L. (1992). Families and early intervention: Diversity and competence. *Journal of Early Intervention,* 16(2), 166–172.

Wenger, A. (1993). Cultural meaning of symptoms. *Holistic Nursing Practice, 7*(2), 22–35.

Wong, J. (1998). Cultural changes in healthcare. *Postgraduate Medicine, 103*(6), 38.

# Resources

## Web Sites

Access to current and extensive information about immigrant and refugee populations is available on the Internet.

Access Project
The Language Services Action Kit: Interpreter Services in Health Care Settings for People with Limited English Proficiency. Available in English and Spanish.
www.accessproject.org/projects.htm

American Academy of Pediatrics
Culturally Effective Pediatric Care
www.aap.org/commpeds/cepc/resources.htm

Center for Applied Linguistics
Cultural profiles and information about educational needs and services for second language students.
www.cal.org

Center for Cross-Cultural Health
www.crosshealth.com/

Ethnomed, University of Washington and Harborview Medical Center
Profiles of specific cultural groups; history, cultural practices, and beliefs.
www.Healthlinks.washington.edu/clinical/ethnomed

Hablamos Juntos. Models for Language Access. Strategies for overcoming language barriers. to effective care. www.hablamosjuntos.org/resourcecenter/models_approaches_tools.asp

Institute of Medicine
Report brief: What Health Care Consumers Need to Know About Racial and Ethnic Disparities in Healthcare (PDF).
www.iom.edu/includes/dbfile.asp?id=4176
Institute of Medicine
Report brief: Unequal Treatment: What Health Care Providers Need to Know About Racial and Ethic Disparities in Healthcare (PDF). www.iom.edu

Interaction American Council for Voluntary International Action
www.interaction.org/refugee/refugees.html/

---

National Association of School Psychologists
The Provision of Culturally Competent Services in the
 School Setting.
 www.nasponline.org/culturalcompetence/provi-
 sion_cultcompsvcs.html

National Council on Interpreting in Health Care
http://www.ncihc.org

Office of Minority Health, U.S. Dept Health and
 Human Services
Available at: http://www.omhrc.gov

School Health Culture Zone
Web site developed by N. McGahn, a school nurse.
http://courses.international.edu/bc680/nmcgahn/

Transcultural Nursing Society
http://www.nursingcenter.com/people/nrsorgs/

U.S. Citizenship and Immigrant Services
Formerly known as U.S. Department of Immigration and
 Naturalization Services (INS).
http://uscis.gov

U.S. Department of Health and Human Services,
 Department of Children and Families, Welfare
 Reform
http://www.acf.dhhs.gov/news/welfare/

## Immunization Resource
Foreign vaccine product list
http:\\www.health.state.mn.us\divs\dpc\adps\
 translte.htm

## Language Line
AT&T Language Line
1 Lower Ragsdale Drive
Monterey, CA 93940
1-800-874-9426
140 languages

## Agencies and Organizations
American Refugee Committee (ARC) International
 Headquarters
2344 Nicollet Avenue South
Suite 350
Minneapolis, MN 55404
pr@archq.org
Bureau of Population, Refugees, and Migration, U.S.
 Department of State
2401 E Street, NW
Suite L-505, SA-1
Washington, DC 20522-0105
www.state.gov/www/global/prm/index.html

Center for Applied Linguistics
1118 22nd Street, NW
Washington, DC 20037
1-202-429-9292
http://www.cal.org/RSC

Center for Victims of Torture
717 East River Road
Minneapolis, MN 55455

Immunization Action Coalition
1573 Selby Avenue
Suite 234
St. Paul, MN 55104
651-647-9131
www.immunize.org

National Institutes of Health (NIH)
www.nih.gov

Office of Global Health, Centers for Disease Control
 and Prevention
1600 Clifton Road, NE
Atlanta, GA 30333

Office of Minority Health Resource Center
PO Box 37337
Washington, DC 20013-7337
1-800-444-6472

Refugee Service Center, Center for Applied Linguistics
1118 22nd Street, NW
Washington, DC 20037
202-429-9292

Transcultural Nursing Society
Madonna University, College of Nursing
36600 Schoolcraft Drive
Livonia, MI 48150
1-888-432-5470

World Health Organization
Headquarters Office
Avenue Appia 20, 1211
Geneva 27, Switzerland
info@who.ch

*Chapter Seventeen*

# Homeless Students With Special Health Needs

Gail Synoground

## Introduction

Homelessness among children is an increasing problem. Its manifestations include poor physical and psychosocial health, lack of academic success, and many other health-related issues. The following three cases illustrate some of the problems this population faces.

Case 1: Recently, a family of three children and their mother was brought to the attention of the local school officials. The children had not been attending school for the past 3 months. The father of the children had been in and out of jail for domestic violence; however, the mother returns to him after each release. Eight-year-old Johnny, who is the youngest of the three children, is being registered at the school today. He is a pale, frail-looking child whose eyes focus on the floor, making very little eye contact. His hair had been crudely cut with very short hairs in places and other areas where the scalp appeared shaved. Live lice were noted along with several scabbed-over and bleeding lesions covering the entire scalp. Occipital lymph nodes were swollen. In observing the rest of the child, it was noted that he had a rash over most of his body. He complained of intense itching, especially at night. Linear threadlike lesions were noted between his fingers. The child had not been seen by a medical professional since he was 3.

Case 2: Ten-year-old Darlene presents continually to the school nurse complaining of stomach pain. Her father has been jailed for domestic violence, and her mother, who appears to be very depressed, is not able to provide basic, emotional, or medical care for her child. Darlene is having difficulty focusing on her schoolwork and is about one grade behind for her age.

Case 3: Six-year-old Mark is the son of a 52-year-old single father. The father was previously married and has two children in their 30s. His first wife passed away. Mark is the product of a brief affair between the father and a woman he met in a bar. Although she delivered the child, she did not wish to keep Mark and left him with the father. Mark was diagnosed as having fetal alcohol syndrome and was labeled a "crack baby" as well. Mark is having problems with anger and frequently disrupts the class with his impulsiveness and frequent outbursts.

All of the children in these cases are living in transitional housing and share many common problems, including homelessness, lack of medical care, disruption in educational pursuits, dysfunctional family life, and uncertainly about their future. The first question that arises is, "Can anything be done for children who spend so little time at any one place?"

School nurses and school personnel are in a good position to work with these youngsters, since the school may provide the most consistent place in a world of constant change and inconsistencies.

### Scope of Problem

Goals of Healthy People 2010 (2000) is to increase the span of healthy life for Americans and reduce the health disparities among the poor and to achieve access to preventive services. Approximately 2 to 3 million people are homeless in any given night. A growing number of homeless people are single women and children. Families with children account for 39% of the homeless population (Deforce & Zehnder, 2001). "The homeless children of today will be the unhealthy, unemployable, destitute and homeless adults of tomorrow" (Norton & Ridenaur, 1995). Children and their families are the largest and fastest growing segment of the homeless population (Huang & Menke, 2001).

Homelessness among single mothers and their children is related to abuse, decreased social supports, limited education, drugs, and alcohol abuse (Bureau of Primary Health Care, 2001a). The average homeless family includes two or three children, most younger than 5 years of age (Huang & Menke, 2001).

Healthcare for these children and their families becomes secondary to survival. Primary to their existence is the need to use their resources and energies to obtain the basic needs of food and shelter. Additionally, many of these families do not appreciate or understand the need for preventive health services. Healthcare becomes crisis-oriented with many homeless families relying on emergency departments for care. This is not only costly, but emergency care facilities rarely have the capacity for follow-up care.

Recent literature has focused on the adolescent segment of the homeless population, particularly adolescent females, stating that they are the most vulnerable and underserved groups within the homeless population Homeless adolescent females are at greater risk for pregnancy and sexually transmitted diseases than their peers.

These young adolescents often find themselves in the position of having to trade sexual favors to meet their basic needs of food, clothing, and shelter (Ensign & Panke, 2002).

The Health Resources and Services Administration (2001b) reported that homeless adolescents had a higher rate of suicide attempts as compared to their peers. This behavior was related to their untreated major depression.

School nurses, because of their experience and knowledge, are in a pivotal position to collaborate with teachers and other staff members in identifying physical and psychosocial problems interfering with developmental and academic progression. However, it is imperative for nurses and others to assess their own attitude and resources toward working with this population. Since these children may be at a given school for only a limited time, the question of investing time and energy does arise. Identifying those services relevant to the needs of homeless children will make a difference in their lives.

A less-than-adequate physical and psychological environment exposes homeless children to an increased risk for lasting physical and mental health problems. Problems span the physical, psychosocial, spiritual, and developmental dimensions, including growth disorders, and a higher incidence of acute and chronic health diseases.

## Pathophysiology

The delivery of health services to this segment of the population requires specific knowledge of the multidimensional health problems facing children, plus the barriers they encounter in accessing and receiving adequate health services.

Therefore, to understand the etiology of health problems identified in homeless children, the school nurse must consider the many unhealthy behaviors and consequences of living in an unstable environment. Health problems affecting the child include the following (HRSC, 2001a,b; Holloway, 2002/2003; Nabors & Weist, 2002):

### Physical Problems

- Higher incidence of acute and chronic health problems, especially infections and communicable diseases
- Increased risk for nutritional deficiencies leading to anemia and growth disorders. Meal times in transitional living quarters are often very regulated, and extra food may not be allowed in the rooms, making it difficult to meet the nutritional needs of children.
- Exposure to sexual abuse, violence, physical abuse, criminal behavior, and substance abuse. Continual exposure predisposes these youngsters to physical, mental health, and behavior problems.
- Preventive healthcare is pursued less frequently than in children from more stable environments; particularly notable is the lack of immunizations.
- Healthcare received in an emergency facility is more likely to be fragmented and oriented to solving only acute problems. Compliance and follow-up care are poor in this population.

- Children are often criticized for their hygiene. Facilities to wash clothes or practice hand washing or other hygienic activities are not available.
- Dental healthcare practices are often nonexistent.

### Developmental Problems

Homeless children have been identified as having more developmental delays, physical and mental health problems, and learning difficulties when compared with children living in stable environments (Huang & Menke, 2001).

A study by Holloway (2002/2003) noted that half of the children in their study were developmentally delayed and experienced emotional and behavioral problems three to four times that expected in the general population.

A study by Riley-Eddins (1995) stated that 61% of children under age 5 had at least one developmental lag, and 44% had two or more lags. The purpose of this study was to examine the health status and utilization of health services of families living in shelters. Findings from this study and others demonstrated the need for delivery of health services to this group; 60% of the children over 5 required medical and psychiatric evaluation, and 55% were performing below average in school.

Each transitional home the child lives in brings with it new restrictions and policies plus very limited living space or play area to accomplish the normal developmental tasks of childhood, such as learning interactive and social skills. Often, because of their own needs and stress level, parents find it difficult to monitor and assess their child's developmental level and needs.

### Psychosocial Problems

Research suggests that children who live in poverty are more likely to experience difficulty in school, become teen parents, and as adults earn less and be unemployed more (America's Children, 1997).

Problems related to mental health include negative attention-seeking behavior, aggressiveness, and learning difficulties. A long-term, safe place where trust can be established is required in order to solve many of these problems. Psychosocial problems common to this population include:

- Disruptions in relationships, losses of friends and possessions
- Lack of consistent routines in performance of daily activities
- Parental depression
- Lack of a male role model (especially in households headed by a female)
- Exposure to family violence and abuse
- Exposure to substance and sexual abuse
- Continual exposure to other families and children with problems

As a result, the environmental effects of homelessness on children often lead to:
- Depression and withdrawal
- Decreased self-esteem
- Aggressive behavior
- Poor impulse control
- Poor attention span
- Poor task persistence, often due to frequent absences from school and changes of schools

All of these problems result in developmental lags and learning difficulties.

## Cognitive

Additionally, homeless children must return to an unhealthy environment after school is dismissed, further exposing them to the many problems associated with meeting academic and basic health need expectations. Studying and completing homework assignments may not be possible because of overcrowding or lack of parental ability to assist the child with school assignments.

## Barriers to Care

Access to healthcare is a very real problem. Many women and their children do not have adequate transportation to a medical facility or, if they are able to take a bus, all the children must accompany her for lack of care. Additionally, many clinics are very busy, which means long waiting periods for patients once they do get there. Homeless children and their families lack the resources to obtain health insurance beyond short-term state/government health coupons. Other barriers may include fear of rejection by health personnel, language barriers, and the inability to navigate the bureaucracy of many health facilities.

## Role of the School Nurse

In developing a healthcare plan for the child facing homelessness, the school nurse needs to consider the following:
- School nurses are in a unique position to assist homeless children and their families for many reasons. They are resourceful and aware of available services and how to access them while being mindful of the economic plight of the families.
- School nurses can provide a broad range of services, including physical assessments, sensory assessments, and case management, and serve as an advocate for the child.
- School nurses, although unable to provide for all of the needs of the homeless child, are able to work collaboratively with agencies and other healthcare providers to offer a wide spectrum of services.

- School nurses can evaluate and assist the school-aged child in achieving a developmental task, such as arranging for the child to achieve independence and industry through school successes. Learning these developmental tasks is often limited because of strict shelter rules and an unstable environment.
- School nurses, through collaboration with school personnel and community resources, are able to increase the child's self-care abilities and knowledge.
- School nurses may be the only medical personnel with whom homeless youngsters have contact.

The length of time a school nurse may have with a homeless child is limited; however, the use of the nursing process will assist in planning and implementing appropriate health promotion, disease prevention, and health maintenance strategies. Nurses in partnership with school personnel, community agencies, parents, and students can play a key role in improving the health of homeless children.

In planning intervention(s) related to a child's health needs, the school nurse must be cognizant of the child's environment. For example, if the child has lice and is excluded from school, the nurse needs to ask the following: (1) Can the child's family can afford the medication? (2) What facilities are there for bathing and washing clothes? (3) Are clean clothes available? and (4) Is it possible for the child and his and her family to carry out all of the instructions to get rid of the lice?

# Individualized Healthcare Plan

## Assessment

*History*
- Family composition. Identify younger children who are not in school but may need services
- Length of time child has been homeless. Has the child ever had a stable environment?
- Average length of stay in each shelter. What relationships has the child been able to establish?
- Number of times moved
- Source of healthcare and when last seen
- Medical history: past, present, acute and chronic infectious diseases
- History of injury/abuse
- Health promotion: immunizations
- Use of prescribed medications, over-the-counter medications, and/or prescribed treatments
- What resources has the family successfully used in the past?

- Knowledge of resources available to the child and family in their current setting
- Review of academic achievements/disruptions
- Financial resources available
- Family goals/hopes/needs

### Physical
- Overall appearance and build
- Height, weight. Is child undernourished, alert, interactive?
- Hygiene (availability of bathing facilities)
- Obvious injuries or health problems
- Dental problems
- Vision and hearing results
- Systems review: any problems noted with each system

### Developmental
Assess developmental level for strengths and lags in social, motor, and language skills. (There are various standardized tools depending on the child's age. The Denver Developmental Screening Tool [DDST] is one tool appropriate for children under 5.)

### Psychosocial
The need to recognize and appropriately refer children with mental health concerns is imperative. The school nurse may wish to team up with counselors or other mental health professionals to make a combined comprehensive assessment. Assessment should focus on those problems associated with homelessness, such as:
- Depression
- Helplessness
- Anxiety
- Interpersonal skills and relationships
- Learning difficulties
- Fears
- Anger
- Distrust
- Inattentiveness

These problems interfere with the child's ability to learn, and even though treatment requires time, identification of these problems is an important first step.

### Environmental
- Facilities at the shelter
- School environment
- Safety issues

### Spiritual
- Life goals, values, beliefs
- Hopelessness

### Academic
- School(s) the student attended in the past
- Academic achievement
- Current or need for special education services
- School attendance pattern
- Child's perception of academic needs/level

### Self-care
- Child/family health-seeking patterns
- Level of child's self-care skills and knowledge
- Knowledge related to body functions and disease processes
- Readiness to learn self-care skills
- Child's perception of being healthy

**Nursing Diagnoses (N.D.)** (NANDA, 2003)

*Physical*

N.D. 1 Imbalanced nutrition: less than body requirements (NANDA 0002) related to economic factors.

N.D. 2 Fatigue (NANDA 00093) related to:
- overwhelming psychological or emotional demand
- increased energy requirements to perform activities of daily living
- excessive social and role demands related to constant change

N.D. 3 Ineffective health management (NANDA 00099) related to:
- inability to seek out or maintain health (health resources)
- lack of knowledge
- alteration in communication skills
- ineffective coping
- lack of material resources
- impairment of support systems

N.D. 4 Disturbed sleep pattern (NANDA 00095) related to:
- environmental distractions in shelter
- overcrowding

N.D. 5 Risk for injury and risk for trauma (NANDA 00035 and 00038) related to
- lack of safety measures
- cognitive or emotional problems
- unsafe environment
- high-crime neighborhood
- exposure to abuse

*Developmental*

N.D. 6 Risk for altered growth and development (NANDA 00112) related to:
- inability to perform self-care or self-control activities (interruption in daily schedules)
- delay in performing self-care activities due to lack of facilities

N.D. 7 Interrupted family processes (NANDA 00060) related to:
- disorganization of family life
- anger, frustration, powerlessness

N.D. 8 Risk for social isolation (NANDA 00053)
related to:
- affectional deprivation
- absence of significant others (father often absent)

N.D. 9 Risk for loneliness (NANDA 00054) related to:
- physical and social isolation (lack of opportunity to form long-lasting relationships)

N.D.10 Diversional activity deficit (NANDA 00097) related to:
- decreased opportunity for stimulation
- lack of environmental diversional activities at the shelters

N.D.11 Risk for situational low self esteem (NANDA 00154) related to:
- decreased opportunity for success and accomplishment

N.D.12 Risk for powerlessness (NANDA 00153) related to broken relationships, frequent moves, unstable environment

*Psychosocial*

N.D.13 Ineffective individual coping skills(NANDA 00069) related to:
- inability to meet basic needs
- alteration in societal participation
- inability to meet role expectation
- inability to ask for help

N.D.14 Relocation stress syndrome (NANDA 00150) related to:
- frequent changes in environment leading to anxiety and uncertainty
- losses, including friends
- decrease in support system

N.D.15 Anxiety (NANDA 00147) related to:

- uncertainty
- conflict about values/goals
- changes in environment
- changes in interaction patterns

### Cognitive
**N.D.16** Knowledge deficit (educational) (NANDA 00127) related to:
- interruption of education
- lack of consistent routines
- absences, frequent

**N.D.17** Impaired verbal communication (NANDA 00051) related to:
- difficulty expressing thought
- lack of opportunity to express concerns

### Self-care
**N.D.18** Health management: Ineffective therapeutic regimen (NANDA 00080) related to:
- decreased resources
- decreased knowledge
- decreased opportunities to integrate activities to maintain health and well-being

## Goals

The student will improve health-enhancing behaviors (N.D. 1–6)
The student will verbalize feelings regarding health issues and homelessness (N.D. 11–15, 17)
The student will develop positive coping skills/strategies (N.D. 12–15)
The student will increase successful completion of educational tasks (N.D. 6, 16)
The student will meet nutritional needs while at school (N.D. 1)
The student will access two available resources to help meet his/her basic needs (N.D. 1,3,5,7–10)
The student will access school health services (nursing, counseling, etc.) to meet basic needs (N.D. 1–6,16)
The student will improve self-care skills: safety measures, self assessment (N.D. 6,18)
The student will develop beginning interest and skill in one recreation activity (N.D. 9–10)
The student will establish relationship with at least one other child: pen pal if he or she moves again (N.D. 8–10, 14)
The student will participate in school and extracurricular activities with peers (N.D. 8–10)
The student will maintain a regular pattern of school attendance (N.D. 16)

## Nursing Interventions

### Physical
- Identify barriers that interfere with families seeking preventive healthcare services. (N.D. 3,7)
- Perform as many assessments as possible, including vision nutritional status, height, weight, hearing, and dental. (N.D. 1–5)
- Identify and prioritize health needs from history and basic health assessment. (N.D. 1–5)
- Assess child's environment for basic needs such as running hot water, soap, clean clothes, sleeping quarters, and recreational opportunities. (N.D. 4–7)
- Develop an individual health record that child can take with him/her. (N.D. 1–5)
- Provide opportunity for child to have immunizations updated. (N.D. 3,18)
- Link student to medical resources for evaluation, care, and follow-up. (N.D. 3,18)
- Teach child basic health survival skills, CPR, first aid, and when and how to call for help. (N.D. 5,18)
- Encourage good hygiene through role modeling and providing basic necessities, such as toothbrush, clean clothes, etc. (N.D. 3–6)
- Allow for adequate rest/sleep periods for sleep deprivation. (N.D. 2)
- Assist parent to obtain free school breakfast and lunch at school (N.D. 1)

- Assist parent in identifying resources and obtaining appropriate clothing for school activities (N.D. 3)
- Collaborate with healthcare provider to assist parent in obtaining needed medications or devices for treatment at reduced cost. (N.D. 3)

*Developmental*
- Encourage social interaction with children. (N.D. 9,10,11,16)
- Encourage child to participate in school extracurricular activities. (N.D. 10,16)
- Assess parents' knowledge and ability to meet child's needs. (N.D. 1–5,7,13–15)
- Identify small goals that the child can accomplish each day to meet developmental tasks, for example, learning proper hand washing, toothbrushing, etc. (N.D. 6,11)
- Assist teachers to identify and provide any academic and support services needed to ensure a positive academic outcome. (N.D. 11–12)

*Psychosocial*
- Develop a team of staff and teachers who are willing to develop intensive short-term relationship with homeless child. (N.D. 8,9,11,16,17)
- Visit the shelters to meet families and personnel to establish a link between school and shelter. (N.D. 7,8,9,16)
- Provide current information on health services available and how to contact various agencies. (N.D. 3,7,13)
- Assist student to identify and access services required to meet needs. (N.D. 1–6,11–13,18)
- Develop a referral and follow-up system to provide continuity of care for these children. (N.D. 3,7)
- Monitor use of services and note if child's needs are being met. (N.D. 1–5,6,8,15)
- Serve as an advocate to the child and the family (N.D. 3,7,16)
- Work with staff and teachers to provide consistency in routines and class activities. (N.D. 16)
- Encourage child to express feelings related to homelessness. (N.D. 8–11,17)
- Encourage child to identify children with whom they would like to correspond. (N.D.)
- Provide a place where child can feel safe; identify at least one consistent staff person child can come to. (N.D. 15–16)

*Cognitive*
- Assist school staff to construct an environment at school where the child can learn self-care and increase self-esteem. (N.D. 6,11,12,16,17)
- Assist student to identify and access services needed to meet needs. (N.D. 1–6,11–13,18)
- Develop a referral and follow-up system to provide continuity of care for these children. (N.D. 3,7)
- Monitor use of services and note if child's needs are being met. (N.D. 1–5,6,8, 15)
- Serve as an advocate to the child and family. (N.D. 3,7,16)
- Work with staff and teachers to provide consistency in routines and class activities. (N.D. 16)
- Encourage child to express feelings related to homelessness. (N.D. 8–11,17)
- Encourage child to identify children with whom they would like to correspond. (N.D. 8,9,14–15)
- Provide a place where child can feel safe; identify at least one consistent staff person to whom child can come. (N.D. 15–16)

*Self-care*
- Identify health resources available to child and family that stress health maintenance and prevention. (N.D. 3,7,13)
- Provide time for child to discuss and problem solve health concerns with nurse. (N.D. 1–6,16)

## Expected Student Outcomes

The student will:
- Identify physical, psychosocial, and developmental needs and describe one way to meet a need in each area. (N.D. 1–5,6–11,13–15)
- Identify and articulate fears and concerns to school nurses or trusted staff member. (N.D. 7,14,15–17)
- Identify two resources to call when needing assistance, for example, food bank and/or clothing bank. (N.D. 1–5,6–10,13)
- Demonstrate proper use of 911. (N.D. 5,7)
- State one person with whom they would like to correspond. (N.D. 8,9,14–15)
- Participate in one extracurricular activity. (N.D. 10)
- Display improved health practices, such as improved hygiene and nutritional practices. (N.D. 3,6,11)
- List accomplishments related to educational and developmental task. (N.D. 6,16)
- Assist in maintaining an updated health record (immunizations, height and weight, vision and hearing). (N.D. 3,7)

- Describe how he or she can perform self-care activities considering environmental limitations. (N.D. 1–6)
- Identify ways to assess shelter environment for safety and make appropriate decisions. (N.D. 1,4,5,7,13)

## Case Study

The following care plan is based on an 8-year-old homeless boy and illustrates many of the complex problems these children present. Although the length of stay in any one school is limited, it is possible to plan strategic interventions with positive outcomes. Note the importance of assessing all dimensions and their effect on total health. Three goals should guide you: (1) teach and encourage self-care, (2) connect child to appropriate resources, and (3) assess as much as you can. You may be the child's only connection to healthcare.

David, an 8-year-old boy, enrolled in the second grade at your school. This is the seventh school he has attended in 3 years. He lives with his mother and two younger siblings (a 3-year-old and an 8-month-old). Currently the family is living in one room in a transitional housing facility. Limited history includes the following: diagnosed with asthma when 5 years old, no follow-up, treated in emergency room settings for flare-ups. There is no record of immunizations but his mom thinks he had "some." He is often kept out of school to help mom care for the siblings. The whereabouts of David's father is unknown. David appears thin and tired and is having difficulty with school assignments.

## Individualized Health Care Plan Homelessness

| Assessment Data | Nursing Diagnosis | Goals | Nursing Interventions | Expected Outcomes |
|---|---|---|---|---|
| Fatigue, pale, malnourished | | David will have required dietary intake for age | Arrange for school breakfast/lunch program. | David will identify resources for finding food. |
| | | David will meet nutritional needs while at school. | Monitor 24-hour dietary intake once a week until weight is stabilized. | David will eat breakfast and lunch at school. |
| | | David will assist in identifying and decreasing physical and psychosocial stressors. | Monitor dietary intake in lunchroom. Work with counselor/social worker and transitional home to obtain food for child and family. | David will maintain progress toward normal height and weight. |
| | | | Plot height/weight on growth grid once a week until stabilized. | David will identify sources of fatigue. |
| | | | Work with school staff to identify increased levels of stress and fatigue. | |
| | | | Provide periods of rest as needed during the school day. | |
| | | | Assist parent to develop an age-appropriate sleep pattern for David (quiet environment, regimented sleep schedule, etc.). | |
| | | | Collaborate with housing facility to offer assistance to the parent in meeting David's needs. | |

| Assessment Data | Nursing Diagnosis | Goals | Nursing Interventions | Expected Outcomes |
|---|---|---|---|---|
| Lack of opportunity to complete developmental tasks, for example, self-care activities<br><br>Inconsistent environmental stimulation | Altered growth and development related to (1) inability to perform self-care or self-control activities (interruption in daily schedule); and/or (2) delay in performing self-care activities due to lack of facilities<br><br>Risk for social isolation related to (1) affectional deprivation; and/or (2) absence of significant others (father often absent)<br><br>Diversional activity deficit related to decreased opportunity for stimulation<br><br>Lack of environmental diversional activities at the shelters | David will increase developmental and language skills<br><br>David will participate in school and extracurricular activities with peers. | Work with councelor/psychologist to determine needs.<br><br>Assist teachers in identifying and providing academic and support services needed.<br><br>Work with PE teacher to identify appropriate activities for child with asthma.<br><br>Assist David to identify possible activities and choose one.<br><br>Assist with transportation needs (if needed)<br><br>Assist David to share information with his mother regarding school activities and obtain needed permission. | David will identify his accomplishments (related to developmental level) each week.<br><br>David participates in school activities and a number of extracurricular activities each week. |
| Homeless-transitional living<br><br>Frequent moves/housing instability<br><br>Interruption of long-term relationship<br><br>Absent father<br><br>Withdrawn<br><br>Stays home to take care of siblings | Relocation stress syndrome related to (1) frequent changes in environment leading to anxiety and uncertainty; (2) losses, friends; and/or (3) decreased support systems | Child will establish positive relationships with adults in the school setting<br><br>David is safe in the school setting.<br><br>David maintains a good school attendance pattern | Assist David to identify 1 or 2 teachers/staff at school that he feels comfortable with and he will connect with every day at school<br><br>Provide name of a child who is willing to be a pen pal for David.<br><br>Assist David to identify a staff adult, male role model, who he can go to and discuss his problems/accomplishments. | David checks in with (identified) school staff member every day<br><br>David identifies (verbalizes) through art work the school as a safe place.<br><br>David will attend school every day unless he is too ill to come. |

| Assessment Data | Nursing Diagnosis | Goals | Nursing Interventions | Expected Outcomes |
|---|---|---|---|---|
| | | | Assist teacher to have David included in class pictures (permission to take the child's picture needs to be cleared with parent, especially if parent has protection issues that may be exposed)<br><br>Assist in arranging for David's celebration of his birthday with class (if appropriate)<br><br>Collaborate with the parent and transitional center to assist David in maintaining a good school attendance pattern.<br><br>Assist in providing needed school supplies (backpack, notebook, pencils, etc.) | |
| Below-level academic skills<br><br>Decreased access to library books or other educational stimuli.<br><br>Decreased opportunity to learn and practice self-care activities. | Knowledge deficit (educational) related to (1) interruption in education; (2) lack of consistent routines; and/or (3) frequent absences | David will increase his academic success.<br><br>David will improve his self-care skills. | Assist teachers in identifying and providing any academic and support services needed.<br><br>Work with teachers to save and showcase child's success.<br><br>Put successful work in booklet form for child to take home or with him to a new school.<br><br>Teach and emphasize self-care skills related to assessing his own health. | Takes pride in showcasing schoolwork.<br><br>Demonstrates self-care skills learned. (Identify specific skills) |

| Assessment Data | Nursing Diagnosis | Goals | Nursing Interventions | Expected Outcomes |
|---|---|---|---|---|
| | | | Provide opportunities for David to access educational resources at school and in the community, such as after-school guided study with a teacher, after-school reading or computer access. | |
| No treatment of sensory screening; having problems reading | Altered health maintenance related to (1) inability to seek out or maintain health resources; (2) lack of knowledge; (3) alteration in communication skills; (4) ineffective coping; and/or (5) impairment of support systems | David will assist to identify ways to correct for sensory deficits. | Assess for vision/hearing deficits. | David will identify how vision/hearing deficits affect academic success. David will identify adults who can assist him if he has problems hearing or seeing. |
| Incomplete history of immunization status. | | David will obtain immunization recommended for age. | Refer for glasses. | |
| Uncontrolled asthma | | David will improve self-care skills regarding asthma (see asthma care plan) | Arrange transportation and someone to accompany child (Families often cancel appointments due to no transportation or fear of rejection). | David will assist in keeping updated immunization record. |
| Source of healthcare emergency room | | | Assist in obtaining financial assistance through community organizations, (Lions Club, etc.) if appropriate. | Student will identify two things he or she needs to do to prevent an asthma episoce. |
| | | | Preferential seating in classroom until deficit is resolved. | |
| | | | Assist student and parent to access source for immunizations for child and family. | |
| | | | See teaching plan on asthma. | |
| | | | Link child up with a child who has successfully controlled his or her asthma. Assist parent to access a source or health care professional to meet the student's asthma care needs. | |

| Assessment Data | Nursing Diagnosis | Goals | Nursing Interventions | Expected Outcomes |
|---|---|---|---|---|
| | | | Provide information to child/parent on possible insurance plans and/or clinics available to low income families. | |
| | | | Assist with finding transportation to and from clinic; identify sources for prescribed medication (work with physician). | |

# References

*America's children: Key national indicators of well being, 1997.* Federal Interagency Forum on Child and Family Statistics. Washington, DC: U.S. Government Document PR 42.8:C 43.

Communications for a Sustainable Future. (n.d.). *Homeless children and youth.* Retrieved January 29, 2004, from http://csf.colorado.edu/homeless/youth.html

DeForge, V., Zehnder S., Ptlene, M., & Carman, M. (2001). Children's perception of homelessness. *Pediatric Nursing 27*(4) 377–383.

Ensign, J., & Panke, A. (2002) Barriers and bridges to care: Voices of female adolescent youth in Seattle, WA. *Journal of Advanced Nursing 37*(2), 166–172

Goals of Healthy People 2010 (2000). National Center for Chronic Disease Prevention and Health Promotion. Retrieved January 2005, from http://cdc.gov/cvh/hp2010/

Holloway, J. H. (2002/2003) Addressing the needs of homeless students. *Educational Leadership, 60*(4), 89–90.

Huang, C. Y., & Menke, E. M. (2001). School-aged homeless sheltered children's stressors and coping behaviors. *Journal of Pediatric Nursing, 16*(2), 102–109.

Nabors, L. A., & Weist, M. D. (2002). School mental health services for homeless children. *Journal of School Health, 72*(7), 269.

NANDA International. (2003). *Nursing diagnosis: Definitions & classifications 2003-2004.* Philadelphia: Author.

*No place to call home.* (2001a). Bethesda, MD: Health Resources and Services Administration (HRSA), Bureau of Primary Health Care (BPHC).

Norton, D., & Ridenour, N. (1995). Homeless women and children: The challenge of health promotion. *Nurse Practitioner Forum, 6,* 29–33.

Riley-Eddins, E. A. (1995). Health status of sheltered homeless families. *Journal of Multicultural Nursing Health, 1*(4), 16–22.

*Understanding the health care needs of homeless youth.* (2001b). Health Program Assistance Letters No. 2001-10. Bethesda, MD: Resources and Services Administration, Bureau of Primary Health Care.

# Bibliography

Committee on Temporary Shelter. (2003). *Homeless facts: Children and homelessness. Some facts.* Retrieved January 29, 2004, from http://www.cotsonline.org/homeless_kids.html

Karr, C. (2003). Homeless children: What every health care provider should know. Retrieved January 29, 2004, from http://wwwnhchc.org/Children/

Kelly, E. (2001). Assessment of dietary intake of preschool children living in a homeless shelter. *Applied Nursing Research, 14*(3), 146–154.

Menke, E. M. (2000). Comparison of the stressors and coping behaviors of homeless, previously homeless, and never homeless poor children. *Issues in Mental Health Nursing, 21,* 691–710.

Morris, R. I., & Butt, R. A. (2003). Parents' perspectives on homelessness and its effects on the educational development of their children. *Journal of School Nursing, 19*(1), 43–50.

Morris, R. I., & Strong, L. (2004). The impact of homelessness on the health of families. *Journal of School Nursing, 20*(4), 221–227.

National Coalition for the Homeless. (2004) Internet resources. Retrieved January 29, 2004, from http://www.nationalhomeless.org/others.html

National Coalition for the Homeless. (2004). Retrieved January 29, 2004, from http://wwwnationalhomeless.org/

National Health Care for the Homeless Council. (2004). Homeless resources on the Web. Retrieved January 24, 2004, from http://www.nhchc.org/links.htm

National Health Care for the Homeless Council. (2003). Because health care is a right, not a privilege. Retrieved January 29, 2004, from http://www.nhchc.org/

National Coalition for the Homeless. (2001a). *Forget me not 2001: Educational materials.* Retrieved January 29, 2004, from http://www.nationalshomeless.org/fmn2001/education.html

Weinreb, L., Wehler, C., Perloff, J., Scott, R., Hosmer., D., & Sagor, L., et al. (2002). Hunger: Its impact on children's health and mental health. *Pediatrics 1106,* e41.

# Resources

National Association for the Education of Homeless Children and Youth (NAEHCY)
512-475-8765
www.naehcy.org

National Center for Homeless Education at SERVE
1-800-308-2145 (Helpline)
homeless@serve.org
www.serve.org/nche

National Coalition for the Homeless
1012 14th Street, NW
Suite 600
Washington, DC 20005-3471
202-737-6444
info@nationalhomeless.org
http://www.nationalhomeless.org

National Health Care for the Homeless Council, Inc.
HCH Clinicians' Network
PO Box 60427
Nashville, TN 37206-0427
615-226-2292
council@nhchc.org
http://www.nhchc.org

National Law Center for Homeless and Poverty (NLCHP)
202-638-2535
www.nlchp.org

## Chapter Eighteen

# Genetics Overview for the School Nurse Developing Individualized Healthcare Plans

Sharon Yearous

## Introduction

The Genetic Diseases Act of 1976 provided the availability of genetic services in each of the 50 United States (Anderson, Black Monsen, Prows, Tinley, & Jenkins, 2000; Lashley, 1998). The provision of genetic services requires that nurses be aware of these resources. The Human Genome Project (HGP) began in 1990 with the intent to map out the location of the 30,000 human genes located on the 23 pairs of chromosomes. The completion of the mapping was achieved in April 2003 (National Human Genome Research Institute, 2004). The explosion of genetic information available in the last 25 years requires that all nurses be knowledgeable of basic genetics.

Gathering health information is an annual and ongoing task of the school nurse. School nurses are often the link to the healthcare system for families in the community. Understanding the anticipated outcomes of genetic disorders allows the school nurse to plan appropriate individualized healthcare plans (IHPs) for students. Genetic disorders are unique in their presentation, and the severity may vary among children. In the development of an IHP for a school-aged child with a genetic disorder, consideration will need to be given to the specific health needs that child faces. Although the underlying genetic disorder will not change for a specific child, the functional level and needs of the child may change throughout a school year or from year to year. It is important to think about the ongoing changes and revisit the IHP often and update it as needed.

When developing the IHP for the child with a genetic disorder, start by gathering information specific to the genetic disorder (see Internet resources listed at end of this chapter). After reviewing the basic information about a genetic disorder, one method the school nurse can use to determine appropriate nursing diagnoses, interventions, and outcomes is to consider the body system(s) that are affected by the genetic disorder. Other chapters in this text may be useful when determining the assessment questions, nursing diagnoses, interventions, and outcomes for the IHP. It is important not to forget about psychosocial aspects of a genetic disorder, which the child (and family) may encounter.

This chapter provides an overview of genetics, reviews the inheritance patterns of genetic disorders, defines the minimum competencies that all nurses should have related to genetics, and provides a review of basic genetic resources that school nurses should be aware of.

## Review of Genetics

A basic understanding of genetics is imperative for all school nurses. There are 23 pairs of chromosomes in humans. Twenty-two of these pairs are called autosomes, and one pair is called sex chromosomes. The autosomes carry a variety of genetic information on genes, and the sex chromosomes determine gender. Two XX sex chromosomes define the female gender, and an XY set of sex chromosomes determines the male gender. Genes are the basic unit of heredity and consist of segments of deoxyribonucleic acid (DNA). There are between 50,000 and 100,000 genes in an individual's makeup. Each parent provides one half of the genetic information to an offspring. A single copy of each autosome and one sex chromosome comes from each parent. Genes that code for a characteristic may be present in a slightly different form than the matching gene from the other parent. These variations in genes are normal and are called alleles. The union of the sperm and egg, each carrying one half of the genetic makeup, unites the genetic information to code for an offspring. If the offspring obtains two genes or alleles that are identical for a given trait, the gene is considered homozygous. If the offspring obtains two genes or alleles that are slightly different, the gene is considered heterozygous. The many possible combinations of genes are what give each individual his or her unique appearance and genetic makeup.

The terms genotype and phenotype refer to the genetic information that is coded in each human. The genotype describes the genetic makeup of an individual; what the person's genes code for. The phenotype describes the physical appearance of an individual. This physical appearance may be visible to anyone or may be biochemically tested for, such as testing for blood types (Lashley, 1998).

## Review of Inheritance Patterns

Genetic disorders occur for a variety of reasons, including chromosomal abnormalities, mutation(s) in a single gene, mutation(s) in more than one gene, the interaction of more than one gene with environmental factors, and the alteration of genetic material by environmental agent(s) (Lashley, 1998). Chromosomal abnormalities include a change in the number of chromosomes or a change in chromosomal structure. Extra chromosomal disorders include Down syndrome (trisomy 21), Patau's syndrome (trisomy 13), and Edwards' syndrome (trisomy 18). A deletion of an entire chromosome (monosomy) is found in Turner's syndrome, in which one of the X chromosomes is missing (45, XO).

Changes in chromosomal structure include deletions, duplications, inversions, and translocations. The deletion refers to the loss of part of a chromosome. This deletion can occur at the end of a chromosome (terminal deletion), or it can occur within a section of the chromosome (interstitial deletion). Examples of chromosomal deletions include 5p- (5 p minus) (cri du chat syndrome), a deletion of the short arm (p arm) of the fifth chromosome; and a loss of genes from chromosome 15, which causes Angelman's syndrome and Prader-Willi syndrome (National Library of Medicine, 2004).

Duplication of chromosomal information occurs when a segment of a chromosome occurs more than the normal number of times. This allows for extra copies of genes. The effects of the duplication vary among individuals. The duplication of chromosome 15 may attribute for hypotonia, mental retardation, seizures, and some indications of autism (National Library of Medicine, 2004).

Inversions occur when a segment of a chromosome becomes rearranged in reverse order. The inversion of chromosomal material may not have a phenotypical presentation if there is not a gain or loss of chromosomal material (balanced inversion) (National Library of Medicine, 2004). On the other hand, unbalanced inversions result in the loss of chromosomal material and almost always result in an abnormal phenotype. Inversions result in a multitude of outcomes, depending on the location and extent of the inversion (National Library of Medicine, 2004).

Translocations occur when the genetic information from one chromosome is transferred to another chromosome (Lashley, 1998). Again, the phenotypical presentation may vary depending on the location and extent of translocation. Down syndrome and cri du chat may be attributed to translocation in some limited cases (National Library of Medicine, 2004).

Single gene mutations are often described as Mendelian disorders. Most commonly, these disorders follow autosomal recessive, autosomal dominant, X-linked recessive, or X-linked dominant inheritance patterns. In an autosomal recessive disorder, each parent carries a mutant gene on one of his or her autosomes. These mutant genes, when both are inherited by an offspring, allow the disorder to appear. There is an equal chance that males and females will be affected by autosomal recessive disorders. Parents who carry the same recessive autosomal gene have a 25% chance of having a child affected with the disorder with each of their offspring. There is a 50% chance that

they will pass this recessive gene on to their offspring (carrier) and a 25% chance that their offspring will not be affected and will not be a carrier. An example of an autosomal recessive disorder is cystic fibrosis.

Autosomal dominant inheritance differs in that only one mutant gene is needed for the genetic disorder to express itself. This mutant gene is again located on an autosome, so males and females are equally affected. Since the offspring obtains one gene (allele) from each parent, there is a 50% chance that every offspring will be affected by the genetic disorder if it has an autosomal dominant inheritance. An example of an autosomal dominant disorder is achondroplasia.

X-linked recessive disorders are those in which males are primarily affected. The mutant gene is located on the X chromosome, which comes from the mother (carrier) in a male offspring (XY). The chances of having an affected male offspring are 50% with each male offspring. There is a 50% chance that any female offspring will become a carrier of the X-linked recessive mutant gene. Hemophilia is an example of an X-linked recessive disorder.

X-linked dominant disorders do not occur as frequently as autosomal recessive, autosomal dominant, or X-linked recessive disorders. X-linked dominant disorders can affect males and females because the mutant gene can be located on either X chromosome of the female or on the X chromosome that the male has. Because the female has another X chromosome, it is thought that the X-linked dominant disorder does not affect the female to the same degree as the male counterparts. An example of an X-linked dominant disorder is fragile X syndrome (Lashley, 1998).

Mulitfactoral inheritance is another form of genetic inheritance. Multifactorial refers to the interaction between several genes and environmental factors. Any child with multiple congenital anomalies should be evaluated for genetic inheritance (Lashley, 1998). The variations and magnitude of all genetic inheritance is too broad to go into further detail in this chapter.

## Genetics Information All School Nurses Should Know

Anderson et al. (2000) stated, "all nurses could enhance the quality of their health care practices and improve patient outcomes by recognizing genetics as essential to a holistic view of personhood and a modern view of healthcare delivery." It is important that we as school nurses continue to increase our knowledge related to genetic conditions and also recognize our limitations. Families and individuals need to be provided with accurate information. The National Coalition for Health Professional Education in Genetics (NCHPEG) has defined a set of core competencies for all health professionals (**see Table 1**). "These competencies outline the minimum knowledge, skill, and attitudes necessary for health professionals in all disciplines...to provide high-quality care for their patients in the era of genomic medicine" (Jenkins, 2002, p. 488). More information about the NCHPEG can be found at http://www.nchpeg.org . The National Association of School Nurses (NASN) is a member of the NCHPEG organization.

The family tree or pedigree is the first step in determining if an inheritance pattern can be identified in a genetic condition. The pedigree is an inexpensive diagnostic and screening tool (Bennett, 1995) that has been noted by the American Medical Association to be the "most important genetic test of all" (as cited in Lea and Monsen, 2003; as cited in Twedell, 2003). The Pedigree Standardization Task Force (PSTF) recommended standardized pedigree nomenclature in 1995 (Bennett et al., 1995) (**see Table 2**). The pedigree construction should include at least three generations (Bennett, 1995; Lea & Monsen, 2003). The pedigree should include the name of the individual collecting the data, the name and relationship of the individual providing the information, and the date the information was obtained. Information collected related to each individual in the family should include date of birth, current health status, and/or reason for death and age at time of death. Other pertinent information related to the condition of question may be included as needed. It is important to note that gathering a family history and pedigree construction may not reveal all inheritance patterns, because some genetic disorders fall into multifactorial inheritance.

Genomics is defined by Lea and Monsen (2003, p. 76) as the "branch of genetics that studies the combined influences of multiple genes and their molecular functions that result in states of health and illness." As the future of genetics in healthcare continues to evolve, Lea and Monsen (2003, p. 76) describe three aspects of genomics that need to be incorporated into nursing practice. These three aspects are:

1. Nurses must "have current knowledge of gene function"; how gene function impacts the "mechanisms, diagnosis, and prevention of disease."
2. Nurses will "need to interpret the concepts of genetic and inherited risks and gene expression."
3. Nurses will "need to coordinate the services of a range of providers," including healthcare providers and commercial organizations that provide testing and/or support services. Support services may include, but are not limited to, a detailed interpretation of the genetic test, information related to inheritance, or counseling.

There are four functions that nurses can fulfill in the area of genetics in their nursing practice. The first of these is to identify clients and families who could benefit from genetic information and evaluation. The second is to provide advocacy for access to genetic information and healthcare. The third function for nurses to incorporate into their practice is to assist with the coordination and collaboration of care with other health professionals. The fourth function is to provide ongoing support through the dimensions of education, physical care, psychosocial care, and spiritual care (Lea, Anderson, & Monsen, 1998).

## The Role of Genetics in School Health

School nurses are not expected to become experts in genetics but rather provide the link that allows students to access appropriate services. It is essential that school nurses identify local and state resources available to accept referrals for genetic services. A listing of general resources is given at the end of this chapter. These resources do not include state and disease-specific resources, although an Internet search will reveal many state and disease-specific resources. The school nurse will need to assess family needs once the referral is made and, upon receiving genetic information, will again need to reassess the family's needs, strengths, and coping. The school nurse can play a crucial role in providing ongoing educational information as appropriate to the child and family. The school nurse can provide reassurance and suggestions for handling disease management as the child progresses through the stages of growth and development. The school nurse will play a vital role in informing educators of the basics of a genetic disorder and can assist in the development of realistic expectations for students with such disorders.

## Ethical and Legal Issues

The recognition and diagnosis of genetic conditions will provide family and healthcare providers with additional information that can optimize a child's outcome. Along with this genetic disease information come several ethical and legal considerations. The Family Educational Rights and Privacy Act (FERPA) allows an educational institution to share pertinent information with school staff who need to know (American School Health Association, 2000). The only information shared with educational personnel should be that which would directly benefit the student in the academic setting. Fibison (2001) noted several ethical and legal considerations that should be considered within the educational setting. These issues include, but are not limited to, respecting the privacy of the child and family in relation to their genetic information, determining who should have access to the student's genetic information, determining screening programs that are appropriate for the school setting, helping to determine to what extent genetic testing is taught in health education curriculum, and determining the role of the school nurse in relation to testing for adult-onset diseases that have a known genetic inheritance, such as some types of breast cancer. Ethical, Legal and Social Issues (ELSI) describes some more of the issues of concern (see Resources for web site).

## Summary

The genetic revolution will continue to offer new information for students, families, communities, and the healthcare arena. It is imperative that school nurses stay in the forefront of the genetic information and become aware of the resources that exist. School nurses do not need to fulfill the role of a genetic counselor, nor are they able to make diagnoses, but they must be knowledgeable of the ever-changing world of genetics and how it can impact students.

## References

American School Health Association. (2000). Guidelines for protecting confidential student health information. Kent, OH: Author.

Anderson, G., Monsen, R. B., Prows, C. A., Tinley, S., & Jenkins, J. (2000). Preparing the nursing profession in a genetic paradigm in health care [Electronic version]. *Nursing Outlook, 48*(1), 23–27.

Bennett, R. L. (1995, December). The genetic family history in primary care. *Genetics Northwest,10*(2-3). Retrieved May 31, 2004, from http://mchneighborhood.ichp.edu/pacnorgg/GNW/GeneticFamilyHx.html

Bennett, R. L., Steinhaus, K. A., Uhrich, S. B., O'Sullivan, C., Resta, R. G., Doyle, D., et al. (1995). Recommendations for standardized human pedigree nomenclature. *American Journal of Human Genetics, 56*(3), 745–752.

Fibison, W. (2001). Future directions in school health care: The genetic revolution. In N. Schwab & M. H. B. Gelfman (Eds.), *Legal issues in school health services: A resource for school administrators, school attorneys, school nurses* (pp. 483–488). North Branch, MN: Sunrise River Press.

National Library of Medicine. (2004, November 29) Genetics Home Reference: Your guide to understanding genetic conditions. Retrieved December 6, 2004, from http://ghr.nlm.nih.gov/ghr

Jenkins, J. (2002). Genetics competency: New directions for nursing. *AACN Clinical Issues, 13*(4), 486-491.

Lashley, F. R. (Cohen). (1998). *Clinical genetics in nursing practice* (2nd ed.). New York: Springer.

Lea, D. H., Anderson, G., & Monsen, R. B. (1998). A multiplicity of roles for genetic nursing: Building toward holistic practice. *Holistic Nursing Practice, 12*(3), 77–87.

Lea, D. H., & Monsen, R. B. (2003). Preparing nurses for the 21st century role in genomics-based health care [Electronic version]. *Nursing Education Perspectives, 24*(2), 75–80.

National Human Genome Research Institute. (2004). Retrieved May 31, 2004, from http://www.genome.gov/10001772

Twedell, D. (2003). Genomics offers opportunities for nurses [Electronic version]. *The Journal of Continuing Education in Nursing, 34*(5), 195–196.

## Resources

Centers for Disease Control: Genomics and Disease Prevention
http://www.cdc.gov/genomics/

Ethical, Legal, and Social Issues
http://www.ornl.gov/sci/techresources/Human_Genome/elsi/elsi.shtml

GeneTests
http://www.geneclinics.org or http://www.genetests.org

Genetic Alliance
http://www.geneticalliance.org/

Genetic Resources on the Web (GROW)
http://www.nih.gov/sigs/bioethics/grow.html

Genetics Home Reference: Your Guide to Understanding Genetic Conditions
http://ghr.nlm.nih.gov/ghr

International Society of Nurses in Genetics
www.isong.org

National Coalition for Health Professional Education in Genetics (NCHPEG)
www.nchpeg.org

National Human Genome Research Institute
http://www.genome.gov

National Organization for Rare Disorders
http://www.rarediseases.org/

Online Mendelian Inheritance in Man (OMIM)
http://www.ncbi.nlm.nih.gov

Rare Genetics Diseases in Children Disabilities Resources Directory:
http://www.med.nyu.edu/rgdc/disable.htm

U.S. Department of Energy of Sciences
http://www.ornl.gov/sci/techresources/Human_Genome/home.shtml

**Table 1. Core Competencies in Genetics Essential for All Health-Care Professionals**

| Purpose | The impetus for developing the ideal competencies related to genetics was to encourage health-care providers to integrate genetics knowledge, skills, and attitudes into routine health care to provide effective care to individuals and families.

The Core Competency and Curriculum Working Group of NCHPEG recommends that all health professionals possess the core competencies in genetics, as identified in this report, to enable them to integrate genetics effectively and responsibly into their current practice.

Competency in these areas represents the minimum knowledge, skills, and attitudes necessary for health professionals from all disciplines (medicine, nursing, allied health, public health, dentistry, psychology, social work, etc.) to provide patient care that involves awareness of genetic issues and concerns.

***Each health care professional should at a minimum be able to:***

• Appreciate limitations of his or her genetic expertise.
• Understand the social and psychological implications of genetic services
• Know how and when to make a referral to a genetics professional. |
|---|---|
| **Background** | During the last decade, the evolution of scientific discoveries from the study of genetics has provided information with potential for tremendous influence on health care. Understanding the role genetics plays in health and disease provides the means to integrate such information into diagnosis, prevention, and treatment of many common diseases and to improve the health of society. Genetic discoveries are already making their way into mainstream healthcare. Patients are beginning to ask providers about genetic services. Primary-care professionals face economic, institutional and professional opportunities and challenges in managing persons at risk for inherited conditions. As outlined by the Institute of Medicine Report on the Future of Public Health (IOM, 1988), public health agencies will have an increasing role in assessing the health needs of populations, working with the private sector in ensuring the quality of genetic tests and services, and evaluating the impact of interventions on medical, behavioral, and psychosocial outcomes. Ultimately, health-care providers, regardless of specialty area, role, or practice setting, will face questions about implications of genetics for their patients. The fast pace of genetic advances and the paucity of professional training in genetics leave many providers without up-to-date answers for their patients. |
| **Implementation** | It is essential that persons and groups responsible for continuing education, curriculum development, licensing, certification, and accreditation bodies for all health-care disciplines adopt these recommendations and integrate genetics content into ongoing education. The competencies provide direction for curriculum content that can be used in the design of seminars, workshops, and academic preparation. There is a need for commitment on the part of all educators to incorporate genetic information into all levels of professional education. Enhanced genetics competency will help us to meet the changing demands of the health-care system and promote human benefit as a result of discoveries in genetics and genetic medicine. Although this list may appear challenging, it is important to prepare for the reality of tomorrow and not only for the needs of today.

This document is a work in progress, because it is likely that the knowledge produced by the Human Genome Project and related activities will create an ongoing need to assess and revise expectations. Although the list is extensive, NCHPEG believes that the recommendations provide a useful tool for organizing the teaching of basic genetics in many educational settings and can be modified for a particular discipline.

Those health professionals involved in the direct provision of genetics services may require additional training to achieve an appropriately higher level of competence. Indeed, there are a number of examples of specific recommendations for training of professionals who require specialized knowledge of genetics (AAFP, 1999; ASCO, 1997; ASHG, 1995; APHMG, 1998; Fine et al, 1996; Hayflick & Eiff, 1998; Jenkins, 2000; Stephenson, 1998; & Taylor-Brown & Johnson, 1998). |

**Table 1. Core Competencies in Genetics Essential for All Health-Care Professionals**

| Recommendations | Note: Throughout this document, the term "clients" includes individuals and their sociological and biological families. |
|---|---|
| **Knowledge** | *All health professionals should understand:*<br>1.1 basic human genetics terminology<br>1.2 the basic patterns of biological inheritance and variation, both within families and within populations<br>1.3 how identification of disease-associated genetic variations facilitates development of prevention, diagnosis, and treatment options<br>1.4 the importance of family history (minimum three generations) in assessing predisposition to disease<br>1.5 the role of genetic factors in maintaining health and preventing disease<br>1.6 the difference between clinical diagnosis of disease and identification of genetic predisposition to disease (genetic variation is not strictly correlated with disease manifestation)<br>1.7 the role of behavioral, social, and environmental factors (lifestyle, socioeconomic factors, pollutants, etc.) to modify or influence genetics in the manifestation of disease<br>1.8 the influence of ethnoculture and economics in the prevalence and diagnosis of genetic disease<br>1.9 the influence of ethnicity, culture, related health beliefs, and economics in the clients' ability to use genetic information and services<br>1.10 the potential physical and/or psychosocial benefits, limitations, and risks of genetic information for individuals, family members, and communities<br>1.11 the range of genetic approaches to treatment of disease (prevention, pharmacogenomics/prescription of drugs to match individual genetic profiles, gene-based drugs, gene therapy)<br>1.12 the resources available to assist clients seeking genetic information or services, including the types of genetics professionals available and their diverse responsibilities<br>1.13 the components of the genetic-counseling process and the indications for referral to genetic specialists<br>1.14 the indications for genetic testing and/or gene-based interventions<br>1.15 the ethical, legal and social issues related to genetic testing and recording of genetic information (e.g., privacy, the potential for genetic discrimination in health insurance and employment)<br>1.16 the history of misuse of human genetic information (eugenics)<br>1.17 one's own professional role in the referral to genetics services, or provision, follow-up, and quality review of genetic services |
| **Skills** | *All health professionals should be able to:*<br>2.1 gather genetic family-history information, including an appropriate multi-generational family history<br>2.2 identify clients who would benefit from genetic services<br>2.3 explain basic concepts of probability and disease susceptibility, and the influence of genetic factors in maintenance of health and development of disease<br>2.4 seek assistance from and refer to appropriate genetics experts and peer support resources<br>2.5 obtain credible, current information about genetics, for self, clients, and colleagues<br>2.6 use effectively new information technologies to obtain current information about genetics<br>2.7 educate others about client-focused policy issues<br>2.8 participate in professional and public education about genetics<br>*Skills 2.9-2.17 delineate the components of the genetic-counseling process and are not expected of all health-care professionals. However, health professionals should be able to facilitate the genetic-counseling process and prepare clients and families for what to expect, communicate relevant information to the genetics team, and follow up with the client after genetics services have been provided. For those health professionals who choose to provide genetic-counseling services to their clients, all components of the process, as delineated in 2.9-2.17, should be performed.* |

**Table 1. Core Competencies in Genetics Essential for All Health-Care Professionals**

| | |
|---|---|
| **Skills** (continued) | 2.9 educate clients about availability of genetic testing and/or treatment for conditions seen frequently in practice<br>2.10 provide appropriate information about the potential risks, benefits, and limitations of genetic testing<br>2.11 provide clients with an appropriate informed consent process to facilitate decision making related to genetic testing<br>2.12 provide, and encourage use of, culturally appropriate, user-friendly materials/media to convey information about genetic concepts<br>2.13 educate clients about the range of emotional effects they and/or family members may experience as a result of receiving genetic information<br>2.14 explain potential physical and psychosocial benefits and limitations of gene-based therapeutics for clients<br>2.15 discuss costs of genetic services, benefits and potential risks of using health insurance for payment of genetic services, potential risks of discrimination<br>2.16 safeguard privacy and confidentiality of genetic information of clients to the extent possible<br>2.17 inform clients of potential limitations to maintaining privacy and confidentiality of genetic information |
| **Attitudes** | *All health professionals should:*<br>3.1 recognize philosophical, theological, cultural, and ethical perspectives influencing use of genetic information and services<br>3.2 appreciate the sensitivity of genetic information and the need for privacy and confidentiality<br>3.3 recognize the importance of delivering genetic education and counseling fairly, accurately, and without coercion or personal bias<br>3.4 appreciate the importance of sensitivity in tailoring information and services to clients' culture, knowledge and language level<br>3.5 seek coordination and collaboration with interdisciplinary team of health professionals<br>3.6 speak out on issues that undermine clients' rights to informed decision making and voluntary action<br>3.7 recognize the limitations of their own genetics expertise<br>3.8 demonstrate willingness to update genetics knowledge at frequent intervals<br>3.9 recognize when personal values and biases with regard to ethical, social, cultural, religious, and ethnic issues may affect or interfere with care provided to clients<br>3.10 support client-focused policies |

From *Core Competencies in Genetics Essential for all Health-Care Professionals* (2001). The National Coalition for Health Professional Education in Genetics (NCHPEG): Lutherville, MD. Available online at http://www.nchpeg.org. Reprinted with permission.

Table 2

Instructions:
— Key should contain all information relevant to interpretation of degree (e.g., define shading)
— For clinical (non-published) pedigrees, include:
   a) family names/initials, when appropriate
   b) name and title of person recording pedigree
   c) historian (person relaying family history information)
   d) date of intake/update
— Recommended order of information placed below symbol (below to lower right, if necessary):
   a) age/date of birth or age at death
   b) evaluation (see Figure 5)
   c) pedigree number (e.g., I-1, I-2 I-3)

| | Male | Female | Sex Unknown | Comments |
|---|---|---|---|---|
| 1. Individual | □ b. 1925 | ○ 30 y | ◇ 4 mo | Assign gender by phenotype. |
| 2. Affected individual | ■ | ● | ◆ | Key/legend used to define shading or other fill (e.g., hatches, dots, etc.). |
| | (partitioned) | (partitioned) | (partitioned) | With ≥2 conditions the individual's symbol should be partitioned accordingly, each segment shaded with a different fill and defined in legend. |
| 3. Multiple individuals, number known | □ 5 | ○ 5 | ◇ 5 | Number of siblings written inside symbol. (Affected individuals should not be grouped.) |
| 4. Multiple individuals, number unknown | □ n | ○ n | ◇ n | "n" used in place of "?" mark. |
| 5a. Deceased individual | ⧄ d. 35 y | ⊘ d. 4 mo | ⬗ | Use of cross (†) may be confuse with symbol for evaluated positive (+). If known, write "d" with age at death below symbol. |
| 5b. Stillbirth (SB) | ⧄ SB 28 wk | ⊘ SB 30 wk | ⬗ SB 34 wk | Birth of a dead child with gestational age noted. |
| 6. Pregnancy (P) | ▨ P LMP: 7/1/94 | Ⓟ 20 wk | ◇ P | Gestational age and karyotype (if known) below symbol. Light shading can be used for affected and defined in key/legend. |
| 7a. Proband | ■ P↗ | ● P↗ | ◈ P↗ | First affected family member coming to medical attention. |
| 7b. Consultand | □ ↗ | ○ ↗ | | Individual(s) seeking genetic counseling/testing. |

Figure 1    Common pedigree symbols, definition, and abbreviations.

Instructions:
—Symbols are smaller than standard ones and individual's line is shorter. (Even if sex is known, triangles are preferred to a small square/circle; symbol may be mistaken for symbols 1, 2, and 5a/5b of Figure 1, particularly on hand drawn pedigrees.)
—If gender and gestational age known, write below symbol in that order.

| | Male | Female | Sex Unknown | Comments |
|---|---|---|---|---|
| 1. Spontaneous abortion (SAB) | △ male | △ female | △ ECT | If ectopic pregnancy, write ECT below symbol |
| 2. Affected (SAB) | ▲ male | ▲ female | ▲ 16 wk | If gestational age known, write below symbol. Key/legend used to define shading. |
| 3. Termination of pregnancy (TOP) | ⧄ male | ⧄ female | ⧄ | Other abbreviations (e.g., TAB, VTOP,Ab) not used for sake of consistency. |
| 4. Affected TOP | ◣ male | ◣ female | ◣ | Key/legend used to define shading. |

Figure 2    Pedigree symbols and abbreviations for pregnancies not carried to term

**Table 2**

| Definitions | Comments |
|---|---|
| 1. relationship line<br>3. sibship line<br>2. line of descent<br>4. individual's lines | If possible, male partner should be to left of female partner on relationship line.<br><br>Siblings should be listed from left to right in birth order (oldest to youngest)<br><br>For pregnancies not carried to term (SABs and TOPs), the individual's line is shortened. |
| 1. Relationship line (horizontal)<br> a. Relationships | A break in a relationship line indicates the relationship no longer exists.<br>Multiple previous partners do not need to be shown if they to not affect genetic assessment. |
| b. Consanguinity | If degree of relationship not obvious from pedigree, it should be stated (e.g., third cousins) above relationship line. |
| 2. Line of descent (vertical or diagonal)<br> a. Genetic | Biologic parents shown. |
| – Twins<br>  Monozygotic  Disygotic  Unknown | A horizontal line between the symbols implies a relationship line. |
| – Family history not available/known for individual | |
| – No children by choice or reason unknown | Indicate reason, if known. |
| – Infertility<br>  vasectomy  tubal<br>  azoospermia  endometriosis | Indicate reason, if known. |
| b. Adoption<br>  in    out    by relative | Brackets used for all adoptions. Social vs. biological parents denoted by dashed and solid lines of descent, respectively. |

Figure 3   Pedigree line definitions

Definitions:
- Egg or sperm donor (D)
- Surrogate (S)
- If the woman is both the ovum donor and a surrogate, in the interest of genetic assessment, she will only be referred to as a donor (e.g., 4 and 5)
- The pregnancy symbol and its line of descent are positioned below the woman who is carring the pregnancy
- Family history can be taken on individuals, including donors, where history is known.

| Possible Reproductive Scenarios | | Comments |
|---|---|---|
| 1. Sperm donor | | Couple in which woman is carrying pregnancy using donor sperm. No relationship line is shown between the woman carrying the pregnancy and the sperm donor. For a lesbian relationship, the male partner can be substituted with a female partner. |
| 2. Ovum donor | | Couple in which woman is carrying pregnancy using donor egg(s) and partner's sperm. |
| 3. Surrogate only | | Couple whose gametes are used to impregnate another woman (surrogate) who carries the pregnancy. |
| 4. Surrogate ovum donor | | Couple in which male partner's sperm is used to inseminate a) an unrelated woman or b) a sister who is carrying the pregnancy for the couple. |
| 5. Planned adoption | | Couple contracts with a woman to carry a pregnancy using ovum of the woman carring the pregnancy and donor sperm. |

Figure 4   Assisted-reproductive-technologies symbols and definitions.

**Table 2**

Instructions:
— Evaluation (E) is used to represent clinical and/or test information on the pedigree.
    a. E is to be defined in key/legend.
    b. If more than one evaluation, use subscript ($E_1$, $E_2$, $E_3$) and define in key. May be written side by side or below each other depending on available space.
    c. Test results should be put in parentheses or defined in key/legend.
    d. If results of exam/family study/testing not documented or unavailable, may use a question mark (e.g., E?).
— Documented evaluation (∗)
    a. Asterisk is placed next to lower right edge of symbol.
    b. Use **only** if examined/evaluated by **you** or **your** research/clinical team or if the outside evaluation has been personally reviewed and verified.
— A symbol is shaded only when an individual is clinically symptomatic.
— For linkage studies, haplotype information is written below the individual. The haplotype of interest should be on left and appropriately highlighted.
— Repetitive sequences, trinucleotides and expansion numbers are written with affected allele first and placed in parentheses.
— If mutation known, identify and place in parentheses.
— Recommended order of information:
    1) age/date of birth or age at death
    2) evaluation information
    3) pedigree number (e.g., I-1, I-2, I-3)

| Definition | Symbol | Scenario | Example |
|---|---|---|---|
| 1. Documented evaluation (∗) | | Woman with normal physical exam and negative fragile X chromosome study (normal phenotype and negative test results). | E − |
| 2. Obligate carrier (will not manifest disease) | | Woman with normal physical exam and premutation for fragile X (normal phenotype and positive test results). | E+ (100n/35n) |
| 3. Asymptomatic/presymptomatic carrier (clinically unaffected at this time but could later exhibit symptoms) | | Man age 25 with normal physical exam and positive DNA test for Huntington disease (symbol filled in if/when symptoms develop). | 25 y  E+ (45n/18n) |
| 4. Uninformative study (u) | Eu | Man age 25 with normal physical exam and uninformative DNA test for Huntington disease ($E_1$) and negative brain MRI study ($E_2$). | 25 y  $E_1$u (36n/18n)  $E_2$− |
| 5. Affected individual with positive evaluation (E+) | E+ | Individual with cystic fibrosis and positive mutation study, although only one mutation has currently been identified. | E+ (ΔF508)    Eu  E+ (ΔF508/u) |
| | | 18 week male fetus with abnormalities on ultrasound and a trisomy 18 karyotype. | 18 wk  E+ (tri 18) |

Figure 5    Pedigree symbolization of genetic evaluation/testing information

## Chapter Nineteen

# Abuse and Neglect

Nancy Manzo-Mattucci

## Introduction

According to The National Center on Child Abuse and Prevention Research, an estimated 1,356 children—nearly four children each day—died in the year 2000 as a result of child abuse and neglect. Over the past 5 years, child fatalities have increased by 8% whereas other incidences of societal violence show a decline (Peddle, Wang, Diaz, & Reid, 2002).

In 1974, the federal government passed P.L. 93-247, the Child Abuse Prevention and Treatment Act (CAPTA); this legislation provides minimum guidelines that states must incorporate in their statutory definitions of child abuse and neglect. These definitions describe the acts and conditions that determine the grounds for state intervention in the protection of a child's well-being (Smith, 2003).

Each state within the United States has developed programs and policies to implement the requirements of CAPTA (Peddle et al., 2002). Although policies vary, all states within the United States mandate that school employees and administrators report child abuse and neglect to child protective services. Any employee, volunteer, student teacher, or student intern who knowingly fails to report suspected cases of child abuse or neglect will be held accountable by local government and licensing agencies of their state (Crenshaw, Crenshaw, & Lichtenberg, 1995).

### Pathophysiology

Horton and Cruise (2001) describe five major types of child maltreatment: physical abuse, sexual abuse, emotional abuse, neglect, and witnessing domestic violence. A child may experience any of the forms of abuse separately, but often more than one type of maltreatment occurs simultaneously.

### Physical Abuse

Physical abuse is inflicting a physical injury upon a child. This may include burning, hitting, punching, shaking, kicking, beating, or otherwise harming a child. The injury may be intentional or may be the consequence of a parent's loss of self-control. There are also occurrences when a parent intends to cause pain but not extensive injuries. The abuser usually acknowledges the wrongful act and attempts to hide the abuse. Children are often coached to give excuses for obvious injuries and some-

times are threatened with further maltreatment if the child reveals the truth to others.

### Sexual Abuse

Sexual abuse is inappropriate adolescent or adult sexual behavior with a child. The act may include sexual contact with the child (e.g., fondling, oral sex, digital penetration, or intercourse). Noncontact sexual acts (e.g., being forced to watch the perpetrator in a sexual act) may also occur. The wide use of the Internet in today's society has expanded the medium for sex offenders, who now have easy access to children and adolescents. It is important to be aware that emotionally needy children with poor boundaries must be closely supervised when using the Internet, because these children are most vulnerable to abusive, leering sex offenders seeking to harm children.

### Emotional Abuse

Emotional abuse involves maltreatment of a child by use of behavior that is rejecting, degrading, terrorizing, isolating, corrupting, exploiting, or denying of emotion. Children and adolescents who suffer other forms of child abuse are also scarred with emotional abuse because is affects them psychologically. Although difficult to detect, it is possible that a child may suffer solely from emotional abuse. Children believe what their parents say to be true, and it affects their self-esteem and self-worth.

### Neglect

Neglect is the chronic failure to provide for a child's basic needs, such as health, hygiene, nutrition, safety, education, and emotional care. Although most cases of neglect are chronic in nature, it is important to note that one single act of negligence may have severe consequences. For example, leaving a young child left unattended in an apartment with burning candles can result in a fire inflicting severe burns or even death, and therefore the child becomes a victim of neglect.

### Witnessing Domestic Violence

This category has recently been recognized as a category of child maltreatment. Children who witness violent altercations at home are unintended victims. Although not physically harmed during the violent episodes, children are often haunted by thoughts and images that they have witnessed. They may experience difficulty sleeping at night and concentrating at school.

## Management

It is imperative that school communities address the issue of child abuse and neglect because children who survive this maltreatment may be at greater risk for problems such as poor academic achievement, drug abuse, teenage pregnancy, and criminal behavior (U.S. Department of Health and Human Services, 2003). Because of their daily interaction with students, teachers are often the first person to notice signs of potential abuse or neglect. There may be a physical marking such as a bruise, burn, or laceration on a student to initiate a referral to the school nurse. A report of suspected child abuse or neglect by a school must be based on collaborative information. One bruise isn't typically considered suspicious unless accompanied by other signs, such as inability to concentrate in school, sudden decline in academic achievement, social withdrawal from peers, or a disclosure of abuse by the victim. Open disclosure by a student is not very common. Children often feel ashamed or embarrassed by their home situation. Internalized feelings that the abuse is brought on by their own shortcomings are common, and children often try to protect the adult who is inflicting the abuse. It is at this time that physical assessment and interviewing skills become important tools for school nurses to identify potential child abuse and neglect situations. School nurses are in a unique position to develop trusting relationships with students under their care because students identify the school nurse as an adult concerned with their health and wellness.

It is important to note that although school personnel are often in the position to detect potential child abuse and neglect owing to their consistent contact with students, they are not professional investigative agents. All potential cases of child abuse and neglect should be immediately reported to child protective agencies (Horton & Cruise, 2001).

The following information is provided to assist the school nurse with assessing for abuse and neglect, handling disclosure, and making appropriate reports to state child protective services. All school personnel also need to be knowledgeable in the management of psychological behaviors related to abuse and neglect, such as grief, fear, anxiety, depression, peer relations, and violent behaviors toward self and others.

When interviewing a child, it is important to be in a private nonthreatening environment. Children are less likely to disclose abuse if they feel that others may overhear their comments. Remain calm and attentive throughout the conversation, and keep an open mind. Refrain from showing emotions of horror or disgust. Acknowledge and validate the child's feelings without guessing or assuming what the student is feeling. Use developmentally appropriate language and be sure to note the child's nonverbal language. Be clear about confidentiality limits at the onset of the interview; if students ask you not to tell anyone their secret, you must be honest.

Explain that if they are being hurt you will have to tell other adults in order to help them. This may cause a child not to disclose abuse initially but may ultimately develop a trusting relationship and prompt a more complete disclosure at a later time. If a child does disclose abusive information, do not have the child repeat the story to other school staff members. Once enough information is gathered to sufficiently suspect abuse, stop the interview and make a call to child protective services. It is important to explain to the child what steps will then be taken. Children can be told that a worker will come out to talk to them. If sexual abuse has been disclosed, you may explain that a police officer may come to speak to them, but assure them that they have done nothing wrong (Horton & Cruise, 2001).

Document the information obtained during the interview in as much detail as possible. Be sure to note non-verbal language. Record the student's name, date of birth, address, parent's name, date, time, and to whom initial disclosure was made. Quote student's statement verbatim about maltreatment; include dates and times of alleged instances of abuse/neglect. Note the student's emotional state during interview (e.g., distress, reluctance, fearful) Document the name of the child protective agency worker that processed intake information. Prepare the written documentation according to school policy and procedures.

Independent initiative is needed on the part of the school nurse to best meet the needs of the child and the abusing family. Collaborative skills must be utilized with professional staff members in the school, other healthcare providers and/or social welfare workers to deal effectively with child-abusing families (Paavilainen, Kurki, & Paunonen, 2000). The ultimate goal of referral for mental health services is to increase the probability of follow-through by the family and treatment for the abused child. School-based mental health services may be a beneficial option when available. It is important to note that school nurses should provide follow-through services for families because of the high probability that services may never be obtained. Provide assistance in finding agencies and mental health professionals. Follow up with telephone reminders, and have guardians sign consent forms to allow the school to communicate with the mental health professionals. Such strategies will assist families to find appropriate professional mental health care, improve and maintain family participation in treatment, and help the student feel supported (Horton & Cruise, 2001).

## Prevention: Primary, Secondary, and Tertiary

Prevention of child abuse and neglect through education is an activity that school nurses, guidance counselors, teachers, and administrators can and should address in the school environment. The ultimate goal of prevention efforts is to support family needs and spare children and parents the emotional and physical trauma related to child abuse and neglect. Horton and Cruise (2001) and Wold (1981) describe the following strategies for primary, secondary, and tertiary prevention of abuse and neglect.

Primary prevention activities are aimed at the general community. Activities that can be implemented or initiated at the school level include:

- DARE (Drug Abuse Resistance Education) Programs
- Community/parent education programs to develop parenting skills with topics such as child development and expectations, discipline techniques, and health, hygiene, and nutritional needs of children
- Sexual-abuse prevention programs offered by local police departments
- School-wide peer mediation or conflict resolution programs

Secondary prevention activities facilitate early detection of maltreatment and target at-risk populations. Activities that can be implemented or initiated at the school level include:

- Training programs for school staff members about detecting and reporting child abuse and neglect

- Student education programs to educate and empower students to identify maltreatment and seek help
- Before- and after-school programs for families in need.
- Parent support groups
- Family life education classes for students

Tertiary prevention activities are specific to families who already have experienced child maltreatment. The goal of tertiary prevention is to decrease the negative consequences of abuse and neglect and prevent further maltreatment episodes. Activities that can be implemented or initiated at the school level include:

- School-based mental health services
- Individual healthcare plans
- School-based anger management, social skills, or self-esteem programs

## Individualized Healthcare Plan

### Assessment

*History*

- Child abuse and neglect within this family
- Parent(s) abused as child/children
- Family crisis or dysfunctional relationships within the family system
- Student-reported incident of child abuse or neglect
- Parent-verbalized role inadequacy frustrations or inability to meet child's needs

*Current Status and Management*

Warning signs of abuse and neglect:

- nervousness around adults
- aggression toward other children or adults
- drowsiness during school hours
- inability to concentrate
- sudden, dramatic changes in personality or activities
- acting-out sexually that is inappropriate for age
- low self-esteem
- depression
- suicide attempts or ideations
- poor personal hygiene
- enuresis
- encopresis
- report of frequent accidents or injuries
- evidence of physical abuse, such as bruises, burns, welts, lacerations, or abrasions
- repeated orthopedic fractures

Assess for physical markings consistent with identifiable characteristics of causative agent:

- cigarette burn
- hanger
- belt buckle
- strap marks
- wooden spoon
- loop from rope or cord
- teeth

- hand, fist, finger
- chain
- iron

Evidence of poor parenting skills:
- inadequate child health maintenance, unsafe home environment, inadequate child-care provisions
- frequently missed scheduled parent-teacher conferences
- inadequate healthcare evidenced by immunization status, untreated illnesses
- frequent unexcused student absenteeism
- poor parent-child interactions
- student-reported sexual contact with an adult
- evidence of pregnancy or sexually transmitted disease

*Self-Care*
- Signs of role reversal, student acting in a parent role to self or others
- Student's ability to carry out person hygiene
- Student's knowledge of personal body safety

*Psychosocial status*
Assess psychological behaviors of student:
- lack of interest in fun activities
- chronic sullen mood
- socially withdrawn from peers
- low self-esteem
- impaired trust
- fearful response to others or situations

*Academic Issues*
- Poor school achievement and failing grades
- Retention and/or referral for special education services
- Truancy and/or increased absenteeism
- Difficulty concentrating on schoolwork
- Behavior problems with peers or staff members
- Lack of parental support and encouragement for school activities
- Teacher concerns regarding student's academic performance, home situation, and socialization

## Nursing Diagnoses (N.D.) (NANDA, 2003)

*Physical*
N.D. 1 Disturbed sleep pattern (NANDA 00095) related to:
- grief
- fear
- anxiety
- depression
N.D. 2 Risk for infection (NANDA 00004) related to:
- traumatized tissue
- sexual penetration or force
- altered nutritional state
- unfulfilled basic needs
N.D. 3 Risk for trauma (NANDA 00038) related to:
- lack of safety precautions and/or parental supervision
- unsafe home environment
- history of physical, emotional, or sexual maltreatment
N.D. 4 Impaired skin integrity (NANDA 00046) related to:
- inflicted trauma
- sexual penetration or force
- altered nutritional state
- hyperthermia/hypothermia

**N.D. 5** Acute pain (NANDA 00132) related to:
- inflicted trauma
- impaired skin integrity
- sexual penetration or force
- severe disciplinary measures
- unsafe home environment
- infection
- altered nutritional state
- unfulfilled basic needs
- hyperthermia/hypothermia

**N.D. 6** Imbalanced nutrition: Less than body requirements (NANDA 0002) related to:
- physical, emotional, or sexual maltreatment
- post-trauma syndrome
- willful neglect
- unfulfilled basic needs

**N.D. 7** Risk for suicide (NANDA 00150) related to:
- history of physical, emotional, or sexual maltreatment
- powerlessness
- fear/anxiety
- depression
- social isolation
- poor family relationships
- inadequate support systems

*Developmental*

**N.D. 8** Delayed growth and development (NANDA 00111) related to:
- inadequate caretaking
- indifference and inconsistent responsiveness of caretaker
- environmental and stimulation deficiencies
- sexual abuse

**N.D. 9** Impaired social interaction (NANDA 00052) related to:
- physical, emotional, or sexual maltreatment
- post-trauma syndrome
- self-concept disturbance
- inadequate support systems
- unfulfilled basic needs
- fear and anxiety

**N.D. 10** Social isolation (NANDA 00053) related to:
- physical, emotional, or sexual maltreatment
- post-trauma syndrome
- self-concept disturbance
- inadequate support systems
- unfulfilled basic needs
- fear and anxiety

**N.D. 11** Ineffective protection (NANDA 00043) related to:
- developmental age
- powerlessness/fear
- altered nutritional state
- impaired parenting
- chronic low self-esteem
- lack of knowledge regarding personal body protection

**N.D. 12** Risk for other directed violence (NANDA 00138) related to:
- history of physical, emotional, or sexual maltreatment
- history of witnessing domestic violence
- cognitive impairment
- negative role-modeling

*Psychosocial*

**N.D. 13** Powerlessness (NANDA 00125) related to:
- physical, emotional, or sexual maltreatment
- self-concept disturbance
- inadequate support systems
- unfulfilled basic needs
- fear and anxiety

**N.D. 14** Anxiety (NANDA 00146) related to:
- physical, emotional, or sexual maltreatment
- post-trauma syndrome
- self-concept disturbance
- inadequate support systems
- powerlessness
- unfulfilled basic needs
- threat of injury or death

**N.D. 15** Fear (NANDA 00148) related to:
- physical, emotional, or sexual maltreatment
- post-trauma syndrome
- self-concept disturbance
- inadequate support systems
- unfulfilled basic needs
- threat of injury or death

**N.D. 16** Chronic low self-esteem (NANDA 00119) related to:
- physical, emotional, or sexual maltreatment
- post-trauma syndrome
- self-concept disturbance
- inadequate support systems
- unfulfilled basic needs
- fear and anxiety

**N.D. 17** Disturbed body image (NANDA 00118) related to:
- physical, emotional, or sexual maltreatment
- post-trauma syndrome
- self-concept disturbance
- inadequate support systems
- unfulfilled basic needs

**N.D. 18** Rape trauma syndrome (NANDA 00142) related to forced sexual maltreatment.

**N.D. 19** Post-trauma syndrome (NANDA 00141) related to:
- physical, emotional, or sexual maltreatment
- witnessing domestic violence

*Cognitive*

**N.D. 20** Impaired parenting (NANDA 00056) related to:
- presence of stressor (e.g., financial problems, legal issues, family crisis)
- role strain
- poor problem-solving skills
- social isolation
- history of being abused
- lack of family relationships
- lack of value of parenthood
- lack of knowledge about child health maintenance and development
- unrealistic expectations for child, self, or others
- poor communication skills
- history of substance abuse
- history of disability or mental illness

**N.D. 21** Ineffective role performance (NANDA 00055) related to:
- family conflict
- stress and conflict
- inadequate support systems
- lack of knowledge regarding role skills
- substance abuse
- role dissatisfaction or overload

## Goals

The student will report any physical, emotional, or sexual maltreatment to a responsible adult. (N.D. 1–21)
The student will identify individually appropriate interventions to promote sleep. (N.D. 1)
The student will show signs of wound healing and improved skin integrity. (N.D. 2, 4, 5)
The student will manage pain/discomfort successfully during school hours. (N.D. 5)
The student will meet nutritional needs while in school. (N.D. 6, 8)
The student will perform physical, social, and/or communicative skills appropriate to chronological age and cognitive abilities. (N.D. 8)
The student will perform self-care and self-control activities appropriate for chronological age. (N.D. 8)
The student will refrain from violent behavior toward self and others while at school. (N.D. 7, 9, 12)
The student will develop and maintain at least two friendships with peers. (N.D. 9, 10, 21)
The student will develop and utilize emergency plan when in presence of danger. (N.D. 11, 20)
The student will develop and maintain positive self-esteem, self-concept, and body image. (N.D. 13–19)
The student will verbalize relief of anxiety and adaptation to body image. (N.D. 13–19)
The student will develop an effective social support system. (N.D. 3, 7, 9, 10, 11, 13–21)
The student will verbalize feelings regarding family relationships, home environment, and maltreatment issues. (N.D. 7, 9, 10, 13–21)
The student will achieve academic success appropriate to chronological age and cognitive abilities. (N.D. 14, 16, 21)

## Nursing Interventions

Report any actual or suspected case of child abuse or neglect to child protective services in accordance with state laws and school district policies. (N.D. 1–21)
Administer analgesics as ordered. (N.D. 5)
Coordinate interview of student by child protective services or police while student is in school if appropriate. (N.D. 1–21)
Explain to student what events will occur after referral is made to child protective services. (N.D. 13–15)
Remain with student to provide support during interview with child protective services when appropriate. (N.D. 13–15)
Perform physical assessment of student and document findings in a confidential file according to school district policy. (N.D. 1–8)
Provide first aid for injuries. (If a child reports sexual maltreatment, do not provide first aid or disturb genital area; it may interfere with investigative procedure.) (N.D. 2–5)
Protect any potential evidence from disturbance (e.g., clothing containing blood, semen, or body fluids, objects used to inflict injury) (N.D. 1–21)
Arrange for medical treatment of injuries. (N.D. 2–5)
Provide emotional support for student. (N.D. 5, 13–19)
Develop and maintain a trusting therapeutic relationship with student. (N. D. 13–19)
Assure student that maltreatment was not his/her fault and encourage verbalization of feelings. (N.D. 8–19)
Provide a safe haven for student in the health suite when the stresses of maltreatment cause anxiety and dysfunctional behavior. (N.D. 7, 10–16, 18, 19)
Teach student health maintenance skills: nutrition, care of wounds, sleep-promoting behaviors, stress management, and personal body protection. (N.D. 1–7)
Assist child with development of emergency plan to use when in a physically dangerous situation. (N.D. 3, 11, 13)
Encourage and assist student to develop peer relationships. (9, 10, 13, 14, 16)
Be knowledgeable of current living situation of student (returned to home, living with relatives, or placed in foster care). (N.D. 14, 15, 19, 20)
Refer student to guidance counselor for counseling sessions when offered as a service. (N.D. 9–19, 21)
Refer student to support group for children dealing with abuse/neglect. (N.D. 9–19, 21)

Refer family to social service programs for additional interventions. (N.D. 11, 20, 21)
Support family involvement in mental health treatment, counseling, and support groups. (N.D. 14, 18–21)
Develop supportive relationship with family. (N.D. 20)
Maintain a nonjudgmental attitude with family. (N.D. 20)
Continue to assess student for further maltreatment after initial incident. (N.D. 3, 11, 20)
Refer student for academic support when grades are affected by home situation. (N.D.14, 16, 21)

## Expected Student Outcomes

The student will:
- Receive family interventions from child protective services. (N.D. 1–21)
- Understand and be able to report any further maltreatment to a responsible adult. (N.D. 1–21)
- Maintain therapeutic trusting relationships with school professionals. (N.D. 9, 11, 13–19)
- Report sleeping comfortably through the night. (N.D. 1)
- Report relief of pain/discomfort during school hours. (N.D. 5)
- Maintain/resolve wound healing. (N.D. 2-6)
- Exhibit appropriate behavior toward others in school. (N.D. 7, 9, 12)
- Develop and maintain peer relationships in school. (N.D. 9, 10, 21)
- Utilize emergency plan in the presence of danger. (N.D. 11)
- Verbalize positive feelings of self. (N.D. 13–19)
- Utilize meditative techniques and breathing exercises to decrease anxiety, fear, and powerlessness. (N.D. 13–19)
- Report a decrease in anxiety, fear, and powerlessness. (N.D. 13–19)
- Participate in school activities with peers. (N.D. 8–19, 21)
- Identify at least three responsible adults to utilize as a support system. (N.D. 3, 7, 9–21)
- Participate in school-based counseling when offered as a service. (N.D. 9–19, 21)
- Achieve and maintain academic success appropriate to age and cognitive abilities. (N.D. 14, 16, 17, 21)

## Case Study

Susie is a 9-year-old student in Ms. White's third grade classroom. She is a quiet child who rarely participates in class and has few friends. Susie often comes to school with dirty, ill-fitting clothing and unkempt hair and she has poor personal hygiene. Susie's grades have always been average, but recently Ms. White has noticed a decrease in her ability to concentrate in class and complete assignments. She is now failing math, reading, and social studies. Today in school Ms. White notices that Susie is limping and walking slowly while traveling to and from classes. When questioned by her teacher, Susie becomes very nervous and stutters to find an answer for why she is limping. Ms. White asks Susie to see the school nurse.

Susie reports to the nurse that she fell and hurt her leg yesterday at home. Upon assessment, the school nurse notes several welts and bruises bilaterally on Susie's posterior calves and thighs. The injuries are suspicious and appear to be inflicted by a wide strap or belt. The school nurse closes her office door and asks Susie how she received the bruises on her legs. While looking down at her wringing hands Susie begins to cry and explains that she didn't mean to upset her mother again. She says that she tries to be good and do everything that her mother expects her to do but sometimes she forgets things, and she promises not to do it again.

The school nurse sits down next to Susie and offers her comfort by holding her hand and explains that she did not do anything to deserve being physically abused by her mother. When questioned further, Susie reports that her mother punishes her by hitting her with a strap. The school nurse explains that she is there to help her and they will have to call a social worker to come and visit with Susie and that she will help her with her family problems.

# Abuse/Neglect Issues

| Assessment Data | Nursing Diagnosis | Goals | Nursing Interventions | Expected Outcomes |
|---|---|---|---|---|
| Welts/bruises noted on bilateral posterior calves and thighs.<br><br>Student limps while walking to class. | Acute pain related to inflicted trauma. | Susie will manage pain/discomfort. | Provide first-aid for injuries.<br><br>Arrange for medical management of injuries.<br><br>Administer analgesics as ordered. | Susie reports a decrease in pain/discomfort. |
| Student reports that mother inflicted injuries with strap. | Impaired parenting related to unrealistic expectations of child. | Susie will develop and utilize emergency plan when in the presence of danger.<br><br>Susie will verbalize feelings regarding maltreatment. | Report incident to child protection services. Follow state law and school policy.<br><br>Remain with Susie during interview and provide emotional support. | Susie receives family intervention services. |
| Student verbalizes inappropriate feelings of guilt related to physical maltreatment. | Chronic low self-esteem related to physical and emotional abuse by parent. | Susie will develop and maintain positive self-esteem. | Explain to Susie that she did not do anything to deserve such maltreatment.<br><br>Refer Susie to support group for children dealing with abuse/neglect.<br><br>Refer Susie to school guidance counselor for one-on-one intervention. | Susie will verbalize feelings of positive self-worth.<br><br>Susie will participate in counseling on a regular basis. |
| Student has few friends and rarely participates in class or school activities. | Social isolation related to post-trauma syndrome and self-concept disturbance. | Susie will develop and maintain at least two friendships with peers. | Provide counseling to develop self-esteem.<br><br>Encourage Susie to participate in school activities.<br><br>Have Susie participate in social skills group with guidance counselor. | Susie develops and maintains peer relationships in school.<br><br>Susie participates in classroom activities and joins one school-sponsored activity.<br><br>Susie's grades will improve within one marking period. |

| Assessment Data | Nursing Diagnosis | Goals | Nursing Interventions | Expected Outcomes |
|---|---|---|---|---|
| Student is failing three subjects. | Ineffective role performance related to stress of dysfunctional family interactions. | Susie will achieve academic success appropriate for age and cognitive level. | Refer student for after-school academic support, if available.<br><br>Utilize peer tutoring and peer support.<br><br>Refer student for child student team evaluation if appropriate.<br><br>Provide Susie with encouragement for hard work and achievement. | Susie's grades will improve within one marking period. |

# References

Crenshaw, W., Crenshaw, L., & Lichtenberg, J. (1995). When educators confront child abuse: An analysis of the decision to report. *Child Abuse & Neglect, 19*(9), 1095–1113.

Horton, C., & Cruise, T. (2001). Child abuse and neglect: *The school's response.* New York: Guilford Press.

NANDA International. (2003). *Nursing diagnoses: Definitions & classification 2003-2004.* Philadelphia: Author.

Paavilainen, E., Kurki, P., & Paunonen, M. (2000). School nurses' operational modes and ways of collaborating in caring for child abusing families in Finland. *Journal of Clinical Nursing, 9,* 742–750.

Peddle, N., Wang, C., Diaz, J., & Reid, R. (2002). *Current trends in child abuse prevention and fatalities: The 2000 fifty state survey.* Retrieved January 29, 2004, from http://www.preventchildabuse.org

Smith, S. (2003). Mandatory reporting of child abuse and neglect. Retrieved February 1, 2004, from http://www.smith-lawfirm.com/mandatory_reporting.htm

U.S. Department of Health and Human Services, Administration on Children, Youth and Families. *Twelve years of child maltreatment 2001* (Washington, DC: US Government Printing Office, 2003). Online summary of findings retrieved January 29, 2004, from http://www.acf.hhs.gov/programs/cb/publications/cm01/outcover.htm

Wold, J. (1981). *School nursing: A framework for practice.* North Branch, MN: Sunrise River Press.

# Bibliography

Besharov, D. J. (1990). *Recognizing child abuse: A guide for the concerned.* New York: The Free Press.

Doenges, M., Moorhouse, M., & Geissler-Murr, A. (2002). *Nurse's pocket guide: Diagnoses, interventions, and rationales* (8th ed.). Philadelphia: Davis.

Kalichman, S. C. (1999). *Mandated reporting of suspected child abuse: Ethics, law and policy.* Washington, DC: American Psychological Association.

Kenny, M. (2001). Child abuse reporting: Teachers' perceived deterrents. *Child Abuse & Neglect, 25*(1), 81–92.

Macdonald, G. (2001). Effective interventions for child abuse and neglect: An evidenced-based approach to planning and evaluating interventions. Oxford, England: John Wiley & Sons.

National Association of School Nurses. (Revised 2003). *Position Statement: Child abuse and neglect.* Scarborough, ME: Author;

Potts, N., & Mandleco, B. L. (2002). *Pediatric nursing: Caring for children and their families.* NewYork: Delmar.

Roberts, A. R. (2000). *Crisis intervention handbook: Assessment, treatment and research.* Oxford, England: Oxford University Press.

Saewyc, E. M., Pettingell, S., Magee, L. L. 2003: The prevalence of sexual abuse among Adolescents in school. *Journal of School Nursing, 19*(5), pp. 266–272.

Wong, D. L., Hockenberry, M. J., Wilson, D., Winkelstein, M. L., Kline, N. E., Hockbery-Eaton, M. (2003). *Wong's nursing care of infants and children* (7th ed.). St. Louis: Mosby.

Yanowitz,, K., Monte, E., & Tribble, J. (2003). Teachers' beliefs about the effects of child abuse. *Child Abuse & Neglect, 27*(5), 483-488.

## Resources

U.S. Department of Health and Human Services
Administration for Children and Families
National Clearinghouse on Child Abuse and Neglect Information
http://nccanch.acf.hhs.gov/index.cfm

Centers for Disease Control
National Center for Injury Prevention and Control
http://www.cdc.gov/ncipc/

U.S. National Library of Medicine
Links to articles regarding child abuse and neglect.
http://www.nlm.nih.gov/medlineplus/childabuse.html

Child Abuse Prevention Services
http://www.kidsafe-caps.org/bullies.html

Child Help USA
http://www.childhelpusa.org/

Cornell Law School Legal Information Institute
Chapter 67: Child Abuse Prevention and Treatment and Adoption Reform
http://www4.law.cornell.edu/uscode/42/ch67.html

National Child Abuse Hotline
    1-800- 4-A-CHILD

Prevent Child Abuse America
    http://www.preventchildabuse.org

# Chapter Twenty

# Attention Deficit Hyperactivity Disorder

Colleen J. Duffy

## Introduction

Attention deficit hyperactivity disorder (ADHD) has recently become a much discussed issue in educational arenas. It is a chronic medical condition with a behavioral component that impacts the child, the child's family, and the child's school. School nurses are on the forefront advocating for the student, educating the family, and assisting the classroom teachers and staff in managing the student's behavior to maximize academic achievements. Although ADHD impacts a student's education, it differs from learning disabilities in that "learning disabilities affect the brain's ability to learn, whereas ADHD interferes with the individual's *availability* for learning" (Sekleman, 2002, p. 272).

## Pathophysiology

Attention deficit hyperactivity disorder causes a disruption in the individual's ability to self-regulate and organize behaviors in response to environmental stimuli (Stein, Efron, Schiff, & Glanzman, 2002). The American Psychiatric Association defines ADHD as "a persistent pattern of inattention and/or hyperactivity-impulsivity that is more frequently displayed and more severe than is typically observed in individuals at a comparable level of development" (2000, p. 85). There are three subtypes of ADHD: (1) ADHD inattentive type, where the child is primarily easily distracted, but generally not impulsive or hyperactive, (2) ADHD hyperactive-impulsive type, where the child has increased activity levels, and (3) ADHD combined type, where the child exhibits mixed behaviors (Lundholm-Brown & Dildy, 2001). The characteristics of ADHD may be displayed differently among individuals, both in terms of demonstrated behaviors and the severity of the behaviors. It is a disorder that is primarily diagnosed in children, but often continues into adulthood. Children affected by ADHD may exhibit distractibility, agitation, aggression, increased activity levels, a diminished ability to follow directions, poor social skills, academic difficulties, and a higher incidence of accidents and injury than other children.

While the exact cause of ADHD is still unknown, several contributing factors have been identified. Genetics, specifically an inherited central nervous system dysfunction involving deficiencies in the neurotransmitters dopamine and norepinephrine, is one suggested cause. This theory notes that a decrease in the aforementioned neurotransmitters leads to problems sustaining attention, and therefore contributes to learning and behavioral difficulties (Sekleman, 2002). Another contributing factor may be traumatic brain injury, sustained at any point in a child's development, including the prenatal period. Maternal substance abuse during pregnancy, prematurity, complications at delivery, lead poisoning, seizure disorders, and thyroid disorders may all contribute to brain injury (Sekleman). An educational-cultural model of ADHD proposed by Ludholm-Brown and Dildy (2001) suggests that factors such as living with a guardian who is a relative or foster parent; insufficient parental supervision, attention, and guidance; a history of neglect or abuse; a change in family structure; poor social relationships; poverty; exposure to violence; sexual promiscuity and profanity; and continued exposure to today's fast-paced entertainment media may all contribute to the behaviors seen with ADHD.

ADHD is diagnosed according to guidelines set forth by the American Psychiatric Association (2000). The guidelines delineate characteristic behaviors that fall under the headings hyperactivity-impulsivity and inattention. A student must demonstrate six or more symptoms of hyperactivity-impulsivity and six or more symptoms of inattention. These should be present for 6 months or longer and be present to such a degree that they are considered maladaptive or are inconsistent with the child's developmental level. They should occur in two or more settings, such as home and school, and in some cases impairment should be noted before 7 years of age. The most important diagnostic criterion is that the symptoms must cause an impairment in functioning, in either the social, occupational, or academic arena. A child may not be diagnosed with ADHD if there is no functional impairment, even if the child meets all of the other criteria. The American Academy of Pediatrics (AAP) (2002) has recommended that the evaluation for ADHD be initiated by the child's pediatrician. Information regarding the age at onset of symptoms, the duration of symptoms, and the degree of impairment should be collected directly from the child's family and school. In addition, the child should be evaluated for potentially coexisting conditions, both physical and mental.

ADHD may occur alone or in conjunction with other disorders. It is often associated with learning disorders and tic disorders such as Tourette's syndrome. It has also been noted that children with a primary diagnosis of conduct disorder (CD), oppositional defiant disorder (ODD), and bipolar disorder (BD) often also have ADHD (Sekleman, 2002). However, it is important to note that a primary diagnosis of ADHD does not mean that a child will also have CD, ODD, or BD.

## Psychosocial Impact

Children diagnosed as having ADHD or other psychiatric disorders often face significant challenges socializing at school and in the community (Panacek & Dunlap, 2003). Children with attention problems have difficulty distinguishing important information from irrelevant information and therefore miss important social and academic cues. The distractible nature of children with ADHD leads others to believe that the child is not paying attention to what he or she is saying or doing, when in fact, the child is trying to pay attention to that and more. Poor social skills, coupled with impulsive behavior, contribute to the alienation of others, rejection by peers, and subsequent low self-esteem (Houck, King, Tomlinson Vrabel, & Wecks, 2002).

In addition to having intrinsic social difficulties, children with ADHD may be placed in separate classrooms or schools, depending on the severity of the disorder, also influencing the child's ability to develop positive social networks. Isolation by way of special education placement may restrict the child from participating in integrated activities, thereby limiting the child's social network and providing the student few opportunities to develop and practice positive and appropriate social skills (Panacek & Dunlap, 2003).

The demands of a child with ADHD also impact the child's family. In some cases, unpredictable behavior may cause a child's parent/guardian to feel like he or she is constantly on guard. It is often difficult for the parent/guardian to maintain quality relationships and equity with the other children in the home. Both these and the changes in routine to accommodate the behavior, trips to the doctor, counselor, school meetings, and so on, can lead to the physical and emotional exhaustion of the caregiver. In addition, the child's poor behavior is often misunderstood and not tolerated by extended family and friends. This may contribute to the social isolation of the family (Fox, Vaughn, Wyatte, & Dunlap, 2002).

Finally, recent changes in disability law have caused school districts to revise protocols that determine student eligibility for special education services and accommodations. If the symptoms of ADHD are severe enough to interfere with the child's education, that child may be eligible for special education services under the Individuals with Disabilities Education Act (IDEA). When the impairment is not severe enough to meet the criteria set forth under IDEA, the child may still be eligible for accommodations under Section 504 of the Rehabilitation Act of 1973. This prohibits schools that receive federal funding from discriminating against the child on the basis of a disability. The school must make appropriate accommodations within the classroom to assist the child in meeting his or her academic potential. Both pieces of legislation may cause great expenses of energy, time and money to personnel within the school district.

## Management

There are a great number of approaches to managing the behaviors of a child with ADHD. Treatment approaches may be nonpharmacologic or pharmacologic in nature. In many cases, a combination of methods brings about the most effective change in behavior. Nonpharmacologic interventions include behavior modification programs, social skills training, and parent and teacher training programs. Pharmacologic treatment involves the use of medication to manage the disorder. Regardless of the chosen method, all approaches should be comprehensive, establish goals, and involve the child, the child's parents/guardians, and the school (Ludholm-Brown & Dildy, 2001). An understanding of the family, their general lifestyle, and environmental considerations will be most helpful in developing an effective treatment plan that the family can implement and follow through with (Fox et al., 2002). Regular communication between the home and school will ensure continuity and consistency in the chosen treatment plan.

Behavior modification may be accomplished in several ways. Caregivers may utilize interventions to elicit positive behaviors and/or token reinforcement systems. Interventions to elicit positive behavior include communicating clear and simple expectations to the child, praising positive behaviors while ignoring negative ones, and utilizing time out for negative behaviors when they become disruptive (Garber, Garber, & Spizman, 1996). Praise for positive behaviors and reprimands for negative behavior should be behavior-specific, administered with each incident of the behavior, and occur immediately following demonstration of the behavior (Flick, 1998). For example, a teacher may praise a child by telling him, "Joseph, I like the way you stayed in your seat and raised your hand to ask for help."

Token reinforcement systems may be implemented at home or in school. They should be simple and target only one or two behaviors at a time. The rules for earning tokens should be positive and simple. Tokens should be given as soon as the desired behavior is demonstrated. There should be a structured time for students to redeem tokens for a meaningful reward or activity (Garber et al., 1996). Reinforcements should be of interest to the child, such as a few extra minutes of computer time or free time, and should be rotated often enough to keep the student interested in earning them (Flick, 1998). A brief example of a token reinforcement plan follows: A child with ADHD has difficulty completing simple assignments during the assigned period. An appropriate goal would be for him to complete the majority of the assignment for each class period. He would then be rewarded with a sticker at the end of each class period that he is able to complete the assignment. He may be given a more meaningful reward, such as 15 minutes of free time at the end of the day, if a specified number of stickers are earned that day. Once the child is able to demonstrate the new behavior on a consistent basis, a new goal is selected and the process is repeated.

Acquiring appropriate social skills may be a challenge for the child with ADHD, but is necessary to assist the child in forming peer relationships and positive interactions with teachers and others. Houck and associates (2002, p.197) propose that social skills should be taught across four domains: emotional understanding, friendship skills, self-control skills, and social problem solving. Children need to learn how to recognize social cues, wait their turn, and recognize specific behaviors that turn others off, such as interrupting conversations or walking away when someone else is speaking. They also need to learn to avoid invading others' personal space, how to keep one's temper in check, and how to transition from one thing to another more smoothly. Finally, the child needs to learn how to interact as part of a group (Garber et al., 1996). The student receives the most benefit when social skills are taught in small groups and ample time is allowed for practice. Positive praise for demonstrations of appropriate skills is also helpful. Children may acquire social skills through playing games and learning to wait one's turn, role playing in various situations, group discussions, video taped interactions, social stories, and walking through actual situations with an elder or more experienced peer.

Parent/guardian training may focus on education about the disorder and treatments, positive parenting techniques, effective disciplinary measures, behavior modification, and communicating with the child's school (Stein et al., 2002). Parents/guardians need to gain an understanding of ADHD, how the child is affected by the disorder, and ways to cope with the child's disorder. Positive parenting techniques will assist the parent/guardian to maintain control of a situation, to minimize frustration with negative behaviors, and to elicit improved behavior from the child. Effective discipline techniques focus on helping the parent/guardian to understand how he or she interacts with the child and how to obtain the best response from the child when intervening to stop problematic behavior (Flick, 1998). The parent/guardian will also learn how to develop and implement behavior modification programs. In addition, the parent/guardian will learn how to work in conjunction with the school to advocate for the child's needs and monitor the child's progress.

Teacher training is one of the most important aspects of managing a child with ADHD, because the classroom is the place where the child spends a significant amount of time each day. Teachers also need to be informed about the disorder, with an emphasis on understanding that the disorder is chronic and will not go away within the course of one school year, though it is possible for the child to make progress in managing his or her behavior and attending to assignments. Classroom management techniques are of prime importance. After a period of observation to assess what distracts the child and what time of day the child works best, the teacher will be prepared to make necessary modifications. Modifications may include minimizing distractions, changing the child's seat, breaking assignments into small manageable parts, and giving more challenging assignments at the time the child works best (Garber et al., 1996). The classroom environment should provide structure for the student, with modifications made as needed. Teachers need to clearly define expectations of the child, share them with the child and parents/guardians, and provide the interventions needed to allow the student to successfully meet these expectations. Teachers should also be familiarized with developing and utilizing token reinforcement systems within the classroom. Methods of communication with the parent/guardian also need to be discussed.

Medication is yet another option to treat children with ADHD. It is not a magic cure and should never be used independently of the methods listed above. The current trend in pharmacologic management involves the use of stimulant medications to improve the child's ability to focus (Sekleman, 2002). Typical stimulant medications include Ritalin, Adderall, and Dexedrine. More recently, longer-acting preparations have been developed and include Concerta, Metadate and Adderall XR. The shorter-acting medications may require the student to receive a dose at school around midday, whereas the longer-acting preparations may allow the child to take only one pill in the morning. Side effects of stimulant medications include headaches, stomach aches, anorexia, weight loss, dizziness, insomnia, and nausea. In some cases medications may exacerbate anxiety and tic disorders (Wilson, Shannon, & Stang., 2004). In addition, children taking stimulant medication may experience "rebound effect," a period of increased irritability and activity as the medication wears off (Sekleman). Within the past year, a new nonstimulant medication has been developed called Strattera. Strattera belongs to another class of medication called selective norepinephrine reuptake inhibitors (SSRIs). The effects of this medication are not seen as readily as in the stimulant medications, because a therapeutic level in the body must be achieved first. Within a month, the child receiving Strattera should demonstrate an improved attention span, less distraction, and decreased hyperactivity with minimal side effects (Wilson et al.).

In cases where the above medications are contraindicated, some clinicians will prescribe second-line medications, including tricyclic antidepressants, clonidine, and guanfacine (Sekleman, 2002). Tricyclic antidepressants do not improve the ability to concentrate and attend as much as stimulant medication, but do appear to be most effective for those children who experience symptoms of anxiety as well (Farrington, 1997). Medications such as clonidine and guanfacine also do not have as much of an effect on attention and distractibility but do show a decrease in hyperactivity (Farrington). Both second-line medications come with more serious side effects than the stimulant medications and therefore require somewhat more monitoring.

The school nurse has a variety of roles when working with a student with ADHD. These roles include assessing the child for any contributing conditions, such as medical problems or visual or hearing difficulties. The school nurse must follow the school medication policy and procedures, administer the medication as prescribed, and monitor for therapeutic effectiveness and side effects (Lundholm-Brown & Dildy, 2001). In addition, the school nurse may sometimes assume the role of case manager, assisting the family in obtaining appropriate care, counseling, making appointments, and following up. The school nurse may need to create and implement an individualized healthcare plan (IHP). Furthermore, the school nurse may need to advocate for the child and the child's family, working with teachers and staff to develop appropriate classroom management techniques, or assist parents/guardians to work with their health maintenance organization or insurance company to obtain or continue coverage of effective treatments.

Although the roles are many, the school nurse does not work independently when caring for a child with ADHD. Perhaps the most important role is participation in the therapeutic treatment team. The school nurse interacts with a variety of professionals and community services to achieve the best possible results for the student. Communication and teamwork with the primary healthcare provider, pediatrician, psychiatrist, neurologist, outside community counselor, psychologist, teacher, school social worker, other school professionals, the child's parents/guardians, and the student are extremely important to coordinated and effective care (Stein et al., 2002). Working as a team ensures that the problematic behaviors and other concerns are being acknowledged and addressed by all who participate in caring for the child. The constant monitoring and interventions by the team assist the child to more readily achieve success at home and in school.

Overall, one of the most important aspects of caring for a child with ADHD is to educate the educators to identify students in need of assistance and to assist in the selection of appropriate interventions for those students (Flick, 1998). Educators need to understand how ADHD can affect their students, that it is a chronic health problem that the student will carry with himself or herself for the rest of his or her life, and that they can assist the student to learn strategies that will assist the student to learn. The school's role, including that of the school nurse, is to make necessary accommodations to meet the needs of the child with ADHD and to help the child to adapt and live with this health condition.

## Individualized Healthcare Plan

### Assessment

*History*
- Pregnancy and delivery: maternal chemical use, illness, stress, type of delivery, complications during delivery
- Age condition was identified, date diagnosis made
- History of abuse or neglect
- Family history: relatives or siblings affected by similar difficulties
- Previous hospitalizations or participation in outpatient programs: reasons, number, length of stay
- Medical history: other acute and chronic illnesses, past and present
- Previous treatments: duration, effectiveness
- Members of current healthcare team: pediatrician, psychiatrist, neurologist, counselor, etc.
- Neighborhood/community: dwelling type (homes, apartments, etc.), community residents (families, elderly, children, adolescents) safety, noise level, local activity
- Financial resources, including health insurance
- Resources tried in past: utilization of support, information, finances
- Mental health concerns
- Developmental milestones: met on normal timeline, delays
- Social, motor and language skills: appropriate for age, delays

*Current Status and Management*
- Overall appearance: stature, hygiene
- Height and weight
- General health
- Nutritional status: diet, dehydration
- Sleep pattern
- Vision status
- Auditory status
- Family life and routine
- Current management plan: counseling, behavior modification, medication

## Self-care
- Decision-making skills
- Locus of control
- Adherence to medication therapy
- Barriers to adherence
- Motivators to adherence
- Problem-solving skills

## Psychosocial Status
- Student's perception of his/her health condition: behaviors and abilities
- Student's perception of strengths and weaknesses
- Composition of family: number of siblings, primary caregiver, others in household
- Family perception of student's difficulties and impact on family unit
- Recent family stressors: death or illness in family, divorce, new family member, recent move, new school, loss of job, financial difficulties, removal of family member from home
- Family resources of support: isolation of student or family, extended family, respite care, community services, religious-based support or services, etc.
- Interactions with peers and adults outside of school

## Academic Issues
- Academic performance
- Academic strengths and weaknesses
- Interaction with staff
- Teacher observations of classroom functioning and behaviors, including interactions with peers and impact of behaviors on other students
- School attendance pattern, including reasons for absences
- Schools attended
- Classroom modifications: preferential seating, organizational strategies, quiet/low-stimulus work or testing area
- Structure of the classroom: mainstream or self-contained class
- Structure of school day: start and end times, classes, recess, classroom changes during the day, passing time between classes
- Involvement with special education services or 504 accommodations

## Nursing Diagnoses (N.D.) (NANDA, 2003)

**N.D. 1** Risk for injury (NANDA 00035) related to:
- impulsivity
- inattention
- inadequate social skills
- increased risk-taking behavior
- difficulty processing sensory input and formulating appropriate response

**N.D. 2** Impaired social interaction (NANDA 00052) related to:
- inadequate social skills
- altered thought processes
- inattention/distraction
- impulsive behaviors

**N.D. 3** Disturbed thought processes (NANDA 00130) related to:
- distractibility
- difficulty processing environmental input
- decreased attention span

**N.D. 4** Disturbed sensory perception (NANDA 00122) related to:
- inability to appropriately process environmental stimuli
- difficulty distinguishing relevant data input
- alteration in auditory or visual acuity
- hypersensitivity or hyposensitivity to sensory input
- decreased ability to organize an appropriate response to stimuli

**N.D. 5** Ineffective role performance (NANDA 00055), individual, related to:
- inattention/distraction
- inappropriate classroom behavior
- inability to follow directions
- altered thought processes
- inadequate social skills
- uncertainty of expectations—home, school, other

**N.D. 6** Risk for situational low self-esteem (NANDA 00120) related to:
- perceived inability to fulfill role expectations
- perceived inability to control behaviors
- inadequate support
- feelings of restlessness/agitation

**N.D. 7** Impaired adjustment (NANDA 00070) related to:
- developmental stage
- denial of problematic behaviors
- multiple transitions—change of educational placement, addition of therapy, etc.
- inadequate support
- reluctance to participate in prescribed therapeutic regimen

**N.D. 8** Ineffective coping (NANDA 00069), individual, related to:
- impulsivity
- perceived lack of control of situation and behavior
- developmental stage
- knowledge deficit—coping skills, social skills, understanding of disability

**N.D. 9** Knowledge deficit (NANDA 00126), individual, related to:
- diagnosis
- interrupted education process
- unfamiliarity with treatment options
- unfamiliarity with available resources—financial, mental health, medical, information, and support
- effective behavior management skills

## Goals

The student will identify roles and responsibilities within the classroom. (N.D. 5-7)

The student will increase his/her appropriate social interactions and positive behavior at home and in the classroom. (N.D. 2-6, 8)

The student will improve ability to filter and process environmental stimuli and select an appropriate response. (N.D. 3, 4)

The student will identify and utilize resources at home and in school that provide support and assist with problem solving. (N. D. 2, 6-9)

The student will learn and utilize positive coping skills. (N.D. 8, 9)

The student will decrease his/her number of visits to the nurse's office for injuries. (N.D. 1, 4)

The student will participate in health assessments and prescribed management plan. (N.D. 5, 7, 8)

## Nursing Interventions

Collect data regarding student's academic progress and behavior in school—initial and ongoing. (N.D. 3-5, 8)

Monitor vision and hearing annually, refer for further evaluation if indicated. (N.D 4).

Identify barriers to obtaining appropriate care. (N.D. 9)

Assist parents/guardians to locate and access resources to evaluate and treat the student. (N.D. 6, 7, 9)

Refer to child study or pupil assistance team, if appropriate. (N.D. 9)

Provide learning opportunities (individual or group) for the student to learn more about ADHD. (N.D. 1, 3)

Provide healthcare provider(s) with feedback regarding academic performance and behavior at school. (N.D. 3-5, 7)

Develop open and communicative relationship with parent/guardian to implement prescribed management plan. (N.D. 7)

Educate parent/guardian regarding diagnosis, treatment options, and follow-up assessments. (N.D. 9)

Identify problem behaviors and assist parents/guardians and teachers to develop a behavior plan to encourage appropriate behaviors and decrease inappropriate behaviors. (N.D. 5-8)

Assist teachers and parents/guardians to provide consistent structure and clear expectations. (N.D. 5, 7, 8)

Collaborate with parents/guardians and teachers to identify motivators that work to change inappropriate behavior and maintain appropriate behaviors. (N.D. 5, 7-9)

Look for appropriate behavior and reward and reinforce. (N.D. 5, 6)

Collaborate with the school psychologist and/or counselor, teach the student self-monitoring techniques, including identifying social cues from peers and adults, techniques to refocus attention, distinguishing between relevant and irrelevant stimuli, and relaxation exercises. (N.D. 3-5, 8).

Educate school staff regarding student expectations and classroom interventions to manage symptoms and behavior, including preferential seating, alternative ways to complete assignments, individualized behavior modification plans, and token reward systems. (N.D 2-8).

Obtain parent/guardian and physician authorization for medication to be given at school and administer medication as prescribed and according to school policy and procedure. (N.D. 1, 7).

Assess the student regularly for side effects of prescribed medications. (N.D. 1, 7, 8).

Provide support and advocate for student as needed. (N.D. 2, 5-8)

Allow the student time to express feelings related to health condition and treatment. (N.D. 2, 6-8)

Assist the student in identifying sources of support within school environment. (N.D. 6-9)

Document student injury and treatment. (N.D 1, 4)

## Expected Student Outcomes

The student will:
- Identify role expectations (e.g., student, son/daughter, team member). (N.D. 5-7)
- Demonstrate a decrease in (specific negative behavior) as reported by the parent and classroom teacher and staff. (N.D. 2, 5, 8)
- Remain seated for classroom instruction and work, (____%) of the time. (N.D. 2, 4, 5)
- Demonstrate on-task, attending behavior for (____ minutes) in classes. (N.D. 3- 5)
- Demonstrate completion of assigned tasks, (____ %) of the time, as reported by classroom teacher and staff. (N.D. 3-5)
- Demonstrate completion and turning in of assigned homework, (____ %) of the time, as reported by parent/guardian and teacher. (N.D. 3, 5)
- Choose appropriate responses to stimuli, (____ %) of the time, as reported by classroom teacher and staff, and parent/guardian. (N.D. 3, 4)
- Demonstrate an organized and appropriate response to stimuli, (____ %) of the time, as reported by classroom teacher and staff. (N.D. 3, 4, 8)
- Identify (specific number) options of appropriate behavior instead of doing (specific inappropriate behavior). (N.D. 1, 2, 5, 6, 8)
- Demonstrate positive, appropriate social interactions with peers at school. (N.D. 2, 5, 6)
- Demonstrate positive, appropriate social interactions with teachers and staff at school. (N.D. 2, 5, 6)
- Describe his/her diagnosis and management plan. (N.D. 6-8)
- Express feelings related to classroom behavior, accomplishments, consequences, adjustment to diagnosis, management plan, etc. (N.D. 5-8)
- Learn and utilize (specific number) positive coping skills. (N.D. 8, 9)
- Participate in management plan. (N.D. 5, 8, 9)
  -Take medication on time without argument (if prescribed)
  -Regularly attend therapeutic counseling sessions (if prescribed)
  -Wear glasses or hearing aids (if prescribed)
  -Attend follow-up appointments, as needed
- Identify resources at school and home that he/she can use to work out a problem. (N.D. 2, 6-9)
- Demonstrate a decrease in the number of visits to the health office for injuries. (N.D. 1, 4)

## Case Study

Joey is a 10-year-old fifth grader at Maple Park Middle School. He was diagnosed with attention deficit hyperactivity disorder last year. He currently receives 10 mg of Adderall at breakfast and at noon. He comes to visit the school nurse for the noon dose of medication. His mother usually gives the morning dose at home. Joey has been out of medicine for the past 3 days. He has become extremely disruptive, talking out of turn, getting up out of his seat without permission, and provoking his peers. He has been involved in two fights during recess and is unable to complete more than one third of an assignment at any given time. He is, however, able to play computer games for hours on end, a tool the teacher has lately utilized to keep Joey's disruption to a minimum. His mother states that Joey's case was closed by the clinic as the result of too many missed appointments. She states that it is difficult for her to get to the appointments because the family has only one car and her husband uses it for work. It is difficult for her to take Joey and his 3-year-old triplet siblings on public transportation to get to the clinic. Joey has also missed several counseling appointments because they conflicted with an after-school band program that Joey participated in. His teacher has had enough of his poor behavior and is having difficulty managing her classroom as a result. She has recommended Joey for an evaluation by the school's pupil assistance committee.

# Attention Deficit Hyperactivity Disorder

| Assessment Data | Nursing Diagnosis | Goals | Nursing Interventions | Expected Outcomes |
|---|---|---|---|---|
| Fighting with peers. | Risk for injury related to impulsivity, inadequate social skills and risk-taking behavior. | Joey will have a decreased number of visits to the health office for injuries.<br><br>Joey will increase appropriate social interactions with peers. | Maintain records of injury and treatment.<br><br>In collaboration with school psychologist/counselor/social worker, role model appropriate social skills.<br><br>Allow Joey time to express feelings related to problematic behavior. | Joey will decrease his number of visits to the health office for injuries.<br><br>Joey will demonstrate improved social skills with peers.<br><br>Joey will identify behaviors that are causing him problems.<br><br>Joey will express his feelings related to problematic behaviors.<br><br>Joey will identify resources for assistance in class. |
| Diagnosed with ADHD.<br>Currently out of medication.<br>Disruptive behavior. | Impaired social interaction related to impulsivity, inadequate social skills, and altered thought processes. | Joey will demonstrate appropriate social interactions and positive behavior within the classroom.<br><br>Joey will identify roles and responsibilities within the classroom. | Provide support and advocate for Joey, as needed.<br><br>Assist Joey to identify symptoms/behaviors that are disruptive to the classroom process.<br><br>Teach Joey self-monitoring techniques, including recognition of social cues, calming techniques, and refocusing techniques.<br><br>Educate school staff regarding expectations and classroom interventions to manage behavior. | Joey will demonstrate a decreased number of negative behaviors.<br><br>Joey will demonstrate positive social interactions with peers and staff at school. |

| Assessment Data | Nursing Diagnosis | Goals | Nursing Interventions | Expected Outcomes |
|---|---|---|---|---|
| | | | Obtain parent and physician authorization for the administration of medication at school. | |
| Disruptive classroom behavior. No medication. Inability to complete assignments. Unable to remain seated. | Ineffective role performance, individual, related to inappropriate classroom behavior, inability to follow directions, and inadequate social skills. | Joey will identify roles and responsibilities within the classroom and ways he can fulfill those roles. Joey will increase positive social interactions. | Collaborate with school social worker to assist Joey to identify his roles and responsibilities as a "student." Collect data regarding behavior on and off of medication. Communicate with healthcare provider and parent regarding disruptive behavior. Educate school staff regarding student expectations and classroom interventions to manage behavior. Assist staff in planning opportunities to practice social interactions. | Joey will identify and fulfill the role of a student – remaining seated and completing assigned tasks. Joey will demonstrate a decrease in negative behaviors. Joey will demonstrate positive, appropriate social interactions with peers. Joey will demonstrate appropriate social skills in class and at recess. |
| Case closed at clinic due to poor attendance. Conflict of needs and activities that promote student's self-esteem and feelings of self-worth. Referred to Pupil Assistance Committee. | Impaired adjustment related to decreased ability of parents to maintain therapeutic treatment plan. | Joey will participate in evaluations and prescribed management plan. Joey will identify and utilize resources in school to assist him in managing his symptoms/behaviors. | Educate parent regarding student's diagnosis, treatment, and follow-up responsibilities. Assist family in identifying barriers to care. Collaborate with school social worker to assist parents to identify healthcare options and access. | Joey will participate in therapeutic management plan. Joey will actively participate in management of symptoms/behaviors at school, with assistance of teachers and school social worker/counselor and others, as needed. |

| Assessment Data | Nursing Diagnosis | Goals | Nursing Interventions | Expected Outcomes |
|---|---|---|---|---|
| | | | Collaborate with school social worker to assist parents to identify and utilize community resources for transportation, child care, etc. | |
| | | | Assist parents in interactions with the Pupil Assistance Committee. | |
| | | | Work with Joey's teachers for release from class/practice if needed to attend counseling/medical appointments. | |
| | | | Assist Joey to obtain missed assigned due to appointments. | |
| | | | Share data collected regarding academic performance and behaviors on and off medication with parents and healthcare providers. | |
| | | | Assist parents to maintain an adequate supply of medication at school and notify parents when there is only 1 week of medication left. | |

# References

American Academy of Pediatrics (AAP) Committee on Quality Improvement, Subcommittee on Attention-Deficit/ Hyperactivity Disorder (2002). Clinical practice guideline: Diagnosis and evaluation of the child with attention-deficit/ hyperactivity disorder. *Pediatrics, 105*(5), 11581170.

American Psychiatric Association. (2000). *Diagnostic and statistical manual of mental disorders* (4th ed., text revision). Washington, DC: Author.

Farrington, E. (1997). Pharmacologic management of ADHD. In J. Vessey (Ed.), *The child with a learning disorder or ADHD: A manual for school nurses* (pp. 3341). Scarborough, ME: National Association of School Nurses.

Flick, G. L. (1998). *ADD/ADHD behavior-change resource kit: Ready-to-use strategies & activities for helping children with attention deficit disorder.* West Nyack, NY: Center For Applied Research and Education.

Fox, L., Vaughn, B. J., Wyatte, M. L., & Dunlap, G. (2002). We can't expect other people to understand: Family perspectives on problem behavior. *Exceptional Children, 68*(4), 437–450.

Garber, S. W., Garber, M. D., & Spizman, R. F. (1996). *Beyond Ritalin.* New York: Harper Perennial.

Houck, G. M., King, M. C., Tomlinson, B., Vrabel, A., & Wecks, K. (2002). Small group intervention for children with attention disorders. *Journal of School Nursing, 18*(4), 196–200.

Ludholm-Brown, J., & Dildy, M. E. (2001). Attention-deficit/ hyperactivity disorder: An educational cultural model. *Journal of School Nursing, 17*(6), 307–315.

NANDA International. (2003). *Nursing diagnoses: Definitions & classification 2003-2004.* Philadelphia: NANDA International.

Panacek, L. J., & Dunlap, G. (2003). The social lives of children with emotional and behavioral disorders in self-contained classrooms: A descriptive analysis. *Exceptional Children, 69*(3), 333–348.

Sekleman, J. (2002). Attention-deficit hyperactivity disorder. *Journal of School Nursing, 18*(5), 270–276.

Stein, M. A., Efron, L. A., Schiff, W. B., & Glanzman, M. (2002). Attention deficits and hyperactivity. In M. L. Batshaw (Ed.), *Children with disabilities* (pp. 389–416). Baltimore, MD: Paul H. Brooks Publishing.

Wilson, B. A., Shannon, M. T., & Stang, C. L. (2004). *Nurse's drug guide 2004.* Upper Saddle River, NJ: Prentice Hall.

# Bibliography

Bergren, M. D. (2002). Child and adolescent mental health Web resources. *Journal of School Nursing, 18*(4), 226–228.

Frame, K. (2003) *Social empowerment training and responsibilities for students with ADHA* (STARS) *curriculum* [Resources]. Scarborough, ME: National Association of School Nurses.

Frame, K. (2004). The STARS program: Social empowerment training for preadolescents with attention deficit hyperactivity disorder (ADHD). *Journal of School Nursing, 20*(5), 257–261.

Houck, G. M., King, M. C., Tomlinson, B., Vrabel, A., Wecks, K. 2002: Small group intervention for children with attention disorders. *Journal of School Nursing, 18*(4), 196–200.

Lundholm-Brown, J., Dildy, M. E. (2001). Attention-deficit/hyperactivity disorder: An educational cultural model. *Journal of School Nursing, 17*(6), 307–315.

National Association of School Nurses. (n.d.). *Addressing the mental health needs of children and adolescence* [Education Program]. Retrieved November 7, 2004, from http://nasn.org/education/education.htm.

Selekman, J. (2002). Attention-deficit/hyperactivity disorder. *Journal of School Nursing, 18*(5), 270–276.

Vessey, J. (1997). *The child with a learning disorder or ADHD* [Manual]. Scarborough, ME: National Association of School Nurses.

## Resources

Children and Adults with
　Attention
　Deficit/Hyperactivity
　Disorder (CHADD)
8181 Professional Place
Suite 150
Landover, MD 20785
1-800-233-4050
301-306-7070
www.chadd.org

The Council for Exceptional
　Children
1110 North Glebe Road
Suite 300
Arlington, VA 22201-5704
1-888-CEC-SPED
703-620-3660
www.cec.sped.org

American Academy of Child and
　Adolescent Psychiatry
3615 Wisconsin Avenue, NW
Washington, DC 20016-3007
202-966-7300
www.aacap.org

National Institutes of Mental
　Health (NIMH)
Office of Communications
6001 Executive Boulevard
Room 8184, MSC 9663
Bethesda, MD 20892-9663
1-866-615-6464
301-443-4513
www.nimh.nih.gov

National Mental Health
　Association (NMHA)
2001 North Beauregard Street
12th Floor
Alexandria, VA 22311
1-800-969-NMHA(6642)
703-684-7722
www.nmha.org

Attention Deficit Disorder
　Association (ADDA)
PO Box 543
Pottstown, PA 19464
484-945-2101
www.add.org

## Chapter Twenty-one

# Anaphylaxis: Severe Allergic Reaction

### Mariann Smith

## Introduction

Allergies in the school-aged population are very common; so common, in fact, that school personnel sometimes tend to trivialize or ignore them (Wynn,1993). However, severe allergic reactions, or anaphylaxis, can occur after insect stings or food intake in susceptible students while at school. These reactions can be life-threatening. The cutaneous, gastrointestinal, respiratory, and cardiovascular systems are often affected. Food allergies are not always obvious, because some foods and spices used as an ingredient can be "hidden" and cause problems for certain individuals even in very small amounts. Prompt treatment is necessary. All school personnel need to be familiar with early recognition, prompt treatment, and prevention measures.

Food allergy, in general, is more prevalent than insect allergy. Current research indicates that up to 6% of the pediatric population is affected by food allergies (NASN, 2001). Mudd and Noone (1995) found that the foods most likely to cause allergic reactions are peanuts, tree nuts, eggs, milk, wheat, and fish; peanut and tree nut allergies account for the most severe reactions. Food allergies are the leading cause of anaphylaxis outside of the hospital setting and account for an estimated 30,000 emergency department visits and 150 to 200 deaths annually (NASN, 2001). A recent study reported on the Food, Allergy & Anaphylaxis Network Web Site (FAAN Information About Anaphylaxis, 2003) showed that teens with a known food allergy and asthma appear to have the highest risk of an anaphylatic reaction because they frequently eat away from home, fail to carry their medications, or ignore or deny symptoms of a reaction.

Because food allergy reactions are so prevalent, related research is receiving more attention. Drug companies are developing and investigating anti-IgE drugs (e.g., Xolair), which bind with the IgE in the bloodstream to block the allergic reaction (FAAN Press Release, 2003). Other research has involved vaccine development, use of activated charcoal to bind with the peanut protein following an accidental ingestion, antigen-specific immunotherapy through genetic engineering, and investigating certain populations to determine if severe food allergies are outgrown (FAAN Research , 2003).

Insects that can cause allergic reaction are from the Hymenoptera species and include honeybees, wasps, yellow jackets, and hornets. Fire ants also have been known to cause severe reactions.

## Pathophysiology

Anaphylaxis is an exaggerated, life-threatening hypersensitivity reaction to a previously encountered allergen. This reaction triggers an incomplete humoral response that allows the allergen to combine with immunoglobulin E (IgE) and causes the release of histamine (Anderson, 1998). The allergy symptoms experienced depend on where in the body the histamine is released. The reaction may be relatively mild (hives, itching, rash, stomach pain, nausea and/or diarrhea) to severe (vascular collapse, bronchospasm, and shock). Severity of past reactions does not necessarily predict how severe subsequent reactions will be; however, there is often a cumulative effect in that each additional encounter with the allergen may result in more severe symptoms.

Anaphylaxis can occur within seconds to minutes from the time of exposure to the sensitizing factor. Occasionally, the student may have a recurrence of symptoms 1 to 2 hours after the initial symptoms have improved. Wynn (1993) stated that this "biphasic" anaphylaxis is difficult to predict; therefore, it is important to continue to monitor the student after the initial reaction.

## Management

Managing the student who has the potential for an anaphylatic crisis involves eliminating the known allergen from the school environment as well as planning for the treatment of any allergic reactions. In the case of food allergies, school personnel need to know the trigger food(s). Teachers need to plan alternative projects involving cooking as well as inform room mothers so appropriate party treats can be provided. The food service department also needs to know the trigger food(s) so appropriate lunch and/or breakfast alternatives can be provided. If the trigger allergen is an insect, school grounds need to be monitored and appropriate pest control maintained. It is also recommended that insect-allergic students planning an outdoor activity be encouraged to wear light-colored, well-fitted clothing and shoes, use unscented grooming products, apply insect repellent, and keep car or bus windows closed while riding or driving (James, 2002).

Treating any allergic reaction involves educating school personnel about symptoms of the allergic reaction and appropriate treatment protocol. School personnel need to know that anaphylaxis is a medical emergency. The emergency care plan (ECP) needs to specify treatment protocol as well as who is responsible for carrying out the plan. It is critical that a source of epinephrine (usually EpiPen) and antihistamines are readily available. If emergency medical personnel are called, school personnel will need to inform them about exposure to the specific allergen, the emergency care plan for the student, and treatment measures that have already been given at school.

## Individualized Healthcare Plan

### Assessment

*History*
- Student's known allergies
- Student's reactions to known allergies
- Symptoms of reactions from mild to severe
- Number of past serious reactions
- Past treatment of reactions from mild to severe and effectiveness of treatment
- Family knowledge about allergic reactions
- Any other health concerns/illnesses
- Past history of allergic episodes at school

*Current Status and Management*
- Current allergy management plan
- Healthcare provider involved in assessment and management
- Assistance needed to implement management plan (e.g., parent, teacher, nurse)
- Knowledge about allergy reactions from mild to severe
- Knowledge about early warning signs of allergy reaction
- Environmental modifications needed at home and school
- Current medications for treatment of an allergic reaction
- Specific food restrictions and requirements

*Self-care*
- Student's ability to avoid allergens (triggers)
- Student's level of knowledge of symptoms and treatment
- Student's ability to alert others to possible reactions and to assist with treatment
- Student's ability to self-medicate
- Student's ability/responsibility to carry medication with him or her (bus, field trips, family activities)
- Student's perception of dangers of a severe reaction
- Compliance with individualized healthcare plan (IHP)

*Psychosocial Status*
- Parent's perception of the dangers of a severe reaction
- Student's perception of the dangers of a severe reaction
- Student's fear of an anaphylactic episode occurring
- Student's feelings regarding outcome of reactions and treatment
- Involvement with support systems
- Peer reactions to anaphylactic episode and treatment
- Feelings of being different and needing food alternatives, etc.
- Age/developmental level

*Academic Issues*
- Past attendance concerns
- Regular vs. special education
- Past patterns of academic performance
- Possible need for 504 plan
- School staff perceptions—information the student and parent feel teachers need to know
- School staff comfort level with a life-threatening situation and what to do if an episode occurs
- Past experiences with school food services (positive and negative)
- Specific modifications in the classroom as needed

- Involvement of school food service department if food allergy is involved
- Involvement of school transportation services if appropriate

## Nursing Diagnoses (N.D.) (NANDA, 2003)

**N.D. 1** Ineffective breathing pattern (NANDA 0032) related to:
- brochospasm
- inflammation of airways

**N.D. 2** Decreased cardiac output (NANDA 00029) related to:
- hypotensive shock
- vascular collapse

**N.D. 3** Effective therapeutic regimen management (NANDA 00082) related to:
- ability to develop and implement IHP and ECP
- ability to seek help from others
- ability to self-medicate when appropriate

**N.D. 4** Deficient knowledge (NANDA 00126) related to:
- allergens
- symptoms of allergic reactions
- ECP

**N.D. 5** Risk for powerlessness (NANDA 00152) related to:
- uncertainty of an allergic reaction/outcome in the school environment

## Goals

The student will identify symptoms of allergic reaction. (N.D. 1, 2, 4)
The student will increase knowledge of trigger allergens. (N.D. 4)
The student will participate in development and implementation of healthcare plans at school. (N.D. 1–5)
The student will be safe in all school environments. (N.D. 1–5)
The student will develop self-medication skills when appropriate. (N.D. 3, 4, 5)
The student will prevent allergic reactions from occurring. (N.D. 3, 4, 5)

## Nursing Interventions

Provide necessary health counseling opportunities for student to participate in self-care (depending on the student's cognitive and/or physical ability). (N.D. 1–5)
- Review symptoms and sources of allergen(s).
- Review treatment methods, including how/when to report allergic symptoms to school personnel.
- Teach proper technique of self-administration of epinephrine.

Provide in-service for school staff (including school bus driver, if appropriate) about allergic reaction/anaphylaxis. (N.D. 1, 2, 4)
- Identify student's known food or insect allergen(s).
- Discuss symptoms of mild to severe allergic reactions, including anaphylaxis.
- Develop specific guidelines for treatment (from mild to severe)—ECP.
- Document each episode of allergic reaction.
- Request that classroom teacher alert room mothers about food allergy and need for alternative party treats.
- Request that classroom teacher use alternative foods in all classroom cooking and other activities.
- Make field trip modifications as needed (e.g., medication must be taken along on all field trips).
- Make extracurricular activities (e.g., dances, carnivals) modifications that are needed.
- Continuously monitor school environment for potential allergens.

Work with food service personnel if allergy is to food. (N.D. 1, 2, 4)
- Determine if a potential allergen is in a food served at school, including ingredients in prepared foods.
- Avoid cross-contamination with allergen.
- Establish a safe environment for student with food allergies.

Work with environmental maintenance personnel if allergy is to insect sting. (N.D. 1,2,4)
- Continuously monitor outdoor environment.
- Eliminate insect from the environment as necessary.

Collaborate with local emergency medical services. (N.D. 3, 5)
- Communicate with EMS staff regarding the potential for an anaphylactic reaction.

- Identify nearest emergency department that will be used.

Develop and implement an allergy ECP. (N.D. 1–5)
- Include mild and severe reaction plans.
- Include student, parents/guardians, appropriate school personnel, and healthcare provider.
- Coordinate school plan with home plan.
- Obtain parent and healthcare provider approval of plan, including orders for medications (antihistamines and/or epinephrine).
- Provide teachers with copies, including an additional copy for the substitute teacher's information folder.
- Make modifications to plan(s) as needed.
- Identify person(s) who have access to medication(s) and know where they are stored and who have been trained to administer the medications.

Monitor medications. (N.D. 3)
- Provide storage for epinephrine and/or antihistamines supplied by parent.
- Check medications frequently for correct dosage per medication order.
- Request new supply of medication if expired and/or used.

Provide health counseling opportunities regarding significance of allergy to student's classmates and friends. (N.D. 4, 5)

Encourage student to wear medical alert bracelet or necklace at all times. (N.D. 3, 5) (Assist parents in obtaining one, if needed.)

## Expected Student Outcomes

The student will:
- Identify his or her symptoms of an allergic reaction (from mild to severe) and share information with appropriate school personnel. (N.D. 1, 2, 4)
- Identify trigger foods or insect(s) that can cause potential severe reaction. (N.D. 4)
- Describe steps to take if an allergic reaction occurs. (N.D. 3, 4)
- Inform school personnel when treatment for an allergic reaction is necessary. (N.D. 3, 5)
- Actively participate in healthcare management and ECP at school. (N.D. 1–5)
- Identify school personnel responsible for helping carry out the healthcare management and ECP. (N.D. 3, 5)
- Demonstrate proper technique of self-medicating when appropriate. (N.D. 3, 4, 5)
- Wear allergy alert bracelet/necklace. (N.D. 3, 5)
- Participate in all school activities with modifications made when necessary. (N.D. 3, 5)
- Interact appropriately with peers in all school settings, including classroom, cafeteria, and playground. (N.D. 3, 5)

## Case Study

Manda is an 8-year-old third-grade student at Place Elementary School. Two weeks ago, Manda and her parents were eating at a new Chinese restaurant when she suddenly started to wheeze, cough, and become cyanotic. Facial swelling occurred immediately, and hives developed on her neck and trunk. An ambulance was called, and Manda was transported to the hospital where she was treated for an anaphylactic reaction. Manda was kept overnight for observation. It was determined that she had suffered an extreme allergic reaction to the peanut oil used in cooking the food at the restaurant. Manda was dismissed with an order to keep an EpiPen Jr. kit with her at all times.

Manda is usually very eager for school to start; however, this year she is apprehensive. She does not want a "shot" at school, and she is afraid that she will not know which foods might contain peanuts. She is also afraid that her classmates will be mad at her if peanut products are banned from the classroom and the lunchroom. The doctor has not determined if peanuts must be ingested before a reaction occurs or if Manda will have a reaction simply because she is in an area where peanuts are present.

# Anaphylaxis

| Assessment Data | Nursing Diagnosis | Goals | Nursing Interventions | Expected Outcomes |
|---|---|---|---|---|
| Manda had severe allergic reaction to peanuts; hospitalized overnight for treatment and observation. | Ineffective breathing pattern related to bronchospasm and inflammation of airways.<br><br>Decreased cardiac output related to hypotensive shock and vascular collapse. | Manda will be able to identify her symptoms of a severe allergic reaction. | Establish trusting, open communication with student to provide health counseling opportunities to review symptoms of reaction.<br><br>Hold in-service with school staff about significance of allergic reaction/anaphylaxis. | Manda will identify her symptoms of an allergic reaction.<br><br>Manda will share information about her allergy with her teachers and other school personnel.<br><br>Manda will tell school personnel when symptoms of an allergic reaction are present. |
| Physician has ordered EpiPen Jr. for use at school. | Effective therapeutic regimen management related to development and implementation of IHP and ECP. | Manda will participate in development and implementation of school healthcare management and ECP in order to prevent and manage anaphylactic reaction. | Develop and implement ECP.<br><br>Collaborate with local emergency medical personnel, as needed.<br><br>Monitor medications to make certain that used or expired medications are replaced. | Manda will describe steps to take if allergic reaction occurs.<br><br>Manda will identify school personnel responsible for helping carry out the school healthcare management and ECP.<br><br>Manda will demonstrate active participation in her school healthcare management and ECP. |
| Manda is hesitant to eat at school because she is not able to recognize peanut as ingredient in other foods. | Deficient knowledge related to possible hidden allergens. | Manda will increase her knowledge about foods containing peanuts or peanut products. | Provide health counseling opportunities for student to identify foods containing peanut ingredients.<br><br>Notify food service personnel of need for alternative food choices. | Manda will identify foods that contain peanut ingredients.<br><br>Manda will avoid eating foods containing peanuts or peanut products. |

| Assessment Data | Nursing Diagnosis | Goals | Nursing Interventions | Expected Outcomes |
|---|---|---|---|---|
| Manda is fearful of another reaction occurring at school and does not want "a shot" at school.<br><br>Manda is not yet ready to self-medicate.<br><br>Manda is afraid that class-mates will not like her because peanut products need to be banned. | Risk for powerlessness relat-ed to uncertainty of an allergic reaction/outcome while at school. | Manda will prevent allergic reactions from occurring.<br><br>Manda will be safe in all school environments.<br><br>Manda will develop self-med-ication skills when appropriate. | Request that classroom teacher alert room mothers about food allergy and need for alternative party treats.<br><br>Request that classroom teacher use alternative foods in all classroom cooking and other activities.<br><br>Provide health counseling opportunities to review treat-ment plan, including how/when to report allergic symptoms to school personnel.<br><br>Encourage student to wear medical alert bracelet or neck-lace at all times.<br><br>Provide health education regarding significance of peanut allergy to student's classmates and friends.<br><br>Provide health education for student to develop ability to self-medicate. | Manda will tell school per-sonnel when symptoms of an allergic reaction are present.<br><br>Manda will demonstrate posi-tive interactions with her peers in all school settings, including classroom, cafete-ria, and playground.<br><br>Manda will participate in all school activities with modifi-cations as needed.<br><br>Manda will demonstrate proper self-administration of epinephrine (EpiPen).<br><br>Manda will wear medical alert necklace at all times. |

# Emergency Care Plan
## Anaphylaxis: Severe Allergic Reaction

Student: _____     Phone: _____

Date: _____     FAX No: _____

Pupil's Name: _____     Physician's Name: _____

I.D. No: _____     Address: _____

Birth Date: _____     Phone: _____

Address: _____     FAX: _____

Phone: _____     Hospital: _____

Parents:
    Mother: _____     Day Phone: _____

    Father: _____     Day Phone: _____

Parent Designee: _____     Day Phone: _____

**Medication Condition:** Severe allergic reaction to peanuts and peanut products

**Location of medication and other supplies:**
    EpiPen Jr. is kept in labeled drawer in locked medicating cabinet in Health Room. Personnel listed below have access to key.

Persons authorized to administer treatment:

School nurse: _____     Nurse Designee: _____

**Signs of emergency:** Hives, itching, swelling, difficulty breathing, cyanosis, hypotension, shock

**Treatment for Severe Allergic Reaction:**
1. Administer epinephrine injection or assist student with self-administration.

2. Call 911, informing emergency personnel that student has severe allergic reaction to peanuts and that epinephrine injection has been given.

3. Call parent or parent designee.

4. Call student's physician to inform of emergency situation.

5. Record administration or self-administration of medication in student's health record (include date, time, source of exposure, treatment, if EMS was called, and signature).

6. Emergency personnel are to transport to _____ or nearest emergency department.

## References

Anderson K. E, Anderson, L. E., & Glanze, W. D. (1998). *Mosby's medical, nursing, and allied health dictionary.* St. Louis, MO: Mosby.

Food Allergy & Anaphylaxis Network (FAAN). (2003). *Food Allergy Research.* Retrieved August 28, 2003, from http://www.foodallergy.org/research.html

Food Allergy & Anaphylaxis Network (FAAN). (2003). *Information About Anaphylaxis.* Retrieved August 28, 2003, from http://www.foodallergy.org/anaphylaxis.html

Food Allergy & Anaphylaxis Network (FAAN). (2003). *Press Release: Xolair, asthma drug gets green light from FDA Advisory Panel. Study on peanut allergy to begin.* Retrieved August 28, 2003, from http://www.foodallergy.org/press_releases/xolair.html

James, S. R., Ashwell, J. W., & Droske, S. C. (2002). *Nursing care of children principles and practice.* (2nd ed., pp. 502–506). Philadelphia: Saunders.

Mudd K. E. & Noone S. A. (1995). Management of severe food allergy. *Journal of School Nursing, 11*(3), 30–32.

National Association of School Nurses (NASN). (2001). *Position Statement: The role of the school nurse in allergy/anaphylaxis management.* Retrieved August 12, 2003, from http://www.nasn.org/positions/allergy.htm

NANDA International. (2003). *NANDA nursing diagnoses: Definitions & classification 2003-2004.* Philadelphia: Author.

## Bibliography

Fleischer, D., Conover-Walker, M. K., Christie, L., Burks, A. W., & Wood, R. A. The natural progression of peanut allergy: Resolution and the possibility of recurrence. *Journal of Allergy and Clinical Immunology, 112*(1), 183–189.

Lewis, K. D., & Bear, B. J. (2002). Manual of school health. (2nd ed). Philadelphia: Saunders.

Li, X., Srivastava, K., Grishin, A., Huang, C., Schofield, B., Burks, W., et al. (2003). Persistent protective effect of heat-killed *Escherichia coli* producing "engineered," recombinant peanut proteins in a murine model of peanut allergy. Journal of Allergy and Clinical Immunology, 112(1), 159–167

Litarowsky, J. A., Murphy, S. O., Canham, D. L. (2004). Evaluation of an anaphylaxis training program for unlicensed assistive personnel. *Journal of School Nursing, 20*(5), 279–284.

National Association of School Nurses (NASN). (2000). *Position Statement: Epinephrine use in life-threatening emergencies.* Retrieved August 12, 2003, from http://www.nasn.org/positions/Epinephrine.htm

Sander, N. (2002). Making the grade with asthma, allergies, and anaphylaxis. Pediatric Nursing, 28(6), 593–598.

School Health Alert's *Clinical Guide for School Nurses* (5th ed.). (2002). Nashville, TN: School Health Alert.

Schwab, N. C., & Polhman, K. J. (2002). Legal and ethical issues: Questions and answers. *Journal of School Nursing, 18*(5), 301–305.

Simonte, S., Ma, S., Mofidi, S., & Sicherer, S. Relevance of casual contact with peanut butter in children with peanut allergy. *Journal of Allergy and Clinical Immunology, 112*(1), 180–182.

Vadas, P., & Perelman, B. (2003). Activated charcoal forms non-IgE binding complexes with peanut proteins. *Journal of Allergy and Clinical Immunology, 112*(1), 175–179.

Weiss, C., Muñoz-Furlong, A., Furlong, T.J., & Arbit, J. (2004). Impact of food allergies on school nursing practice. *Journal of School Nursing, 20*(5), 268–278.

Wynn, S. (1998). *Anaphylaxis: The extreme allergic emergency.* Port Washington, NY: Center Laboratories.

## Resources

American Academy of Allergy,
  Asthma, & Immunology
611 East Wells Street
Milwaukee, WI 53202
414-272-6071
1-800-822-2762
www.aaaai.org

American Academy of Pediatrics
141 Northwest Point Boulevard
Elk Grove Village, IL 60007-1098
847-434-4000
1-800-842-7777
www.aap.org

American College of Allergy,
  Asthma, & Immunology
85 West Algonquin Road
Suite 550
Arlington Heights, IL 60005
847-427-1200
www.allergy.mcg.edu

Food Allergy & Anaphylaxis
  Network
11781 Lee Jackson Highway
Suite 160
Fairfax, VA 22033-3309
1-800-929-4040
www.foodallergy.org

National Association of School
  Nurses (NASN)
Western office:
1416 Park Street
 Suite A
Castle Rock, CO 80109
1-866-627-6767
www.nasn.org
Eastern office:
PO Box 1300
Scarborough, ME 04070-1300
1-877-627-6476

# Chapter Twenty-two

# Anxiety Disorder

### Lorali Gray

## Introduction

Anxiety is an experience that is universal. However, an individual can develop an anxiety disorder if successful adaptation does not occur (Wilson & Kneisl, 1996). Moreover, anxiety disorders are the most common mental illnesses experienced by children and adolescents (Velting, Setzer, & Albano, 2004). Additionally, in the United States, recent epidemiologic studies estimate that 12% to 20% of youth are affected by this disorder (Achenbach, Howell, McConaughy, & Stanger, 1995 Gurley, Cohen, Pine & Brook, 1996; Shaffer et al., 1996, in Velting et al., 2004). Several types of anxiety disorders are common to children and adolescents:

- *Separation anxiety disorder.* This disorder is seen most often in children aged 6 to 9. These children generally exhibit intense anxiety when separated from their caregiver. They may refuse to attend school, cling to their parents, experience nightmares, and present with stomachaches and headaches. They appear to have a need to be with their parents (National Mental Health Association, 2004).
- *Specific phobias.* These phobias often occur in children ages 6 to 9; however, they are more common in young children. Specific phobias cause an inappropriate level of fear related to a specific object or situation. In addition, children are irrational in their behavior and reaction (Anxiety Disorders Association of America, 2004).
- *Generalized anxiety disorder (GAD).* Seen in middle childhood and adolescence, children with GAD have recurring worries that are difficult to control. They tend to be eager to please and may be "perfectionists." In addition, they may experience difficulty concentrating and be restless, tired, tense, or irritable (National Mental Health Association, 2004).
- *Social anxiety disorder (SAD).* SAD is more common in the teenage years rather than in childhood. Most teens with this disorder have a fear of social situations that may require them to perform, speak, or be in front of others. They often have associated sweating, blushing, rapid heart rate, or shortness of breath. Additionally, they tend to avoid these situations rather than confront them, often owing to low self-esteem or a lack of assertiveness (National Mental Health Association, 2004).
- *Panic disorder.* This disorder results in an intense feeling of impending doom and the fear of dying, lasting just minutes or hours. It is more common in adolescence than childhood. It can strike repeatedly, suddenly, and without any warning, intensifying the anxiety. Physical symptoms associated with panic disorder include chest pain, rapid heart rate, shortness of breath, sweating, dizziness, and abdominal discomfort (National Alliance for the Mental Ill, 2004)
- *Obsessive-compulsive disorder (OCD).* Typically, OCD begins in childhood or adolescence and manifests itself in frequent "obsessions," uncontrollable thoughts or "compulsions," a ritual or routine that attempts to eliminate the thought. The obsessions and compulsions eventually disrupt the child's ability to function normally and cause a great deal of anxiety (National Mental Health Association, 2004).
- *Post-traumatic stress disorder (PTSD).* Children and adolescents both can suffer from PTSD. It usually follows an unexpected traumatic event. According to the Anxiety Disorders Association of America (2004), there are three main symptoms of PTSD: reliving the event, avoidance and emotional numbing, and physiological arousal.

As seen in **Figure 1**, whatever the type of disorder, anxiety may affect all areas of the child's or adolescent's life and is characterized by behavioral, cognitive, and psychological symptoms. Onset may be sudden, or the disorder may take years to develop (Wilson & Kneisl, 1996).

### Pathophysiology

The development of an anxiety disorder involves interactions between behavioral, psychosocial, and physiologic factors (Wilson & Knesil, 1996). Additionally, some experts also believe that biological and environmental factors play a part in its development (Anxiety Disorders Association of America, 2004). Figure 2 illustrates the physiologic response to anxiety.

**Figure 1. The holistic impact of anxiety.**

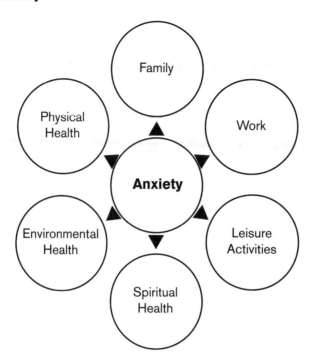

From *Psychiatric Nursing* (5th ed.), (p. 377), by H. S. Wilson and C. R. Kneisl, 1996, Menlo Park, CA: Addison-Wesley. Copyright 1996 by Addison-Wesley Nursing. Adapted with permission.

**Figure 2. The physiologic response to anxiety.**

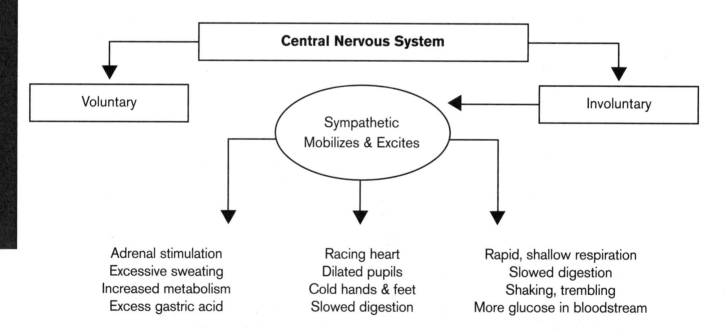

From *Psychiatric Nursing* (5th ed.), (p. 368), by H. S. Wilson and C. R. Kneisl, 1996, Menlo Park, CA: Addison-Wesley. Copyright 1996 by Addison-Wesley Nursing. Adapted with permission.

  Furthermore, the research identifies several theories that address possible causes of anxiety disorders (Wilson & Kneisl, 1996).

### Genetic Theories

Through research, it has been found that there is a familial predisposition for anxiety disorders. According to Gross and Hen (2004), a person's lifelong susceptibility to anxiety is determined by both genetic and environmental influences on early development. Recent twin studies have also shown that the likelihood to develop an anxiety disorder is due to genetic factors (Gordon & Hen, 2004). For children who have a parent with an anxiety disorder, there is a greater risk that they will also develop an anxiety disorder (Barloon, 1993 in Wilson & Kneisl, 1996).

### Psychosocial Theories

In these theories, anxiety is viewed as a psychological conflict. It is believed that the person fears experiencing forbidden impulses. The real source of the anxiety needs to be discovered and dealt with by bringing the unconscious conflict into consciousness (Wilson & Kneisl, 1996).

### Behavioral Theories

According to some learning theorists, anxiety is seen as a learned response that can be changed with behavior modification. These theorists tend to avoid the use of medication because they believe it may interfere with the ability to learn modification behaviors (Wilson & Kneisl, 1996).

### Humanistic Theories

The humanistic approach includes the sociocultural, intrapersonal, environmental, and biological factors when assessing, diagnosing, and planning interventions for the child with an anxiety disorder (Wilson & Kneisl, 1996). The humanistic perspective helps to understand the complex biological, sociocultural, environmental and intrapersonal factors involved with anxiety disorders.

### Other Theories

Current research has also examined the impact of trauma occurring early in life and its involvement in the neurodevelopmental aspect of pathologic anxiety states. Additionally, neurobiological studies have looked further into the role the amygdala plays in both the expression and acquisition of conditioned fear and anxiety (Cummins & Ninan, 2002).

## Diagnosis

Many children and adolescents with anxiety disorders are often not recognized or treated. Furthermore, it can be difficult to determine if a child's behavior is related to a disorder or to developmental adjustments. It was once thought that anxiety was just a mild deviation from a child's normal development, a "stage" or "phase" that caused exaggerated fear or worry (Walkup & Ginsburg, 2002). Consequently, misdiagnosis and undertreatment are common, costing the United States more than $42 billion a year (Anxiety Disorders Association of America, 2004). Anxiety may be experienced along with other clinical syndromes such as mood disorders, depression, or schizophrenia. Therefore, anxiety disorders demand a careful evaluation and often involve a multimethod approach (March & Albano, 1996 in Velting et al., 2004).

Because of an increased universal use of diagnostic interviews, the diagnosis can be more reliable (Saavedra & Silverman, 2002). Diagnosis involves a complete medical examination as well as information that is gathered by the clinician across multiple contexts and from a variety of sources, such as the child, parents, teachers, and peers. There are four basic modalities for assessing the child with anxiety: clinical interviews, self-reporting/rating scales, diaries, and fear hierarchies and behavioral observation (Velting et al., 2004).

## Management

According to Clark (1999), anxiety disorders are a serious mental health concern that have significant short- and long-term morbidity that requires effective treatment. Anxiety disorders of childhood and adolescence can cause functional impairment, poor school performance, social/behavioral concerns, adjustment difficulty, and significant suffering (National Alliance for the Mentally Ill, 2004). Therefore, treatment and management are tailored to the individual's needs. With professional help, the majority of children or adolescents with this disorder can be treated effectively. Early treatment can prevent feelings of low self-esteem, loss of friendships, and social and academic difficulties (American Academy of Child and Adolescent Psychiatry, 2003).

Treatment and management of anxiety disorders include multiple modalities. However, careful diagnosis and the determination of coexisting conditions are critical in the determination of proper treatment. A comprehensive diagnostic evaluation by a physician will determine the specific treatment plan for a given child (National Alliance for the Mentally Ill, 2004). In addition, anxiety with moderate to severe symptoms and functional impairment may require both psychotherapy and drug therapy as a maximal initial intervention (Clark, 1999).

According to the Anxiety Disorders Association of America (2004), a number of effective treatments are currently used:

- Many therapists use a combination of both cognitive and behavioral therapy. With *cognitive-behavior therapy* (CBT), children will be actively involved in their own recovery by learning skills that will be useful for a lifetime.
- *Cognitive therapy* helps children change their thinking patterns and has been found to be effective with panic disorders and social anxiety disorders. The goal is for children to overcome their fears through a change in their thinking about the fear or physical symptoms they are experiencing.
- *Behavior therapy* seeks to change the child's reaction or behavior to a situation that causes the anxiety. This type of therapy helps children to cope with the difficult situation and gives them a sense of control. In addition, deep breathing and relaxation are used as an aid to anxiety management (National Institute of Mental Health, 2000).

- *Psychotherapy* involves children talking with a mental health professional to learn how to express their feelings and deal with their anxiety. This is considered an adjunct therapy to CBT.
- In some instances, the child may benefit from *medication*. Antidepressants and anxiolytics may be used in conjunction with other therapies. Generalized anxiety disorder has a high rate of comorbidity with major depressive disorder (62%) and dysthymia (37%). Therefore, antidepressants may be helpful (Flynn & Chen, 2003). **Table 1** identifies anxiety medications used in children and adolescents.

**Table 1. Anxiety Medications Used With Children and Adolescents**

| Drug Class | Brand Name | Gereric Name | Target Anxiety Disorder |
|---|---|---|---|
| Anticonvulsants | Neurontin | Gabapentin | SAD |
| Azaspirones | BuSpar | Buspirone | GAD |
| Benzodiazepines | Ativan<br>Centrax<br>Dalmane<br>Klonopin<br>Halcion<br>Librium<br>Paxipam<br>Restoril<br>Serax<br>Tranxene<br>Valium<br>Xanax | Lorazepam<br>Prazepam<br>Flurazepam<br>Clonazepam<br>Triazolam<br>Chloridazepoxide<br>Halazepam<br>Temazepam<br>Oxazepam<br>Clorazepate<br>Diazepam<br>Alprazolam | GAD, SAD, panic disorder |
| Beta Blockers | Inderal<br>Tenormin | Propanolol<br>Atenolol | SAD |
| Monoamine Oxidase Inhibitors (MAOIs) | Eldepryl<br>Marplan<br>Nardil<br>Parnate | Selegiline<br>Isocarboxazid<br>Phenelzine<br>Tranylcypromine | Panic disorder, SAD, PTSD |
| Selective Seretonin Reuptake Inhibitors (SSRIs) | Celexa<br>Luvox<br>Prozac<br>Zoloft | Citalopram<br>Fluvoxamine<br>Fluoxetine<br>Sertraline | Panic disorder, OCD, SAD, GAD |
| Tricyclic Antidepressants (TCAs) | Adapin<br>Anafranil<br>Aventyl<br>Elavil<br>Janimine<br>Ludiomil<br>Norpramin<br>Pamelor<br>Pertofrane<br>Sinequan<br>Surmontil<br>Tofranil<br>Vivactil | Doxepin<br>Clomipramine<br>Nortriptyline<br>Amitriptyline<br>Imipramine<br>Maprotiline<br>Desipramine<br>Nortriptyline<br>Desipramine<br>Doxepin<br>Trimipramine<br>Imipramine<br>Protriptylin | Panic disorder, PTSD, OCD (Anafranil only) |
| Other Antidepressants | Desyrel<br>Effexor<br>Serzone | Trazodone<br>Venlafaxine<br>Nefazodone | Panic disorder, OCD, SAD, GAD |

GAD = generalized anxiety disorder; OCD = obsessive-compulsive disorder; PTSD = post-traumatic stress disorder; SAD = social anxiety disorder. Adapted from *Anxiety Medications and Kids* , *2003,* Silver Spring, MD: Anxiety Disorders Association of America. Copyright 2003 by Anxiety Disorders Association of America (www.ADAA.org). Adapted with permission.

Other interventions and strategies that support treatment include the following:

- *School support.* The child with an anxiety disorder needs support within the school setting. Modifications may need to be made to their current program to accommodate their needs.
- *Family therapy.* Support from the family of the child with an anxiety disorder is critical to recovery. Often parents will also have a history of an anxiety disorder; therefore family counseling may helpful.
- *Stress management and meditation.* Both of these modalities may help children to calm themselves

and enhance the effects of therapy. Aerobic exercise may also be of value (National Institute of Mental Health, 2000).

Anxiety disorders affect a significant number of children and adolescents. If these disorders are not recognized and treated, those affected are at risk for educational underachievement, impaired functioning, mood disorders, depression, alcohol and drug abuse, and a decreased level of support (Velting et al., 2004).

## Individualized Healthcare Plan

### Assessment

*History*
- Child's medical and developmental history
- Known allergies
- Medication history
- Family history of anxiety or mental health disorders
- Age at onset of symptoms
- Source of the anxiety
- Recent life-altering events
- Major losses
- History of present condition: student description of his/her symptoms
- Past impairment in social and academic functioning?
- Medical interventions or treatments
- Other treatment modalities being used
- Medication
- Medical and educational assessments
- Sociodemographic information: where he/she lives (house, apartment, etc.), relationship to persons he/she lives with (parents, foster parents, other relatives, etc.), peers his/her age in the neighborhood, local access to mental healthcare
- Financial issues, including health insurance
- Chemical/substance use or abuse

*Current Status and Management*
- Healthcare providers, mental health specialists
- Current anxiety management plan
- Current medications: effects and side effects
- Sleep pattern
- Nutritional pattern
- Energy level: decreased/increased, fatigue, hyperactivity
- Participation in activities of daily living
- Child's current level of functioning: cognitive, social/emotional
- Current developmental needs: maturational or situational
- Symptoms, including somatic complaints/symptoms, difficulty concentrating, irritability, apprehension/fearfulness, confusion
- Current level of distress: risk of suicide
- Thought processes: age-appropriate, coherent, realistic, rational, and oriented
- Possible alcohol abuse or self-medicating behaviors
- Student vital signs and weight

## Self-care
- Student's knowledge of anxiety disorder and its impact on self-care and school activities
- Knowledge of possible stressors
- Knowledge of medication and side effects and who to report effects and side effects to
- Current self-management: hygiene, sleep, nutrition, medication, school work
- Current participation in anxiety management plan
- Independence and dependence on others
- Decision-making skills
- Problem-solving skills

## Psychosocial Status
- Student's strengths and abilities
- Student's perception of his/her health condition
- Parent's perception of the health condition
- Student's response to the diagnosis
- Student's current coping strategies: effectiveness
- Parent's and other family members' current coping strategies: effectiveness
- Support systems: home, community, school, etc.
- Social functioning: impairment
- Social activities or activities with peers
- Impact of anxiety on family, social and school relationships

## Academic Issues
- Academic performance and achievement: past and current
- Educational implications of anxiety: decreased productivity and academic performance, disruptions to normal school routine and activities, inability to complete work due to constant worry and anxiety, difficulty concentrating, eagerness to please but critical of own performance, etc.
- Attendance pattern: reasons for absences
- Modifications needed in the school environment or educational program: small-group testing, alternate assignments (taped speech instead of standing in front of a class), alternate passing time in hallways, access to quiet, private space when needed to decrease anxiety, etc.
- Need for educational support or accommodations: special education, 504 plan

## Nursing Diagnoses (N.D.) (NANDA, 2003)

**N.D. 1** Deficient knowledge (NANDA 00126) related to:
- Recent diagnosis of anxiety disorder
- Lack of understanding of the disorder
- Management of treatment and medication regimen

**N.D. 2** Fear (NANDA 00148) related to:
- Inability to predict or control symptoms
- Feeling of panic and impending doom during anxiety episodes
- Feelings of distress

**N.D. 3** Risk for low self-esteem (NANDA 00153) related to:
- Academic difficulties
- Poor school attendance
- Shame and embarrassment
- Feelings of worthlessness
- Fatigue
- Social withdrawal

**N.D. 4** Ineffective individual coping (NANDA 00069) related to:
- Lack of or inadequate coping strategies
- Possible substance abuse and self-medicating behaviors
- Interrupted sleep
- Irritability and restlessness
- Worrying
- Possible associated depression
- Knowledge deficit of school resources

**N.D. 5** Ineffective role performance (NANDA 00055) related to:
- Isolation from social activities or peers
- Decreased productivity and school performance
- Dependence on others
- Impact of anxiety on family, social, and school relationships
- Poor school attendance

**N.D. 6** Disturbed sleep pattern (NANDA 00095) related to:
- Insomnia
- Nightmares or night terrors
- Panic attacks during the nighttime
- Other somatic complaints

**N.D. 7** Hopelessness (NANDA 00124) related to:
- Symptoms of depression
- Inadequate coping strategies
- Chronic anxiety
- Fear and apprehension

**N.D. 8** Disturbed thought processes (NANDA 00130) related to:
- Sensory alterations
- Reduced ability to solve problems
- Poor concentration and attention
- Impaired judgment
- Impaired abstract reasoning
- Possible distortion of the meaning of a situation
- Disrupted personality
- Unrealistic or distorted perception
- High level of anxiety

## Goals

The student will describe his/her symptoms of anxiety, in his/her own words, and what impact symptoms have on activities of daily living. (N.D. 1)

The student will identify symptoms that indicate his/her own anxiety. (N.D. 1)

The student will increase his/her knowledge about anxiety disorders and his/her anxiety management plan. (N.D.1)

The student will increase his/her knowledge about common physiologic, emotional, and cognitive features of anxiety. (N.D. 1, 4)

The student will increase participation in school activities. (N.D. 2, 3, 5)

The student will use positive coping strategies to deal with anxiety episodes. (N.D. 4)

The student will identify triggers or sources of anxiety and fear. (N.D. 2, 4, 7)

The student will maintain a good school attendance pattern. (N.D. 3, 5)

The student will maintain a normal uninterrupted sleep pattern. (N.D. 6)

The student will develop and maintain healthy sleep patterns. (N.D. 6)

The student will maintain a healthy relationships with his/her family members. (N.D. 5)

The student will establish and maintain healthy peer relationships. (N.D. 3, 5)

The student will identify symptoms of depression. (N.D. 3, 4, 6, 7, 8)

The student will increase his/her knowledge about the proper use, expected benefits, and side effects of his/her prescribed medication. (N.D. 1)

The student will identify his/her support system at home, at school, and within the community. (N.D. 4, 7)

The student will experience and report fewer somatic complaints. (N.D. 2, 4)

The student will decrease frequency of acute anxiety episodes at school/home. (N.D. 2, 4, 7)

The student will maintain academic performance and achievement. (N.D. 3, 8)

The student will increase his/her ability to concentrate and complete school work. (N.D. 3, 8)

The student will participate in activities with peers in school activities and after-school activities. (N.D. 3, 5)

The student will increase his/her ability to cope with symptoms of anxiety and panic. (N.D. 4, 7)

## Nursing Interventions

Assist the education team in assessing the learning needs of the student. (N.D. 1)

Assist the education team alerting the student of any changes to the usual school day before it happens. Examples: (N.D. 3, 5, 8)
- I will be gone tomorrow to a meeting, so you will be having a substitute teacher.
- We will be switching activities in physical education class tomorrow from volleyball to basketball.
- We will have a test on Friday on Chapter 3—Revolutionary War. Write it down in your planner.

Discuss anxiety disorder with the student: Determine the student's understanding of the disorder and his/her symptoms and what further information the student needs and wants to know. (N.D. 1, 8)

Educate the student about his/her condition and management plan, including medication. (N.D. 1)

Assist the student in identifying the goals of his/her anxiety management plan. (N.D. 1)

Collaborate with educational staff in implementing instructional strategies and classroom accommodations as needed. (ND 1)
- Modify/adapt curriculum to better fit student's learning style.
- Post daily schedule/assignments, so the student knows what to expect.
- Set and keep a schedule, as much as possible.
- Encourage student to check in with teacher (or teacher with student) to make sure assignments are written down correctly.

Suggest that the student keep a journal of anxiety episodes. (N.D. 3, 8)

Assist the student identifying his/her strengths and abilities. (N.D. 1, 3, 4)

Assist the student identifying previous and current effective coping strategies. (N.D. 1, 3, 4)

Identify effective coping mechanisms that are not presently being used. (N.D. 1, 4)

Assist the student in identifying precipitating events or sources of their anxiety or fear. (N.D. 1, 4)

Assist the student to verbalizing his/her thoughts and feelings. (N.D. 4)

During acute anxiety or panic episodes at school:
- Assess the level of distress. (N.D. 2, 4, 7, )
- Assess the student's perception of what is occurring. (N.D. 3, 5, 8)
- Assess the student's thought process. (N.D. 8)
  -coherent
  -oriented
  -rational thought process
  -decision-making ability
  -problem-solving capability
- Reduce external stimulation by providing a private, quiet, safe place for the student to go, with supportive supervision.

Assist student in identifying and setting up a support network at home, at school, and within the community. (N.D. 1, 4, 5)

Assist student and parents/guardians to identify the effects of the anxiety disorder on the entire family. (N.D. 1)

If medication needs to be administered during the school day: (N.D. 2, 3, 7, 8)
- Obtain parent/guardian and healthcare provider authorization.
- Obtain medication supply, in properly labeled container.
- Document medication given.

Assist student and parents/guardians to identify and utilize healthcare providers for management of the student's anxiety disorder: evaluation, follow-up appointments, further symptom management, concerns and problems, refilling prescribed medications.

Collaborate with parents/guardians, student, and healthcare providers. (N.D. 5)
- Facilitate communication.
- Monitor effectiveness of medication and therapies during the school day.
- Monitor and document student symptoms during the school day.

Collaborate with parents/guardians and healthcare providers (psychiatrist, psychologist, therapist, etc) in managing symptoms at school. (N.D. 2, 4, 5)

Teach and reinforce use of adaptive, effective coping mechanisms. (N.D. 1, 4)

Provide emotional support, caring, empathy, and a listening ear. (N.D. 3, 7)

Identify, with the student, measures that reduce anxiety. (N.D. 1, 4)

Assist the student in learning and utilizing problem-solving skills. (N.D. 2, 3, 4, 7)

Monitor for risk of suicide. (N.D. 2, 4, 7, 8)

Assist student to identify somatic complaints associated with his/her anxiety. (N.D. 5, 7, 8)

Collaborate with school psychologist/counselor/social worker; refer student for counseling or further evaluation, if indicated. (N.D. 4, 7, 8)

Discuss and reinforce the importance of maintaining a good nutritional pattern and regular exercise. (N.D.1, 4, 6)

Teach the student relaxation exercises, and assist him/her to use them to reduce stress and anxiety symptoms. (N.D. 1, 2, 4, 6, 7)

Provide assistance to a student experiencing anxiety or panic symptoms in school (see **Table 2**). (N.D. 2, 4)

**Table 2. Nursing Interventions for Working With Students With Anxiety or Panic Episodes**

| Strategy | Rationale |
|---|---|
| Stay with the student. | Being left alone may further increase the anxiety. |
| Maintain a calm, serene, nonjudgmental manner. | Knowing that the nurse is calm and in control may be reassuring and calming to the student. This will enlist the student's confidence in the nurse. |
| Use a firm and authoritative voice. | Conveys the nurse's ability to provide external controls. |
| Use short, simple sentences. | Because the student's perceptual field is disrupted, the student will experience difficulty focusing and concentrating. |
| Move the student to a quieter, smaller, and less stimulating environment. | Prevents further disruption of the perceptual field by sensory stimuli. |
| Focus the student's diffuse energy on a repetitive or physically tiring task. | Repetitive tasks or physical exercise can help drain off excess energy. |
| Administer antianxiety medication, if prescribed during school hours. | Antianxiety medication may help reduce anxiety. |
| Assess the student's ability to stay at school. Is student in need of further immediate medical care? Does student need to go home? | Depending on the IHP and the physician's recommendations, the student may need medical care or need to be removed from the current situation by the family. |
| Assist the student in understanding that his/her present state has occurred because of the contributing event or panic. | This will help make the anxiety/panic more understandable and less frightening and facilitates hope and coping. |

Adapted From *Psychiatric Nursing* (5th ed.), (p. 379), by H. S. Wilson and C. R. Kneisl, 1996, Menlo Park, CA: Addison-Wesley. Copyright 1996 by Addison-Wesley Nursing.

## Expected Student Outcomes

The student will:
- List physiologic, emotional, and cognitive features of anxiety disorder. (N.D. 1)
- Accurately describe his/her anxiety disorder. (N.D. 1)
- List components (medication, counseling, therapy, relaxation exercises, etc.) of his/her anxiety management plan. (N.D. 1, 4, 7)
- Demonstrate a good school attendance pattern, missing less than days per year due to illness or symptoms related to anxiety. (N.D. 3, 5)
- Participate in school activities, beyond the school day (athletics, chess club, class parties, drama club, etc). (N.D. 3, 5)

- Identify persons in his/her (family, school, community) support system he/she can use for assistance in dealing with anxiety symptoms. (N.D. 4, 5, 7)
- Identify possible triggers or precipitating events to increase in anxiety symptoms or episodes. (N.D. 1, 2)
- Describe how anxiety symptoms have impacted his/her life at school, at home, and in the community. (N.D. 1).
- Describe his/her feelings of nervousness and anxiety to (teachers or identified support persons) when they occur at school. (N.D. 3, 4, 7)
- Demonstrate a healthy sleep pattern, as evidenced by appearing rested at school and as reported by parent/guardian. (N.D. 4, 6)
- Identify symptoms of depression. (N.D. 1, 2, 7)
- Identify support persons at school (school counselor, nurse, psychologist, social worker, teachers and other staff members) who can help in a crisis or as a resource. (N.D. 2, 4)
- Demonstrate active participation in school activities. (N.D.3, 4, 5, 7)
- Demonstrate an ability to concentrate, (____%) of the time, in the classroom setting, as reported by student and teachers. (N.D. 3, 5, 8)
- Complete classroom assignments, (____%) of the time, as reported by student and teachers. (N.D. 3, 5, 8)
- Complete and turn in homework assignments, (____%) of the time, as reported by student and teachers. (N.D. 3, 5, 8)
- Demonstrate reduced episodes or symptoms of anxiety (for example, tachycardia, chest pain, fear of dying) at school. (N.D. 2, 7)
- Demonstrate reduced episodes or symptoms of anxiety at home, as reported by student and parents/guardians. (N.D. 2, 6, 7)
- Demonstrate the use of effective coping strategies (name the strategy). (N.D. 4)
- Demonstrate effective management of panic or anxiety episodes. (N.D. 2, 4, 7)
- Name and describe (number, ex: 2) somatic symptoms he/she has experienced related to his/her anxiety. (N.D. 4,6,8)
- Name somatic symptoms that have decreased in frequency and/or intensity. (N.D. 4, 6, 8)
- Report symptoms of physiologic, emotional, or cognitive distress as well as perceptual changes or somatic discomforts to teachers. (N.D. 4, 7, 8)
- Sleep hours a night, uninterrupted, as reported by student and parent. (N.D. 4, 6)
- Demonstrate appropriate, healthy interactions with peers in the school setting. (N.D. 5)
- Demonstrate appropriate, healthy interactions with family members, as reported by student and parents/guardians. (N.D. 5)
- Demonstrate appropriate interactions with teachers and school staff. (N.D. 5)
- Name the medication he/she is taking to reduce symptoms of anxiety. (N.D. 1)
- Identify positive effects of the medication on his/her anxiety symptoms. (N.D. 1)
- Identify (possible/actual) side effects of the medication. (N.D. 1)

# Case Study

Emma is a 15-year-old high school student recently diagnosed as having an anxiety disorder. A year ago, she began experiencing frequent onset of anxiety and panic, shortness of breath, chest pain, sweaty palms, and a fear of dying. These episodes would happen suddenly and without warning to the point where she started avoiding school and any place an attack had previously occurred. It was also noted that visits to the school nurse and counselor were increasing as she constantly anticipated an "attack" and reported feeling helpless and worthless and thinking she was losing her mind. Her anxiety became so severe it started to interfere with her daily social and academic activities. Because of this, her attendance at school started to suffer and her life became extremely restricted. Her worries became exaggerated and excessive. Eventually her friendships, schoolwork, and family relationships also suffered. Emma is an above-average student who strives to please and holds herself to strict academic standards, which she is no longer able to meet. Her perceptions are distorted and unrealistic, creating difficulty in her ability to attend and concentrate. It became obvious that she did not have any strategies for coping with her anxiety. Subsequently, she feels guilty and ashamed and as if she has failed. It is difficult for her family to accept that she is having problems in school.

Emma's mother also lives with an anxiety disorder that often cripples her ability to keep a job and live her life. She can understand the challenges Emma is facing; however, it takes all the energy she can muster to deal with her own worries. Unfortunately, she is not much support to Emma. Her father works full-time and tries the best he can to support two family members with a mental illness. Her brother is very quiet and often keeps to himself to avoid the tension and conflict that occurs within the family.

Emma's management plan includes a combination of cognitive and behavioral therapy along with the antidepressant Zoloft. The school nurse and counselor are instrumental in keeping Emma in school, supporting her in attending her therapy sessions, and monitoring the effects of her medication.

## Anxiety Disorder

| Assessment Data | Nursing Diagnosis | Goals | Nursing Interventions | Expected Outcomes |
|---|---|---|---|---|
| Recent diagnosis of anxiety disorder.<br><br>Symptoms of anxiety and panic for a year. | Deficient knowledge related to recent diagnosis of anxiety disorder, and minimal understanding about her anxiety management plan. | Emma will demonstrate an increased knowledge of anxiety disorder and her anxiety management plan.<br><br>Emma will identify signs and symptoms of anxiety and fear. | Assist Emma in learning about anxiety disorders, her anxiety management plan.<br><br>Assist Emma in learning and describing the implications her diagnosis has for school, social, and academic interactions.<br><br>Discuss with Emma why the symptoms occur and what interventions can be used to decrease the severity or length of the symptoms.<br><br>Assist Emma to learn about the medication she is taking, its benefits, and side effects. Discuss with Emma the importance of taking her medication as prescribed. | Emma will describe her anxiety disorder.<br><br>Emma will list the components of her management plan.<br><br>Emma will describe 3 physiologic, 3 emotional, and 3 cognitive features of anxiety that she experiences.<br><br>Emma will describe what occurs during an anxiety or panic episode.<br><br>Emma will identify 2 things that make the symptoms decrease or go away.<br><br>Emma will list the medication she is currently taking and identify and describe benefits and side effects. |
| Sudden and unpredictable onset of symptoms: anxiety, panic, shortness of breath, chest pain, sweaty palms, fear of dying.<br><br>Constantly anticipating "attacks".<br><br>Emma feels like she is losing her mind. | Fear, related to inability to predict or control symptoms, feeling of panic and impending doom during anxiety episodes, and feelings of distress. | Emma will decrease frequency of fear and anxiety episodes at school. | Assist in setting up a safe location during the school day for Emma to go to calm down and use relaxation techniques learned in therapy (per her management plan).<br><br>Provide supportive measures to assist Emma to decrease her fear, anxiety, and panic when it occurs. | Emma will describe how she feels when symptoms of anxiety occur.<br><br>Emma utilizes school staff for assistance during an anxiety or panic episode.<br><br>Emma will demonstrate effective management of an anxiety or panic episode at school. |

| Assessment Data | Nursing Diagnosis | Goals | Nursing Interventions | Expected Outcomes |
|---|---|---|---|---|
| No evident coping strategies. Feelings of shame, guilt, and failure. Holds self to strict academic standards. Continually striving to please. Feels helpless, worthless. | Ineffective individual coping, related to stress regarding possible school failure, developmental level/understanding, stressors that exacerbate symptoms, anxiety, possible associated depression, and knowledge deficit of school resources. | Emma will learn and use positive, effective coping strategies to deal with anxiety episodes. Emma will identify triggers or sources of anxiety and fear. Emma will identify her support system at school, at home, and within her community. | Assist Emma to identify coping strategies she uses, effective and ineffective. Assist Emma to learn effective coping strategies. Reinforce the use of effective coping strategies. Assist Emma in identifying the triggers and sources of her anxiety and fear. Assist Emma to identify persons who can be a support to her at school, at home, and in the community. Assist Emma to identify: • Aspects of her life she has control over • Aspects of her life she does not have control over and how she can use supportive persons to help her with both Determine Emma's risk for depression and suicide. | Emma will identify 2 ways to express her needs. Emma will identify 3 coping strategies that can be utilized when experiencing symptoms of anxiety or fear. Emma will demonstrate 2 effective coping strategies that reduce her anxiety. Emma will identify 2 school-related situations/activities that cause known distress. Emma will identify 3 school staff members who can help her in a crisis or as a resource for assistance. Emma will identify 2 family members she can use for support and assistance. Emma will identify 2 community members she can use for support and assistance. |
| Poor school attendance. Symptoms interfering with daily social and academic activities. Restricted life due to avoidance behaviors. | Ineffective role performance, related to isolation from social activities or peers, decreased productivity and school performance, dependence on others, impact of anxiety on family, social and school relationships, and poor school attendance. | Emma will increase her school attendance pattern. Emma will increase social interactions with friends. | With assistance from parents and teachers, identify Emma's current level of distress at school and in classes. | Emma will demonstrate a good school pattern (less than 5 days missed due to illness or symptoms related to anxiety). Emma will actively participate with peers in classroom activities. |

| Assessment Data | Nursing Diagnosis | Goals | Nursing Interventions | Expected Outcomes |
|---|---|---|---|---|
| | | | With assistance from parents and teachers, identify Emma's current level of distress at school and in classes.<br><br>Assist Emma in identifying and setting up a support network at home, at school, and within her community she can use for assistance. | Emma will participate in one school activity with peers beyond the school day (name the activity).<br><br>Emma will demonstrate appropriate healthy interactions with peers in the school setting.<br><br>Emma will identify 2 ineffective avoidance behaviors she has used and what occurred because she uses them. |
| Distorted, unrealistic, and exaggerated perceptions of her situation.<br><br>Difficulty attending and concentrating on schoolwork.<br><br>Excessive, exaggerated worry.<br><br>Somatic complaints. | Disturbed thought processes, related to sensory alterations, reduced ability to solve problems, poor concentration and attention, possible distortion of the meaning of a situation, and unrealistic or distorted perception, and high level of anxiety. | Emma will increase her ability to concentrate and complete schoolwork.<br><br>Emma will maintain academic performance and achievement.<br><br>Emma will experience and report fewer perceptual changes, somatic complaints, and sensory alterations. | Assist the educational team in assessing the educational needs of Emma.<br>• Emma's perception of her learning and ability to learn:<br>• strengths<br>• weaknesses<br>• how she learns best<br>• what she needs assistance with<br>• Emma's thought processes:<br>-coherent<br>-rational cognitive process<br>-oriented to role and expectations<br>-decision-making ability<br>-problem-solving capability<br><br>Assist teachers to make modifications in the classroom as needed:<br>• preferential seating | Emma will demonstrate an increased ability to concentrate in the classroom setting.<br><br>Emma will complete schoolwork assigned in class and homework.<br><br>Emma will identify and effectively demonstrate 2 problem-solving strategies that reduce symptoms and assist her to be successful in classes.<br><br>Emma will identify when she is experiencing somatic symptoms and how anxiety maybe related to the symptom(s). |

| Assessment Data | Nursing Diagnosis | Goals | Nursing Interventions | Expected Outcomes |
|---|---|---|---|---|
| | | | • study/work time in library to assist in decreasing distractions<br>• clarifying questions and assignment criteria to be followed<br>• repeating or restating directions, so Emma understands them<br><br>Suggest Emma keep a journal of all anxiety episodes.<br><br>Assist Emma in identifying problem-solving strategies that decrease symptoms.<br><br>Ask Emma to describe her somatic symptoms.<br><br>Assist Emma in learning and using problem-solving skills. | Emma will name 2 somatic symptoms she has experienced related to her anxiety.<br><br>Emma utilizes problem-solving skills to decrease somatic symptoms. |

# Anxiety Disorders in Adolescents: A Self–Test

How much stress or worry is considered too much? Complete the following self-test by checking "yes" or "no" next to each question. If you are concerned about a possible anxiety disorder, show the results to your healthcare professional.5009

## As a teenager, are you troubled by:

| | |
|---|---|
| Repeated, unexpected "attacks" during which you suddenly are overcome by intense fear or discomfort for no apparent reason, or the fear of having another panic attack? | ○ Yes ○ No |
| Persistent, inappropriate thoughts, impulses or images that you can't get out of your mind (such as preoccupation with getting dirty or with worry about the order of things)? | ○ Yes ○ No |
| Distinct and ongoing fear of social situations involving unfamiliar people? | ○ Yes ○ No |
| Excessive worrying about a number of events or activities? | ○ Yes ○ No |
| Fear of places or situations where getting help or escape might be difficult, such as in a crowd or on an elevator? | ○ Yes ○ No |
| Shortness of breath or racing heart for no apparent reason? | ○ Yes ○ No |
| Persistent and unreasonable fear of an object or situation, such as flying, heights, animals, blood, etc.? | ○ Yes ○ No |
| Being able to travel alone, without a companion? | ○ Yes ○ No |
| Spending too much time each day doing things over and over again (i.e., hand washing, checking things, or counting)? | ○ Yes ○ No |

## More days than not, do you:

| | |
|---|---|
| Feel restless? | ○ Yes ○ No |
| Feel easily fatigued or distracted? | ○ Yes ○ No |
| Experience muscle tension or problems sleeping? | ○ Yes ○ No |

## More days than not, do you feel:

| | |
|---|---|
| Sad or depressed? | ○ Yes ○ No |
| Disinterested in life? | ○ Yes ○ No |
| Worthless or guilty? | ○ Yes ○ No |
| You have experienced changes in your sleeping or eating habits? | ○ Yes ○ No |
| You relive a traumatic event through thoughts, games, distressing dreams, or flashbacks? | ○ Yes ○ No |
| Your anxiety interferes with your daily life? | ○ Yes ○ No |

Based on *Diagnostic and Statistical Manual of Mental Disorders* (4th ed.), 1994, Washington, DC: American Psychiatric Association. From Anxiety Disorders Association of America Web site. Retrieved January 15, 2004, from http://www.adaa.org/Public/selftest_ADA.htm. Adapted with permission.

| | | |
|---|---|---|
| If you think your child may have an anxiety disorder, please answer the following questions and show the results to your child's healthcare professional. | ○ **Yes** | ○ **No** |
| Does the child have a distinct and ongoing fear of social situations involving unfamiliar people? | ○ **Yes** | ○ **No** |
| Does the child worry excessively about a number of events or activities? | ○ **Yes** | ○ **No** |
| Does the child experience shortness of breath or a racing heart for no apparent reason? | ○ **Yes** | ○ **No** |
| Does the child experience age-appropriate social relationships with family members and other familiar people? | ○ **Yes** | ○ **No** |
| Does the child often appear anxious when interacting with his/her peers and avoid them? | ○ **Yes** | ○ **No** |
| Does the child have a persistent and unreasonable fear of an object or situation such as flying, heights, animals, blood, etc.? | ○ **Yes** | ○ **No** |
| When the child encounters the feared object or situation, does he/she react by clinging, freezing, or having a tantrum? | ○ **Yes** | ○ **No** |
| Does the child cry, have tantrums, or refuse to leave a family member or other familiar person when he/she must? | ○ **Yes** | ○ **No** |
| Does the child worry excessively about his/her competence and the quality of that performance? | ○ **Yes** | ○ **No** |
| Does the child spend too much time each day doing things over and over again (i.e., hand washing, checking things, or counting)? | ○ **Yes** | ○ **No** |
| Has the child experienced a decline in classroom performance, refused to go to school, or avoided age-appropriate social activities? | ○ **Yes** | ○ **No** |
| Does the child have exaggerated fears of people or events (i.e., burglars, kidnappers, car accidents) that might be difficult, such as in a crowd or on an elevator? | ○ **Yes** | ○ **No** |
| Does the child experience a high number of nightmares, headaches or stomachaches? | ○ **Yes** | ○ **No** |
| Does the child repetitively re-enact with toys scenes from a disturbing event? | ○ **Yes** | ○ **No** |
| Does the child redo tasks because of excessive dissatisfaction with less-than-perfect performance? | ○ **Yes** | ○ **No** |

Based on *Diagnostic and Statistical Manual of Mental Disorders* (4th ed.), 1994, Washington, DC: American Psychiatric Association. From Anxiety Disorders Association of America Web site. Retrieved January 15, 2004, from http://www. adaa.org/Public/selftest_ADA.htm. Adapted with permission.

# References

American Academy of Child and Adolescent Psychiatry. (2003). *The anxious child.* Retrieved January 15, 2004, from www.aacap.org/publications/factsfam/anxious.htm

Achenbach, T.M., Howell, C.T., McConaughy, S.H. & Stanger, C. (1995). Six-year predictors of problems in a national sample of children and youth: I. Cross-informant syndromes. *Journal of the American Academy of Child and Adolescent Psychiatry, 34,* 336-347.

Anxiety Disorders Association of America. (2004). *Anxiety disorders information: A guide to treatment.* Retrieved January 15, 2004, from www.adaa.org

Anxiety Disorders Association of America. (2004). *Brief overview of anxiety disorders.* Retrieved January 15, 2004, from www.adaa.org

Clark, D. (1999). New developments in the drug treatment of common adolescent mental disorders. *Brain waves: A neurological update for school nurses.* Seattle, WA: University of Washington School of Medicine, Department of Psychiatry.

Cummins, T. K., & Ninan, P. T. (2002). The neurobiology of anxiety in children and adolescents. *International Review of Psychiatry, 14,* 114–128.

Flynn, C. A., & Chen, Y. C. (2003). Antidepressants for generalized anxiety disorder. *American Family Physician, 68*(9), 1757–1759.

Gordan, J. A., & Hen, R. (2004). Genetic approaches to the study of anxiety. *Neuroscience, 27,* 193–222.

Gross, C., & Hen, R. (2004). The developmental origins of anxiety. *Neuroscience 5,* 545–552.

Gurley, D., Cohen, P., Pine, D.S., & Brook, J. (1996). Cognitive-behavioral and pharmacological treatment of generalized anxiety disorder: A preliminary meta-analysis. *Behavior Therapy, 28,* 285-305.

NANDA International. (2003). *Nursing diagnoses: Definitions & classifications 2003-2004.* Philadelphia: Author.

National Alliance for the Mentally Ill. (2004). *Anxiety disorders in children and adolescents.* Retrieved January 15, 2004, from www.nami.org

National Institute of Mental Health. (2000). *Anxiety disorders.* Bethesda, MD: Author.

National Mental Health Association. (2004). *Anxiety disorders.* Retrieved January 15, 2004, from www.nmha.org

Saavedra, L., & Silverman, W. (2002). Classification of anxiety disorders in children: What a difference two decades make. *International Review of Psychiatry, 14,* 87–101.

Walkup, J. T., & Ginsburg, G. S. (2002). Anxiety disorders in children and adolescents. *International Review of Psychiatry, 14,* 85–86.

Wilson, H. S., & Kneisl, C. R. (1996*). Psychiatric nursing* (5th ed.). Menlo Park, CA: Addison-Wesley.

Velting, O. N., Setzer, N. J., & Albano, A. M. (2004*).* Update on and advances in assessment and cognitive-behavioral treatment of anxiety disorders in children and adolescents. *Professional Psychology: Research and Practice 35,* 42–54.

# Bibliography

Adelman, H., & Taylor, L. (1997-2000). *Nursing assessment of school age youth. Psychosocial screening.* (Home Study Module No. 3). Scarborough, ME: National Association of School Nurses.

Bergren, M. D. (2002). Child and adolescent mental health Web resources. *Journal of School Nursing, 18*(4), 226–228.

Beidel, D. (1998). *Special focus on anxiety disorders in children, adolescents and young adults.* Silver Spring, MD: Anxiety Disorders Association of America (ADAA).

*Clinical Guidelines for School Nurses* (2002). *School health alert* (5th ed.). Nashville, TN: Author.

Delaney, K. R., Belmonte-Mann, F. (2001). Identifying the mental health needs of preschool children. *Journal of School Nursing, 17*(4), 222–226.

Denehy, J. (2002). Supporting children through these uncertain times. *Journal of School Nursing, 18*(1), 1–2.

Denehy, J. (2002). The mental health needs of children and adolescents. *Journal of School Nursing, 18*(4), 189–190.

DeSocio, J., Hootman, J. (2004). Children's mental health and school success. *Journal of School Nursing, 20*(4), 189–196.

Hootman, J., Houck, G. M., King, M. C. (2002). A program to educate school nurses about mental health interventions. *Journal of School Nursing, 18*(4), 191–195.

Hyman, S. E., & Rudorfer, M. V. (2000). Anxiety disorders. In: D. C. Dale, D. D. Federman (Eds.), *Scientific American Medicine: Vol. 3.* New York: Healtheon/WebMD Corp., Section13, Subsect, VIII.: Research and Practice

March, J. S., & Albano, A. M. (2002). Anxiety disorders in children and adolescents. In D. Stein & E. Hollander (Eds.), *Textbook of anxiety disorders* (pp. 415–427). Washington, DC: American Psychological Association.

National Association of School Nurses. (n.d.). *Addressing the mental health needs of children and adolescence* [Education Program]. Retrieved November 7, 2004, from http://nasn.org/education/education.htm

National Association of School Nurses. (2000). *Issue Brief: Mental health and illness.* Scarborough, ME: Author.

National Association of School Nurses. (Revised 2000). *Position Statement: Mental health of students.* Scarborough, ME: Author.

National Association of School Nurses. (2003). *Issue Brief: Bully peer.* Scarborough, ME: Author.

Schniering, C. A., Hudson, J. L., & Rapee, R. M. (2000). Issues in the diagnosis and assessment of anxiety disorders in children and adolescents. *Clinical Psychology Review, 20,* 453–478.

Wong, D. L., Hockenberry, M. J., Wilson, D., Winkelstein, M. L., & Kline, N. E. (2003). *Wong's nursing care of infants and children* (7th ed.). St. Louis, MO: Mosby.

## Resources

American Academy of Child and Adolescent Psychiatry (AACAP)
PO Box 96106
Washington, DC 200090
www.aacap.org

American Psychiatric Association
1000 Wilson Boulevard
Suite 1825
Arlington, VA 22209-3901
703-907-7300
www.psych.org.main.html

American Psychological Association (APA)
750 First Street, NE
Washington, DC 20002-4242
202-336-5500
www.apa.org

Anxiety Disorders Association of America (ADAA)
8730 Georgia Avenue
Suite 600
Silver Spring, MD 20910
301-231-9350
www.adaa.org

Association for Advancement of Behavior Therapy
395 Seventh Avenue
New York, NY 10001
212-647-1890
www.aabt.org

Center for Mental Health Services (CMHS)-US

Department of Health and Human Services, Knowledge Exchange Network (KEN)
PO Box 42490
Washington, DC 20015
1-800-789-2647
www.mentalhealth.org

Depression and Related Affective Disorders Association (DRADA)
600 North Wolf Street
Meyer 3-181
Baltimore, MD 21287-7381
410-955-4647

ERIC Clearinghouse—Disabilities and Gifted Education
1920 Association Drive
Reston, VA 20191
1-800-328-0272
703-264-9494 (fax)
http://ericec.org

National Alliance for the Mentally Ill (NAMI)
200 North Glebe Road
Suite 1015
Arlington, VA 22203-3754
703-516-7991 (TDD)
www.nami.org

National Anxiety Foundation
3135 Custer Drive
Lexington, KY 40517
1-800-755-1576
http://lexington-on-line.com/naf.html

National Center for PTSD
U.S. Department of Veterans Affairs
116 VA Medical and Regional Office Center
215 Main Street
White River Junction, VT 05009
802-296-5132
www.ncptsd.org

National Institute of Mental Health (NIMH)
Anxiety Disorders Education Program
Office of Communications and Public Liaison
6001 Executive Boulevard
Room 8184, MSC 9663
Bethesda, MD 20892-9663
1-88-88-ANXIETY
www.nimh.nih.gov

National Library of Medicine
Clinical Trials Database
www.clinicaltrials.gov

National Mental Health Association (NMHA)
2001 North Beauregard Street
12th floor
Alexandria, VA 22311
703-684-7722
www.nmha.org

Obsessive Compulsive (OC) Foundation
337 Notch Hill Road
North Brandford, CT 06471
203-315-2190
203-315-2196 (fax)www.ocfoundation.org

*Chapter Twenty-three*

# Asthma

Jacalyn Peck Dougherty

## Introduction

Asthma is a serious, chronic respiratory disease characterized by airway inflammation and recurrent episodes of airway swelling, constriction, and excessive formation of mucus. As one of the most common chronic illnesses in children, it is responsible for significant physical, social, and economic burdens for students and their families. These burdens are often underestimated and sometimes unrecognized. They include missed school days (Newacheck & Halfon, 2000) and missed time from class; missed time at work for parents and caregivers; physician office and emergency department visits; costly hospitalizations (National Center for Health Statistics, 2004; Weiss, Sullivan, & Lytle, 2000); and curtailed activities, lifestyle changes, and adaptations made by affected children and family members to accommodate the disorder, particularly when asthma is poorly controlled (American Lung Association, 1998). Although rare, asthma is also responsible for deaths in children, with the highest childhood mortality rates occurring in adolescence (Akinbami & Schoendorf, 2002). These deaths are largely preventable with proper treatment.

Asthma affects children and adults of all ages, all races, and both males and females. More males than females have the disorder in childhood and adolescence; more females than males have asthma in adulthood (Institute of Medicine, 2000). Ethnic minorities, especially African Americans and Puerto Rican Hispanics, and poor children living in urban areas tend to be disproportionately affected (National Institutes of Health, 1997; Akinbami & Schoendorf, 2002). The higher prevalence of asthma in African American children and adults reflects the confounding of race and conditions associated with lower socioeconomic status, such as crowded housing; recurrent exposure to agents and situations that contribute to asthma episodes, such as dust mites, roaches, pollution, mold, and respiratory infections; and lack of access to healthcare, all factors that have been associated with greater asthma morbidity and mortality.

About 12% of the population of children 17 years and younger—or 6.4 million children from birth up to 18 years of age—were reported to have asthma in 2002, and almost 6% of these children experienced an asthma episode (or attack) in the previous year (National Center for Health Statistics, 2004). Given the prevalence of asthma and the fact that individuals with even relatively mild disease are at risk for experiencing a life-threatening asthma episode, school nurses need to be familiar with this chronic condition and its appropriate management. Moreover, the many environmental factors that promote chronic airway inflammation and trigger acute respiratory distress underscore the importance of providing continuity in healthcare services between healthcare provider offices, the home and community settings like day-care centers, and the school environment. School nurses, public health nurses working in schools, and school-based or school-linked health center nurse practitioners serve a vital role in ensuring this continuity toward the goal of keeping children with asthma safe, in school, and ready to learn. And, although asthma can't be cured, it can and should be well controlled so that students are afforded every opportunity for optimal physical, emotional, social, and academic development.

## Pathophysiology

Asthma can develop at any age, but 50% to 80% of children with asthma develop symptoms before age 5 (American Academy of Allergy, Asthma, and Immunology [AAAAI], 2003). Although most children with asthma have allergies, children with allergies don't necessarily have asthma. The diagnosis of asthma in children is complicated by the lack of consensus by physicians about the criteria for defining its onset (Institute of Medicine, 2000), the hesitation of providers to confer a chronic disease "label" on children, younger children's inability to express verbally the symptoms they are experiencing, the difficulty in obtaining objective measures of lung function (e.g., spirometry, peak expiratory flows) in those younger than five, and the lack of continuity in healthcare providers seen by those at greatest risk. Thus, school nurses are likely to have children in their school who have symptoms of this condition, but no formal diagnosis.

The diagnosis of asthma is also complicated by the fact that it is highly variable in how it manifests; some children wheeze only occasionally or in conjunction with respiratory infections and generally remain symptom-free between episodes. Many young wheezers "outgrow" their tendency to wheeze with colds as their airways become larger. In contrast, other children, particularly those with allergies, eczema, wheezing in the absence of colds, and a family history of asthma (AAAAI, 2003), persist with recurrent episodes of wheezing, shortness of breath, chest tightness, and coughing, the four classic signs and symptoms of a worsening of the chronic condition.

The diagnosis of asthma may become more apparent when a recurring pattern of "bad" or "lingering" chest colds becomes evident or with repeated episodes of bronchitis, bronchiolitis, pneumonia, or hospitalizations for respiratory infections. In others, a pattern of wheezing and difficulty breathing in conjunction with physical activity or exercise unfolds. However, it is important to note that some children with asthma don't wheeze; rather, they present only with recurrent coughing. These individuals may be identified by eliciting a careful history that yields a finding of persistent coughing, especially at night or early in the morning. These students may also appear fatigued at school because they haven't slept well.

Although the exact cause of chronic asthma is unknown, three major factors have been linked with whether or not individuals *develop* this disorder. These are genetic susceptibility, exposure to respiratory infections early in life, and contact with certain agents in the environment that either predispose individuals to asthma development or, in contrast, provide a degree of protection against its development (Institute of Medicine, 2000, AAAAI, 2003). First, *genetic endowment* plays a role in both the extent to which individuals are sensitive or resilient to allergens and to infections, in their ability to adapt to environmental conditions, and in the extent to which their immune systems react when allergenic or irritating substances are encountered. As noted earlier, those with a history of allergy and asthma in the immediate family are more likely to develop symptoms of asthma than are others without such a history.

Second, asthma has been linked in preliminary research to particular *respiratory infections in early life.* For example, research suggests that young children who experience respiratory syncytial virus infections may be more prone to subsequent asthma development. Although the exact mechanism is not known, it is thought that the virus may trigger cellular changes in the airway lining that contribute to increased airway sensitivity and chronic inflammation. However, it may also be the case that children who are predisposed to asthma are more susceptible to the effects of respiratory viruses than are those without this genetic predisposition.

Third, research also strongly suggests that *exposure to tobacco smoke* and to *dust mite antigens* in the early years contributes to the development of asthma in young children and also is associated with worsening symptoms in those with known disease (Institute of Medicine, 2000). Other data suggest that contact with some agents, like endotoxins encountered by those living on farms, being in close proximity to animals, having older siblings who "share" colds with younger siblings, and being in day care, may confer a degree of protection against developing asthma. One explanation proposed for this is that the stimulation of the body's immune system through a gradual exposure to endotoxins lessens the chance of the body's overreaction to these agents when they are encountered later on.

## Chronic Airway Inflammation

The three factors noted above that have been associated with the development of asthma—genetic susceptibility, certain respiratory infections early in life, and contact with particular environmental agents in the early years—contribute to chronic airway inflammation. This inflammation, in turn, results in increased airway sensitivity, or hyperreactivity. When susceptible individuals are exposed to various factors and agents, called triggers, that irritate the already-sensitive airways, a cascade of effects occurs. First, these triggers (discussed subsequently) cause further airway inflammation. Next, constriction of the muscles surrounding the bronchi, bronchioles, and lungs occurs, and third, there is excessive production of thickened mucus. These effects result in narrowed airways, limited air exchange, and difficulty breathing that are characteristic of asthma episodes.

Although asthma is considered a reversible disease because episodes typically resolve either spontaneously or with treatment, researchers have recently posited that the chronic inflammation associated with unrecognized or undertreated asthma may lead to gradual and permanent alterations in the airways in some individuals (National Institutes of Health, 2003). The inflammatory process may result in structural changes in the airway, termed airway remodeling, that cannot be reversed with therapy (Institute of Medicine, 2000). Thus, controlling airway inflammation and preventing asthma episodes are essential components of asthma management to prevent irreversible damage.

## Asthma Severity

School nurses are well aware of the great variability in how asthma manifests. Some individuals, especially those whose asthma is poorly controlled, have continual symptoms and frequent episodes of severe respiratory distress; others may experience only periodic, relatively mild episodes of breathing problems when exposed to certain irritants, allergens, or physical exercise, or when they develop a respiratory viral infection. School nurses should be aware of a student's level of asthma severity because severity ratings aid in prioritizing those in greatest need for intervention and those most at risk for asthma episodes.

Four categories of severity were published in 1997 by the Expert Committee of the National Asthma Education and Prevention Program to assist healthcare providers in determining treatment requirements for children and adults with asthma or suspected asthma (National Institutes of Health, 1997). These fall along a continuum—**mild intermittent, mild persistent, moderate persistent,** and **severe persistent** asthma. Ratings are determined by the frequency of day and nighttime asthma symptoms (cough, wheezing, shortness of breath, rapid breathing, chest tightness, and being awakened at night by these symptoms) and by pulmonary function testing. As shown in **Table 1**, a child whose pattern of daytime asthma symptoms is two or fewer times a week, or whose nighttime symptoms occur two or fewer times a month, would be considered to have **mild intermittent asthma**. A child with clinical symptoms more than twice a week would be considered to have either **mild, moderate,** or **severe persistent asthma**, with higher severity levels linked to increasing day and nighttime symptom frequency and declining pulmonary function.

Pulmonary function of the airways and lungs is measured by spirometry and peak flow measurements. These tools provide an indication of airflow obstruction that reflects the presence of inflammation. Spirometry is done in clinicians' offices and assesses the amount of air a person is able to forcefully exhale from the lungs following a deep breath, termed forced expiratory volume in one second ($FEV_1$), and forced vital capacity (FVC) (AAAAI, 2003). $FEV_1$ and $FEV_1/FVC$ values are compared to standardized, predicted values for children of the same age and racial group. Along with symptom patterns, they are used to assess asthma severity.

Spirometry is also used as a diagnostic tool to measure the reversibility of airway obstruction following treatment with an inhaled short-acting bronchodilator in those suspected of having asthma. A significant improvement in $FEV_1$ values after bronchodilator treatment reflects reversibility of inflammation and suggests the presence of asthma. In addition, as shown in the fifth column of Table 1, comparisons can be made between day and evening lung functioning. Asthma symptoms tend to be worse in the early morning, so morning testing occurs soon after awakening. An afternoon or evening measurement is then used to assess evening functioning. A diurnal variation of <20% is suggestive of **mild intermittent** asthma; a variation of 20% or more is suggestive of **persistent** asthma.

Peak flow meters are also used to assess pulmonary function. They are portable, hand-held devices that vary in style and design and measure maximum or "peak" expiratory volume of air forcefully and very quickly exhaled from the lungs, or peak expiratory flow (PEF). Like spirometers, peak flow meters reflect the degree of airway compromise due to inflammation, but primarily of the large airways. They are not intended for use in diagnosing asthma, but rather for monitoring airway status to ascertain severity (1) before treatment is started, which informs initial treatment requirements; (2) after treatment is initiated to monitor the response to treatment so that adjustments can be made, if needed; and (3) after optimal therapy is attained to determine what level of treatment is needed to maintain control of the individual's asthma.

Although peak flow values can be compared against established norms by age, sex, and height to help determine asthma severity, variation in peak flow meter readings by brand and in published referenced values have led to the suggestion that peak flows be compared to the child's "personal best" (AAAAI, 2003) rather than standardized norms. A personal best, as the name indicates, is the highest value obtained over a period of 2 to 3 weeks taken from two to four measurements performed daily when the asthma is in "good control" (excluding markedly higher or outlying values that might have been associated with spitting or coughing). Comparing subsequent readings to the student's personal best provides information about the child's present airway status (or degree of inflammation present).

For monitoring asthma status, peak flows can be used in two ways. First, measurements can be taken first thing in the morning, before any medication is used, and compared to the child's personal best (AAAAI, 2003). Eighty to 100% of the child's personal best indicates the asthma is in good control and medications should be continued as usually prescribed; 50% to 80% of the child's personal best indicates the asthma is not in good control and a short-acting bronchodilator is needed and/or that medications need to be changed or increased; <50% of personal best indicates an asthma emergency that requires immediate treatment with a short-acting bronchodilator as well as a call or visit to the doctor or emergency department.

Peak flow measurements can also be assessed in the morning before medication is taken, and then again in the evening (after a short-acting bronchodilator, when prescribed, is used). A comparison between the two values showing a difference of >20% between the evening and morning reading is indicative of poor asthma control and the need to reevaluate the child's asthma treatment.

## Management

Four components for effective asthma management have been suggested by the AAAAI following recommendations made by the Expert Panel of the National Asthma Education and Prevention Program (National Institutes of Health, 1997; AAAAI, 2003). These components are appropriately applied to the management of asthma in children by school nurses and other school health professionals. They include:

1. assessing and monitoring;
2. controlling factors that contribute to symptoms and asthma severity;
3. using medications to make the airways less sensitive and responsive to asthma triggers while using the least amount of medication to minimize side effects; and
4. educating the child, family, and others about asthma and its effective management.

As a chronic disease, asthma requires ongoing assessment and monitoring of symptoms and pulmonary function, analogous to the monitoring of blood sugar required for children with diabetes. Because children spend a significant portion of their day in school and in school-related activities, some of this monitoring needs to be done at school by school nurses, teachers, physical educators and coaches, and other school staff, like psychologists and social workers. In addition, because various factors that aggravate asthma symptoms are commonly found in

**Table 1. Levels of Asthma Severity**

| Classification | Days with Symptoms | Nights with Symptoms | For Children >5 yr Who Can Use a Spirometer or Peak Flow Meter | |
|---|---|---|---|---|
| | | | FEV$_1$ or PEF (% predicted normal) | PEF Variability |
| Severe persistent | Continual | Frequent | $\leq 60\%$ | $>30\%$ |
| Moderate persistent | Daily | $\geq 5$/month | $>60\%$ to $<80\%$ | $>30\%$ |
| Mild persistent | $>2$/week | 3 to 4/month | $\geq 80\%$ | 20% to 30% |
| Mild intermittent | $\leq 2$/week | $\leq 2$/month | $\geq 80\%$ | $<20\%$ |

FEV$_1$, forced expiratory volume in 1 second; PEF, peak expiratory flow.

Note: The above chart was developed by a consensus of experts in asthma care as a general guide for classifying asthma severity. Not all patients fit precisely into this classification system.
From *Pediatric Asthma Promoting Best Practice: Guide for Managing Asthma in Children* (p. 31), by American Academy of Allergy, Asthma and Immunology, 2003, Milwaukee, WI: Author. Adapted with permission.

schools and en route to and from school, as well as in the home environment, school nurses play an important role in helping students and school faculty and staff to identify these triggers and to help students avoid or control exposure to these triggers. Further, because asthma is a common disorder that affects millions of schoolchildren, the potential for a severe asthma episode exists in a notable proportion of our school populations. Thus, school nurses need to be familiar with medications used to manage acute episodes, as well as with long-acting asthma medications that help to prevent or control these acute episodes. Finally, educating students with asthma, their parents, classmates, and school personnel about the disease is critical to the early recognition and treatment of symptoms and is essential for promoting children's self-efficacy in managing their own illness.

Asthma experts and researchers have noted that national guidelines for effective management of asthma in both children and adults are often not implemented (National Institutes of Health, 1997). This results in unacceptable rates of morbidity and mortality across all ages due to asthma. However, these rates could be significantly reduced if people were better educated about the guidelines and worked toward their implementation. With conscientious application of the guidelines designed to promote more effective asthma management in children (AAAAI, 2003; National Institutes of Health, 1997), we could expect the following in our students:

- normal or near-normal lung function
- freedom from symptoms of coughing, wheezing, difficulty breathing, and chest tightness, and ability

to sleep through the night without being awakened by asthma
- no acute episodes of asthma that require a healthcare provider, emergency department, and urgent care visits, or hospitalizations
- ability to participate in normal school and day-care activities, including play, sports, and exercise
- not missing school or school activities on account of asthma symptoms
- no missed time from work for parents and caregivers on account of the child's asthma
- use of medications that have as few side effects as possible
- minimal use (less than once a day on average) of a short-acting beta$_2$-agonist

Because children typically spend a significant portion of their day at school and in school activities, students with asthma, their parents and caregivers, school personnel, and health providers should understand these expectations for good asthma control and expect nothing less.

## Assessing and Monitoring

In addition to routine observation of a child's clinical signs and symptoms of asthma, it is well within the scope of school nurses' practice to use peak flow meters at school to monitor those with a known asthma diagnosis. Such monitoring is particularly important with children with moderate and severe persistent asthma. The information gathered about lung function, especially when documented alongside students' self-reports of current asthma symptoms and exposure to things that exacerbate asthma, can provide useful data about current airway status. This can help determine whether airway inflammation has improved in response to pharmacologic treatment and to trigger avoidance and control, or has worsened in response to inadequate treatment or exposure to factors that aggravate the illness. Peak flow results can also be used to help children learn to link subjective symptoms of respiratory function with a more objective index of airway status.

Further, during asthma episodes, peak flow meters can be used to assess initial severity of an episode and the student's response to treatment specified in the student's individualized healthcare plan (IHP) or school emergency treatment protocol or guideline. In addition, school nurses may want to use peak flow meters with students who have not been diagnosed with asthma but are absent frequently or often visit the health office with complaints of respiratory problems. Linking peak flow meter readings with the child's history and physical examination findings can be particularly useful in planning and initiating appropriate referrals to local healthcare providers.

Knowing the factors that place students at highest risk for death from asthma is important in helping to prioritize students most in need of monitoring at school. Risk factors for asthma mortality (Akinbami & Schoendorf, 2002; AAAAI, 2003, p. 85; Castro, Schechtman, Halstead, & Bloomberg, 2001) include:

- Past history of sudden severe exacerbations
- Prior intubation for asthma
- Prior admission to intensive care unit for asthma
- ≥2 hospitalizations for asthma in past 12 months
- ≥3 emergency department visits for asthma in past 12 months
- Use of >1 canister/month of inhaled short-acting beta$_2$-agonist
- Current long-term use of oral corticosteroids
- Difficulty perceiving airflow obstruction or its severity
- Low socioeconomic status and urban residence
- African American ethnicity
- Adolescent age-group
- Illicit drug use
- Serious psychiatric disease or psychosocial problems

In school settings, school nurses, nonlicensed assistive personnel, asthma care delegates, teachers, coaches, and other school personnel responsible for students should be taught to monitor clinical signs and symptoms of asthma. School personnel should also know how to assist a child to use a peak flow meter to assess airway status during acute episodes in the process of properly implementing the student's emergency care plan (ECP). In addition, readable and easily understood protocols that identify signs and symptoms of respiratory distress and the emergency procedures that school personnel should follow in managing these episodes should be posted in classrooms and common areas.

## Controlling Factors That Exacerbate Asthma: Avoiding and Controlling Triggers

The second component of effective asthma management, avoiding and controlling factors that make asthma symptoms worse, is very important to asthma control and can be challenging because of the ubiquitousness of asthma triggers. *Triggers* are those things that exacerbate asthma symptoms and can be categorized as allergens, irritants, and other factors (e.g., physical exercise, respiratory illnesses, weather, strong emotional reactions, and miscellaneous factors like gastroesophageal reflux disease [GERD]). *Allergens* provoke allergic reactions in individuals sensitized to them; *irritants* are substances that irritate the airways of all people, but are particularly troublesome to individuals with asthma because of the increased sensitivity of their airways. *Other factors* have an adverse impact on individuals' airways through a variety of mechanisms. For example, the rapid breathing that accompanies vigorous physical activity, especially in cold, dry air, contributes to drying of the airways, irritates the airway lining, and causes bronchoconstriction. With sinusitis, upper airway inflammation may contribute to inflammation of the lower airway. With GERD, it is suspected that microaspiration of stomach contents into the airways, particularly during sleep, and a vagal response from the lower end of the irritated esophagus, contribute to asthma symptoms. **Table 2** lists common triggers.

Asthma triggers vary from individual to individual, and different children react to different factors and in varying degrees to these factors. Triggers vary as well within the same person. For example, a child's asthma symptoms may be mild when she or he is exposed to a single factor or when the exposure is of short duration. The same child may have a more severe reaction when exposed at another time, when exposed to more than one trigger simultaneously, or when in longer contact with the offending substance(s). In addition, evidence of sensitivity to a trigger may not become immediately apparent; some individuals experience a delayed reaction to substances to which they have become sensitized. This occasionally makes it especially difficult to discern the cause of the exacerbation.

Finally, in cases where students might be exposed to triggers that they know exacerbate their asthma but can't avoid (e.g., attending an important family event at a home where cats are present), symptoms can be prevented or minimized with proper pharmacologic intervention. For example, with expected but unavoidable exposure to allergens, the use of nonsteroidal anti-inflammatory medications (either cromolyn sodium or nedocromil sodium) 5 to 30 minutes before expected exposure might be prescribed (AAAAI, 2003).

**Table 2. Common Asthma Allergens and Irritants**

| Type of Trigger | Trigger Characteristics | Individual and School Actions to Prevent Symptoms |
|---|---|---|
| Allergens: Pollens (weeds, grasses, trees, grain dust, alfalfa) | Biological substances (such as proteins in pollen) perceived by the body as foreign; allergens cause an immune-mediated reaction upon exposure to them | • Ensure heating, ventilation, air conditioning (HVAC) systems are maintained and filters cleaned or changed regularly<br>• Monitor pollen count during relevant seasons; avoid exercising outdoors during early to mid morning or exercise indoors when pollen counts high<br>• Avoid grass mowing during school hours; avoid sitting in grass<br>• Pay attention to pollen counts before opening windows for "fresh air"<br>• For children on farms with chores, have them wash face and hands and change clothing before coming indoors |
| Mold | • Molds are ubiquitous microscopic fungi found on plant and animal matter<br>• Molds produce spores that grow on nearly any surface when they land on wet or damp surfaces | • Keep school indoor humidity between 30% and 50%<br>• Identify and fix leaks and other sources of moisture<br>• Vent shower and bathroom areas; scrub off mold and dry<br>• Clean spills immediately<br>• Regularly check for sources of mold and mildew and initiate control measures<br>• Encourage school's use of EPA's Indoor *Air Quality Tools for Schools: Managing Asthma in the School* Environment tool kit and *Mold Remediation in Schools and Commercial Buildings* materials |
| Furry and feathered animals, feathers | • Animal dander (skin flakes), saliva, urine | • Remove furred and feathered animals from home and classroom<br>• Keep animals away from fabric-covered furniture, carpets<br>• Keep cages away from vents and ducts<br>• Clean cages regularly |
| Cockroaches and other pests | • Feces, secretions, and body parts of roaches; feces, urine, and saliva of mice, rats | • Remove pests with bait traps or boric acid; use traps vs. spray pesticides when possible<br>• Repair sites where pests gain access to school<br>• Clean food areas well; keep food in airtight containers; remove access to water<br>• Clean kitchens, dining, and food surfaces regularly<br>• Keep garbage away from building<br>• Encourage school's use of EPA's *Integrated Pest Management* program |

**Table 2. Common Asthma Allergens and Irritants**

| Type of Trigger | Trigger Characteristics | Individual and School Actions to Prevent Symptoms |
|---|---|---|
| Dust mites | • Feces and body parts of microscopic insects that reside in mattresses, pillows, bedcovers, carpets, fabric-covered furniture, clothes, stuffed toys<br>• Predominately in regions of the country with high humidity and in homes and schools with >50% indoor humidity. | • Keep environment clean, dust-free; keep humidity <30% to <50%<br>• Avoid carpet in classroom when possible; vacuum carpeted areas frequently<br>• Reduce upholstered furniture in classrooms<br>• Wash stuffed toys weekly; store in plastic bags<br>• At school, wash cot blankets, covers weekly in hot water (≥130°); at home, use allergen-impermeable covers for pillow, mattress, bedsprings |
| Irritants:<br>  Tobacco smoke | • From smoking directly; breathing in smoke from burning cigarettes, pipes, cigars; inhaling smoke exhaled by smokers | • Ensure that school smoke-free zones are in place and smoking bans are enforced<br>• Keep children away from smoky venues, smoky cars<br>• Offer smoking prevention and smoking cessation for students and staff |
| Air pollution, fumes, coal dust, chalk dust, house dust | • Air contamination from indoor and outdoor air pollution | • Avoid exposure to idling busses, high-traffic areas, wood stoves, wood fires, malfunctioning gas appliances, unvented kerosene or gas space heaters<br>• Avoid outdoor or midday play on high-pollution, high-ozone days, crop spraying, lawn applications, during fire storms or when air quality poor for other reasons; use air conditioning, change filters as needed<br>• Keep children away when areas are being vacuumed<br>• Clean chalkboard and erasers when students not around<br>• Avoid using curtains; damp-dust mini-blinds and roller shades frequently<br>• Store books behind doors<br>• Schedule school repairs, renovations, painting, roofing when schools not in session or noncontact days |
| Strong odors from perfumes, paints, cleaning agents, pesticides | • Strong chemical odors irritate the airways | • Use natural cleaning agents (e.g., cider vinegar, baking soda, club soda)<br>• Use cleaning agents in well-ventilated area; replace caps of cleaning agents quickly<br>• Avoid perfumes, scented powders, hair sprays |
| Dry-erase markers, glue, paste, chemicals | • Chemicals and strong odors emitted from school supplies | • Use in well-ventilated areas<br>• Replace caps quickly<br>• Vent science and cooking labs |

**Table 2. Common Asthma Allergens and Irritants**

| Type of Trigger | Trigger Characteristics | Individual and School Actions to Prevent Symptoms |
|---|---|---|
| Volatile organic compounds emitted (VOCs) from new furnishings (upholstery, rugs) | • Substances emitted from new products can irritate the airways | • Use vinyl, leather, or wood furniture when possible |
| Physical activity and exercise | • Faster breathing during physical activity tends to dry airways, causing further irritation to hypersensitive airways | • Premedicate with beta2-agonist 5 to 15 minutes prior to exercise<br>• Warm up before exercise<br>• Cover nose and mouth with scarf on cold days<br>• Modify activity if needed during recovery from acute episodes or if child experiencing symptoms |
| Respiratory illnesses, colds, sinusitis | • Viral infections of respiratory system irritate the airway<br>• Inflammation and mucus associated with upper airway infections and sinusitis can irritate lower respiratory tract | • Promote careful hand washing throughout school<br>• Avoid exposure to individuals with respiratory illness when possible<br>• Get sinusitis treated<br>• Request annual flu vaccine (unless allergic to eggs) |
| Weather: exposure to cold air, wind, sudden changes in the weather, temperature changes | • Sudden or marked changes in temperature may irritate the airways (e.g., going from heated inside air to cold outside air; from air-conditioning to hot air outside)<br>• Wind may dry airways as well as carry pollens and dust | • Try for gradual transition indoors and outdoors<br>• Wear scarf over nose, mouth on cold days<br>• Avoid outside activity on windy days |
| Strong emotional reactions that result in hard laughing, crying, fast breathing | • These activities can dry and irritate sensitivairways, increasing inflammation and bronchoconstriction | • Collaborate with mental health staff as needed to provide services for children who are anxious, stressed, easily upset |
| Miscellaneous: GERD, foods, medications | • Microaspiration of stomach contents into the airways, especially at night, and vagal stimulation of lower esophagus by stomach acid may trigger asthma symptoms<br>• Children who have allergies to foods or medications may experience asthma symptoms with ingestion | • Refer children with asthma symptoms for care, especially when history of reflux, nighttime symptoms<br>• Ensure appropriate school staff aware of food allergies or medications, especially with history of severe reactions |

Asthma

## Pharmacologic Interventions

Asthma medications are an essential component of effective asthma management, and the correct combination of medications can effectively control the symptoms of asthma. Asthma medications belong to two broad categories: long-term "controller," or "maintenance," medications, and quick-relief, or "rescue," medications. Long-term control medications are designed to control asthma symptoms by preventing or reducing airway inflammation, by relaxing the smooth muscles around the airway, or by interrupting the inflammatory process in the airway before it can develop. They are **not** intended to provide quick relief of asthma symptoms and should never be used for this purpose. Quick-relief medications, on the other hand, are designed to provide fast relief for asthma episodes and as a preventive medication before exercise or before unavoidable exposure to asthma triggers.

Examples of long-acting anti-inflammatory medications include inhaled corticosteroids (e.g., Advair Diskus, Flovent); inhaled nonsteroidal anti-inflammatory medications (e.g., cromolyn, nedocromil); and oral systemic steroids (e.g., prednisone). Examples of long-acting bronchodilating medications include inhaled bronchodilators (e.g., Foradil, Serevent Diskus); oral theophylline (e.g., Uniphyl, Quibron-TSR); or omalizumab (Xolair). Other long-acting medications that act by interrupting the inflammatory process before it begins include leukotriene receptor antagonists (e.g., Accolate, Singulair, Zyflo). At this time, only one medication (Advair Diskus) contains both an anti-inflammatory and a long-acting bronchodilator. Note the importance of informing students, parents, and school personnel that the oral and inhaled corticosteroids used in asthma therapy are not those that are sometimes misused by athletes (i.e., anabolic steroids). Rather, they are naturally occurring hormones in the body that reduce inflammatory processes. Further, the AAAAI (2003) recommends that children with persistent asthma use a daily long-term control medication to lessen inflammation and airway hyperreactivity. Inhaled "controller" corticosteroids are the medications preferred for this purpose.

Examples of quick-relief medications include a number of short-acting inhaled bronchodilators, such as albuterol (Proventil, Ventolin), levalbuterol (Xopenex), metaproterenol (Alupent), pirbuterol (Maxair Autohaler), and an anti-cholinergic medication, ipratropium bromide (Atrovent). (The latter may have additive benefits to inhaled beta$_2$-agonists used in severe exacerbations or as a possible alternative bronchodilator for children who cannot tolerate inhaled beta$_2$-agonists well) (AAAAI, 2003). In addition, when oral corticosteroids are used for a short period (usually 3 to 10 days) to quiet inflammation and lessen the duration of an asthma episode, this is termed an oral prednisone "burst." It is considered in this context to be a quick-relief medication.

The severity of asthma dictates the level of pharmacologic intervention needed to gain control of asthma symptoms. Some physicians begin with aggressive therapy with a regimen at a level higher than that suggested by the initial severity rating in order to quickly control inflammation, and they then step down treatment to the minimum therapy needed to maintain control (AAAAI, 2003). Others begin with a medication regimen that corresponds to the initial asthma severity rating and step up medications as needed until control is achieved. All children with asthma, regardless of severity, should have a short-acting beta$_2$-agonist for use in exacerbations or for preventive use. In addition, generally all children with persistent asthma (mild, moderate, and severe) should be receiving inhaled corticosteroids (low-dose for mild persistent asthma, higher doses for moderate and severe persistent asthma). (Note that inhaled corticosteroids should always be administered with a spacer and administration is followed by rinsing out the mouth to avoid developing oral thrush and to avoid swallowing any residue that may be left in the mouth.) Further, in addition to inhaled anti-inflammatory medication, children with moderate or persistent asthma typically need a second controller medication (generally a long-acting beta$_2$-agonist) to maintain good asthma control.

Since pharmacologic treatment regimens vary depending on the status of the student's level of asthma severity and degree of control, school nurses need to be aware that treatment regimens may change as the asthma becomes better controlled. Monitoring the child's symptoms and peak flows during the school day provides useful information to parents and the medical provider about the child's response to treatment. It also helps to inform about the effectiveness of medication as the child goes about her usual day at school, where she may be more active or exposed to asthma triggers not encountered at home. Such data may provide an indication of the child's ability to tolerate certain medications, an important consideration when side effects commonly influence an individual's willingness to adhere to a prescribed treatment. Side effects, of course, vary by both type of medication and by brand and may include the following: oral thrush or hoarseness with inhaled corticosteroids; increased appetite with oral corticosteroid "bursts"; dry mouth or bad taste associated with inhaled nonsteroidal medications cromolyn sodium and nedocromil; tachycardia, tremors, and nervousness with inhaled short-acting beta$_2$-agonists and with inhaled and oral long-acting beta$_2$-agonists; (rare) liver dysfunction with leukotriene modifiers; and tachycardia, tremors, nervousness, insomnia, seizures, headaches, and heartburn with methylxanthines (theophylline).

Finally, antibiotics may be needed for children whose sinusitis may be contributing to asthma, and immunotherapy or desensitization therapy may be a consideration for those with allergies.

## Asthma Action Plans

**Asthma Action Plans** are written, individualized plans developed jointly by the student, parent or caregiver, and the healthcare provider. Asthma Action Plans typically include the following:

- Student's name, age, and date of birth
- Emergency contact information for parents or guardians and for the healthcare provider and local emergency services or 911
- Allergies and asthma triggers
- Signs and symptoms of an asthma episode (or, "attack")
- Asthma medications (both "quick-relief" and long-term control or "maintenance"), including names of medications, routes of administration, and dosages
- Actions to be taken for reported signs and observed symptoms of asthma. These actions are linked with peak flow measurements to indicate asthma status. (A stoplight analogy is typically used, with values that are 80% to 100% of the child's personal best considered in the "Green zone," meaning "GO! Continue what you are doing" in terms of preventive medication, controller medication, and trigger avoidance. Values 50% to 80% of normal are considered in the "Yellow zone," suggesting "Caution," and the need to use a "quick-relief" medication to open the airways and to possibly begin a short course of oral corticosteroids (e.g., prednisone "burst") to lessen inflammation. Values ≤50% reflect the "Red zone," meaning "Stop! Danger! Take your quick-relief medication and immediately call your doctor, or if symptoms are life-threatening, immediately go to the emergency room or call 911."
- The medical care provider's signature if the plan is to be used as a medical order.

The student's healthcare provider should request that the parents share a copy of the Asthma Action Plan with the school nurse. If the school nurse has not been provided with an Asthma Action Plan, he/she can either ask a parent to obtain one from the medical provider or develop one with a parent and student based on the information he/she does have (e.g., medication orders from the medical provider, known allergies, contact information). The school nurse can then, with permission of the parent, send the plan to the provider for review and for a signature. The Asthma Action Plan is used by the school nurse to complete the student's IHP, which includes an ECP component. Getting written permission from the parent to allow the school nurse and physician to communicate about the child's illness is also important.

## Education About Asthma

The ability to self-manage one's asthma is a critical component of maintaining effective asthma control. Perhaps the most essential aspect of the student's education involves his or her ability to understand and use an Asthma Action Plan. Individual teaching with students with asthma and their parent or caregiver is essential to obtaining and maintaining good asthma control. Efforts must be made to involve both the parent and the child in learning about the child's asthma and to reinforce developmentally appropriate self-care strategies at every opportunity. In addition, several effective programs (see resources listed in **Table 3**) have been developed by asthma- and health-related organizations, such as the American Lung Association, the Allergy and Asthma Foundation of America, and the American Academy of Family Physicians, to teach groups of children of varying age levels about asthma and about the importance of not smoking. Because school nurses are often in environments with limited time and few human and material resources, it is important that they establish collaborative efforts with community agencies and organizations and with other school and community colleagues to offer these educational programs whenever possible.

Whether students are taught individually or in groups, they should be taught several essential concepts and demonstrate an appropriate level of understanding of these concepts. These should be reflected in the student's IHP and include:

- Mechanisms underlying chronic asthma and asthma exacerbations
- Symptoms of asthma episodes
- Avoidance and control of asthma triggers
- What Asthma Action Plans are and how to use them, including actions for emergencies
- What ECPs are and how to use them
- How to use a peak flow meter and record PEF values and symptoms (or lack of symptoms)
- Types of, indications for, dosages of, and side effects of prescribed asthma medications
- Correct use and care of medication delivery devices (metered dose inhalers, dry powder inhalers (DPIs), nebulizers, spacers)
- Rights and responsibilities for self-carrying of preventive/emergency medicines at school

An important aspect of managing students with asthma at school and ensuring that they are kept safe and healthy involves being aware of the extent to which they and their families are able or willing to comply with written plans for asthma management. To optimize adherence, in addition to addressing knowledge deficits about asthma and its management, the school nurse should work with other school personnel to determine if other threats to a student's compliance with treatment may be operating. Some considerations include poor perception of asthma symptoms or of severity of asthma episodes (e.g., poor perceivers); perceived ineffectiveness of medication; perceived unacceptability of medication side effects; denial of need for treatment; oppositional or rebellious behavior; secondary gains from illness; and inability to physically or financially access medication. Involving other school personnel (e.g., teachers to report on observed behaviors, social workers to assist with financial barriers to obtaining medication, psychologists to evaluate and treat oppositional behaviors) can have huge benefits both in determining reasons for noncompliance and in addressing relevant issues.

Asthma Action Plan  —use to create→  IHP (c̄ Emergency Care Plan) included

**Table 3. Selected Asthma Resources**

| Organization/Association | Useful Materials | Target Audience |
|---|---|---|
| Allergy and Asthma Network/Mothers of Asthmatics http://www.aanma.org | *Breatherville* online and print educational materials. Especially useful is routinely updated table of asthma medications (see "Pharmacy") | Parents, children with asthma, health professionals |
| American Academy of Allergy, Asthma, and Immunology (AAAAI) http://www.aaaai.org | Allergy and Asthma School Nurse Tool Kit<br><br>Pediatric Asthma Promoting Best Practice. A Guide for Managing Asthma in Children<br><br>Especially useful is routinely updated table of asthma medications | School and public health nurses<br><br>Health professionals<br><br>Health professionals, parents |
| American Academy of Family Physicians http://www.aafp.org | Tar Wars: Tobacco-Free Education for Today and the Future curriculum | Teachers to educate students in 3rd & 4th and 5th & 6th grades about smoking |
| American Academy of Pediatrics http://www.aap.org | Position statements<br><br>Asthma Action Plans | Health professionals<br><br>Parents |
| American Association of School Administrators http://www.aasa.org | School Governance & Leadership, Asthma Wellness: Keeping Children with Asthma in School and Learning | School administrators, teachers |
| American Lung Association (ALA) http://www.lungusa.org | A is for Asthma<br><br>Open Airways<br><br>Asthma 101<br><br>Asthma Friendly Schools Toolkit | Preschool and early elementary<br><br>8- to 11-year-olds<br><br>Teachers and school staff<br><br>Community members, ALA staff, school personnel |
| Asthma and Allergy Foundation of America (AAFA) http://www.aafa.org | Asthma Care Training for Kids<br><br>Power Breathing<br><br>Meeting in a Box (ABCs of Asthma, Getting the Most From Your Meds, Tools of Asthma Management, Asthma Management at School) | 7- to 12-year-olds and parents<br><br>Adolescents<br><br>For health professionals to educate students, parents, school staff about asthma |
| Centers for Disease Control and Prevention, Division of Adolescent and School Health http://www.cdc.gov/nccd-php/dash | Strategies for Addressing Within a Coordinated School Health Program | General public, school personnel, health professionals |
| National Association of School Nurses http://www.nasn.org | Managing Asthma Triggers<br><br>School Nurse<br><br>Asthma Management Program | School nurses<br><br>School nurses |

**Table 3. Selected Asthma Resources**

| Organization/Association | Useful Materials | Target Audience |
|---|---|---|
| National Association of State Boards of Education http://www.nasbe.org | Fit, Healthy, and Ready to Learn policy guide book | School boards and administrators |
| National Asthma Education and Prevention Program, National Heart, Lung, and Blood Institute http://www.nhlbi.nih.gov | Managing Asthma: A Guide for Schools  Asthma and Physical Activity in the School  Asthma Awareness Curriculum for the Elementary Classroom | General public, school personnel, health professionals  As above, especially coaches  Teachers |
| Starbright Foundation http://www. starbright.org | Quest for the Code (CD-ROM game) | Preadolescent and adolescents |
| U.S. Environmental Protection Agency http://www.epa.gov/iaq | Indoor Air Quality: Tools for Schools  Pest Control in the School Environment: Adopting Integrated Pest Management  Mold Remediation in Schools and Commercial Buildings | School personnel  School personnel, particularly building and facilities supervisors  School personnel, particularly building and facilities supervisors |

# Individualized Healthcare Plan

## Assessment

*History*

Past history

- Age of onset of asthma symptoms; age at diagnosis
- Past history of allergies, eczema
- Previous respiratory illnesses (bronchitis, bronchiolitis, reactive airway disease, pneumonia)
- Exposure to parental smoking in early years
- Intubations, ICU admission for asthma, 911 calls
- Hospitalizations and emergency department visits for respiratory illnesses past 12 months
- Frequency of unscheduled healthcare provider visits due to asthma
- Family history
- Ethnicity, socioeconomic status, location of residence, parental educational level
- Family history: allergies, asthma, hay fever

*Current Status and Management*

- Ability to access healthcare and obtain medication
- Present asthma care provider
- Asthma management plan
- Level of asthma severity (mild intermittent, mild persistent, moderate persistent, severe persistent)
- "Personal best" PEF; PEF values associated with Green, Yellow, Red zones
- Current medication(s), type, dose, response, adherence, side effects, self-carrying
- Frequency and severity of asthma exacerbations
- Pattern of onset of asthma signs and symptoms, early warning signs of asthma episodes
- Triggers of asthma episodes (particularly upper respiratory tract infections, exercise, exposure to certain allergens, such as cats, molds, cigarette smoke)
- Avoidance of triggers or control of exposure to triggers
- Level of participation in play, school and classroom activities, and sports
- Stopping or avoiding physical activity due to asthma symptoms

*Self-care*
- Current knowledge and understanding of asthma (e.g., etiology and physiology of chronic asthma and acute exacerbations, Asthma Action Plans, peak flow meter use, recognition of asthma triggers, asthma signs and symptoms, early warning signs of episodes, proper use of and indications for medications, care and use of medication devices)
- Self-care skills (e.g., self-medication, degree of adherence to Asthma Management Plan, recognition and avoidance or control of triggers, developmentally appropriate actions to take for attaining and maintaining good asthma control, problem solving)
- Motivation for and barriers to compliance with treatment regimen

*Psychosocial Status*
- Impact on family routines, activities, dynamics, economics
- Family, peer, and community support systems
- Cognitive, emotional, and social development; temperament
- Child's past response and current adaptation to having a chronic illness

*Academic Issues*
- Past and current academic achievement
- Absences from school, missed time from class due to asthma
- School health services needed—peak flow and symptoms monitoring, medications
- School environment issues—asthma triggers at school and en route to and from school; accommodations needed to avoid or control triggers (e.g., removal of furry or feathered pets from classroom, pretreatment prior to exercise)
- Curriculum modifications—allowances for making up missed schoolwork due to asthma; expectation that asthma is not an excuse not to participate in physical exercise; alterations to physical education activities; avoiding outdoor exposure under certain conditions (e.g., recovery from acute episode, extremely cold or windy weather, high pollution or high pollen-count day)

## Nursing Diagnoses (N.D.) (NANDA, 2003)

*Disease Management Issues*
**N.D. 1** Ineffective airway clearance (NANDA 00031) associated with chronic inflammation causing bronchoconstriction and excessive mucus production
**N.D. 2** Impaired gas exchange (NANDA 00082) related to:
- airway inflammation, bronchoconstriction, and excessive mucus production
**N.D. 3** Activity intolerance (NANDA 00092) and risk for activity intolerance (NANDA 00094) related to:
- exacerbation of symptoms associated with exercise-induced bronchospasm
**N.D. 4** Disturbed sleep pattern (NANDA 00095) associated with asthma symptoms

*Self-management of condition*
**N.D. 5** Deficient knowledge (NANDA 00126) about asthma and asthma self-care
**N.D. 6** Noncompliance (NANDA 00079) with treatment regimen related to:
- Knowledge deficit about trigger avoidance and control, and medication regimen
- Lack of understanding of why treatment important
- Poor perception of symptoms
- Perceived ineffectiveness of medication
- Perceived unacceptability of medication side effects
- Denial of need for treatment
- Oppositional or rebellious behavior
- Secondary gain from illness
- Inability to physically or financially access medication
**N.D. 7** Ineffective therapeutic regimen management (NANDA 00078) evidenced by poor control of asthma symptoms
**N.D. 8** Effective therapeutic regimen management (NANDA 00082) evidenced by good control of asthma symptoms

*Adaptation and coping*

**N.D. 9** Anxiety (NANDA 00146) related to:
- experiencing a chronic childhood illness and experiences with exacerbations of asthma symptoms

**N.D. 10** Chronic low self-esteem (NANDA 00119) related to:
- experiencing a chronic illness and experiences with exacerbations of asthma symptoms

## Goals

*Disease management*

The student will use an identified healthcare provider for asthma care services. (N.D. 1-4)

The student will assist in the development of an Asthma Action Plan with the parent and healthcare provider. (N.D. 1-4)

The student will assist in the development of the IHP and ECP, based on the Asthma Action Plan (if available). (N.D. 1-4).

The student will comply with written plans (IHP with ECP, which are based on the student's Asthma Action Plan) for asthma management to attain or maintain good asthma control evidenced by: (N.D. 1-4)
- normal or near-normal lung function
- avoidance of asthma symptoms (coughing, wheezing, difficulty breathing, chest tightness)
- full participation in school activities, including play, sports, and exercise
- avoidance of acute asthma exacerbations that require nonroutine healthcare provider, emergency, and urgent care visits, 911 calls, or hospitalization
- avoidance of school absences, missed time from class, and fatigue due to asthma
- minimal reliance on quick-relief (short-acting beta$_2$-agonist) medication to control asthma symptoms

The student will have his/her needed asthma medication available and easily accessible at school. (N.D. 1-4)

The student will communicate with parent(s)/guardian(s), the school nurse, health office staff, school personnel, and healthcare provider about his/her asthma. (N.D. 1-4)

The student will increase his/her ability to identify and manage environmental triggers. (N.D. 1-4)

The student will avoid experiencing nighttime asthma symptoms (night wakening due to coughing, wheezing, breathing difficulty, chest tightness) and fatigue during the day due to night wakening. (N.D. 1-4)

*Self-management of condition*

The student will increase his/her knowledge about asthma and skills in asthma self-management, including the importance of adherence to the Asthma Action Plan and IHP to avoid asthma episodes and possible long-term harm to airways. (N.D. 5, 6)

The student will increase his/her understanding of the link between adherence to asthma management plan and decreased risk of long-term harm to airways. (N.D. 6).

The student will increase his/her awareness of factors that both promote and interfere with compliance with asthma management plan and strategies to help manage threats to compliance. (N.D. 6)

The student will increase his/her skills in self-management of asthma and in recognizing an ineffective asthma management plan vs. poor compliance as a factor in poor control of symptoms. (N.D. 7)

The student will increase his/her self-management skills to attain and maintain current good control of asthma (e.g., is able to recognize asthma symptoms and increasing asthma severity, uses a peak flow meter and monitors results, avoids and controls triggers, uses medication(s) as prescribed, and effectively communicates with family members, healthcare providers, and school personnel about asthma). (N.D. 8)

*Adaptation and coping*

The student will acquire an enhanced sense of well-being through greater confidence and competence in controlling asthma symptoms and preventing acute exacerbations. (N.D. 9, 10)

The student will demonstrate appropriate problem solving, communication, and healthy, adaptive coping skills for managing chronic asthma and asthma exacerbations. (N.D. 9, 10)

The student will describe own abilities and any limitations associated with having asthma realistically and accurately. (N.D. 9, 10)

## Nursing Interventions

*Disease management issues*

Assist the parents/guardians to find a primary healthcare provider/asthma care specialist for asthma care services if the student is not under the care of a healthcare provider for asthma. (N.D. 1-4)

Obtain an Asthma Action Plan from the parents/guardians and the healthcare provider. (N.D. 1-4)

In conjunction with the student and parent, develop an IHP and ECP based on the student's Asthma Action Plan. (Note: If an Asthma Action Plan is not available from the parent/guardian or provider, develop a Plan with the student and parent based on information that is available [e.g., student biographical information, parent and emergency contact information, health history including allergies, level of severity, medication orders or requests for medication administration at school, peak flow meter results to compare to established standards or "personal best"] and send Plan to the healthcare provider's office for review and signature with request to return signed copy to the school). (N.D. 1-4)

Identify the student's level of asthma severity by monitoring peak flows and asthma signs and symptoms to help in establishing priority for intervention. (N.D. 1-4)

Establish a schedule with the student and parent/guardian to attain or maintain good asthma control and to assess the effectiveness of the IHP through regular monitoring of the following: lung function, asthma symptoms, asthma exacerbations, nonroutine healthcare visits, visits for respiratory emergencies, school absences, missed time from class, fatigue due to night awakening, and reliance on quick-relief medication (short-acting beta$_2$-agonist) for control of asthma symptoms. (N.D. 1-4)

Periodically assess the effectiveness of the IHP, ECP, and Asthma Action Plan. (N.D. 1-4)

Maintain accurate records related to monitoring and treating the student's asthma. (N.D. 1-4)

Identify and obtain necessary medications, medication devices, and asthma supplies for the student (e.g., nebulizer, mouthpiece, tubing, back-up inhaler). (N.D. 1-4)

Obtain medication administration authorization from the parent/guardian and physician/healthcare provider. (N.D. 1-4)

Ensure that quick-relief medication is easily and quickly available to the student through one or more of the following: (N.D. 1-4)
- self-carried medication
- easy accessibility to medicine by school staff responsible for the student's asthma care at school
- proper instruction of school personnel about exact location in school of the student's asthma medication and supplies

Assess the student's developmental and emotional readiness for self-carrying of quick-relief medication. (N.D. 1-4)

Obtain necessary releases/agreement for self-carrying signed by the student, parent/guardian, healthcare provider, and/or school nurse (as needed depending on school policy/procedure). (N.D. 1-4)

Obtain parental permission or release for school nurse and healthcare provider to communicate about the student's asthma status and establish a mechanism for this. (N.D. 1-4)

Post an easily understandable school-wide Guideline for Managing Respiratory Distress Emergencies or the school's first-aid guidelines in school classrooms and common areas and review them with school personnel. (N.D. 1-4)

Provide an ECP to school personnel who work with the student, which includes what to observe and how to appropriately respond to increasing levels of symptom severity. (N.D. 1-4)

Educate teachers and other school personnel about the student's asthma, monitoring of student's symptoms, and means to implement the asthma management plan, as specified in the IHP including: (N.D. 1-4)
- expectations for good asthma control
- specific ways to remove or minimize exposure to asthma triggers in the classroom, during school, and en route to and from school
- strategies to prevent exercise-induced asthma episodes by pretreatment with beta$_2$-agonist, use of warm-up exercises, wearing a scarf on cold days, staying indoors on extremely cold days
- how to recognize signs and symptoms of asthma exacerbation and specific actions to take and what to do for increasing levels of asthma episode severity
- proper use of and access to quick-relief medications prior to exercise and at the first onset of asthma symptoms, including school policy and procedures for self-carrying and self-treatment with quick relief inhalers
- good asthma control should result in no nighttime wakening due to asthma symptoms and avoidance of daytime fatigue.

Educate the school community through direct teaching and use of in-service training, bulletin boards, school announcements, and parent newsletters about the following: importance of careful hand washing, avoiding the spread of upper respiratory tract viruses, annual flu vaccination, not smoking, avoidance of second-hand smoke, and enforcement of smoking bans. (N.D. 1-4)

Assist teachers to plan for accommodations needed for various field trips, off-site activities, making up schoolwork missed during exacerbations, and adapting physical education activities during onset of asthma episodes, during recovery from exacerbations, during episodes of upper respiratory tract infections, on high-pollen count or high pollution days, and during adverse weather (extreme cold, windy days). (N.D. 1-4)

Teach or review tasks designated to health assistants/asthma care delegates/nonlicensed personnel responsible for monitoring and treating the student and establish plan for periodic review of task performance. (N.D. 1-4)

### Self-management of condition

Identify learning needs of the student and family about asthma and self-care management and develop plan to address identified asthma knowledge deficits through one-to-one instruction and participation in group asthma education class (e.g., *Open Airways*). (N. D. 5)

Educate the student and family about: (N.D. 5)
- characteristics of good control of asthma, including information that good asthma control should result in no nighttime wakening due to asthma symptoms and in a reduction or avoidance of daytime fatigue
- etiology and physiology of chronic and acute asthma, including terms and definitions related to illness, role of inflammation in asthma, importance of controlling inflammation, and when student should be kept home
- early recognition of signs and symptoms of an asthma exacerbation, interpretation of peak flow meter results, and actions to take to manage asthma symptoms that correspond to asthma episode severity (based on ECP and/or Asthma Action Plan that uses a stoplight analogy Green = Go, good control; Yellow = Caution, add medication; Red = Danger, get help immediately)
- student's asthma triggers and specific strategies to avoid or control exposure to them (e.g., removal of cat from home, staying indoors on high-pollen-count days, removing furry or feathered animals from classroom)
- rights and responsibilities for self-carrying of inhaler medication

Assist the student to identify motivators for participating in self-care and develop and implement plan that reinforces self-care efforts. (N.D. 6)

Assist the student in identifying factors that might interfere with compliance with therapeutic regimen and develop specific strategies for dealing with these barriers to compliance. (N.D. 6)

Regularly monitor and reward adherence to asthma management plan, including medication compliance (e.g., proper use of long-term controllers and quick-relief medications) and avoidance and control of triggers (e.g., pretreating with beta$_2$-agonist to prevent asthma episodes, staying inside and using air-conditioner on high pollution days, avoiding allergens). (N.D. 6)

Discuss with the student and parents/guardians the possible side effects of medication and importance of monitoring and reporting these, because they may interfere with adherence to the asthma management plan and self-care plans. (N.D. 6)

Periodically assess and monitor whether the student is able to accurately recognize asthma symptoms and increasing asthma severity, correctly use a peak flow meter and interpret results, avoid and control triggers, use medication(s) as prescribed, and effectively communicate with family, healthcare providers, and school personnel about his/her asthma. (N.D. 7)

For students requiring intensive case management, particularly those with moderate or severe persistent asthma, use the "Is the Asthma Action Plan Working?" tool to assess treatment effectiveness. (N.D. 7)

Reinforce the student's strengths and accomplishments in asthma self-management. (N.D. 8)

Provide the student with opportunities for increasing responsibility for asthma management and for making decisions regarding his/her asthma management. (N.D. 8)

### Adaptation and coping

Monitor the student's attendance patterns, reasons for absences, academic performance, peer relationships, and overall emotional well-being for declines in functioning, and refer as needed to mental health team members. (N.D. 9, 10)

Involve the student (and parent/guardian when possible) in a group asthma education program to reinforce individual teaching and to offer the support of group members. (N.D. 9, 10)

Provide privacy to the student when he/she is uncomfortable using or taking medication in front of others and use role-playing to help the student be more comfortable with having to take medication around peers. (N.D. 9, 10)

Provide opportunities for the student to make decisions regarding his/her asthma management. (N.D. 9, 10)

Asthma

Communicate regularly with the parent/guardian of the student with asthma to answer questions and to provide reinforcement for the student's and family's compliance with the asthma management plan. (N.D. 9, 10)

Emphasize the student's strengths and abilities. (N.D. 9, 10)

Encourage the student's participation in sports, school, and peer activities to promote a sense of school engagement and sense of belonging. (N.D. 9, 10)

Provide opportunities for the student to take on responsibility and control of identified factors in his/her life, such as relaying information to teachers, parents, and healthcare provider, proposing alternate physical education activities during recovery from exacerbations, and recording peak flow meter values. (N.D. 9, 10)

Model the importance of focusing on the child rather than on his/her condition by referring to the student as a "student with asthma" rather than as "an asthmatic" or "an asthmatic student." (N.D. 10)

## Expected Student Outcomes

The student will:

- Identify persons, including healthcare providers, who assist him or her with their asthma care. (N.D. 1-4)
- Have an Asthma Action Plan on file in the school health office to be used in developing an IHP and ECP. (N.D. 1-4)
- Demonstrate proper peak flow technique. (N.D. 1-4)
- Use a peak flow meter and record findings daily for two consecutive weeks to obtain a "personal best" and/or to establish a level of asthma severity (if needed). (N.D. 1-4)
- Participate in regular monitoring of asthma status through recording peak flows and signs and symptoms in an asthma diary or log. (N.D. 1-4)
- Demonstrate avoidance or minimization of exposure to asthma triggers in the classroom and in and around school. (N.D. 1-4)
- Premedicate before physical exercise and use other pre-exercise measures to prevent exercise-induced bronchospasm. (N.D. 1-4)
- Identify and follow ECP when symptoms occur. (N.D. 1-4)
- Assist in making sure that necessary medications (including a back-up inhaler in the school health office) and asthma care devices and supplies are easily accessible and available (e.g., carried in his/her pocket, not in his/her locker). (N.D. 1-4)
- Identify responsibilities for self-carrying of medication. (N.D. 1-4)
- Describe indications for and proper use of self-carried medication. (N.D. 1-4)
- Demonstrate proper technique for using asthma medications and medication delivery devices (e.g., metered dose inhalers, dry powder inhalers, nebulizers, spacers) (N.D. 1-4)
- Identify components of his/her ECP and actions to take for self-management of an asthma episode. (N.D. 1-4)
- Identify major concepts in his/her IHP related to: (N.D. 1-4)
  -asthma assessment and monitoring
  -avoiding or controlling exposure to asthma triggers
  -medications (including indications, types, frequency, routes of administration, dose, side effects)
  -full participation in school activities
  -avoidance of absences and missed class time due to asthma
  -avoidance of fatigue associated with night wakening
  -avoidance of reliance on quick-relief medications for asthma control
- Demonstrate careful hand-washing technique and describe means to avoid exposure to individuals with colds. (N.D. 1-4)
- State two reasons individuals with asthma should not smoke or be around those who smoke or are smoking. (N.D. 1-4)
- Identify why annual flu vaccine is important for individuals with asthma. (N.D. 1-4)
- Describe/demonstrate what to do for managing asthma during field trips. (N.D. 1-4)
- Describe/demonstrate what to do for making up missed schoolwork due to asthma exacerbations. (N.D. 1-4)
- Describe/demonstrate what to do to adapt physical education activities during asthma episodes, during recovery from exacerbations or upper respiratory tract infections, on days when allergies are severe, or for adverse weather considerations (e.g., extremely cold or windy days). (N.D. 1-4)
- Identify persons at school who can assist them to monitor and follow their asthma management plan and Asthma Action Plan. (N.D. 1-4)
- Experience no fatigue associated with asthma symptoms that awaken the student or keep the student awake at night. (N.D. 1-4)

- Describe the contents of the Asthma Action Plan and ECP and steps to take to self-manage asthma episodes. (N.D. 5)
- Identify at least five indices of good asthma control. (N.D. 5)
- Describe (at a developmentally appropriate level) what asthma is, what causes chronic asthma and acute episodes, the role of inflammation in the illness, and symptoms that indicate that he/she should stay home from school. (N.D. 5)
- Identify symptoms of asthma. (N.D. 5)
- Identify early indications of an asthma exacerbation. (N.D. 5)
- Demonstrate how to use and interpret a peak flow. (N.D. 5)
- Identify specific actions to take based on symptoms and peak flow results. (N.D. 5)
- Identify his/her asthma triggers and list strategies for how to avoid these or how to control exposure to them. (N.D. 5)
- Identify and describe responsibilities for self-carrying of medication and demonstrate safe use of self-carry medications (N.D. 5)
- Discuss the importance of adherence to asthma management plan to avoid airway harm and risk of acute exacerbation. (N.D. 6)
- Identify factors that motivate compliance. (N.D. 6)
- Identify factors that might interfere with compliance and identify several strategies for dealing with these. (N.D. 6)
- Identify possible side effects of medication and agree to communicate with adults if he/she believes the medications are not being tolerated well. (N.D. 6)
- Come to the school health office and participate daily in monitoring of his/her peak flows and/or asthma symptoms and effectiveness of self-management efforts. (N.D. 6)
- Ask for and accept assistance when needed. (N.D. 6)
- Identify to parents and/or school personnel how medication makes them feel and suspected untoward reactions to medications that might interfere with compliance. (N.D. 6)
- Periodically review with the school nurse and parent the effectiveness of his/her asthma management using self-reports of ability to comply with the asthma management plan and indices of good asthma control. (N.D. 7)
- Periodically review with the school nurse and parent the tool "Is the Asthma Action Plan Working?" and self-reports of ability to comply with the asthma management plan when students have less than optimal control or moderate to severe asthma. (N.D. 7)
- Participate with the school nurse, parent/guardian, and healthcare provider to adjust plans (IHP, ECP, Asthma Action Plan) as needed. (N.D. 7, 8)
- Report an enhanced sense of overall emotional well-being and sense of control of his/her asthma. (N.D. 9, 10)
- Establish friend or peer support systems through participation in group asthma class. (N.D. 9, 10)
- State preferences in regard to how and where he/she wants to take or use medicine. (N.D. 9, 10)
- Participate in role-playing to discuss peer responses to student's having to take medication. (N.D. 9, 10)
- Demonstrate an increase in self-management skills by appropriate and responsible choices for asthma self-management evidenced by: (N.D. 8-10)
  -avoiding day and night symptoms
  -experiencing fewer asthma episodes that require unexpected doctor or emergency visits, hospitalizations, or 911 calls
  -being able to fully participate in physical and other school activities with peers
- Communicate with school personnel regarding asthma status. (N.D. 9, 10)
- Identify own strengths and limitations in regard to what he/she can and can't do in regard to having asthma. (N.D. 9, 10)

# Case Study

Francine is a 9-year-old girl in the fifth grade who has just transferred to Smoky Hill Elementary. In talking with her father when he comes to enroll her in school, you find out she started having trouble breathing when she started soccer last year and when running at recess. She was seen by a pediatric nurse practitioner at her primary healthcare doctor's office and was diagnosed as having exercise-induced asthma. She was given a prescription for an albuterol metered dose inhaler (MDI) and taught to take two puffs (waiting 1 minute between puffs) 5 to 15 minutes before soccer practice and recess. She is also to warm up before starting physical activity. If she was having an asthma episode, she was also supposed to take two puffs and repeat this dose in 15 minutes if her symptoms weren't gone. Francine's father also remembers that her breathing was "tested with a machine she blew into," but he doesn't recall any information about this. Francine doesn't have a current Asthma Action Plan. Her father isn't aware if her level of asthma severity was ever determined.

Francine's father states that albuterol seemed to help his daughter's asthma initially, but her asthma now seems to be getting worse and her symptoms more frequent, especially with a move to a drier climate. He thinks that Francine will continue to have asthma episodes at school, but generally isn't too worried because her coughing and wheezing seem to resolve fairly quickly with the use of the MDI. Francine has never been hospitalized for asthma, but was seen in urgent care earlier this year for wheezing with a bad cold. Because you are aware that even those with mild asthma could experience a serious asthma episode, you ask the father to meet with you the next day to talk further about Francine's asthma. Several issues were discussed:

1. Francine has typically been a good student at her old school, but her grades were starting to fall, mostly because she says she was often tired during class. Her father says he's noticed she seems to be coughing more at night and early in the morning.

2. Yesterday, during her first afternoon in her new school, she noticed that her new teacher had on a lot of perfume, which Francine really liked, but it also seemed to "bother" her breathing.

3. Francine says the family doesn't have any pets, but comments that she gets "stuffed up" and her eyes water when they visit her grandmother's home. They'll be going there on Thanksgiving Day for a big family reunion. Her grandmother has two cats.

4. Francine doesn't yet have a primary care provider, but her father says he plans to find a pediatrician soon. She will need a refill of her quick-relief medications before too long because she's using her albuterol inhaler more since moving here, about seven or eight times a week.

5. The hallways in the wing where Francine's classroom and the gymnasium are located are to be painted in early December.

In her previous school, carrying asthma inhalers wasn't allowed, and Francine had to go down to the school health office to use the inhaler to pretreat before each recess. Her father would like to know if this school has a self-carry policy so that Francine can use her inhaler in the classroom instead of having to miss a part of class.

## Asthma

| Assessment Data | Nursing Diagnosis | Goals | Nursing Interventions | Expected Outcomes |
|---|---|---|---|---|
| Increasing frequency and severity of asthma symptoms; wheezing and difficulty breathing with exercise and physical activity. | Ineffective airway clearance associated with chronic inflammation causing bronchoconstriction and excessive mucus production. | Francine will assist in the development of the IHP and Emergency Care Plan based on the Asthma Action Plan, including determining asthma severity. | Assist family to find a primary healthcare/asthma care provider for Francine and request an Asthma Action Plan from the parent or provider. | Francine and her family identify a new asthma care provider. |
| Does not have an Asthma Action Plan on file at present. | Risk for impaired gas exchange related to airway inflammation, bronchoconstriction, and excessive mucus production | Francine will participate in monitoring own asthma and share findings with her parent and healthcare provider. | With Francine and parent, develop IHP and ECP based on the Asthma Action Plan. (If Action Plan not available, develop one with information available and send to provider for review and signature). | Francine has an Asthma Action Plan on file in the school health office. |
| Poor asthma control (asthma episodes >2/ week and night awakening from asthma symptoms >2/ month); over-reliance on quick-relief medication to relieve symptoms. | Francine and her family will have identified a local healthcare provider for her asthma care and will assist in obtaining an Asthma Action Plan. | Francine will adhere to asthma management plans to attain and maintain good asthma control with minimal reliance on quick-relief medication. | Teach proper peak flow technique and, along with symptom observation, use to identify severity level and to determine "personal best." | Francine participates in planning the IHP and ECP meeting on _____ (date).<br><br>Francine demonstrates proper peak flow technique.<br><br>Francine participates in determining asthma severity and "personal best" by coming to clinic each noon for 2 weeks to do peak flows and records results. |
| | | Francine will talk with parent, healthcare provider about treatment for triggers she can't avoid (e.g., her grandmother's cats at Thanksgiving). | Assist Francine in regularly monitoring asthma status (lung function, asthma symptoms, exposure to triggers, and response to medications). | Francine regularly monitors asthma status, records peak flows and signs and symptoms in asthma diary or log, and reports frequency and effectiveness of albuterol inhaler use. |
| | | Francine will be involved in periodic assessment of written plans.<br><br>Francine will have needed asthma medication available and easily accessible. | Share results of initial monitoring with parent and healthcare provider so that asthma management plan can be adjusted as needed. | Francine and her parent will share records and discuss information with primary care/asthma care provider. |
| | | Francine communicates with her parent(s), the school nurse, health office staff, school personnel, and the healthcare provider about her asthma.<br><br>Francine will increase her ability to identify and manage environmental triggers. | Assist Francine in implementing the IHP (avoiding and controlling triggers; using medication as directed; and using peak flows and asthma symptoms to direct treatment as indicated in the Asthma Action Plan). | |

| Assessment Data | Nursing Diagnosis | Goals | Nursing Interventions | Expected Outcomes |
|---|---|---|---|---|
| | | | Educate Francine and parent about need for long-term controller. | Francine will: |
| | | | | • identify her major asthma triggers (cats, strong odors, exercise) |
| | | | Discuss with administrative staff the need to defer hallway painting until holiday break. | • describe strategies to avoid or control exposure to triggers (e.g., teacher asked to avoid perfume) |
| | | | Encourage parents to discuss with healthcare provider treatment options for unavoidable trigger exposure at Thanksgiving and other events. | • pretreat with her albuterol inhaler 2 puffs 5 to 15 minutes before recess and soccer practice |
| | | | | • wear scarf over mouth on cold days, warm up prior to exercise |
| | | | With Francine, periodically assess the effectiveness of the IHP and Asthma Action Plan. | • identify actions to take for increasing severity of asthma symptoms |
| | | | Obtain necessary medications devices, and supplies. | Francine will premedicate prior to exposure to triggers she cannot avoid. |
| | | | Assess Francine's developmental and emotional readiness for self-carrying quick-relief medications. | |
| | | | Obtain necessary releases/agreement for self-carrying signed by Francine, her parent, and the healthcare provider per school policy. | Francine participates in evaluating effectiveness of asthma management plan every 3 to 4 months using "Is the Asthma Action Plan Working?" |
| | | | Ensure back-up quick-relief medication is easily and quickly available to Francine and that school personnel know exactly where Francine's medication and supplies are kept in the school. | Francine has her inhaler with her at all times in school, on field trips, and on the bus. Francine has a back-up inhaler at school in the school health office. |
| | | | | Francine describes indications for and proper use of self-carried medications. |

| Assessment Data | Nursing Diagnosis | Goals | Nursing Interventions | Expected Outcomes |
|---|---|---|---|---|
| | | | Obtain parental permission/release for school nurse and healthcare provider to communicate about Francine's asthma status and establish mechanism for this. | Francine identifies responsibilities for self-carrying of medication (e.g., informing responsible adult of use and when symptoms persist even with use, not sharing inhaler). |
| | | | With school staff, identify potential triggers in the classroom/school environment and remove them or minimize Francine's exposure (and that of other students with asthma) to them. | Francine will tell parents and school staff when she is having:<br>• asthma symptoms<br>• side effects from medication<br>• problems avoiding triggers |
| | | | Post an easily understandable school-wide Protocol/Guideline for Managing Respiratory Distress Emergencies or the school's emergency first-aid guidelines in school classrooms and common areas, and review with school personnel. | Francine identifies things in the school environment that may trigger her asthma.<br><br>Francine identifies components of her ECP and actions to take for self-management of an asthma episode. |
| | | | Provide an ECP for school staff who work with Francine and educate about components of the plan (e.g., what to observe, actions to follow for increasing levels of symptom severity, when to call 911). | Francine identifies major aspects of care in her IHP, including the assessment and monitoring of her asthma symptoms, avoiding and controlling triggers, medication use, and expectations for good control (e.g., full participation in school activities, no absences and missed class time due to asthma, no fatigue associated with night wakening, good control of symptoms with minimal use of short-acting inhalers). |

| Assessment Data | Nursing Diagnosis | Goals | Nursing Interventions | Expected Outcomes |
|---|---|---|---|---|
| | | | Educate school staff who work with Francine about monitoring Francine's asthma symptoms and asthma management plan as specified n the IHP (including expectations for good asthma control; removing/minimizing exposure to triggers in the classroom and en route to and from school; importance of pre-exercise treatment regimen; recognizing asthma exacerbations and actions for emergencies; proper use of quick-relief medications; self-carrying policy and procedures).<br><br>Educate the school community through direct teaching and various media about the importance of careful hand washing, avoiding spreading of respiratory viruses, annual flu vaccination, not smoking, avoiding secondhand smoke, enforcing smoking bans, and maintaining good indoor air quality.<br><br>Introduce Francine to asthma care delegatees/nonlicensed personnel and identify their role in her asthma care. Teach or review tasks for Francine's care designated to asthma care. Establish plan for periodic review of task performance. | Francine will:<br>• demonstrate good hand washing technique<br>• describe ways to avoid exposure to others with colds<br>• state two reasons individuals with asthma should not smoke or be around those who are smoking<br>• state importance of annual flu vaccination.<br><br>Francine identifies adults in school who can assist her with asthma management. |

**Asthma**

| Assessment Data | Nursing Diagnosis | Goals | Nursing Interventions | Expected Outcomes |
|---|---|---|---|---|
| Physical activity results in asthma symptoms during sports and playground play. | Risk for activity intolerance related to exacerbation of symptoms associated with exercise-induced bronchospasm. | Francine will participate fully in normal school and day-care activities, including play, sports, and exercise. | Assist teachers to plan for accommodations as needed including:<br>• use of inhaler and warm-up activities before exercise<br>• adapting physical education activities during asthma episodes, during recovery from exacerbations or upper respiratory tract infections, on days when allergies are severe, or for adverse weather considerations (e.g., extremely cold or windy days)<br>• adaptations needed for various field trips and off-site activities<br>• making up school work missed during exacerbations. | Francine participates in developing a plan for asthma care at school, including use of inhaler before exercise; adapting physical education activities due to exacerbations, upper respiratory tract infections, severe allergy days, weather; field trips; and making up missed school-work due to asthma episodes.<br><br>Francine actively participates in physical activities at school, with modifications made as needed. |
| Night wakening from asthma symptoms causing daytime fatigue and risk to academic performance. | Risk for disturbed sleep pattern associated with asthma symptoms. | Francine will avoid experiencing nighttime symptoms (night wakening due to coughing, wheezing, breathing difficulty, chest tightness) and fatigue during the day due to this. | Educate parents that good asthma control should result in no nighttime wakening due to asthma symptoms and that proper monitoring and treatment will help student avoid fatigue and enhance learning. | Francine will experience no nighttime symptoms that disturb sleep.<br><br>Francine will decrease daytime fatigue due to disturbed sleep. |
| Increasing frequency and severity of symptoms, lack of long-term controller medication, lack of awareness of asthma severity; no Asthma Action Plan. | Deficient knowledge about asthma and asthma self-care. | Francine will increase her knowledge about asthma and self-management skills, including importance of adherence to asthma management plan and Asthma Action Plan to avoid acute asthma episodes and possible long-term harm to airways. | Identify the learning needs of Francine and her parents about asthma and self-care management. Develop a plan to address identified knowledge deficits. Educate Francine and parents about:<br>• indices of good asthma control<br>• etiology and physiology of chronic and acute asthma<br>• terms and definitions related to asthma | Francine participates in one-to-one instruction about asthma and attends group asthma program.<br><br>Francine identifies/describes/demonstrates:<br>• steps to take to self-manage chronic asthma and asthma episodes<br>• five indices of good asthma control |

| Assessment Data | Nursing Diagnosis | Goals | Nursing Interventions | Expected Outcomes |
|---|---|---|---|---|
| | | | | • role of inflammation and importance of its control<br>• when Francine should be kept home<br>• early recognition of exacerbations<br>• interpreting peak flows<br>• actions to take that align with symptom severity based on the ECP and/or Asthma Action Plan using stoplight analogy<br>• asthma triggers and specific strategies to manage them (e.g., staying indoors on high pollen-count days, keeping humidity low, removing furred or feathered animals from classroom)<br>• rights and responsibilities for self-carrying of inhaler medication | • what asthma is (at a developmentally appropriate level)<br>• what causes chronic asthma and acute episodes<br>• the role of inflammation in asthma<br>• symptoms indicating when to stay home from school<br>• her asthma symptoms<br>• early indications of exacerbation<br>• how to use and interpret peak flows<br>• specific actions to take based on symptoms and peak flow results<br>• her asthma triggers<br>• strategies for managing triggers<br>• responsibilities for self-carrying of medication<br>• safe, proper use of self-carry medications. |
| Poor asthma control, likely due to knowledge deficit about importance of good asthma control, trigger avoidance and control, and medication regimen, but need to gather more information about student and family. | Risk for noncompliance with treatment regimen associated with knowledge deficit about asthma. | Francine will increase her understanding of the link between adherence to the asthma management plan and a decreased risk of long-term harm to airways.<br><br>Francine will increase her awareness of factors that both promote and interfere with compliance with asthma treatment and strategies to help manage barriers to compliance. | Educate Francine and family about asthma and self-management and about importance of adherence to asthma management plans to avoid exacerbations and possible long-term harm to airways. Continue to gather data to rule out other compliance issues (e.g., poor symptom perception; perceived ineffectiveness of medication or unacceptability of side effects denial of need for treatment; oppositional or rebellious behavior; secondary gain from illness; inability to physically or financially access medication). | Assist Francine in developing strategies to deal with barriers to compliance. Develop and implement a plan that reinforces Francine's self-care efforts.<br><br>Francine describes the importance of adherence to the treatment plan to avoid airway harm and risk of acute episodes.<br><br>Francine will:<br>• have no or minimal day and nighttime asthma symptoms<br>• participate fully in school activities |

| Assessment Data | Nursing Diagnosis | Goals | Nursing Interventions | Expected Outcomes |
|---|---|---|---|---|
| | | | Assist Francine to identify motivators for self-care activities and factors that might interfere with compliance (e.g., side effects of medication, peer pressure).

Assist Francine in developing strategies to deal with barriers to compliance.

Develop and implement a plan that reinforces Francine's self-care efforts. | Francine will demonstrate a good attendance pattern.

Francine will experience no ER visits, hospitalizations, or 911 calls due to asthma.

Francine identifies at least 3 factors that foster compliance with asthma self-care plans.

Francine identifies 3 factors that might interfere with compliance with asthma self-care plan.

Francine identifies several strategies for dealing with barriers to compliance. |
| More frequent asthma symptoms, and greater developmental capacity for self-other comparisons places child at greater risk for anxiety and self-esteem issues. | Anxiety/Risk for anxiety related to experiencing a chronic childhood illness and experiences with exacerbations of asthma symptoms.

Risk for chronic low self-esteem related to experiencing a chronic illness and experiences with exacerbations of asthma symptoms. | Francine will develop an enhanced sense of well-being through greater confidence and competence in controlling asthma and in preventing acute exacerbations. | Monitor Francine's attendance patterns, academic performance, peer relationships, and overall emotional well-being for declines in functioning.

Refer Francine as needed to mental health team members.

Involve Francine (and parent when possible) in group asthma education program to reinforce one-to-one teaching and to potentially offer member support. | Francine reports an enhanced sense of subjective overall emotional well-being and sense of control of own asthma.

Francine develops friend or peer support systems through participation in group asthma class.

Francine demonstrates appropriate interactions with peers at school. |

# Emergency Care Plan
## Asthma

Date: _____

Student: _Francine Doe_____

Date of birth: _____

Parent(s)/Guardian(s): _Fred & Claire Doe____
_____
_____

Primary Care Provider: _Alberta Teitelbaum__

Specialist: _____

Contact: _____

School: _Smoky Hill Elementary_____

Grade: _____5_____

Home telephone: _555-1213_____

Father's work: _____

Mother's work: _555-1214_____

Telephone: _555-1212_____

Telephone: _____

Medical Diagnosis: _Asthma – triggered by exercise, respiratory infections, paint fumes_____

Persons Authorized to Administer Treatment: _____

| Symptom | Action |
|---|---|
| Coughing for prolonged periods<br><br>Wheezing or musical sounds in chest; unusual noises with breathing<br><br>Shaking chills with or without fever<br><br>Shortness of breath, difficulty breathing<br><br>Tightness in chest<br><br>Anxious expression<br><br>Stopping activity, not wanting to walk fast or run<br><br>Hunching over to breathe | 1. **Have Francine use her Quick-relief "Rescue" medication:**<br>**Albuterol MDI : 2 puffs, 1 minute between each puff, at onset of asthma symptoms**<br>2. Remove Francine from trigger—stop activity participation, remove from area of allergen.<br>3. If symptoms are not quickly relieved, Francine should go immediately to school health office accompanied by another student or adult. Do not sent her alone. **OR** Call school health office personnel (ext. 2424) to come to her.<br>4. Have someone stay with Francine and monitor her breathing. Speak calmly and reassuringly. Encourage Francine to relax, sitting up in a comfortable position. Encourage slow, deep breathing.<br>5. If symptoms are not relieved after 20 minutes, repeat medication dose (#1)<br>**Albuterol MDI : 2 puffs, 1 minute between each puff**<br>6. Contact parents. |

| Symptom | Action |
|---------|--------|
| Struggling to breathe, sucking in of skin<br><br>Bluish discoloration of lips, nails, between ribs from breathing in hard; pallor in students of color; unusual noises with breathing<br><br>Sweaty, clammy skin<br><br>Not wanting to lie down<br><br>Declining level of consciousness<br><br>Talking in short, clipped sentences | 1. **Call 911. Transport to nearest emergency room.**<br>2. Notify school health office personnel.<br>3. Contact parent. |

**Signatures:**

School Nurse_____ Date_____

Parent/guardian (if required)_____ Date_____

# References

Akinbami, L. J., & Schoendorf, K. C. (2002). Trends in asthma prevalence, health care utilization, and mortality. *Pediatrics, 110*(2), 315–322.

American Academy of Allergy, Asthma, and Immunology (2003). *Pediatric asthma promoting best practice: Guide for managing asthma in children.* Milwaukee, WI: Author.

American Lung Association. (1998). Executive summary: The American Lung Association asthma survey. Retrieved October 21, 2002, from http://www.lungusa.org/asthma/merk_summary.html

Castro, M., Schechtman, K.B., Halstead, J., & Bloomberg, G. (2001). Risk factors for asthma morbidity and mortality in a large metropolitan city. *Journal of Asthma, 38*(8), 625–635.

Institute of Medicine, Committee on the Assessment of Asthma and Indoor Air (2000). Clearing the air: Asthma and indoor air exposures. Washington, D.C.: National Academy Press.

NANDA International. (2003). *Nursing diagnoses: Definitions & classification 2003-2004.* Philadelphia, PA: Author.

National Association of School Nurses. (in press). *School nurse asthma management program (SNAMP) resource manual for school-based asthma management.* Castle Rock, CO: Author.

National Center for Health Statistics. (2004, September 28). *Asthma.* Retrieved October 7, 2004, from http://www.cdc.gov/nchs/fastats/asthma.htm

National Institutes of Health. (1997). *Expert panel report 2: Guidelines for the diagnosis and management of asthma* (NIH publication 97-4051). Rockville, MD: Author.

National Institutes of Health. (2003). *Expert panel report 2: Guidelines for the diagnosis and management of asthma, update on selected topics 2002* (NIH publication 027-50741). Rockville, MD: Author.

Newacheck, P. W., & Halfon, N. (2000). Prevalence, impact and trends in childhood disability due to asthma. *Archives of Pediatric and Adolescent Medicine, 15*(3), 287–293.

Weiss, K., Sullivan, S. D., & Lytle, C. S. (2000). Trends in the cost of illness for asthma in the U.S., 1985-1994. *Journal of Allergy and Clinical Immunology, 106*(3, part 1), 493–499.

# Bibliography

Baker, V.O., Friedman, J., & Schmitt, R. (2002). Asthma management: Part I: An overview of the problem and current trends. *Journal of School Nursing, 18*(3), 128–137.

Baker, V. O., Friedman, J., & Schmitt, R. (2002). Asthma management, Part II: Pharmacologic management. *Journal of School Nursing, 18*(5), 257–269.

Berg, J., Tichacek, M. J., & Theodorakis, R. (2004). Evaluation of an educational program for adolescents with asthma. *Journal of School Nursing, 20*(1), 29–35.

Borgmeyer, A., Jamerson, P., Gyr, P., Westhaus, N., & Glynn, E. (2005). The school nurse role in asthma management: Can the action plan help? *Journal of School Nursing, 21*(1), 23–30.

Epstien, B. L. (2001). Childhood asthma and indoor allergens: The classroom may be a culprit. *Journal of School Nursing, 17*(5), 253–257.

Harris, L. (2002). Asthma education for middle school students and staff. *Journal of School Nursing, 18*(2), 117–121.

National Association of School Nurses. (n.d.). *Asthma resources.* Retrieved November 7, 2004, from http://nasn.org/resources/disasterpreplinks.htm

National Association of School Nurses. (n.d.). *Managing asthma triggers* [Education Program]. Retrieved November 7, 2004, from http://nasn.org/education/education.htm

National Association of School Nurses. (n.d.). *School nurse asthma management program (SNAMP)* [Education Program]. Retrieved November 7, 2004, from http://nasn.org/resources/asthma.htm

National Association of School Nurses. (Revised 1999). *Position Statement: The use of asthma inhalers in the school setting.* Scarborough, ME: Author.

National Association of School Nurses. (2002). *Issue Brief: Asthma management in the school setting.* Scarborough, ME: Author.

National Association of School Nurses. (Adopted 2004). *Position Statement: Rescue medications in school.* Scarborough, ME: Author.

Neuharth-Pritchett, S., & Getch, Y. Q. (2001) Asthma and the school teacher: The status of teacher preparedness and training. *Journal of School Nursing, 17*(6), 323–328.

Nies, M. A., Bickes, J. T., Schim, S.M., & Johnson, A. L. (2002) Model for community health nursing care: Application to an integrated asthma intervention program. *Journal of School Nursing, 18*(2), 74–78.

Synoground, G., & Thiele, J. (1997-2000). *Nursing assessment of school age youth. Respiratory functions.* (Home Study Module Number 2). Scarborough, ME: National Association of School Nurses.

Praeger, S., & Zickler, C. (2002). *Care of students with asthma in schools: Applications of professional school nursing practice standards* [Manual]. Scarborough, ME: National Association of School Nurses.

Velsor-Friedrich, B., Vlasses, F., Moberley, J., & Coover, L. (2004) Talking with teens about asthma management. *Journal of School Nursing, 20*(3), 140–148.

## Resources

Allergy and Asthma Network/Mothers of Asthmatics (AANMA)
2751 Prosperity Avenue
Suite 150
Fairfax, VA 22031
703-573-7794 (fax)
1-800-878-4403
http://www.aanma.org

American Academy of Allergy, Asthma, and Immunology (AAAAI)
555 East Wells Street
Suite 1100
Milwaukee, WI 53202-3823
414-272-6071
1-800-822-2762 (Patient Information Line)
http://www.aaaai.org

American Academy of Family Physicians (AAFP)
PO Box 11210
Shawnee Mission, KS 66207-1210
1-800-274-2237
http://www.aafp.org

American Academy of Pediatrics (AAP)
141 Northwest Point Boulevard
Elk Grove, IL 60007
847-434-4000
847-434-8000 (fax)
http://www.aap.org

American Academy of School Administrators (AASA)
801 North Quincy Street
Suite 700
Arlington, VA 22203-1730
703-528-0700
703-841-1543 (fax)
http://www.aasa.org

American Lung Association (ALA)
61 Broadway
Sixth Floor
New York, NY 10006
212-315-8700
http://www.lungusa.org

Asthma and Allergy Foundation of America (AAFA)
1233 20th Street, NW
Suite 402
Washington, DC 20036
202-466-7643
202-466-8940 (fax)
1-800-727-8462 (hot line)
http://www.aafa.org

Centers for Disease Control and Prevention
Division of Adolescent and School Health
1600 Clifton Road
Atlanta, GA 30333
800-311-3435
http://www.cdc.gov/nccdphp/dash

National Association of School Nurses (NASN)
Eastern Office
PO Box 1300
Scarborough, ME 04070
207-883-2117
1-877-627-6476
http://www.nasn.org

National Heart, Lung, and Blood Institute (NHLBI)
NHLBI Health Information Center
PO Box 30105
Bethesda, MD 20824-0105
301-592-8573
240-629-3246 (fax)
http://www.nhlbi.nih.gov

U.S. Environmental Protection Agency
Office of Radiation and Indoor Air
Indoor Air Environments Division
1200 Pennsylvania Avenue, NW
Washington, DC 20460
202-343-9370
202-343-2394 (fax)
http://www.epa.gov/iaq

Asthma

## Chapter Twenty-four

# Autism Spectrum Disorders (Pervasive Developmental Disorders)

### Jeanette H. Williams

## Introduction

Autism spectrum disorders (ASD), also known as pervasive developmental disorders (PDDs) consist of a group of disorders that have some similar characteristics. Included in this category in the *Diagnostic and Statistical Manual of Mental Disorders,* fourth edition text revision *(DSMR-IV-TR),* of the American Psychiatric Association (APA) (APA, 2000) are autism, Asperger's syndrome, Rett syndrome, PDD not otherwise specified (NOS), and childhood disintegrative disorder (Heller's syndrome). It is estimated that the prevalence rate for PDDs is between 45 and 60 children in 10,000 (Chakrabarti & Fombonne, 2001; Hyman, Rodier, & Davidson, 2001).

Common symptoms include delays and deviance in social skills, impaired communication, lack of imaginative skill, and behavioral problems (APA, 2000; Volkmar, Lorc, Klin, & Cord, 2002; Edelson, 1999). Many of these children have limited cognitive ability. Autism is the best known of this group of disorders.

Treatment of these disorders is primarily educational and behavioral and needs to be multidisciplinary, intensive, and continuous (Cumine, Leach, & Stevenson, 2000).

## Pathophysiology

### Autism

Kanner (1943) added the diagnosis of autism to the psychiatric literature in 1944, more than 60 years ago. He described it as a syndrome defined by behaviors and a characteristic history. *Harvard Mental Health Letter* (1997) described it as a neurodevelopmental disorder with neuropathic, neurochemical, and genetic components (Sheehan, 2004). It is a spectrum disorder with varying degrees of severity. It can be a severe and incapacitating, lifelong developmental disability.

The prevalence of autism is currently estimated to be 15 to 17 children in 10,000 (Chakrabarti & Fombonne, 2001). Approximately 75% of children with autism are boys (Harvard Mental Health Letter, 1997; Edelson, 1999). However, affected females are likely to have more severe symptoms and lower intelligence (APA, 2000; National Institute of Mental Health [NIMH], 2004). Many theories as to causes of autism exist, including vaccine, particularly measles, mumps, and rubella (MMR); food allergies (gluten and casein); and environmental caus-

es. In 2004, a report by the Institutes of Medicine (IOM) concluded that there is no association between autism and vaccines such as MMR that contain thimerosal as a preservative (CDC Vaccines and Autism Fact Sheet, 2004). Much research is still being conducted.

Signs of the disorder include delayed or absent communication, impairment of social interaction, restrictive and repetitive behavior, interest and activities, and resistance to changes in schedule or environment (Sheehan, 2004). Some signs may appear in the early months. Infants with autism do not like to cuddle and may shrink from touch (Harvard Mental Health Letter, 1997). Symptoms may be subtle during infancy and go unnoticed, but it is apparent before age 30 months that something is wrong. Children with autism have little interest in other people, do not maintain eye contact, and may not distinguish their parents from strangers (Harvard Mental Health Letter). They have a narrow and restrictive range of interests (APA, 2000). Approximately 80% of autistic children have mental retardation. An IQ of between 35 and 50 is common (Volkmar et al., 2002). Children with autism are attracted to objects rather than people. They may have a range of behavioral symptoms, including violent and extreme reaction to a slight change, hyperactivity, short attention span, impulsivity, and aggressiveness. Sleeping and eating disorders may also be present. Their play is ritualistic and repetitive. Imaginative play may be absent or impaired. They have a narrow and restricted range of interests. Language may be absent, or development of language is delayed (APA, 2000; Harvard Mental Health Letter, 1997). Children with autism have a high threshold for pain, hypersensitivity to sound and/or touch, exaggerated reactions to light or odors, a lack of fear in response to real dangers, and a variety of self-injurious behaviors (head banging or finger, hand, or wrist biting) (APA , 2000). A wide variety of neurologic disorders have been reported in children with autism, including cerebral palsy, maternal rubella, toxoplasmosis, tuberous sclerosis, cytomegalovirus infection, demyelinating disease, lead encephalopathy, meningitis, encephalitis, severe brain hemorrhage, phenylketonuria, and many types of epilepsy. Delahunty (2002) reports that more than 10% of children with autism having some degree of hearing loss. Twenty-five percent of children with autism develop seizures as adults (Harvard Mental Health Letter, 1997).

### PDD-NOS

This disorder is described as severe and pervasive impairment in the development of reciprocal social interaction or verbal and nonverbal communication, and the presence of stereotyped behavior, interests, and activities. However, the criteria for a specific PDD diagnosis are not met (National Information Center for Children and Youth with Disabilities [NICHCY], 1995; Towbin, Mauk, & Batshaw, 2002). PDD-NOS has also been called atypical autism or mild autism (Levine, 1996; Towbin et al.).

Autism and PDD-NOS share many of the same characteristics. Both are neurologic disorders that affect a child's ability to communicate, understand language, play, and relate to others (NICHY, 1995). Children with PDD have abnormal responses to sensations. Any one or a combination of senses or responses may be affected: sight, hearing, touch, balance, smell, taste, reaction to pain. Speech and language are absent or delayed, and these children relate to people abnormally.

### Rett syndrome

Rett syndrome is an X-linked, dominant, genetic disorder, almost exclusively affecting females, that is caused by mutation in the gene *MeCP2* (Amir et al., 1999). It is a progressive neurologic disorder characterized by loss of purposeful hand use, progressive spasticity of lower extremities, seizures, acquired microcephaly, and mental retardation (Ellaway & Christodoulou, 1999; Hagberg, Hanefeld, Percy, & Skjeldal, 2002).

An essential feature of the condition is regression after a relative period of normal functioning. Normal development takes place until 6 to 18 months of age. Deceleration of head growth, developmental delays, and characteristic hand wringing and mouthing of the hands occurs between 6 months and 4 years. Acquired verbal communication skills are lost, and there is a regression in ambulation skills and stability. There may also be breathing problems, including apnea episodes, hyperventilation, and forced expiration of air. The child with Rett syndrome becomes irritable, has frequent crying episodes, and has difficulty sleeping. Regression in cognition, motor skills, and social development occurs throughout life (Gorum, 1999).

### Asperger syndrome

Persons with Asperger syndrome (or disorder) share many behavior and social features of autism, including severe deficits in social interaction, a restricted pattern of activities, and repetitive stereotyped behaviors, but without the significant delays in the acquisition of language, cognitive functioning, development of self-help skills, adaptive behavior, or curiosity about the environment (APA , 2000, Klin, Volkmar, & Sparrow, 2000). Asperger syndrome is sometimes referred to as a high-functioning autistic disorder.

Children with Asperger syndrome have significantly stronger verbal skills than nonverbal skills. They usually have strong abilities for learning facts, spelling, and vocab-ulary, but have difficulty with forming concepts, problem solving, and complex verbal and reading comprehension (Towbin et al., 2002). They exhibit significant impairment in social skills and nonverbal communication, which makes it difficult for them to form friendships and long-term personal relationships (Bashe & Kirby, 2001). Motor delays or motor coordination problems may be seen in the preschool period.

### Childhood disintegrative disorder

In this rare disorder, the child's development is normal until somewhere between 3 and 5 years of age (Hendry, 2000). Then the child's developmental skills decline rapidly. The child loses social, language, play, and motor skills and may lose bowel and bladder control. The decline does stabilize, leaving the child with behavior and skills that resemble autism (Towbin et al., 2002). The child exhibits restricted repetitive and stereotyped behaviors and mannerisms (Levine, 1996; APA, 2000; Kutscher, 2002; Haiti, 2002).

## Management

Management of ASD is primarily educational and behavioral, with medications used as needed for associated problems (seizures, behaviors, etc.) Services for children vary greatly depending on the community and the quality of programs available in the school district. The programs may vary but should always be highly structured and geared to the child's developmental level of functioning (Towbin et al., 2002). The following paragraphs describe some of the therapies being used for children with ASD.

Facilitated communication is an educational intervention based on the theory that children with autism cannot control their movements to communicate what they think and feel. The child works with a facilitator who isolates the index finger of the child and teaches him or her how to type responses. In this way, the child learns to communicate. The program has met with both praise and criticism (Harvard Mental Health Letter, 1997).

Applied behavior analysis (ABA) is an intensive behavior modification program being used. It requires dedication and makes heavy demands on the parents and school systems. Therapy is home-based and school-based. The children are enrolled as early as age 3 years in an intense program for most of their waking hours. The program is aimed at changing the child's environment and patterns of reinforcement. According to a 1987 article written by Dr. Ivar Lovaas and published in the *Journal of Counseling and Clinical Psychology,* 47% of a group of 19 children with ASD were functioning normally in intellectual and academic areas following ABA training. Nine of the children had completed first grade in a regular classroom (Harvard Mental Health Letter, 1997).

Much controversy exists as to the effectiveness of this treatment, and research has been extremely limited. More studies are being done, and children are being followed up over a period of time to determine the long-term success of the program (Harvard Mental Health Letter, 1997; Bell,

1996). Early replications of research report gains in IQ, language, and adaptive and social skills (Autism Society of America, 2003).

TEAACH (Treatment and Education of Autistic and Related Communication Handicapped Children) is a structured, modified environmental program with emphasis on visual learning. Gains in function, development, and improved ability to adapt and generalize skills have been reported. The program was developed by the University of North Carolina (Autism Society of America, 2003).

Floor Time targets personal interaction to help develop appropriate skills for the child. This method sees the child as integrated and does not treat individual pieces (speech, motor, etc) (Autism Society of America, 2003).

Social Stories is a program developed in 1991 by Carol Gray. It is designed to help students understand social clues and rules (Autism Society of America, 2003).

Medical management of the child with ASD has centered on controlling the associated problems that develop because of the condition. If seizures develop, seizure medication is indicated. Neuroleptic drugs can be used to reduce behavioral symptoms. Anticholinergic drugs may be used to treat the extrapyramidal symptoms that are some-times a side effect of some neuroleptic drugs (e.g., haloperidol). Children with ASD should be carefully screened for hearing, lead poisoning (due to pica or long-term oral motor stage), vision, and nutrition (Delahunty 2002).

Serotonin reuptake inhibitors (SRIs) have been studied somewhat, but evidence supporting their use is minimal (Scahill, 2003). Secretin (an intestinal hormone) has been studied, but it does not alleviate core symptoms. Three controlled studies researched by Lloyd (June 2001) did not report benefits for children given secretin. Scahill (2003) also reports that there is no evidence the drug works. Megavitamin therapy has been tried. Special diets and nutritional supplements are being tried by many parents.

Education, counseling, and extended family support are necessary to help parents raising a child with an ASD. Having a child with ASD significantly affects all family members. Families need support groups and access to new findings and research to help them cope with the concerns, questions, and problems they incur daily while living with a child with one of these conditions (Sigman & Capps, 1997). Respite care should be available to families, especially in severe cases, to ensure that they may continue to care for the child in the home.

## Individualized Healthcare Plan

### Assessment
*History*
- Age and developmental level
- At what age was the diagnosis made?
- Diagnosis, severity of condition, and prognosis
- Growth and weight gain pattern
- Medications
- Illnesses
- Injuries
- Seizures (may or may not be present)

*Current Status and Management*
- Current developmental level of student, including:
  -physical
  -cognitive, evidence of mental retardation
  -social
  -communication/language skills
- Student's temperament/behavior
- Student's ability to interact with peers and adults
- Student's current height and weight
- Student's current vision status
- Student's current hearing status
- Healthcare providers involved in management of child's condition (neurologist, psychiatrist, psychologist, pediatrician)
- Seizures (may or may not be present)
- Medications: effectiveness and side effects
- Eating habits/nutritional pattern
- Sleeping habits

*Self-care*
- Student's perception of health
- Self-care skills
- Decision-making skills
- Parents' perception of student's condition

*Psychosocial Status*
- Student's temperament
- Student's perception of stressors
- Student's fears, anxieties
- Student's coping skills (effective and ineffective)
- Student's interest in recreational/social activities
- Level of family functioning
- Parents' coping skills (effective and ineffective)
- Family education and counseling; modifications in family environment
- Family resources, socioeconomic, extended family, friends
- Availability and involvement of support systems
- Involvement with peers outside of school

*Academic Issues*
- Educational providers involved in management of child's education (teacher, occupational therapist, physical therapist, speech and language therapist, school nurse)
- Review of special education assessments/interventions
- Behavior management plan
- Classroom modifications necessary for child's participation in class
- Parents' and teachers' knowledge of specific PDD condition affecting student
- Student's comfort level in the school setting and on field trips

## Nursing Diagnoses (N.D.) (NANDA, 2003)

**N. D. 1** Delayed growth and development (NANDA 00111) related to:
- delay in performing skills (motor, social, expressive) typical of age group
- inability to perform self-care, self-control activities

**N.D. 2** Disturbed thought processes (NANDA 00130) related to:
- inaccurate interpretation of environment
- inappropriate non-reality-based thinking

**N.D. 3** Disturbed sensory perception (NANDA 00122) related to:
- decreased ability to control sensory input
- decreased ability to choose which sensory data to consider relevant
- incomplete processing of sensory inputs (auditory, kinesthetic, tactile, olfactory)

**N.D. 4** Anxiety (NANDA 00146) related to disturbed thought processes

**N.D. 5** Deficient knowledge (NANDA 00126) related to:
- mental retardation
- disturbed thought processes
- disturbed sensory perception

**N.D. 6** Ineffective coping (NANDA 00069) related to:
- lack of goal-directed behavior
- inability to organize information

**N.D. 7** Impaired verbal communication (NANDA 00051) related to:
- inability to speak
- difficulty establishing and maintaining effective communication pattern

**N.D. 8** Risk for injury (NANDA 00035) related to affective orientation and developmental age

**N.D. 9** Risk for self-directed violence (NANDA 00140) related to mental health

**N.D. 10** Impaired social interaction (NANDA 00052) related to:
- inability to communicate
- dysfunctional interaction with peers, family, and others

**N.D. 11** Deficient diversional activity (NANDA 00097) related to lack of interest
**N.D. 12** Risk for disturbed sleep pattern disturbance (NANDA 00095) related to chronic health condition
**N.D. 13** Imbalanced nutrition: less than body requirements (NANDA 00002) related to lack of interest in food
**N.D. 14** Bathing/hygiene self-care deficit (NANDA 00108) related to impaired ability to perform activity

## Goals

The student will increase and utilize cognitive skills and emotional strengths. (N.D. 1–6)
The student will improve his/her ability to interpret sensory input. (N.D. 3)
The student will utilize effective strategies to increase comfort level in school setting. (N.D. 4).
The student will utilize positive coping strategies with assistance from family members. (N.D. 4, 6.)
The student will verbally and nonverbally demonstrate increase in comfort level in the school setting and on field trips. (N.D. 4–6)
The student will communicate effectively with peers and staff. (N.D. 7)
The student will remain safe in the school environment. (N.D. 8)
The student will decrease episodes of violent behavior. (N.D. 9)
The student will increase/maintain effective, appropriate family interactions. (N.D. 10).
The student will participate in social/recreational activities with peers. (N.D. 10. 11)
The student will maintain normal sleep pattern. (N.D. 12)
The student will maintain normal growth pattern. (N.D. 13)
The student will wash hands at appropriate times. (N.D. 14)

## Nursing Interventions

Refer special education team if student is not receiving services. (N.D. 1–7)
Consult and collaborate with education staff to provide for a safe, consistent, routine environment. (N.D. 1–7)
Explore what causes anxiety and fears in student and collaborate with staff and family to eliminate or minimize these situations or stimuli. (N.D. 4)
Respect and support effective family interaction and coping. (N.D. 6)
Collaborate with staff to promote effective methods of communication for student. (N.D. 7)
Provide for a safe environment with adequate personnel and enclosed areas as deemed appropriate. (N.D. 8, 9)
Identify and utilize effective calming techniques. (N.D. 1–9)
Use a calm, reassuring approach when working with the student. (N.D. 1–10)
Identify factors leading to outbursts of violent behavior. (N.D. 5, 9)
Use appropriate physical restraints, as necessary, according to school district policy. (N.D. 8, 9)
Refer for medical consultation with the child's healthcare provider if self-injurious behavior or violence toward others is exhibited. (N.D. 8, 9).
Reinforce positive behaviors demonstrated by the student in collaboration with teachers and other educational specialists. (N.D. 9)
Reinforce effective communication demonstrated by student in collaboration with teacher and speech clinician. (N.D. 10)
Collaborate with educational staff/parents to identify social/recreational interests of child. Encourage student to explore various activities and participate. (N.D. 10, 11).
Consult with parents/physician regarding sleep patterns. Assist parents in exploring strategies for dealing with the sleep-pattern issues (medication, calming techniques). (N.D. 12)
Offer variety of foods and encourage child to try new foods. (N.D. 13)
Monitor growth pattern in collaboration with parent and physician. (N.D. 13)
Provide instruction and practice in hand-washing technique and when to wash hands. Monitor student for compliance. (N.D. 14)
Provide educational opportunities for parents regarding PDD and specific syndrome of student in collaboration with special education staff. (N.D. 1–14)
Consult with staff, physician, and parents as needed. (N.D. 1–14).
Be available and provide resources for parents for education, counseling, support groups, and respite care. (N.D. 1–14)
Encourage parents to attend behavior management classes for parents of children with PDD. (N.D. 10, 11)

## Expected Student Outcomes

The student will:
- Demonstrate (specific motor skill[s]). (N.D. 1)
- Demonstrate effective expressive language skills. (N.D. 1, 7)
- Exhibit appropriate social behavior in the (classroom, hallway, lunchroom, etc.). (N.D. 1, 8, 9, 10)
- Accurately interpret (number, specific stimulus) environmental stimulus. (N.D. 2, 3)
- Demonstrate (specific) effective coping strategies that reduce anxiety. (N.D. 4)
- Verbally and nonverbally demonstrate increase of comfort level in the (school setting, on field trips, etc.). (N.D. 4–6)
- Demonstrate increased use of expressive language skills when communicating with (staff , peers). (N.D. 7)
- Demonstrates increased use of receptive language skills when communicating with (staff, peers). (N.D. 7)
- Communicate effectively, verbally, and nonverbally with staff. (N.D. 7)
- Communicate effectively, verbally, and nonverbally with peers. (N.D. 7)
- Express he/she feels safe in the school environment. (N.D. 8, 9)
- Demonstrate a decrease in inappropriate behavioral episodes. (N.D. 8, 9)
- Demonstrate appropriate interaction with family members, as reported by parents. (N.D. 10)
- Demonstrate positive social behaviors with family members. (N.D. 10).
- Develop and participate in minimum of two social/recreational activities. (N.D. 10, 11)
- Demonstrate maintenance/improvement of sleep pattern, as reported by parent. (N.D. 12)
- Demonstrate good nutritional intake during the school day. (N.D. 13)
- Wash hands independently at appropriate times. (N.D. 14)

## Case Study

Jamie is a 7-year-old girl who attends Windsor Elementary School. She has a diagnosis of PDD-NOS from her neurologist. She is in the second grade and is doing fairly well academically. She has an educational diagnosis of language impairment and receives therapy from the therapist 5 hours a week.

Jamie has few friends and usually plays alone at recess. This does not seem to bother her, and she seems very content at amusing herself. She does not like to try new foods and is a poor eater. She is below the fifth percentile in weight for her age. She is easily upset by the unexpected or by a change in any routine. She sometimes refuses to participate in new activities introduced in physical education and prefers to do the same thing over and over.

Her parents are very concerned about her lack of friends and her reluctance to try new activities. They also worry about her outbursts when her routine is changed.

## Individualized Education Program
## Recommendations for Student With Pervasive Developmental Disorder

Student's name: _____ Jamie _____

Jamie should be weighed monthly until her weight falls within the fifth percentile.

Nurse will consult with parents regarding Jamie's nutritional requirements.

Nurse will consult with parents regarding available resources, support groups, etc.

Nurse will collaborate with educational staff regarding ways to help Jamie interact with peers and form friendships.

**Weekly School Nursing Time Required**

Total weekly nursing: indirect services needs = 30 minutes per week

# Autism Spectrum Disorders

| Assessment Data | Nursing Diagnosis | Goals | Nursing Interventions | Expected Outcomes |
|---|---|---|---|---|
| Jamie's fear, anxieties.<br><br>Jamie is easily upset by change in routine. | Anxiety related to disturbed thought processes.<br><br>Ineffective coping related to lack of goal-directed behavior and inability to organize information. | Jamie will increase emotional strengths and utilize coping strategies to alleviate anxiety and increase comfort level in the school setting.<br><br>Jamie will utilize positive, appropriate behavior in the school setting and at home. | Consult and collaborate with staff to provide safe consistent routine environment.<br>• Minimize/remove stimuli that cause anxiety/fear.<br>• Use a calm, reassuring approach when working with the student.<br>Provide resources for education, counseling, support groups, and respite care.<br>Assist family to increase/maintain family functions (parenting, family interactions).<br>Assist family to utilize positive coping strategies in dealing with Jamie's behavior.<br>Assist parents to increase knowledge of condition.<br>Assist parents to utilize positive coping strategies. | Jamie will demonstrate, verbally and nonverbally, an increase in comfort level and/or decrease in anxiety level in the school setting.<br><br>Jamie will demonstrate (1) effective coping strategy that reduces anxiety.<br><br>Jamie will demonstrate positive, appropriate behaviors in school.<br><br>Jamie will demonstrate positive, appropriate behaviors at home, as reported by his parents. |
| Jamie's lack of friends and interaction with peers. | Impaired social interaction related to inability to communicate and dysfunctional interaction with peers, family, and others. | Jamie will interact effectively with peers in the school. | Encourage Jamie to explore various activities and participate in activity with other students and community settings.<br><br>Collaborate with educational staff/parents in how to involve her in group activity. Consult with parents about having student join after-school activities (Brownies, sports, etc.). | Jamie will communicate with peers.<br><br>Jamie will develop friendly relationship with two peers.<br><br>Jamie will demonstrate appropriate behavior when interacting with peers<br>• at school<br>• during after school activity |

| Assessment Data | Nursing Diagnosis | Goals | Nursing Interventions | Expected Outcomes |
|---|---|---|---|---|
| Jamie's interest in recreational/social activities. | Deficient diversional activity related to lack of interest. | Jamie will participate in social/recreational activity with peers. | Collaborate with educational staff/parents to identify social recreational interest of child. | Jamie will participate in minimum of two social, recreational activities. |
| Jamie's weight is abnormally low for age and height. | Imbalanced nutrition: less than body requirements. | Jamie will increase and maintain normal growth and weight. | Weigh Jamie monthly. Consult with parents regarding nutritious high-calorie foods and likes and dislikes. Educate parents about Jamie's nutrition requirements to maintain growth and development. Consult with occupational therapist regarding food textures. Allow Jamie to eat with peers in quiet calm area at lunch. Assist in providing for nutritional activities at school—small snacks with high nutrition and calories. | Jamie will move to 5th percentile or above and maintain height and weight at that level. |

# References

American Psychiatric Association. (2000). *Diagnostic and statistical manual of mental disorders* (4th ed., text revision). Washington, DC: Author.

Amir, R. E., Van den Veyver, I. B., Wan, M., Tran, C. O., Francke, U., & Zoghbi, H. Y. (1999). Rett syndrome is caused by mutations in X-linked MeCP2 encoding methyl-CpG-binding protein 2. *Nature Genetics, 23,* 185–188.

Autism Society of America. (2003). *Autism treatments: Current interventions in autism—A brief analysis.* Retrieved September 24, 2003, from http://www.autism-society.org

Autism Society of America. (2004). *Common characteristics of autism.* Retrieved August 25, 2004, from http://www.autism-society.org

Bell P. (1996 Winter). Autism: Even the experts debate treatment. *Pacesetter,* 9–11.

Chakrabarti, S., & Fombonne, E. (2001). Pervasive developmental disorders in preschool children. *Journal of the American Medical Association, 285,* 3093–3099.

Centers for Disease Control (2004). *Vaccines and autism: Important conclusions from the institute of medicine – Information for health care professionals.* Retrieved May 17, 2005 from http://www.cdc.gov/nip/vacsafe/concerns/autism/vacc-austism-iom_hcp.pdf

Cumine, V., Leach, J., & Stevenson, G. (2000). *Resource materials for teachers—Autism in the early years: A practical guide.* London: David Fulton.

Delahunty, C. (2002). Medical management of pervasive developmental disorder. In B. L. Maria (Ed.), *Current management in child neurology* (2nd ed., pp. 200–205). London: Decker.

Edelson, S. M. (1999). *Rett syndrome.* Salem, OR: Center for the Study of Autism. Retrieved September 22, 2003, from http://www.autismorg.rett.html

Ellaway, C., & Christodoulou, J. (1999). Rett syndrome: Clinical update and review of recent genetic advances. *Journal of Paediatrics and Child Health, 35,* 419–426.

Gardner, M. R. (2001). Understanding and caring for the child with Asperger syndrome. *Journal of School Nursing, 17*(4), 178–184.

Gorun, C. R. (1999). Rett syndrome. In M. J. Arnold & C. K. Silkworth. *The school nurse's source book of individualized healthcare plans* (Vol. 2, pp. 331–341). North Branch, MN: Sunrise River Press.

Grandin, T. (1996). *Teaching tips for children and adults with autism.* Fort Collins, CO: Colorado State University.

Hagberg, B., Hanefeld, F., Percy, A., & Skjeldal, O. (2002). An update on clinically applicable diagnostic criteria in Rett syndrome. *European Journal of Paediatric Neurology, 6,* 293–297.

Hait, E. (2002). *Childhood disintegrative disorder.* MedlinePlus Medical Encyclopedia. Retrieved September 21, 2003, from http://www.nim.nih.gov/medlineplus/ency/article/001535.htm

Harvard Mental Health Letter. (1997). *Autism.* Retrieved January 5, 1999, from http://www.mentalhealth.com/mag/

Hendry, C. N. (2000). Childhood disintegration disorder: Should it be considered a distinct diagnosis? *Clinical Psychology Review, 20,* 77–90.

Hyman, S. L., Rodier, P. M., & Davidson, P. (2001). Pervasive developmental disorders in young children. *Journal of the American Medical Association, 285*(24), 3141–3142.

Kanner, L. (1943). Autistic disturbances of affective contact. *Nervous Child, 2,* 217–280.

Klin, A., Volkmar, F., & Sparrow, S. (Eds.). (2000). *Asperger syndrome.* New York: Guilford Press.

Kutscher, M. L. (2002). *Autistic spectrum disorders: Sorting it out.* Retrieved September 21, 2003 from http:www.pediatricneurology.com/autism.htm

Levine, K. (1996). Pervasive developmental disorders: *PDD-NOS, Asperger's disorder and autism parent information booklet.* Boston: Institute for Community Inclusion/UAP.

Lloyd, J. W. (2001). *Autism and secretin.* University of Virginia. Retrieved 9/3/2003 from http://curry.edschool.virginia.edu/sped/projects/ose/information/seretin.html

Luther, E. H., Canham, D. L., Young Cureton, V. (2005). Coping and social support for parents of children with autism. *Journal of School Nursing, 21*(1), 40–47.

NANDA International. (2003). *Nursing diagnoses: Definitions & classification 2003–2004.* Philadelphia: Author.

National Information Center for Children and Youth with Disabilities. (NICHCY) (1995). *Autism/PDD.* Washington, DC: Author.

National Institute of Mental Health (NIMH). (2004). *Autism Spectrum Disorders.* Retrieved May 7, 2005, from http://www.nimh.nih.gov/publicat/autism.

National Institutes of Neurological Disorders and Stroke (NINDS). (2001). *NINDS autism information page.* Retrieved August 24, 2004, from http://www.ninds.nih.gov/health_and_medicaldisorders/autismshortdoc.htm

Scahill, L. (2003). Taking a hard look at pharmacotherapy. What hasn't worked? What might? *Academy briefings Autism: New frontiers in research & discovery.* Retrieved September 3, 2003, from http://www.nyas.org/aeb/autism/report_07.html

Sheehan, M. (2004). Autism. In P. J. Allen & J. A. Vessey (Eds), *Primary care of the child with a chronic condition* (4th ed.). St. Louis, MO: Mosby.

Sigman, M., & Capps L. (1997). *Children with autism: A developmental perspective* (p. 86). Cambridge, MA: Harvard University Press.

Towbin, K. E., Mauk, J. E., & Batshaw, M. L. (2002). Pervasive developmental disorder. In M. L. Batshaw. *Children with disabilities* (5th ed.). Baltimore: Paul H. Brooks.

Volkmar, F. R., Lorc, C., Klin, A., & Cord, E. (2002). Autism and the pervasive developmental disorders. In M. Lewis (Ed.). *Child & adolescent psychiatry* (3rd ed., pp. 587–596). Philadelphia: Lippincott Williams & Wilkins.

## Bibliography

American Psychological Association. (2001). *Publication manual of the American Psychological Association* (5th ed.). Washington, DC: Author.

Edelson, S. (1999) *Overview of autism*. Salem, OR: Center for the Study of Autism. Retrieved September 20, 2003, from http://www.autism.org/contents.html#toc

B. J. Freeman. (1996). *Diagnosis of the syndrome of Autism: Questions parents ask*. Retrieved February 20, 1998, from http://www/autism–society.org/packages/getstart_diagnosis.html

Centers for Disease Control. (2004). *Vaccines & autism: Important conclusions from a recent report from the institute of medicine – Information for parents*. Retrieved May 17, 2005 from http://www.cdc.gov/nip/vacsafe/concerns/autism/vacc-autism-iom_parent.pdf

Hootman, J. (1996). *Nursing diagnosis: Application in the school setting*. Scarborough, ME: National Association of School Nurses.

Indiana Resource Center for Autism. (n.d.). *Characteristics of the person with autism*. Bloomington, IN: Indiana University.

Johnson, M., Bulechek, G., Dochterman, J. M., Maas, M., & Moorhead, S. (2001). *Nursing diagnosis, outcomes and interventions*. St. Louis, MO: Mosby.

Kline, F. M., Silver, L. B., & Russell, S. C. (2001). *The educator's guide to medical issues in the classroom*. Baltimore: Paul H. Brooks.

Neuwirth, S. (1997). *Autism*. National Institute of Mental Health, Publication 97-4023. Retrieved September 13, 2003 from http://www.nimh.nih.gov/publicat/autism.cfm

Volkmar, F. R., Klin, A., Siegel, B., Szatmari, P., Lord, C., Campbell, M., et al. (1994). Field trial for autistic disorder in DSM-IV. *American Journal of Psychiatry*, *151*(9), 1361–1367. Retrieved September 21, 2003, from http://info.med.yale.edu/chldstdy/autism/cdd.html

Autism Spectrum Disorders (Pervasive Developmental Disorders)

# Resources

Asperger Syndrome Support
    Newsletter
Mark Bebbengton, Editor
National Autistic Society
276 Willesden Lane
London, England NW2 5RB

Autism Research Institute
4182 Adams Avenue
San Diego, CA 92116
619-281-/165
619-563-6840 (fax)
http://www.autismresearchinsti-
    tute.com

Autism Society of America
7910 Woodmont Avenue
Suite 650
Bethesda, MD 20814-3067
301-657-0881
1-800-3-AUTISM
http://www.autism-society.org

Center for the Study of Autism
3904 Southeast Clinton Street
Portland, OR 97202
(Auditory training research)

Centers for Disease Control and
    Prevention
1600 Clifton Rd,
Atlanta, GA 30333
1-800-CDC-INFO immunization
    information hotline
http://www.cdc.gov/nip/vacsafe/co
    ncerns/autism/

Council for Exceptional Children
11920 Association Drive
Reston, VA 20191-1589
703-620-3660
1-800-641-7824

Cure Autism Now
5455 Wilshire Boulevard, #715
Los Angeles, CA 90036
323-549-0500

Division TEACCH
(Treatment and Education of
    Autistic and Related
    Communication Handicapped
    Children)
Campus Box 7180
310 Medical School Wing E
University of North Carolina at
    Chapel Hill
Chapel Hill, NC 27599-7180
919-966-2173

Illinois Society for Autistic Citizens
2200 South Main Street
Suite 317
Lombard, IL 60148

Indiana Resource Center for
    Autism
Institute for the Study of
    Developmental Disabilities
Indiana University
2853 East Tenth Street
Bloomington, IN 47408-2601
812-855-6508

International Rett Syndrome
    Association
9121 Piscataway Road
Suite 2B
Clinton, MD 20735
301-856-3334
1-800-818-7388
http://www.rettsyndrome.org

National Alliance for Autism
    Research
414 Wall Street, Research Park
Princeton, NJ 08540
609-430-9160
1-888-777-622
http://www.naar.org

National Information Center for
    Children and Youth With
    Disabilities
PO Box 1492
Washington, DC 20013-1492
1-800-695-0285
http://www.nichcy.org

National Institute of Neurological
    Disorders and Stroke
PO Box 5801
Bethesda, MD 20824
301-496-5751
1-800-352-9424
http://www.ninds.nih.gov

PDD/Asperger Syndrome Support
    Group
49 Ascolese Road
Trumbull, CT 06611-2330
kkr74a@prodigy.com

Progress ACCESS
Southwest Missouri State
    University
901 South National Avenue
Springfield, MO 65804
417-836-6755
(Has large lending library)

Temple Grandin, PhD
2915 Silver Plume Drive, #C3
Fort Collins, CO 80526
(Autistic adult)

University of California at Los
    Angeles
Department of Psychology
1282A Franz Hall
PO Box 951563
Los Angeles, CA 90095-1563
310-825 2319

## Chapter Twenty-five

# Bipolar Disorder

Cheryl R. Brubaker

## Introduction

Extreme shifts in mood, energy, and functioning characterize bipolar disorder, also known as manic-depressive illness (National Institute of Mental Health [NIMH], 2003). Disruption in the biochemistry, structure, and/or activity of the brain results in neurobiological imbalances. This imbalance of brain systems undermines a variety of cognitive functions and intrudes on work, school, family, and social life for the individual with this disorder. Without effective treatment, those with bipolar disorder commit suicide in nearly 20% of cases (NIMH). The effects of bipolar disorder can create devastation in the lives of individuals and their families, but diagnosis can and should be a turning point for developing strategies for treatment, education, and coping (Child and Adolescent Bipolar Foundation, 2002).

Early Greek physicians described mania and melancholia observed in patients. Mania and melancholia have been observed and described through history in both adults and children. In 1952, the American Psychiatric Association published the first *Diagnostic and Statistical Manual of Mental Disorders*, which described "manic-depressive reaction." From this time, and until the mid-1990s, it was the opinion of most researchers and psychiatrists that manic-depressive illness was not possible in preadolescents (Child and Adolescent Bipolar Foundation timeline, 2002). This has proved to be a myth (Papolos & Papolos, 2003). The signs of bipolar disorder can begin to emerge very early, even in infancy.

### Pathophysiology

Evidence does suggest that bipolar disorder beginning in childhood or early adolescence may be more severe and present differently than illness with a later onset (NIMH, 2003). Children rarely fit the recognizable pattern of adult bipolar disorder (Papolos & Papolos, 2003). No one symptom identifies a child as having bipolar disorder, but if hyperactivity, irritable and shifting moods, and prolonged temper tantrums co-occur, along with a family history of mood disorders and/or alcoholism, the index of suspicion should be high (Papolos & Papolos, 2003).

Mania is defined as "a mental disorder characterized by excessive excitement" (Taber's Cyclopedic Medical Dictionary, 2001) and the diagnostic criteria for a manic episode include a "distinct period of abnormally and persistently elevated, expansive, or irritated mood" (American Psychiatric Association, 2004). During this episode of mood disturbance, at least three of the following symptoms must have persisted and been present: inflated self-esteem or grandiosity; decreased need for sleep or increased energy; pressured speech or excessive/increased talkativeness; flight of ideas or racing thoughts; distractibility; increased goal-directed activity or psychomotor agitation; excessive involvement in pleasurable activities that have a high potential for negative consequences or disregard of risk (American Psychiatric Association). Hypersexuality with inappropriate or precocious sexual behavior may be a feature as well (NIMH, 2000). Children may have particularly rapid cycling or changing of moods that last a few hours to a few days. Explosive, lengthy, and often destructive rages can occur, as well as separation anxiety; defiance of authority; bedwetting and encopresis; night terrors; strong and frequent cravings (often for carbohydrates and sweets); excessive involvement in multiple projects and activities; hypersensitivity to tactile, visual, or auditory stimuli; problems with peers; temperature dysregulation or intolerance; daredevil behaviors, delusions, and hallucinations (Papolos & Papolos, 2003; Child and Adolescent Bipolar Foundation, 2002).

Depression is characterized by a sustained period of depressed mood or loss of interest or pleasure in usually pleasurable activity and subjective feelings of sadness, emptiness, irritability, or hopelessness. Depression also may be accompanied by weight loss or gain, an increase or decrease in appetite, insomnia or hypersomnia, psychomotor agitation or retardation, fatigue or loss of energy; feelings of worthlessness or excessive or inappropriate guilt; diminished ability to think or concentrate or indecisiveness; and recurrent thoughts of death or suicide (NIMH, 2000; American Psychiatric Association, 2004). Children usually have an ongoing, continuous mood disturbance that is a mix of mania and depression. This rapid and severe cycling between moods produces chronic irritability and few clear times of wellness between episodes of illness (Child and Adolescent Bipolar Foundation, 2002).

When bipolar disorder begins before or soon after puberty, it is often characterized by a continuous, rapid-cycling, irritable, and mixed symptom state with marked changes in mood and energy that may co-occur with disruptive behavior disorders, particularly attention deficit hyperactivity disorder (ADHD) or conduct disorder, or may have features of these disorders as initial symptoms (NIMH, 2000). A child or adolescent who appears to be depressed and exhibits ADHD-like symptoms that are very severe, with excessive temper outbursts and mood changes, should be evaluated by a psychiatrist or psychologist with experience in bipolar disorder, particularly if there is a family history of the illness or alcoholism (Papolos & Papolos, 1999; NIMH). Diagnosis usually follows months or years of the child's mood instability, school difficulties, and damaged relationships with family and friends (Child and Adolescent Bipolar Foundation, 2002). It is not known how many children and adolescents are affected by bipolar disorder, but some recent studies indicate it may range from 0.6% to the same 1% prevalence as in adults (Marley, 2004). It is suspected that a significant number of children diagnosed with ADHD in the United States have early-onset bipolar disorder instead of, or along with, ADHD. Up to one third of the children and adolescents diagnosed as having depression may actually be experiencing early-onset bipolar disorder (Child and Adolescent Bipolar Foundation, 2002).

Bipolar disorder clearly has a genetic component; identical twins, for example, have about a 70 percent risk for the disorder if the sibling has bipolar disorder, but there are environmental factors. In every generation since World War II, there has been a higher incidence and an earlier age of onset of bipolar disorder and depression, with children experiencing their first episode of illness 10 years earlier than their parents' generation did (Child and Adolescent Bipolar Foundation, 2002). Diagnosis is based on the behavior of the child over time, the family history, response to medications, developmental stage, and current information. Unfortunately, there is no clinical test that can be obtained that yields a definitive result and diagnosis, but this may become possible in the future as the ability to measure neurochemicals and scan brain structures becomes more refined.

## Management

Bipolar disorder is a neurobiologic disturbance in the balance of central nervous system functions. The mainstay of treatment is the use of mood stabilizers. It is difficult to determine which medication regimen will work for any individual child, and it is often a trial-and-error process. All medications used have side effects, which means the risks and benefits of any medication must be carefully evaluated (Papolos & Papolos, 2003). The use of antidepressants and stimulants can, in many cases, worsen symptoms in a child with bipolar disorder. Because many children with bipolar disorder may be misdiagnosed with depression or attention deficit disorder, it is important to be aware of the potential impact of antidepressants or stimulants and report observations about medication response to the primary care provider.

The first mood stabilizer discovered was lithium, which was first approved by the Food and Drug Administration in 1974 as a prophylactic agent for the treatment of acute mania (Papolos & Papolos, 2003). In adults, it is considered the gold standard for treatment of bipolar or cyclic mood disorders; however, it is known to be less efficacious in those with rapid cycling and therefore may not be the best choice for children. Some children do have a good response to lithium alone or in combination with other drugs, and it has a particularly strong effect against suicidal behavior in those with bipolar disorder (Papolos & Papolos, 2003). Blood levels must be monitored on initiation of treatment and then every 4 to 6 months, which may present some difficulties for use in children. The blood draw must be timed at about 12 hours after the last dose (a trough level). Lithium comes in liquid and pill forms, and dose is determined by weight. It is important to be aware of the side effects and the signs of lithium toxicity, as well as the potential interactions with other medications or substances. Discontinuation of the drug must be done gradually over at least 15 to 30 days to prevent a sharp increase in suicide risk (Papolos & Papolos, 2003).

A variety of anticonvulsant medications have been found to have a mood-stabilizing effect and are being used and evaluated in the treatment of bipolar disorder (Papolos & Papolos, 2003). There is benefit in those who cycle rapidly. Currently, only Depakote is approved for use in bipolar adults, and the other anticonvulsants are not approved for use as mood stabilizers. The medications being used for the "off label" treatment of bipolar disorder include: Tegretol (carbamazepine), Depakote (divalproex sodium), Neurontin (gabapentin), Lamictal (lamotrigine), Topamax (topiramate), and Gabitril (tiagabine). Again, all have side effects and it is important to be aware of them, as well as the signs of toxicity and the potential interactions with other medications or substances.

Calcium channel blockers are another group of agents receiving attention as a potential mood stabilizer for some patients. This group of agents includes verapamil, Nimotop (nimodipine), and DynaCirc (isradipine). It is unlikely that children will be prescribed these agents, but it is important to know that grapefruit and grapefruit juice should not be consumed by any person taking a calcium channel blocker (Papolos & Papolos, 2003).

Antipsychotic medications can be useful in the treatment of bipolar disorder, especially when a child is experiencing heightened mania, psychotic symptoms, or uncontrolled rages and aggression. The list of antipsychotic medications is extensive. Children seem to be more sensitive to the movement disorder side effects, such as dystonic reactions, akinesia, tardive dyskinesia, and others, and may therefore need lower doses than adults (Papolos & Papolos, 2003). Important facts to be aware of are the side effects, signs of toxicity, and interaction potential with other agents.

Benzodiazepines such as Klonopin (clonazepam), Ativan (lorazepam), and Restoril (temazepam) are used to decrease arousal systems and thereby diminish anxiety, agitation, and activity and promote sleep. Catapres (clonidine) is a drug often used to treat tic disorders, ADHD, pervasive developmental disorders, and aggression but should be used very cautiously until bipolar disorder has been ruled out, because it can cause depression in children with mood disorders (Papolos & Papolos, 2003). Tenex (guanfacine), similar to clonidine, may also cause depression in children with bipolar disorder. If a child appears to be unstable or irritable and is receiving clonidine or guanfacine, the use should be evaluated. Abrupt discontinuation of either medication can result in rebound hypertension (Papolos & Papolos, 2003). Any child taking either medication requires regular blood pressure monitoring.

Other therapies and medications are being researched, and new modalities for treatment may become standards. Omega-3 fatty acids from concentrated fish oils show promise, in some studies, for stabilization of mood swings in children. It is important to know that cod liver oil is potentially toxic in large doses and omega-3 oils are nontoxic. Flaxseed oil is not equivalent and has been shown to promote hypomania in some patients (Papolos & Papolos, 2003). Light therapy shows promise and is being researched in children with bipolar disorder who have rapid cycling. Electroconvulsive therapy has been successful in children and adolescents. The child will generally have no memory of the period surrounding the treatment, so information and experiences from the days or weeks prior to the treatment may not be retained in memory, and the memory loss may persist for some months (Papolos & Papolos, 2003).

The treatment team consists of the family, the primary care providers, psychiatrists, psychologists, and therapists of the child or adolescent. An important element of management is observation for side effects, signs of toxicities, and the behaviors, moods, and responses of the child. Ongoing assessment is critical to successful management for children and adolescents with bipolar disorder. A mood cycle chart is a record of the assessment details for a child and is an invaluable tool for the provider making the diagnosis and prescribing medications or treatments, as well as the therapist conducting psychotherapy. The patient and the family can gain insights for managing the cycles by keeping a cycle chart and recording observations as well. A sample chart is given in **Figure 1**, but there are a variety of charts available, and they can be adapted to the individual needs of each child.

Academic management is critical for students with bipolar disorder. An entire team consisting of the teacher, special education teacher, school nurse, occupational therapist, physical therapist, speech and language therapist, counselor, social worker, administrator, and parent(s) may be necessary to meet the educational needs of the student. School attendance is often an issue for the student with bipolar disorder and can lead to the student falling behind academically. It is important to utilize assessments done prior to the onset of signs or symptoms of bipolar disorder to provide a good baseline measure for illness-related changes (Trudeau, 2000). It is also important to find the student's optimum learning style (e.g., auditory, visual, kinesthetic) as well as the teacher's willingness to allow flexibility in the format of work product that would best represent the student's understanding of concepts (Trudeau).

A student who has had a break in school attendance related to the onset of bipolar disorder benefits from a gradual or partial reintegration to school rather than returning with a full academic load. Predictable and consistent daily routines are ideal for recovering students (Trudeau, 2000). The student may worry about ostracism or harassment by peers, and these concerns should be addressed proactively by parents, therapists, and school staff. Instances of bullying or ridicule about psychiatric hospitalization or diagnosis should be dealt with swiftly and seriously in a manner consistent with racial or sexual harassment (Trudeau). The emergence of psychotic symptoms at school should be handled as discreetly as possible. Consider the assignment of a peer mentor. Consider allowing a recovering bipolar student to mentor younger peers. Assignment of responsibility may be important to developing self-competency.

Teachers and staff should encourage a self-help philosophy through advocating for a life-management perspective including self-challenge, self-acceptance, honesty, and especially humor. An additional strategy for success is to consider pacing academic work over, for example 1.5 academic years for each grade rather than "hoping" the student will be able to complete the work if he or she remains stable, particularly if there are frequent absences or hospitalizations (Trudeau, 2000).

Teachers should be educated about medication, because in the evaluation of work product and performance, the limitations of residual symptoms and medication side effects must be considered (poor penmanship due to hand tremor, awkward gait or rapid weight gain in physical education, dry mouth and increased fluid intake necessitating frequent bathroom trips, heightened sensitivity to light and noise are all common in students treated with psychotropic medications.) (Trudeau, 2000). Medication and treatment nonadherence difficulties often occur around school and holiday transitions. Adaptive behavior skills should be assessed as measured by tools like the Vineland Adaptive Behavior Scale to identify deficits or problems that parents and/or teachers have attributed to "motivational" factors (Trudeau).

Any prior special education plans (individualized education programs [IEPs]), student accommodation plans (504 plans), and behavior intervention plans need to be reviewed, and classroom modifications required to enhance the student's educational outcomes and success should be incorporated. 504 plans or IEPs for students should emphasize development of strengths and to follow creative projects equally with addressing any academic needs. Any special transportation needs must be addressed. Support services that may be required, such as social work services or school psychologist services, are made a part of any educational plan for the student.

The family and education staff should all have an awareness of the ramifications of bipolar disorder and any medications used and how these impact the stu-dent. The most important goal for an educator of a bipolar student is to keep the student interested in learning and feeling welcome at school (Trudeau, 2000).

**Figure 1. Sample of a mood chart.**

**DAILY MOOD CHART**

| Name:<br>Student No.<br>DATE AND HOURS OF SLEEP LAST NIGHT | CLASS PERIOD | DOWN | | | OK | UP | | | OTHER<br>0 = none<br>1 = mild<br>2 = moderate<br>3 = severe | | | Comments |
|---|---|---|---|---|---|---|---|---|---|---|---|---|
| | | Not able to work | Problem, but able to work | No problem working | No Symptoms Mood not definitely elevated or depressed | No problem working | Problem, but able to work | Not able to work | Irritability | Anxiety | Psychotic systems | |
| | Previous Evening | | | | | | | | | | | |
| | 1st period | | | | | | | | | | | |
| | 2nd period | | | | | | | | | | | |
| | 3rd period | | | | | | | | | | | |
| | 4th period | | | | | | | | | | | |
| | Lunch | | | | | | | | | | | |
| | 5th period | | | | | | | | | | | |
| | 6th period | | | | | | | | | | | |
| | Previous Evening | | | | | | | | | | | |
| | 1st period | | | | | | | | | | | |
| | 2nd period | | | | | | | | | | | |
| | 3rd period | | | | | | | | | | | |
| | 4th period | | | | | | | | | | | |
| | Lunch | | | | | | | | | | | |
| | 5th period | | | | | | | | | | | |
| | 6th period | | | | | | | | | | | |
| | Previous Evening | | | | | | | | | | | |
| | 1st period | | | | | | | | | | | |
| | 2nd period | | | | | | | | | | | |
| | 3rd period | | | | | | | | | | | |
| | 4th period | | | | | | | | | | | |
| | Lunch | | | | | | | | | | | |
| | 5th period | | | | | | | | | | | |
| | 6th period | | | | | | | | | | | |
| | Previous Evening | | | | | | | | | | | |
| | 1st period | | | | | | | | | | | |
| | 2nd period | | | | | | | | | | | |
| | 3rd period | | | | | | | | | | | |
| | 4th period | | | | | | | | | | | |
| | Lunch | | | | | | | | | | | |
| | 5th period | | | | | | | | | | | |
| | 6th period | | | | | | | | | | | |
| | Previous Evening | | | | | | | | | | | |
| | 1st period | | | | | | | | | | | |
| | 2nd period | | | | | | | | | | | |
| | 3rd period | | | | | | | | | | | |
| | 4th period | | | | | | | | | | | |
| | Lunch | | | | | | | | | | | |
| | 5th period | | | | | | | | | | | |
| | 6th period | | | | | | | | | | | |
| SATURDAY | | | | | | | | | | | | |
| SUNDAY | | | | | | | | | | | | |

Check box that indicates the predominate mood for the time/period

Bipolar Disorder

# Individualized Healthcare Plan

## Assessment

### History

- Growth and weight gain pattern
- At what age was the diagnosis made?
- Diagnosis, severity of condition, and prognosis
- Hospitalizations
- Student's past sleeping and eating patterns or cycles
- Student's past behavioral/mood patterns or cycles
- Student's past participation in development and implementation of treatment plan
- Family communication
- Family roles and responsibilities
- Family sociocultural values
- Family resources and support systems (e.g., economic, social, community, spiritual, cultural, extended family)
- Past personal and family changes, stresses, crises, losses
- Past family developmental stage
- Family coping patterns
- Previous history of affective or mood disorders
- Medications and treatment regimens
- Family history of mental health conditions, mood disorder, and/or substance abuse/chemical dependency
- History of suicide attempts, ideation, threats

### Current Status and Management

- Age and developmental level
- Student's general health status and most recent physical examination
- Recent personal and family changes, stresses, crises, losses
- Current family developmental stage
- Family education and counseling
- Current general health: sleep pattern, decreased/increased need for sleep, night terrors
- Current general health: energy level, decreased/increased energy level
- Speech pattern: pressured speech or excessive/increased talkativeness
- Flight of ideas or racing thoughts
- Distractibility
- Short-term memory: good/poor
- Activity level: increased/decreased activity
- Psychomotor agitation or retardation
- Increased risk-taking behavior or excessive involvement in pleasurable activities that have a high potential for negative consequences
- Inappropriate or precocious sexual behavior
- Explosive, lengthy, or destructive rages
- Separation anxiety
- Defiance of authority
- Enuresis and/or encopresis
- Strong and/or frequent food cravings and type (often sweets or carbohydrates)
- Hypersensitivity to tactile, visual, or auditory stimuli (e.g., rips out tags from shirts)
- Self-esteem: deflated/inflated
- Problems with peers
- Aggressive behavior
- Frustration tolerance: low
- Low threshold for anxiety and phobias
- Overreaction to stressful events (either positive events or negative)
- Temperature dysregulation or intolerance
- Delusions or hallucinations
- Loss of interest in usually pleasurable activity
- Growth pattern: weight loss/gain
- Appetite: decreased/increased
- Feelings of worthlessness or excessive/inappropriate guilt

- Diminished ability to concentrate or make decisions
- Poor judgment
- Morbid preoccupations
- Recurrent thoughts of death or suicide and/or evidence of self-injuring behavior
- Frequency of mood shifts/cycles, rapid or abrupt shifts of mood and energy
- Inconsistency in school performance/decreased school performance
- Current treatment and/or medication
- Student's communication skills
- Student's communication style in stressful and nonstressful conditions

*Self-care*
- Student's perception of health
- Student's awareness of moods/cycles
- Current perspectives and ability regarding self-management
- Student's decision-making skills and variation in decision-making ability in various settings/environments
- Student's locus of control
- Student's ability to interact productively with peers, family, school staff, and others
- Student's coping skills

*Psychosocial Status*
- Current coping strategies: effective/ineffective
- Student's general temperament and coping ability
- Student's perception of abilities and/or disabilities
- Student's communication style in stressful and nonstressful conditions
- Student's fears, anxieties
- Student's family interaction
- Parent's perception of student's condition
- Student's usual support available and resources (parents, school, community)
- Student's perceptions of peers, family, community supports
- Student's participation in activities with peers: sports, church classes (outside of the school day), support groups
- Student's participation in family activities
- Family functioning and coping ability/skills
- Family perception of stressors, current situation, and outlook for the future
- Family resources and supports (socioeconomic, extended family, friends, support groups) and availability of these support systems

*Academic Issues*
- Medications needed at school
- Support services needed at school
- Classroom modifications needed to enhance student's educational outcomes and success
- Past and current academic performance
- School attendance pattern: reasons for absences
- Special education or 504 accommodation needs
- Behavior management needs
- Transportation needs

## Nursing Diagnoses (N.D.) (NANDA, 2003)

**N.D. 1** Effective therapeutic regimen management (NANDA, 00082).
- Related to:
- Social supports
- Empowerment
- Perceived benefits
- Family pattern of healthcare
- Trust of regimen and/or healthcare personnel
- Family strengths

**N.D. 2** Ineffective therapeutic regimen management (NANDA, 00078).
- Related to:
- Perceived barriers
- Social support deficit(s)
- Powerlessness
- Perceived susceptibility
- Perceived benefits
- Mistrust of regimen and/or healthcare personnel
- Knowledge deficit
- Family pattern of healthcare
- Family conflict
- Excessive family or personal demands
- Economic difficulties
- Decisional conflicts
- Complexity of therapeutic regimen or the healthcare system
- Perceived seriousness
- Inadequate number and types of cues to action

**N.D. 3** Readiness for enhanced therapeutic regimen management (NANDA, 00162).
Related to:
- Social supports
- Empowerment
- Perceived benefits
- Family pattern of healthcare
- Trust of regimen and/or healthcare personnel
- Family strengths
- Perceived barriers
- Social support deficit(s)
- Perceived susceptibility
- Knowledge deficit
- Decisional conflicts
- Complexity of therapeutic regimen or the healthcare system

**N.D. 4** Disturbed sleep pattern (NANDA, 00095).
Related to:
- Racing thoughts
- Circadian asynchrony
- Depression
- Daylight/darkness exposure
- Excessive stimulation
- Separation anxiety

**N.D. 5** Sleep deprivation (NANDA, 00096).
Related to:
- Circadian asynchrony
- Sustained excessive stimulation
- CNS hypersomnolence
- Sleep terror/night terrors

**N.D. 6** Disturbed sensory perception (specify: visual, auditory, kinesthetic, gustatory, tactile, olfactory) (NANDA, 00122).
Related to:
- Altered sensory perception
- Psychological stress
- Altered sensory reception, transmission, and/or integration
- Biochemical imbalances for sensory distortion (e.g., illusions, hallucinations)
- Biochemical imbalance

**N.D. 7** Deficient knowledge (specify) (NANDA, 00126).
Related to:
- Lack of exposure
- Lack of recall
- Information misinterpretation

- Cognitive limitation
- Lack of interest in learning
- Unfamiliarity with information resources

**N.D. 8** Readiness for enhanced knowledge (specify) (NANDA, 00161).
Related to:
- Participation in health management plan
- Anxiety management
- Depression management

**N.D. 9** Disturbed thought processes (NANDA, 00130).
Related to:
- Disturbance in the balance of brain systems that subserve various cognitive functions

**N.D. 10** Powerlessness (NANDA, 00125).
Related to:
- Healthcare environment
- School environment
- Interpersonal interaction
- Lifestyle of helplessness

**N.D. 11** Ineffective role performance (student) (NANDA, 00055).
Related to:
- School/class demands
- Peer or teacher conflicts
- Absences from school

**N.D. 12** Impaired social interaction (NANDA, 00052).
Related to:
- Knowledge/skill deficit about ways to enhance mutuality
- Sociocultural dissonance
- Communication barriers
- Altered thought processes
- Self-concept disturbance

**N.D. 13** Ineffective sexuality patterns (NANDA, 00065).
Related to:
- Variant sexual preferences
- Altered thought processes
- Biochemical imbalances of brain systems
- Self-concept disturbance

**N.D. 14** Ineffective coping (NANDA, 00069).
Related to:
- Inadequate level of perception of control
- Inadequate resources
- Maturational crisis
- Disturbance in pattern of tension release
- Inability to conserve adaptive energies
- Disturbance in pattern of appraisal of threat
- Altered thought processes
- Biochemical imbalances of brain systems

**N.D. 15** Readiness for enhanced coping (NANDA, 00158).
Related to:
- Effective management of symptoms
- Participation in activities with peers
- Social involvement
- Support system available

**N.D. 16** Risk for self-directed violence (NANDA, 00140).
Related to:
- Depressed mood
- Anxious mood
- Poor impulse control
- Uncontrolled anger

**N.D. 17** Risk for suicide (NANDA, 00150). Poor support systems

Related to:

- Feelings of loneliness
- Feelings of hopelessness
- Feelings of helplessness
- Social isolation
- Legal or disciplinary problems
- Cluster suicides

**N.D. 18** Social isolation (NANDA, 00053).

Related to:

- Alterations in mental status
- Inability to engage in satisfying personal relationships
- Unaccepted social values
- Inappropriate or unaccepted social behavior
- Inadequate personal resources
- Immature interests
- Factors contributing to the absence of satisfying personal relationships (e.g., delay in accomplishing developmental tasks)

## Goals

The student will effectively communicate feelings to appropriate others (e.g., counselor, school nurse, teacher, parents). (N.D. 2, 3, 10, 12, 14–18)

The student will use positive, effective coping mechanisms to decrease stresses. (N.D. 2, 3, 10, 11, 14–18)

The student will develop and/or enhance an internal locus of control. (N.D. 1–3, 10, 11, 13–15, 17, 18)

The student will participate in managing his/her healthcare. (N.D. 1–3, 7, 8, 10–15)

The student will develop and maintain meaningful social interactions with peers. (N.D. 10, 12, 18)

The student will participate in classroom and other school activities, with modifications as necessary. (N.D. 7, 10, 11, 18)

The student will participate in activities with peers. (N.D. 11, 12, 18)

The student will increase awareness of self and his/her abilities. (N.D. 1–3, 7, 8, 10–15, 18)

The student will maintain appropriate behavior in the school setting. (N.D. 9, 11, 13)

The student will [increase, attain, maintain, progress toward] an age-normal sleep pattern. (N.D. 4, 5)

The student will appropriately advocate for self and self-care. (N.D. 1-5, 9–11, 14, 15)

The student will increase ability to concentrate and complete academic tasks in the classroom setting. (N.D. 5, 6, 9)

The student will seek help or assistance from others and accept assistance from others. (N.D. 1–5, 10, 14-18)

The student will maintain a consistent and regular school attendance pattern. (N.D. 1-3, 5, 9, 11, 12, 14, 18)

The student will demonstrate academic progress and success consistently and regularly. (N.D. 1–6, 9–11, 14, 15, 18)

The student will follow up with primary care provider and/or specialists and therapists as needed, with assistance from family. (N.D. 2–7, 9, 10, 13, 14, 16–18)

## Nursing Interventions

Establish a relationship with the student, which conveys sincere interest, acceptance, caring, positive attitudes, and support. (N.D. 2, 6, 7, 9-14, 16–18)

Encourage school personnel to utilize active listening to encourage communication and convey an understanding attitude to the student. (N.D. 2, 6, 7, 9, 10–14, 16–18)

Maximize student and family participation in decisions regarding the support and structure provided in the school environment. (N.D. 1–6, 9–18)

Assist the family to identify resources and assistance they are willing to accept in the management of bipolar disorder. (N.D. 2–18)

Assist the family to identify resources and assistance they are willing to accept in the management of suicidal ideation and/or behavior. (N.D. 16, 17)

Establish support networks within the school for student. (N.D. 2, 6, 7, 9–14, 16–18)

Assist in establishing/utilizing school crisis team to respond to students in distress or in an emergency situation. (N.D. 6, 9-4, 16–18)

Assist in establishing multidisciplinary prevention/education strategies for school-wide implementation. (N.D. 2, 6, 9–14, 16–18)

Assist the student to identify options and strategies for responding to mood swings or behavior impulses. (N.D. 1–18)

Assist student and parent to identify and remove barriers to sleeping at night. (N.D. 4, 5)

Assist student to identify effective coping strategies that increase his/her ability to sleep at night. (N.D. 4, 5)

Assist student to identify effective coping strategies that increase his/her ability to stay awake and work during the school day. (N.D. 4, 5)

Assist the student to implement options/strategies for responding to swings in mood or behavior impulses. (N.D. 1–3, 6–18)

Facilitate student exploration and awareness of self. (N.D. 1–3, 6–18)

Assist the student to articulate perception of self and health status. (N.D. 1–3, 9–18)

Assist the student to articulate perception of the impact of bipolar disorder on self and family. (N.D. 1–18)

Encourage the student to express feelings, views, concerns, and self-perceptions to appropriate support persons. (N.D. 2, 6, 9–18)

Encourage the student to ask questions regarding health, health planning and management, and prognosis. (N.D. 2, 6, 7, 9–18)

If medication is part of the student's current mental health management plan, encourage and assist parent to keep a constant supply of medication available for the student. (N.D. 1–18)

Encourage parent to reorder when there is one week of medication left to avoid running out. (N.D. 1–18)

If medication is given at school, call parent to reorder medication when there is one-week supply left. (N.D. 1–17)

Assist parent to get medication authorization completed if medication will need to be given at school. (N.D. 1–5, 8, 9, 13–17)

Monitor for medication side effects at school. (N.D. 1–18)

Facilitate communication between the student, family, school multidisciplinary team, and community providers. (N.D. 1–18)

Assist the student to explore activities with peers that are enjoyable and appropriate. (N.D. 10–13, 18)

Assist the student, family, teachers, and providers to understand the importance of social interactions with peers by discussing: school guidelines for attendance; modifications needed in the classroom; daily and weekly schedules; environmental considerations; extracurricular activities; home interactions with neighbors, family and extended family; indoor and outdoor play; community activities and organizations. (N.D. 3, 10–13, 18)

Assist the student to develop social skills in individual and/or group learning situations. (N.D. 10–13, 18)

Assist the student to explore and articulate ways that he/she is alike or different from peers and ways to remove any barriers to interacting with peers. (N.D. 10–13, 18)

Assist the student to explore ways the student can interact with peers at school, home, and in the community. (N.D. 10–13, 18)

Assist teachers and family to implement school/classroom modifications that will enhance student success. (N.D. 1–12, 14, 15, 18)

Arrange for staff education/in-service on the classroom management of behaviors that are disruptive to the learning environment as needed. (N.D. 4–6, 9–18)

Assist the student to identify strengths and weaknesses. (N.D. 1–3, 10–15)

Assist the student to identify ways to utilize strengths to compensate for weaknesses. (N.D. 1–3, 10–18)

Assist the student to identify and remove barriers to learning and to effective coping. (N.D. 2–15)

Assist the student to identify signs or evidence of effective coping, effective problem solving, such as assignments completed, done well, and handed in on time; being "in control" of school responsibilities; participation in activities (school, athletic, church, community, with peers). (N.D. 10, 11, 14, 15)

Assist the student to identify signs or evidence of ineffective coping: inability to problem solve; anxiety; destructive behavior; inability to complete school assignments or similar role expectations; feeling overwhelmed; decreased social contact or participation. (N.D. 2–18)

Assist the student to identify coping behaviors that have been productive and helpful in the past. (N.D. 1–18)

Assist the student to identify positive and effective coping behaviors: seeking information; identifying cause(s) of feelings of anxiety/stress; setting realistic, short-term, achievable goals; exploring and learning new methods to create calm, positive feelings (relaxation techniques, reducing environmental stimuli); asking for assistance if needed. (N.D. 1–17)

Facilitate the development of a plan/contract in which the student can identify and utilize previously agreed-on strategies or a "menu of reasonable choices" for management of anticipated problems. (N.D. 2–18)

Encourage revising the collaborative plan/contract as needed to get improved results. (N.D. 2–6, 9–18)

Assist staff to identify, with the student, the "costs" associated with the reasonable options and choices versus the "costs" associated with inappropriate choices. (N.D. 1–3, 9–15)

Assist the student to identify circumstances when it might be important to ask for assistance from others. (N.D. 1–5, 10–18)

Encourage the student to accept assistance from others when needed and provide positive reinforcement when the student is able to ask for and/or accept assistance. (N.D. 1–18)

Explore dimensions of potential problems, examine possible solutions, and assist the student in taking concrete action. (N.D. 1–18)

Provide health education opportunities either individually or in groups that address problem-solving techniques, stress-reducing activities, decision-making skills. (N.D. 1–3, 7, 8, 10, 14–18)

Provide opportunities for the student to make decisions and participate in self-care. (N.D. 1–5, 10, 11, 14, 15)

Provide positive reinforcement to the student when appropriate, positive, and constructive coping methods have been utilized. (N.D. 1–18)

Provide positive reinforcement to the student when he/she makes appropriate decisions and participates in self-care. (N.D. 1–3, 10, 11, 13, 14, 16)

Assist the student to identify ways to feel empowered. (N.D. 10, 11, 13–18)

Assist the student to identify things that are within his/her ability to control and things that are not within his/her ability to control. (N.D. 2, 3, 10–18)

Assist the student to select aspects of concern that he/she can do something about and create a manageable perspective on it. (N.D. 2, 3, 10, 14–18)

Assist the student to explore possible solutions to concerns and/or gain comfort with a process to handle the concern. (N.D. 2, 3, 10, 14–18)

Assist staff to model effective communication with the student. (N.D. 1–3, 7-11, 18)

Assist student to identify family, friends, and professionals who are in a position to provide a positive influence on the student and assist to form a psychological support system that may buffer the student from stress or emotional overarousal. (N.D. 1–3, 5, 9–18)

Utilize a student-rated self-report daily mood chart to facilitate efficient and rapid assessment of depressed, elevated, irritable, or anxious moods, as well as their duration and severity when needed. Report this information to the provider/physician and family as needed and requested. (N.D. 2–18)

Explain all school and healthcare procedures, rules, and options to the student and family as requested or indicated. (N.D. 1–3, 6, 9, 11)

Encourage and allow time for the student and family to ask questions. (N.D. 1–18)

Assist the student and family to identify and clarify roles and responsibilities within the school, the family, and the community. (N.D. 1–18)

Assist the student and family to formulate a plan(s) that would reduce stress or enhance coping with stress. (N.D. 2–5, 10, 14–17)

Assist school personnel to keep the student, family, and providers (with release of information from parents) informed about the student's health and academic status. (N.D. 1–5, 11, 12, 14–18)

Identify and remove as many barriers to self-care as possible. (N.D. 1–3, 7, 8, 10, 11, 14, 15)

Provide school staff with ongoing in-service and resources on symptoms and management of bipolar disorder as requested/needed. (N.D. 5–18)

Assist the student and family in obtaining ongoing counseling in collaboration with the medical management provider(s). (N.D. 1–18)

Establish a medication protocol as prescribed by the healthcare provider/physician, as needed in the school setting. (N.D. 1–18)

In the case of any suicide risk or attempt, assess injuries and institute appropriate emergency care and activation of emergency medical services. (N.D. 16, 17)

In the case of any suicide risk or attempt, stay with the student until in the direct care of the parents and/or other healthcare personnel. (N.D. 16, 17)

Assist the school multidisciplinary team (nurse, counselor, social worker, teachers, administrators, etc.) to develop a system of supports for the student that will allow for a "safe" place to ventilate feelings and "decompress" when needed to prevent acting out or outbursts. (N.D. 2, 5, 6, 8–18)

Collaboration with the school crisis team as needed. (N.D. 16, 17)

Assist the family and student in accessing follow-up care for the student as indicated. (N.D. 2–6, 9–18)

# Expected Student Outcomes

The student will:

- Describe self-perceptions and current health status realistically. (N.D. 1–18)
- Communicate feelings and concerns to appropriate others (e.g., teachers, parents, school counselor, physician, school nurse). (N.D. 2, 6, 9–18)
- List signs of effective coping and decision making. (N.D. 4–18)
- Demonstrate effective coping strategies. (N.D. 14, 15)
- List signs of ineffective coping and the need for adjustment/changes in responses. (N.D. 2, 4–6, 9–18)
- Identify current sources of stress and those sources that can be changed. (N.D. 2–18)
- Identify sources of stress that cannot be changed and ways to enhance coping with these stresses. (N.D. 2–18)
- Report a lessening of the intensity of the emotional distress experienced. (N.D. 2, 4–6, 8–18)
- Demonstrate an age-appropriate sleep pattern (as reported by parent). (N.D. 4, 5)
- Demonstrate less fatigue and drowsiness during the school day. (N.D. 4, 5)
- Demonstrate increased concentration and less distractibility in the classroom (as reported by teachers). (N.D. 5, 6, 9)
- Demonstrate implementation of an effective coping strategy that increases his/her ability to sleep at night (as reported by student and parent). (N.D. 4, 5)
- Demonstrate implementation of an effective coping strategy that increases his/her ability to stay awake during the school day. (N.D. 4, 5)
- Identify aspects in his/her life that he/she has some control over. (N.D. 10)
- Obtain additional community counseling with assistance from his/her family as needed. (N.D. 2–6, 8–18)
- Identify individuals who are appropriate resources and support (at school, at home, and in the community). (N.D. 1–18)
- Seek out appropriate support persons during times of stress or crisis as needed. (N.D. 9–18)
- Demonstrate appropriate decision making. (N.D. 1–5, 9–18)
- Participate in self-care. (N.D. 1–5, 9–11, 14–16)
  - List activities that are appropriate and enjoyable that can be shared with peers. (N.D. 10–13)
  - Name his/her friends. (N.D. 12, 18)
  - Identify his/her barriers to social contact and ways to decrease barriers. (N.D. 12, 13, 18)
  - List ways he/she may effectively interact with peers. (N.D. 12, 13, 18)
  - Demonstrate effective interaction with peers (in class, in hallways, in activities, etc.) (N.D. 12, 13, 18)
  - Participate in activities with peers at school, at home, and in the community. (N.D. 12, 13, 18)
  - Identify strengths and weaknesses. (N.D. 1–3, 7, 8, 10–12, 14–18)
  - Demonstrate use of his/her strengths (identify specific strengths) to compensate for weaknesses. (N.D. 1–3, 7, 8, 10–12, 14–18)
  - Define the menu of reasonable choices to utilize in a variety of specific situations or circumstances. (N.D. 1–18)
  - Demonstrate ability to act on these appropriate choices. (N.D. 1–18)
  - Demonstrate avoidance of negative interactions with others. (N.D. 9–15)
  - Demonstrate [a decrease in, no] aggressive acting-out of anger feelings. (N.D. 9–18)
  - Utilize constructive methods to cope with feelings of anger. N.D. 1–3, 6–17)
  - Demonstrate positive, effective interactions (staff, peers, and family members). (N.D. 1–18)
  - Describe circumstances when he/she might need assistance from others. (N.D. 1–3, 10–15, 18)
- Ask for assistance appropriately when needed. (N.D. 1–5, 10–12, 14–18)
- Accept assistance from others, as needed. (N.D. 1–5, 10, 11, 14–18)
- Attend school regularly (less than ___ days absent per year). (N.D. 1–15, 18)
- Participate in regular classroom activities, with modification as necessary. (N.D. 1–5, 8–15, 18)
- Follow medication plan at home and school. (N.D. 1–5, 8, 9, 11, 13–15, 16, 17)
- Not attempt suicide. (N.D. 16, 17)
- Report that he/she feels (heard, understood, accepted, supported). (N.D. 1–3, 6, 9, 10, 12, 14–18)

Bipolar Disorder

# Case Study

Barry is a 14-year-old high school student who was diagnosed as having bipolar disorder 3 years ago. Barry is personable and is able to show good attention and focus for short periods of time. He is a gifted student but has repeated difficulties with peer and adult interactions escalating to a crisis. He experiences auditory and visual hallucinations and cycles abruptly and rapidly over a few hours rather than days, weeks, or months. Barry can, at times, experience a very low frustration tolerance that can lead to explosive rages. He often experiences anxiety and overreacts to changes/stressful events. He demonstrates poor impulse regulation and can be aggressive with others. When he is experiencing mania, he will ditch class. Barry will, at times, go 2 to 4 days without sleep, resulting in decreased stress tolerance and frustration tolerance and an increased tendency to make poor choices and demonstrate poor judgment. Barry experiences racing thoughts during manic cycles, and pressured speech is evident at these times, as well as ego inflation and invincibility. During these times, he feels his understanding is superior to that of his classmates and that he has no need to complete work assignments. He can be disrespectful to adults, oppositional, and provoking to his peers.

During depressive cycles, Barry feels listless and hopeless and verbalizes feelings of worthlessness, but he has never had concrete suicidal/homicidal ideation or plans. Barry does dwell on thoughts of death and graphic gore often, which are expressed in his writing and drawing. He often displays psychomotor agitation and distractibility in the classroom. Barry has difficulty with short-term memory, and this impacts his academic performance. He has difficulty expressing his feelings and frustrations but has demonstrated some improvement by removing himself appropriately from frustrating situations and seeking the "safe" zone of the school health room.

Barry has been taking Depakote, 30 mg every morning, after school, and bedtime, and Risperdal, 1 mg every morning and every evening, so he does not take medication at school. He is compliant about taking his medications, and he has the desire to do what it takes to manage his disorder. His family is a cohesive, supportive unit that is committed to providing the services Barry needs to manage his disorder and to succeed. Barry has been experiencing increasing difficulty with the transition to high school, and a team decision has been made to place Barry in the health room as an aide during fourth period. This is to provide the school nurse and Barry an opportunity to document the pattern of Barry's mood cycles daily and establish some plans for constructively managing the rapid cycling.

# Bipolar Disorder

| Assessment Data | Nursing Diagnosis | Goals | Nursing Interventions | Expected Outcomes |
|---|---|---|---|---|
| Barry experiences low frustration tolerance, low threshold for anxiety, and phobias at times. Barry may experience excessive lethargy or activity in cycles through the school day. | Disturbed thought processes. The student has disruptions in cognitive operations and activites related to: disturbance in the balance of brain systems. | Barry will attend school consistently and regularly. Barry will increase his ability to concentrate and complete academic tasks in the classroom. | Establish a relationship with Barry, which conveys sincere interest, acceptance, caring, positive attitudes and support. School personnel should utilize active listening to encourage communication and convey an understanding attitude to Barry. Assist Barry, family, teachers, and providers to understand the social interactions with peers by discussing: school guidelines for attendance; modifications needed in the classroom; daily and weekly schedules; environmental considerations; extracurricular activities; home interactions with neighbors, family and extended family; indoor and outdoor play; community activities and organizations. | Barry will describe self-perceptions and current health status realistically. Barry will communicate feelings and concerns to appropriate others. Barry experiences a lessening of the intensity of emotional distress. Barry attends school regularly, fewer than four days absent per semester, and does not ditch class. Barry participates in regular classroom activities, with modification as necessary. Barry demonstrates an increase in his ability to concentrate and focus his attention on academic tasks in the classroom, to 75% of the time. Barry demonstrates an increase in completing academic tasks in the classroom setting, to 75% of the time. |

*Chapter Twenty-five: Bipolar Disorder*

| Assessment Data | Nursing Diagnosis | Goals | Nursing Interventions | Expected Outcomes |
|---|---|---|---|---|
| Barry often experiences over-reaction to stressful events (either positive or negative events) at times. Barry experiences rapid, abrupt shifts of mood and energy. | | Barry will demonstrate academic progress and success consistently and regularly. | Maximize student and parent participation in decisions regarding the support and structure provided in the school environment.<br><br>Identify resources and assistance the student and parent are willing to accept in the management of bipolar disorder.<br><br>Encourage teachers to give Barry frequent reinforcement for positive, appropriate behavior and for academic accomplishments.<br><br>Identify, with Barry and teachers, effective strategies for dealing with feelings of being stressed, and assist Barry to implement them as needed. | Barry will identify individuals who are appropriate resources and support at school, at home and in the community.<br><br>Barry asks for assistance appropriately when needed. Barry accepts assistance from others as needed. |
| Barry demonstrates poor impulse regulation with resultant aggressive impulses, rage attacks, and increased participation in risky behaviors. | | Barry will increase awareness of self and abilities.<br><br>Barry will maintain appropriate (non-violent) behavior in school. | Assist Barry to identify positive and effective coping behaviors: seeking information; identifying cause(s) of feelings of anxiety/stress; setting realistic, short-term, achievable goals; exploring and learning new methods to create calm, positive feelings (relaxation techniques, reducing environmental stimuli); asking for assistance f needed. | Barry will list signs of effective coping and decision making.<br><br>Barry will list signs of ineffective coping and the need for adjustment/changes in responses.<br><br>Barry will demonstrate effective coping strategies in the classroom and school setting.<br><br>Barry will identify current sources of stress and those sources that can be changed. |

| Assessment Data | Nursing Diagnosis | Goals | Nursing Interventions | Expected Outcomes |
|---|---|---|---|---|
| | | | Assist Barry to identify things that are within his ability to control and things that are not within his ability to control.<br><br>Help Barry select aspects of concern that he can do something about and create a manageable perspective on it.<br><br>Help Barry to explore possible solutions to concerns and/or gain comfort with a process to handle the concern. | Barry will identify sources of stress that cannot be changed and ways to enhance coping with these stresses.<br><br>Barry will demonstrate appropriate (non-violent) behavior in school, 90% of the time. |
| Barry experiences racing thoughts and flights of ideas, talkativeness, and having diminished interest and loss of pleasure doing previously enjoyable activities. | | Barry will participate in classroom and other school activities, with modifications as necessary. | Facilitate the development of a plan/contract in which Barry can identify and utilized pre-agreed upon strategies or a "menu of reasonable choices" for management of anticipated problems.<br><br>Assist staff to identify with Barry the "costs" associated with the reasonable options and choices versus the "costs" associated with inappropriate choices. | Barry will list what the menu of reasonable choices is to respond to a variety of situations or circumstances.<br><br>Barry will demonstrate choosing an effective problem-solving strategy, implementing the strategy, and effectively resolving the problem, 75% of the time. |
| Barry at times will go 2 to 4 days without sleep, resulting in poor judgement/decision making, poor concentration and poor short-term memory. | | Barry will develop and enhance his internal locus of control. | Encourage revising the collaborative plan/contract as needed to get improved results.<br><br>Encourage Barry to process information and make choices from the "menu of reasonable choices" that will enhance student success. | Barry will implement appropriate behavioral choices. |

| Assessment Data | Nursing Diagnosis | Goals | Nursing Interventions | Expected Outcomes |
|---|---|---|---|---|
| | | | Provide assistance, if needed, for Barry to implement an appropriate choice that enhances positive behavior and academic success. | |
| Barry often displays psychomotor agitation and distractibility. | | | Explore dimensions of potential problems, examine possible solutions, and assist Barry in taking concrete action. | Barry will not demonstrate aggressive acting out of anger feelings. |
| | | | Provide health education opportunities, either individually or in groups, that address problem-solving techniques, stress-reducing activities, decision-making skills. | Barry will utilize constructive, positive methods to cope with feelings of anger. |
| | | | | Barry will demonstrate positive, effective interactions with staff, peers and family. |
| | | | Provide opportunities for Barry to make decisions and participate in self-care. | Barry will not demonstrate negative interactions with peers and school staff. |
| | | | Provide positive reinforcement to Barry when appropriate, positive, and constructive coping methods have been utilized. | Barry, with assistance from his parents, will follow through with and actively participate in his mental health treatment plan, including medications, counseling appointments and re-evaluation appointments. |
| | | | Provide positive reinforcement to Barry when he makes appropriate decisions and participates in self-care. | |

**Bipolar Disorder**

| Assessment Data | Nursing Diagnosis | Goals | Nursing Interventions | Expected Outcomes |
|---|---|---|---|---|
| | | | Utilize a student-rated self-report daily mood chart to facilitate efficient and rapid assessment of depressed, elevated, irritable or anxious moods as well as their duration and severity when needed. Report this information to the provider/physician and family as needed and requested.<br><br>Assist Barry and his parents to follow through with maintenance of his mental health treatment plan, including counseling appointments, maintenance of medication supply, and re-evaluation appointments. | |
| Barry has a tendency towards sleep/wake reversals and cycling through periods of needing less sleep or having difficulty sleeping and periods of needing more sleep.<br><br>Barry, at times, will go 2 to 4 days without sleep. | Disturbed sleep pattern related to: racing thoughts, circadian asynchrony, depression, daylight/ darkness exposure. | Barry will use positive, effective coping mechanisms to decrease stresses.<br><br>Barry will increase progress toward an age-normal sleeping pattern.<br><br>Barry will participate in classroom and other school activities, with modifications as necessary if fatigue or problems staying awake occur during the school day. | Assist Barry to identify and remove barriers to rest and sleep.<br><br>Assist Barry to identify signs or evidence of effective coping with sleep/resting problems.<br><br>Assist Barry to identify signs or evidence of ineffective coping: inability to problem solve; anxiety; destructive behavior; inability to complete school assignments or similar role expectations; feeling overwhelmed; decreased social contact or participation. | Barry will list signs of effective coping and decision making regarding his sleeping problems.<br><br>Barry will list signs of ineffective coping and the need for adjustment/changes in responses.<br><br>Barry will demonstrate implementation of an effective coping strategy that increases his ability to sleep at night, as reported by parent and Barry. |

| Assessment Data | Nursing Diagnosis | Goals | Nursing Interventions | Expected Outcomes |
|---|---|---|---|---|
| | | | | Barry will demonstrate implementation of an effective coping strategy that increases his ability to decrease fatigue and stay awake during the school day. |
| | | | | Barry will decrease the number of nights he goes without sleep, as reported by Barry and his parents. |
| | | | | Barry will decrease the number of days he experiences fatigue and sleepiness at school. |
| | | Barry will be able to appropriately advocate for self and self-care regarding sleep problems or inability to sleep at night or stay awake during school. | Assist Barry to identify coping behaviors that have been productive and helpful in the past. | Barry will identify current sources of stress and those sources that can be changed. |
| | | | Assist Barry to identify positive and effective coping behaviors: seeking information; identifying cause(s) of feelings of anxiety/stress; setting realistic, short-term, achievable goals; exploring and learning new methods to create calm, positive feelings (relaxation techniques, reducing environmental stimuli); asking for assistance if needed. | Barry will identify sources of stress that cannot be changed and ways to enhance coping with these stresses. |
| Barry experiences racing thoughts and flights of ideas, talkativeness, and having diminished interest and loss of pleasure doing previously enjoyable activities. | | | Assist Barry to implement effective coping strategies that assist him with appropriate self care, especially regarding attaining and maintaining an appropriate sleep pattern. | Barry will report he feels there are options and that he has some control over his response to stressful situations. |

# References

American Psychiatric Association (2004). *Practice guideline for the treatment of patients with bipolar disorder (revised)*. Retrieved April 27, 2004, from http://www.psych.org/psych_ pract/treatg/pg/bipolar_revise-book_4.cfm

Arnold, M., & Silkworth, C. (1999). *The school nurse's source book of individualized healthcare plans: Issues and applications in school nursing practice* (Vol. II). North Branch, MN: Sunrise River Press.

Child and Adolescent Bipolar Foundation. (2002). *About early-onset bipolar disorder (timeline)*. Retrieved August 28, 2003, from http://www.bpkids.org/learning/about_historical.htm

Child and Adolescent Bipolar Foundation. (2002). *About early-onset bipolar disorder*. Retrieved April 26, 2004, from http://www.bpkids.org/printing/about.htm

National Institute of Mental Health (2000). *Child and adolescent bipolar disorder: An update from the National Institute of Mental Health*. Retrieved April 27, 2004, from http://www.nimh.nih.gov/publicat/bipolarupdate.cfm

National Institute of Mental Health (2003). *Bipolar disorder research at the National Institute of Mental Health*. Retrieved August 28, 2003, from http://www.nimh.nih.gov/publicat/ bipolarresfact.cfm

Marley, M. (2004, April). *Bipolar disorder in children and adolescents*. Paper presented at the meeting of the University of New Mexico, School Based Health Clinics, Albuquerque.

NANDA International (2003). *Nursing diagnoses: Definitions & classification*. Philadelphia: Author.

Papolos, D. & Papolos J. (2003). *The bipolar child: The definitive guide to childhood's most misunderstood disorder*. New York: Broadway Books.

*Taber's Cyclopedic Medical Dictionary* (19th ed.). (2001). Philadelphia: Davis.

Trudeau, T. (2000). *Educator's guide to receiving bipolar students after hospitalization*. Retrieved April 26, 2004, from http://www.bpkids.org/printing/015.htm

# Bibliography

Bergren, M.D. (2002). Child and adolescent mental health Web resources. *Journal of School Nursing, 18*(4) 226–228.

Denehy, J. (2002). The mental health needs of children and adolescents. *Journal of School Nursing, 18*(4), 189–190.

DeSocio, J., Hootman, J. (2004). Children' mental health and school success. *Journal of School Nursing, 20*(4), 189–196.

Frame, K. (2004). *Depression in school-age youth: The role of the school nurse* [Manual]. Scarborough, ME: National Association of School Nurses.

Hootman, J., Houck, G.M., King, M.C. (2002). A program to educate school nurses about mental health interventions. *Journal of School Nursing, 18*(4), 191–195.

National Association of School Nurses. (n.d.). *Addressing the mental health needs of children and adolescence* [Education Program]. Retrieved November 7, 2004, from http://nasn.org/education/education.htm

National Association of School Nurses. (2000). *Issue Brief: Mental health and illness*. Scarborough, ME: Author.

National Association of School Nurses. (Revised 2000). *Position Statement: Mental health of students*. Scarborough, ME: Author.

*Psychosocial screening* (Home Study Module Number 3). Scarborough, ME: National Association of School Nurses.

Bipolar Disorder

## Resources

Bristol-Meyers Squibb Company
345 Park Avenue
New York, NY 10154-0037
212-546-4000
Sponsors Web site "About Bipolar
    Disorder" located at:
    http://bipolar.about.com/
"About Bipolar Disorder" has a
    wide variety of support
    resources available and a dedi-
    cated crew of volunteers who
    share their time and energy on
    forums and in chat rooms.
    Meet the guides and volunteers,
    keep yourself informed about
    issues, updates, and changes at
    the site, and explore the
    resources.

American Academy of Child and
    Adolescent Psychiatry
3615 Wisconsin Avenue, NW
Washington, DC 20016-3007
202-966-7300
www.aacap.org

Child and Adolescent Bipolar
    Foundation (CABF)
1000 Skokie Boulevard
Suite 425
Wilmette, IL 60091
847-256-8525
www.bpkids.org

Center for Mental Health Services
Substance Abuse and Mental
    Health Services Administration
    (SAMHSA)
PO Box 42557
Washington, DC 20015
1-800-789-2647
www.mentalhealth.org

Depression and Bipolar Support
Alliance (DBSA)
730 North Franklin Street
Suite 501
Chicago, IL 60610-7224
1-800-826-3632
www.dbsalliance.org

Depression and Related Affective
Disorders Association (DRADA)
2330 West Joppa Road
Suite 100
Lutherville, MD 21093
410-955-4697
www.drada.org

National Institute of Mental Health
(NIMH)
Office of Communications
6001 Executive Boulevard
Room 8184, MSC 9663
Bethesda, MD 20892-9663
1-866-615-6464
www.nimh.nih.gov
Information about bipolar disorder
at: http://www.nimh.nih.gov/health-
information/bipolarmenu.cfm

Parents of Behaviorally Different
Children (PBDC)
7101 Cardenas NE
Suite 202
Albuquerque, NM 87110
1-800-273-7232
http://www.pbdconline.org/
This nonprofit organization was
formed by families of children and
adolescents with neurobiological,
emotional, and behavioral differences. It was originally founded to
provide a forum for families and to
provide a collective voice to implement improvements to services and
service delivery systems.

## Chapter Twenty-six

# Brain Injury, Traumatic

MaryAnn Tapper Strawhacker

## Introduction

Traumatic brain injury (TBI) is the most likely cause of death or permanent disability in children and adolescents. Each year among children 14 years of age and younger, TBI claims 3,000 deaths, 29,000 hospitalizations, and 400,000 emergency department visits. Young people between the ages of 15 and 24 years and those over age 75 are the two age groups at greatest risk for TBI. By gender, males are two times more likely to sustain a TBI than females (National Center for Injury Prevention and Control, 2003).

In public schools, approximately 13,000 children receive services each year related to TBI (Youse, Le, Cannizzaro, & Coelho, 2002). Many of these children require special education. TBI is defined in the Individuals with Disabilities Education Act as "...an acquired injury to the brain caused by an external physical force resulting in total or partial functional disability or psychosocial impairment, or both, that adversely affects a child's educational performance...." Excluded from this definition are brain injuries that are congenital, degenerative, or resulting from birth trauma (National Information Center for Children and Youth With Disabilities, 2002).

## Pathophysiology

TBI is commonly divided into two major types of primary injury: open and closed. Open TBI means an opening has been created from the outside, through the skull and dura. Damage from this type of injury tends to be localized to the region of the brain penetrated. Closed head injury is the most common type of injury, and although the dura has not been penetrated, injury tends to be diffuse owing to a variety of mechanisms. Secondary damage resulting from sources such as infection, lack of oxygen, edema, and increased intracranial pressure may compound the effects of both types of primary TBI (Youse et al., 2002).

Four common types of brain injury that can be detected through medical testing are skull fracture, contusion, diffuse axonal injury, and hematoma. Skull fracture is a break or crack in the skull and can be depressed when fragments of the bone press into brain tissue. Skull fracture may also cause contusions and areas of bleeding, resulting from bruising of brain tissue. Cells may be dam-

aged to the point of death, resulting in permanent function loss, or may be partially damaged and capable of repair. In coup-countercoup injuries, there are actually two contusions. The force of the impact is so great that a contusion results both at the point of impact and 180 degrees away on the opposite side of the brain. Contusions with severe TBIs tend to occur in the frontal and temporal lobes and in the brainstem. This occurs when the head is in motion and then suddenly stops, causing the brain to smash against the skull. Injury occurs when the brain contacts rough areas on the skull's inner surface. Injuries to the axons (nerve cells) are called diffuse axonal injury and are the result of shearing force. Twisting movements during injury can cause the axon to stretch to the point of pulling apart, resulting in cell death (Christensen, 2001; Brain Injury Association of America (BIA), 2003). Finally, hematomas are the result of damage to a major blood vessel within the brain and cause bleeding in or around the brain. Bleeding between the skull and dura results in an epidural hematoma, whereas bleeding between the dura and the arachnoid membrane results in a subdural hematoma. Within the brain, bleeding results in an intracerebral hematoma. Surgery may be required in about half of those with severe brain injuries to remove hematomas and contusions or repair damage (National Institute of Neurological Disorders and Stroke [NINDS], 2002).

### Severity of TBI

The severity of TBI is determined by a combination of clinical measures, including use of the Glasgow Coma Scale (GCS), length of unconsciousness, and length of amnesia after the event. The GSC was developed by neurosurgeons as an objective way to detect improvement or deterioration in intensive-care patients with TBI. The GCS measures the best response on a series of three subtests for eye, verbal, and motor responses. Scores range from a perfect 15 to a score of 3, denoting no response (Christensen, 2001). Research has demonstrated initial Glasgow score, in combination with other measures, is a significant prognostic factor for outcome in children with TBI (Pillai, Praharaj, Mohanty, & Kolluri, 2001). The second measure is loss of consciousness or time spent in a coma. The end of a coma is marked by the time when the child is able to respond to environmental stimuli, although this definition varies by setting. The final predictor of TBI severity is post-traumatic amnesia (PTA). This is defined as the period of amnesia or memory impairment after the initial injury and may be marked by confusion, disorientation, and agitation (Christensen). Using these three clinical measures, brain injury is divided into three levels: mild, moderate, and severe (BIA, 2003).

Almost 75% of all traumatic brain injuries fit the definition of **mild**, meaning loss of consciousness was less than 1 hour (Semrud-Clikeman, 2001). There may be no loss of consciousness, however, and the child just appears dazed or confused. Also, PTA must be less than 1 hour and GCS score must be 13 to 15 for an injury to be defined as mild (Christensen, 2001). Common symptoms for at least 1 week after mild injury include headache, dizziness, and fatigue (Ponsford et al., 1999). Other symptoms may include sleep disturbance; irritability; sensitivity to noise or light; balance problems; decreased concentration, attention span, and speed of thinking; memory problems; nausea; depression; anxiety; and emotional mood swing. Tests or scans of the brain appear normal (BIA, 2003). By 3 months after injury, symptoms have usually resolved with no significant cognitive impairments (Ponsford et al., 1999). For up to 15% of children, symptoms may persist even beyond 1 year and are called postconcussion syndrome (Bazarian, Wong, Harris, Leahey, Mookerjee, & Dombovy, 1999).

Mild brain injury occurring during athletics is a primary concern for school-aged children. The Standardized Assessment of Concussion was developed to detect and track mild brain injury in athletes. The instrument is easy to use, requires little training, and yields a reliable score to guide coaches and trainers in deciding when a player can safely return to play (McCrea, Kelly, & Randolph, 1997).

**Moderate** traumatic brain injury requires loss of consciousness for a time not greater than 24 hours, GCS score of 9 to 12, and PTA of 1 to 24 hours. Symptoms are similar to those with mild traumatic brain injury; however, they are more likely to persist for several months (Semrud-Clikeman, 2001). Students with a moderate TBI may have a headache that persists or gets worse, ongoing nausea and vomiting, seizures, difficulty arousing, dilation of one or both pupils, abnormal speech, loss of coordination, and/or behavioral changes (NINDS, 2002). Students with moderate TBI tend to more closely resemble those with mild and not severe TBI (Semrud-Clikeman). Recovery may require treatment but generally is satisfactory, or compensatory strategies can be learned to balance deficits (BIA, 2003). Signs of moderate to severe brain injury require immediate medical attention. Brain scans may show abnormal findings such as hematomas or contusions (Semrud-Clikeman).

**Severe** brain injury is defined by either loss of consciousness or PTA greater than 24 hours and a GCS score of 3 to 8. Roughly half of all children brought to the emergency department with severe brain injuries will die (Semrud-Clikeman, 2001). Of those who survive, poor outcomes are associated with initial GCS score of 3 to 5, absent verbal response, and presence of subarachnoid hemorrhage, among other measures (Pillai et al., 2001). Post-traumatic epilepsy occurs in 5% to 7% of closed brain injury and up to 11% with severe TBI. The risk for seizures after penetrating TBI is much greater (Christensen, 2001). Parents of children with severe TBI report lower health-related quality of life (HRQL) measures relative to behavior, mental health, general health, and family impact. Also, communication skills, daily living skills, and general adaptive functioning were rated lower for severely brain-injured adolescents. Risk factors for poor HRQL include family social disadvantage and prior existence of problems in areas such as behavior or academic achievement. In one study, 67% of families with a severely brain-injured child used mental health counseling sometime after injury (Stancin et al., 2002).

Students with severe TBI demonstrate selective long-term deficits in social problem-solving skills, which may account for poor social and academic outcomes (Janusz, Kirkwood, Yeates, & Taylor, 2002). At 6 and 12 months after injury, comparing children with mild to those with severe TBI, greater deficits were seen for the severely injured group on memory tasks (Catroppa & Anderson, 2002). Children with prior learning problems who sustain a TBI display worse memory abilities, suggesting less cognitive reserve (Farmer et al., 2002). Two years after injury, children with severe TBI demonstrated a significant difference on tasks requiring sustained attention, especially on complex tasks requiring speed, accuracy, and decision making, when compared with children who sustained a mild TBI (Catroppa & Anderson, 2003). Long-term follow-up of students with severe TBI demonstrates significantly lower reading recognition, spelling, and arithmetic scores than those with less severe injury. Also, a large majority of severely injured students had either received special education assistance or failed a grade (Ewing-Cobbs, Fletcher, Levin, Iovino, & Miner, 1998). In addition, the younger the child was at the time of injury, the greater the likelihood of receiving special education services (Hux, Marquardt, Skinner, & Bond, 1999). A number of studies have demonstrated that brain damage early in life is associated with long-term deficits and intellectual impairments (Stein & Hoffman, 2003). Not only is the injury a disruption to normal growth and development but it also may cause regression to an earlier stage of development. Although students with severe brain injury can improve, physical, cognitive, or behavioral impairments are often permanent (BIA, 2003). Postinjury progress can be influenced by family environment. In particular, social disadvantage is a predictor of more adverse behavioral consequences and less favorable changes in some outcome measures (Taylor et al., 2002). Despite the fact that the vast majority of recovery occurs in the first 12 to 18 months, recovery in children may continue for up to 6 years after injury (Semrud-Clikeman, 2001).

## Location of Injury

Unfortunately, the general public and healthcare professionals without expertise in brain injury commonly have inaccurate and inadequate knowledge. One misconception is that a complete recovery is possible after severe TBI. Other areas where lack of understanding is common include daily variability in task performance, behavioral sequelae, and cognitive sequelae. Injuries seldom follow discrete boundaries. However, the location of permanent injury within the brain determines whether resultant disabilities will be visible or hidden, physical or psychological, or a combination (Swift & Wilson, 2001)

The **frontal** lobes are responsible for complex thinking; anticipating, planning and initiating action; executing behavioral sequences; personality; and self-regulation (Uomoto, 2000). Frontal lobes also assist with coordinated fine movements, motor aspects of speech, and social skills (Christensen, 2001). Because of integration functions, the frontal lobes have many connections to other brain parts. This is the part of the brain thought to be responsible for self-awareness and regulation of behavior (Uomoto). In severe TBI with contusions, damage often occurs in the frontal lobe, temporal lobe, and brainstem (Christensen).

Major functions associated primarily with short-term memory and motor function occur in the **temporal** lobe. The left temporal lobe is believed to process verbal information and the right, visual information. Together with the limbic system, the temporal lobe is thought to be responsible for working memory, the ability that facilitates completion of many everyday tasks (Uomoto, 2000).

**Occipital lobes**, located at the rear of the brain, are responsible for visual perception, interpretation, and recognizing visual input. However, visual-spatial organizational ability is interpreted in the **parietal lobes**. Usually the right lobe is more responsible for analyzing and organizing spatial information, whereas the left lobe is important for executing arithmetic problems, comprehending speech, reading, and writing. (Uomoto, 2000). The parietal lobes are also responsible for goal-directed voluntary movements, integration of senses, and manipulation of objects (Centre for Neuro Skills, 2004).

Beneath the cortex are the limbic system, brainstem, and cerebellum. The **limbic system** is essential to regulate emotion, manipulate and store information, and distribute information to recent memory. Working together with higher-level brain structures, it accomplishes complex actions and reactions. Damage to the limbic system may occur directly to one of the structures involved, or the system may malfunction on account of lost connections. Located at the brain's base is the **brainstem**. Its importance is in regulation of basic body functions such as heart rate, breathing, and sleep-wake cycles (Uomoto, 2000). It also helps regulate balance and movement. The **cerebellum** is located at the base of the skull and is responsible for coordination of fine movements, balance and equilibrium, and memory for motor reflex acts (Centre for Neuro Skills, 2004).

## Management

Even with mild brain injuries, it is crucial to prevent additional injury. Second-impact syndrome occurs when the student suffers a second traumatic brain injury before symptoms from the first injury have fully resolved. The second injury has a greater likelihood of causing widespread damage and edema. Emergency medical treatment is needed immediately for second-impact syndrome because death can occur rapidly (BIA, 2003). Unfortunately, mild brain injuries may be unreported to school staff, making it important to carefully assess history of previous injuries and follow up with students suspected of a mild brain injury.

Students with moderate to lower-end severe injuries are likely to be hospitalized for a short term but may not receive any rehabilitation assessment or services. Subtle deficits may not be recognized until a student returns to school and demonstrates difficulties with attention, memory, concentration, organization, or planning. Educational modifications may be needed on a long-term or short-term basis to help these students succeed academically and vocationally (Savage, Pearson, McDonald, Potoczny-Gray, & Marchese, 2001). Referrals may also be needed to assist families to locate necessary services to manage lingering symptoms and facilitate adaptation to permanent disabilities.

Permanent disabilities are most likely to result from severe brain injuries. Rehabilitation has proven to reduce the level of disability, required supervision, and occupational/educational impairment (Ashley & Persel, 1999). It is important to note that many long-term outcomes of rehabilitation services are stable over time (Ashley, Persel, & Krych, 1997). Rehabilitation is vital to attain maximal age-appropriate community functioning and may require a variety of specialists, including physical therapists, occupational therapists, rehabilitation nurses, psychologists, speech and language pathologists, and social workers. An individualized rehabilitation program is designed, usually during hospitalization, and may continue on an outpatient basis until therapy goals are reached. Coordinating a student's educational program with outpatient therapies can be challenging, especially when plans are frequently revised to reflect skill mastery (NINDS, 2002). The school nurse is the ideal liaison between the medical and educational communities to facilitate transition between settings and monitor progress toward full-time school reentry.

Medications may also be required to manage physical and behavioral effects of TBI (NINDS, 2002). Physical symptoms may include headaches, muscle contractures, seizures, incontinence, and paralysis, among others. Behavioral effects may include, but are not limited to, interruptions in the sleep-wake cycles, inattention, depression, behavioral outbursts, aggression, and impulsivity. Medications are directed at symptom relief or management. Commonly prescribed medication classifications include antipsychotics, psychostimulants, beta blockers, anticonvulsants, and antidepressants (Senelick & Ryan, 1998). Medication monitoring during the school day is essential to maximize effectiveness while minimizing side effects.

### School Reentry

Planning for school reentry should begin once the child's health status is stable. Planning must consider student safety and address school community concerns, while maintaining confidentiality. Request that the parent or guardian sign a release to permit sharing of information between the school and medical providers. If the student remains hospitalized, try to arrange for a school representative to attend staffings or discharge planning meetings. If the student is homebound, schedule a planning meeting with staff, parents, and, if appropriate, the student prior to reentry. The school needs information from the physician or hospital to adequately prepare for a severely injured student's return. Medical orders for activity restrictions and outpatient therapies provide important information when planning for reentry. Medical records will also provide vital information regarding the student's cognitive functioning, gross and fine motor skills, communication and language skills, and current psychosocial functioning level (Tyler & Mira, 1999).

## Individualized Healthcare Plan

### Assessment

#### History

- Source of brain injury (motor vehicle accident, fall, sports, abuse, gunshot, other)
- Region of brain affected and type of injury
- Duration of unconsciousness
- Length of post-traumatic amnesia
- Glasgow Coma Scale rating upon presentation to emergency department and changes throughout hospitalization
- Age when injury occurred
- Physical and cognitive abilities prior to the accident
- Difficulty with behavior or impulsivity noted prior to the accident
- Presence of other health concerns prior to the accident
- Date of last complete physical examination
- Last date for professional vision and hearing examinations

#### Current Status and Management

- Effects of injury on normal developmental milestones
- Challenges to mobility, such as balance, muscle weakness, and residual paralysis
- Observed changes in mood, affect, behavior, memory, organization, or psychosocial functioning since the accident
- Changes noted in stamina or tolerance since the accident
- Changes noted in five senses since accident (hearing, vision, taste, smell or touch)
- Changes noted in health status since the accident
- Residual disability related to brain injury
- Level of supervision required to monitor safety needs with both decision making and mobility
- Need for activity restrictions
- Use of prescription and over-the-counter medications
- Use of alternative medicine (herbal, homeopathic, vitamin and mineral supplements, etc.)
- Use of adaptive aids, equipment, or devices
- Accessibility of school building, including restrooms
- Ability to participate in standard emergency building evacuation plans and potential need for modifications
- Daily transportation needs between school and home and for field trips
- Supplies, medication, or equipment needed during the school day
- Need for ongoing community services such as therapy or rehabilitation
- Nutritional status and need for supplements or caloric adjustments

*Self-care*
- Personal hygiene needs (toileting, bathing, grooming, and dressing)
- Medications/treatments/procedures administered independently at home and with supervision
- Self-management skills currently taught at home (medication administration, procedures, and other)
- Student's ability to monitor his/her own health status
- Student's ability to ask for assistance when needed
- Student's ability to make decisions and exercise judgment
- Changes in self-care needs during transitions through grade levels, building changes, and in preparation for adult living

*Psychosocial Status*
- Family and student's perception of overall health status
- Family and student's ability to cope with changes after brain injury
- Family and student's ability to address circumstances surrounding the accident (guilt, blame, shame, remorse, and grief)
- Presence of other family major life stressors (other family members killed or injured, divorce, job loss, or other)
- Reaction of friends and family after the accident and effect on student/family
- Concerns regarding peer interactions or with student's social skills
- Changes in mood or coping style since the accident
- Disclosure of student's disability with peers and peer response
- Participation in extracurricular and community activities
- Existence of social support network within the extended family or community
- Community resource(s) currently in use and remaining unmet needs

*Academic Issues*
- Past school attendance record
- Student's academic history prior to and since the accident, noting any decline in scores/grades
- Plans for present or future employment, including vocational training needs
- Modifications, accommodation, adaptations required for the student during the school day
- Additional modifications, accommodation, adaptations needed during the school day
- Existence of 504 plan or individualized education program (IEP) to address health and educational needs at school
- Required staff training to address student needs
- Need for behavior management plan at school

## Nursing Diagnoses (N.D.) (NANDA, 2003)

N.D. 1 Fatigue (NANDA 00093) related to:
- ongoing recovery after injury
- depression
- reduced physical stamina

N.D. 2 Impaired memory (NANDA 00131) related to:
- neurologic damage

N.D. 3 Imbalanced nutrition: more than body requirements (NANDA 00001) related to:
- increased intake
- decreased caloric demands
- sedentary lifestyle
- impaired mobility

N.D. 4 Toileting self-care deficit (NANDA 00110) related to:
- impaired mobility
- cognitive impairment

N.D. 5 Risk for injury (NANDA 00035) related to:
- impaired physical mobility
- impulsivity
- impaired problem-solving abilities
- uncontrolled movements of seizures
- visual perceptual changes

**N.D.6** Risk for noncompliance with prescribed treatment (NANDA 00079) related to:
- denial of need for medication/ therapy
- memory impairment
- perceived ineffectiveness of medication/therapy
- time involvement with therapy
- cost of therapy
- loss of control

**N.D. 7** Ineffective coping (NANDA 00069) related to:
- impulsivity
- inadequate social support
- ineffective parental coping

**N.D. 8** Ineffective role performance (NANDA 00055) related to:
- absence from school due to therapy and rehabilitation
- impaired coping
- cognitive deficits (such as memory loss or poor organizational skills)
- mood disturbance
- impaired self-esteem
- transition into new environment

**N.D 9** Risk for other-directed violence (NANDA 00138) related to:
- impulsivity
- neurologic impairment

**N.D. 10** Impaired social interaction (NANDA 0052) related to:
- failure to recognize social cues
- flat affect
- perseveration of ideas
- impulsivity
- impaired social boundaries
- neurologic impairment
- impaired self-esteem

**N.D. 11** Disturbed sensory perception (NANDA 00122) related to:
- visual distortion (double vision, field deficits)
- impaired hearing
- delays in central processing

**N.D. 12** Impaired adjustment (NANDA 00070) related to:
- neurologic impairment
- recent disability
- lack of limitation awareness
- lack of support (family or peer)
- transition into new environment

**N. D. 13** Knowledge deficit (NANDA 00126) related to:
- implications of TBI on learning
- implications of TBI on future health needs
- effects of repeat injuries
- medication management

**N. D. 14** Acute pain (NANDA 00132) related to:
- failure to intervene early in the pain process
- effects of physical therapy

**N. D. 15** Impaired physical mobility (NANDA 00085) related to:
- effects of residual paralysis
- muscle weakness
- poor balance
- visual disturbances
- weight gain

## Goals

The student will demonstrate improved physical activity tolerance. (N.D. 1, 3, 14, 15)

The student will assist with identifying modifications required during the school day on account of TBI. (N.D. 1–5, 7–12, 14, 15)

The student will attend school/class and participate with modifications made as needed. (N.D. 1–5, 7–12, 14, 15)

The student will attend his/her 504/IEP meetings and participate in team decision making and academic goal setting. (N.D. 1–15)

The student will progress toward adapting to living with the effects of TBI. (N.D. 1–15)

The student will collaborate with primary caregiver, school staff, and healthcare providers to identify and prioritize therapy goals (i.e., physical, occupational, speech, cognitive, behavioral) and develop an action plan. (N. D. 2–4, 6–12, 14, 15)

The student will follow the school routine schedule. (N.D. 2, 8, 12)

The student will maintain a body mass index (BMI) below the 95th percentile of BMI index by age and sex. (N.D. 3, 15)

The student will remain free from injury. (N.D. 5, 9, 15)

The student will demonstrate compliance with prescribed medications/treatments/therapy. (N.D. 6, 14, 15)

The student will identify a source of social support outside immediate family. (N.D. 7–10, 12)

The student will demonstrate use of adaptive coping skills. (N.D. 7–10, 12, 14)

The student will demonstrate improved self-esteem. (N.D. 8, 10)

The student will recognize and honor social boundaries of others. (N.D. 10)

The student will develop compensatory strategies for sensory deficits. (N.D. 11, 15)

The student will use knowledge of his/her brain injury to self-advocate with peers and staff. (N.D. 12, 13, 15)

The student will demonstrate mastery of self-medication management. (N.D. 13, 15)

The student will report decreased level of pain after therapeutic intervention(s). (N.D.14)

The student will demonstrate improved physical mobility in the school setting. (N. D. 14, 15)

The student will demonstrate increased muscle strength. (N. D. 15)

The student will, in collaboration with primary caregiver and providers, develop a mutually agreeable treatment plan. (N.D. 1–15)

## Nursing Interventions

*Student/Family Interventions*

Obtain a signed release of information to obtain pertinent medical records and to share information with the medical provider. (N.D. 1–15)

Obtain parental and student permission to share relevant medical information with school personnel who have a legitimate need to know. (N.D. 1–15)

Establish a preferred mode of scheduled communication with parents/ guardians to facilitate coordination of medical treatment and to monitor the student's social and emotional adjustment. (N.D. 1–15)

Facilitate student participation in the therapeutic plan. (N.D. 1–15)

- determine student's current level of participation
- set participation goals with student and primary caregiver
- explore strategies with the student to progress towards goal attainment
- breakdown treatment plan into discrete teachable components
- maintain consistency in student performance of self-help skills through written protocol and support staff training
- encourage the student to participate in monitoring progress toward goal attainment
- evaluate plan and modify, in collaboration with student and family, as needed for goal attainment
- provide ongoing feedback to primary caregiver regarding student's progress towards goal attainment
- provide positive reinforcement to student
- assist student in developing realistic therapeutic expectations

Establish a mode of communication with parents/guardians to facilitate coordination of medical treatment and to monitor the student's social and emotional adjustment. (N.D. 1–4)

In collaboration with the medical providers, family, and student, develop a school reentry plan. (N.D. 1–15)

Arrange a tour of the empty building and a walk-through of the student's schedule prior to reentry. (N.D. 2, 5, 8, 12, 15)

Modify the school environment to promote safety. (N.D. 5, 11, 15)
- remove environmental hazards (barriers in hallways, uneven mats, broken furniture)
- encourage use of hand rails on stairs
- arrange furniture to promote easy access

Provide support and encouragement to student. (N.D. 1–4, 6–10, 12, 14, 15)

Assist student to identify and implement effective memory strategies to arrive at the health office at scheduled times and to perform self-care skills. (N.D. 2)

Review school emergency evacuation procedures and determine need for special adaptations for student's disability. (N.D. 2, 5, 8, 11, 15)

In collaboration with the educational team, promote social skill enhancement. (N.D. 2, 7–10, 12)
- assist student to identify strengths and challenges with interpersonal skills after TBI
- assist student to identify target skills to be shaped
- teach student to interpret facial expression and nonverbal cues as part of the total communication message
- collaborate with other disciplines to design an intervention to teach identified skills
- provide opportunities to practice developing skills in real-life situations
- provide positive reinforcement when targeted skills are observed
- involve peers in social skills training when appropriate
- utilize and adult mentor to support and practice skill attainment
- encourage student to self-evaluate effectiveness of social skills intervention

Refer family to counseling resources as needed to facilitate the student and family's adaptation to living with the effects of TBI. (N.D. 2, 6–10, 12, 14, 15)

Assist student to develop personal health goals. (N.D. 3, 6–10, 12–14)
- determine student's awareness of personal health needs and implications
- facilitate exploration of student's strengths and weaknesses
- assist student prioritize health needs
- incorporate student's values and beliefs when developing goals
- assist student to develop realistic attainable goals
- record goals in clear, measurable terms
- establish baseline functioning for identified goals

Reinforce or provide additional TBI education to the student/family. (N.D. 3–10, 13–15)
- assess the student/ primary caregiver's knowledge of TBI
- determine readiness and ability of caregivers/student to learn the necessary skills
- review the known pathophysiological processes with the student at a developmentally appropriate level
- provide current BI resources as needed
- reinforce teaching with the student/primary caregiver on an ongoing basis

Collaborate with private therapy services to utilize similar strategies across settings and to provide reinforcement teaching. (N. D. 5, 7–12,14, 15)

In collaboration with the educational team, assist student to manage negative behavior. (N. D. 5, 6–10, 12)
- document types of negative behavior across settings
- determine the function of negative behaviors
- communicate expectations for behavior in dominant learning mode for student (verbal, pictorial, or written)
- break down instructions into parts containing three steps or less
- allow student to complete one set of directions before being given another
- set consistent rules across settings
- refrain from arguing or bargaining over established rules or limits
- provide clear and consistent consequences for behavior
- assist student in problem-solving possible positive alternatives to past negative behavior
- establish routines within the health office to facilitate compliance with treatment
- provide environmental cues that will facilitate attention to task
- redirect attention away from source of agitation
- reduce environmental stimuli
- use external means to help calm student (music, solitude, dim lighting)
- reinforce positive efforts at self-control
- teach and model appropriate expression of feelings
- teach and model appropriate social skills

- assess environment for dangerous items and remove them from the area

Provide medication management. (N.D. 5–7, 9, 10, 13–15)
- determine medication required and administer per physician's orders
- assess student's ability to self-medicate
- assist student to identify effective medication strategies to manage pain related to PT
- monitor effectiveness of medications
- monitor for adverse drug effects
- review with the student/family appropriate use of over-the-counter as well as prescription medications
- discuss use of herbals and alternative therapies that may interact with over-the-counter or prescription medication
- monitor student's medication/treatment compliance
- assist to identify and remove barriers to medication compliance
- collaborate with other healthcare providers regarding medication treatment results and the need for adjustments
- problem solve with other healthcare providers regarding issues related to noncompliance

Develop trusting open communication with the student, encouraging verbalization of feelings of anger, frustration, depression, concerns, and fears. (N.D. 6–10, 12–14)

Facilitate development of adaptive coping skills. (N. D. 7–10, 12, 14, 15)
- appraise student's adjustment after TBI and its impact on family and peers
- provide age-appropriate explanations of diagnosis and its links to current functional difficulties
- encourage realistic hopefulness towards regaining lost skills
- evaluate student's decision-making abilities
- seek to understand the student's perspective
- encourage gradual reentry into former activities while following medical recommendations
- support use of adaptive defense mechanisms
- plan situations to allow maximum student autonomy
- identify and promote constructive outlets for anger and frustration
- facilitate access to potential sources of social support
- instruct student in self-calming strategies
- facilitate student's adaptation to living with a disability
- collaborate with mental health professionals to promote continuity between settings

Promote self-esteem enhancement. (N.D. 7, 8, 10, 12)
- facilitate an environment that encourages self-esteem
- assist student to identify the impact of TBI on self concept
- assist student to examine negative self perceptions and reasons for self criticism
- monitor self-critical statements
- assist student to identify self-destructive behaviors
- facilitate contact with peers during periods of absence
- facilitate self-expression with peers
- provide social-skills training
- monitor student for signs of social isolation
- assist student to identify strengths and reinforce examples of those strengths when observed
- convey confidence in student's abilities for self care

Promote optimal growth and development. (N.D. 8, 10, 12)
- build trust with the student and parents (guardians)
- teach student how to ask for help when needed and refuse help politely when not needed
- adapt age-appropriate risk-avoidance instruction to intellectual abilities (reproduction, AIDS, drug and alcohol awareness)
- encourage goal setting
- while on physical activity restrictions, promote use of safe exercise such as walking or use of a stationary bike
- refer to mental health professional or school counselor as needed

Determine precipitating factors for pain and its impact on learning and activity level. (N.D. 1, 7, 8, 14, 15)

Assist student to anticipate precipitating pain factors and to engage in strategies or interventions to avoid pain exacerbations. (N.D. 14, 15) Develop a menu of pain-relief strategies based on etiology of pain (muscular, bone, headache, other). (N.D. 14, 15)

Obtain medical orders for BI management at school when applicable. (N.D. 1, 3–6, 14)

Educate school staff as to the effects of traumatic brain injury on memory. (N.D. 2) Provide BI educational materials to designated school personnel and allow time for questions. (N.D. 7–12)

Assist teacher(s) to monitor student's activity tolerance and make adjustments in scheduling as needed. (N.D. 1, 7–10, 14, 15)

With parent and student permission, provide opportunities for student/ family/ nurse to educate classmates regarding BI. (N.D. 7–12)

Refer student to building student assistance team or 504 coordinator as needed. (N.D. 1, 2, 7–12, 15)

Collaborate with the educational team to identify potential required health accommodations such as: (N.D. 1–15)

- shortened school day to minimize fatigue
- two sets of texts, in case student forgets to bring books home
- use of a daily planner as a memory guide
- assigned seating closest to instruction to facilitate attention
- peer buddy to facilitate transitions between classes
- alternate pass times to minimize stimuli or enhance safety
- alternate activities during recess or physical education class
- encourage rest periods at school as needed to ease transition into school

## Expected Student Outcomes

The student will:

- Participate in usual activities without signs of fatigue. (N.D. 1, 15)
- Improve school attendance with accommodations as needed. (N.D. 1–5, 7, 9, 10, 11, 14, 15)
- Navigate hallways between classes with minimal directions from staff. (N.D. 2)
- Engage in safe regular exercise while restricted from PE/recess. (N.D. 1, 3, 15)
- With adult assistance, select healthy choices from the school cafeteria menu. (N. D. 3)
- Assist with transfers from wheelchair to toilet. (N.D. 4, 15)
- Demonstrate use of safe technique when using adaptive mobility equipment (wheelchair, walker, crutches). (N.D. 5, 15)
- Come to the health office daily to take prescribed medications. (N.D. 6)
- Demonstrate effective use of at least one coping skill during times of frustration. (N.D. 7–10, 12, 14)
- Describe himself/herself as an active part of the school community. (N.D. 8–10, 12)
- Attend his/her school health planning meetings. (N.D. 8, 12)
- Identify and utilize existing community resources as needed. (N.D. 2–4, 7–15)
- Participate in development of the behavior management treatment plan. (N.D. 6–10, 12)
- Demonstrate a reduction in self-critical comments. (N.D. 7, 8, 10, 12)
- Obtain counseling as needed. (N.D. 1–14)
- With adult assistance, identify early signs and symptoms of depression. (N.D. 7, 8, 12, 14)
- Utilize community resources to assist with reintegration into school. (N.D. 2, 4, 7–12)
- Demonstrate use of consistent therapeutic strategies across all settings. (N.D. 7–10, 12, 14, 15)
- Experience an increased level of comfort, allowing active participation in school activities. (N.D. 14)

## Case Study

Emma is a 15-year-old high school student who suffered a severe traumatic brain injury 1 month ago as the result of a car accident. Emma lives at home with her parents and younger brother. According to her mother, Emma was unconscious for 5 days and has no memory of events that occurred the week prior to the accident or the first week of hospitalization. Medical records confirm frontal and temporal lobe contusions with an initial Glasgow Coma Score score of 4 in the emergency department. While an inpatient, Emma is receiving physical therapy (PT), occupational therapy (OT), and speech therapy. Her anticipated discharge is in 2 weeks with return to school the following week. She will continue to have outpatient OT and PT services to assist with managing her residual short-term memory deficits and double vision. Prior to the accident, Emma took stimulant medication daily for impulsivity and difficulty concentrating.

## Tramatic Brain Injury

| Assessment Data | Nursing Diagnosis | Goals | Nursing Interventions | Expected Outcomes |
|---|---|---|---|---|
| Parents report Emma is sleeping 10 to 14 hours per day and complains of constant tiredness. Prior to the accident Emma participated in chorus, volleyball, and dance team. Discharge planning meeting is scheduled in 2 weeks. | Fatigue related to ongoing recovery after injury. | Emma will attend class with modifications as needed. | 1. Obtain signed release of information to facilitate communication between medical providers and school. 2. Collaborate with medical providers to develop a school reentry plan. 3. Encourage gradual reentry into former school activities. 4. Collaborate with the educational team to identify potential accommodations or modifications needed at school to minimize fatigue such as schedule changes, shortened school day, dropping a class, or resting during the school day. 5. Refer Emma to educational assessment teams as needed to receive services. 6. With parent's and Emma's permission, educate peers regarding the effects of traumatic brain injury. | Emma will participate in usual activities without signs of fatigue. Emma will improve school attendance with accommodations as needed. |
| Visited Emma while inpatient. She had difficulty remembering names of other students. Parents report she has difficulty with remembering when therapies are scheduled and what was done the previous day. | Impaired memory related to neurological damage. | Emma will be able to follow the routine school schedule. | 1. Arrange a tour of the empty building and a walk-through following Emma's schedule prior to reentry. 2. Assist Emma to identify and implement effective memory strategies to prompt coming to the health office at scheduled times. 3. Educate school staff as to the effects of traumatic brain injury on memory. | Emma will navigate the hallways between classes with minimal directions from staff. |

| Assessment Data | Nursing Diagnosis | Goals | Nursing Interventions | Expected Outcomes |
|---|---|---|---|---|
| Parents report Emma had quit taking her stimulant medication a few weeks prior to the accident. She complained the medication made her feel sick to her stomach and wasn't helping.<br><br>Parents have requested that Emma take her morning dose of stimulant medication at school to make sure she is compliant. | Risk for noncompliance with prescribed treatment related to perceived ineffectiveness of medication therapy. | Emma will demonstrate compliance with prescribed medications. | 1. Develop trusting, open communication with Emma, encouraging verbalization of feelings of anger, frustration, depression, concerns, and fears.<br>2. Facilitate participation in the therapeutic plan by assisting Emma to develop realistic medication goals and expectations.<br>3. Establish preferred mode of scheduled communication with parents to facilitate coordination of medication management.<br>4. Contact parents weekly to report progress with medication compliance.<br>5. Monitor Emma for adverse drug effects.<br>6. Assist to identify and remove barriers to medication compliance.<br>7. Collaborate with other healthcare providers regarding medication treatment results and the need for adjustments.<br>8. Problem-solve with other healthcare providers regarding issues related to noncompliance. | Emma will come to the health office daily to take prescribed medication.<br><br>Emma will verbalize change in perception toward effectiveness of medication therapy. |

| Assessment Data | Nursing Diagnosis | Goals | Nursing Interventions | Expected Outcomes |
|---|---|---|---|---|
| Parents are concerned Emma will have difficulty adjusting to her yearlong physical activity restrictions. Initially, in the hospital, Emma had frequent visitors. Her parents believe the visits have become infrequent, because she failed to recognize some classmates and had difficulty carrying on conversation.<br><br>Private occupational therapist and speech therapist are partnering together to improve working memory and conversation strategies. | Risk for impaired adjustment related to recent disability. | Emma will progress toward adapting to living with the effects of TBI. | 1. Refer family to counseling resources as needed to facilitate Emma's and the family's adaptation to living with the effects of TBI.<br>2. Assist Emma to develop personal health and rehabilitation goals.<br>3. Facilitate development of adaptive coping skills.<br>4. With parent's and Emma's permission, provide opportunities for student/family/ nurse to educate classmates regarding TBI.<br>5. Weekly appraise Emma's adjustment after TBI and its impact on peers and make referrals to school counselor as needed.<br>6. Support use of adaptive defense mechanisms.<br>7. Encourage realistic hopefulness toward regaining lost skills.<br>8. Monitor Emma for signs of isolation.<br>9. Plan situations to allow Emma maximum autonomy.<br>10. Identify and promote constructive outlets for anger and frustration.<br>11. Facilitate access to potential sources of social support. | Emma will utilize community resources to assist with reintegration into school.<br><br>Emma will describe herself as an active part of the school community.<br><br>Emma will, with adult assistance, identify early signs and symptoms of depression. |

# References

Ashley, M. J., & Persel, C. S. (1999). Traumatic brain injury recovery rates in post-acute rehabilitation of traumatic brain injury: Spontaneous recovery or treatment. *Journal of Rehabilitation Outcomes Measurement, 3*(4), 15–21.

Ashley, M. J., Persel, C. S., & Krych, D. K. (1997). Long-term outcome follow-up of postacute traumatic brain injury rehabilitation: An assessment of functional and behavioral measures of daily living. *Journal of Rehabilitation Outcomes Measurement, 1*(4), 40-47.

Bazarian, J. J., Wong, T., Harris, M., Leahey, N., Mookerjee, S., & Dombovy, M. (1999). Epidemiology and predictors of post-concussive syndrome after minor head injury in an emergency population. *Brain Injury, 13*(3), 173–189.

Brain Injury Association of America. (n.d.). *Types of brain injury.* Retrieved October 17, 2003, from http://www.biausa.org/Pages/types_of_brain_injury.html

Catroppa, C., & Anderson, V. (2002). Recovery in memory function in the first year following TBI in children. *Brain Injury, 16*(5), 369–384.

Catroppa, C., & Anderson, V. (2003). Children's attentional skills 2 years post-traumatic brain injury. *Developmental Neuropsychology, 23*(3), 359–374.

Centre for Neuro Skills. (n.d.). Traumatic brain injury resource guide. Retrieved October 6, 2004, from http://neuroskills.com/index.shtml?main=/main.html

Christensen, J. R. (2001). What is traumatic brain injury? In L. Schoenbrodt, (Ed.), *Children with traumatic brain injury: A parents' guide.* Bethesda, MD: Woodbine House.

Ewing-Cobbs, L., Fletcher, J. M., Levin, H. S., Iovino, I., & Miner, M. E. (1998). Academic achievement and academic placement following traumatic brain injury in children and adolescents: A two-year longitudinal study. *Journal of Clinical and Experimental Neuropsychology, 20*(6), 769–781.

Farmer, J. E., Kanne, S. M., Haunt, J. S., Williams, J., Johnstone, B., & Kirk, K. (2002). Memory functioning following traumatic brain injury in children with premorbid learning problems. *Developmental Neuropsychology, 22*(2), 455–469.

Hux, K., Marquardt, J., Skinner, S., & Bond, V. (1999). Special education services provided to students with and without parental reports of traumatic brain injury. *Brain Injury, 13*(6). 447–455.

Janusz, J. A., Kirkwood, M. W., Yeates, K. O., & Taylor, H. G. (2002). Social problem solving skills in children with traumatic brain injury: Long-term outcomes and prediction of social competence. *Child Neuropsychology (Neuropsychology, Development and Cognition: Section C), 8*(3), 179–194.

McCrea, M., Kelly, J., & Randolph, C. (1997). *The Standardized Assessment of Concussion (SAC).* Alexandria, VA: Brain Injury Association.

NANDA International. (2003). *Nursing diagnosis: Definitions & classification 2003-2004.* Philadelphia: Author.

National Center for Injury Prevention and Control (CDC). (2003, October 8). *Traumatic brain injury.* Retrieved October 17, 2003, from http://www.cdc.gov/ncipe/facts/tbi.htm

National Center for Injury Prevention and Control. (2003). *Report to Congress on mild traumatic brain injury in the United States: Steps to prevent a serious public health problem.* Atlanta, GA: Centers for Disease Control and Prevention.

National Information Center for Children and Youth with Disabilities. (2002, August). *Traumatic brain injury.* Retrieved October 17, 2003, from http://www.nichy.org

National Institute of Neurological Disorders and Stroke. (2002, October 10). Traumatic brain injury: Hope through research. Retrieved November 10, 2003, from http://www.ninds.nih.gov/health_and_medical/pubs/tbi.htm

Pillai, S., Praharaj, S. S., Mohanty, A., & Kolluri, V. R. (2001). Prognostic factors in children with severe diffuse brain injuries: A study of 74 patients. *Pediatric Neurosurgery, 34*(2), 98–103.

Ponsford, J., Willmontt, C., Rothwell, A., Cameron, P., Ayton, G., Nelms, R., et al. (1999). Cognitive and behavioral outcome following mild traumatic head injury in children. *Journal of Head Trauma Rehabilitation, 14*(4), 360–372.

Savage, R. C., Pearson, S., McDonald, H., Potoczny-Gray, A., & Marchese, N. (2001). After hospital: Working with schools and families to support the long term needs of children with brain injuries. *NeuroRehabilitation, 16*, 49–58.

Semrud-Clikeman, M. (2001). Traumatic brain injury in children and adolescents: Assessment and intervention (S. Elliott & J. Witt, Eds.). New York: Guilford Press.

Senelick, R. C., & Ryan, C. E. (1998). *Living with brain Injury: A guide for families.* Birmingham, AL: HealthSouth Press.

Stancin, T., Drotar, D., Taylor, H. G., Yeates, K. O., Wade, S. L., & Minich, N. M. (2002). Health-related quality of life of children and adolescents after traumatic brain injury. *Pediatrics, 109*(2), E34.

Stein, D. G., & Hoffman, S. W. (2003). Concepts of CNS plasticity in the context of brain damage and repair. *Journal of Head Trauma Rehabilitation, 18*(4), 317–341.

Swift, T. L., & Wilson, S. L. (2001). Misconceptions about brain injury among the general public and non-expert health professionals: An exploratory study. *Brain Injury, 15*(2), 149–165.

Taylor, H. G., Yeates, K. O., Wade, S. L., Drotar, D., Stancin T., & Minich, N. (2002). A prospective study of short- and long-term outcomes after traumatic brain injury in children: Behavior and achievement. *Neuropsychology, 16*(1), 15–27.

Tyler, J. S., & Mira, M. P. (1999). Traumatic brain injury in children and adolescents: A sourcebook for teachers and other school personnel (2nd ed.). Austin, TX: Pro-Ed.

Uomoto, J. M. (2000). Application of the neuropsychological evaluation, In R. T. Fraser & D. C. Clemmons, (Eds.), *Traumatic brain injury rehabilitation: Practical vocational, neuropsychological, and psychotherapy interventions.* New York: CRC Press.

Youse, K. M., Le, K. N., Cannizzaro, M. D. & Coelho, C. A. (2002). Traumatic brain injury: A primer for professionals. *ASHA Leader, 7*(12), 4–7.

## Bibliography

Allen, P. J., & Vessey, J. A. (2004). *Primary care of the child with a chronic condition* (4th ed.). St. Louis, MO: Mosby.

Blosser, J. L., & DePompei, R. (2003). Pediatric traumatic brain injury: Proactive intervention (2nd ed.). Clifton Park, NY: Delmar Learning.

Crawford, P., Mitchell, R., & Ikeda, J. (2000). Childhood overweight: A fact sheet for professionals. Berkley, CA: Cooperative Extension Department of Nutritional Sciences, University of California.

Elovic, E. (2000). Use of provigil for underarousal following TBI. *Journal of Head Trauma Rehabilitation, 15*(4), 1068–1071.

Keyser-Marcus, L., Briel, L., Sherron-Targett, P., Yasuda, S., Johnson, S., & Wehman, P. (2002). Enhancing the schooling of students with traumatic brain injury. *Teaching Exceptional Children, 34*(4), 62–67.

Lewis, J. K., Morris, M. K., Morris, R. D., Krawiecki, N., & Foster, M. A. (2000). Social problem solving in children with acquired brain injuries. *Journal of Head Trauma Rehabilitation, 15*(3), 469–483.

McCloskey, J. C., & Bulechek, G. M. (Eds.). (2000). *Nursing interventions classification (NIC)* (3rd ed.). St. Louis, MO: Mosby Yearbook.

National Safe Kids Campaign. (2002, May). *A national study of traumatic brain injury and wheel-related sports.* Retrieved October 17, 2003, from http://wwwlsafekids.org

Ruoff, J.. (2001). *The student with a brain injury: Achieving goals for higher education.* Washington, DC: American Council on Education.

Schlund, M. W. (2002). Effects of acquired brain injury on adaptive choice and the role of reduced sensitivity to contingencies. *Brain Injury, 16*(6), 527–535.

Turkstra, L. S., McDonald, S., De Pompei, R. (2001). Social information processing in adolescents: Data from normally developing adolescents and preliminary data from their peers with traumatic brain injury. *Journal of Head Trauma Rehabilitation, 16*(5), 469–483.

# Resources

## Web sites

Brain Injury Association of New Jersey
*Brain injury: A Guide for School Nurses*
*Brain Injury: A Guide for Educators*
http://www.bianj.org/hwch_pubs.html

Center for Neuro Skills
*The Traumatic Brain Injury Resource Guide*
http://www.neuroskills.com

Health Resource Center
*Secondary Education*
1-800-544-3284
202-833-5696 (fax)
http://www.heath.gwu.edu/

I. M. Brainy, Brain Injury Awareness and Prevention Kit
http://www.biausa.org/Pages/biam2003/imbrainy.html

MEDLINEplus Health Information
Brain Injury Resource Site
http://www.nlm.nih.gov/medline-plus/headandbraininjuries.html

The TBI Help Desk for Caregivers
http://www.tbihelp.org/

University of Iowa Virtual Hospital
*Acute Brain Injury: A Guide for Families and Friends* (2000)
http://www.vh.org/navigation/vh/topics/pediatric_patient_head_and_brain_injuries.html

## Organizations

Brain Injury Association
105 North Alfred Street
Alexandria, VA 22314-3010
1-800-444-6443
familyhelpline@biusa.org
http://www.biausa.org

Brain Injury Society
1901 Avenue North
Suite 5E
Brooklyn, NY 11230
718-645-4401
718-469-4100 (fax)
bisociety@aoll.com
http://www.bisociety.org

Head Injury Hotline
212 Pioneer Building
Seattle, WA 98104-2221
206-621-8558
brain@headinjury.com
http://www.headinjury.com

National Rehabilitation Information Center (NARIC)
1010 Wayne Avenue
Silver Spring, MD 20910-5633
1-800-346-2742
301-562-2401 (fax)
naricinfo@kra.org
http://www.naric.com

Research and Training Center on the Community Integration of Individuals with TBI (RTC/TBI)
One Gustave L. Levy Place
Box 1240
New York, NY 10029
212-241-7917
http://www.mssm.edu/tbinet

Brain Injury, Traumatic

*Chapter Twenty-seven*

# Brain and Spinal Cord Tumors

Katherine M. Sommer

## Introduction

Central nervous system (CNS) tumors in children can occur in the brain and/or the spinal cord. These tumors are relatively rare, with an estimated incidence in 2002 of 3,110 new cases in the United States among children and adolescents (aged 0 to 19 years) (CBTRUS, 2002). However, CNS tumors are the most common solid tumor diagnosed in children and adolescents. The etiology of CNS tumors in children is still mostly unknown. The only risk factors reliably identified for development of CNS tumors in childhood are ionizing radiation exposure and some specific genetic or familial disorders (Bestak, 2001). Improvements in survival for children with CNS tumors have been realized with advances in surgical outcomes as well as in chemotherapy and radiation treatment regimens. Nonetheless, the majority of deaths from pediatric cancers is due to CNS tumors (Bestak; Strother et al., 2002). Those children who survive typically experience significant morbidity from long-term sequelae of treatment. The diagnosis, treatment, and follow-up for children with CNS tumors require the support of a multidisciplinary team, and because many of these children attend school at least intermittently, involvement of the school nurse and other school staff in planning the care for these children in the academic setting is paramount.

## Pathophysiology

CNS tumors have generally been defined by the tissue or cell type they resemble under the microscope and/or by the location of the tumor. Classification systems for CNS tumors have suffered from a lack of consensus over the years (Strother et al., 2002), and this is still the case, although progress to standardize classification is slowly being made. The use of the terms *benign* and *malignant* can be somewhat misleading in regard to CNS tumors because even a "benign" tumor can cause significant morbidity or even prove fatal. In general, the nature of a particular tumor depends on its histology (tumor type), its mitotic activity (amount of cell division), and, equally important, its location in the CNS. Benign CNS tumors tend to cause local damage, whereas malignant tumors, which make up greater than half of all pediatric CNS tumors (Ryan-Murray & Petriccione, 2002), can invade normal brain structures more aggressively and can also spread within the CNS.

It is very rare for a malignant CNS tumor to spread outside of the CNS.

### Anatomy

It is helpful to have knowledge of CNS anatomy and physiology in order to understand the impact that a particular tumor may have on a child's functioning (**Figures 1 and 2**). When discussing location of CNS tumors, clinicians generally refer to five anatomical categories: supratentorium (cerebrum/cerebral hemispheres), infratentorium (posterior fossa), diencephalon (thalamus and hypothalamus), optic pathway, and spinal cord. The tentorium is a thick band of dura mater that separates the posterior fossa from the cerebral hemispheres. Tumors located above the tentorium are referred to as supratentorial, and those below are infratentorial. The cerebral hemispheres contain the frontal, parietal, temporal, and occipital lobes; the lateral and third ventricles; and the corpus callosum, which divides the two sides of the brain. The diencephalon refers to the central structures in the brain, which include the thalamus, hypothalamus, and the pituitary and pineal glands. The posterior fossa contains the cerebellum, the brainstem (pons and medulla), and the fourth ventricle. The optic pathway consists of the eyes, optic nerves, and optic radiations (fibers), which extend to the occipital cortex. The spinal cord connects the brain to the body via the spinal nerves, which are considered part of the peripheral nervous system. The spinal cord generally ends at the level of the first or second lumbar vertebra (Netter, 2003).

### Signs and Symptoms

The presenting signs and symptoms of CNS tumors in children are dependent on the location of the tumor, type of tumor, and the age of the child (Ryan-Murray and Petriccione, 2002). CNS tumors may cause symptoms by putting pressure on neighboring tissue, by invading into and damaging normal structures, and/or by blocking the cerebrospinal fluid (CSF) pathways. These effects can be quite variable, and the rapidity of symptom onset can be slow and insidious, or seem to come out of the blue. The history of symptom progression can often give a clue to the behavior of the tumor, with a rapid or acute onset suggesting a more aggressive type of tumor. Presenting signs and symptoms include headache, vomiting, ataxia and

**Figure 1. The tentorium.**

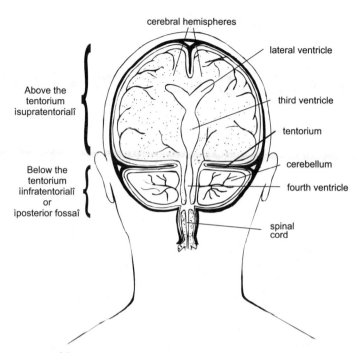

From *A primer of brain tumors: A patient's reference manual* (8th ed.). [Online]. Retrieved May 16, 2004, from http://www.abta.org/buildingknowledge5.htm. Reprinted with permission of the American Brain Tumor Association.

**Figure 2. Cross section of the brain.**

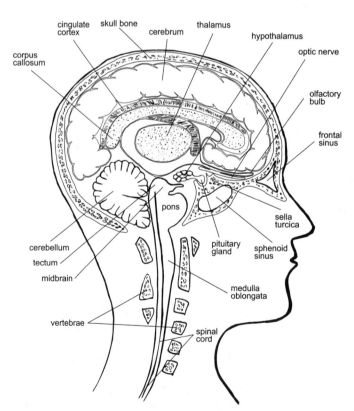

From *A primer of brain tumors: A patient's reference manual* (8th ed.). [Online]. Retrieved May 16, 2004, from http://www.abta.org/buildingknowledge5.htm. Reprinted with permission of the American Brain Tumor Association.

incoordination, seizures, weakness (usually focal), visual changes, mental status changes, personality changes, academic difficulties, speech and language dysfunction, swallowing difficulties, memory problems, hormonal imbalance, water imbalance, and sensory changes. See **Table 1** for an expanded review of presenting signs and symptoms based on the location of the tumor.

Adapted with permission from *Nursing Care of Children and Adolescents With Cancer* (3rd ed.)(2002) (pp. 503–523), C. R. Baggott, K. P. Kelly, D. Fochtman, and G. V. Foley (Eds.), Philadelphia: Saunders, with permission from Elsevier; and "Pediatric Brain Tumors: An Overview," by P. K. Duffner, M. E. Cohen, and A. Freeman, 1985, *Cancer, 35,*

pp. 287–301, with permission from Lippincott Williams & Wilkins; Supplemented with information from and *A primer of Brain Tumors: A Patient's Reference Manual* (25th anniversary ed.), 1998, Des Plaines, IL: American Brain Tumor Association, with permission from ABTA. Supplemented with information from *A Primer of Brain Tumors: A Patient's Reference Manual* (8th ed.) [Online]. Retrieved 5/16/2004 from http://www.abta.org/building-knowledge5.htm; "Transient Loss of Speech After Removal of Posterior Fossa Tumors—One Aspect of a Larger Neuropsychological Entity: The Cerebellar Cognitive Affective Syndrome," by M. Sadeh and I. Cohen, 2001, *Pediatric Hematology & Oncology, 18,* pp. 423–426; and

**Table 1. Presenting Signs and Symptoms of Childhood CNS Tumors According to Location**

| 1A. General Symptoms | | |
|---|---|---|
| Headache | May be intermittent; can be worse in the morning and improve during the day; may awaken a child during the night; can worsen with cough, exercise or bending over | |
| Seizures | May be generalized or focal, depending on the tumor location | |
| Mental status changes | May manifest with disturbance of memory, speech, communication, and/or concentration. Behavior, mood, or personality changes may also occur. In some cases, somnolence may progress to coma. | |
| Increased intracranial pressure (ICP) | Is due to tumor growth, hydrocephalus (blockage of cerebrospinal fluid flow), and/or edema. Symptoms often include nausea and vomiting, headache, drowsiness, visual changes, papilledema (swollen optic nerves), mental status changes, and eventually decreased level of consciousness, with potential for brain herniation in extreme cases—this is a life-threatening surgical emergency. | |
| **1B. Location-Specific Symptoms** **Posterior Fossa** **Tumor Location** | **Normal Function** | **Common Symptoms** |
| Fourth ventricle | Location of the chemoreceptor trigger zone, along the floor of the 4th ventricle, adjacent to the cerebellum | Nausea and vomiting are cardinal features, along with other symptoms of cerebellar tumors. |
| Cerebellum | In conjunction with the thalamus and cerebral cortex, controls fine and gross motor coordination and balance; also has a role in coordination of speech, and thought to play a role in coordination of behavior and other thought processes. Several cranial nerves exit from the brainstem in this area. | Clumsiness, ataxia (uncoordinated walk), dizziness, tremor, difficulty with coordinated speech, diplopia (double vision), nystagmus (jerky eye movements), signs of increased ICP |
| Brainstem | Controls basic life functions (heart rate, blood pressure, respiratory rate), reticular formation within the brainstem controls eating/sleeping patterns, wakefulness, and attention. The cranial nerves (except for the optic nerves) originate in the brainstem and control many critical functions. | Vomiting, ataxia, headache, cranial nerve palsies (hearing loss, head tilt, swallowing problems/drooling, facial droop, hoarse voice), personality changes, long-tract signs (hemiparesis, spastic gait, hyperreflexia, positive Babinski sign [upgoing toes]), increased ICP as a late development |

| Cerebral Hemispheres Tumor Location | Normal Function | Common Symptoms |
|---|---|---|
| Frontal lobe | Motor strip controls voluntary movement on the opposite side of the body, dominant hemisphere controls language and writing, intellectual function, thought processes, behavior, memory. | One-sided paralysis, seizures, short-term memory loss, impaired judgment, personality changes (disinhibition), urinary frequency and urgency, gait disturbance, communication problems |
| Occipital lobe | Understanding visual images and meaning of written words | Visual disturbances, seizures |
| Parietal lobe | Receives and interprets sensations, including pain, temperature, touch, pressure, size, and shape; body part awareness, proprioception (sensation of body location in space); hearing, reasoning, memory | Seizures, language disturbance if dominant hemisphere, loss of ability to read, spatial disorders, loss of ability to do math calculations, difficulty distinguishing left from right |
| Temporal lobe | Understanding sounds and spoken words; emotion and memory; depth perception and sense of time | Seizures, loss of ability to recognize sounds or source of sounds; visual impairments, emotional lability |

| Midline Structures Tumor Location | Normal Function | Common Symptoms |
|---|---|---|
| Thalamus (deep within the hemispheres, adjacent to the lateral ventricles) | Process messages to and from the cerebrum; "gateway" to the cerebral cortex | Any combination of symptoms inherent in cerebral tumors, except seizures |
| Hypothalamus/pituitary | Regulate many hormonal functions in the body, as well as water balance and appetite/satiety; also thought to have a role in temperature control | Diabetes insipidus, syndrome of inappropriate antidiuretic hormone, growth acceleration or failure, precocious puberty, appetite disruption. Often accompanied by visual changes due to proximity to optic chiasm. Symptoms of increased ICP. |
| Optic nerves/chiasm | Transmit visual stimuli to the occipital cortex | Visual disturbances, visual loss; other symptoms of hypothalamic tumors |
| Pineal gland (located at the rear of the third ventricle) | Thought to regulate the biologic rhythm of the body; produces melatonin | Symptoms of increased ICP, especially headache, vomiting, and diplopia; abnormal eye movements (due to proximity with specific cranial nerves) |

| Spinal Cord Tumor Location | Normal Function | Common Symptoms |
|---|---|---|
| Cervical, thoracic, or lumbar | Transmission of motor and sensory impulses to and from the brain. (Please refer to Spinal Cord Injury chapter for more detailed information regarding functional ability. | Localized pain (worse in recumbent position), motor or gait disturbance, spasticity, sensory changes, extremity weakness, mild scoliosis or kyphosis; urethral or anal sphincter dysfunction is less common. The symptoms are highly dependent upon the level of the lesion in the cord. |

Brain and Spinal Cord Tumors

*Tumors of the Pediatric Central Nervous System* (pp. 14–21), R.F. Keating, J.T. Goodrich, and R.J. Packer (Eds.), 2001, New York: Thieme Medical.

## Types of CNS Tumors

As discussed previously, CNS tumors are usually defined by the cell type that they resemble under the microscope, and occasionally by the location of the tumor. **Figure 3** demonstrates the distribution of CNS tumors by histology (cell type) in the pediatric population.

**Figure 3**

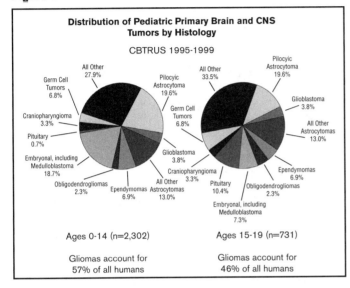

**Figure 3.** Distribution of CNS tumors by cell type in the pediatric population. From *Statistical report: Primary brain tumors in the United States, 1995-1999.* Central Brain Tumor Registry of the United States. Retrieved May 16, 2004, from http://www.cbtrus.org/2002/2003report.pdf. Reprinted with permission from CBTRUS (2002).

## Glial Tumors/Gliomas

The largest category of CNS tumors in children is the gliomas. Gliomas arise from glial cells, which make up the supportive tissue of the brain. The most common type of glial cell is astrocytes, followed by oligodendrocytes, and ependymal cells.

Astrocytomas are the most common type of CNS tumor in children and adolescents and can occur in any location within the CNS. Astrocytomas comprise the majority of the intracranial and spinal cord tumors in children. A specific grading system is used to classify these tumors. Grades I and II are called "low-grade" because they tend to behave in a more benign fashion—slower-growing and less invasive. Grades III and IV are called "high-grade" because they are faster growing and more invasive. Grade I astrocytomas are also called pilocytic astrocytomas, or juvenile pilocytic astrocytomas (JPA). JPAs are most often found in the cerebellum, and account for 80% to 85% of the low-grade tumors in this area (Strother et al., 2002). Cerebellar JPAs are considered the most benign of all childhood CNS tumors

because of the lack of invasiveness and the surgical accessibility. Estimated 10-year relative survival for pilocytic astrocytoma in children is approximately 90% (CBTRUS, 2002). Grade II, or fibrillary, astrocytomas are less common and tend to be more infiltrating. These also have a predilection for the posterior fossa and are considered to be low-grade tumors. Grade III astrocytomas are often referred to as anaplastic astrocytomas because of their microscopic anaplastic (cells lacking differentiation) features. Grade IV astrocytomas are also known as glioblastoma multiforme and carry a dismal prognosis, with an estimated 10 year relative survival rate of approximately 16% (CBTRUS, 2002). Grade III and IV astrocytomas, more commonly found in the cerebral hemispheres, are considered high-grade tumors because of their characteristic invasion into adjacent tissue and tendency to spread more widely and rapidly within the brain, and even occasionally to organs outside the CNS (Strother et al., 2002).

Brainstem gliomas (BSG) are defined by their location in the CNS, which is the critical factor in the outcome for patients with this type of tumor. These tumors can be low-grade or high-grade, infiltrating or focal. Biopsy or surgery is often not possible due to the location in the brainstem; however, low-grade astrocytomas of the brainstem may extend outside of the brainstem, allowing for surgical biopsy or debulking, and tissue diagnosis. Many times the onset of symptoms may be clues to the nature of the tumor, with a rapid onset of symptoms often indicating a higher-grade tumor. Outcome for patients with high-grade BSG is very poor; however, some low-grade BSGs that are surgically accessible carry a good prognosis (Strother et al., 2002)

Ependymomas are technically considered a type of glioma, but due to the unique nature of this type of tumor, it is typically discussed as a separate entity. These tumors arise from the ependymal lining of the ventricular system and are most commonly found in the posterior fossa; however, they can occur anywhere along the lining of the CSF pathways. Ependymomas can spread within the CNS but tend to recur locally. They are usually considered microscopically benign but have garnered the phrase "malignant by location" due to the difficulty in obtaining a total surgical resection and the tendency for recurrence. There is a subset of ependymomas that have more anaplastic features, but a correlation between histology and clinical outcome has not been well established (Strother et al, 2002; Weitman & Cogen, 2001).

Other gliomas include craniopharyngioma, optic glioma, oligodendroglioma, ganglioglioma, and choroid plexus tumors. Craniopharyngiomas are low-grade tumors found in the central structures of the brain, in the area above the sella turcica, which is below the pituitary, hypothalamus, and the optic chiasm (where the optic nerves cross). These tumors have significant morbidity due to the critical function of the structures in that area.

Optic pathway gliomas can occur anywhere along the optic tracts and also are typically low-grade tumors. Patients with the autosomal dominant disorder, neurofibromatosis type I, are at increased risk of developing optic gliomas.

Oligodendrogliomas and gangliogliomas (which are actually glial/neuronal tumors) typically occur supratentorially, and both of these are generally considered low-grade but sometimes behave more aggressively.

Choroid plexus tumors arise from the choroid plexus, which is located within the ventricles, and is responsible for producing CSF. Choroid plexus papilloma is more common than its malignant counterpart, the choroid plexus carcinoma. The prognosis for choroid plexus papilloma is quite good with surgical removal alone.

### Embryonal Tumors

Embryonal tumors, the second most common type of CNS tumor in children (CBTRUS, 2002), arise from more immature or primitive cell types that are poorly differentiated. Classification of these tumors continues to stir controversy in pediatric neuro-oncology circles. In general, tumors that arise from immature cell types tend to be malignant and aggressive. This holds true for embryonal CNS tumors in children, which include medulloblastoma, primitive neuroectodermal tumor (PNET), pineoblastoma, and other less common embryonal tumors (Strother et al., 2002).

Medulloblastomas get their name from the location in which they occur, near the medulla of the brainstem, adjacent to the cerebellum. These are the most common type of malignant brain tumor in children, and they account for 15% to 20% of all pediatric brain tumors (Strother et al., 2002; ABTA, n.d.). Medulloblastomas have a propensity to spread within the CNS by way of the CSF, causing diffuse seeding of tumor along the CSF pathways in the brain and spinal cord (ABTA, n.d.). Metastatic nodules of tumor along the spinal cord are commonly referred to as "drop mets." Spread outside the CNS is rare but has been documented with varying frequency (Strother et al., 2002). Survival for children with medulloblastoma has improved in recent years, with advances in treatment regimens and surgical techniques. For children with "low-risk" localized tumors and near-total surgical removal, the 5-year survival rate ranges from 55% to 79% (Strother et al., 2002). Outcome is lower for those with tumor spread at diagnosis or with significant residual tumor after surgery.

PNET is microscopically identical to medulloblastoma but occurs outside of the posterior fossa. Similarly, pineoblastoma is a PNET of the pineal gland. Because the extent of surgical removal is a significant factor in outcome and the areas in which PNETs occur are either hard to reach surgically or are critical for ongoing function, it is not surprising that survival for patients with supratentorial PNET is lower.

### Germ Cell Tumors

Germ cell tumors are an altogether different category of CNS tumors and may occur as primary tumors within the CNS, typically arising from midline structures in the brain. Germ cell tumors also occur outside of the CNS, in the testes or ovaries, chest or abdomen. CNS germ cell tumors are thought to arise from germ cells that abnormally migrated to the brain (instead of the gonads) during embryogenesis (Strother et al., 2002). There are a number of different CNS germ cell tumors, some considered to be benign and some more malignant. These tumors are unique in that many of them secrete substances into the CSF or the bloodstream that can be measured in a laboratory; a-feto-protein (a-FP) and b-human chorionic gonadotropin (b-HCG) are considered tumor markers for germ cell tumors. Elevation of these markers may eliminate the need for surgical biopsy. Most CNS germ cell tumors can be very sensitive to radiation and chemotherapy; thus aggressive surgical intervention is rarely used (Strother et al., 2002).

### Spinal Cord Tumors

Spinal cord tumors comprise between 4% and 10% of all pediatric primary CNS tumors. Astrocytomas are by far the most common spinal cord tumor in children, followed by ependymomas and a few others. The majority of pediatric spinal cord tumors are low-grade and amenable to surgery, despite a significant percentage of them being intramedullary (within the cord) (Muszynski, Constantini, & Epstein, 2001).

There are other, less prevalent types of CNS tumors in children, but discussion of these is beyond the scope of this chapter. The reader is referred to the bibliography if there is a need to obtain information on an uncommon CNS tumor.

## Management

### Surgery

Maximum surgical resection is the goal for most CNS tumors in children. For the majority of tumor types, there is a direct correlation between extent of resection and prognosis. An exception to this generalization is most germ cell tumors, which respond so well to radiation and chemotherapy that surgical resection is often unnecessary (Strother et al., 2002). Extent of surgical resection is always balanced with the potential for functional deficits; therefore, it is not unusual for some children to have a second operation, following chemotherapy and/or radiation therapy, to remove residual tumor. Advanced surgical technologies, such as the operating microscope, various image-guided surgical systems, and brain mapping, have improved surgical outcomes in recent years. Shaving a large area of the scalp prior to craniotomy is less common these days, and most children will have only the immediate area around the incision shaved.

Some children will have a ventriculoperitoneal (VP) shunt placed to manage hydrocephalus before and/or after surgery. The risk of ventriculitis (infection in the ventricles) is increased for children receiving immunosuppressive steroids or chemotherapy within the first few months following VP shunt placement.

Surgical morbidity varies depending on the location of the tumor. Midline tumors, such as optic gliomas, craniopharyngiomas, and pineal tumors, carry significant risk for morbidity, including visual loss and endocrinopathies such as growth failure, hypothyroidism, diabetes insipidus, precocious puberty, gonadal failure, and hyperphagia (increased appetite), as well as possible mental status changes such as difficulty with memory, personality changes, and mood disturbance (Strother et al., 2002). Functional deficits from cerebral tumors vary based on location and are related to the function of the particular area of the cortex. Some patients with cerebral tumors continue to receive antiepileptic medication, especially if there were seizures preoperatively (Strother et al.). (The reader is referred to the chapter on neurology for further information regarding children with seizure disorders). Thalamic tumors pose another surgical challenge, owing to the processing function of the thalamus; thus resection of these tumors may result in a myriad of deficits, as described in Table 1.

Resection of tumors in the posterior fossa, the most common location for pediatric CNS tumors, may result in varying degrees of deficits, depending on what structures are nearby and the invasiveness of the tumor. Tumors near the brainstem may result in a number of cranial nerve palsies (Table 1). Cerebellar tumors are associated with the greatest success of all the pediatric CNS tumors in achieving maximum resection (Medlock, 2001); however, children with these tumors (benign or malignant) are likely to have some degree of ataxia persisting long after surgery (Sønderkær et al., 2003).

A less common, but significant, constellation of symptoms following surgery for infratentorial tumors has been described in the literature as "cerebellar mutism," "posterior fossa syndrome," or, more recently, "cerebellar cognitive affective syndrome." Symptoms may include transient loss of speech, emotional lability, impairment of executive function, and visual-spatial problems (Sadeh & Cohen, 2001). It is thought to occur from disruption of the cerebellum during surgery. The condition is temporary, although it can persist for weeks to months, with dysarthria (halting, uncoordinated speech) as an intermediate phase (Seiff & Goodrich, 2001).

Surgery for spinal cord tumors has made significant advances in recent years, and it is not unusual for low-grade intramedullary tumors to be completely resected, with excellent long-term survival. Higher-grade tumors tend to be more invasive, increasing the difficulty in achieving a complete resection, and increasing the chance of postoperative morbidity. Scoliosis and kyphosis are common following surgery, and a second surgery to correct these problems may be necessary (Muszynski et al., 2001). Surgery is not indicated for metastatic nodules from intracranial primary tumors, because this is an indication of widespread dissemination of tumor. In this circumstance, the disease may be treated with radiation and/or chemotherapy.

By the time a child returns to school following surgery, acute postoperative pain has usually resolved. However, there may be some chronic pain issues that develop, depending on the child's specific circumstances.

## Corticosteroids

Corticosteroids (also known as glucocorticoids) are commonly used in the management of children with CNS tumors. Dexamethasone is typically used to reduce edema and symptoms of increased intracranial pressure at the time of diagnosis and through the immediate postoperative period. It is usually tapered off over a week's time, unless the child has been taking it for a longer period of time preoperatively, which would necessitate a more gradual taper (Seiff & Goodrich, 2001). Dexamethasone is also commonly used during radiation therapy for prevention or management of radiation-induced symptoms such as nausea, vomiting, headache, or drowsiness. Patients with progressive malignant tumors may be placed on corticosteroids for extended periods of time to help with symptom management. Hydrocortisone, less potent than dexamethasone, is usually used at the end of a long-term corticosteroid taper or for stress-steroid dosing (short-term high-dose steroids during periods of increased stress on the body such as surgery or infection). Side effects of high-dose or prolonged corticosteroid use are well known, including gastrointestinal irritation, immunosuppression and increased risk for infection, compromised wound healing, osteonecrosis (permanently interrupted blood supply to the ends of the long bones, often requiring hip or knee replacement), mood swings, restlessness or agitation, and weight gain due to increased appetite and fluid retention (Seiff & Goodrich, 2001). Only some of these side effects can be prevented or managed; therefore, the benefits and risks are carefully considered.

## Radiation Therapy

Radiation therapy has been used for many decades in the treatment of childhood CNS tumors. Radiation uses high-energy photon and electron beams that cause tissue damage by effects on the DNA molecule (Vines, Bertsch, & Goldwein, 2001). Some of this DNA damage is repairable, but most often it is irreversible. With advances in computer technology, radiation beams can be more effectively targeted to a desired area, allowing for more focused treatment, and increased likelihood that normal tissues are spared. Radiation is typically given in small daily doses called "fractions," over a period of 4 to 6 weeks, depending on the total dose to be administered. A specialized type of radiation, stereotactic radiation, is a high-dose, precisely focused radiation treatment administered in a one-time single dose. It is reserved for that are relatively small and not readily amenable to surgery. The side effects of stereotactic radiation are similar to those from conventional radiation, but there is a higher incidence of tumor necrosis, which may require surgical intervention after all.

Some young children require sedation or anesthesia for their treatments on account of the positioning requirements and the need to lie perfectly still. Most school-aged children are able to receive their treatments without sedation; however, if part of their treatments require a prone position, this may be more difficult for some children without sedation.

The role of radiation therapy in pediatric CNS tumors has changed over the years, with efforts to reduce doses or eliminate radiation altogether, especially for very young children or for supratentorial tumors. This has come about as more has been learned about the long-term effects of radiation therapy in children, especially the cognitive effects. Radiation tends to be reserved for higher-grade or malignant tumors, or for lower-grade tumors that are subtotally resected and at high risk for morbidity with tumor progression. Children with medulloblastoma receive radiation to the whole brain and spinal column, with an additional boost dose to the posterior fossa.

Acute side effects of cranial radiation include fatigue, anorexia (poor appetite), nausea and vomiting, headache, dry or reddened skin at the site of radiation, external otitis, and alopecia (which is sometimes permanent, especially with higher doses). Craniospinal radiation may also cause esophagitis and low blood counts (due to suppression of bone marrow in the vertebral bodies). A common delayed acute side effect of cranial radiation is known as somnolence syndrome; it is characterized by increased sleepiness, which may be profound, occurring between 4 and 8 weeks following the completion of radiation and lasting from 10 days to more than 5 weeks. No focal neurologic abnormalities have been identified with this syndrome (Vines et al., 2001). Dexamethasone is sometimes used to ameliorate the effects of this phenomenon.

Late effects of radiation therapy for CNS tumors in children are significant and may occur from months to years after treatment has been completed. Long-term sequelae of cranial radiation include neurocognitive deficits, endocrine dysfunction, lack of organ maturation, hearing loss, cataracts, dental defects/caries, radiation necrosis, vascular abnormalities, secondary tumors, and alopecia. With spinal radiation, there is also risk for bone marrow changes, cardiovascular and lung damage, as well as damage of the spinal cord resulting in sensory and/or motor deficits (Vines et al., 2001; Strother et al., 2002).

A recent longitudinal analysis of pediatric medulloblastoma survivors supported the findings that younger age at the time of radiation and higher total radiation dose to the cerebrum were associated with poorer intellectual outcome. This study also confirmed the hypothesis that children with medulloblastoma show a decline in intelligence (IQ) scores due to inability to acquire new information and skills at a rate similar to their healthy peers of the same age, rather than a loss of previously learned information (Palmer et. al., 2001).

### Chemotherapy

The role of chemotherapy in the treatment of childhood CNS tumors continues to evolve through cooperative clinical trials at the institutional and national level, as well as through international collaboration. Over the last 20 years, clinical trials have demonstrated the effectiveness of chemotherapy for children with newly diagnosed and recurrent malignant CNS tumors, especially medulloblastomas and high-grade gliomas. The use of chemotherapy has also been established with some benign CNS tumors. Improvements in survival have been shown for some tumor types when chemotherapy is used adjunctively with radiation therapy. In some cases, chemotherapy has reduced or even eliminated the need for radiation therapy (Nicholson & Packer, 2001).

Chemotherapy regimens vary depending on the type of tumor and sometimes on the extent of residual tumor following surgery. Most utilize multiple drugs and involve intravenous (IV) chemotherapy; some utilize oral chemotherapy in addition to or in place of IV chemotherapy. The treatment may be given over a number of months at specified intervals to allow for recovery of blood cell counts and other side effects. Some treatments may be given in an outpatient setting, and some require intermittent hospitalization. Most treatment plans have a written plan of treatment called a "road map" or "schema," which lays out the plan for treatment in a day-by-day or week-by-week fashion.

Many children requiring chemotherapy have an implanted vascular access device, also commonly referred to as a "port," for safe infusion of chemotherapy, IV fluids, transfusions, and other medications. These devices may also be used for blood sampling. With the use of topical anesthetics now readily available, accessing these ports with a special needle is virtually painless. When the port is not in use, it is infused with heparin and the needle is removed, leaving only a small bump under the skin. Most ports are surgically implanted in the upper chest, over the bony rib cage, and the end of the catheter is tunneled under the skin and ends in or near the right atrium of the heart. Another type of central IV catheter, called a right atrial catheter, typically has two lumens, with the catheter extending out of the skin and remaining there for the duration of treatment. This type of catheter requires more maintenance, with dressing changes and daily heparinization, and its use is generally reserved for regimens requiring more intensive treatment and supportive care. The reader is referred to cancer chapter for more information on supportive care.

Despite having a better reputation than radiation when it comes to late effects, chemotherapy is not without sequelae. Most people are familiar with the acute side effects of chemotherapy such as nausea, vomiting, and hair loss, all of which are reversible side effects. Nausea and vomiting can often be prevented with the newer antiemetic agents now available. There are other acute and long-term side effects that may be less known to the average person. Some of these are drug class–specific, and others are more universal. (See cancer chapter.)

Because chemotherapy in general targets rapidly growing cells, the logical untoward effects on normal tissues are seen in the bone marrow, the gastrointestinal tract, and the hair follicles. Side effects in these areas are usually acute, resulting in low blood counts and increased risk for infection, mouth sores, and alopecia. The peak of these short-term effects usually occurs 10 to 14 days following each treatment. It is often thought that the biggest risk for infection in patients with a low white blood cell count is germs from others, but to the contrary, the greatest risk is from bacteria that come from the patient's own body (skin or gastrointestinal tract) and enter the bloodstream through compromised tissue or central venous catheter.

Other side effects from chemotherapy result from direct effects on tissues. Many chemotherapeutic agents cause irritation of the chemoreceptor trigger zone in the brain, resulting in nausea and vomiting that is immediate or delayed. Chemotherapy drugs may have effects on the bladder (bleeding), kidneys (renal damage resulting in electrolyte imbalance), liver (elevated enzymes, or even more severe dysfunction), gonads (infertility, delayed or precocious puberty), skin (photosensitivity, pigment changes), heart (decreased ejection fraction), or lungs (fibrosis). A few of the agents often used in CNS tumors also may cause sensorineural hearing loss or neurologic effects such as peripheral nerve weakness (including foot-drop, constipation, droopy eyelids) and paresthesias (tingling, numbness, pain), or damage to white matter in the brain (which is thought to contribute to learning difficulties). Some of these organ-specific effects may be permanent, such as hearing loss, heart damage, kidney damage, infertility, lung damage, and neurologic deficits (Kaplan & Jenkins, 1998). Other side effects are self-limited or preventable/reversible with medication or other interventions, such as fluid hydration.

Peripheral blood stem-cell rescue is a treatment regimen that involves taking stem cells from the patient and saving them to be given back to that patient to "rescue" the bone marrow after high-dose chemotherapy. This treatment is used in infants and very young children, to avoid or delay radiation therapy, and is also being studied in relapsed patients as a "salvage" treatment. This is a high-morbidity treatment, with increased risk for life-threatening complications.

### Follow-up Care

Following completion of surgery or treatment, patients are monitored with magnetic resonance imaging (MRI) scans of the tumor area to watch for recurrence or progression. History taking and physical examination, with a thorough neurologic examination, are perhaps even more important than MRI for detecting not only tumor recurrence or progression, but also for detecting lingering effects of surgery or treatment. The interval of this follow-up care is usually determined by the clinical trial and/or the risk for that particular patient of tumor recurrence or progression. In the first year following treatment, follow-up is usually every 3 to 6 months, and in years thereafter, less frequently if the patient's status is stable. Many pediatric tertiary centers have comprehensive clinics for treatment and follow up of children with CNS tumors in which the patient and family can see multiple specialists at the same visit. Long-term follow-up or late-effects clinics are also important for assisting patients and families who may be dealing with significant long-term effects of treatment.

For children with CNS tumors, especially those who received cranial radiation, periodic testing by a pediatric neuropsychologist affiliated with a pediatric oncology program is ideal and may be a helpful adjunct to the testing and support provided by the child's school district. Early detection of cognitive, academic, and psychosocial difficulties is desirable, and the parents and school staff often see problems first, because these are the people who know the child best. Barriers to care (such as lack of insurance coverage, transportation issues) may interfere with the patient's ability to participate in regular follow-up with the CNS tumor program, so the observations of parents and school staff become even more important in detecting difficulties that the child may have following treatment. Accommodations to assist the student in compensating for or overcoming deficits should be implemented, as part of an individualized healthcare plan (IHP), 504 plan, or individualized education plan (IEP). Consideration should be given to extended-school-year opportunities, if available, for those students who struggle to retain skills over the summer months.

# Individual Healthcare Plan

## Assessment

*History*

- When was the tumor diagnosed?
- What type of tumor does the student have?
- Where is/was the tumor located?
- What were the presenting symptoms?
- What is the grade of the tumor? (If applicable)
- Is the tumor localized or are there metastases?
- What is the student's prognosis, if known?
- Were there any predisposing factors?
- What was the student's health and growth/development prior to the tumor?
- When and what type of surgery (if any) did the student have?
- What was the extent of the surgical resection?
- What, if any, were the surgical complications?
- Were there any functional deficits following surgery? Have they resolved?
- Did the student receive physical, occupational, or speech therapy? Are these ongoing?
- How long was the student hospitalized at the time of diagnosis and/or surgery? What was the frequency/duration of hospitalization(s) following initial discharge?
- What was the student's school attendance pattern?
- What were the significant events or procedures during the hospitalization?
- Does the student have a VP shunt? Is it unilateral or bilateral?
- Did/will the student receive radiation therapy? When? To what site? At what dose?
- Did/will the student receive chemotherapy? When? What drugs? What route? Outpatient or inpatient?
- What side effects have been experienced?
- Does the student have a central line? What type is it? When was it placed?
- Does the student have a gastrostomy or nasogastric tube? Are there tube feedings?
- Does the student have a home-care company or home-care nurse?
- Who is caring for the student at home?
- What is the family structure? Are there siblings?

*Current Status and Management*

- Current status of the tumor/response to treatment
- Treatment/follow-up plan; radiation therapy, chemotherapy, surgery; road maps of treatment
- Current functional status, including ambulation, feeding/swallowing, coordination (fine motor, gross motor, balance), strength, mobility, sensation, speech, vision, hearing, bowel and bladder function, ability to manage activities of daily living (ADLs)
- Baseline height and weight
- Baseline vital signs
- Baseline respiratory and cardiac assessment
- Baseline abdominal assessment (especially quality and extent of bowel sounds)
- Baseline neurologic assessment
- Baseline skin and mucous membrane assessment
- Current pain assessment
- Current and ongoing spine assessment (observe for scoliosis/kyphosis in student with spinal cord tumor)
- Assess for side effects of radiation (if applicable):
- Short-term: fatigue, anorexia (poor appetite), nausea and vomiting, headache, dry or reddened skin, external otitis, alopecia, esophagitis, low blood counts, somnolence
- Long-term: alopecia, short stature, growth failure, precocious puberty/gonadal failure, thyroid dysfunction, hearing loss, dental problems/caries, cognitive dysfunction/academic difficulties
- Assess for side effects of chemotherapy (if applicable):
- Gastrointestinal: nausea, vomiting, anorexia, diarrhea, constipation, jaundice (impaired liver function), abdominal pain, difficulty swallowing
- Skin/mucous membranes: mouth sores, rashes, bruising or other discoloration, alopecia, sensitivity to sunlight, signs of dehydration

- Bone marrow suppression: low platelets (bruising, petechiae), low hemoglobin (pallor, tachycardia, systolic murmur, fatigue, shortness of breath), low white blood cell (WBC) count (may see mouth sores with low WBC)
- Infection/sepsis (from low WBC): fever, chills, hypotension, fainting
- Respiratory/cardiovascular: shortness of breath, wheezing, crackles, irregular heart rate, hypertension, chest pain, heart murmur/rub
- Genitourinary/renal: urinary frequency, dysuria, gross hematuria, abdominal or flank pain, hypertension, edema, secondary amenorrhea
- Musculoskeletal/neurologic: cramping, weakness, tripping/falling, difficulty with stairs, paresthesias, vision changes, hearing loss, headaches
- Treatment/procedure orders
- Activity orders
- Medications
- Diet/feedings
- Central venous catheter care
- Gastrostomy/nasogastric tube care

## Self-care
- Student's ability and motivation to participate in ADLs in school and at home
- Limitations to student participating in self-care
- Student's willingness to accept assistance when necessary
- Student's knowledge of side effects and ability to manage side effects
- Student's understanding of warning signs indicating the need to seek medical care
- Does the student wear a medical alert bracelet?

## Psychosocial Status
- Student's knowledge of tumor, surgery, treatment plan, and prognosis for survival
- Student's perception of functional status, prognosis for recovery of deficits
- Parent(s)' perception of student's functional status, prognosis for recovery
- Current emotional status, interaction with peers, family, and adults
- Student's developmental level
- Current coping strategies for student and family
- Peer group knowledge about the diagnosis and treatment
- Student's feelings regarding real and potential reaction of peers and family
- Student's feelings about the tumor or about having cancer (if tumor is malignant)
- Past and current participation in activities within the family, peer group, school, and extracurricular setting
- Level of involvement of support services/support persons/groups
- Evidence of depression and/or grieving

## Academic Issues
- Academic performance pattern
- Attendance pattern
- Instructional setting history (homebound, hospital instruction, other)
- Current cognitive status, including ability to comprehend, ability to communicate, or other nuances that may be helpful to ascertain (any neuropsychological reports)
- School health services required: medications, special procedures
- Physical environment issues: wheelchair access if necessary, access to elevator
- Classroom and school accommodations needed: schedule modification; assistance with moving between classes; help with lunch, locker, toileting; access to computer, library, media center; availability of peer and paraprofessional assistance
- Curriculum accommodations: workload, performance expectations, make-up time, type of activities (lab, small group, independent), method of testing (written, oral, having tests read, computer tests, essay, multiple choice), adaptive physical education
- Extracurricular accommodations: plan for attendance at school-sponsored after-school events
- Need for a written 504 accommodation plan
- Special education services—past and current needs

- Special transportation needs
- Emergency evacuation plan

## Nursing Diagnoses (N.D.) (NANDA, 2003)

(The reader is referred to the spinal cord injury chapter for diagnoses related to spinal cord tumors and the neurology chapter for diagnoses related to seizures.)

**N.D. 1** Activity intolerance (NANDA 00092) related to:
- generalized weakness
- fatigue
- medication side effects
- radiation side effects

**N.D. 2** Impaired physical mobility (NANDA 00085) related to:
- neuromuscular impairment
- sensoriperceptual impairment
- medication side effects

**N.D. 3** Impaired walking (NANDA 00088) related to:
- ataxia
- neuromuscular impairment
- medication side effects

**N.D. 4** Risk for disuse syndrome (NANDA 00040) related to:
- neuromuscular impairment

**N.D. 5** Unilateral neglect (NANDA 00123) related to:
- hemianopsia (from cerebral or optic nerve damage)

**N.D. 6** Disturbed sensory perception: visual, auditory, tactile (NANDA 00122) related to:
- injury to nerve or brain tissue from tumor and/or surgery

**N.D. 7** Impaired verbal communication (NANDA 00051) related to:
- injury to nerve or brain tissue from tumor, radiation, and/or surgery
- visual/auditory impairment

**N.D. 8** Disturbed thought processes (NANDA 00130) related to:
- injury to brain tissue from tumor, radiation therapy, and/or surgery
- medication side effects (steroids)

**N.D. 9** Ineffective protection (NANDA 00043) related to:
- immunosuppression from treatment
- bone marrow suppression
- neurosensory impairment
- impaired skin integrity
- inadequate nutrition

**N.D. 10** Risk for infection (NANDA 00004) related to:
- immunosuppression from treatment
- inadequate primary defenses (surgical wounds, central venous catheter, VP shunt)
- inadequate secondary defenses (leukopenia, decreased inflammatory response)

**N.D. 11** Risk for injury (NANDA 00035) related to:
- impaired mobility
- ataxia
- sensory deficit
- thrombocytopenia (low platelet count)

**N.D. 12** Decreased intracranial adaptive capacity (NANDA 00049) related to:
- increased intracranial pressure from VP shunt malfunction or tumor progression

**N.D. 13** Risk for impaired skin integrity (NANDA 00046) related to:
- immobility
- medication side effects
- radiation side effects
- inadequate nutrition
- percutaneous catheter(s) (central venous catheter, gastrostomy tube)

**N.D. 14** Self-care deficit related to functional and/or cognitive limitations:
- feeding (NANDA 00102)
- bathing/hygiene (NANDA 00108)

- dressing/grooming self-care deficit (NANDA 00109)
- toileting self-care deficit (NANDA 00110)

**N.D. 15** Fatigue (NANDA 00093) related to:
- medication side effects
- radiation side effects
- anemia
- malnutrition
- inadequate sleep

**N.D. 16** Nausea (NANDA 00134) related to:
- chemotherapy/medication side effects
- radiation therapy
- CNS tumor
- increased intracranial pressure

**N.D. 17** Imbalanced nutrition: Less than body requirements (NANDA 00002) related to:
- anorexia
- nausea/vomiting
- mucositis (mouth sores)
- ineffective swallowing

**N.D. 18** Risk for constipation (NANDA 00015) related to:
- medication side effects
- inadequate activity
- change in eating patterns
- neurologic impairment

**N.D. 19** Diarrhea (NANDA 00013) related to:
- chemotherapy
- inflammation
- infectious process

**N.D. 20** Impaired oral mucous membrane (NANDA 00045) related to:
- chemotherapy
- leukopenia
- radiation therapy

**N.D. 21** Impaired dentition (NANDA 00048) related to:
- chemotherapy
- chemotherapy/medication side effects
- radiation therapy
- ineffective oral hygiene
- nutritional deficit

**N.D. 22** Risk for imbalanced fluid volume (NANDA 00025) related to:
- medication side effects
- vomiting or diarrhea
- diabetes insipidus
- syndrome of inappropriate antidiuretic hormone

**N.D. 23** Impaired swallowing (NANDA 00103) related to:
- neurologic impairment
- impaired oral mucous membrane

**N.D. 24** Ineffective airway clearance (NANDA 00031) related to:
- neurologic impairment
- medication/chemotherapy side effects
- radiation therapy

**N.D. 25** Pain, acute (NANDA 00132) or chronic (NANDA 00133), related to:
- effects of tumor, surgery, or treatments
- medication side effects

**N.D. 26** Disturbed sleep pattern (NANDA 00095) related to:
- hospitalization
- medication/treatment effects
- delayed sleep phase

**N.D. 27** Risk for disproportionate growth (NANDA 00113) related to:
- hyperphagia, fluid retention from corticosteroids
- inadequate oral intake from nausea, vomiting, anorexia, impaired swallowing
- growth hormone deficiency

**N.D. 28** Risk for delayed development (NANDA 00112) related to:
- cranial radiation
- chemotherapy
- sensory impairment (visual and/or auditory)
- tumor/surgical effects

**N.D. 29** Deficient knowledge (NANDA 00126) of tumor and its treatment related to:
- lack of exposure/access to information
- inadequate recall of information
- cognitive limitation related to tumor

**N.D. 30** Impaired adjustment (NANDA 00070) related to:
- intense emotions and stressors
- lack of optimism
- inadequate support to adapt to diagnosis

**N.D. 31** Ineffective coping (NANDA 00069) related to:
- situational crisis
- uncertainty of prognosis
- inadequate social support

**N.D.32** Impaired social interaction (NANDA 00052) related to:
- impaired communication skills
- cognitive/behavioral impairment
- physical limitations
- frequent or prolonged absence from school

**N.D. 33** Social isolation (NANDA 00053) related to:
- physical limitations
- cognitive/behavioral impairment
- alteration in physical appearance
- frequent or prolonged absence from school

**N.D. 34** Risk for situational low self-esteem (NANDA 00153) related to:
- tumor diagnosis and functional impairment
- side effects of treatment (changes in appearance)
- diminished social interaction/social isolation

**N.D. 35** Ineffective health maintenance (NANDA 00099) related to:
- cognitive impairment
- impaired communication skills
- inability to cope with illness

**N.D. 36** Ineffective therapeutic regimen management (NANDA 00078) related to:
- knowledge deficit/complexity of regimen
- cognitive impairment
- mistrust of healthcare system
- inadequate support
- powerlessness/inability to cope with illness

**N.D. 37** Risk for powerlessness (NANDA 00152) related to:
- functional impairment
- knowledge deficit
- low self-esteem

**N.D. 38** Hopelessness (NANDA 00124) related to:
- social isolation
- physiologic deterioration
- possible poor prognosis

**N.D. 39** Death anxiety (NANDA 00147) related to:
- ineffective coping
- fears/knowledge deficit
- morbid prognosis of disease

**N.D. 40** Interrupted family processes (NANDA 00060) related to:
- crisis of diagnosis and treatment
- shift in family roles
- modification in family finances

## Goals

The student will attend school when able and participate in classroom activities, including physical education, with appropriate modifications as necessary. (N.D. 1–7, 15, 25, 26)

The student will adjust energy expenditure during the school day relative to activity tolerance level. (N.D. 1, 15, 26)

The student will maintain independent mobility when able and utilize assistance when necessary to remain mobile in the school setting. (N.D. 2, 3, 6, 25)

The student will maximize functional status by fully utilizing his/her body as able and participating in physical, occupational, and/or speech therapy as ordered. (N.D. 2–7, 14, 35, 36)

The student will improve self-care skill(s) [specify skill(s)]. (N.D. 14)

The student will remain free from physical injury. (N.D. 9, 11)

The student will participate in the development of an emergency evacuation plan (EEP). (N.D. 1-3, 6)

The student will successfully communicate and receive information in the school setting, using accommodations as indicated for speech/language, auditory, or visual impairment. (N.D. 6, 7)

The student will succeed academically in accordance with developmental level and cognitive abilities. (N.D. 6–8, 28)

The student will increase knowledge of tumor, treatment, side effects, and long-term issues. (N.D. 29, 35, 36)

The student will maintain a regular bowel pattern. (N.D. 18)

The student will experience minimal nausea, vomiting, diarrhea, or mucositis. (N.D. 16, 19, 20)

The student will experience safe swallowing of appropriate liquids and/or solids. (N.D. 23, 24)

The student will experience minimal to no pain during the school day. (N.D. 25)

The student will obtain adequate sleep so he/she may participate fully in expected activities or tasks. (N.D. 26)

The student will maintain an appropriate weight during treatment, and maintain normal growth pattern. (N.D. 16, 17, 19, 20, 22, 23, 27)

The student will maintain oral/dental health. (N.D. 9, 10, 14, 20, 21, 35, 36)

The student will identify and act appropriately upon symptoms requiring medical attention. (N.D. 9, 10, 12, 13, 16, 18–20, 22–26, 35, 36)

The student will participate in the development and management of an emergency care plan (ECP) for management of serious complications such as infection, bleeding, or increased intracranial pressure. (N.D. 10, 12, 36)

The student will participate in development of and efforts to maintain his/her health and treatment plan(s). (N.D. 35, 36)

The student will adjust to living with a chronic or life-threatening illness. (N.D. 30)

The student will appropriately cope with the stressors related to his/her illness. (N.D. 31)

The student will receive adequate social support to adjust and cope with his/her illness. (N.D. 32–36, 38)

The student will maintain peer relationships and activities. (N.D. 32–34)

The student will maintain or increase self-esteem vis-à-vis his/her alteration in physical appearance and/or functional status. (N.D. 34, 37, 38)

The student will experience some sense of hope and empowerment within the school setting. (N.D. 37, 38)

The student will feel supported to discuss fears of death or end-of-life issues. (N.D. 39)

The student will be supported to accommodate to changes in the family system. (N.D. 40)

## Nursing Interventions

Initiate appropriate homebound/hospital instruction if student meets criteria and is in need of services. (N.D. 1)

Assist with arranging special transportation to and from school if indicated. (N.D. 2, 3, 6)

Participate in communication between school, hospital/clinic, and home in regard to management of health condition or related issues within the school setting. (N.D. 1–40)

Maintain regular communication with student and family regarding management of health condition and related issues. (N.D. 35, 36, 40)

Educate and support staff with regard to student diagnosis, treatment, and effects, functional and/or cognitive limitations, and end-of-life issues if necessary. (N.D 1–40)

Identify and monitor (as appropriate) student's level of functioning in regard to physical, sensory, cognitive, academic, psychosocial, and emotional status through record review, interview, and direct assessment, and communicate status to appropriate school personnel or others as necessary. (N.D. 1–40)

Monitor student's height and weight if indicated, and notify parent/guardian or appropriate healthcare personnel of significant changes or deviation from expected values. (N.D. 27)

Identify student's level of ability in accomplishing ADLs. (N.D. 14)

Develop IHP(s) to establish management of the student's health-related needs in the school setting. (N.D. 1–40)

Develop an ECP to establish management of emergency health situations in the school setting, including criteria for calling 911. (N.D. 9–12, 24)

Develop an EEP to establish procedures for evacuating student from the school, should the need arise. (N.D. 11)

Assess school environment for situations that pose potential injury risk to student, and facilitate modifications to improve student safety. (N.D. 9, 11)

Make arrangements for assistance and/or modifications if necessary for student participation in daily school activities, such as paraprofessional support, schedule modification, alternate passing times, assistive devices, railings/grab bars, wheelchair accessibility, and elevator access as needed. (N.D. 1–3, 6-11, 14, 23–26)

Participate with school guidance personnel and/or the multidisciplinary student support team to determine student eligibility and/or needs related to Section 504 accommodation plan or individualized education plan. (N.D. 6–8, 28)

Advocate for extended-school-year opportunities to facilitate academic skill retention, if indicated. (N.D. 8, 28)

Function in a collaborative role as necessary with occupational therapy (OT), physical therapy (PT), speech therapists, audiologists, deaf/hard-of-hearing teachers, and vision specialists in monitoring and supporting student to improve functional status and adapt to school environment. (N.D. 1–9, 11, 23)

Work with student and staff as appropriate to maximize student's independence with ADLs, and provide or arrange for assistance as necessary, e.g., paraprofessional support. (N.D. 14)

Provide, or delegate appropriately, health-related services and/or procedures that the student may require in the school setting, including medication administration, symptom management, vital sign monitoring, sensory assessment, enteral feedings, oral hygiene, or other specialized procedures as necessary. (N.D. 9, 10, 12–14, 21)

Allow for rest periods, snacks, or oral fluids in the health office as needed. (N.D. 1, 15, 17, 26)

Allow for frequent and easy access to restroom as necessary. (N.D. 16, 18, 19)

Assess student's understanding of diagnosis, prognosis, treatment, side effects, and when to seek medical attention. (N.D. 29)

Reinforce and augment education that student has received about diagnosis, treatment, side effects, and management of his/her health needs. (N.D. 29, 30, 35–37)

Monitor student's ability level to manage his/her health condition, and provide instruction/support to student to increase self-management skills. (N.D. 29, 35, 36)

Assess and monitor student's psychosocial/emotional status and provide support and referral as indicated. (N.D. 30–34, 37–39)

Utilize active listening with student and family, and encourage expression of fears, anxieties, concerns, loss, and grief. (N.D. 30, 31, 37–40)

Encourage student to identify strengths and positive experiences, and reinforce the student's positive self-appraisals. (N.D. 34, 37, 38)

Assist student with maintaining and/or promoting appropriate peer relationships through direct support of student and collaboration with family, staff, and healthcare personnel. (N.D. 32–34, 37, 38)

Encourage student to share questions and feelings regarding diagnosis, treatment, limitations, appearance, and peer/family relationships with school staff, peers, healthcare team, and family. (N.D. 29–40)

Discuss with student/family having a staff person from the healthcare team (Child Life Specialist, nurse, or social worker) visit the school to provide information and guidance to students and staff with regard to diagnosis, treatment, and its impact on the student, family, peers, and others. (N.D. 29–34, 37–40)

Support student and family with adaptation, coping, and changes in school and family processes related to diagnosis and/or treatment; provide for referral as indicated. (N.D. 30, 31)

## Expected Student Outcomes

The student will:

- Have an appropriate IHP, ECP, and EEP in place for management of care in the school setting. (N.D. 1–40)
- Attend school when able and/or will receive hospital or homebound instruction as indicated. (N.D. 1)
- Demonstrate appropriate activity level modifications relative to tolerance, as evidenced by utilizing the health office for brief rest periods or naps if necessary, or using a wheelchair for longer distances. (N.D. 1, 15, 26)
- Become progressively more mobile in the school setting, by demonstrating improved mobility skill(s) [specify skill(s)]. (N.D. 2, 3, 6, 25)

- Utilize assistive devices (such as a walker or wheelchair) to maximize mobility in the school setting. (N.D. 2, 3, 6, 25)
- Show improved functional status through active participation in PT, OT, and/or speech therapy regimens. (N.D. 2–7, 14, 35, 36)
- Demonstrate improved self-care skill(s) [specify skill(s)]. (N.D. 14)
- Explain ways to protect himself/herself from injury in the school setting. (N.D. 9, 11, 29)
- Describe the plan for emergency evacuation from the school building. (N.D. 1–3)
- Demonstrate intelligible communication through his/her speech and/or use of assistive devices. (N.D. 6, 7)
- Demonstrate academic success in accordance with developmental level and cognitive abilities, as shown by remaining at grade level, retaining knowledge and skills, mastering new concepts and skills to full capability, and receiving team and/or resource instruction to achieve educational goals if necessary. (N.D. 6–8, 28)
- Show improved understanding of diagnosis, treatment and effects, and longer term issues by being able to tell the story of his/her diagnosis and treatment, and being able to verbalize side effects and how they affect his/her life. (N.D. 29, 35, 36)
- Defecate with ease and regularity. (N.D. 18)
- Experience no (or minimal) episodes of nausea, vomiting, diarrhea, or mucositis in the school setting. (N.D. 16, 19, 20)
- Have no episodes of aspiration in the school setting. (N.D. 23, 24)
- Exhibit minimal to no signs of discomfort during the school day. (N.D. 25)
- Express satisfaction with the amount and quality of sleep he/she is receiving. (N.D. 26)
- Eat lunch and drink beverages without emesis. (N.D. 16, 17, 19, 20, 22, 23, 27)
- Exhibit appropriate weight and height for age based on standardized growth charts with consideration given for short-term treatment effects. (N.D. 27)
- Remain free from dental caries or gingivitis and experience no more than the expected amount of mucositis. (N.D. 9, 10, 14, 20, 21, 35, 36)
- Explain symptoms requiring immediate medical attention, seek attention of an adult when experiencing unusual symptoms, and follow treatment plan to minimize symptoms. (N.D. 9, 10, 12, 13, 16, 18–20, 22-26, 35, 36)
- Demonstrate compliance with treatment plan. (N.D. 29, 35, 36)
- Show satisfactory adjustment to living with a chronic or life-threatening illness by being able to participate in academic, social, and/or community activities. (N.D. 30)
- Exhibit successful coping skills for dealing with the stresses of his/her health condition and accompanying effects, such as participating in support group(s), confiding in a trusted friend or adult, or seeking assistance when unable to handle things. (N.D. 31)
- Express satisfaction with and demonstrate benefit from the amount of social support he/she is receiving. (N.D. 32–36, 38)
- Exhibit maintenance and/or development of appropriate peer relationships in the school setting. (N.D. 32–34)
- Express ways to cope with peer response to alterations in his/her appearance or functioning, and show successful implementation of these coping strategies. (N.D. 34, 37, 38)
- Express hope(s) and appraisal(s) of strengths to peers and/or staff members. (N.D. 34, 37, 38)
- Express desires, concerns, or fears regarding possible end-stage events in the school setting. (N.D. 39)
- Show successful accommodation to changes in the family system by being able to identify who to go to with fears/worries, who is responsible for transportation, and who to contact with and urgent concern. (N.D. 40)

# Case Study

Jeremy is a 9-year-old boy who will be starting 4th grade at Pine Valley Elementary School in the fall. Jeremy was diagnosed as having medulloblastoma, a malignant brain tumor, in late June. He underwent a poster fossa craniotomy for removal of the tumor from the fourth ventricle, near the cerebellum. He also required placement of a VP shunt. Prior to the diagnosis, Jeremy had developed some difficulty with balance and could no longer ride his bike or rollerblade because he was experiencing some falls. He also complained of morning headaches and went on to develop vomiting as well. His parents also noticed that his eye movements looked a little jerky. His symptoms progressively worsened, and his pediatrician ordered an MRI, which detected the tumor. Jeremy was previously a healthy young boy who enjoyed sports, the outdoors, and playing with his friends. He had no problems academically and received satisfactory grades.

Jeremy's tumor was totally removed, and he had no evidence of spread to the rest of the brain or spine. His spinal fluid was also free of tumor cells. He had postoperative posterior fossa syndrome, with absent speech followed by dysarthria, and left-sided weakness. He had emotional outbursts that were very troubling to his parents. His physical deficits also included fine motor incoordination, ataxia, and nystagmus. He had postoperative diplopia, which resolved. Jeremy received inpatient rehabilitation, including PT, OT and speech therapy. He currently receives these therapies as an outpatient twice a week. He is ambulating with a walker, and uses a wheelchair only for longer distances. Jeremy needs some assistance with getting on and off the toilet, but once he is on, he is independent in his toileting needs. He is right-handed, and is able to write, albeit slowly.

Jeremy received an implanted port for vascular access for chemotherapy treatments and blood work. It is located under the skin of his left upper chest. He began daily (Monday through Friday) radiation treatments in early August and will complete his radiation on September 10. He needed sedation early on during radiation therapy but now is able to stay still on his own. He also receives weekly intravenous (IV) push chemotherapy with vincristine during this radiation therapy phase. He will then have a 4-week break before he begins the maintenance phase of his treatment. This will involve stronger chemotherapy, administered in the hospital or clinic every 3 to 4 weeks for approximately 1 year. He will receive cisplatin (IV), cyclophosphamide (IV), vincristine (IV), and lomustine (oral) on a schedule to allow for recovery of blood cell counts in between cycles of chemotherapy. Cisplatin can cause kidney dysfunction with electrolyte imbalance, permanent sensorineural hearing loss, tingling in fingers and toes, and severe nausea and vomiting. Cyclophosphamide can cause nausea and vomiting as well as hemorrhagic cystitis. It also may result in infertility. Lomustine can cause nausea and vomiting as well as lung damage. Vincristine can cause nerve weakness, constipation, jaw pain, and numbness or tingling in fingers or toes. Sometimes neurologic sequelae from vincristine may persist for the long term. All of the chemotherapy drugs cause low blood cell counts except vincristine.

The radiation treatments caused Jeremy to feel tired, with headaches and nausea. He has restarted treatment with a low dose of dexamethasone to counteract these effects, but the dexamethasone is causing some mood swings and also has increased his appetite. Jeremy has gained about 10 pounds since the start of radiation therapy. Jeremy's blood cell counts are slightly low following the spinal radiation he received, though he has not required any transfusions.

Jeremy is having some issues with constipation from the vincristine, and he takes daily laxatives to keep his bowel movements regular. The vincristine has also caused some nerve weakness in his legs, making it more difficult for Jeremy to dorsiflex at the ankle. This has resulted in a plateau in his physical therapy progress. Jeremy is beginning to lose his hair as well, and this is somewhat distressing to him, because he is worried about how his friends will treat him. He had a few friends visit him when he was in the hospital, but now that he is busy with radiation treatments every day and is more fatigued, he has not had much contact with his pals.

Jeremy lives at home with his parents Mindy and John, 5-year-old sister Jenna, and their dog, Max. Jenna will be starting full-day kindergarten this fall. Jeremy's mom and dad were both working outside the home prior to the diagnosis, but now Mindy is home on a leave of absence to care for Jeremy. The family plans for her to return to work once Jeremy is done with radiation, and then when he starts his chemotherapy phase, his parents plan to alternate time off to be with him for his treatments. The medical insurance coverage leaves them with significant out-of-pocket expenses, so his parents are worried about finances. They have one set of grandparents who live locally and can help out with meals and child care. They are also well connected in their church community and in their neighborhood.

Jeremy has been well informed about his treatments and side effects by staff at the hospital and clinic and has made a special bond with Kirsten, the Child Life Specialist, who has spent a lot of time with Jeremy, helping him process at his own level what has happened and will happen to him. He needs reinforcement of new information to assimilate it into his reality. He has resisted taking medications, and his mother has some frustrations with this at home. They have a chart that they use at home to help motivate him to accomplish his daily tasks, and he receives "rewards" from the clinic prize box when he fills up his stickers for the week.

Jeremy is aware that this illness does cause some kids to die but that chances are good that he will survive. His parents have been open with him if he asks questions, but have not made a point to initiate discussions in this area, and they wish for others to respect and adhere to this approach. They have also utilized counseling through the hospital psychologist and social worker to help them deal with the emotional roller coaster they have been on over the last couple of months. His parents have some trepidation about starting the chemotherapy phase of the treatment, because of their own experience with John's father, who received chemotherapy for adult lymphoma and had many side effects.

Jeremy had baseline neurologic testing prior to the start of radiation therapy and, in general, his scores fell in the average range.

Jeremy's parents visited the school (which is on a single level) earlier this week, and in meeting with them, several health-related concerns were identified.

- Jeremy will need accommodations for safety and convenience when moving from one area of the school to another, especially if he needs to carry something with him.
- Jeremy may need assistance getting on and off the bus.
- An EEP and an ECP will need to be established.
- Jeremy will need extra time to complete written assignments and may benefit from receiving class notes printed or typed.
- Jeremy will need assistance with toileting until he regains enough strength and balance to become independent.
- Jeremy will need ready access to a handicap-equipped bathroom, to maximize bowel regularity.
- Jeremy will need help to open his milk carton or other sealed container(s), due to weakness and incoordination of his hands.
- Jeremy may need a healthy snack mid-morning and/or mid-afternoon to satisfy real hunger caused by dexamethasone.
- Jeremy's exposure to contagious persons should be avoided or minimized.
- Jeremy may need to have vital signs monitored during the chemotherapy phase, especially temperature and blood pressure.
- Homebound instruction may be needed on an intermittent basis once the chemotherapy phase starts.
- Additional make-up time and/or alternate assignments may be necessary to accommodate for frequent absences.
- Jeremy would like Kirsten, the Child Life Specialist from the clinic, to come to the school and talk with his teacher and classmates about his diagnosis and treatment. He thinks that this will help them understand and support him.
- Effective communication between health services and the family regarding bowel pattern, vital signs, oral intake, or symptoms of concern will be essential.
- Jeremy should receive PT, OT, and speech therapy as indicated in the school setting, when he is in attendance.

# Brain and Spinal Cord Tumors

| Assessment Data | Nursing Diagnosis | Goals | Nursing Interventions | Expected Outcomes |
|---|---|---|---|---|
| Jeremy will miss school for treatments and possibly for side effects.<br><br>Jeremy is easily fatigued.<br><br>He has left-sided weakness, and ambulating increases his energy expenditure.<br><br>Jeremy has experienced fatigue from radiation therapy and needs a short nap mid-morning and late afternoon to get through the day. | Activity intolerance related to: (1) weakness; (2) fatigue; (3) radiation side effects (NANDA 00092)<br><br>Fatigue related to: radiation side effects | Student will have an appropriate school attendance pattern.<br><br>Student will modify activity level based on tolerance. | Provide for rest periods as needed during the school day.<br><br>Facilitate student's participation in adaptive physical education.<br><br>Encourage student to listen to his body signals to rest.<br><br>Initiate homebound instruction as indicated. | Student will attend school when able and participate in classroom activities, including physical education as tolerated.<br><br>Student will show progress with activity tolerance when expected, as evidenced by walking between classes instead of using a wheelchair or walker.<br><br>Student will demonstrate appropriate modifications in his activity level, as evidenced by napping during the day when fatigued. |
| Jeremy has weakness of his left arm, hand, and leg.<br><br>Jeremy has difficulty with dorsiflexing his feet at the ankles.<br><br>Jeremy has a broad-based gait and has difficulty maintaining his balance and coordination when walking.<br><br>Jeremy uses a walker to ambulate. | Impaired physical mobility related to: (1) left-sided weakness; (2) vincristine side effects. (NANDA 00085)<br><br>Impaired walking related to: (1) ataxia; (2) left-sided weakness; (3) vincristine side effects | Student will maintain independent mobility when able and utilize assistance when necessary to remain mobile in school.<br><br>Student will maximize functional status by fully utilizing his body as able and participating in PT/OT as ordered. | Encourage student in the use of his walker, and arrange for assistance as necessary in moving about the school. He may need an adult to accompany him until it is determined that he can be fully independent, or can walk with a peer.<br><br>Arrange for another student or staff member to carry his belongings.<br><br>Arrange for assistance getting on and off the bus at school.<br><br>Facilitate student's participation in PT/OT sessions. | Student will become progressively more mobile in the school setting, eventually eliminating the need for a walker.<br><br>Student will successfully utilize his walker to maximize his mobility.<br><br>Student will show improved functional status through participation in PT/OT regimens. |

| Assessment Data | Nursing Diagnosis | Goals | Nursing Interventions | Expected Outcomes |
|---|---|---|---|---|
| Jeremy's speech sounds halting, and sometimes he jumbles up his words. | Impaired verbal communication (dysarthria) related to: posterior fossa craniotomy | Student will successfully communicate in the school setting. | Facilitate student's participation in speech therapy sessions. | Student will demonstrate intelligible communication in the school setting, through his speech and/or use of assistive devices. |
| | | | Work with speech pathologist(s) to determine if student needs a communication board or other assistive devices at school. | |
| Jeremy has had some emotional outbursts, especially when he is frustrated or something unexpected happens. | Disturbed thought processes related to: (1) posterior fossa surgery; (2) dexamethasone; (3) anger, fear, powerlessness | Student will maintain an appropriate behavioral pattern in the school setting. | Provide opportunities for the student to express feelings and frustrations, or to blow off steam in an appropriate way. | Student will express his concern(s) or frustration(s) to adults in a respectful way. |
| | | | Prepare student ahead of time for new procedures or occurrences. | Student will recognize when his is feeling out of control, and ask for a break or a time-out. |
| | | | Educate staff regarding student's issues, and work together with teachers, guidance counselors, and parents to develop a behavior plan that is appropriate and feasible. | |
| Jeremy's immune system is suppressed from the dexamethasone and may be further suppressed when his blood cell counts drop during the chemotherapy phase. | Ineffective protection related to: (1) immunosuppression; (2) potential bone marrow suppression; (3) potential impaired skin integrity | Student will maintain primary and secondary defenses as much as possible. | Notify student's parents of disease outbreaks in the classroom or school setting. | Student will experience minimal episodes of unpreventable illness and no episodes of preventable illness. |
| His port and VP shunt are potential sources of infection. | Risk for infection related to: (1) immuno-suppression; (2) implanted port, VP shunt; (3) potential leukopenia | | Educate staff regarding the student's vulnerabilities and how to promote good hand washing and overall hygiene in the school setting. | Student will demonstrate good hand washing, oral hygiene, and skin care, and will avoid peers who are ill. |
| His platelet count may drop during the chemotherapy phase. | | | Reinforce with student ways to stay protected from infection or other insults to his system, and how to recognize early signs that warrant attention, such as fever, chills, lightheadedness; headache; bruises or bloody noses; or skin sores or redness. | Student will seek the attention of an adult when he experiences unusual symptoms |

| Assessment Data | Nursing Diagnosis | Goals | Nursing Interventions | Expected Outcomes |
|---|---|---|---|---|
| Jeremy's functional deficits as outlined above put him at increased risk of injury from falls, or from being bumped into. | Risk for injury related to: (1) left-sided weakness; (2) ataxia; (3) footdrop; (4) potential thrombocytopenia | Student will remain free from physical injury. | Assess school environment for situations that pose a potential injury risk to student, and facilitate modifications to improve student safety. Especially observe for changes in levels of walking surfaces that may impede moving over them with a walker, or for tight spaces in the classroom that may interfere with movement. Work with staff, teachers, and student to create a safer environment. | Student will explain ways to protect himself from injury in the school setting. Student will experience no falls in the school setting. |
| Jeremy could develop reddened skin in the radiation field. He may also develop skin breakdown or infection around the implanted port. | Risk for impaired skin integrity related to: (1) radiation therapy; (2) implanted port | Student will show appropriate skin care in the school setting. | Assess student periodically for skin breakdown in the at-risk areas, and reinforce education with student regarding symptoms of concern, such as redness, swelling, drainage, pain, or peeling skin. Encourage student to care for skin as directed. | Student will identify and act appropriately upon symptoms of skin breakdown. Student will use good hand washing and apply lotion or cream as needed to skin. |
| Jeremy has difficulty getting onto and off of the toilet due to weakness and balance/coordination problems. Jeremy has difficulty opening tightly sealed packages due to fine motor weakness and incoordination. | Self-care deficit (feeding, toileting) related to: (1) fine motor impairment; (2) ataxia; (3) weakness (NANDA 00102, 00110) | Student will improve self-care skills of feeding and toileting. | Provide assistance to student with getting onto and off of the toilet, or arrange for that assistance. Work with PT/OT staff to help student gain strength and learn to use assistive equipment (i.e., grab bars) in bathroom. Arrange for a staff person or another student to open milk cartons or other containers at lunchtime, until such a time when student is able to do this | Student will ask for assistance at lunch if he is having difficulty with opening containers. Student will ask for help with transfers to and from the toilet. Student will eventually be able to toilet independently and to eat independently. |

| Assessment Data | Nursing Diagnosis | Goals | Nursing Interventions | Expected Outcomes |
|---|---|---|---|---|
| Jeremy currently has occasional nausea and will expect to experience more when he starts the chemotherapy phase.<br><br>He currently takes oral ondansetron, an antiemetic, once daily in the morning, and PRN.<br><br>He also takes daily dexamethasone during radiation (to help control nausea), as well as famotidine, an antacid. | Nausea related to: (1) radiation therapy; (2) chemotherapy (future) | Student will show results of successful management of nausea.<br><br>Student will maintain adequate oral intake. | Administer PRN or schedule medications as ordered.<br><br>Encourage oral intake, and monitor as appropriate.<br><br>Provide for comfort and privacy should the student become ill at school. | Student will experience minimal nausea in the school setting.<br><br>Student will be able to eat his lunch and drink his beverage without emesis. |
| Jeremy has had trouble with constipation while receiving weekly vincristine, and now has a daily bowel movement with administration of Miralax twice daily at home. | Risk for constipation related to: (1) vincristine side effect; (2) inadequate activity; (3) dehydration | Student will maintain a regular bowel pattern. | Provide for privacy in toileting if student desires to have bowel movements in the health office restroom.<br><br>Encourage oral fluid intake. | Student will defecate with ease and regularity and maintain this pattern in the school setting.<br><br>Student will participate in activity as tolerated.<br><br>Student will drink at least 2 to 3 glasses of fluids during the school day. |
| Jeremy has an increased appetite while taking dexamethasone, and craves fatty, salty foods. He has gained 10 pounds over the last month.<br><br>He may have weight loss during the chemotherapy phase.<br><br>He may also develop growth failure in the years following radiation therapy. | Risk for disproportionate growth related to: (1) hyperphagia; fluid retention; (2) potential inadequate intake from nausea; (3) future growth hormone deficiency | Student will maintain an appropriate weight during treatment and grow when expected to do so. | Work with parents to provide healthy snacks in the health office as needed.<br><br>Encourage/educate student regarding healthy food choices.<br><br>Encourage student to exercise as tolerated.<br><br>Monitor weight and height if indicated, and notify parent of significant changes or deviation from expected values. | Student will exhibit an appropriate weight and height for age, with consideration given for short-term treatment effects.<br><br>Student will lose steroid-induced weight gain once steroids are discontinued.<br><br>Student will maintain height velocity according to the standardized growth charts. |

**Brain and Spinal Cord Tumors**

| Assessment Data | Nursing Diagnosis | Goals | Nursing Interventions | Expected Outcomes |
|---|---|---|---|---|
| Children who receive radiation to the whole brain are expected to lose IQ points due to an inability to acquire new information and skills at a rate similar to their peers. | Risk for delayed development related to: cranial radiation | Student will succeed academically in accordance with developmental level and cognitive abilities. | Participate with school guidance personnel and/or the multidisciplinary student support team to determine student eligibility and/or needs related to an IEP/Special Education.<br><br>Work with parents, clinic staff, and school personnel to increase staff knowledge regarding student's abilities and disabilities. | Student will demonstrate academic success in accordance with developmental level and cognitive abilities as evidenced by remaining at grade level appropriate for age, receiving educational support such as resource or team classes, continuing to gain skills or knowledge up to full capability, maintenance of previously acquired skills/knowledge, and a feeling of success in school. |
| Jeremy needs reinforcement of new information regarding tumor/treatment until it holds significant meaning for him. | Deficient knowledge of tumor and its treatment related to: (1) inadequate recall of information; and (2) limited exposure to information | Student will increase knowledge of tumor, treatment, and side effects. | Obtain access to information that student was given, and assess student's understanding of that information.<br><br>Reinforce education in the areas that the student still needs experience with, especially the need for medication compliance and symptom recognition and management. | Student will show an improved understanding of diagnosis, treatment, and effects by being able to tell his story to others, and by verbalizing side effects of treatment and how they affect his life, and what he can do about it. |
| Jeremy has expressed concern about how his peers will perceive him. | Risk for situational low-self esteem related to: (1) functional impairment; (2) changes in appearance; (3) diminished social interaction | Student will maintain or increase self-esteem vis-à-vis his alteration in physical appearance and functional status. | Assess and monitor student's psychosocial/emotional status and provide support and referral as indicated.<br><br>Utilized active listening with student, and encourage expression of fears, anxieties, concerns, loss, and grief.<br><br>Encourage student to share questions and feelings with staff, peers, healthcare team, and family. | Student will express ways to cope with peer response to alterations in his appearance and functioning.<br><br>Student will express hope(s) and appraisal(s) of strengths to peers and/or staff members.<br><br>Student will participate in "school visit" for staff and students. |

| Assessment Data | Nursing Diagnosis | Goals | Nursing Interventions | Expected Outcomes |
|---|---|---|---|---|
| | | | Encourage student to identify strengths and positive experiences, and reinforce the student's positive self-appraisals. | Student will participate in "school visit" for staff and students. |
| | | | Arrange for Child Life Specialist to visit the school to provide information to students and staff, if in accordance with student and family desires. | |
| Jeremy has shown resistance to taking medications at home. | Ineffective therapeutic regimen management related to: (1) knowledge deficit/complexity of regimen; (2) inability to cope with illness; (3) powerlessness ( | Student will participate in efforts to maintain his health and follow the treatment plan. | Monitor student's ability level to manage his health condition, and provide instruction/support to increase self-management skills. | Student will demonstrate understanding and compliance with treatment plan, as evidenced by taking medications, and verbalization of rationale for medications or treatments. |
| | | | Collaborate with parents to utilize a similar approach to medication compliance as in the home setting, and communicate progress to parents. Support efforts of positive reinforcement, such as a sticker chart. | |
| The initial time of diagnosis and beginning treatment have been overwhelming to the family. There is fear of treatment effects. | Interrupted family processes related to: (1) crisis of diagnosis and treatment; (2) shift in family roles; (3) modification in family finances | Student and family will be supported to accommodate to changes in the family system. | Establish open and regular communication with the family. | Student and family members will verbalize feeling supported in their struggles and challenges. |
| The roles in the family have changed (mother is unemployed), and the family finances are strained. | | | Support student and family (including younger sibling) with adaptation, coping, and changes in school and family processes related to diagnosis and treatment. Provide for referral as indicated. | Student and family will access/accept community support services such as counseling or support groups as needed. |
| There is a good support system available to the family. | | | | Student and sibling will identify who in the family is responsible for transportation, who to call in case of an urgent concern, and who they can go to with their fears and worries. |

# Emergency Care Plan
## CNS Tumor

Date: _____          School: _____

Student: _____          Grade: _____

Date of birth: _____

Parent(s)/Guardian(s): _____          Home telephone: _____

_____          Father's work: _____

_____          Mother's work: _____

Primary Care Provider: _____          Telephone: _____

Specialist: _____          Telephone: _____

Contact: _____

Medical Diagnosis: _____

Persons Authorized to Administer Treatment: _____

_____

| Symptom | Action |
|---|---|
| Fever: Temperature ≥101°F<br><br>OR<br><br>Shaking chills with or without fever | 1. Check blood pressure (see next box below).<br>2. Notify parent ASAP.<br>3. Administer antipyretic as ordered: Acetaminophen (15 mg/kg) ____mg PO.<br>4. Apply topical anesthetic cream to implanted port site if ordered:EMLA/ELA-MAX cream to port site one hour prior to use, cover with occlusive dressing.<br>5. Give oral fluids if alert and able to swallow.<br>6. Keep student in health office on cot rest and monitor until parent arrives. |
| Blood pressure ≤80/40 (or other parameters as ordered_____)<br><br>AND/OR<br><br>Student appears ill, lethargic, and decreased level of consciousness<br><br>OR<br><br>Fainting | 1. Call emergency response team (911).<br>2. Notify parent ASAP.<br>3. Cot rest and continue to monitor until team arrives.<br>4. Encourage oral fluids if alert and able to swallow.<br>5. Begin CPR if indicated by ABCs and continue until ambulance arrives. |

| Symptom | Action |
|---|---|
| Severe headache<br><br>OR<br><br>Persistent vomiting (more than once in a 30-minute period) | 1. Perform brief neurologic assessment (Can student state his name, location, and date/time?).<br>2. Check temperature, blood pressure (see boxes on previous page).<br>3. Notify parent ASAP.<br>4. Cot rest and continue to monitor until parent arrives.<br>5. Follow symptom guidelines as above for notification of emergency services. |
| Implanted port is accessed and heparin-locked (there is a needle [with short tubing attached] resting in the port through the skin, but the tubing is not connected to an IV bag or other device)<br><br>AND<br><br>Tubing is leaking blood, cap comes off tubing, student complains of pain, or needle comes out of port | 1. Put on gloves and examine tubing and port area.<br>2. Clamp tubing above any leak.<br>3. Do not replace any lost cap.<br>4. Do not remove needle, even if port area looks swollen, red, or otherwise abnormal.<br>5. If needle is out of skin, then dispose of needle and tubing together in a sharps container.<br>6. Notify parent ASAP. |
| Seizure activity | 1. Call emergency response team (911) unless student has a written plan that states otherwise.<br>  2. Notify parent ASAP. |

**Signatures:**

School Nurse_____ Date_____

Parent/guardian (if required)_____ Date_____

# Emergency Evacuation Plan
## CNS Tumor

**Student:** Jeremy Anderson      **School:** Pine Valley Elementary
**Disability Area:** Physically Impaired      **Grade:** 4
**Medical Diagnosis:** Medulloblastoma      **Teacher:** Ms. Kate Johnson

**Student Assessment:** Jeremy is physically impaired from his brain tumor. Specifically, he has left-sided weakness and difficulty maintaining his balance and coordination while walking. He also suffers from fatigue and generalized weakness. He uses a walker for ambulation. He uses a wheelchair for longer distances. He is unable to negotiate stairs at this time.

**Building Assessment:** Pine Valley Elementary is a one-story building, with no stairs to negotiate to enter or exit the building. There are several doorway thresholds to negotiate before leaving the building. A wheelchair is always kept in the health office.

**Plan:** For emergency evacuation from the school building, the school nurse or health assistant will take the wheelchair to Jeremy's classroom to transport him out of the building.
- The assistant principal or administrative assistant will go to Jeremy's classroom to escort the other children out of the building.
- Jeremy's teacher will remain with Jeremy in the classroom until the wheelchair arrives.
- The school nurse or health assistant will evacuate Jeremy from the building in the wheelchair by way of the front school door or the south exit, whichever is less congested.
- If Jeremy is in the gymnasium or cafeteria at the time of the evacuation, then his teacher may escort him (with his walker) out of the building with the rest of the class, since there are emergency exits in both areas.

**Signatures:**

School Nurse_____ Date_____

Building Principal_____ Date_____

# References

American Brain Tumor Association. (n.d.). *A primer of brain tumors: A patient's reference manual* (8th ed.) [Online]. Retrieved May 16, 2004, from http://www.abta.org/buildingknowledge5.htm

American Brain Tumor Association. (1998). *A primer of brain tumors: A patient's reference manual* (25th anniversary ed.). Des Plaines, IL: Author.

Bestak, M. (2001). Epidemiology of brain tumors. In R. F. Keating, J. T. Goodrich, & R. J. Packer (Eds.), *Tumors of the pediatric central nervous system* (pp. 14–21). New York: Thieme Medical.

CBTRUS (2002). *Statistical report: Primary brain tumors in the United States, 1995-1999.* Central Brain Tumor Registry of the United States. Retrieved May 16, 2004, from http://www.cbtrus.org/2002/2003report.pdf

Duffner, P. K., Cohen, M. E., & Freeman, A. (1985). Pediatric brain tumors: An overview. *Cancer, 35,* 287–301.

Kaplan, C. A., & Jenkins, N. B. (1998). Chemotherapy In M J Hockenberry-Eaton & K. L. Dahl (Eds.), *Essentials of pediatric oncology nursing: A core curriculum.* Glenview, IL: Association of Pediatric Oncology Nurses.

Medlock, M. D. (2001). Infratentorial astrocytoma. In R. F. Keating, J. T. Goodrich, & R. J. Packer (Eds.), *Tumors of the pediatric central nervous system* (pp. 199–205). New York: Thieme Medical.

Muszynski, C. A., Constantini, S., & Epstein, F. J. (2001). Astrocytoma. In R. F. Keating, J. T. Goodrich & R. J. Packer (Eds.), *Tumors of the pediatric central nervous system* (pp. 14–21). New York: Thieme Medical.

Netter, F. H. (2003). *Atlas of human anatomy* (3rd ed.) Teterboro, NJ: Icon Learning Systems.

Nicholson, H. S. & Packer, R. J. (2001). Chemotherapy. In R. F. Keating, J. T. Goodrich, & R. J. Packer (Eds.), *Tumors of the pediatric central nervous system* (pp. 168–183). New York: Thieme Medical.

NANDA International. (2003). *Nursing diagnoses: Definitions & classification 2003-200.* Philadelphia: Author.

Palmer, S. L., Goloubeva, O., Riddick, W. E., Glass, J. O., Gajjar, A., Kun, L., et al. (2001). Patterns of intellectual development among survivors of pediatric medulloblastoma: A longitudinal analysis. *Journal of Clinical Oncology, 19*(8), 2302–2308.

Ryan-Murray, J., & Petriccione, M. M. (2002). Central nervous system tumors. In C. R. Baggott, K. P. Kelly, D. Fochtman, & G. V. Foley (Eds.), *Nursing care of children and adolescents with cancer* (3rd ed.) (pp. 503–523). Philadelphia: Saunders.

Sadeh, M., & Cohen, I. (2001). Transient loss of speech after removal of posterior fossa tumors—One aspect of a larger neuropsychological entity: The cerebellar cognitive affective syndrome. *Pediatric Hematology & Oncology, 18,* 423–426.

Seiff, M. E., & Goodrich, J. T. (2001). Postoperative considerations. In R. F. Keating, J. T., Goodrich & R. J. Packer (Eds.), *Tumors of the pediatric central nervous system* (pp. 477–501). New York: Thieme Medical.

Sønderkær, S., Schmiegelow, M., Carstensen, H., Nielsen, L. B., Muller, J., & Schmiegelow, K. (2003). Long-term neurological outcome of childhood brain tumors treated by surgery only. *Journal of Clinical Oncology, 21*(7), 1347–1351.

Strother, D. S., Pollack, I. F., Fisher, P. G., Hunter, J. V., Woo, S. Y., Pomeroy, S. L., et al. (2002). Tumors of the central nervous system. In P. A. Pizzo, & D. G. Poplack (Eds.), *Principles and practice of pediatric oncology* (4th ed.) (pp. 751–824). Philadelphia: Lippincott Williams & Wilkins.

Vines, E., Bertsch, H. F., & Goldwein, J. (2001). Radiotherapy. In R. F. Keating, J. T. Goodrich & R. J. Packer (Eds.), *Tumors of the pediatric central nervous system* (pp. 135–167). New York: Thieme Medical.

Weitman, D. M., & Cogen, P. H. (2001). Infratentorial ependymoma. In R. F. Keating, J. T. Goodrich, & R. J. Packer (Eds.), *Tumors of the pediatric central nervous system* (pp. 232–238). New York: Thieme Medical.

## Bibliography

Deasy-Spinetta, P., & Irvin, E. (Eds.). (1993). *Educating the child with cancer* [Booklet]. Bethesda, MD: The Candlelighters Childhood Cancer Foundation. (Available from The Candlelighters Childhood Cancer Foundation, 7910 Woodmont Avenue, Suite 460, Bethesda, MD 20814-3015; 1-800-366-2223, 301-657-8401)

Keene, N., Hobbie, W., & Ruccione, K. (2000). *Childhood cancer survivors: A practical guide to your future.* Sebastopol, CA: O'Reilly & Associates.

Leukemia & Lymphoma Society. (n.d.). *Back to school for the child with cancer: The Trish Greene back to school program for the child with cancer.* [Brochure]. White Plains, NY: Author. (Available from the Leukemia & Lymphoma Society, Information Resource Center, 1311 Mamaroneck Avenue, White Plains, NY 10605; 1-800-955-4572; www.leukemia-lymphoma.org)

This brochure lists many additional resources related to school re-entry.

PACER Center. *Who we are* [Brochure]. Minneapolis, MN: Author. (Available from PACER Center, 8161 Normandale Boulevard, Minneapolis, MN 55437-1044; 952-838-9000, 952-838-0190 (TTY), 952-838-0199 (fax); pacer@pacer.org; www.pacer.org)

PACER Center is the Parent Advocacy Coalition for Educational Rights, a national center based in Minnesota.

Shaminski-Maher, T., Cullen, P., & Sansalone, M.; N. Keene (Ed.). (2002). *Childhood brain and spinal cord tumors: A guide for families, friends & caregivers.* Sebastopol, CA: O'Reilly & Associates.

Watterson, J., Oliver, J., & Carlson-Green, B. (1999). *Helping your child: A manual for parents of children with brain tumors* [Booklet] and *Teaching the child with a brain tumor* [Booklet]. St. Paul, MN: Children's Health Care—St. Paul. (Available from Children's Hospitals and Clinics, Department of Hematology/Oncology, 347 North Smith Avenue, St. Paul, MN 55102; 651-220-6732)

## Resources

American Brain Tumor Association
http://www.abta.org

CancerCare
http://www.cancercare.org/CancerCareServices

Cancervive
http://www.cancervive.org/

Children's Brain Tumor Foundation
http://www.cbtf.org

CureSearch (from the National Childhood Cancer Foundation and the Children's Oncology Group)
http://www.curesearch.org

National Cancer Institute
http://www.cancer.gov/cancertopics/types/childhoodcancers
 and
http://www.cancer.gov/cancerinformation/cancertype/braintumor/

Pediatric Brain Tumor Foundation of the United States
http://www.pbtfus.org/

The Childhood Brain Tumor Foundation
http://www.childhoodbraintumor.org

## Chapter Twenty-eight

# Burns

Patricia S. Latona

## Introduction

More than 1 million burn injuries occur every year. More than 45,000 burn injuries require hospitalization. An estimated total of 4,500 people die every year from fire and burn injuries (Burn Incidence and Treatment in the US: 2000 Fact Sheet). Burns are the second most common cause of accidental death in children, second only to motor vehicle accidents.

The incidence of burn injury, hospitalization, and death has shown a decrease over the past two decades. The injury rate has declined from 2 million per year to approximately 1 million per year. Hospitalizations and deaths related to burn injuries have declined 50% since 1971 (Burn Incidence and Treatment in the US: 2000 Fact Sheet). This decline is due to numerous factors. Fire and burn prevention education, management of burn patients in specialized centers, regulation of consumer products, and implementation of occupational safety standards have impacted this trend of burn incidence. (However, burns continue to remain the second leading cause of death among children.) With the decrease in mortality rate, more children survive to return to school and to their communities.

Treatment of a major burn injury is very intense and complicated. Hospitalization is determined by the age of the victim, the depth and size of the burn, the location of the burn, the cause of the burn, and the presence of associated injuries. Recovery time varies from several weeks with a minor burn to several years with a major burn. The majority of burns can be treated in an outpatient setting (Morgan, Bledsoe, & Barker, 2000).

## Pathophysiology

The skin is the largest organ of the body, and at some point it interfaces with all major systems of the body. Therefore, the pathology of a major burn injury presents a multitude of complicated medical problems and issues.

The skin is basically divided into three layers. The outer layer is the epidermis, which is composed of epithelial cells. These cells re-epithelialize. The middle layer is the dermis. Within the dermis are some epithelial cells, hair follicles, sebaceous glands, sweat glands, melanin cells, blood vessels, nerve fibers, and lymphatic vessels. Beneath the dermis is the hypodermis. The hypodermis contains fat, smooth muscle, and areolar tissue.

### Causes of Burns

Burn treatment and management depend on the cause of the burn. Most burns are caused by thermal, chemical, and electrical injuries. Radiant heat injuries and tar injuries are seen less frequently.

Thermal burns are caused by dry heat (flame, hot surface, or object) or moist heat (hot liquid). The degree of injury is directly related to the total time of exposure and temperature. Thermal burns comprise the majority of all burn injuries. There are marked changes in the vascular and metabolic responses of the body.

Electrical injuries comprise 3% to 5% of all burn unit admissions (Wright, 2001). These injuries vary with the type of circuit, voltage, amperage, resistance of the body, pathway of current through the body, and the duration of contact with the current. Lightning injuries account for more than 500 electrical deaths per year. (Wright, 2001). Electrical injuries have an entrance wound as well as an exit wound. Frequently, an electrical injury also has a thermal injury at the exit point. This occurs because the victim's clothing ignites. Loss of consciousness often occurs, and cardiopulmonary resuscitation at the scene is frequently required. Treatment and follow-up continue for several years after injury. Electrical injuries require massive fluid recuscitation, cardiac assessment, complicated multisystem stabilization, and possible amputation.

A chemical injury is caused by the thermal energy produced when a chemical reacts with the body's tissue. These burns are progressive and can cause extensive injury. Tissue damage continues until the agent has been removed or neutralized. There is a potential for systemic toxicity as well as local damage. Chemical agents that are exposed to the eyes or ingested are of great concern.

### Burn Wound Description

The description of burn wounds includes their size and depth. Size is estimated using a modified Lund and Browder chart. The extent of the burn is expressed as a percentage of total body surface area (Wong, Hockenberry, Wilson, Wilkelstein, & Kline, 2003).

Burn depth is classified as superficial, partial thickness, or full thickness. Previous classification referred to the depth as first-, second-, or third-degree burns (sometimes fourth).

Superficial (first-degree) burns are usually of minor signficance. The skin remains intact. There is usually erythema and significant pain.

Partial thickness (second-degree) burns involve the first layer of skin (epidermis) and part of the second layer of skin (dermis). They appear red or mottled, contain blisters, and are wet and weeping. They are extremely painful. They usually heal within 2 to 3 weeks with a variable amount of scarring (Wong et al., 2003).

Full thickness (third-degree) burns involve injury to the deep dermis and the hypodermis. They appear dark and are covered with eschar (dead skin tissue). Healing involves separation of eschar, debridement of the wound, and wound closure through skin grafting and other surgical interventions. This process can take months and can result in considerable scarring. (Wong et al., 2003).

## Management

Destruction of the skin by a major burn injury causes numerous physiologic and hemodynamic changes throughout each of the body's systems. Some of the changes occur immediately, whereas others occur as the burn wound progresses.

Burn wound physiology and care have been divided into three phases of burn management. The first phase is the emergent phase (shock phase), the second phase is the acute phase (fluid remobilization phase), and the third phase is the rehabilitation phase (recovery phase).

During the emergent phase, there is massive edema formation and a decrease in blood volume. Increased capillary permeability combined with an increase in hydrostatic pressure causes loss of water, protein, and electrolytes from the circulating volume into the interstitial spaces. Adequate fluid volume replacement is necessary to maintain vital organ function. This phase lasts anywhere from 36 to 48 hours (Wong et al., 2003).

During the acute phase, fluid shifts from the interstitial space back into the cardiovascular space. When this occurs, there is massive diuresis. Management of the burn wound and prevention of complications such as infection and respiratory, circulatory, gastrointestinal, and central nervous system problems become imperative during this phase. Wound closure and prevention of complications are the goals during this phase.

The final and most important phase is the rehabilitative phase. It begins once wound coverage has been completed. During this phase, final preparations for reentry into the burn child's community are made. This phase includes use of pressure bandages and splints, occupational therapy, physical therapy, and psychological and social support for dealing with issues and concerns regarding the burn injury and reintegration back into the family, school, and community.

Next to the home, school is the most important social event for a child. Preparation for school reentry begins during the acute phase of hospitalization. The process of returning to the community and resuming life outside the hospital can be frightening for the child and his or her family, especially if the injury leaves the child visibly changed and/or different from other children (Blakeney et al., 1998).

It is critical for the school nurse to establish herself or himself as the school contact person for the student's school reentry program as soon after the injury has occurred as possible. The school nurse can then assist in developing a school reentry program that includes:

1. Inclusion of the student and family in the planning and implementation of the school reentry program
2. Information on burn injury and management to staff and students
3. Specific information regarding the student
4. Information regarding psychosocial issues that the student may be experiencing. (Blakeney et al., 1998)
5. The needed adaptations or modification in their school environment and assignment requirements

The school presentation should include discussion of topics such as the cause of the injury; history of the hospitalization; scars; splints, assistive devices, pressure garments, and other appliances; activity level and tolerance limitations; how individuals can help the student transition; and emphasis on how the child may have changed on the outside, but is the same on the inside. Note: Special care must be taken to explain that accidents happen and they can be prevented, versus blaming the child and his or her parents for the injury.

Teachers, staff members, and the student's peers may be very anxious. This anxiety is realistic; however, it can be decreased by assisting them to learn about burns and to discuss any questions or concerns they may have that will assist them in the school reentry program. Utilizing the staff from the burn center can assist in providing accurate information and answers to questions and concerns. Some burn centers use individualized videotapes in addition to written literature. Allowing the students to view pressure garments, splints, assistive devices, and other appliances will help them understand the complexity of burn care and wound management.

The student may qualify for special education services. A referral by the school nurse to the student assistance team may be necessary.

There is great risk for caregiver role strain related to the injury and/situational crisis. Demographics, parenting skills, substance abuse, pre-existing family issues/relations, and stress can significantly affect the burn victim's successful recovery. See resources for further information and support.

Assisting the student and his or her family to access and utilize community services such as counseling, support groups and/or burn camps is also crucial. The student's participation in community services could assist the student to maintain or enhance his or her self-esteem by addressing some of the psychosocial aspects of having a burn injury.

# Individualized Healthcare Plan

## Assessment

*History*

Prehospitalization (previous history)
- Preexisting health conditions
- Surgeries
- Medications
- Allergies
- Height and weight

History related to the burn injury
- Date and time of burn
- Cause of burn

How the burn occurred
- Where the burn occurred (open versus closed space)
- Loss of consciousness
- Other associated injuries
- Areas of body burned and thickness of burns
- Date of admission; date of discharge
- Surgeries (how many and what for)
- Treatment
- Complications
- Medical/psychological problems during hospitalization
- Height/weight upon discharge

*Current Status and Management*
- Status of burn wounds (healed areas, open areas, treatments, etc.)
- School reentry program (objectives, activities, timeline)

Healthcare providers

Physician(s)

School reentry coordinator

Nurse (from hospital/burn center)

Contact for current and further questions or concerns
- Activity: restrictions, encouraged
- Appliances (splints, assistive devices, etc.)
- Pressure garments
- Medications
- Nutritional status (appetite/diet requirements)

Sleep pattern, need for additional rest

*Wound Status*

Wound stage or classification (standard used by hospital)

Wound edges

Necrotic tissue (color, consistency, adherence, amount present, and location)

Wound exudate (location, consistency, adherence, amount present, and location)

Surrounding tissue (color, induration, and edema)

Granulation tissue and epithelialization (size, amount, and location)

*Self-Care*
- Self-care abilities
- Desire to do self-care
- Motivators to do self-care
- Barriers to self-care
- Areas to encourage self-care
- Compliance with treatment management plan
- Decision-making skills

*Psychosocial Status*
- Student's concerns regarding returning to school
- Student's perception of body image
- Family status/concerns regarding returning home, to school, peer activities, athletics, and other activities
- Student's concerns regarding peers' reaction to burn injury

*Academic Issues*
- Past academic performance
- Current academic performance; need for academic assistance in the classroom
- School attendance pattern: pre-injury, hospital school program, homebound instruction
- Adaptive equipment needed
- Modifications needed: school day, schedule, homework, classroom assignments
- Activity limitations
- School environment: transportation needs
- Special precautions (e.g., exposure to sun, cold, etc)

## Nursing Diagnoses (N.D.) (NANDA, 2003)

**N.D. 1** Impaired skin integrity (NANDA 00046) related to:
- burn injury resulting in hypertropic scarring
- photosensitivity
- diminished/absent sweat glands
- dryness
- pruritus
- temperature sensitivity

**N.D. 2** Risk for infection (NANDA 00004) related to loss of skin integrity

**N.D. 3** Risk for injury (NANDA 00035) related to:
- impaired tissue integrity
- psychologic/physiologic stress reaction to severe trauma
- immobility

**N.D. 4** Chronic pain (NANDA 00133) related to:
- burn injury
- immobility
- treatment

**N.D. 5** Delayed growth and development (NANDA 00111) related to:
- inability to perform self-care appropriate with age
- delay/difficulty in performing skills typical for age group due to hospitalization and inability to attend school
- effects of burn injury

**N.D. 6** Altered nutrition, less than body requirements (NANDA 00002) related to:
- increased metabolic needs
- decreased appetite

**N.D. 7** Disturbed body image (NANDA 00118) related to:
- changes in appearance secondary to severe trauma from burn injury
- perception of appearance
- activity limitations and restrictions

**N.D. 8** Impaired physical mobility (NANDA 00085) related to:
- range-of-motion limitations
- searing

**N.D. 9** Activity intolerance (NANDA 00092) related to:
- prolonged hospitalization/period of inactivity
- impaired joint movement

**N.D. 10** Dressing/grooming self-care deficit (NANDA 00108) related to:
- range-of-motion limitations
- scarring

**N.D. 11** Bathing/hygiene self-care deficit (NANDA 00108) related to:
- range-of-motion limitations
- scarring

**N.D. 12** Disturbed sensory perception (NANDA 00122) related to:

- trauma of burn injury
- environmental stimuli
- stress
- protective isolation
- altered sensory function and/or integration

**N.D. 13** Risk for imbalanced body temperature (NANDA 00005)
**N.D. 14** Risk for imbalanced fluid volume (NANDA 00025)

## Goals

The student will minimize scar and contracture formation. (N.D. 8, 9)
The student will increase flexibility, strength, and endurance. (N.D. 8)
The student will increase independence and self-care skills. (N.D. 5, 10, 11)
The student will utilize school and community resources for support. (N.D. 5)
The student will effectively manage pain/discomfort successfully during the school day. (N.D. 4)
The student will achieve and maintain good nutritional and hydration intake. (N.D. 6, 14)
The student will increase his/her physical activity tolerance. (N.D. 9)
The student will utilize assistive devices as needed. (N.D. 3, 9)
The student will demonstrate improved body image. (N.D. 7)
The student will increase independent mobility in the school environment. (N.D. 8)
The student will increase participation in self-care activities. (N.D. 5, 10, 11)
The student's skin will show signs of wound healing and improved skin integrity. (N.D. 1)
The student will maintain good skin integrity. (N.D. 1)
The student will prevent infection of burn wounds. (N.D. 2)
The student will meet height and weight requirements as prescribed. (N.D. 6)
The student will recognize signs and symptoms of imbalanced body temperature. (N.D. 13)

## Interventions

The Student will interact appropriately with others and with the environment. (N.D. 12)
Apply prescribed lotion (cold) that contains water and lipids to newly healed skin. (Avoid creams, lanolin, fragrances, and nonessential ingredients.) (N.D. 1)
Refrigerate lotions and apply them cold. (N.D. 1)
Assist in providing appropriate school environment that will increase humidity in the air of classroom(s). (N.D. 1)
Assist student to avoid direct sunlight for 6 or more months to prevent sunburn and hyperpigmentation. (N.D. 1)
Encourage student to wear a hat and long sleeves when out in sun. (N.D. 1)
Assist student to apply sunscreen to newly formed skin prior to participating in outdoor activities. (N.D. 1)
Modify student schedule in order to limit outdoor activities to early morning and late afternoon. (N.D. 1, 13)
Assist student to avoid extreme changes in temperature. (N.D. 1)
Administer antihistamines in conjunction with topical antipruritics for itching as prescribed. (N.D. 1)
Encourage good hygiene practices. (N.D. 1)
Assist and encourage student to actively participate in self-care. (N.D. 1)
Educate family to support student in participation in self-care. (N.D. 1)
Monitor compliance with compression therapy plan. (N.D. 1)
Assist student to maintain compliance with compression therapy plan in the school setting. (N.D. 1)
Monitor skin integrity for signs and symptoms of infection. (N.D. 2)
Monitor skin integrity for signs of wound healing. (N.D. 1)
Assist student to notify his/her parents if signs or symptoms of infection occur. (N.D. 2)
Assist student to use assistive devices and/or adapted equipment as prescribed. (N.D. 3)
Assist in providing for proper positioning during all school activities to prevent contractures. (N.D. 3)
Assist student and family to comply with prescribed exercise program. (N.D. 3)
Monitor effectiveness of splints. (N.D. 3)
Monitor student's range of motion with occupational and physical therapy staff. (N.D. 3)
Refer to assessment team if needed for academic-related issues/concerns, if they develop. (N.D. 3)
Assist student to learn positive strategies to reduce stress. (N.D. 3)
Assist the student to practice using the strategies when experiencing stress at school. (N.D. 3)
Monitor need for and effectiveness of pain medication. (N.D. 4)
Obtain authorization for medications to be provided during the school day. (N.D. 1, 4)

Assist parents to maintain supply of medication at school. (N.D. 1, 4)

Administer pain medication, as prescribed. (N.D. 4)

Coordinate therapy procedures, with minimal classroom disruption. (N.D. 4)

Anticipate energy requirements and assist teachers to plan schedule to maximize energy for academic activities. (N.D. 4)

Provide/plan rest periods, as needed. (N.D. 4)

Promote time and guidance for self-help activities. (N.D. 4)

Assist student to identify strategies that increase comfort/decrease pain (clothing, positioning, movement, etc.). (N.D. 4)

Encourage student to verbalize thoughts, feelings, and concerns with family, healthcare providers, and school staff. (N.D. 7, 12)

Encourage and/or assist teacher to discuss academic and other issues with student and family. (N.D. 5)

Encourage student to keep a journal of negative and positive reactions of others toward him or her. (N.D. 7, 12)

Encourage student and family to participate in school and community events. (N.D. 5)

Encourage student and family to participate in rehabilitative follow-up visits. (N.D. 5)

Encourage student and family to utilize community-based services and resources for counseling and support groups. (N.D. 5)

Assist student to have available high-calorie, high-protein meals and snacks and foods that the student likes, as needed. (N.D. 6)

Assist student to eat meals and snacks during times that the student desires to eat and as prescribed. (N.D. 6)

Assist student to maintain adequate hydration
- fluids readily available
- refrigerator available (N.D. 14)

Assist in encouraging the student to socialize with peers during meals. (N.D. 6)

Monitor height and weight as needed/requested. (N.D. 6)

Convey positive feedback to the student with honesty and sincerity. (N.D. 7)

Promote peer interactions and cooperative activities with peers. (N.D. 7)

Assist other students to address their questions and concerns appropriately, utilizing their parents, teachers, counselors, and administrators as needed. (N.D. 7)

Prepare peers regarding child's appearance. (N.D. 7)

Encourage the student and parents to discuss issues surrounding body image. (N.D. 7)

Encourage the student to participate in support groups and activities with other children with burn injuries (burn camps). (N.D. 7)

Discuss activity limitations with the student's teachers. Assist them to modify activities based on the student's needs and abilities. (N.D. 3, 8, 9)

Discuss, develop, and plan for making up work when the student is unable to attend class or is absent. (Follow-up visits with healthcare providers and/or further treatment may occur during the school day.) (N.D. 5)

Hold in-service for staff regarding the student's return to school, prior to student's return. (N.D. 1–14) Include:
- The student's burn injury
- The student's treatment and recovery
- Expectations for further health-related interventions
- Student and parents' concerns
- Teachers' concerns
- Resources available and how to access them
- Possible/current academic concerns/needs

## Expected Student Outcomes

The student will:
- Demonstrate good wound healing. (N.D. 1, 2)
- Remain free from wound infection. (N.D. 3)
- Demonstrate good skin integrity. (N.D. 1)
- Demonstrate (a specific positive strategy) that reduces stress. (N.D. 3)
- Report freedom from pain during the school day. (N.D. 4)
- Request and appropriately utilize medication for pain/discomfort during the school day. (N.D. 4)
- Use nonmedication strategies to decrease discomfort/pain. (N.D. 4)
- Identify and describe their needs. (N.D. 5)

- Maintain nutritional intake to meet caloric needs. (N.D. 6)
- Maintain fluid intake to meet fluid requirements. (N.D. 14)
- Demonstrate appropriate weight gain. (N.D. 6)
- Participate in activities with family, peers, and community. (N.D. 5, 7)
- Participate in planning and implementation for school reentry. (N.D.5-10)
- Refrigerate lotions and apply cold. (N.D. 1)
- Demonstrate good hygiene. (N.D. 1, 11)
- Demonstrate an increase in activity tolerance (specific criteria: i.e., half-day attendance to full-day school attendance). (N.D. 9)
- Participate in classroom/school activities with peers. (N.D. 7)
- Describe himself/herself in positive terms. (N.D. 7)
- Describe his/her abilities and areas where he/she feels assistance is needed. (N.D. 7, 10)
- Increase participation in self-care skills (specific skills). (N.D. 10)
- Demonstrate independence in: (specific skill). (N.D. 10)
- Eliminate possible sources of infection. (N.D. 2)
- Demonstrate (academic, physical) performance to level of ability. (N.D. 8)
- Participate in follow-up care. (N.D. 5)
- Demonstrate improved range of motion (specify joints). (N.D. 8,9)
- Request assistance from adults and peers in the classroom, for physical/academic needs as needed. (N.D. 5)
- Discuss feelings and concerns regarding his/her appearance/peer reactions/adults reactions with (parent, school nurse, counselor, physician, teacher). (N.D. 7)
- Demonstrate good school attendance pattern. (N.D. 5, 9)
- Correctly interpret information from others (ex: healthcare provider, teachers, parents, etc.)
- Demonstrate appropriate interaction with peers and teachers. (N.D. 12 identify (number) of risks related to impaired sensory function/intergration in the environment at school. (N.D. 12)
- Identifies (number) of symptoms of imbalanced body temperature. (N.D. 13) maintains normal body temperature (N.D. 13)
- Wears clothing appropriate to the weather. (N.D. 13)

## Case Study

Samantha is an 8-year-old girl who sustained burns over 25% of her body when she was playing with a lighter. She had partial and full-thickness burns to her face, neck, chest, and right arm and hand. She was hospitalized at a university hospital burn center for 4 weeks. She had three skin graft surgeries.

Samantha had no pending medical problems upon discharge. She has lost 12 pounds from her preburn weight. Range of motion of the right hand, wrist, elbow, and arm is limited. She has extreme pruritus. A splint has been applied to her neck to prevent contracture and a pressure garment to her chest and right arm.

Samantha is on her regular diet and takes a supplement between meals at 10 a.m., 2 p.m., and 8 p.m. Snacks and fluids are encouraged. She is able to resume full activity, but she hesitates to participate. Samantha's graft sites have healed completely, and the partial-thickness burn areas have healed. She frequently complains of pruritus. Due to right hand involvement, Samantha needs assistance in all activities, including eating.

Samantha participated in an in-hospital educational program with teacher-coordinated academics provided by her school. Her academic progress has been good. Samantha and her family are very anxious about her reentry to school and community. Her mother wants Samantha to be home-schooled until she is completely healed.

# Burns

| Assessment Data | Nursing Diagnosis | Goals | Nursing Interventions | Expected Outcomes |
|---|---|---|---|---|
| Recent burn injury 25% burn (partial and full-thickness) to face, neck, chest, and right arm and hand.<br><br>Hospitalized 4 weeks; three skin graft surgeries; graft sites completely healed.<br><br>Extreme pruritus; pressure garment to be worn to cover chest and right arm. | Impaired skin integrity related to burn injury resulting in hypertrophic scarring, photosensitivity, diminished/absent sweat glands, dryness, pruritus, and temperature sensitivity. | Samantha's wounds will show progressive signs of wound healing and improved skin integrity.<br><br>Samantha will prevent infection of burn wounds. | Apply prescribed refrigerated lotion to skin.<br><br>Assist Samantha to limit outdoor activities to early morning and late afternoon.<br><br>Assist Samantha to apply sunscreen to newly formed skin before going outside for activities.<br><br>Encourage Samantha to wear a hat and long sleeves when out in the sun.<br><br>Administer antihistamines in conjunction with topical antipruritics for itching as prescribed.<br><br>Monitor compliance with compression therapy plan. | Samantha's burn wounds and skin will progress toward total healing and skin closure.<br><br>Samantha will maintain skin integrity by:<br>• applying sunscreen before going outside<br>• wearing a hat and long sleeves when out in the sun<br>• utilizing measures that prevent itching. |
| 12-pound weight loss from preburn to now.<br><br>Regular diet-with supplements at 10 a.m., 2 p.m., and 8 p.m.<br><br>Possibility to develop hypovolemia.<br><br>Samantha hesitates to participate in activities; burn to right hand requires assistance in all activities to include eating. | Altered nutrition, less than body requirements due to increased metabolic needs and decreased appetite.<br><br>Risk for imbalanced fluid volume.<br><br>Impaired physical mobility due to impaired joint movement and searing. | Samantha will achieve and maintain adequate nutritional intake.<br><br>Samantha will meet height and weight requirements for age.<br><br>Samantha will maintain adequate hydration.<br><br>Samantha will minimize scar/contracture formation.<br>Samantha will increase flexibility, strength, and endurance. | Assist Samantha to have available high-calorie, high-protein meals and snacks and foods that she likes, as needed.<br><br>Assist Samantha to eat meals and snacks during times that she desires to eat and as prescribed.<br><br>Assist in encouraging the student to socialize with peers during meals.<br><br>Monitor height and weight as indicated/requested. | Samantha will maintain nutritional intake to meet caloric needs.<br><br>Samantha demonstrates weight (maintenance/gain).<br><br>Samantha demonstrates adequate fluid intake and hydration.<br><br>Samantha will utilize assistive devices to accomplish academic/self-care tasks at school. |

| Assessment Data | Nursing Diagnosis | Goals | Nursing Interventions | Expected Outcomes |
|---|---|---|---|---|
| | | Samantha will participate in classroom activities with modifications made as needed. | Assist Samantha to consume adequate fluids. Assist Samantha to anticipate and recognize increased flui needs.<br><br>Discuss activity limitations with Samantha's teachers. Assist them to modify activities based on Samantha's needs and abilities.<br><br>Refer to assessment team, if indicated. | Samantha will demonstrate physical mobility functioning to the level of her ability. |
| Samantha and family very anxious about her reentry to school and community.<br><br>Mother wants student to be home-schooled.<br><br>No activity limitations per discharge plan; Samantha has made good progress. | Ineffective role performance (student) related to burn injury, hospitalization, and missing school for a month. | Samantha will utilize school and community resources for support.<br><br>Samantha will participate in planning and implementing her return to school. | Encourage student to verbalize thoughts, feelings, and concerns with family and staff.<br><br>Encourage and assist teacher to discuss academic and other issues with student and family.<br><br>Encourage and facilitate Samantha and her family involvement in planning and implementing Samantha's return to school: Timeline; Modifications; Health needs, Nutritional needs, Parent concerns, Teacher concerns; Feedback needed with parents (daily at first then move to weekly). | Samantha actively participates in planning and implementation for school reentry.<br><br>Samantha will participate in activities with family, peers, and community.<br><br>Samantha demonstrates a good school attendance pattern.<br><br>Samantha will participate in classroom school activities with peers. |

| Assessment Data | Nursing Diagnosis | Goals | Nursing Interventions | Expected Outcomes |
|---|---|---|---|---|
| | | | Samantha's return to school: Timeline; Modifications; Health needs, Nutritional needs, Parent concerns, Teacher concerns; Feedback needed with parents (daily at first then move to weekly).<br><br>Encourage Samantha and her family to participate in school and community events.<br><br>Encourage Samantha and family to participate in rehabilitative follow-up visits. | |
| Student and family very anxious about student's appearance and peer response. | Disturbed body image related to scaring from burn injury on face, neck, arm, and hand. | Samantha will demonstrate improved body image. | Samantha will be assisted to transition from hospital to school/community setting without difficulty.<br><br>Encourage Samantha to verbalize her thoughts and feelings with her parents and healthcare providers. | Samantha will describe herself in positive terms.<br><br>Samantha will discuss feelings and concerns regarding her appearance with and the reaction of peers and adults with her parents and school nurse. |

# Burn Injury Discharge
# Instructions to School

Student's name: _____

Student's school: _____


History of burn: _____

    Date_____

    Cause_____

    Open space fire/Closed space fire_____

    Loss of consciousness_____

    Percent of body burn_____

Hospitilization dates_____


Physical abilities_____

Physical limitaitons/restrictions_____


Student may attend school    ☐ Part-time    ☐ Full-time    ☐ Home school

Student requires tutor    ☐ Yes    ☐ No


Medications_____
_____


Treatments_____
_____
_____


Diet_____    Nutritional needs_____

Special equipment needs/Appliances_____
_____
_____


Pressure garments_____

Skin care_____
_____


Student may participate in P.E.    ☐ Yes    ☐ No

P.E. limitations_____


Student may participate in contact sports    ☐ Yes    ☐ No

Physical therapy needs_____

Occupational therapy needs_____


Authorized signatures:

Date:_____    Telephone number:_____

# References

Blakeney, P., Meyer, W., Robert, R., Desai, M., Wolf, S., & Herndon, D. (1998). Long-term psychosocial adaptation of children who survive burns involving 80% or greater total body surface area. *Journal of Trauma: Injury, Infection, and Critical Care, 44*(4), 625–634.

*Burn incidence and treatment in the US: 2000 fact sheet.* Retrieved February 21, 2004, from http://www.ameriburn.org/pub

Morgan, E. D., Bledsoe, S. C., & Barker, J. (2000). Ambulatory management of burns. *American Family Physician, 62*(9), 2015–2026.

NANDA International. (2003). *Nursing diagnoses: Definitions & classification 2003-2004.* Philadelphia: Author.

Wong, D. L., Hockenberry, M. J., Wilson, D., Winkelstein, M. L., & Kline, N. E. (2003). Conditions that produce fluid and electrolyte imbalance In D. L. Wong (Ed.), *Nursing care of infants and children* (7th ed.) (pp. 1227–1254). St Louis, MO: Mosby.

Wright, R. K. (2001). *Electrical injuries.* Retrieved March 2, 2004, from http://www.emedicine.com/emerg/topic162.htm

# Bibliography

Alisa Ann Ruch Burn Foundation. (2001). *Back to school: Re-entry program for burn injured children.* San Francisco: Author.

Bates-Jensen, B. (1999). Chronic wound management. *Nursing Clinics of North America, 34*(4), 799–845.

Bishop, B., & Gilinsky, V. (1995). School reentry for the patient with burn injuries: video and/or on-site intervention. *Journal of Burn Care and Rehabilitation, 16,* 455–457.

Cahners, S., Dumont, J., O'Connor, M., & McLoughlin, E. (1976). *The Burned Child's Return to School.* Boston: Shriner's Burn Institute.

Consumer Product Safety Commission. *Don't let children put caps for toy guns in their pockets.* CPSC Document 5009. Retrieved February 21, 2004, from http://www.cpsc.gov/CPSCPUB/PUBS/5009.pdf

Carpenito-Moyet, L. J. (2004). *Handbook of nursing diagnosis* (10th ed.). Philadelphia: Lippincott.

Consumer Product Safety Commission, Office of Information and Public Affairs. (1993). *Miracle recreation offers deck covering to prevent burns on bare metal playground decks.* Retrieved February 21, 2004, from http://www.cpsc.gov/CPSCPUB/PUBS

Consumer Product Safety Commission. *Young children and teens burned by hair curling irons.* CPSC Document 5029. Retrieved February 21, 2004, from http://www.cpsc.gov/CPSCPUB/PUBS/5029.pdf

Dowd, M. D. (1999). Childhood injury prevention at home and play. *Current Opinion in Pediatrics, 11*(6), 578.

Dressler, D. P., & Hozid, J. L. (2001). Thermal injury and child abuse: The medical evidence dilemma. *Journal of Burn Care and Rehabilitation, 22,* 180–185.

Joholske, J., & Greene, M. A. (2003). *2002 fireworks annual report.* Retrieved February 21, 2004, from http://www.cpsc.gov/library/2002fwreport.PDF

Mancususo, M. G., Bishop, S., Blakeney;, P., Robert, R., & Gaa, J. (2003). Impact on the family: psychosocial adjustment of siblings of children who survive serious burns. *Journal of Burn Care and Rehabilitation, 24,* 110–118.

Marsh, E. (2002). Interventions for clients with burns. In D. Ignatavicius, & M. L. Workman (Eds.), *Medical surgical nursing critical thinking for collaborative care* (pp 1555–1586). Philadelphia: Saunders.

Pidcock, F. S., Fauergbach, J. A., Ober, M., & Carney, J. (2003). The rehabilitation/school matrix: A model for accommodating the noncompliant child with severe burns. *Journal of Burn Care and Rehabilitation, 24,* 342–346.

Rosenstein, D. L. (1987). A school reentry program for burned children. Part I: Development and implementation of a school reentry program. *Journal of Burn Care and Rehabilitation, 8,* 319–324.

## Resources

Alisa Ann Rush Burn Foundation
665 Third Street
Suite 345
San Francisco, CA 94107
415-495-7223
415-495-7224 (fax)
1-800-755-BURN (survivor assistance)
www.aarbf.org

American Burn Association
ABA Central Office-Chicago
625 North Michigan Avenue
Suite 1530
Chicago, IL 60611
312-642-9260
312-642-9130 (fax)
www.ameriburn.org

Burn Institute
3702 Ruffin Road
Suite 101
San Diego, CA 92123
858-541-2277
www.burninstitute.org

The Phoenix Society for Burn Survivors, Inc.
2153 Wealthy Street SE
Suite 215
East Grand Rapids, MI 49506
616-458-2773
616-458-2831 (fax)
1-800-888-2876 (burn survivors)
www.phoenix-society.org

Shriners International Headquarters
2900 Rocky Point Drive
Tampa, FL 33607-1460
813-281-0300
www.shrinersshg.org

# Chapter Twenty-nine

# Cancer

## Tambra R. Dahlheimer

## Introduction

The word "cancer" holds meaning for many people. But this meaning usually comes from our knowledge of or experience with an adult with cancer. Cancer in children is much more rare, and therefore our experience with and knowledge of it may be limited. Pediatric and adolescent cancer cases make up only 2% (Rasco, 1998a) of the cancer cases in the United States and around the world. The American Cancer Society (2004a) estimates that "about 9200 children under the age of 15 in the United States will be diagnosed with cancer in 2004" (p. 1). Leukemia is the most common type of childhood cancer (Smith & Gloeckler Reis, 2002). Central nervous system tumors and lymphoma are also high on the list (U.S. Cancer Statistics Working Group, 2003). Despite advances in diagnosis and treatment, cancer continues to be the second leading cause of death among children aged 1 to 14 (Reis et al., 2004; Ruccione, 1998).

Treatment outcomes have improved in part because of the collaboration of dedicated pediatric treatment centers and advances in technology, but also because of the development of national cooperative groups that study cancer (Rasco, 1998a; Schwartz, A, 2003). Because childhood cancer is so rare, cooperation in research has been essential, and thus significant improvements in survival have been possible.

The uses of combination chemotherapies and multi-modal therapies have changed the care of pediatric malignancies. Holistic care and changes in supportive management of these children have also positively affected outcomes, and many children are surviving these cancers. During treatment they are less likely than ever to be hospitalized and are more likely to be attending school. In fact, owing to improvements in treatments, the childhood cancer mortality rate has decreased by nearly 50% since 1975 (American Cancer Society, 2003). The 5-year survival rate for childhood cancer is 80.4% among white children and slightly less at 71.8% for African American children (Ries et al., 2004).

For these reasons, the school nurse may be involved with children in the school setting who are undergoing treatment or have completed treatment for many types of pediatric cancers. Nurses need to be aware of pathophysiology, principles and side effects of treatments, and sup-

portive care strategies, as well as prognosis and palliative care issues if necessary.

## Pathophysiology and Treatment

Cancer is a disease in which abnormal cells grow in an uncontrolled way. It begins when the system that directs the growth and development of cells fails. The body is usually able to control the development of cells so that they mature properly. When cancer develops, this process hasn't worked well (Barr et al., 2001). The body has allowed changes to occur in the genetic material inside the cell. Researchers are looking at many possible factors that may contribute to the development of pediatric cancers (American Cancer Society, 2001). There are many types of pediatric and adolescent cancers that may affect the school-aged child.

### Leukemia

Leukemia is a cancer of the blood-forming cells. Leukemia is most often a cancer of the white blood cells but can involve other blood cell types as well. These cell precursors can infiltrate bone marrow, peripheral blood, and other organs.

There are three types of pediatric leukemia:

1. Acute lymphoblastic leukemia (ALL), which is the most common and accounts for 75% to 80% of all childhood leukemia
2. Acute myeloid leukemia (AML), which accounts for 20% to 25% of childhood leukemia but cause about 30% to 50% of leukemia deaths
3. Chronic myeloid leukemia, which is only about 5% of leukemia (Rahman, 1998) and is rare in children and will not be discussed in this chapter

Over 2,400 new cases of ALL are diagnosed each year in the United States (Westlake & Bertolone, 2002). The peak age at onset is 4 years. Caucasians are more likely to be diagnosed with ALL than African Americans or Asian Americans, and males more often than females. There is a known genetic predisposition for ALL with trisomy 21, Fanconi's anemia, Bloom syndrome, and ataxia-telangiectasia. Children born to mothers of advanced age or those with a history of fetal loss may also be predisposed. Also at risk are identical twins. Twenty-five percent of identical twins who have a twin with ALL will go on to develop the disease. Some environmental factors may influence the likelihood of developing leukemia, such as radiation, chemotherapy for other cancers and certain chemicals (American Cancer Society, 2004a). Symptoms of ALL may include anemia, fatigue, pallor, fever, enlarged spleen or liver, swollen lymph nodes, and, in some persons, bone pain. Children will also show symptoms of low platelet count, such as petechia, easy bruising, prolonged bleeding with epistaxis, or wounds.

Treatment is decided based on the child's individual prognostic factors (Rahman, 1998) and risk category. More intensive therapy is given to children with high-risk disease (children who are diagnosed when they are age 10 or older and/or have a white blood cell count of over 50,000), and their outcomes are generally poorer than children with low-risk disease (American Cancer Society, 2001). Central nervous system prophylaxis is used early and throughout therapy, and combination chemotherapy is used to maintain remission. Treatment is given in three basic phases. Induction therapy is given first to eliminate as many leukemia cells as possible. The number of spinal tap procedures the child has during this phase of therapy is dependent on whether there is evidence of disease in the spinal fluid. About 3% of those diagnosed will have central nervous system disease (Westlake & Bertolone, 2002). Consolidation therapy follows to kill the remaining leukemia cells and to protect the central nervous system from leukemia through medicines that are given into the spinal fluid. Finally, maintenance therapy, as its name implies, is given to "maintain" the remission. It is usually well tolerated. Spinal taps with chemotherapy infusions into the spinal fluid continue in this phase.

Nearly all children achieve an initial remission (Westlake & Bertolone, 2002), but some will relapse during or after therapy. Since the 1970s, survival for children with ALL has improved. The 5-year survival rate for ALL is 80% (Westlake & Bertolone). Relapsed disease, however, is more difficult to treat, and chance of cure is less likely (Westlake & Bertolone).

AML is a cancer of the myeloid stem cells that infiltrate the peripheral blood, bone marrow, and other organs. The presenting symptoms for AML are swollen lymph nodes, fever, pallor, and anorexia and weight loss. Weakness and fatigue are also common. Presenting symptoms do differ somewhat from ALL in that children with AML may have a sore throat or recurrent infections, respiratory symptoms, or gastrointestinal symptoms. Also, gingival hypertrophy and chloromas, which are localized tumors of malignant cells, are symptoms unique to AML (Rahman, 1998). Treatment consists of much more in-hospital time and is quite intense. Many of these children will undergo bone marrow transplant if they have a matched sibling donor. Children without donors will continue chemotherapy (Golub & Arceci, 2002) or may receive unrelated donor marrow. The survival rates are dependent on which therapy is used and range from 40% to 60%. Survival is improved with matched sibling donor transplant (American Cancer Society, 2001).

## Hodgkin's Disease

Hodgkin's lymphoma is a cancer of the lymphoid system. It accounts for 5% of the cancers diagnosed in children younger than 15 years of age in the United States. The highest incidence is in teenagers and young adults, and it is actually considered rare in children under the age of 5 years. It is also known to occur more frequently in boys (Liebhauser, 2002). The American Cancer Society (2004b) estimates that about 7,880 new cases of Hodgkin's disease will occur in the United States in 2004. Of these, about 10% to 15% will be in children younger than 16 years (p. 4).

The cause of Hodgkin's disease is unknown, but some studies show an increased risk in close relatives. Hodgkin's disease is also more common in people with genetic or acquired immunodeficiency (Liebhauser, 2002). The association of Epstein-Barr virus with Hodgkin's lymphoma has been studied, but the relationship is not yet completely understood (Hodgkins & Donaldson, 2002).

Diagnosis is usually confirmed with a biopsy. Hodgkin's disease has several histologic types: lymphocyte predominant (LP), mixed cellularity (MC), lymphocyte depleted (LD), and nodular sclerosing (NS). The lymphocyte predominant type is more common in younger children and usually presents as localized disease (Liebhauser, 2002). It often involves the lymph nodes in the neck and under the arms and has the best prognosis (American Cancer Society, 2004b). Mixed cellularity most frequently presents with more advanced disease. Lymphocyte depleted is associated with poor prognosis but is rare in children, whereas nodular sclerosing is the most common type and carries a better prognosis.

Staging of Hodgkin's disease is determined by the extent of the disease at diagnosis (Liebhauser, 2002). Stage I is the involvement of a single lymph node region or one area of an organ outside the lymphoid system (American Cancer Society, 2004b). Stage II is the involvement of two or more lymph node regions or lymphoid structures on the same side of the diaphragm. If both sides (above and below) of the diaphragm are involved, it is considered stage III. Stage IV occurs if there is spread to one or more of the extralymphatic sites. Nearby lymph nodes may or may not be involved. The stages are further subdivided into A and B symptoms. "B" symptoms include weight loss, night sweats, and fever. "A" symptoms are the absence of any of these symptoms. About 60% of children with Hodgkin's lymphoma have stage I or II disease.

Treatment is primarily radiation and/or chemotherapy. Individualized therapy depends on age, stage, symptoms, and tumor burden (Liebhauser, 2002; Van Sycle, 1998a). Advanced stages of the disease (III or IV) and the presence of "B" symptoms have an unfavorable effect on prognosis. Other poor prognostic factors include an elevated erythrocyte sedimentation rate (ESR) throughout treatment, the LD subtype, and "bulky" disease (a lymph node with the largest dimension great than 10 cm) (Van Sycle, 1998a). The 5-year survival rate for children with stage I or stage II disease is as high as 85% to 95%

(Liebhauser, 2002). However, advanced stage disease still has about a 70% to 90% 5-year survival rate.

School nurses need to be aware that hospitalization is more likely for treatment of more advanced disease and may necessitate more missed days of school. Communication with the oncology healthcare providers is important when developing an individualized healthcare plan (IHP) that includes medications needed at school for possible nausea after chemotherapy, how to respond to oncologic emergencies while in school, and pain relief measures. School nursing staff should be aware that children receiving chemotherapy who experience fever need to be evaluated by a doctor. The nurse should notify parents immediately. Pediatric patients who receive radiation may experience late effects, such as a decrease in their final height, lung dysfunction, or increased risk of a second cancer (Liebhauser, 2002).

### Non-Hodgkin's Lymphoma

Non-Hodgkin's lymphoma is a cancerous solid tumor. In non-Hodgkin's lymphoma, lymphoid cells spread in a haphazard, erratic, and aggressive pattern. These cells can be found in the lymph nodes and lymphoid tissue such as the spleen, but can also infiltrate bone marrow and cerebrospinal fluid. Non-Hodgkin's lymphoma is the most common solid tumor in childhood and accounts for 60% of all childhood lymphomas (Van Sycle, 1998b). Many of the same etiologic factors play a role in the development of non-Hodgkin's lymphoma that occur in Hodgkin's lymphoma. Geographic, immunologic, viral, and genetic factors are likely to be involved. Childhood non-Hodgkin's lymphoma can be categorized into three main types. The first is small, noncleaved cell, which accounts for almost half of all childhood non-Hodgkin's lymphoma. Most of these start in the abdomen. This type includes Burkitt and non-Burkitt subtypes. The second type, lymphoblastic lymphoma, is similar to leukemia. In fact, the two are distinguished from one another by noting the percentage of immature cancer cells that are found in the bone marrow. If it is greater than 25%, it is considered leukemia instead of lymphoma. Finally, the large cell type is known to be found in extranodal sites (such as the skin, lungs, bones, and brain) (Hussong, 2002). This type accounts for about 15% to 20% of childhood non-Hodgkin's lymphoma (Van Sycle, 1998b).

Symptoms usually relate to the location of the primary tumor. Children with mediastinal disease will have respiratory symptoms, whereas those with abdominal tumors will have nausea, vomiting, or intestinal obstructions. The symptoms will progress rapidly and are associated with the location of the tumor.

Non-Hodgkin's lymphoma responds well to chemotherapy. Radiation is used only in special situations (Hussong, 2002) . Survival has increased to an overall rate of 80% with the use of several chemotherapy agents.

### Neuroblastoma

Neuroblastoma is the second most common solid tumor in childhood and the fourth most common childhood malignancy (Sulivan, 1993). There are about 550 new cases per year in the United States. Ninety-seven percent of cases will present before age 10. Neuroblastomas are derived from neural crest cells that develop into the sympathetic nervous system. The most common site is the abdomen, specifically the adrenal gland. Neuroblastoma is known as the "silent tumor" because about two thirds of children will present with widespread metastatic disease. It is usually seen in the bone marrow, bone, liver, and lymph nodes (Frothingham,1998; Dadd, 2002).

There is no known cause. Studies have looked at the possibility of increased risk due to maternal exposure to alcohol, certain drugs, and hair coloring. They have also looked at paternal exposure to electromagnetic fields. The tumor cells show some genetic abnormalities that are considered prognostic. The first is a deletion of the short arm of chromosome 1. It is associated not only with advanced disease but also with poor prognosis. MYCN (or n-MYC) is a proto-oncogene that is found on chromosome 2. Thirty percent of nueroblastomas are found to have multiple copies of this gene (or are said to have MYCN amplification) which is predictive of poor outcome (Dadd,2002). The DNA content of the cell can also affect outcome. Symptoms of neuroblastoma will vary depending on where along the sympathetic nerve pathway the tumor arises and where it has spread. Tumor markers, VMA and HVA, will be excessive in the urine. These urinary catecholamines are measured at diagnosis and throughout and after therapy to monitor the disease.

Treatment is based on age and stage identified by the International Neuroblastoma Staging System (Frothingham,1998; Dadd, 2002). The stages are 1, 2 (A or B), 3, 4, and 4S. Stage 1 is localized and easily excised, and stage 4 is disseminated to various parts of the body. Stage 4S is most often observed and not treated. It may show spontaneous regression. Treatment is used in specific cases. For the other stages, multimodal therapy, including chemotherapy, surgery, radiotherapy, peripheral blood stem cell transplant, and immune modulators, will be used. The majority of children with neuroblastoma have excellent survival rates, with the exception of children with high-risk disease (higher disease stage, greater than 12 months at diagnosis, and grossly abnormal laboratory levels). Five-year survival in high-risk disease in only 22% to 30%, but in lower risk groups it is 80% to 98% (Dadd).

### Rhabdomyosarcoma

There are about 250 new cases of rhabdomyosarcoma diagnosed in the United States each year. Rhabdomyosarcoma can be diagnosed at any age, but 65% of cases are diagnosed before the age of 6 years. A second age peak is noted at 10 to 18 years of age, when the remaining cases usually occur. Rhabdomyosarcoma is a cancer of the muscle cell and can affect many different parts of the body (CancerBACUP 2003). The child may be alerted to seek medical care by seeing the mass, or they may have an interruption of a normal body function depending on the site of the rhabdomyosarcoma. The head and neck is the most common site. The genitourinary tract is the second most common site, accounting for 22% of rhabdomyosarcomas. A tumor starting in an extremity is usually tender. It can be mistaken for a hematoma after an injury especially in school age children. There can often be a delay in diagnosing rhabdomyosarcoma in the extremity because it is most often found in adolescents to whom injuries to the extremities are frequent. School nurses need to evaluate sports injuries carefully and refer for continued complaints of discomfort in the same extremity or area of the extremity.

Treatment combines the use of radiation, chemotherapy, and surgery for the best outcomes. Five-year disease-free survival with multimodal therapy is 70%. There are concerns about late effects with this disease. Radiation, depending on the site to which it is given, can cause cataracts, hormonal imbalances, fibrosis, growth retardation, bowel obstruction, and hematuria. Loss of function in the affected area can occur following surgery. Optimally, surgery will remove the entire tumor while preserving function, but this is not always possible. Other effects, such as kidney problems, infertility, and second malignancies, are all possibilities for childhood survivors of rhabdomyosarcoma (Kotsubo, 2002; Rasco, 1998b).

## Wilms' Tumor

Wilms' tumor is a tumor of the kidney accounting for only 6% of all childhood cancers in the United States (Drigan & Androkites, 2002). Eighty percent of these tumors occur before age 5 years (Rasco, 1998c). Usually the initial presenting sign is an asymptomatic abdominal mass in a well-appearing child. These tumors are usually very large with a fragile covering. Some children may also have fever, blood in their urine, pain, or high blood pressure as presenting symptoms. Familial cases are about 1.5% of Wilms' tumor cases (Drigan & Androkites, 2002) and are associated with certain anomalies such as congenital absence of the iris, genitourinary malformations, hemihypertrophy, Beckwith-Weidemann syndrome, and others.

The two histologic categories of Wilm's tumor are favorable and unfavorable or anaplastic. Anaplastic cells divide more rapidly and are more aggressive. These tumors are usually found in older children. Most are favorable tumors (85%) and have an excellent prognosis. Seven percent of children with Wilms' tumor have involvement of both kidneys.

Surgery is important for staging and as initial treatment. The surgeon needs to completely remove the tumor and needs to do it without accidentally opening the gelatinous cover and spilling its contents. Surgical management in bilateral disease is to preserve as much normal kidney tissue as possible. This is important for maintaining adequate kidney function. The National Wilms' Tumor Study Group has developed staging that ranges from stage I to

IV depending on clinical, surgical, and pathological features of the tumor. They have long studied this tumor and treatment options. Treatment is based on stage and consists of chemotherapy with the addition of radiation in some cases. The overall cure rate for all stages is 80% to 90% (Rasco, 1998c).

## Bone Tumors

### Osteogenic Sarcoma

Osteogenic sarcoma accounts for about 60% of malignant bone tumors in children less than 15 years of age. The most common primary sites are the long bones (Betcher, Simon, & McHard, 2002). Although the etiology is unknown, several factors are associated with the development of osteogenic sarcomas. The first is genetic. The retinoblastoma gene and p53, the tumor suppressor gene located on chromosome 17, have been implicated so that children who have retinoblastoma or Li-Fraumeni syndrome, which is a rare inherited disorder (Genetics Home Reference, 2004), are more likely to develop osteogenic sarcoma. High-dose radiation exposure is also known to have caused osteogenic sarcoma.

Children who develop osteogenic sarcoma will most frequently have pain or the area, and may have a mass. Activity usually increases the pain. Limping or a refusal to walk could also occur. Ten to twenty percent of patients will have metastasis at diagnosis, most commonly to the lung. Of these, only 10-20% will have long-term survival. Sixty-five percent of patients without metastasis may be cured (McHard, 1998 and Betcher et al., 2002). Surgery is the mainstay of treatment, but chemotherapy also plays an active role.

### Ewing's Sarcoma

Ewing's sarcoma is primarily a malignant tumor of the bone. However, it can also arise in soft tissue. Seventy percent are diagnosed in patients less than 20 years of age. It most commonly affects bones of the humerus, femur, pelvis, and tibia.

Symptoms may be present for several months before diagnosis and may come and go. The most common symptoms are pain and swelling in the soft tissue around the bone. Chemotherapy is imperative treatment for Ewing's sarcoma. Surgery and/or radiation are important local control measures. If surgical removal of the tumor is possible without unacceptable loss of function, it should be performed. The extent of disease at diagnosis is prognostic (McHard & Rasco, 1998). Cure rates for local disease are estimated to be 50% to 70%, whereas cure rate with metastatic tumors is less than 20%.

Surgical management of both osteogenic sarcoma and Ewing's sarcoma tumors is most commonly accomplished with limb salvage or amputation. Limb salvage will allow children and adolescents a more functional extremity. There are, however, complications to consider, such as immediate and long-term infections or possible nonunion of the bones. Response to chemotherapy and the extent and resectability of the tumor are also considered as the surgeon decides how to proceed. Amputation is considered more often for tumors in expendable locations such as ribs or fingers. Compliance issues are also considered. Families that cannot handle the complex wound management or intensive physical therapy that may be necessary with the other options may choose amputation. In both tumors, the amount of tumor necrosis at the time of surgery is predictive of outcome (Betcher et al., 2002). Patients with less than 10% viable (capable of living) tumor in their surgical specimens will do better than those with more viable tumor.

## Other Cancers

Although the cancers described here are not the only ones found in children, they are the most common. Some cancers that occur rarely in children include liver tumors, germ call tumors (ovarian or testicular), thyroid cancers, sarcomas, and melanoma. These cancers are beyond the scope of this chapter. Refer to the bibliography at the end of this chapter for additional resources.

## Additional Issues for All Pediatric Cancers

### Central Lines

Central lines are placed by surgeons at the start of therapy to more easily deliver chemotherapy and other intravenous medications, draw blood samples, and administer transfusions. There are two categories of central lines—partially implanted or totally implanted. The Port-a-Cath is an example of the totally implanted line and is completely hidden inside the subcutaneous tissue. It is accessed with a needle through the skin on the chest. The right atrial catheter has tubing that is partially external.

There is an external site on the chest ,which can be a source of infection (Barr et al., 2001) .

### Immunizations

Children who are being treated for cancer should not be given live virus vaccines such as measles, mumps, rubella (MMR), oral OPV, and the chickenpox vaccine. These can usually be given 3 months after therapy has been completed. If transplantation is part of the child's therapy, it is better to wait 6 to 12 months after therapy has been completed. Pnuemovax and influenza can and should be given to students undergoing therapy. However, before any immunizations are given, the student needs to check with his or her oncology care provider (Barr et al., 2001).

### Chickenpox

The child with cancer is vulnerable to chickenpox. If the child is exposed to chickenpox, the school nurse should notify the parent right away. Medical care should be sought immediately and gamma globulin administered to minimize the possibility of an outbreak.

### Mouth Sores

Mouth sores can be a very painful complication of chemotherapy. Often children who have mouth sores repeatedly with therapy will be placed on a preventative medication, such as glutamine. At school, the child should be allowed to make food choices that will not cause further injury or pain but will provide nutritional requirements to maintain weight. The mouth should be cleansed well after meals.

# Individualized Healthcare Plan

## Assessment

### History
- When was the cancer diagnosed?
- What kind of cancer does the child have?
- What were the presenting symptoms?
- Were there any predisposing factors?
- What is the stage of the disease?
- Is there any metastasis?
- When did treatment begin?
- What type of treatment is the child undergoing?
- Has the child had any surgeries?
- Does the child have a central line?
- Has the child had chemotherapy? Which medicines?
- Has the child had any radiation? When? To what site? At what dose?
- Has there been response to treatment?
- Is the child in remission or have there been periods of remission?
- Who is caring for the child?
- What is the family structure?
- Has the child been hospitalized related to this cancer? When? How frequently is the child hospitalized? What happened during the hospital stays?
- Are there disabilities associated with this cancer?
- Are there any other health problems prior to diagnosis?

- Are there any growth or other developmental delays?
- What is the child's attendance record?

### Current Status
- Treatment regimen: Surgery, chemotherapy, and/or radiation plan: The road map of the treatments
- Baseline height and weight
- Baseline respiratory and cardiac assessment
- Baseline neurologic assessment
- Baseline skin and mucous membrane assessment
- Current pain assessment
- Monitor vital signs (temperature, blood pressure, pulse rate and rhythm, and respiration rate and quality
- Observe for side effects of chemotherapy:
  - Gastrointestinal: nausea, vomiting, diarrhea, constipation, jaundice from impaired liver function, abdominal pain related to possible pancreatitis, and poor or no appetite
  - Skin/mucous membranes: mouth sores, rashes, bruising or other discoloration of skin, alopecia, sensitivity to sunlight, signs of dehydration
  - Low platelet count (bruising, bleeding)
  - Low white cell count (immunosuppression resulting in frequent infections) and low hemoglobin (pale, tired, increased heart rate)
  - Cardiac: Changes in energy and stamina, irregular heart rate, signs of cardiac failure
  - Also observe for renal and respiratory changes
  - Monitor for neurologic complications (paresthesias, neuropathies, decreased reflexes, and muscle weakness)
- Observe for side effects of radiation (effects will depend on the site)
  - Brain: monitor for headaches, and nausea and vomiting; neurologic changes (lightheaded, changes in consciousness) can also occur
  - Eyes: observe for lens opacity or changes in vision
  - Digestive tract: dry mouth, mouth sores, difficulty eating and swallowing, nausea and vomiting, tenderness of the liver, cramping, diarrhea
  - Cardiac: postirradiation pericarditis symptoms, which can include fever, dyspnea, chest pain, and a pericardial rub
  - Urinary tract: hypertension, protein in urine, edema, urinary frequency, and pain or difficulty with urination
  - Reproductive organs: sterility or infertility
  - Bones: growth problems, hematologic problems
  - Skin: erythema, radiation burns, hair loss (may be permanent with high doses)
- Treatment orders
  - Activity
  - Medications
  - Diet
  - Central venous catheter care
- Student's description of and definition of cancer

### Self-care
- Can the student demonstrate understanding of condition and treatment?
- Can the student demonstrate understanding of warning signs indicating the need to seek medical care?
- Physical and cognitive ability to understand need for and administer medicines and other care when needed (i.e., pain relief measures or medications, chemotherapy, and antinausea medicines)
- Does the student wear Medic Alert bracelet?
- Does the student maintain a reasonable diet, and is the student able to make modifications when needed?
- Does the student understand the need for assistance with academics and/or personal care issues?

### Psychosocial Status
- How is the student/family coping?
- What is the student/family's
  - Level of understanding and acceptance
  - Support system
  - Evidence of depression/grieving
  - Developmental level
  - Feelings about having cancer

- Has the diagnosis been shared with peer group? What was the reaction?
- Has the child experienced disruption of activities? Sports? Socialization?
- Has child experienced concerns about peer's reactions?
- Does child participate in after-school programs? Social activities? Community events or activities?

*Academic Issues*
- School attendance
- Academic performance pattern
- Current cognitive status
  - Ability to comprehend and communication
  - Neuropsychological testing
- Regular education and special education issues
- Need for 504 plan
- Health needs during the school day: medications, special procedures
- Participation in after-school activities and the need for accommodations
- Classroom, school, and/or curriculum modifications
  - Student schedule changes
  - Physical environment (wheelchair or elevator needs)
  - Toileting assistance if needed
  - Help with lunch
  - Computer access
  - Library access
  - Need for peer assistance
  - Home/hospital tutoring needs

## Nursing Diagnoses (N.D) (NANDA, 2003)

**N.D 1** Risk for infection (NANDA 00004) related to:
- immunosuppression related to therapy
- inadequate primary defenses (central line, invasive procedures, surgical wounds)
- leukopenia and/or altered inflammatory response
- malnutrition

**N.D 2** Nausea (NANDA 00134) related to:
- chemotherapy medication side effects
- radiation side effects

**N.D 3** Impaired oral mucous membrane (NANDA 00045) related to:
- chemotherapy side effects
- immunosupression/ leukopenia
- radiation side effects

**N.D 4** Fatigue (NANDA 00093) related to:
- anemia
- inadequate sleep
- medication and/or radiation side effects
- disease state
- malnutrition

**N.D 5** Risk for activity intolerance (NANDA 00092) or impaired physical mobility (NANDA 00085) related to:
- low blood cell counts
- fatigue
- medication and/or radiation side effects
- alteration in activities of daily care and self-care
- amputation
- knowledge deficit

**N.D 6** Constipation or the risk for constipation (NANDA 00015) related to:
- disease process
- medication side effects
- inadequate activity
- changes in eating patterns

**N.D 7** Diarrhea (00013) related to:
- physiologic changes associated with disease
- adverse effects of therapy

**N.D 8** Risk for imbalanced fluid volume (NANDA 00025) related to:
- surgeries
- side effects and fluid therapy associated with chemotherapy administration or radiation
- vomiting and diarrhea associated with medicines

**N.D 9** Impaired adjustment (NANDA 00070) related to:
- lack of acceptance of cancer diagnosis
- inadequate support to adapt to diagnosis
- intensity of emotions and stressors
- lack of optimism

**N.D 10** Decreased cardiac output (NANDA 00029) related to:
- medications
- fever, infection with potential for shock

**N.D 11** Ineffective coping (NANDA 00069) related to:
- uncertainty of prognosis
- inadequate social support
- situational crisis

**N.D 12** Risk for delayed development (NANDA 00112) related to:
- chronic illness
- therapy side effects

**N.D 13** Ineffective health maintenance (NANDA 00099) related to:
- lack of knowledge regarding cancer pathophysiology
- lack of resources
- inability to cope with illness
- impaired communication skills
- cognitive impairment

**N.D 14** Imbalanced nutrition: less than body requirements (NANDA 00002) related to:
- anorexia related to medicines
- nausea/vomiting associated with chemotherapy
- mouth sores

**N.D 15** Chronic (NANDA 00133) or acute (NANDA 00132) pain related to:
- cancer
- surgery
- side effects or medications or radiation

**N.D 16** Impaired skin integrity (NANDA 00046) or risk for impaired skin integrity related to:
- central line
- side effects of medications and/or radiation
- alteration in nutritional state
- immobility

**N.D 17** Impaired social interaction (NANDA 0052) related to:
- frequent and/or prolonged school absences
- decreased self-esteem related to body changes
- physical limitations/fatigue

**N.D 18** Death anxiety (NANDA 00147) related to:
- morbid nature of disease
- poor prognosis of individual diagnosis
- fear/knowledge deficit
- ineffective coping

**N.D 19** Risk for injury (NANDA 00035) related to:
- low platelet count
- central line

**N.D 20** Ineffective protection (NANDA00043) related to:
- immunosuppression from treatment
- bone marrow suppression
- impaired skin integrity
- inadequate nutrition

**N.D 21** Self-care deficit related to functional limitations:
- Feeding 00102 (NANDA 00102)
- Bathing/hygiene (NANDA 00108)
- Dressing /grooming self-care deficit (NANDA 00109)
- Toileting self-care deficit (NANDA 00110)

**N.D 22** Impaired dentition (NANDA 00048) related to:
- medication side effects
- malnutrition/anorexia
- radiation side effects
- ineffective oral hygiene

**N.D 23** Disturbed sleep pattern (NANDA 00095) related to:
- hospitalization
- medication/treatment effects
- delayed sleep phase

**N.D 24** Delayed growth and development (NANDA 00111) related to:
- effects of medication/radiation

**N.D 25** Deficit knowledge (NANDA 00126) of cancer and its treatment related to:
- cognitive limitations
- lack of information

**N.D 26** Social isolation (NANDA 00053) related to:
- physical limitations
- frequent or prolonged absences from school
- alteration in physical appearance

**N.D 27** Risk for situational low self-esteem (NANDA 00153) related to:
- cancer diagnosis functional impairment
- side effects of treatment (changes in appearance)
- diminished social interaction/social isolation

**N.D 28** Ineffective therapeutic regime management (NANDA 00078) related to:
- depression
- lack of knowledge
- fatigue/weakness

**N.D 29** Risk for powerlessness (NANDA 00152) related to:
- knowledge deficit
- low self-esteem
- lack of control over therapy

**N.D 30** Hopelessness (NANDA 00124) related to:
- social isolation
- possible poor prognosis

**N.D 31** Interrupted family processes (NANDA 00060) related to:
- crisis of the diagnosis and treatment
- shift in family roles
- potential stress on family finances

## Goals

The student will increase his/her knowledge of signs and symptoms of infections to promote early intervention and treatment. (N.D. 1, 3, 10, 16, 25, 28)

The student will increase his/her knowledge of the cancer and its treatment. (N.D. 2, 4-8, 12–14, 25, 28)

The student will improve skills to manage cancer, its treatments, and side effects. (N.D. 1–8, 12, 14, 17)

The student will manage age-appropriate treatments, medications, and diet needs in the school setting. (N.D. 2, 3, 6–8, 12, 14, 16, 17, 21)

The student will participate in regular school class activities, including physical education class, with modifications made as necessary. (N.D. 4, 5, 15, 17)

The student will have a good school attendance pattern. (N.D. 1–5, 17)

The student will maintain adequate intake by preventing nausea when possible. (N.D. 2, 14)

The student will maintain peer relationships and activities. (N.D. 4, 5, 9, 11, 17, 30)

The student will assist in the development of the emergency care plan (ECP) and the IHP. (N.D. 1, 10, 13, 16)

The student will have a normal elimination pattern. (N.D. 6–8)

The student will not have pain. (N.D. 3, 15)
The student will be free of mouth sores. (N.D. 3, 14, 22)
The student will adjust to living with a chronic illness. (N.D. 11, 18, 26, 27)
The student will have decreased anxiety about condition and appearance in the school setting. (N.D. 17)
The student will progress in discussing death and dying issues and other concerns. (N.D. 18)
The student will be free of injury. (N.D. 19, 20)
The student will be alert and attentive in school. (N.D. 4, 15, 23)
The student will discuss his/her feelings and concerns about the disease. (N.D. 9, 11, 17, 18, 24, 26, 27, 29, 30-31)

## Nursing Interventions

Discuss with student (N.D. 1–31)
- What cancer is
- Current therapy
- How low blood counts may affect activity and risk for infection
- Warning signs of infection
- Importance of seeking care if signs of infection
- Medic Alert bracelet if needed
- Medication side effects
- Avoidance of over-the-counter medications that contain aspirin or affect platelet function
- Nutrition
- Supportive care measures
- Coping skills
- Emotional issues and frustrations
- Death and dying issues

Assess student for side effects of chemotherapy and radiation if applicable. (See Current Status section for list of possible side effects.) (N.D. 1–5, 8, 10, 14, 16, 17)

Develop an ECP with the student and his/her guardians and healthcare provider for the care of fever, bleeding, and other effects of treatment and also when 911 is to be called. (N.D. 1–8. 14–17)

Provide rest periods as needed in the health office. (N.D. 4, 5, 23)

Allow student to complete mouth care in the health office after meals. (N.D. 1, 3, 14)

Notify or assist student to notify parents if he/she has signs/symptoms of infections or regarding infectious diseases exposures/outbreaks, such as chickenpox. (N.D. 1, 19, 20)

Participate in the development of a 504 plan or individualized education plan (IEP). (N.D. 1–8, 14–17)

Refer to Special Education if appropriate. (N.D. 12)

Assist in modifying educational program as needed. (N.D. 1–8, 14–17)
- Plan for makeup work for school days absent.
- Help coordinate homebound or hospital-based education if much missed school secondary to inpatient therapy or extended illness.
- Modify physical education requirements for fatigue or low counts periods.
- Provide in-service education to staff about cancer, ECP, and symptoms to be reported to school nurse and/or parents.
- Monitor school attendance.
- Increase transition time between classes if needed.
- Assist with mobility and activities of daily living.

Participate in transition planning. (N.D. 11, 12, 17, 26, 31)

Assess student and family level of knowledge regarding cancer and current treatment. (N.D. 9, 14, 31)

Obtain orders and authorization for any treatments, medication, and/or any special diet requirements from healthcare provider and parents. (N.D. 2, 6–8, 16, 17, 28)

Consult with dietitian regarding dietary needs, and arrange for appropriate meals. (N.D. 8, 14)

Monitor compliance with treatment. (N.D. 13, 21, 28)

Monitor temperature and vital signs when symptoms occur. (N.D. 1–4, 6, 7, 10, 15, 16)

Monitor height and weight. (N.D.12, 14)

Assist to increase self-care and independence. (N.D. 13, 21, 28)

Monitor frequency of nausea and vomiting and hydration status. (N.D. 2)

Monitor for signs of electrolyte imbalance. (N.D. 7, 8, 14)

Ensure privacy and confidentiality. (N.D. 11, 13, 21, 27, 28, 29)

Assist in obtaining medical releases to allow information to be shared between healthcare provider and school. (N.D. 1–18, 31)

Facilitate ongoing communication between healthcare provider, teachers, guardians, and student regarding current status and needs of the student. (N.D. 1–18, 31)

Assist student in communicating disease process and therapy effects with his/her peers if the student wishes. (N.D. 17, 26, 27, 29, 30)

Provide emotional support. (N.D. 17, 26, 27, 29, 30)

Provide comfort measures. (N.D. 2–7, 15)

Assess for factors affecting social interaction. (N.D. 11, 17, 27))

Changes in physical appearance (surgery, amputation, hair loss, catheter)

Fatigue

Extended hospitalizations

Assess for factors affecting learning. (N.D. 4, 5, 12)

Neuropsychological effects of chemotherapy

Coordination problems

Vision and/or hearing problems

Refer to appropriate resources and/or support groups. (N.D. 11, 17, 26, 30, 31)

## Expected Student Outcomes

The student will:

- Demonstrate an age-appropriate understanding of his/her cancer diagnosis and treatment through discussions with the school nurse and return demonstrations of treatments and medication administration. (N.D. 1–9, 13–17, 28)
- Achieve functioning to age-appropriate level of ability. (N.D. 4, 5, 13, 15, 24, 31)
- Participate in all school activities with modifications if needed. (N.D. 4, 5, 26)
- Assist in planning the IHP and ECP. (N.D. 9, 13, 29, 31)
- Comply with medical treatment plan in school. (N.D. 1-10, 12, 14–17, 21, 28)
- Demonstrate proper technique of self-medication in compliance with orders and school policy. (N.D. 2, 4, 6–8, 10, 15, 16, 21, 28)
- Remain free of infection. (N.D. 1, 20)
- Have intact mucous membranes. (N.D. 3, 20, 22)
- Maintain clean, intact central line site. (N.D. 16, 20)
- Recognize early warning signs of infections and seek appropriate care. (N.D. 1, 20-21, 26, 28)
- List and recognize side effects of medicines. (N.D. 1–5, 8, 10, 14, 16, 17, 21, 25, 28)
- Assist with planning self-care, activities of daily living, and any modifications needed. (N.D. 13, 21, 28)
- Recognize and verbalize symptoms of fatigue and be able to modify situation as needed. (N.D. 4, 5, 23, 31)
- Inform teacher/school nurse of needs and/or symptoms. (N.D. 1–5, 8, 10, 14, 16, 17)
- Maintain current weight and adequate growth patterns. (N.D. 8, 12, 14, 24)
- Develop coping mechanisms by participating in support groups and/or be able to identify support systems. (N.D. 9, 17, 26, 27, 29–31)
- Verbalize feelings with the school nurse, peers, or other identified staff person. (N.D. 9, 11, 17, 18, 27, 29, 30)
- Wear Medic Alert bracelet if needed. (N.D. 1, 10, 13)
- Feel comfortable in the school setting as evidenced by participation in programs at school, and verbalization of adjustment, increased self-esteem, and stressors with school staff. (N.D. 9, 13, 17, 27, 29, 30)
- Have minimal or no pain. (N.D. 1, 3, 6, 7, 15, 16)
- Interact with peers in an appropriate way. (N.D. 9, 13, 17, 27, 29, 30)
- Participate in transition planning. (N.D. 9, 18, 28, 31)
- Utilize modification for mobility and access if needed. (N.D. 5, 19)

# Case Study

Jane is a 7-year-old girl who was brought to the doctor after a 1-week history of fever, lethargy, and bruising. She was diagnosed was having acute lymphoblastic leukemia after a bone marrow biopsy. Her spinal fluid was free of disease. She was hospitalized for 4 days to begin induction chemotherapy. A central line was placed to more easily administer her chemotherapy. She will not receive radiation. She was discharged and completed 1 month of steroid therapy. She is currently in remission, beginning her second month of therapy. She will be missing school for weekly spinal taps this month, and doctors expect an occasional hospitalization for fever during times of more intensive chemotherapy. She has needed occasional blood and platelet transfusions.

Jane's family appears to be coping well with the diagnosis and treatment. Jane also has an older brother and several close friends. She sometimes tires on the playground but has otherwise been participating in full class days when she is here. She has missed 10 days of school on account of her diagnosis. Her teachers describe her as a good student.

Currently Jane is without fever, and vital signs are stable. She has thinning hair but has not yet lost all of it. She is at the 75th percentile for height, and her weight is at the 40th percentile for age. She has one small mouth sore, which she notes is improving. She has occasional back pain, especially on the day following her procedures, but otherwise she feels well. She is currently experiencing some problems with constipation. She has learned how to swallow her medications and has antinausea medicine at school.

Cancer

## Leukemia

| Assessment Data | Nursing Diagnosis | Goals | Nursing Interventions | Expected Outcomes |
|---|---|---|---|---|
| Jane is a 7-year-old girl who was diagnosed with acute lymphoblastic leukemia. | Ineffective health maintenance due to lack of knowledge regarding cancer pathophysiology. | The student will increase knowledge of her cancer diagnosis and treatment. | Discuss with student what cancer is, current therapy, how low blood cell counts may affect activity and risk for infection and warning signs of infection.  Demonstrate medication administration and treatments. | The student will accurately discuss an understanding of her cancer diagnosis.  The student will demonstrate proper technique of self-medication and will be able to provide return demonstrations of all treatments that are needed in the school setting.  The student will recognize and describe early warning signs of infections and seek appropriate care. |
| She will be missing school for weekly spinal taps this month, and doctors expect an occasional hospitalization for fever during times of more intensive chemotherapy.  She has missed 10 days of school on account of her diagnosis.  Jane has several close friends.  She has thinning hair but has not yet lost all of it.  She sometimes tires on the playground but has otherwise been participating in full class days when she is here. | Fatigue due to anemia, malnutrition, poor sleep, medication side effects, and/or disease state.  Impaired social interaction due to school absences/attendance pattern, decreased self-esteem related to body changes, fatigue.  Ineffective coping due to uncertainty of prognosis, inadequate social support, and/or situational crisis. | The student will participate in regular school class activities, including physical education class, with modifications made as necessary.  The student will have a good school attendance pattern.  The student will maintain peer relationships and activities.  The student will feel comfortable in the school setting.  The student will develop coping mechanisms and verbalize feelings. | Participate in the development of a 504 plan, IEP, and/or IHP.  Assist in modifying educational program as needed.  Monitor school attendance.  Provide emotional support.  Provide information about support programs within the school setting and community.  Provide rest periods as needed in the health office.  Refer family to support group.  Encourage activities with peers. | The student will turn in all required work and will maintain current grades or academic status.  The student will participate in all school activities with modifications if needed.  The student can identify her friends and will participate in activities with them.  The student will participate in support programs at school and will verbalize adjustment, increased self-esteem, and stressors with school staff.  The student will verbalize her feelings. |

| Assessment Data | Nursing Diagnosis | Goals | Nursing Interventions | Expected Outcomes |
|---|---|---|---|---|
| A central line was placed to more easily administer her chemotherapy. | Risk for infection due to immunosuppression related to therapy, invasive procedures, and inadequate primary defenses (central line). | Maintain clean central line site. | Development of the ECP (including plan for chest injury or care in case of damage to the central line) and the IHP. | The student will maintain a clean, intact central line site that is free from infection.<br><br>The student will assist in the development of the ECP and IHP. |
| Currently Jane is without fever, and vital signs are stable. | Risk for infection due to immunosuppression related to therapy. | The student will increase her knowledge of signs and symptoms of infections to promote early intervention and treatment. | Monitor temperature and vital signs when symptoms appear. | The student will be free of infection.<br><br>The student will notify school nurse when she has symptoms. |
| Jane is in the 75th percentile for height, and her weight is at the 40th percentile for age. | Risk for delayed development due to chronic illness and/or therapy.<br><br>Imbalanced nutrition: less than body requirements due to poor appetite related to medicines and nausea associated with chemotherapy. | The student will manage diet needs in the school setting.<br><br>The student will maintain adequate intake by preventing nausea when possible. | Discuss nutrition with student.<br><br>Monitor weight.<br><br>Collaborate with dietary staff to provide foods that are palatable to Jane. | The student will maintain current weight and good growth patterns. |
| Jane is currently experiencing some problems with constipation. | Constipation due to medication effects.<br><br>Risk for constipation due to cancer, medications, inadequate activity, and poor diet. | The student will not have constipation. | Educate student regarding food choices that assist in elimination.<br><br>Encourage fluid intake.<br><br>Educate student regarding expected side effects of medications. | The student will have a normal stool pattern.<br><br>The student will list expected side effects of medications. |

*Chapter Twenty-nine: Cancer*

| Assessment Data | Nursing Diagnosis | Goals | Nursing Interventions | Expected Outcomes |
|---|---|---|---|---|
| Jane has one small mouth sore, which she notes is improving. | Impaired oral mucous membrane due to chemotherapy, immunosuppression. | The student will be free of mouth sores. | Allow student to complete mouth care in the health office after meals. | The student will have intact mucous membranes.<br><br>The student will be independent in oral hygiene regimen. |
| Jane has occasional back pain, especially the day following her procedures. | Chronic pain due to cancer. | The student will not have pain. | Provide comfort measures. | The student will have minimal or no pain. |
| She has learned how to swallow her medications and has antinausea medicine at school. | Nausea due to chemotherapy. | The student will maintain adequate intake by preventing nausea when possible.<br><br>The student will manage medications and diet needs in the school setting. | Discuss side effects of medications with the student.<br><br>Monitor nausea and vomiting.<br><br>Monitor for weight loss or signs of electrolyte imbalance. | The student will maintain weight and meet nutritional needs.<br><br>The student will have minimal or no nausea or vomiting.<br><br>The student will demonstrate proper technique of self-medication. |

# References

American Cancer Society. (2001). *Overview: Leukemia—children's.* Retrieved April 26, 2004, from http://www.cancer.org/docroot/CRI/CRI_2_1x.asp?dt=24

American Cancer Society. (2003). *Minnesota cancer facts and figures.* Retrieved March 26, 2004, from http://www.cancer.org/downloads/COM/mn%20facts%20and%20figures.pdf

American Cancer Society. (2004a). *Childhood cancer: General statement.* Retrieved May 15, 2004, from http://documents.cancer.org/135.00/135.00.pdf

American Cancer Society. (2004b). *Hodgkin's disease in children.* Retrieved March 26, 2004, from http://documents.cancer.org/6889.00/6889.00.pdf

Barr, R., Crockett, M., Dawson, S., Eves, M., Whitton, A., & Weirnikowski, J. (2001). *Childhood cancer information for the patient and family.* Hamilton, Ontario: Decker.

Betcher, D., Simon, P., & McHard, K. (2002). Bone tumors. In C. Rasco Baggott, K. Patterson Kelly, D. Fochtman, & G. Foley (Eds.), *Nursing care of children and adolescents with cancer* (3rd ed.). Philadelphia: Saunders.

CancerBACUP (2003). *Rhabdomyosarcoma in children.* Retrieved May 4, 2004, from http://www.cancerbacup.org.uk/Cancertype/Childrenscancers/Typesofchildrenscancers/Rhabdomyosarcoma

Dadd, G. (2002). Neuroblastoma. In C. Rasco Baggott, K. Patterson Kelly, D. Fochtman, & G. Foley (Eds). *Nursing care of children and adolescents with cancer* (3rd ed). Philadelphia: Saunders.

Drigan, R., & Androkites, A. (2002). Wilms' tumor. In C. Rasco Baggott, K. Patterson Kelly, D. Fochtman, & G. Foley (Eds.). *Nursing care of children and adolescents with cancer* (3rd ed). Philadelphia: Saunders.

Frothingham, B. (1998). Neuroblastoma. In M. Hockenberry-Eaton (Ed.), *Essentials of pediatric oncology nursing: A core curriculum* (pp. 32–35). Glenview, Illinois: Association of Pediatric Oncology Nurses.

Golub, T., & Arceci, R. (2002). Myeloid diseases. In C. Rasco Baggott, K. Patterson Kelly, D. Fochtman, & G. Foley (Eds.). *Nursing care of children and adolescents with cancer* (3rd ed). Philadelphia: Saunders.

Hudson, M., & Donaldson, S. (2002). Hodgkin's disease. In P. Pizzo & D. Poplack, (Eds.). *Principles and practice of pediatric oncology* (4th ed.). Philadelphia: Lippincott, Williams & Wilkins.

Hussong, M. R. (2002). Non-Hodgkin's lymphoma. In C. Rasco Baggott, K. Patterson Kelly, D. Fochtman, & G. Foley (Eds.). *Nursing care of children and adolescents with cancer* (3rd ed). Philadelphia: Saunders.

Kotsubo, C. (2002). Rhabdomyosarcoma. In C. Rasco Baggott, K. Patterson Kelly, D. Fochtman, & G. Foley (Eds.). *Nursing care of children and adolescents with cancer* (3rd ed). Philadelphia: Saunders.

Liebhauser, P. (2002). Hodgkin's disease. In C. Rasco Baggott, K. Patterson Kelly, D. Fochtman, & G. Foley (Eds.). *Nursing care of children and adolescents with cancer* (3rd ed). Philadelphia: Saunders.

Li-Fraumeni syndrome. (2004). In *Genetics home reference: Your guide to understanding genetic conditions.* Retrieved August 31, 2004, from http://www.ghr.nlm.nih.gov/ghr/disease/lifraumenisyndrome

McHard, K. (1998) Osteosarcoma. In M. Hockenberry-Eaton (Ed.), *Essentials of pediatric oncology nursing: A core curriculum* (pp. 36–38). Glenview, Illinois: Association of Pediatric Oncology Nurses.

McHard, K., & Rasco, C. (1998). Ewings sarcoma of bone and soft tissue and peripheral primitive neuroectodermal tumors. In M. Hockenberry-Eaton (Ed.), *Essentials of pediatric oncology nursing: A core curriculum* (pp. 38-41). Glenview, Illinois: Association of Pediatric Oncology Nurses.

NANDA International. (2003). *Nursing diagnoses: Definitions & classification 2003-2004.* Philadelphia: Author.

Rahman, S. (1998). Leukemia. In M. Hockenberry-Eaton (Ed.), *Essentials of pediatric oncology nursing: A core curriculum* (pp. 15–20). Glenview, Illinois: Association of Pediatric Oncology Nurses.

Rasco, C. (1998a). Overview of childhood cancer. In M. Hockenberry-Eaton (Ed.), *Essentials of pediatric oncology nursing: A core curriculum* (pp. 12). Glenview, Illinois: Association of Pediatric Oncology Nurses.

Rasco, C. (1998b). Rhabdomyosarcoma. In M. Hockenberry-Eaton (Ed.), *Essentials of pediatric oncology nursing: A core curriculum* (pp. 45–48). Glenview, Illinois: Association of Pediatric Oncology Nurses.

Rasco, C. (1998c). Tumors of the kidney. In M. Hockenberry-Eaton (Ed.), *Essentials of pediatric oncology nursing: A core curriculum* (pp. 41–45). Glenview, Illinois: Association of Pediatric Oncology Nurses.

Ries L. A. G., Eisner M. P., Kosary C. L., Hankey B. F., Miller B. A., Clegg L., et al. (Eds.). (2004). Bethesda, MD. Retrieved April 11, 2004, from *SEER cancer statistics review, 1975-2001, National Cancer Institute.* http://seer.cancer.gov/csr/1975_2001/

Ruccione, K. (1998). Epidemiology of childhood cancer. In M. Hockenberry-Eaton (Ed.), *Essentials of pediatric oncology nursing: A core curriculum* (pp. 12–15). Glenview, Illinois: Association of Pediatric Oncology Nurses.

Schwartz, A. (2003). Oncology. In C. Rudolph & A. Rudolph (Eds.), *Rudolph's pediatrics* (21st ed). New York: McGraw-Hill.

Cancer

Smith, M., & Gloeckler Ries, L. (2002). Childhood cancer: Incidence, survival and mortality. In P. Pizzo & D. Poplack (Eds.). *Principles and practice of pediatric oncology* (4th ed.). Philadelphia: Lippincott Williams & Wilkins.

Sullivan, M. (1993) Nueroblastoma. In G Foley, D. Fochtman, & K. Hardin Mooney (Eds.). *Nursing care of the child with cancer* (2nd ed). Philadelphia: Saunders.

U.S. Cancer Statistics Working Group. (2003). *United States cancer statistics: 2000 incidence.* Atlanta, GA: Department of Health and Human Services, Centers for Disease Control and Prevention and National Cancer Institute.

Van Sycle, K. (1998a). Hodgkin's disease. In M. Hockenberry-Eaton (Ed.), *Essentials of pediatric oncology nursing: A core curriculum* (pp. 23–27). Glenview, Illinois: Association of Pediatric Oncology Nurses.

Van Sycle, K. (1998b). Non-Hodgkin's lymphoma. In M. Hockenberry-Eaton (Ed.), *Essentials of pediatric oncology nursing: A core curriculum* (pp. 20–23). Glenview, Illinois: Association of Pediatric Oncology Nurses.

Westlake, S. ,& Bertolone, K. (2002). Acute lymphoblastic leukemia. In C. Rasco Baggott, K. Patterson Kelly, D. Fochtman, & G. Foley (Eds.). *Nursing care of children and adolescents with cancer* (3rd ed). Philadelphia: Saunders.

## Bibliography

Ablin, A. (Ed.) (1997). *Supportive care of children with cancer* Baltimore: Johns Hopkins University Press.

Adams, D. W. (1993) .*Coping with childhood cancer* (new revised edition). Hamilton, Ontario: Kingbridge.

Brunning, N. (1985). *Coping with chemotherapy.* New York: Baltimore Books.

Hockenberry-Eaton, M. (Ed.). (1998). Essentials *of pediatric oncology nursing: A core curriculum.* Glenview, Illinois: Association of Pediatric Oncology Nurses.

Hodder, H., & Keen, N. (2002). *Childhood cancer: A parent's guide to solid tumor cancers* (2nd ed.). Sebastopol, CA: O'Reilly & Associates, Inc.

Keen, N. (2002). *Childhood leukemia: A guide for families, friends, & caregivers* (3rd ed.). Sebastopol, CA: O'Reilly & Associates, Inc.

Pizzo, P., & Poplack, D. (Eds.). (2002). *Principles and practice of pediatric oncology* (4th ed.). Philadelphia: Lippincott Williams & Wilkins.

Rasco Baggott, C., Patterson Kelly, K., Fochtman, D., & Foley, G. (Eds). (2002). *Nursing care of children and adolescents with cancer* (3rd ed.). Philadelphia: Saunders.

Rudolph, C., & Rudolph, A. (Eds.). Rudolph's *Pediatrics* (21st ed.). New York: McGraw-Hill.

Watterson, J., Carlson-Green, B., & Oliver, J. (1999). *Helping your child. A manual for parents of children with leukemia..* St. Paul: Children's Hospitals and Clinics—St. Paul.

Watterson, J., Carlson-Green, B., & Oliver, J. (1999). *Teaching the child with Leukemia.* St. Paul: Children's Hospitals and Clinics—St. Paul.

## Resources

Association of Pediatric Oncology
4700 W Lake Avenue
Glenview, IL 60025
847-375-4724
877-734-8755 (fax)
http://www.apon.org

Candlelighter Childhood Cancer
Foundation
PO Box 398
Kensington, MD 20895-0498
1-800-366-2223
301-962-3521 (fax)
http://www.candlelighters.org

MedlinePlus
http://www.nlm.nih.gov/medline-plus

National Childhood Cancer
Foundation
CureSearch
4600 East W Highway
Suite 600
Bethesda, MD 20814-3457
http://www.curesearch.org

OncoLink
Abramson Cancer Center
University of Pennsylvania
3400 Spruce Street
2 Donner Building
Philadelphia, PA 19104-4283
215-349-5445 fax
http://www.oncolink.upenn.edu

Outlook: Life Beyond Childhood
Cancer
http://www.outlook-life.org

## Chapter Thirty

# Cardiovascular Disorders

Andrea D. Posey and Emelyn L. Hudson

## Introduction

Cardiovascular diseases affect many children worldwide. These pathophysiological processes can be categorized as congenital or acquired. Congenital conditions commonly require surgical intervention for correction or palliative care. Acquired cardiovascular diseases are those conditions that the patient develops after birth and can be seen in the normal heart or the heart with congenital defects. Acquired cardiovascular conditions in children include heart rate and conduction problems, hypertension, atherosclerosis, cardiomyopathy, and chest pain. Cardiovascular disease in children can compromise activity tolerance and endurance due to decreased oxygenation. Nursing management often includes identification, teaching, and support of children with these problems and their families.

## Pathophysiology
### Congenital Heart Disease

The American Heart Association (AHA) estimates that over 1 million Americans have a congenital heart defect (AHA, 2004). The incidence of congenital heart disease is 8 in 1,000 live births (Tak & McCubbin, 2002).

Congenital diseases are usually structural abnormalities of the heart that are present at birth, often due to a genetic defect, or environmental factors such as maternal alcohol consumption, drug abuse, diabetes, viruses, or other teratogens. These abnormalities are categorized into two groups: cyanotic and noncyanotic. Because these heart defects often compromise hemodynamic status, they are also classified according to the level and type of hemodynamic compromise the child experiences (**Figure 1**).

### Cyanotic Defects

Cyanotic disorders are those in which the patient has a right-to-left shunt. Desaturated blood from the right side of the heart is mixed with oxygenated blood from the left side of the heart and is pumped throughout the body. The patient may or may not exhibit cyanosis. The severity of cyanosis depends upon how much desaturated blood is shunted. Some indications of a right-to-left shunt are hypoxemic spells during infancy, a right-sided aortic arch visible on a chest x-ray, or a systolic ejection murmur heard at the upper left sternal border. **Table 1** describes several cyanotic heart defects. Treatment for these defects is usually surgical correction during infancy (Corno, 2000).

---

**Figure 1. Cyanotic and noncyanotic heart defects.**

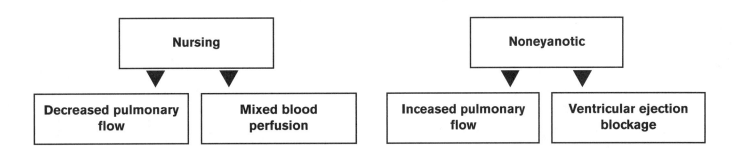

---

**Table 1. Description of Cyanotic Heart Defects**

| Disorder | Signs and Symptoms | Diagnostic Tests | Treatment |
|---|---|---|---|
| Tetrology of Fallot<br><br>Four components are:<br>• ventricular septal defect (VSD)<br>• pulmonary stenosis<br>• right ventricular hypertrophy<br>• an overriding aorta, which means that the aorta lies directly over the ventricular septal defect | Infant hypoxemic episodes that include:<br>• sudden-onset cyanosis<br>• systolic murmur<br>• sudden-onset dyspnea<br>• changes in level of consciousness<br>• decrease in intensity | Chest x-ray<br><br>Echocardiography<br><br>Electrocardiogram (ECG)<br><br>Cardiac catheterization | Surgical correction<br><br>Beta-blocking agents |
| Pulmonary atresia with VSD<br><br>No pulmonary valve exists; therefore, blood can't flow from the right ventricle into the pulmonary artery and on to the lungs. | Symptoms range from asymptomatic to severe hypoxemia, depending on the collateral circulation. | Echocardiography<br><br>Cardiac catheterization | Surgical correction |
| Hypoplastic left heart syndrome<br><br>The mitral and aortic valves are tiny or absent, as well as the left ventricle and the first part of the aorta. | • Mild cyanosis at birth<br>• Rapid onset of shock with the ductus closed.<br>• Little or no adventitious heart sounds | Chest x-ray<br><br>ECG<br><br>Echocardiography | Infusion of PGE1 to maintain patent ductus<br><br>Surgical correction/heart transplant |
| Transposition of the great vessels<br><br>The aorta originates from the right ventricle and the pulmonary artery from the left ventricle. | Cyanosis at birth<br><br>No respiratory distress<br><br>Systolic murmur<br><br>More common in males | Chest x-ray<br><br>Echocardiogram<br><br>Cardiac catheterization | Early surgical correction |
| Truncus arteriosis<br><br>Only one artery originates from the heart and forms both the aorta and the pulmonary artery. | Early congestive heart failure | Chest x-ray showing a "boot-shaped" heart<br><br>Echocardiography<br><br>Angiography | Surgical correction<br><br>Anticongestive treatment |

## Noncyanotic Defects

Noncyanotic heart defects include those in which the blood flows from the high-pressure left side of the heart to the lower-pressure right side of the heart (**Table 2**). This is termed left-to-right shunting. When left-to-right shunting occurs through an opening along the septum or an opening along the great vessels, increased volume in the right ventricle causes an increase in pulmonary blood flow. This leads to pulmonary overload and eventually congestive heart failure. Obstructive defects are also classified as noncyanotic defects. An obstructive defect is one in which the blood flow within the vessel is inhibited by a stenosis. The pressure in the artery before the obstruction is increased on account of the obstruction, and pressure within the artery beyond the obstruction is decreased. Many of the obstructions occur near valves and are classified as valvular, subvalvular, and supravalvular.

Signs and symptoms of obstructive defects may be hypertension, bounding upper extremity pulses, and decreased or absent lower extremity pulses. Lower extremities will be cool to the touch. Children may exhibit exercise intolerance, chest pain, and orthostatic hypotension. The treatments for these noncyanotic disorders are surgical closure of the opening, resection of the affected vessel, or an enlargement of the stenosis.

### Table 2. Noncyanotic Heart Defects

| Increased Pulmonary Flow | Obstructive |
|---|---|
| Atrial septal defect | Coarctation of the aorta |
| Ventricular septal defect | Aortic stenosis |
| Patent ductus arteriosus | Pulmonic stenosis |
| Atrioventricular canal | |

## Cardiomyopathy

Dilated cardiomyopathy can be congenital or acquired. It is seen annually in an incidence of 4 to 8 cases per 100,000 people in the United States and Europe (AHA, 2004). The most common form is idiopathic, which may occur from a genetic defect, and less common is cardiomyopathy from myocarditis. Signs and symptoms of cardiomyopathy include the symptoms of congestive heart failure, decreased exercise tolerance, failure to thrive, and tachypnea. If untreated, the heart will continue to dilate and the heart muscle will become weak and unable to pump effectively. The child will experience a decrease in peripheral perfusion, rales and a gallop upon thoracic auscultation, and hepatomegaly. Treatment options are supportive therapies such as medications to unload the heart (e.g., digoxin, diuretics, beta-blocking agents). Heart transplantation is a consideration if the heart does not respond to pharmacologic treatment (Wong, Hockenberry, Wilson, Winkelstein, & Kline, 2003).

## Acquired Cardiovascular Disorders

Acquired cardiovascular disorders are those that occur after birth and are not congenital. They are a sequela to diseases such as rheumatic heart disease, endocarditis, and Kawasaki disease.

## Rheumatic Fever

This inflammatory process is associated with a beta-hemolytic streptococcal infection of the pharynx. The most significant complication of this infection is rheumatic heart disease. The pathophysiology of rheumatic fever includes the formation of Aschoff bodies, which cause swelling and hemorrhagic lesions. These lesions may be found in the heart, vasculature, brain, pleura, and joints. One clinical sign of rheumatic heart disease is carditis, which involves the endocardium, pericardium, and myocardium. Most frequently, the mitral valve is affected, resulting in mitral regurgitation and a systolic murmur at the apex of the heart. Polyarthritis, chorea, and erythema marginatum (a pink rash and occasionally hard nodules under the skin) on the chest and upper extremities are also major clinical signs of rheumatic fever. Therapy includes pharmacologic treatment with penicillin to terminate the beta-hemolytic streptococcal infection. Salicylates are used to decrease inflammation and reduce pain, and bed rest is required until the acute phase of the infection has passed.

## Bacterial Endocarditis

This infection occurs on the valves or the endocardium. The most common organisms that lead to endocarditis are *Streptococcus viridians, Staphylococcus aureus,* and *Candida albicans. Haemophilus* species have also been documented in cases of endocarditis (Feder, Roberts, Salazar, Leopold, & Toro-Salazar, 2003). The infecting microbes usually enter the circulation from an external site that is already infected, such as a urinary tract infection, through the mouth following dental work, or as a result of a nosocomial infection acquired during a surgical procedure. The bacteria tend to grow where the blood flow is restricted or turbulence leaves deposits or vegetations of fibrin or platelets. These vegetations may break off and travel to other organs, such as the spleen or kidney.

Signs and symptoms of endocarditis may be subtle and include a chronic low-grade fever, heachaches, weight loss, malaise, and diaphoresis. A new murmur may be heard upon thoracic auscultation, and if the condition has been prolonged, splenomegaly may occur. As the vegetations embolize throughout the body, splinter hemorrhages, Janeway spots (small bruises on the palms of the hands and soles of the feet) or petechiae on the oral mucosa may also be seen.

Treatment is usually an anti-infective agent such as penicillin, or other antibiotic that is specific to the invading organism. If the bacterial endocarditis is not successfully treated with pharmacologic measures, other interventions, such as replacing damaged heart valves or surgically removing the infected areas, may be needed.

## Kawasaki Disease

Also known as mucocutaneous lymph node syndrome, Kawasaki disease usually strikes children under 4 years of age, most commonly males (Rozin, Koehler, Shakir, Ladham, & Wecht, 2003). It is characterized by fever, rash, hand and foot edema, lymphadenopathy in the neck, and inflammation of the lips and oropharynx. The disease process is usually self-limiting and rarely serious in the acute phase, but the long-term effects on the heart are serious. The disease causes widespread inflammation of small blood vessels, which progresses to larger vessels. This inflammation damages the vessels, causing them to weaken and dilate, resulting in coronary artery aneurysms. As the disease subsides, the vessels attempt to return to a normal diameter. Sometimes, the vessels become constricted with calcium deposits and thrombi from sluggish blood flow.

Cardiac involvement of Kawasaki disease includes the potential for myocardial infarction. The infarction is a result of a stenotic occlusion by an aneurysm. In children, myocardial infarction presents differently from in adults. Children may have abdominal pain, pallor, crying, restlessness, vomiting, and finally shock. Older children may complain of chest pain (Wong et al., 2003).

Treatment for Kawasaki disease includes high-dose intravenous immunoglobulin during the acute phase. Aspirin is also given as an anticoagulant during the acute phase. If coronary artery damage occurs, warfarin as well as aspirin may be given indefinitely. In the long term, these children are encouraged to practice a heart-healthy lifestyle. (Wong et al., 2003).

## Cardiac Dysrhythmias

The most common cardiac dysrhythmias in children are supraventricular tachycardia (SVT) and bradycardia (Wong et al., 2003). SVT is an abnormally fast heart rate that originates in the atria. The heart rate is regular and can exceed 200 beats per minute; the body is unable to compensate for such a rapid heart rate, and thus the child may experience signs and symptoms of congestive heart failure, dizziness, palpitations, chest pain, diaphoresis, and irritability. The initial episode of SVT occurs before age 1 year in 60% of the children who have SVT. Thirty percent of these children will have recurrent episodes (Tortoiello et al., 2003). First-line treatments for SVT include vagal maneuvers or the administration of intravenous adenosine (Wong et al., 2003). Long-term treatments include pharmacologic interventions such as digoxin and beta blockers as well as the implantation of an internal cardioverter-defibrillator (Love et al., 2001).

Bradydysrhythmias are characterized by an abnormally slow heart rate and may be sinus bradycardia or some form of heart block. The rates are slow and may be regular or irregular. Bradycardia in children is commonly due to an increase in vagal tone or due to hypoxia or acidosis. Sinus bradycardia not related to the above causes may be seen in children who have had extensive repair to the atria. Heart blocks that lead to bradycardia may also occur after cardiac surgery. Temporary pacemakers are used postoperatively to treat these arrythmias, and they normally resolve after the tenth postoperative day (Wong et al., 2003). If the bradydysrhythmias do not resolve, a permanent pacemaker may be placed.

## Hypertension

Hypertension is defined as a consistent elevation in blood pressure that exceeds the high-normal limits. Essential hypertension occurs with no known cause, and secondary hypertension occurs as the result of an identifiable etiology (Wong et al., 2003). Normally, blood pressure in children is much lower than in adults and rises with age. Clinicians consider growth and development when evaluating blood pressure. This individualization allows growth extremes to be considered (AHA, 2004).

In children, 80% to 85% of secondary hypertension is due to renal disease such as pyelonephritis, polycystic kidneys, or urinary tract infection. Only 5% of secondary hypertension is due to endocrine disorders, such as Cushing's syndrome or pheochromocytoma (Mehta, 2001). In older children and adolescents, hypertension may occur from obesity, high cholesterol, or smoking. The incidence of hypertension is higher in children in which there is a family history of elevation. African Americans also have a higher incidence of hypertension than other races (Wong et al., 2003).

Clinical signs of hypertension include headaches, dizziness, or changes in vision. In children who cannot communicate pain or dizziness, irritability or behavioral changes may signal hypertensive episodes.

Treatment of hypertension in children is multifocal. First, the underlying cause is treated. This may include changes in diet, increased exercise, and smoking cessation. If lifestyle changes fail to produce the desired results, medications such as angiotensin-converting enzyme (ACE) inhibitors or calcium channel blockers may be used to reduce blood pressure (California Pacific Medical Center, 2003; Wong et al., 2003).

## Management

Management of cardiovascular disorders focuses on supporting the child and family and treating the disorder, either pharmacologically or invasively. This is a multidisciplinary effort, and the family must work with the team of healthcare professionals to plan and implement appropriate interventions and treatment regimens. Members of the healthcare team include cardiologists, cardiovascular surgeons, nursing staff, radiology and catheterization laboratory staff, dietitian, cardiac rehabilitation staff, respiratory therapist, home healthcare nurses, and the school nurse. Management includes the following:

- Respiratory care: Children with congestive heart failure may require respiratory interventions such as oxygen therapy in the more acute phases.

- Family teaching: Families will require much instruction about their child's diagnosis, treatment regimen, and emergency care.
- Nutrition: Emphasis must be placed on eating a heart-healthy diet. The family and child should be given information about what constitutes an acceptable diet and be given assistance with finding these foods.
- Activity tolerance: The child with a cardiac disorder may have decreased cardiac output and require planning of activities to reduce exertion and fatigue.
- Medication administration: Medications are often required to support the child with cardiovascular disease. The school nurse may administer some of theses medications, assess for side effects, and teach the child and family.

- Risk for infection: The child with a carditis-type cardiovascular disease may be at higher risk for a recurrent episode. Dentists should be made aware of the child's issues, and prophylactic antibiotics should be prescribed prior to any dental procedures.

Psychosocial care: The older child with a cardiovascular disorder may feel different from his or her peers due to the inability to keep up in sports, dietary restrictions, or implanted devices. Psychosocial support should concentrate on building positive attitudes and increasing self-esteem. Support for the family should also be included as part of psychosocial care (Wong et al., 2003).

## Individualized Healthcare Plan

### Assessment
*History*
- Student history of cardiac disease: congenital defect, enlarged heart, arrhythmias, murmur, stenosis or insufficiency of valves, septal defects, coronary heart disease, congestive heart failure, angina, myocardial infarction, hypertension, diabetes, hypercholesterolemia, a history of stroke (cerebral vascular accident)
- Family history of cardiac disease: family members with any of the above described illnesses (note relation to the client, specific problem, age at onset, age at death, disease/cause of relative's death)
- Risk factors: congenital heart disease; rheumatic fever; thyroid disease; hypertension; diabetes; obesity; tobacco use; hypercholesterolemia; excessive caffeine, alcohol, or drug abuse
- Healthcare: providers, insurance, facilities utilized

*Current Health Status and Management*
- Current diagnoses
- Current healthcare providers
- Current healthcare management plan
- Current symptoms
  -Cardiac
    -Chest pain: location; radiation; quality; rating on scale of 1 to 10 (10 being the worst); duration; cause that brings it in, relieves it; associated symptoms, such as nausea, vomiting, sweating
    -Irregular heart beat, palpitations, heart pound or beat too fast, heart skip or jump
    -Dizziness
    -Swollen ankles
    -Heart murmur
  -Respiratory: cough, dyspnea, shortness of breath, expiratory grunt
  -Clubbing of fingers
- Vital signs: heart rate and rhythm, blood pressure, respiratory rate
- General appearance: color
- Behavior and functioning
- Physical endurance
- Exercise tolerance
- Growth pattern: weight and height
- Sleep pattern
- Nutritional pattern: meals, snacks, hydration
- Medications at home and school (name, dosage, route, time, purpose)
- Current development levels: cognitive, speech/language, physical

*Self-care*
- Student's level of understanding of his/her heart condition, treatment regimen, diet regimen, and activity limitations
- Student's level of self-care skills

- Student's decision-making and problem-solving skills
- Student's personal strengths
- Student's current level of self-care and self-care goals for the future

*Psychosocial Status*
- Student's view of health condition
- Student's priorities
- Student's participation with school club or athletic activities past and present
- Community and church activities past and present
- Student's support systems: family, friends, and others
- Student and family strengths and resources
- Student and family support/liaison needs
- Sibling considerations
- Social/cultural issues: extended family members, religion, culture

*Academic Issues*
- Academic performance and achievement: past and current
- Safety issues: special electric and climate considerations
- Maintenance of, storage of, and access to equipment
- Privacy considerations and preparation of peers
- Student's health needs during the school day: medications, monitoring, oxygen, rest, healthcare required
- Transportation needs
- School attendance pattern: past, present, anticipation for frequent absences

## Nursing Diagnosis (N.D.) (NANDA, 2003)

N.D. 1 Risk for decreased cardiac output (NANDA 00029) related to:
- structural defect
- myocardial dysfunction

N.D. 2 Activity intolerance (NANDA 00092) related to:
- imbalance between oxygen supply and demand

N.D. 3 Delayed growth and development (NANDA 00111) related to:
- inadequate oxygen and nutrients to tissues
- social isolation
- frequent absences from school

N.D. 4 Risk for infection (NANDA 00004) related to:
- debilitated physical status
- reduced body defenses
- pulmonary congestion

N.D. 5 Risk for injury (complications) (NANDA 00035) related to:
- cardiac condition and therapies
- presence of streptococcal organisms
- susceptibility to recurrence of rheumatic fever
- bacterial endocarditis
- operative procedure

N.D. 6 Ineffective breathing pattern (NANDA 00032) related to:
- pulmonary congestion

N.D. 7 Risk for fluid volume imbalanced (NANDA 00025) related to:
- cardiac condition
- fluid accumulation (edema)

N.D. 8 Impaired gas exchange (NANDA 00030) related to:
- diminished oxygen needed for impaired tissue perfusion

N.D. 9 Impaired tissue perfusion (NANDA 00024) related to:
- reduced blood flow
- decreased blood volume
- reduced vascular tone

**N.D. 10** Fear (NANDA00148) or anxiety (NANDA 00146) related to:
- hospitalizations
- diagnostic procedure
- surgical procedure
- emergency care
- intensive care unit

## Goals

The student will maintain good/improved vital signs (heart rate, respiratory rate, blood pressure), within his/her normal limits, during the school day. (N.D. 1, 9)

The student will maintain/increase activity tolerance levels. (N.D. 2)

The student will maintain growth for weight and height. (N.D. 3)

The student will participate in school and classroom activities, with modifications made as needed. (N.D. 3)

The student will maintain academic performance and progress. (N.D. 3)

The student will utilize measures to prevent infections. (N.D. 4)

The student will utilize measures to prevent complications. (N.D. 5)

The student will utilize positive, effective coping strategies. (N.D. 5, 10)

The student will increase his/her knowledge of his/her health condition. (N.D. 1, 2, 4, 5, 6, 7, 8)

The student will increase his/her self-care skills. (N.D. 5)

The student will recognize signs of complications early. (N.D. 5)

The student will comply with medical management plan. (N.D. 5)

The student will experience minimal or no complications or discomfort. (N.D. 5)

The student will increase his/her knowledge and understanding of his/her medical management plan. (N.D. 6, 10)

The student will maintain good respiratory function during the school day. (N.D. 6)

The student will maintain effective breathing pattern during the school day. (N.D. 8)

The student will assist in maintaining proper fluid balance during the school day. (N.D. 7)

The student will prevent additional respiratory or cardiac stress at school and on field trips. (N.D. 8, 9)

The student will utilize effective strategies that reduce fear and anxiety. (N.D. 10)

The student will utilize health and educational resources for information and support, as needed. (N.D. 10)

## Nursing Interventions

Collaborate with parent/guardian in obtaining and sharing health information to meet the healthcare needs of the student during the school day. (N.D. 1–10)
- Obtain parental and student permission for the release of information.
- Obtain health history records from parents and healthcare providers.
- Obtain and clarify health and education information, as needed.
- Assist the student and parent/guardian to develop a list of names of healthcare, education, and resources providers who can provide information and assistance.
- Medication authorization from parent and healthcare provider
- Activity limitations and encouraged activities (N.D. 2)

Administer medication, as prescribed. (N.D. 1)
- Assist student to take medication at prescribed time—required time/least disruption to school schedule.
- Assist parent/guardian and student to maintain a supply of medication at school.
- Develop delegation plan for administration of medication on field trips.

Observe for signs of hypokalemia or hyperkalemia. (N.D. 1, 5)

Assist student, parent, teacher (especially physical education teacher) in determining appropriate physical activity. (N.D. 2)

Allow student to set his/her own pace and self-limit his/her activities. (N.D. 2, 3)

Allow for rest periods during the school day, as needed. (N.D. 2, 4)

Assist student in selecting activities appropriate to age, health condition, and abilities. (N.D. 2, 3)

Monitor the student's activity tolerance and endurance during the school day. (N.D. 2)

Avoid extremes of environmental temperature, because hypothermia and hyperthermia increase the need for oxygen. (N.D. 2)

Respond promptly to expressions of distress. (N.D. 2)

Emphasize to school staff and family that student has same need for socialization as peers. (N.D. 2, 3)

Assist the student and parent/guardian to plan for anticipated absences from school due to the student's health condition, (such as planned surgery or diagnostic testing). (N.D. 3)

Assist parent/guardian to provide well-balanced, highly nutritious diet to achieve adequate growth (N.D. 3, 4)
- Snacks during the school day
- Bag lunch/school lunch

Assist parent and healthcare provider in monitoring height and weight; plot on growth charts to determine growth trend. (N.D. 3)

Monitor school population for infectious diseases: (N.D. 4)
- Report presence of an infectious disease to parent/guardian.
- Determine if there was exposure or not.
- Determine any steps that might be needed to protect the student from acquiring an infection.

Reinforce to the student and family the need for antibiotic prophylaxis for dental work and invasive procedures. (N.D. 4, 5)

Reinforce the need to detect complications early. (N.D. 5)

Assist student to identify signs and symptoms of possible complications. (N.D. 5)

Assist student to identify adults (at school, at home, and in the community) that he/she can go to for assistance if signs or symptoms of complications are present. (N.D. 5)

Encourage student to follow medical management plan at school and at home. (N.D. 5)

Explain to student and family the importance of ongoing long-term health supervision. because student is susceptible to recurrent rheumatic fever. (N.D. 5)

Teach skills needed for self-care (administration of medications, eating techniques, interventions to conserve energy and those directed toward relief of frightening symptoms, signs that indicate complications, and where and whom to contact for help and support). (N.D. 5, 10)

Maintain fluid restriction, if ordered. (N.D. 7)

Monitor for evidence of increased or decreased edema. (N.D. 7)

Assist the student with skin care for edema, if needed. (N.D. 7)

Administer oxygen, as prescribed, to ensure adequate tissue oxygenation. (N.D. 8)

Discuss with parent/guardian (and student, if appropriate) their fears and concerns regarding child's cardiac defects and physical symptoms, because these frequently cause anxiety/fear. (N.D. 10)

Assist the student to identify coping strategies that reduce fear and anxiety and assist the student to implement them. (N.D. 10)

Encourage family to participate in care of student to better facilitate good healthcare management and effective coping. (N.D. 10)

Encourage family members to include others in student's care to prevent their own exhaustion and prevent interruption of care. (N.D. 10)

Provide educational opportunities for the student and parent/guardian to learn more about the health condition. (N.D. 10)

Assist the parent/guardian and other family members to obtain instruction in CPR and other community resources, as needed. (N.D. 10)

Assist the student to explore his/her feelings regarding his/her health condition and medical management plan, including surgical interventions. (N.D. 10)

Encourage student to verbalize concerns/feelings to others (parents, healthcare providers, etc.). (N.D. 10)

Reassure student, as appropriate, using empathetic communication. (N.D. 10)

Assist student to identify barriers and motivators to compliance with his/her medical management plan. (N.D. 10)

Develop emergency care plan for possible emergency situations, as needed. (N.D. 1, 6, 8, 9)

Assist school personnel in understanding and implementing special health needs at school. (N.D. 1–8)

Provide in-service training for staff working with the student. (N.D. 1, 6, 8, 9)
- CPR training/certification
- Accessory equipment (purpose, mechanics of equipment, alternative for power failure)
- Signs that indicate problems, complications, or distress and the actions to be taken when observed (emergency care plan)

Provide the appropriate licensed health staff in the educational setting to meet the health needs of the student. (N.D. 1, 6, 8, 9)

## Expected Student Outcomes

The student will:
- Demonstrate normal (defined) heart rate and circulation (specific criteria) during the school day. (N.D. 1)
- Demonstrate adequate urinary output (specific criteria) during the school day. (N.D. 1, 7)
- Identify (number, specific) activities he/she is able to do at school and at home. (N.D. 2, 3)
- Demonstrate active participation in activities at school within activity tolerance. (N.D. 3)
- Actively participate in activities with peers in (classes, at recess). (N.D. 2, 3)
- Demonstrate age-appropriate sleep pattern (specify: hours per night), as reported by parent/guardian and student. (N.D. 2, 6)
- Demonstrate adequate growth pattern (specific criteria) (N.D. 3)
- Utilize prevention measures (specify, for example: hand washing, antibiotics before dental appointments, etc.) to assist in preventing infection. (N.D. 4)
- Demonstrate compliance with (specific part of) medical management plan. (N.D. 1, 2, 5–9)
- Demonstrate (specify) measures that prevent complications or discomfort (N.D. 5)
- Demonstrate respiratory rate and rhythm within normal limits (specific criteria) during the school day. (N.D. 6, 8)
- Student will rest quietly, (as prescribed, as needed) (N.D. 2, 6, 8)
- Demonstrate effective fluid balance measures (specific measures) during the school day. (N.D. 7)
- Demonstrate good ventilation and oxygenation (specific criteria) during the school day (N.D. 8)
- Demonstrate good circulation (specific criteria) during the school day. (N.D. 1, 8)
- Identify (number) of signs of complications that might occur. (N.D. 5)
- Inform (teacher, health office staff) if signs of complications occur at school. (N.D. 5)
- Inform parents if signs of complications occur at home, (as reported by parent) (N.D. 5)
- Accurately describe his/her health condition (age-appropriate description). (N.D. 1, 2, 4–10).
- Identify (number) of components of medical management plan that he/she does daily at home and school. (N.D. 1–10)
- Accurately describe the procedure/surgery he/she is going to have (age-appropriate). (N.D. 10)
- Discuss their fears and anxieties with (parents, school staff). (N.D. 10)
- Demonstrate ability to perform self-care (specific skill being measured). (N.D. 10)
- Demonstrate use of effective coping strategies (specific strategies) that reduce fear and anxiety. (N.D. 10)

## Case Study

James is a 6-year-old boy who will be entering the first grade at Northern Elementary School in the fall. James is a quiet, reserved student who has a history of progressive cardiomyopathy. He is currently on the list awaiting a heart transplant.

James will be placed in a regular first-grade class and in the past has demonstrated an academic ability appropriate for his age. James does not regularly participate in physical activity and prefers to stay inside during recess. He is on several medications that need to be taken during the school day.

James and his parents will visit the school and meet with teachers and the school nurse to discuss pertinent health issues:

1. James experiences shortness of breath with moderate exercise. The parents and student are concerned about participation in physical education and recess activities.
2. James is on several heart medications that need to be administered during the school day. His parents are concerned that he might experience adverse effects from the medications and that these effects might affect his academic performance.
3. Occasionally, James experiences a dysrhythmia due to his cardiomyopathy. James is usually aware of dysrhythmia when it occurs. In the past, the dysrhythmia has been transient and self-limiting. However, emergency care procedures need to be in place.

James is on a prescribed cardiovascular diet and fluid restriction. To minimize his congestive failure symptoms, James must strictly adhere to this diet.

# Cardiovascular Disorders

| Assessment Data | Nursing Diagnosis | Goals | Nursing Interventions | Expected Outcomes |
|---|---|---|---|---|
| James has progressive cardiomyopathy. | Activity intolerance related to cardiac insufficiency secondary to cardiomyopathy. | James will maintain optimal activity level in the school setting. | Request physician direction for activity level: encouraged activities and activity restrictions. | James will identify three signs that he is exceeding his exercise tolerance. |
| James has shortness of breath and fatigue with moderate exercise. | Impaired gas exchange related to congestive failure. | James will recognize signs and symptoms of complications early and inform appropriate adults. | Collaborate with physician, parents, and teachers to establish exercise activities that meet encouraged and restricted activities. | James will participate in physical education , with modified activities. |
| James prefers to stay inside at recess. | Ineffective breathing pattern related to dyspnea secondary to cardiomyopathy. | James will participate in school activities with peers, with modifications made as needed. | Assist teachers to modify activities, as needed. | James will go outside with peers at recess. |
| James doesn't participate in physical education activities. | | | Assist teachers to assess for signs and symptoms of increasing shortness of breath and fatigue. | James will tell his teacher if he is having shortness of breath. James will identify and describe his symptoms. |
| | | | Assess lung sounds with symptoms of increasing respiratory difficulty. | James will identify when to et the teacher or school nurse know that his is having difficulty breathing or excessive fatigue. |
| | | | Discuss with James:<br>• the signs and symptoms of increasing fatigue and shortness of breath<br>• what the symptoms mean<br>• the need to stop activity if the symptoms occur<br>• James will participate in activities, with peers, at school. | |
| James is on several cardiac medications. He and his family are unable to discuss the reasons for and actions of these medications. As a result, James occasionally skips doses. | Fear and anxiety related to medications.<br><br>Knowledge deficit related to need for medication resulting in noncompliance with taking medication. | James will increase knowledge about cardiovascular problems and medical management plan.<br><br>James will take medications as prescribed.<br><br>James will maintain academic performance and progress. | In collaboration with healthcare providers, teach James and his parents about his medications and why they are needed. | James will identify (3) important effects of his medication and why they are important.<br><br>James will identify (3) important adverse effects that need to be reported to his parents, teachers, or the school nurse. |

| Assessment Data | Nursing Diagnosis | Goals | Nursing Interventions | Expected Outcomes |
|---|---|---|---|---|
| Parent concern regarding medication effects on academic performance. | | | Provide in-service for school personnel about James's medications and side effects, especially if they could affect his academic performance.<br><br>Assist James and his parents to utilize resources for information, discussion, and support regarding cardiovascular disease and medications.<br><br>Teach James about any adverse effects of his medications and the need to report them if they occur. | James demonstrates accurate reporting of symptoms to parents, teachers, or school nurse. |
| James reports that he occasionally feels his heart racing or pounding. This makes him feel dizzy.<br><br>James had episodes of dysrhythmias in the past due to cardiomyopathy.<br><br>They have been transient and self-limiting. | Decreased cardiac output related to altered cardiac function secondary to dysrhythmias. | James will notify his teacher or the school nurse when he feels his heart racing or pounding.<br><br>James will describe how he feels when he has dysrhythmias.<br><br>The school will have in place an emergency care plan. | Develop an emergency care plan in collaboration with James, his parents, and healthcare providers.<br><br>Teach James:<br>• signs and symptoms to report<br>• what these symptoms mean<br>• how to report his signs and symptoms to parents, teachers, and school health staff.<br><br>Provide in-service for school staff who work with James:<br>• signs and symptoms of dysrythmia<br>• emergency care plan<br><br>James will describe:<br>• how his dysrhythmias make him feel<br>• when to notify the teacher or the school nurse | James reports an episode of racing or pounding heart to parent, teacher, or school health staff immediately. |

| Assessment Data | Nursing Diagnosis | Goals | Nursing Interventions | Expected Outcomes |
|---|---|---|---|---|
| Prescribed cardiovascular diet and fluid restriction; daily meals consist of sugary cereals and high-fat meals. | Knowledge deficit pertaining to cardiovascular dietary guidelines.<br><br>Fear and anxiety related to unfamiliarity with information resources. | James will increase his knowledge about his cardiovascular diet and fluid restriction.<br><br>James will follow his prescribed diet during the school day.<br><br>James will maintain a healthy weight. | Review the elements of James's diet with James and parents.<br><br>Discuss with James and his family why the prescribed diet is crucial to James's health.<br><br>Assist James and his parents in developing an appropriate menu for school lunches and snacks in terms that meet the criteria for James's cardiovascular diet and fluid restrictions.<br><br>Assist James's parents in finding resources for nutritional discussion to further promote heart health. | James will assist in developing a menu of heart-healthy foods that he likes to eat and are part of his diet and fluid restrictions, for school lunches and snacks.<br><br>James will adhere to his dietary guidelines during the school day.<br><br>James will maintain weight within normal limits for height. |

# References

American Heart Association. (2004). Retrieved March 4, 2004, from www.americanheart.org/presenter.jhtml?indentifi-er=12052

California Pacific Medical Center. (2003). Evaluation and management of hypertension in children and adolescents. Retrieved February 21, 2004, from http://www.cpmc.org/advanced/pediatrics/physicians/pedspage1003cardiac.html

Corno, A. F. (2000). Surgery for congenital heart disease. *Current Opinion in Cardiology, 15*(4), 238–243.

Feder, H. M., Roberts, J. C., Salazar, J. C., Leopold, H. B., & Toro-Salazar, O. (2003). HACEK endocarditis in infants and children: Two cases and a literature review. *Pediatric Infectious Disease Journal, 22*(6), 557–562.

Hockenberry, M. & Wong, D. (2004). *Wong's clinical manual of pediatric nursing* (6th ed.). Philadelphia: Mosby.

Love, B. A., Barrett, K. S., Alexander, M. E., Bevilacqua, L. M., Epstien, M. R., Triedman, J. K., et al. (2001). Supraventricular arrhythmias in children and young adults with implantable cardioverter defibrillators. *Journal of Cardiovascular Electrophysiology, 12*(10), 1097-101.

Mehta, K. (2001). Hypertension in children. Retrieved February 21, 2004, from http://www.pediatriconcall.com/fordoctor/DiseasesandCondition/hypertension.asp

NANDA International. (2003). *NANDA nursing diagnoses: Definitions and classification, 2003-2004.* Philadelphia: Author.

Rozin, L. M., Koehler, S. A., Shakir, A., Ladham, S., & Wecht, C. H. (2003). Kawasaki disease: A review of pathologic features of stage IV disease and two cases of sudden death among asymptomatic adults. *American Journal of Forensic Medicine and Pathology, 24*(1), 45–50.

Tak, Y. R., & McCubbin, M. (2002). Family stress, perceived social support and Coping following the diagnosis of a child's congenital heart disease. *Journal of Advanced Nursing, 32*(9), 190–198

Tortoiello, T. A., Syder, C. S., Smith, E. O., Fenrich, A. L., Friedman, R. A., & Kerttesz, N. J. (2003). Frequency of recurrence among infants with supraventricular tachycardia and comparison of recurrence rates among those with and without preexcitation and among those with and without response to digoxin and/or propanolol therapy. *American Journal of Cardiology, 92*(9), 1045–1049.

Wong, D. L., Hockenberry, M. J., Wilson, D., Winklestien M. L., & Kline, N. E. (2003). *Wong's nursing care of infants and children* (7th ed.). St. Louis, MO: Mosby.

# Bibliography

Braunwald, E. (1992). *Heart disease: A textbook of cardiovascular medicine* (4th ed., pp. 1404–1415). Philadelphia: Saunders.

Burns, C. E., et al. (2000). *Pediatric primary care: A handbook for nurse practitioners,* Philadelphia: Saunders.

Carpenito, L. J. (2002). *Nursing diagnosis: Application to clinical practice* (9th ed.). Philadelphia: Lippincott.

Gravanis, M. B. (1997). *Cardiovascular disorders: Pathogenesis and pathophysiology* (pp. 241–250). St. Louis, MO: Mosby.

Martin Memorial Health Systems. *Cardiovascular disorders.* Retrieved March 4, 2004, from http://www.mmhs.com/clinical/peds/english/cardiac/sitemap.htm

National Heart, Lung, and Blood Institute. *Heart and vascular diseases.* Retrieved March 4, 2004, from http://www.nhlbi.nih.gov/health/public/heart/index.htm

National Association of School Nurses, American Academy of Pediatrics, and the American Heart Association. (Adopted 2004). *Joint Position Statement: Response to cardiac arrest and selected life-threatening medical emergencies: The medical emergency response plan for schools.* Scarborough, ME: Author.

National Association of School Nurses. (Adopted 2002). *Position Statement: Automatic external defibrillators in the school setting.* Scarborough, ME: Author.

National Association of School Nurses. (Revised 2000). *Position Statement: Do not resuscitate.* Scarborough, ME: Author.

Thede, J., & Iverson, C. (1997-2000). *Nursing assessment of school age youth. Cardiovascular health.* (Home Study Module Number 4). Scarborough, ME: National Association of School Nurses.

Vessey, J. A., Ben-Or, K. M., Dionne J., Krapac, N. E., Cobb, N., Poltrack, M., et al. (2001). Evaluating the value of screening for hypertension: An evidence-based approach. *Journal of School Nursing, 17*(1), 44–49.

Williams, R. A. (Ed.). (1999) *The athlete and heart disease: Diagnosis, evaluation and management.* Philadelphia: Lippincott Williams & Williams.

Woods, S. L., Sivarajan Froelicher, S., Motzer, S. A. (2000). *Cardiac nursing* Philadelphia: Lippincott Williams & Wilkins.

## Resources

American Academy of Pediatrics
141 Northwest Point Boulevard
Elk Grove Village, IL 60007-1098
1-847-434-4000
1-847-434-8000 (fax)
http://www.aap.org

American Heart Association
7272 Greenville Avenue
Dallas, TX 75231
1-800-242-8721
http://www.americanheart.org

Children's Health Information
  Network
1561 Clark Drive
Yardley, PA 19067
215-493-3068
http://www.tchin.org

Congenital Heart Anomalies:
  Support, Education,
  Resources
2122 Wilkins Road
Swanton, OH 43558
419-825-5575
http://www.csun.edu/~hfmth006/
  chaser/

National Health Information
  Center
PO Box 1133
Washington, DC 20013
1-800-336-4797
http://www.health.gov/nhic

National Heart, Lung, and Blood
  Institute
National Institutes of Health
31 Center Drive
Building 31
Baltimore, MD 20892
301-496-4236
http://www.nhlbi.nih.gov

Young at Heart
1281 Forest Avenue
Palo Alto, CA 94301
650-231-8882
toobionic@aol.com

Cardiovascular Disorders

*Chapter Thirty-one*

# Celiac Disease

Carole Ellerbe Moore

## Introduction

Celiac disease (CD) is a chronic, genetic condition that persists throughout life. It is triggered by the ingestion of gluten and is managed by adherence to a gluten-free diet. CD is an example of an autoimmune disease for which early diagnosis and treatment with a gluten-free diet can prevent severe complications. CD is one of the most common but underdiagnosed diseases in the United States.

## Pathophysiology

CD is an autoimmune inflammatory disease of the small intestine, triggered by the ingestion of gluten-containing grains (including wheat, rye, and barley) in genetically susceptible individuals. Malabsorption results from injury to the mucosa of the small intestine after gluten ingestion (Nelsen, 2002). CD is associated with human leukocyte antigen (HLA) DQ2 and DQ8 haplotypes (Fasano et al., 2003). The combination of genes and environment (gluten) produces the intestinal damage that characterizes CD. Unlike allergy responses that are IgE-mediated, the autoimmune reaction in CD involves plasma cells that produce IgA and IgG. The intense local inflammatory reaction in the small intestine results in mucosal damage and flattening of the villi, which are the hallmarks of CD. This leads to malabsorption of nutrients, including vitamins, minerals, protein, carbohydrates, and fats. CD is extremely variable in its manifestations as well as age at onset. Even though CD typically causes damage to the mucosa of the small intestine, approximately 50% of individuals do not have any gastrointestinal symptoms at initial presentation of the disease. In many cases, the presenting symptoms are anemia, dermatitis herpetiformis, lethargy, unexplained weight loss, and, in children, short stature (Hill, 2003).

Recent epidemiologic studies have demonstrated that CD is much more common in the United States than previously recognized, affecting one in 133 people in not-at-risk groups. Not-at-risk groups include blood donors, schoolchildren, as well as individuals seen in outpatient clinics for routine checkups (Fasano et al., 2003). Recent data suggests that CD occurs frequently in individuals with gastrointestinal symptoms, as well as first- and second-degree relatives. Particularly significant is the high prevalence of CD among people without gastrointestinal symptoms who have common disorders, including type 1 diabetes, anemia, arthritis, osteoporosis, infertility, and Down syndrome (Fasano et al.). For example, the prevalence of CD in persons with Down syndrome is approximately 1 in 14, or 7%. Screening is recommended through blood antibody tests for children with Down syndrome at age 3 years, even in the absence of gastrointestinal symptoms (Zachor, Mroczek-Musulman, & Brown, 2000). Substantial morbidity is associated with symptomatic CD, due to weight loss, anemia, chronic malabsorption, bone disease, and general weakness. Manifestations of CD in persons without symptoms include reduced bone density, iron and folate deficiencies, and associated autoimmune diseases (Green & Jabri, 2003).

Infants and young children often have symptoms such as diarrhea, abdominal pain and distention, and failure to thrive. Loose, foul-smelling stools are typical. Vomiting, anorexia, fatigue, and constipation are also common (Green & Jabri, 2003). Older children often have nongastrointestinal symptoms, such as short stature, anemia, or neurologic symptoms such as gluten ataxia. CD that is asymptomatic is common in children and has been associated with growth failure, lymphoma, cerebellar ataxia, osteoporosis, and other autoimmune disorders (Hoffenberg et al., 2003). The diagnosis of CD is often not considered in the absence of diarrhea. Therefore, diarrhea remains the most common presenting symptom. Delays in diagnosis are very common; most individuals in the United States with CD have symptoms for 11 years prior to diagnosis (Green & Jabri, 2003).

CD is also identified because of other manifestations, such as dermatitis herpetiformis, a pruritic vesicular rash, most commonly found on extensor surfaces (knees and elbows) and the scalp. Almost all individuals with dermatitis herpetiformis have CD. Some individuals with CD seek care with symptoms of peripheral neuropathy, epilepsy, dental enamel defects, dyspepsia, or aphthous stomatitis (Green & Jabri, 2003).

Diagnosis is achieved primarily through small intestinal biopsy and serologic tests. Small intestinal clinical evaluation and biopsy are performed through upper gastrointestinal endoscopy, focusing on enlarged crypts, increased numbers of intraepithelial lymphocytes, and presence of villous atrophy (Hoffenberg et al., 2003). Serologic tests detecting CD autoimmunity include IgA endomysial and tissue transglutaminase autoantibody assays (Hoffenberg et al.). Celiac disease is strongly associated with genetic markers, human leukocyte antigen (HLA) molecules DQ2 and DQ8. HLA typing, done by blood testing or oral mucosal swab, also aids in identifying persons who are at risk of developing CD. This is of particular interest because of close genetic association between CD and other conditions, including type 1 diabetes, selective IgA deficiency, autoimmune thyroid disease, Sjögren's syndrome, Addison's disease, systemic lupus erythematosus, and alopecia areata. Individuals with these conditions may exhibit similar genotypes and are at risk for developing CD (Nelsen, 2002).

## Management

### Diet

The primary treatment for CD is strict lifelong adherence to a gluten-free diet (Hill, 2003). Gluten is the primary protein in wheat. Similar proteins are found in rye and barley, so these must also be avoided. Oats are controversial, because although oats themselves may not be toxic, most commercial oat products in the United States are contaminated with other grains, such as wheat. Foods included in the gluten-free diet are breads or baked goods prepared from corn, rice, potato, or soy flours or cornmeal; rice, noodles, and pasta; all meats, chicken, and fish; milk and unprocessed cheese; dried beans, nuts, and peanut butter; potatoes, rice, tapioca, and corn, as well as fruits and vegetables.

Foods to avoid include breads, baked goods, cereals, or pasta prepared from wheat, barley, or rye; creamed or breaded vegetables; and salad dressings, gravies, sauces, and soups prepared with gluten-containing ingredients. Caution should be used in restaurants and commercial kitchens to eliminate foods that are cross-contaminated with gluten during production. Current food labeling laws in the United States do not require information needed to determine if products are gluten-free, because the source of each ingredient is not identified. For example, hidden gluten may be found in some types of modified food starch, caramel color, emulsifiers, and flavorings. Contacting food manufacturers is usually helpful in determining gluten-free status.

Success with the gluten-free diet is enhanced through careful examination of food labels, obtaining lists of gluten-free items from manufacturers, and involvement in local and national support groups. The bibliography at the end of this chapter includes many excellent books and cookbooks on gluten-free cooking. The resources section contains a list of several vendors of gluten-free food products as well as national organizations supporting CD research and individuals with CD.

In the school setting, collaboration with food services and parents centers on determining which cafeteria foods are gluten-free and prevention of cross-contamination. Parents of younger children may keep a small supply of frozen gluten-free cupcakes and pizza for classroom celebrations and pizza parties. Collaboration with parents includes maintaining a supply of nonperishable gluten-free snacks in the classroom, as well as a supply of nonperishable gluten-free foods to store with supplies for campus emergencies. It is important to consider the need for gluten-free products when preparing for disasters or other campus emergencies. The school nurse should be a resource by sharing information and identifying sources of gluten-free foods that are favorites of children, such as pizza, cookies, spaghetti, cake mixes, and breads. Referral of families to local and national CD support groups also enhances compliance with and normalization of the gluten-free diet.

In addition, management of CD in the school setting should include giving children liberal bathroom privileges as needed and rest periods if fatigued.

### Medications and Other Considerations

Some individuals will need supplements such as calcium, vitamin D and other fat-soluble vitamins, iron, multivitamins, magnesium, and other nutrients (Nelsen, 2002). Gluten-free status of all medications should be checked with the manufacturers. Most individuals have a rapid response to the gluten-free diet as the intestinal mucosa heals. People who are extremely ill may require hospitalization for intravenous fluids and electrolytes; some may require treatment with steroids.

# Individualized Healthcare Plan

## Assessment

### History
- Age and developmental level
- Method and date of diagnosis
- Previous hospitalization for CD
- General course with CD
- Others in immediate family with CD
- Other health concerns or related disorders
- Involvement in support group by child and family
- Compliance with gluten-free diet
- History of growth and weight gain

### Current Status and Management
- Child's healthcare providers (primary care provider, gastroenterologist, dietitian)
- Ordered treatment (gluten-free diet, nutritional supplements, medications)
- Toleration of treatment (dietary restrictions, medication side effects)
- Symptoms child experiences after dietary exposure to gluten
- Symptom (including diarrhea and abdominal pain) management at home
- Activity restrictions or limitations
- Nutritional status
- Height, weight, and body mass index

### Self-care
- Self-monitor gluten-free status of foods
- Self-monitor activity level if fatigued
- Assistance with personal hygiene if diarrhea present after gluten exposure

### Psychosocial Status
- Family/child's coping skills after child's diagnosis of CD
- Disruption of usual activities
- Peer awareness of diagnosis and response
- Teasing from peers
- Family/child involvement in local or national CD support group
- Family/child knowledge level concerning where to access information on gluten-free status of foods and other materials, and vendors of gluten-free food products

### Academic Issues
- School staff knowledge level regarding CD and the gluten-free diet (GFD)
- School attendance record
- Reasons for absences
- Medications that may need to be given at school
- Child's academic history. Change in performance since diagnosis of CD and treatment with GFD
- Schedule or activity modifications needed during the school day and/or after-school activities
- Child eating only food from home or also food from school cafeteria and classroom
- Designated storage area for GF snacks
- Supply of GF treats from home for special class parties/celebrations
- Need for unlimited bathroom privileges
- 504 plan need

## Nursing Diagnoses (N.D.) (NANDA, 2003)

**N.D. 1** Imbalanced nutrition: less than body requirements (NANDA 00002) related to inability to absorb nutrients

**N.D. 2** (Risk for) Diarrhea (NANDA 00013) related to:
- dietary contamination with gluten
- malabsorption

**N.D. 3** Risk for activity intolerance (NANDA 00094) related to:
- fatigue
- anemia
- general weakness

**N.D. 4** Deficient knowledge (NANDA 00126) related to unfamiliarity with information about CD and the gluten-free diet

**N.D. 5** (Risk for) Disturbed body image (NANDA 00118) related to:
- exacerbation of CD symptoms
- small stature
- weight loss
- weakness

**N.D. 6** (Risk for) Situational low self-esteem (NANDA 00120) related to:
- fatigue
- altered body appearance, weight loss, small stature
- exacerbation of CD symptoms

**N.D. 7** (Risk for) Noncompliance (NANDA 00079) related to:
- knowledge deficit
- denial of need for GFD
- poor problem-solving skills

**N.D. 8** Readiness for enhanced nutrition (NANDA 00163) related to:
- adherence to GFD
- interest in enhanced nutrition

## Goals

The student will demonstrate increased knowledge about CD and the GFD. (N.D. 4, 8)

The student will comply with the GFD. (N.D. 4, 7)

The student will be involved in choosing appropriate gluten-free foods in the school setting. (N.D. 1, 2, 6-8)

The student will demonstrate improved nutritional status. (N.D. 1, 2, 8)

The student will attend school and participate with modifications made as needed. (N.D. 3)

The student will demonstrate increased tolerance for physical activities. (N.D. 3)

The student will maintain positive self-esteem and body image. (N.D. 5, 6)

The student will seek community support for self and family. (N.D. 4, 8)

## Nursing Interventions

Provide nutritional counseling regarding (N.D. 1,4 , 7, 8)
- healthy food choices
- reading labels to determine gluten-free status
- student preferences
- methods of modifying/supplementing school lunches and snacks to provide adequate food intake

Provide student and family with current educational materials and resources about CD and the GFD. (N.D. 4, 8)

Obtain written parental permission to share CD diagnosis and need for GFD with school personnel. (N.D. 1, 2, 3)

Collaborate with student, family, and other school personnel to (N.D. 1, 2, 3)
- explore need for 504 plan
- participate in development of 504 plan
- implement 504 plan

Provide nutritional therapy in collaboration with child's healthcare team by monitoring intake and ensuring availability of variety of gluten-free foods in the school lunch program, classroom, and after-school activities. (N.D. 1, 4, 7, 8)

Provide educational materials about CD and the GFD to school personnel. (N.D. 1–8)

Collaborate with and educate school food services personnel regarding how to determine if foods are gluten-free, label reading, hidden gluten. (N.D. 1, 2, 7)

- cross-contamination with gluten in food preparation
- establishing safe environment for students with CD

Provide encouragement and support to student by (N.D. 18)
- referring family to local and national CD support groups and summer camps
- facilitating open communication with student

Notify school personnel of necessary modifications regarding (N.D. 18)
- modified physical education program
- unlimited restroom privileges
- need for gluten-free snacks during school day
- modified school lunch to comply with GFD
- coordination of academic assignments as needed
- physical activity level alterations during periods of exacerbation
- need for hand washing after handling gluten (art supplies, home economics supplies)

Monitor student's attendance in collaboration with teacher or attendance secretary. (N.D. 3)

Promote healthy self-esteem by (N.D. 6)
- encouraging student to share feelings about impact of CD on self-concept, requirements of the GFD, and feedback from peers
- assisting student in problem-solving difficult social situations due to GFD
- encouraging student to identify personal strengths and weaknesses
- assisting student in developing strategies to educate peers about CD and need for GFD

Promote development of healthy body image through (N.D. 5)
- discussing student's perceptions of body image
- discussing student's body changes since diagnosis of CD (weight, energy level, presence of symptoms)
- identifying coping strategies utilized by student

## Expected Student Outcomes

The student will:
- Demonstrate understanding of CD and the GFDF. (N.D. 4, 8)
- Recognize symptoms of gluten exposure. (N.D. 4)
- Take action to manage symptoms of gluten exposure. (N.D. 4)
- Reduce number of gluten-induced diarrhea episodes. (N.D. 2)
- Choose gluten-free items daily for school snacks and lunch. (N.D. 1, 4, 7, 8)
- Improve school attendance pattern with accommodations as needed. (N.D. 3)
- Participate in school activities with modifications as necessary. (N.D. 3)
- Verbalize positive feelings about self and body. (N.D. 5, 6)
- Identify and utilize resources about CD in the community. (N.D. 4, 8)

## Case Study

Emily Downs is a 12-year-old student at Royal Oaks Middle School who was diagnosed as having celiac disease 6 months ago. She was referred to a pediatric gastroenterologist after experiencing persistent diarrhea, flatulence, heartburn, anemia, and a weight loss of 10 pounds within the last 18 months. Emily had previously been diagnosed with irritable bowel syndrome and hypothyroidism. She missed 18 school days earlier in the school year due to diarrhea and general weakness. After testing, which included upper GI series, endoscopy with small bowel biopsy, serologic IgA endomysial and tissue transglutaminase autoantibody assays, and HLA typing, the diagnosis was made. Emily's aunt has type 1 diabetes, one grandmother was diagnosed as having lupus, and her father has chronic diarrhea.

Emily was placed on a gluten-free diet, and symptoms improved within 1 week. Her body mass index now falls in the 18th percentile for her age and gender. Emily and her family have become involved in local and national celiac support organizations, and Emily plans to attend a summer camp for children with celiac disease in the area next summer. She and her family utilize knowledge gained from the support groups to choose gluten-free products at the grocery store and obtain a wide variety of gluten-free foods from vendors through mail order. They enjoy preparing gluten-free food at home with the help of cookbooks.

Emily takes Synthroid daily as well as iron, calcium, and multivitamin supplements. She is very active in the school choir and soccer team but has missed several practices recently due to fatigue. The school nurse met with Emily and her parents to discuss Emily's diagnosis and need for a gluten-free diet at school, and to develop a health-care plan that would accommodate Emily's needs at school. Emily expressed interest in increasing her level of nutrition. She states that she makes appropriate, healthy, gluten-free food choices when away from home.

**Celiac Disease**

| Assessment Data | Nursing Diagnosis | Goals | Nursing Interventions | Expected Outcomes |
|---|---|---|---|---|
| Weight loss of 10 pounds in last 18 months; current BMI 18th percentile. | Imbalanced nutrition: less than body requirements related to inability to absorb nutrients. | Emily will be involved in choosing appropriate gluten-free foods at school. | Provide nutritional counseling:<br>• healthy food choices<br>• reading labels to determine gluten-free status<br>• student preferences<br>• methods of modifying/supplementing school lunches and snacks to provide adequate food intake<br><br>Provide nutritional therapy:<br>• monitor food intake<br>• ensure availability of variety of gluten-free foods<br>Collaborate with and educate school food service personnel:<br>• how to determine if foods are gluten-free, label reading, hidden gluten sources<br>• cross-contamination with gluten in food preparation<br>• establish safe environment<br><br>Provide Emily and family with list of gluten-free foods in the school lunch program. | Emily will choose gluten-free snacks and lunches in the lunchroom daily. |
| Emily has missed 18 school days this year and several soccer games and choir performances due to fatigue. | Risk for activity intolerance related to fatigue, anemia, and general weakness. | Emily will attend school and participate with modifications as needed.<br><br>Emily will show increased tolerance for activities. | Obtain written parental permission to share CD diagnosis with school personnel. | Emily will miss no more than 9 days with accommodations as needed.<br><br>Emily will participate in 4 out of 5 days of choir and soccer with modifications as necessary. |

| Assessment Data | Nursing Diagnosis | Goals | Nursing Interventions | Expected Outcomes |
|---|---|---|---|---|
| | | | Provide educational materials about CD and the GFD to school personnel. Implement 504 plan (which includes modifications in physical education, participation in school sports and other extracurricular activities, and academic assignments), in collaboration with other school personnel. | |
| | | | Monitor Emily's attendance on weekly basis, in collaboration with teacher or attendance secretary. | |
| | | | Provide encouragement and support to the student; facilitate open communication. | |
| Emily expresses interest in increasing level of nutrition. | Readiness for enhanced nutrition related to adherence to GFD and interest in enhanced nutrition. | Emily will comply with GFD.  Emily will demonstrate increased knowledge about CD and the GFD. | Provide Emily and family with current educational materials and resources about CD and the gluten-free diet. | Emily will demonstrate understanding of the GFD and will choose gluten-free items daily for school snacks and lunch. |
| Emily makes appropriate, healthy, gluten-free food choices. | | | Provide encouragement and support to Emily, including referral to local and national CD support organizations and summer camps. | Emily will utilize resources from local and national CD support organizations. |

# References

Fasano, A., Berti, I., Geraduzzi, T., Not, T., Colletti, R. B., Drago, M. S., et al. (2003). Prevalence of celiac disease in at-risk and not-at-risk groups in the United States. *Archives of Internal Medicine, 163*(3), 286–292.

Green, P. H., & Jabri, B. (2003). Coeliac disease. *The Lancet, 362*(9381), 383–391.

Hill, I. D. (2003). Celiac disease—a never-ending story? *The Journal of Pediatrics, 143*(3), 289–291.

Hoffenberg, E. J., MacKenzie, T., Barriga, K. J., Eisenbarth, G. S., Bao, F., Haas, J. E., et al. (2003). A prospective study of the incidence of childhood celiac disease. *The Journal of Pediatrics, 143*(3), 308–314.

NANDA International. (2003). *Nursing diagnoses: Definitions & classification 2003-2004*. Philadelphia: Author.

Nelsen, D. A., Jr. (2002). Gluten-sensitive enteropathy (celiac disease): More common than you think. *American Family Physician, 66*(12), 2259–2266.

Zachor, D. A., Mroczek-Musulman, E., & Brown, P. (2000). Prevalence of celiac disease in Down syndrome in the United States. *Journal of Pediatric Gastroenterology and Nutrition, 31*(3), 275–279.

# Bibliography

Barera, G., Bonfanti, R., Viscardi, M., Bazzigaluppi, E., Calori, G., Meschi, F., et al. (2002). Occurrence of celiac disease after onset of type 1 diabetes: A 6-year prospective longitudinal study. *Pediatrics, 109*(5), 833–838.

Danowski, L., Brand, L. G., & Connolly, J. (2003). Gluten-free diets, coeliac disease and associated disorders. *Family Practice, 20*(5), 607–611.

Dennis, M., & Case, S. (2004). Going gluten-free: A primer for clinicians. *Practical Gastroenterology, 28*(4), 86–104.

Farrell, R. J., & Kelly, C. P. (2002). Celiac sprue. *New England Journal of Medicine, 346*(3), 180–188.

Fasano, A., & Catassi, C. (2001). Current approaches to diagnosis and treatment of celiac disease: An evolving spectrum. *Gastroenterology, 120*, 636–651.

Fasano, A. (2003). Celiac disease—how to handle a clinical chameleon. *New England Journal of Medicine, 348*(25), 2568–2570.

Korn, D. (2002). *Wheat-free, worry-free: The art of happy, healthy, gluten-free living*. Carlsbad, CA: Hay House. (A book for adults and families.)

Korn, D. (2001). *Kids with celiac disease: A family guide to raising happy, healthy, gluten-free children*. Bethesda, MD: Woodbine House. (A book for parents.)

Kruszka, B. (2003). *Eating gluten free with Emily*. Philadelphia: Xlibris Corp. (A book for children.)

Lowell, J. P. (1996). *Against the grain: The slightly eccentric guide to living well without gluten or wheat*. New York: Henry Holt. (A book for adults and families.)

Luchtefeld, W., Burton, M. S., & Donavon, P. (2003). The importance of a gluten-free diet. *Nurse Practitioner, 28*(7), 47–49.

Michael, M. (2003). Recognizing and managing celiac disease in primary care. *Journal of the American Academy of Nurse Practitioners, 15*(3), 108–114.

Sanderson S. L. (2002). *Incredible edible gluten-free food for kids: 150 family-tested recipes*. Bethesda, MD: Woodbine House. (A cookbook.)

Wasburn, D., & Butt, H. (2003). 125 best gluten-free recipes. Toronto, Ontario: Robert Rose. (A cookbook.)

Wong, D. L., Hockenberry, M. J., Wilson, D., Winkelstein, M. L., & Kline, N. .E. (2003). *Wong's nursing care of infants and children* (7th ed.). St. Louis, MO: Mosby.

# Resources

**Gluten-Free Food Vendors**

Authentic Foods
1850 West 169th Street
Suite B
Gardena, CA 90247
310-366-7612
www.authenticfoods.com

Dietary Specialties
10 Leslie Court
Whippany, NJ 07981
1-888-640-2800
www.dietspec.com

Ener-G Foods
5960 First Avenue South
PO Box 84487
Seattle, WA 87124800-331-5222
www.ener-g.com

Gluten Solutions
3810 Riviera Drive
Suite 3
San Diego, CA 92109
1-888-845-8836
www.glutensolutions.com

Kinnikinnick Foods
10940-120 Street
Edmonton, Alberta, Canada
T5H3P7
877-503-4466
www.kinnikinnick.com

The Gluten-Free Pantry
PO Box 840
Glastonbury, CT 06033
1-800-291-8386
www.glutenfree.com

**National Celiac Disease Support Organizations**

Celiac Disease Foundation
13251 Ventura Boulevard
Suite 1
Studio City, CA 91604
818-990-2354
www.celiac.org
Offers support and general information about celiac disease and increased awareness among the general public, and provides link between clinical research and patient care.

Celiac Sprue Association
PO Box 31700
Omaha, NE 68131
1-877-CSA-4CSA
www.csaceliacs.org
Provides educational resources to people with celiac disease and their families; has network of 80 chapters throughout the United States.

Gluten Intolerance Group of North America
15110 10th Avenue SW
Suite A
Seattle, WA 98166
206-246-6652
www.gluten.net
Provides education and support to people with gluten intolerance. Hosts summer camp for children with celiac disease.

## Chapter Thirty-two

# Cerebral Palsy

Annette L. Perschke and Nancy Manzo-Mattucci

## Introduction

Cerebral palsy (CP) is a "disorder of movement and posture that results from an insult to or anomaly of the immature nervous system" (Shapiro & Capute, 1999). More specifically, Johnston (1998) describes CP as a "clinical diagnostic term referring to a group of upper motor neuron (UMN) syndromes secondary to disorders of early brain development." CP is often considered a nonprogressive neurologic disorder, but this terminology can be misleading. Despite the fact that the cerebral injury does not change over time, the *clinical picture* does change as the child matures.

Historically, CP was recognized in ancient and biblical times, but Sir William John Little is credited with the "first medical descriptions of a puzzling disorder that struck children in the first years of life, causing stiff, spastic muscles in their legs and to a lesser degree, their arms" (Cerebral Palsy, 2001). Later in the 19th century, William Osler published his lectures on CP, in which he classified the disorder "based on neuroanatomy, etiology, and extremity involvement" (Hoon & Johnston, 2002). Osler (1987) proposed that "the upper corticospinal tract, extending from the cells of the cortex to the gray matter of

the cord" was central to understanding the anatomical origins of CP.

Twentieth century advances in neuroimaging have allowed for a more extensive and complex understanding of CP. Similarly, treatment options have expanded to include new pharmacologic and surgical interventions that address concerns of spasticity, tone, and pain.

### Pathophysiology

The pathophysiology related to CP defies a single, concise explanation, but understanding basic neuromuscular pathways aids in the understanding of CP. Motor function is brought about by one of two pathways. One pathway is the reflex arc. The second pathway is that which initiates "at the cerebral cortex and other centers in the brain through the various nerve pathways of the central nervous system (CNS)" (Hockenberry, 2003). This pathway consists of UMN and lower motor neurons (LMN). The UMN pathway starts at the cerebral cortex and terminates at the anterior horn. The LMN pathway "involves the cells of the anterior horns, its axons and the peripheral nerves branches" (Hockenberry). Faulty development of or insult to the CNS can lead to the development of CP.

**Table 1. Characateristics of Two Basic Types of Cerebral Palsy**

| Spastic (Pyramidal) | Nonspastic (Extrapyramidal) |
|---|---|
| Spastic hemiplegia:<br>    Spasticity mainly on one lateral side of the body. | Choreoathetoid:<br>    Involuntary slow, irregular, writhing movements of muscle groups, usually distal in origin. |
| Spastic diplegia:<br>    Spasticity seen more in legs than arms, but not exclusive to legs. | Bradykinesia:<br>    Slowing or reduction of movements |
| Spastic quadriplegia:<br>    Spasticity seen in all four extremities; can also involve neck and trunk muscles. | Dystonic:<br>    Involuntary twisting or jerking or sustained extremities; can also abnormal posture. |
| Bilateral hemiplegia:<br>    Spasticity in both legs or both arms | |

## Classifications

Just as there are multiple explanations regarding the etiology of CP, the description and categorizing of CP can be quite complex as well. One simple way to is to appreciate *how* CP affects the body and therefore *what type of dysfunction* CP brings about. This is what is meant by physiolgic classification. Furthermore, the spastic type of CP can be described in more detail based on *what parts* of the body are affected. This is known as topographical classification. **Table 1** describes the two basic types of CP, while topographically describing spastic CP. Nonspastic CP is not described topographically, but rather is specified according to the type of movements involved.

## Incidence

CP is the most common form of movement disorder affecting children. Despite medical and diagnostic advances that have impacted the specialty areas of prenatal, obstetric, and neonatal practice, the prevalence of CP has remained constant at about 2 per 1,000 live births in the United States. According to the United Cerebral Palsy Association, there are more than 500,000 Americans with CP. The economic impact from such a disability is staggering. A 2004 *Morbidity and Mortality Weekly Report* indicates that the average lifetime costs for a person with CP is estimated to be about $921,000 (Honeycutt, Dunlap, Chen, al Homsi, Grosse, & Schendel, 2004).

## Etiologies

Birth asphyxia has been traditionally associated with the onset of CP. Recent large studies, however, indicate that only a small percentage of cases can be attributed to birth asphyxia. "Birth complications, including asphyxia, are now estimated to account for about 6% of congenital cerebral palsy cases" (Cerebral Palsy, 2001).

Prematurity and low birth weight are risk factors associated with CP. "The association, however, is not absolute, because only 10% of infants weighing less than 1,500 g develop cerebral palsy, and, similarly, only 10% to 28% of children with cerebral palsy weighed less than 1,500 g at birth" (Wollack & Nichter, 2002). Adding further insight into the association of prematurity and CP, the Collaborative Perinatal Project, funded by the National Institutes of Health and involving 45,000 children, revealed that most children with CP were born full-term and experienced uncomplicated labor and delivery. "In 80% of cases, features were identified pointing to antenatal factors causing abnormal brain development" (Johnston, 2004). Intrauterine exposure to infection, ischemic events in utero, endocrine or metabolic disorders, as well as thrombophilic disorders, can also be cause for a child to develop CP.

## Management

Despite the lack of specific explanations as to why a child develops CP, the goals for managing a child with CP are broadly defined. According to Hockenberry (2003), "the broad aims of habilitative therapy are to (1) establish locomotion, communication and self-help; (2) gain optimum appearance and integration of motor function; (3) correct associated defects as early and effectively as possible; (4) provide educational opportunities adapted to the individual child's needs and capabilities; and (5) promote socialization experiences with other affected and unaffected children." Optimizing motor function, treating pain and spasticity, and assisting with associated cognitive, speech, oral motor, and other associated problems dictate the involvement of a specialized team of health professionals.

Realizing that each plan is individualized, maximizing motor function to promote locomotion, communication, and self-help is of primary importance. Devices ranging from orthotics to wheelchairs can be used to promote movement. Medications commonly used to treat spasticity include benzodiaepines, GABA-agonists such as baclofen, and dantrolene sodium (a phenytoin derivative). Furthermore, Hoon and Johnston (2002) suggest that "for patients with localized spasticity, botulinum toxin has been effectively utilized to improve gross and fine motor abilities." Dystonia, associated with extrapyramidal CP, may be treated with levodopa, carbamezepine, or trihexyphenidyl. Medical-surgical interventions may be used to treat spasticity that is not corrected by pharmacologic means. Neurosurgical approaches to controlling spasticity include the use of a subcutaneous implanted device to deliver baclofen intrathecally. Selective dorsal rhizotomy is another neurosurgical procedure, whereby specific dorsal rootlets are surgically severed in a discriminate manner. Orthopedic surgery may be indicated to "correct contracture or spastic deformities, to provide stability for an uncontrollable joint, and to provide for balanced muscle power" (Hockenberry, 2003). Soft tissue surgeries, such as surgically dividing the affected tendon (tenotomy), have been used to treat spasticity in the Achilles tendon and hip girdle area.

Facilitating communication is of primary importance as the child grows from infancy to preschool and beyond. Speech and language therapy may be utilized to enhance communication skill; the use and optimization of oral communication skills is preferred. Children whose lack of motor capabilities prevents oral communication may benefit from the use of such devices as adaptive computers, visual scanning systems, and pictorial communication boards.

Visual, cognitive, and behavioral deficits, if present, will need to be addressed by healthcare and educational specialists. "Significant behavior problems may substantially interfere with the development of a child with CP;

their early identification and management are important, and the assistance of a psychologist or psychiatrist may be necessary. Learning and attention deficit disorders, and mental retardation are assessed and managed by a psychologist and educator" (Johnston, 2004).

With use of a team approach, the child with CP can be further assisted by maintaining a healthy appearance and working to coordinate motor function capabilities. Occupational therapy, physical therapy, and nutritional services, among others, can provide such resources. These therapies, along with medical or surgical intervention, not only help to make the most of a child's abilities, but can also aid in the correction of deformities or contractures.

Last, but just as important, a comprehensive habilitation plan includes socialization and education at the appropriate level. Enabling the child to socialize with other children, regardless of abilities, facilitates exploration and understanding of self, others, and the world at large.

## Individualized Healthcare Plan

### Assessment
*History*
Low birth weight, prematurity, infections, congenital malformations, coagulopathies, cerebral vascular accidents, anoxia, and inflammatory mediators have all been cited as possible etiologic factors in the development of CP. In fact, "recent epidemiological studies indicate that most cases [of CP] are related to prenatal disorders of genetic and environmental origin" (Hoon & Johnston, 2002). In light of this understanding, it is imperative that the assessment of the parent(s) and child include a thorough review of the prenatal, gestational, and antenatal periods.
- Maternal gynecologic history including
  -presence of infection
  -preeclampsia
  -delivery complications
  -problems with the placenta
  -maternal endocrine disturbances.
- Presence of siblings with or without health concerns
- Specific prenatal/birth history information pertaining to child with or suspected of having CP such as
  -birth weight
  -gestational age
  -incidence of infection
  -hemorrhage
  -anoxia
  -congenital abnormalities
- Developmental progression of milestones, including motor skills and reflexes
- Presence of any feeding or swallowing difficulties or persistent tongue thrusting
- Presence of any difficulties with diapering due to increased muscle tone
- Presence of any concerns regarding irritability or excessive colic
- Difficulties or concerns regarding oral communication and/or language skills

*Motor Examination*
It is essential to remember that an infant's neurologic system is immature, and volitional (purposeful) movements are not seen until later, thereby inhibiting the very early diagnosis of CP through clinical evaluation.

"If the pediatrician sees generalized decreases in movement, asymmetrical findings, or a neurodevelopmental exam which approximates that of an infant of one-half the child's chronological age, the examination is abnormal" (Shapiro & Capute, 1999). In summary, the diagnosis of CP is based on an assessment of the child's developmental level and functional and physical capabilities (Allen & Vessey, 2004), whereas a comprehensive medical history may assist in the identification of possible etiologic factors.
- Tone, strength, symmetry of muscle movement
- Primitive reflexes (ex: Moro reflex, stepping reflex, asymmetric tonic neck reflex, which normally extinguishes early on in infancy)
- Deep tendon reflexes (ex: Babinski or other pathological reflex)
- Observation of spontaneous movements noting quality, quantity, symmetry
- Developmental milestones
- Posture
- Transitioning of positions
- Ambulation
- Upper extremity grasp, release, reach, ability to transfer object, and ability to pick up small and large items.

## Current Status and Management

According to the Centers for Disease Control, "approximately 10,000 infants born each year develop cerebral palsy" (Allen & Vessey, 2004). The overall management and treatment goals are to optimize mobility, muscle function, communication, and independence with activities of daily living. Considerations for managing the student with CP include the following:

- Promote and allow for mobility within environment.
- Promote use of assistive devices and adaptive equipment.
- Administration of prescribed medications or treatments.
- Promote and maintain safe environment, including emergency evacuation plans (EEPs).
- Encourage and promote communication abilities.
- Maintain adequate nutrition and hydration.
- Assess and promote skin integrity.
- Encourage independence with self-care activities.
- Advocate for and promote appropriate learning environment
- Promote continency, if appropriate. Otherwise, monitor and assist with bowel and bladder needs.
- Actively support other medical conditions as necessary (seizure disorder, asthma, sensory defects).
- Provide information to other professionals within school environment regarding the child's needs. Act as consultant as needed.
- Provide psychological and social support to child and family. Refer for additional support services as indicated.

## Self-Care

- Student's cognitive, psychomotor, and behavioral abilities to promote participation in self-care activities
- Student's knowledge and understanding of the disorder
- Student's motivation and willingness to participate in planning and carrying out self-care activities
- Family's understanding of, and ability to promote, self-care, if an appropriate goal
- Student's ability to apply adaptive equipment and/or use assistive devices
- Level of mobility with consideration for the amount of assistance needed; include transfers
- Environmental assets and barrier relating to self-care (home, school, community)
- Family and student resources: assess insurance, community, other financial resources or drains, time constraints, or demands
- Safe environment: Can student keep self from harm, or is patient dependent on others?

## Psychosocial Status

- Student's level of cognition and psychomotor capabilities
- Student's current level of contact and interaction with family, friends, peers, and adults
- Student's current level of involvement in community, family, school, and social activities
- Student's level of motivation
- Student's perception of the disorder and how it affects him or her
- Student's ability to cope with difficulties
- Student's or family history of mental health or behavioral issues
- Student's available resources (support groups, transportation services, etc.)
- Student's level of independence and mobility
- Ability of family or caregiver(s) to support student in activities

## Academic Issues

- Evaluate past and current academic achievement and services.
- Refer for Child Study Team evaluation for perceptual or cognitive impairments.
- Mainstream student with disabilities in a regular education environment whenever possible.
- Provide for home-based instruction for time lost from school.
- Provide support to staff when placing a student with disabilities in a regular education classroom.
- Evaluate need for modified physical education classes.
- Evaluate need for assistive technology devices.
- Develop an EEP.
- Evaluate student's accessibility into school building and on playground.
- Evaluate need for personal assistant during school hours.
- Consider potential for diagnosis/surgical procedures of CP to impact learning and academic schedule.

## Nursing Diagnoses (NANDA, 2003)

**N.D. 1** Impaired physical mobility (NANDA 00085) related to:
- neuromuscular impairment

**N.D. 2** Risk for impaired skin integrity (NANDA 00046) related to:
- impaired mobility
- orthotics

**N.D. 3** Risk for injury (NANDA 00035) related to:
- physical disability
- neuromuscular impairment
- perceptual and cognitive impairment

**N.D. 4** Feeding self-care deficit (NANDA 00102) related to:
- physical disability
- difficulty swallowing

**N.D. 5** Bathing/hygiene self-care deficit (NANDA 00108) related to:
- physical disability

**N.D. 6** Dressing/grooming self-care deficit (NANDA 000109) related to:
- physical disability

**N.D. 7** Toileting self-care deficit (NANDA 00110) related to:
- physical disability

**N.D. 8** Impaired urinary elimination (NANDA 00016) related to:
- sensory motor impairment

**N.D. 9** Bowel incontinence (NANDA 00014) related to:
- sensory motor impairment
- immobility
- decreased fluid intake

**N.D. 10** Impaired verbal communication (NANDA 00051) related to:
- cognitive impairment

**N.D. 11** Disturbed body image (NANDA 00118) related to:
- perception of disability

**N.D. 12** Impaired social interaction (NANDA 00052) related to:
- physical disability
- impaired mobility
- communication problems

**N.D. 13** Delayed growth and development (NANDA 00111) related to:
- neuromuscular impairment
- perceptual and cognitive impairment

## Goals

The student will have access to and from classes with use of devices and assistance from others as appropriate. (N.D. 1)

The student will maintain skin integrity. (N.D. 2)

The student will remain safe and free of injuries while in school. (N.D. 1, 3)

The student will maintain optimal positioning in wheelchair, desk, or other devices. (N.D. 1–3)

The student will utilize splints, braces, and specialized equipment as directed. (N.D. 1–3)

The student will evacuate the building in a safe and efficient manner in an emergency situation and remain free of injury. (N.D. 1, 3)

The student will participate and remain safe in modified physical education classes as documented in individualized education plan (IEP). (N.D. 1, 3, 13)

The student will assist with self-care activities as age and capabilities permit. (N.D. 4–7)

The student will not experience bladder distention during school day. (N.D. 7, 8)

The student will not experience bowel incontinence or constipation during school day. (N.D. 7, 9)

The student will notify caregiver immediately for assistance with toileting/hygiene needs. (N.D. 7–9)

The student will communicate needs and express ideas with staff, peers, and others. (N.D. 10, 12, 13)

The student will use adaptive devices appropriately. (N.D. 1, 11, 13)

The student will verbalize acceptance of self and physical limitations. (N.D. 11–12)

The student will develop relationships with peers and staff members. (N.D. 12)
The student will participate in age-appropriate school and social activities. (N.D. 12)
The student will perform motor, social, and/or expressive skills as age and capabilities permit. (N.D. 13)

## Nursing Interventions

Develop and implement individualized healthcare plan (IHP).
Develop and implement an EEP for student. (N.D. 1, 3)
Encourage and assist student to change position at least every 2 hours. (N.D. 1–3)
Refer for, and coordinate, physical and occupational therapy services. (N.D. 1–7)
Assist student to position extremities in functional position and maintain neutral position of head. (N.D. 1–3)
Encourage student to assist with movement and exercises using unaffected extremities to support or move weaker side. (N.D. 1–3)
Refer student for adaptive physical education class. (N.D. 1, 2, 13)
Develop plan for (self or assisted) catheterization with student, parents, and personal assistant if appropriate. (N.D. 7, 8)
Train and evaluate personal assistant in clean catheterization procedure. (N.D. 7, 8)
Develop plan for bowel elimination with student, parents, and personal assistant. (N.D. 7, 9)
Encourage student to increase fluid intake. (N.D. 7, 8, 9)
Allow use of health office/bathroom for toileting/hygiene needs. (N.D. 5–9)
Refer student for speech and language evaluation/therapy. (N.D. 10, 13)
Assist teachers and child study team in evaluating need for assistive technology devices for communication. (N.D. 10, 13)
Avoid doing things for the student that he/she can do alone, but provide assistance as necessary. (N.D. 4–7, 11, 13)
Maintain a firm and supportive attitude with student. Allow student ample time to accomplish tasks. (N.D. 4–7, 11, 13)
Assess student's need for assistance with assistive technology (e.g., pencil with adaptive grip, laptop computer, mouth stick or head pointer, voice recognition software, adaptive eating devices). (N.D. 1, 4, 10, 13)
Provide positive feedback for efforts and accomplishments. (N.D. 11-13)
Encourage student to verbalize feelings of self and physical disabilities. (N.D. 11, 12)
Acknowledge and accept feelings of dependency, grief, and hostility. (N.D. 11, 12)
Refer student to school guidance counselor for individual counseling. (N.D. 11, 12)
Encourage student to verbalize feelings of discomfort about social interactions. (N.D. 12)
Determine student's use of coping skills that affect his/her ability to be involved in social interactions. (N.D. 12, 13)
Refer student for special education evaluation when appropriate. (N.D. 13)
Participate in multidisciplinary conferences with parents to evaluate progress in school. (N.D. 1–13)
Ensure that IHP and IEP include appropriate transition planning activities. (N.D. 1–13)
Assist and educate family with special education process and implementation of interventions while student is in the home setting. (N.D. 1–13)

## Expected Student Outcomes

The student will:
- Quickly and safely evacuate the building in an emergency situation with assistance from designated personnel. (N.D. 1, 3)
- Maintain optimal positioning as evidenced by absence of contractures and maintenance of skin integrity. (N.D. 1, 2)
- Demonstrate techniques/behaviors that enable optimal participation in activities. (N.D. 1, 4–7, 10, 13)
- Establish a method of communication in which needs can be expressed. (N.D. 10)
- Demonstrate techniques to meet self-care needs. (N.D.4–7)
- Perform self-care activities within level of own ability. (N.D. 4–7)
- Demonstrate achievement in modified physical education classes as evidenced by passing grade and participation in activities. (N.D. 1, 3, 13)
- Catheterize every 4 to 6 hours (self or with assistance). (N.D. 7–9)
- Follow bowel elimination plan during school day. (N.D. 7, 9)
- Maintain healthy body image as evidenced by verbalization of acceptance of self and participation in school

activities with peers. (N.D. 11, 12)
- Maintain relationships with peers at school. (N.D. 12)
- Participate in classroom and extracurricular activities. (N.D 12)
- Demonstrate use of motor, social, and/or expressive skills as age and capabilities permit. (N.D. 10, 13)

## Case Study

Joey Black is a new 5th-grade student with spastic cerebral palsy. His cerebral palsy is manifested by left-sided hemiplegia. Joey's muscle tone is tight, and he has stiff and jerky movements. He often has a hard time moving from one position to another or letting go of something in his left hand. Joey is able to walk, although he does look awkward and has a limp. He uses a walker to travel throughout the school building during the day. He has permission to use the elevator to reach the second floor classrooms.

Joey's speech is affected by the cerebral palsy, but he does not have any learning disabilities. His speech is slurred, and he often has difficulty expressing his ideas in class and speaking to other students. He likes to listen to music, play on the computer, and watch basketball.

Joey has been acting out in class and has had a difficult time adjusting to his new school. His teacher reports that he has not made many friends yet. The school nurse met with Joey to discuss his behaviors. Initially, Joey refused to talk to the nurse, but after she engaged him with some discussion about his favorite basketball team, he began to open up and talk. Joey verbalized, "One of the hardest things about having a disability is that some people tease me simply because I walk and talk differently. They think that because I have trouble moving, I am stupid and I don't have feelings. It's hard to make new friends; I miss my old friends from my last school."

# Cerebral Palsy

| Assessment Data | Nursing Diagnosis | Goals | Nursing Interventions | Expected Outcomes |
|---|---|---|---|---|
| Diagnosis: spastic cerebral palsy manifested by left-sided hemiplegia, with stiff and jerky movements. Joey has an awkward gait and a limp. | Impaired physical mobility related to neuromuscular impairment. | Student will have access to and from classes with use of assistive devices (walker, wheelchair).<br><br>Student will participate and remain safe in modified physical education classes as documented in IEP. | Student utilizes walker to travel through school.<br><br>Student has permission to use elevator to access 2nd floor.<br><br>Refer student for adaptive physical education class. | Student will demonstrate techniques/behaviors that enable optimal participation in activities.<br><br>Student will demonstrate achievement in modified physical education classes as evidenced by passing grade. |
| Joey has been acting out in class and has had a difficult time adjusting to his new school. His teacher reports that he has not made many friends yet. | Impaired social interaction related to physical disability and impaired mobility and move to a new school. | Student will verbalize acceptance of self and physical limitations.<br><br>Student will develop relationships with peers and staff members. | Refer student to school guidance counselor for individual counseling.<br><br>Encourage student to verbalize feelings of discomfort about social interactions.<br><br>Determine student's use of coping skills that affect his/her ability to be involved in social interactions. | Student maintains relationships with peers at school.<br><br>Student participates in classroom and extracurricular activities.<br><br>Acknowledge and accept feelings of dependency, grief, and hostility. |
| Diagnosis: spastic cerebral palsy manifested by left-sided hemiplegia, with stiff and jerky movements. Joey has an awkward gait and a limp. | Risk for injury related to physical disability, neuromuscular impairment, and perceptual and cognitive impairment. | Student will remain safe and free of injuries while in school.<br><br>Student will evacuate the building in a safe and efficient manner in an emergency situation. | Develop and implement an emergency evacuation plan for student.<br><br>Refer for and coordinate physical and occupational therapy services. | Student will quickly and safely evacuate the building in an emergency situation with assistance from designated personnel. |
| Joey's speech is slurred, and he often has difficulty expressing his ideas in class and speaking to other students. | Impaired verbal communication related to cerebral palsy. | Student will communicate needs and express ideas with staff, peers, and others. | Refer student for speech and language evaluation/therapy.<br><br>Assist teachers and child study team in evaluating need for assistive technology devices for communication. | Student will establish a method of communication in which needs can be expressed.<br><br>Student will demonstrate use of motor, social, and/or expressive skills as age and capabilities permit. |

# Emergency Evacuation Plan
# For Students with Disabilities

Date: _____     Disability: Physically impaired: uses walker
Student: Joey Black _____     School: Oakwood Elementary _____
Date of birth: 3-12-1993 _____     Teacher: Mrs. Jones, Room 7 _____

## Student Hisotry:

Joey Black is a 5th-grade student with cerebral palsy (mild-moderate) with left-sided hemiplegia since birth. Joey's speech is slurred, and he has difficulty expressing himself. He does not have any learning disabilities. Joey's muscle tone is tight, causing his movements to be stiff and jerky. He has difficulty walking and utilizes a walker to travel throughout the school building. He has permission to use the elevator to reach the second-floor classrooms. Use of the elevator is prohibited during emergency evacuation of the school building.

## Evacuation Plan from the 1st floor:

- Joey will require assistance evacuating the building safely in an emergency situation.
- Joey will exit the building from either the classroom exit door (rooms 7 through 10), or via the front doors from special area classrooms with assistance from Ms. Wright, the teacher's assistant, and the chief custodian. If Ms. Wright is not in the building, the school nurse or guidance counselor will be notified immediately via walkie-talkie to assist him along with the chief custodian.

## Evacuation Plan from the 2nd floor:

- Joey will exit his classroom and go to the main staircase. The school nurse, teacher's assistant, and/or other designated personnel will assist him down the stairs. In cases of extreme danger, Joey will be carried down the stairs to evacuate the building.
- Once safely outside, Joey will return to his class for role call.

## The following staff members have been instructed and are available to assist in an emergency situation:

❑ Administrator: _____

❑ Classroom Teacher: _____

❑ Special Area Teacher: _____

❑ Teacher Assistant: _____

❑ Guidance Counselor: _____

❑ Chief Custodian: _____

❑ Other: _____

# References

Allen, P. J., & Vessey, J. A. (2004). *Primary care of the child with a chronic condition* (4th ed.). St. Louis, MO: Mosby.

Hockenberry, M. J; D. Wilson, M. L. Winkelstein, & N. E. Kline (Eds.). (2003). *Wong's nursing care of infants and children* (7th ed.) (pp. 1832–1843). St. Louis, MO: Mosby.

Honeycutt, A., Dunlap, L., Chen, H., al Homsi, G., Grosse, S., Schendel D. (2004, 30 January). Economic costs associated with mental retardation, cerebral palsy, hearing loss, *and vision impairment—United States, 2003. In Morbidity and Mortality Weekly Review [Online].* Retrieved August 11, 2004, from http://www.cdc.gov/mmwr/preview/mmwrhtml/mm5303a4.htm

Hoon, A. H., & Johnston, M. V. (2002). Cerebral palsy. In Asbury, Arthur K., McKhann, Guy M., McDonald, W. Ian, Goadsby, Peter J., McArthur, Justin C. (Eds.), *Diseases of the Nervous System.* Cambridge, Cambridge University Press

Johnston, M. V. (1998). Can a mother's infection damage her baby's brain? *Neurology Network Commentary, 2,* 305–311.

Johnston, M. V. (2004). Encephalopathies. In R. E. Behram, R. M. Kliegman, & H. B. Jenson (Eds.), *Behram: Nelson Textbook of Pediatrics* (17th ed.). Philadelphia: Saunders.

NINDS Cerebral Palsy Information Page. (2001 July). Retrieved March 10, 2004, from http://www.ninds.nih.gov/health_and_medical/disorders/cerebral_palsy.htm

NANDA International. (2003). *Nursing diagnoses: Definitions and classification 2003-2004.* Philadelphia: Author.

Osler, W. (1987). *The cerebral palsies of children.* London: Mac Keith Press.

Shapiro, B. K., & Capute, A. J. (1999). Cerebral palsy. In J. A. McMillan, C. D. DeAngelis, R. D. Feigin, & J. B. Warshaw (Eds.), *Oski's pediatrics; Principles and practice* (pp. 1910–1917). Philadelphia: Lippincott Williams & Wilkins.

Wollack, J. B., & Nichter, C. A. (2002). Static encephalopathies. In C. D. Rudolph & A. M. Rudolph (Eds.), *Rudolph's pediatrics* (21st ed.). New York: McGraw-Hill.

# Bibliography

Arnold, M., & Silkworth, C. (Eds.) (1999). *The school nurse's source book of individualized healthcare plans* (Vol. II). North Branch, MN: Sunrise River Press.

Doenges, M., Moorehouse, M., & Geissler-Murr, A. (2002). *Nurse's pocket guide: Diagnosis, interventions, and rationales* (8th ed.). Philadelphia: Davis.

# Resources

Cerebral Palsy Facts
http://cerebralpalsyfacts.com

Individuals with Disabilities
Education Act (IDEA '97)
www.ed.gov/offices/OSERS/Policy/IDEA/index.html

National Dissemination Center
for Children with Disabilities
PO Box 1492
Washington, DC 20013
1-800-695-0285
nichcy@aed.org
http://www.nichcy.org

National Institute of
Neurological Disorders and
Stroke
http://www.ninds.nih.gov/health_and_medical/disorders/cerebral_palsy.htm

United Cerebral Palsy
Association
1660 L Street, NW
Suite 700
Washington, DC 20036
1-800-872 - 5827
ucpnat@ucpa.org
http://www.ucp.org

Worldwide Education and
Awareness for Movement
Disorders
204 West 84th Street
New York, NY 10024
wemove@wemove.org
http://www.wemove.org/pediatirc/

## Chapter Thirty-three

# Cystic Fibrosis

### MaryAnn Tapper Strawhacker

## Introduction

Cystic fibrosis (CF) is an autosomal recessive genetic disorder of the exocrine glands, affecting an estimated 30,000 children and adults in the United States. CF occurs in about one of every 3,200 live Caucasian births and one of every 3,900 live births of all Americans (Cystic Fibrosis Foundation [CFF], 2003). Median age at diagnosis is 6 months. Those with less severe types of mutations are often diagnosed at a later age. With improved treatments and earlier diagnosis, median survival age has increased to 33.4 years (Cystic Fibrosis Foundation Patient Registry, 2002).

In 1989, the gene responsible for CF was identified on chromosome 7. Localized to 250,000 base pairs of genomic DNA on 7q, the protein coded in this region is named cystic fibrosis transmembrane regulator (CFTR). The most common genetic mutation is $D F_{508}$ resulting in an absence of phenylamine residue at position 508 on the CFTR protein (Beers & Berkow, 1999). CRFT protein functions as a channel, within select cell membranes, to transport chloride ions outside the cell. When altered, as in CF, fluids in secretions are insufficient and can result in plugging and dysfunction at an organ level (Davis, 2001). The CF mutation does not interfere with synthesis or integration into the cell. Mutations resulting in reduced or absent CFTR protein tend to have more severe pulmonary and pancreatic disease. Mutations simply altering the function of CFTR may spare pancreatic involvement (Beers & Berkow). Over 1,000 different mutations in the CFTR gene have been identified to date (Wagener & Headley, 2003). The number of mutations accounts at least in part for the wide variety of clinical presentations associated with CF.

### Pathophysiology

Respiratory disease is the most recognized symptom of CF and also the primary cause of morbidity and mortality. The severity of lung disease increases with age. Defects in CFRT lead to thickened mucus, causing obstruction in the small airways. Together with chronic infection and airway inflammation, this defect produces lung damage (Wagener & Headley, 2003). Frequent monitoring and aggressive treatment of pulmonary exacerbations are associated with better outcomes. Respiratory cultures growing *Psuedomonas aeruginosa* and some strains of *Burkholderia cepacia* may suggest a poorer outcome (Orenstein, Winnie, & Altman, 2002). Eventually, chronic impaired oxygen absorption causes muscle walls of the pulmonary arteries to thicken, resulting in pulmonary hypertension and right ventricular heart enlargement (Beers & Berkow, 1999). Complications of CF may also include pneumothorax and hemoptysis. Any sudden increase in respiratory distress or blood in the sputum equal to 240 ml per 24-hour period should be treated as a medical emergency (McMullen & Bryson, 2004). The leading cause of death, according to the CF Foundation Patient Registry (2002), is cardiorespiratory (79.7%).

Pancreatic insufficiency and damage result from obstruction of the pancreatic ducts by thick secretions. Insufficient pancreatic enzymes lead to foul-smelling, bulky stools and malnutrition, causing slowed growth and development (The National Institutes of Diabetes and Digestive and Kidney Diseases, 1997). Pancreatic disease is also progressive throughout life and may produce CF-related diabetes (CFRD) in up to 15%. CFRD has features of both type 1 and 2 diabetes but is a separate condition (Hardin, Brunzell, Sheissel, Schindler, & Moran, 1999). Usual onset is in the second or third decade. CFRD may present with weight loss and increased urination and thirst, or be asymptomatic (Zeitler, Travers, & Kappy, 1999). Those with the $D F_{508}$ defect may have a higher incidence of CFRD (Rosenecker, Eichler, Barmeier, & von der Hardt, 2001). Although estimates of occurrence vary, recent CF Foundation data report a chronic CFRD prevalence of 2.7% among those under age 18 (CF Foundation Patient Registry, 2002). Strangulation of the islet of Langerhans, caused by CF-related damage, decreases secretion of both insulin and glucagon, making ketoacidosis rare (Davis, 2001). CRFD has been linked with poorer lung function, lower age per weight ratio, and decreased survival rates (Koch et al., 2001).

Nutritional status plays an important role not only in growth and development, but also in pulmonary function. Nutritional intervention may slow pulmonary decline (Zemel, Jawad, FitzSimmons, & Stallings, 2000). Also, body wasting is a significant predictor of poor 5-year CF survival rates (Sharma et al., 2001). One study demonstrated that although deficits occur in both adipose and muscle tissue, the deficits in muscle tissue were greater (Stapleton, Kerr, Gurrin, Sherriff, & Sly, 2001). Delayed sexual development is also attributed to malnutrition (Zeitler et al., 1999). Students with CF experience malabsorption of fats and protein in addition to increased caloric demands (Orenstein et al., 2002).

CF is known to affect the reproductive system. Infertility rate for males is over 95% due to obstruction or abnormal development of the vas deferens (CF Foundation, 2003). Cervical mucous and menstrual abnormalities reduce fertility in females but do not necessarily prevent conception (Beers & Berkow, 1999). Contraception or abstinence education is important to provide during sexual maturation. Pregnancy may pose additional health risks for the teen with CF and requires careful monitoring of both mother and child.

## Management

CF treatment is a three-pronged approach: aggressively treat respiratory infections, promote airway clearance, and provide adequate nutritional support. Optimal nutrition management usually requires the expertise of a clinical dietitian to monitor growth and caloric intake. Pancreatic enzyme supplements are prescribed before meals and snacks to help digest fats and proteins. Fat-soluble vitamin supplements may also be prescribed. Children with CF require 25% to 50% more calories than standard age, gender, or height recommendations (Davis, 2001). Some students may experience gastroesophageal reflux symptoms. Burning and regurgitation may further complicate the ability to consume adequate calories due to decreased appetite and desire to eat. (McMullen & Bryson, 2004). High-caloric-density foods and snacks are the first line of defense to deliver adequate calories. Some students may drink commercial formulas to boost nutrition. A small percentage may require nighttime tube feedings to achieve adequate growth (Davis).

Airway clearance should be a routine activity for students with CF. Clearance techniques are performed prior to eating and should always be followed by encouraging the student to cough. Sometimes bronchodilators or mucolytic medications are given prior to treatments. However, corticosteroids and inhaled antibiotics should be given after the treatment, once secretions have been cleared, to allow maximum absorption (Wagener & Headley, 2003). Standard airway clearance treatment is chest physiotherapy (CPT). Most students perform CPT outside school hours, unless they have severe respiratory involvement or are recovering from an exacerbation. Either a cupped hand or a plastic percussion device is used to perform CPT, by clapping onto the chest over the lung fields. The student assumes a variety of positions to facilitate movement of mucus from smaller to larger airways, where it can be expectorated. Some students may perform front and side percussion independently and need assistance only with the posterior chest wall. The child may also put on a vestlike device that that helps vibrate loose secretions. A more portable device is called a flutter valve. It is a relatively small hand-held plastic device, containing a ball bearing. The student exhales into the device, creating a vibration that helps to break up mucus, making it easier to expectorate (Wagener & Headley). Regular exercise is an important intervention to promote improved lung function and may assist with mucus clearance. Exercise for at least 30 minutes, three times per week, is a good starting point once a physician has assessed the student and made recommendations (Wagener & Headley).

Chronic infection and inflammation associated with pulmonary involvement require aggressive treatment. In addition to standard medications (inhalants, antibiotics, and steroids) research continues to refine and develop new treatments. Inhaled tobramycin (TOBI) to help delay or even reduce progressive chronic obstructive lung disease (Wagener & Headley, 2003; Rosenfeld et al., 2001) and ibuprofen to reduce chronic inflammation (CFF, 2002) are two examples. Another newer inhaled drug is dornase alfa (Pulmozyme), which breaks up extra DNA fragments in mucus of CF patients, making it less viscous (Orenstein et al., 2002). One of the more recent clinical trials uses Azithromycin as a prophylaxis, three times per week. Results are promising in CF patients chronically infected with *Pseudomonas aeruginosa* (CFF, 2002). Early identification of potential exacerbations is also crucial. Persistent cough, chest crackles, exercise intolerance, reduced appetite, failure to gain weight, increased sputum production, and fever may be signs of an impending exacerbation and require careful monitoring (Wagener & Headley).

Aside from physiologic aspects, the disease also has psychosocial implications. Physical differences such as short stature, slight build, and clubbing of fingers may impact body image as well as self-esteem. These differences may also put the student at risk for teasing and bullying. Inability to keep pace with peers during recess or physical education class may isolate the student, limiting opportunities for building friendships. Under normal circumstances, time spent before and after school performing treatments and general fatigue may limit participation in extracurricular activities and opportunities for peer interaction. Exacerbations intensify the amount of time spent performing health-related tasks and decrease energy. Hospitalization adds to feelings of isolation from peers and decreases opportunities for shared experiences with classmates. Research has found that exacerbations within the last 6 months were strongly associated with declines in both psychosocial and physical measures of self-health perception (Britto et al., 2002). Students with severe CF may see declines in health status as early as during the middle school years, the same time peers often view themselves as invincible. Living with the reality of having a life-shortening condition takes a toll on emotional health. Students with CF are more likely to demonstrate depression, anxiety, lower self-worth, and emotional disorders when compared to peers (Berge & Patterson, 2004). The school nurse should monitor the student for these complications and refer the family to a mental health professional when indicated.

# Individualized Healthcare Plan

## Assessment

### History

- Age at child's diagnosis
- Presenting symptoms at diagnosis (gastric, respiratory, other)
- Average number of yearly exacerbations
- Average number of days hospitalized per year
- Diagnosis of pancreatic insufficiency or liver involvement
- History of severe complications such as pneumothorax or hemoptysis
- Diagnosed with related health concerns such as asthma, diabetes, or reflux
- Date of last complete physical examination
- Consistency of growth pattern (height and weight percentile over time)

### Current Status and Management

- Names and roles of regular healthcare providers (physicians, specialists, practitioners)
- Number of specialists managing the student's CF
- Participation in CF clinical trial studies past or present (focus of study and details)
- Daily medications and those used on an as-needed basis
- Required medications during the school day
- Use of over-the-counter medications
- Use of alternative medical therapies (herbal, homeopathic, other)
- Type of chest physiotherapy (CPT) student uses and schedule both at home and at school
- Supplies/medications/equipment needed during the school day
- Preferred method of notification when medication refills are needed at school
- Past and present use of a peripheral line or an infusiport
- Frequency of dietary consultation and growth monitoring
- Sexual maturation signs (on schedule or delayed)
- Daily dietary habits (eats regularly, skips meals, varied intake)
- Required dietary supplements or snacks during the school day
- Required nighttime feedings (nasogastric or gastrostomy tube)
- Average hours of uninterrupted sleep per night
- Participation in school and community activities
- Environmental restrictions (dust, mold, other)
- Current level of physical fitness and tolerance
- Incidence of shortness of breath or significantly decreased oxygen saturation with exertion
- Use of oxygen for activities
- Effectiveness of preventative treatments in decreasing respiratory exacerbations
- Date and results of last routine sputum cultures
- History of chronic organism overgrowth such as *Pseudomonas aeruginosa* or *Burkholderia cepacia*
- Usual signs of an oncoming exacerbation
- Changes noted in the general health/ activity level/tolerance before, during, or after an exacerbation
- Tolerance of treatment, including medication side effects
- Resources available to provide items needed for care
- Difficulties meeting the financial burden of treatment

### Self-care

- Medications/treatments/procedures independently administered at home and need for supervision
- Student's ability to carry and administer own pancreatic enzymes or inhaled medications, as prescribed and when needed
- Self-management skills currently learning at home
- Student's ability to self-regulate dietary intake and activity level
- Ability to recognize early signs and symptoms of respiratory distress or oncoming exacerbation

### Psychosocial Status

- Perception of general health status
- Coping strategies and effectiveness in dealing with the demands of routine treatments and exacerbations
- Difficulties experienced in complying with ordered treatments

- Application for public assistance programs to defray costs
- Disruption of activities due to an exacerbation in the recent past
- Level of diagnosis disclosure with the teachers/peer group and response
- Concerns related to peer's reactions toward symptoms or diagnosis
- Extracurricular activity participation with peers
- Problems with teasing or bullying at school or in the community
- Ability to identify a support system within the extended family or community
- Community resource(s) currently utilized and unmet need for resources

### Academic Issues

- Past school attendance record, including patterns of absences and excuse
- Average number of school days missed yearly
- Student's academic history
- Participation in yearly school-wide measures of academic achievement
- Current modifications made for the student during the school day
- Additional modifications needed during the school day
- Presence of a 504 or individualized education plan (IEP) to address health and educational accommodations at school
- Training required by school staff to meet student needs
- Provisions made for CF management at school

## Nursing Diagnoses (N.D.) (NANDA, 2003)

**N.D. 1** Ineffective airway clearance (NANDA 00031) related to:
- excessive mucus production
- retained secretions
- chronic infection
- chronic inflammation
- refusal to cough and/or use CPT therapies at school
- inadequate fluid intake
- pulmonary exacerbation

**N.D. 2** Risk for activity intolerance (NANDA 00094) related to:
- impaired gas exchange
- pulmonary exacerbation
- inability to acknowledge early signs of fatigue

**N.D. 3** Imbalanced nutrition: less than body requirements (NANDA 00002) related to:
- inadequate intake
- increased caloric demands
- decreased digestion and absorption of nutrients
- pulmonary exacerbation

**N.D. 4** Risk for deficient fluid volume (NANDA 00028) related to:
- extreme exertion during hot humid weather conditions
- failure to ingest adequate fluids

**N.D. 5** Ineffective therapeutic regimen management (NANDA 00078 ) related to:
- knowledge deficit
- denial of early warning signs of pulmonary exacerbation
- lack of financial resources
- complexity of regimen
- multiple changes in medications/treatments
- lack of social support system
- inconsistent primary caregiver
- multiple caregiver demands
- family conflict

**N.D. 6** Risk for noncompliance with prescribed treatment (NANDA 00079) related to:
- denial of need for medication/treatment
- perceived ineffectiveness of medication/treatment
- time involvement
- cost of treatment

- undesirable side effects of medication
- knowledge deficit

**N.D. 7** Ineffective coping (NANDA 00069) related to:
- severity of exacerbation
- fear of future exacerbations
- stress imposed by CF and its management
- altered role performance
- inadequate social support
- ineffective parental coping

**N.D. 8** Ineffective role performance (NANDA 00055) related to:
- absence from school due to CF
- inadequate coping
- frequent exacerbations
- inadequate support system
- impaired self-esteem

**N.D 9** Chronic low self-esteem (NANDA 00119) related to:
- disturbed body image
- activity intolerance
- perceived negative feedback from peers
- ineffective coping
- altered role performance
- inadequate support system

**N.D. 10** Disturbed body image (NANDA 00118) related to
- delayed puberty
- medication side effects
- gastrostomy placement
- impaired nutritional status
- activity intolerance
- excessive gas production and fatty foul-smelling stools

**N.D. 11** Risk for acute infection (NANDA 00004) related to:
- ineffective airway clearance
- chronic inflammation of airways
- introduction of new pathogen
- antibiotic resistance

## Goals

The student will follow airway clearance procedures at school, as outlined in protocol. (N.D. 1, 5, 6,)

The student will demonstrate improved airway clearance. (N.D. 1)

The student will demonstrate effective hand-washing techniques. (N.D. 1, 11)

The student will comply with infection control measures. (N.D. 1, 5, 6, 11)

The student will demonstrate improved physical activity tolerance in the school setting. (N.D. 2, 9, 10)

The student will demonstrate improved nutritional status. (N.D. 2, 3, 5, 6, 10)

The student will consume adequate fluid during the school day. (N.D. 1, 4, 5, 6)

The student and primary caregiver, in collaboration with the physician, will develop a mutually agreeable school treatment plan. (N.D. 1–10)

The student will attend school/class and participate with modifications made as needed. (N.D. 1–10)

The student will comply with prescribed therapeutic regimen. (N.D. 1, 3–6, 10)

The student will be able to identify a source of social support within the school community (N.D. 5, 6–9).

The student will assist with identifying modifications required during the school day due to CF (N.D. 1–11).

The student will attend his/her 504/IEP meetings and participate in team decision making (N.D. 2–9).

The student will progress toward adapting to living with a chronic condition. (N.D. 2, 3, 5–10)

The student will seek treatment for signs of pulmonary exacerbation. (N.D. 1–3, 5–8, 11)

The student will demonstrate improved self-esteem. (N.D. 7–9)

## Nursing Interventions

Obtain a signed release of information to obtain pertinent medical records and orders and to share information with the medical provider. (N.D. 1–11)

Contact physician after all absences, due to exacerbations, to verify current orders. (N.D. 1–11)

Parent and physician will be notified when signs of a potential impending exacerbation are observed at school, such as persistent cough, chest crackles, exercise intolerance, reduced appetite, failure to gain weight, increased sputum production, and fever. (N. D. 1–3, 11)

Obtain parental and student permission to share relevant medical information with school personnel. (N.D. 1–11)

In collaboration with the medical provider, family, and student, develop a school CF treatment plan. (N.D. 1–11)

Establish a preferred mode of scheduled communication with parents/guardians to facilitate coordination of medical treatment and to monitor the student's social and emotional adjustment. (N.D. 1–11)

Develop trusting open communication with the student, encouraging verbalization of feelings of anger, frustration, depression, concerns, and fears. (N.D. 1–3, 5–10)

Provide support and encouragement to student. (N.D. 1–11)

Designated staff will be given training regarding CF, need for accommodations, and potential educational implications. (N.D. 1–11)

Provide CF educational materials to designated school personnel and allow time for questions. (N.D. 1–11)

Facilitate student participation in the therapeutic plan. (N.D. 1–11)
- Determine student's current level of participation.
- Set participation goals with student and primary caregiver.
- Explore strategies with the student to progress toward goal attainment.
- Break down treatment plan into discrete teachable components.
- Maintain consistency in student supervision through written protocol and support staff training.
- Encourage the student to participate in monitoring progress toward goal attainment.
- Evaluate plan and modify, in collaboration with student, as needed for goal attainment.
- Provide ongoing feedback to primary caregiver regarding student's progress toward goal attainment.
- Provide positive reinforcement to student.
- Assist student to develop realistic therapeutic expectations.

Assist student to develop personal health goals. (N.D. 1–11)
- Determine student's awareness of personal health needs and implications.
- Facilitate exploration of student's strengths and weaknesses.
- Assist student to prioritize health needs.
- Incorporate student's values and beliefs when developing goals.
- Assist student to develop realistic attainable goals.
- Record goals in clear, measurable terms.
- Establish baseline functioning for identified goals.

Promote management of therapeutic plan. (N.D. 1–11)
- Determine student's level of dependency on family.
- Identify family's expectations for management.
- Assess need for reinforcement teaching.
- Assist student/primary caregiver to identify strengths and challenges with current management strategies.
- Collaborate with student and primary caregiver to set goals for school management.
- Support student and primary caregiver through active listening.
- Assist to resolve conflicts between the student and family that serve as barriers to treatment.

Collaborate with the student, family, and other school personnel to: (N.D. 1–11)
- Determine need for an accommodation plan.
- Participate in plan development.
- Implement the plan.
- Evaluate effectiveness of the plan.

Collaborate with the educational team to identify the need for health accommodations such as: (N.D. 1–7, 11)
- Two sets of texts
- Access to assignments when absent
- Seating assigned to allow easy access to exits
- Permission to eat snacks during class
- Unrestricted restroom privileges
- Wiping classroom hard surfaces with antimicrobial solution on a daily basis

- Placement in air-conditioned classroom where available
- Permission to self-limit physical activity

Assist teacher(s) to monitor student's activity tolerance and make adjustments in scheduling as needed. (N.D. 1, 2, 7–9)

With parental permission, provide opportunities for student/family/nurse to educate classmates regarding CF. (N.D. 1, 2–4, 6, 7–11)

Reinforce or provide additional CF education to the student/family. (N.D. 1–11)
- Assess the student/primary caregiver's knowledge of CF.
- Determine readiness and ability of caregivers/student to learn the necessary skills.
- Review the known pathophysiologic processes with the student at a developmentally appropriate level.
- Provide current CF resources as needed.
- Reinforce teaching with the student/primary caregiver on an ongoing basis.

Promote effective airway clearance. (N.D. 1, 2, 5, 6, 11)
- In collaboration with student, parent, and physician, develop a protocol to describe correct technique for CPT, inhaled medications, coughing, and infection-control measures.
- Teach designated staff to assist student per protocol with airway clearance procedures.
- Auscultate breath sounds to obtain normal baseline and as needed to determine effectiveness of airway clearance techniques.
- Perform CPT at school per ordered after acute exacerbations.
- Reinforce cough techniques taught in clinic.
- Encourage student to cough throughout the school day to expel excess mucus.
- Reinforce infection-control techniques of good hand washing and use of tissues when expelling mucus.
- Administer inhaled medications as ordered and observe student's technique as needed to ensure correct use.
- Encourage adequate fluid intake to keep secretions less viscous.
- Designated staff will be trained to recognize signs and symptoms of respiratory distress and to notify the school nurse immediately if symptoms of distress are observed at school.

Develop an incentive program and facilitate its implementation to encourage compliance with treatment regimen. (N.D. 1, 3–6)

Provide medication management. (N.D. 1, 5, 6)
- Determine medication required and administer per physician's orders.
- Assess student's ability to self-medicate.
- Monitor effectiveness of medications.
- Monitor for adverse drug effects.
- Review with the student/family appropriate use of over-the-counter as well as prescription medications.
- Review medication administration technique for inhaled and parenteral routes
- Discuss use of herbal and alternative therapies that may interact with over-the-counter or prescription medication.
- Monitor student's medication/treatment compliance and assist in removing existing barriers.
- Provide consultation with other healthcare providers regarding results of treatment and necessary modifications.

Facilitate self-medication administration when appropriate and in accordance with district policy. (N.D. 1, 5, 6)

Provide nutritional support. (N.D. 3)
- Discuss nutritional requirements.
- Discuss food intolerances.
- Discuss student's food preferences.
- Collaborate to identify increased calorie meals and snacks to be offered at school.
- Discuss ways to modify and/or supplement school lunches to provide adequate intake.
- Discuss ways to increase fluid intake during the school day.
- Assist student to set personal nutrition goals.
- Monitor weight as ordered and notify physician and parent.
- Assist family to locate financial resources, if needed, to provide nutritional supplements.

Provide nutritional therapy in collaboration with the student's medical team by monitoring intake, facilitating nutritious snacks, and ensuring availability of well-tolerated foods in the school lunch program. (N.D. 3, 9)

Assist student and family to minimize disruption of daily life due to CF management. (N.D. 1–8)
- Determine impact of cultural practices and beliefs on management.
- Determine, in association with the student and primary caregiver, the scope of disruption.
- Assist family to adapt prescribed treatment into their lifestyle.
- Assist focus to shift to the student's strengths and not on CF.

- Encourage participation in age-appropriate activities.
- Encourage parents to set age-appropriate limits and expectations.
- Discuss strategies for managing exacerbations.
- Identify and promote use of adaptive coping mechanisms.
- Assist student and primary caregiver to advocate for needs in a variety of settings.
- Encourage student and family to seek and maintain a social support network.
- Assist to locate and utilize existing community resources as needed.
- Make referrals to outside agencies as appropriate.

Refer family to counseling resources as needed to facilitate the child's adaptation to living with a chronic condition. (N.D. 5–10)

Assist student in adapting to the stress of CF disease and management. (N.D. 5–10)
- Provide an attitude of unconditional acceptance.
- Assist student to develop an objective appraisal of his/her health status.
- Assist student to identify personal strengths and challenges.
- Explore past methods of dealing with stress.
- Discuss alternative responses to stress.
- Encourage constructive outlets for expression of frustration and anger.
- Facilitate acceptance of others' limitations.
- Evaluate student's decision-making ability.
- Teach new coping and problem-solving skills.
- Introduce student to an adult mentor, with family approval, that successfully manages a chronic heath condition.
- Encourage the use of spiritual resources as appropriate.
- Introduce student to applicable community and Internet resources.

Promote self-esteem enhancement. (N.D. 7–10)
- Facilitate an environment that encourages self-esteem.
- Assist student to identify the impact of CF on self-concept.
- Assist student to examine negative self perceptions and reasons for self-criticism.
- Monitor self-critical statements.
- Assist student to identify self-destructive behaviors.
- Assist student in problem-solving situations made difficult because of CF.
- Encourage increased level of self-care and responsibility.
- Facilitate contact with peers during periods of absence.
- Encourage student to discuss the impact of peer group on self-worth.
- Facilitate self-expression with peers.
- Provide social skills training.
- Monitor student for signs of social isolation.
- Assist student to identify strengths and reinforce examples of those strengths when observed.
- Convey confidence in student's abilities for self-care.

## Expected Student Outcomes

The student will:
- Use effective cough maneuvers during the school day to clear airways. (N.D. 1)
- Wash his/her hands routinely before eating, after toileting, and after handling secretions. (N.D. 1, 11)
- Improve school attendance with accommodations as needed. (N.D. 1–3, 8, 11)
- Demonstrate an understanding of effects of CF on various body systems and utilize that knowledge to make health management decisions. (N.D. 1–6, 10)
- Participate in usual activities without signs of fatigue. (N.D. 2, 8)
- Consume recommended daily calories during the school day. (N.D. 3, 6)
- Take pancreas enzymes daily with meals and snacks. (N.D. 3, 5, 6)
- Achieve or exceed expected gains in proportionate height and weight. (N.D. 3, 10)
- Maintain signs of adequate hydration. (N.D. 1, 4)
- Consume daily recommended ounces of fluids. (N.D. 1, 4, 6)
- Describe himself/herself as an active part of the school community. (N.D. 8, 9)
- Attend his/her school health planning meetings. (N.D. 1-11)
- Learn to connect with other students with CF through electronic means. (N.D. 7–9)
- Demonstrate use of adaptive coping skills. (N.D. 7)
- Identify and utilize existing community resources as needed. (N.D. 7–10)

- Demonstrate a reduction in self-destructive behavior. (N.D. 7–10)
- Self-administer medications in compliance with prescribed orders and district policy/procedures. (N.D. 1, 5, 6, 8)
- Participate in development of the CF treatment plan. (N.D. 1–8)
- Comply with medically prescribed treatment. (N.D. 6)
- Demonstrate a reduction in self-critical comments. (N.D. 7–10)
- Obtain counseling as needed. (N.D. 7–10)
- Identify early signs and symptoms of pulmonary exacerbations (N.D. 1–3, 11)
- Utilize community resources to assist with therapeutic management. (N.D. 5)
- Maintain consistent treatment strategies across all settings. (N.D. 1, 3, 5)

## Case Study

Rachael Burk is a 14-year-old eighth grader in public schools. She demonstrates average aptitude on standardized testing. This semester, Rachael missed 16 days of school due to complications of CF. Rachael is small for her age (5% for height and <1% for weight) and has shown only early signs of puberty (Tanner II). Rachael requires pancreatic enzyme tablets before eating, but she fails to come to the health office three or four times per week to get her medicine. She often forgets to come in to pick up her snack as well. Pulmonary treatments are usually performed at home; however, she does carry and use an inhaler as needed for wheezing. Periodically she requires reinforcement to use her inhaler correctly. Teachers report that Rachael often leaves class to cough in the hallway. Rachael has no siblings or extended family in the region. She lives with her mother in subsidized housing. Ms. Burk is recently unemployed and has difficulty paying for high-calorie snacks and formulas, so instant breakfast drink is being used. The family has applied for public assistance but is waiting for approval.

Rachel spent the last 3 weeks hospitalized for a *Pseudomonas* infection. She is recovering at home and is expected to return to school next week. Rachael is having difficulty consuming adequate fluid and calories at home during her recovery. At her follow-up clinic visit she had lost 3 pounds and grown 0.25 inches. The possibility of nighttime nasogastric feedings should her intake not improve has been discussed with the family. The doctor has requested that Rachael be weighed once a week at school. The school nurse and school counselor made a home visit shortly after Rachael returned from the hospital. She confided that she is not eager to return to school. She does not feel like part of the social group when she returns to school after extended absences. She also confided that some of the teachers "hassle her" about the number of days she is absent; consequently, she does not want to leave class to take medicine or get snacks. When questioned, she reported that only a few friends from elementary are aware of her CF diagnosis. Teachers have reported in the past that peers have mixed reactions to Rachael's absences. Both she and her mother agreed it may be time to share more information about CF with some of her peers and all her teachers.

# Cystic Fibrosis

| Assessment Data | Nursing Diagnosis | Goals | Nursing Interventions | Expected Outcomes |
|---|---|---|---|---|
| • Mother reports difficulty with inadequate fluid and caloric intake at home. If intake fails to improve, Rachael may require nighttime feedings<br>• Mother provides snacks and high-calorie beverages for use at school when able.<br>• Finances have been tight since unemployed. High-calorie formula is now replaced with instant breakfast drink.<br>• Mother has applied for financial assistance to cover treatment costs.<br>• Rachael had lost 3 pounds at last clinic visit and grew 0.25 inches. Currently 5% for height and >1% for wt. on growth chart. Rated at Tanner II in development. Physician requests weekly weightings at school. | Imbalanced nutrition: less than body requirements related to inadequate absorption of nutrients and inadequate intake. | Rachael will demonstrate improved nutritional status, gaining at least 2 pounds during the current school year. | 1. Obtain a signed release of information to obtain pertinent medical records and to share information with the medical providers (physician and dietitian).<br>2. Collaborate with student, parents, and dietitian to identify increased calorie meals and snacks to be offered at school.<br>3. Provide nutritional therapy in collaboration with the student's medical team by monitoring intake, facilitating nutritious snacks, and ensuring availability of well-tolerated foods in the school lunch program.<br>4. Assist Rachael to set personal nutrition goals.<br>5. Develop an incentive program and facilitate its implementation to encourage compliance with enzyme supplements and fluids/snack intake.<br>6. Monitor weight as ordered and notify physician and parent.<br>7. Assist family to locate financial resources to provide nutritional supplements. | Rachael will consume 70% of her minimum recommended daily calories during the school day. |

| Assessment Data | Nursing Diagnosis | Goals | Nursing Interventions | Expected Outcomes |
|---|---|---|---|---|
| • Rachael does well using her inhaler but sometimes needs reinforcement for proper technique.<br>• Teachers report Rachael often leaves class to cough in the hallway. | Ineffective airway clearance related to excessive mucus production. | Rachael will follow airway clearance procedures at school, as outlined in protocol. | 1. In collaboration with student parent, and physician, develop a protocol describing correct technique for CPT, inhaled medications, coughing, and infection control measures.<br>2. Teach designated staff to assist student per protocol with airway clearance procedures.<br>3. Auscultate breath sounds to obtain normal baseline and as needed to determine effectiveness of airway clearance techniques.<br>4. Perform CPT at school per ordered after acute exacerbations.<br>5. Reinforce cough techniques taught in clinic.<br>6. Encourage Rachael to cough throughout the school day to expel excess mucus.<br>7. Reinforce infection control techniques of good hand washing and use of tissues when expelling mucus.<br>8. Administer inhaled medications as ordered and observe Rachael's technique quarterly to promote proper use.<br>9. Encourage adequate fluid intake to keep secretions less viscous. | Rachael will use effective cough maneuvers during the school day to clear her airways. |

| Assessment Data | Nursing Diagnosis | Goals | Nursing Interventions | Expected Outcomes |
|---|---|---|---|---|
| | | | 10. Designated staff will be trained to recognize signs and symptoms of respiratory distress and to notify the school nurse immediately if symptoms of distress are observed at school.<br>11. Physician will be contacted after all absences, due to exacerbations, to verify current orders.<br>12. Parent and physician will be notified when signs of a potential impending exacerbation are observed at school. | |
| • Teachers report peers have mixed reactions to Rachael's absences.<br>• Rachael fails to come to the health office for snacks and enzyme tablets 3 or 4 times per week.<br>• Rachael says some of the teachers "hassle her" about the number of days she has been absent so she doesn't want to ask to leave class to take medicine or get snacks. | Ineffective coping related to inadequate social support. | Rachel will be able to identify a least one peer and one adult source of social support within the school community. | 1. Develop trusting, open communication with the student, encouraging verbalization of feelings of anger, frustration, depression, concerns, and fears.<br>2. Provide daily support and encouragement to Rachael when she comes for enzyme tablets.<br>3. Establish a preferred mode of scheduled communication with parents/guardians to facilitate coordination of medical treatment and to monitor the student's social and emotional adjustment. | Rachael will demonstrate use of adaptive coping skills. |

| Assessment Data | Nursing Diagnosis | Goals | Nursing Interventions | Expected Outcomes |
|---|---|---|---|---|
| • Only a few friends from elementary are aware of CF diagnosis. Mother and Rachael have agreed it may be time to share more CF information with some of her peers and all of her teachers.<br>• Rachael reports she doesn't feel like part of the social group when she returns to school after extended absences. | | | 4. Provide opportunity for Rachael and school nurse to educate selected classmates regarding CF.<br>5. Designated staff will be given training regarding CF, need for accommodations, and potential educational implications.<br>6. Collaborate with the educational team to identify the need for health accommodations.<br>7. Refer family to counseling resources as needed to facilitate Rachael's adaptation to living with a chronic condition. | |

# References

Beers, M. H., & Berkow, R. (Eds.). (1999). *The Merck Manual* (17th ed., pp. 2366–2371). Whitehouse Station, NJ: Merck Research Laboratories.

Berge, J. M., & Patterson, J. M. (2004). Cystic fibrosis and the family: A review and critique of the literature. *Families, Systems, & Health, 22*(1), 74–100.

Britto, M. T., Kotagal, U. R., Hornumg, R. W., Atherton, H. D., Tsevat, J., & Wilmott, R. W. (2002). Impact of recent pulmonary exacerbations on quality of life in patients with CF. *Chest, 121*(1), 64–72.

Cystic Fibrosis Foundation. (2002). *Facts for CF care providers.* Bethesda, MD: Author.

Cystic Fibrosis Foundation. (2003). *What is CF.* Retrieved July 15, 2003, from http://www.cff.org/about_cf/what_is_cf

Cystic Fibrosis Foundation Patient Registry. (2002). *2001 Annual data report to the center directors.* Bethesda, MD: Author.

Davis, P. M. (2001). Cystic fibrosis. *Pediatrics in Review, 22*(8), 257–264.

Hardin, D.S., Brunzell, C., Shcissel, K., Schindler, T., & Moran, A. (1999). *Managing cystic fibrosis related diabetes (CFRD).* Bethesda, MD: Cystic Fibrosis Foundation.

Koch, C., Rainisio, M., Madessani, U., Harms, H., Hodson, M., Mastella, G., et al. (2001). Presence of cystic fibrosis-related diabetes mellitus is tightly lined to poor lung function in patients with cystic fibrosis: Data from the European epidemiologic registry of cystic fibrosis. *Pediatric Pulmonology, 32,* 343–350.

McMullen, A. H. & Bryson, E. A.( 2004). Cystic fibrosis. In P. J. Allen & J. A. Vessey (Eds.), *Primary care of the child with a chronic condition* (4th ed., pp.404–425). St. Louis, MO: Mosby.

National Institutes of Diabetes and Digestive and Kidney Diseases. (1997). *Cystic fibrosis research directions.* Retrieved April 17, 2003, from http://www.niddk.nih.gov/health/endo/pubs/cystic/cystic.htm

NANDA International. (2003*). Nursing diagnosis: definitions & classification 2003-2004.* Philadelphia: Author.

Orenstein, D. M., Winnie, G. B., & Altman, H. (2002). Cystic fibrosis: A 2002 update. *Journal of Pediatrics, 140*(2), 156–164.

Rosenecker, J., Eichler, I., Barmeier, H., & von der Hardt, H. (2001). Diabetes mellitus and cystic fibrosis: Comparison of clinical parameters in patients treated with insulin versus oral glucose lowering agents. *Pediatric Pulmonology, 32,* 351–355.

Rosenfeld M., Gibson R., McNamara S., Emerson J., McCoy K., Shell R., et al. (2001). Serum and lower respiratory tract drug concentrations after tobramycin inhalation in young children with cystic fibrosis. *Journal of Pediatrics, 139*(4), 572–577.

Sharma, R., Florea, V. G., Bolger, A. P., Doehner, W., Florea, N. D., Coats, A. J., et al. (2001). Wasting as an independent predictor of mortality in patients with cystic fibrosis. *Thorax, 56,* 746–750.

Stapleton, D., Kerr, D., Gurrin, L., Sherriff, J., & Sly, P. (2001). Height and weight fail to detect early signs of malnutrition in children with cystic fibrosis. *Journal of Pediatric Gastroenterology and Nutrition, 33,* 319-325.

Wagener, J. S., & Headley, A. A. (2003). Cystic fibrosis: Current trends in respiratory care. *Respiratory Care, 48*(3), 234–247.

Zeitler, P. S., Travers, S., & Kappy, M. S. (1999). Advances in the recognition and treatment of endocrine complications in children with chronic illness. *Advances in Pediatrics, 46,* 101–149.

Zemel, B. D., Jawad, A. F., FitzSimmons, S., & Stallings, V. A. (2000). Longitudinal relationship among growth, nutritional status, and pulmonary function in children with cystic fibrosis: Analysis of the Cystic Fibrosis Foundation national CF patient registry. *Journal of Pediatrics, 137*(3), 374–380.

# Bibliography

Abbott, J., Conway, S., Etherington, C., Fitzjohn, J., Gee, L., Morton, A., et al. (2000). Perceived body image and eating behavior in young adults with cystic fibrosis and their healthy peers. *Journal of Behavioral Medicine, 23*(6), 501–517.

Abrams, S. A. (2001). Chronic pulmonary insufficiency in children and its effects on growth and development. *Journal of Nutrition, 131*(3):938S–941S.

Anthony, H., Paxton, S., Bines, J., & Phelan, P. (1999). Psychosocial predictors of adherence to nutritional recommendations and growth outcomes in children with cystic fibrosis. *Journal of Psychosomatic Research, 47*(6), 623–634.

Aurora, P., Whitehead, B., Wade, A., Bowyer, J., Withmore, P., Rees, R. G., et al. (1999). Lung transplantation and life extension in children with cystic fibrosis. *Lancet, 354*(9190), 1591–1593.

Johnson, M., Maas, M., & Moorhead, S. (Eds.). (2000). *Nursing outcomes classification (NOC)* (2nd ed.). St. Louis, MO: Mosby Yearbook.

Cystic Fibrosis

Kercsmar, C. M. (1998). The respiratory system. In R. . Behrman & R. M. Kliegman (Eds.), *Nelson essentials of pediatrics* (3rd ed., pp. 478–481). Philadelphia: Saunders.

McCloskey, J. C. & Bulechek, G. M. (Eds.). (2000). *Nursing interventions classification (NIC)* (3rd ed.). St. Louis, MO: Mosby Yearbook.

Schechter, M., Shelton, B., Margolis, P., & Fitzsimmons, S. (2001). The association of socioeconomic status with outcomes in cystic fibrosis patients in the United States. *American Journal of Respiratory Critical Care Medicine, 163*(6), 1331–1337.

Tapper Strawhacker, M., & Wellendorf, J. (2004). Caring for children with cystic fibrosis: A collaborative clinical and school approach. *Journal of School Nursing, 20*(1), 5–15.

Wong, D. L. (Ed.). (2003). *Whaley & Wong nursing care of infants and children* (6th ed.). St. Louis, MO: Mosby.

## Resources

Cystic Fibrosis Foundation
6931 Arlington Road
Bethesda, MD 20814
301-951-4422
1-800-344-4823
http://www.cff.org/home/

Cystic Fibrosis Worldwide
56 Central Street
Hudson, MA 01749
http://www.cfww.org/

# Chapter Thirty-four

# Depression and Suicide

Barbara Erickson and Julie Young-Burns

## Introduction

Depression was once thought to occur only rarely in childhood and adolescence. Current research, however, indicates that this age-group experiences depression at a rate similar to that of adults (National Institute of Mental Health [NIMH], 2000. Children who are depressed will often exhibit different behaviors from those seen in adults, resulting in the depression going unrecognized. As childhood depression has become better understood, however, it has been more frequently diagnosed and treated. The increased prevalence of depression is only partially explained by this improved awareness. Researchers have reported there is also an increasing incidence of depression in the childhood and adolescent years. Environmental factors are thought to be behind this increase, with poverty, family dysfunction, the unrealistically high expectations and pressures placed on children, and exposure to violence through victimization being highly contributory (Ingersoll & Goldstein, 2001). Environmental factors, however, only partially explain the complexities of what causes depression. Researchers have found that depression is correlated with neurobiological factors, heredity, difficult temperament, certain medical conditions, childhood trauma causing hypersecretion of corticotropin-releasing factor, untreated depression in a parent, and child abuse or neglect (Emslie, Mayes, & Hughes, 2000; NIMH, 2000; Lott, 1999; Ingersoll & Goldstein, 2001). When children become depressed, many areas of life are likely to be affected. The school nurse, working with other team members in the school and community, has an important role to play in the recognition of depression's devastating effects for the child and in the formulation of a therapeutic plan of intervention.

As the prevalence rate has increased for depression in the child and adolescent years, it follows that the suicide rate has also risen. Depression is the single biggest risk factor for suicidal behavior. Suicidal risk increases as a child enters adolescence, with suicide being the third leading cause of death in this age group (Chlebus, 2004). Adolescent suicide is frequently an impulsive act. Substance abuse, particularly alcohol, is correlated with suicidal behavior and contributes to risk. Alcohol use has the effect that judgment is impaired, inhibition is lowered, and impulsivity and depressive symptoms are increased. It is not unusual to find a suicidal victim to be intoxicated (Ingersoll & Goldstein, 2001). The school nurse, functioning both as a provider of care for a depressed and potentially suicidal child or adolescent and as a resource for educational awareness about suicide, has a crucial role to perform.

### Pathophysiology

Depression is not just a state of mind, nor is it a weakness of character. It is best described as a disorder that may occur in children or adults, resulting in depressed mood, significant irritability, or loss of interest and pleasure in activities for at least 2 weeks. This diagnosis of depression has been standardized in the *Diagnostic and Statistical Manual of Mental Disorders (DSM-IV-TR)* with a listing of key symptoms that have been agreed upon as being characteristic of the disorder. The *DSM-IV-TR* criteria for depression also require that an individual have at least four of the following symptoms: marked change in appetite, significant weight loss or gain, insomnia or hypersomnia, psychomotor retardation or agitation, fatigue, lack of libido, feelings of hopelessness, worthlessness, or excessive guilt, decreased concentration, and recurrent thoughts of death or suicide (*DSM-IV-TR*). Although both children and adults are assessed using these same criteria, children with depression will frequently exhibit marked irritability rather than the sadness seen with adults. To those not familiar with the signs of depression in children, the depressed child may just seem chronically cranky, argumentative, or disruptive. Children are often less able to label their emotions and to articulate their needs than adults. These factors have contributed to delays in seeking professional help for a depressed child, or, of even greater concern, to not seeking help at all. Research indicates that it is early diagnosis and treatment that is most successful in the treatment of childhood depression (NIMH, 2000).

The *DSM-IV-TR* guidelines stipulate the specific criteria required for each of the several depressive disorders. What is termed major depressive disorder is the diagnosis given when full criteria are present. Dysthymic disorder, another of the depressive disorders, is characterized as a lower level of depression that has become chronic, lasting at least 1 year. These and several other depressive disorders comprise the category of unipolar depression. A separate but related diagnostic category is that of bipolar disorder, for which only a brief description will be given here.

Bipolar disorder includes the symptoms of major depressive disorder but is additionally characterized by unstable mood with a depressive episode being followed by a period of hypomania or full mania. The manic episode is experienced by some as a heightened mood or euphoria and by others as heightened irritability. It is often a self-destructive period, when ability to modulate behavior is diminished. An individual with bipolar disorder might participate in reckless activities, such as significant overspending and sexual promiscuity. The disorder is also characterized by explosive outbursts, aggressiveness, grandiosity, hyperactivity, and other behaviors that signal a loss of self-control. Children and adolescents may develop bipolar disorder, but, rather than exhibiting distinct episodes of depression followed by mania, will have an unpredictable mixture of lowered and heightened mood throughout the day (Biederman et al., 2003). Between 20% and 40% of children diagnosed with unipolar depression will later go on to develop bipolar depression (NIMH, 2000). All of these disorders have significant negative impact on the life of a child, affecting multiple areas, including relationships, self-worth, academics, physical and emotional well-being, and health-related decision making.

The 8.3% prevalence rate for depression in children is similar to that found in adults. Younger children have a lower rate, at about 2.5%, whereas adolescents have the highest rate. In the childhood years, girls and boys have about the same prevalence rate, but by adolescence, girls with depression outnumber boys by two to one (Emslie et al., 2000). Adolescent girls are particularly vulnerable to depression, with some studies finding a dramatic increase in prevalence rate from ages 14 to 16 of up to 16% (Ingersoll & Goldstein, 2001). The suicide prevalence rates have also varied according to age, with the highest rates occurring during adolescence. In this age group, it is reported that about 7% of those diagnosed with major depressive disorder will commit suicide (NIMH, 2000). Several factors will increase suicidal risk, including having a first-degree relative commit suicide; being diagnosed with more than one psychiatric disorder; having a gay, lesbian, or bisexual orientation; being a member of a racial minority; and experiencing family dysfunction (Chlebus, 2004).

Children and adolescents with depression experience impairment in numerous areas of life. General health may be compromised in areas of disordered sleep, appetite problems, loss of energy, and a variety of somatic complaints. Headaches, stomachaches, and other physical complaints are associated with depression and with other psychiatric disorders. One recent study found that among children with recurrent abdominal pain, 79% had an anxiety disorder and 43% had a diagnosis of depression (Campo, Bridge, & Ehmann, 2003). Psychosocial impairment associated with depression may also be present.

The depressed child often develops decreased concentration, slowed thinking, and a loss of motivation. School performance frequently deteriorates, further lowering self-esteem that often has already dwindled with the onset of depressive symptoms. Children experiencing school difficulties need to reach out for help, but depression often creates cognitive distortions that cause them to feel isolated and negative toward others. The child may misinterpret the intentions of those who would try to help.

Strained relationships with family, friends, staff, and peers at school and in the community are frequent in depression, enhancing feelings of isolation and rejection. Temper outbursts, aggressiveness, and defiant disruptive behaviors may also occur, resulting in negative interpersonal consequences. Adolescents who are depressed may have particular difficulty with antisocial actions and choices, which become expressions of their extreme irritability. Substance abuse is also seen in these individuals, which further compromises judgment and ability to function. Some adolescents with depression will socially withdraw, and others fall into a pattern of constantly needing to be with friends (Ingersoll & Goldstein, 2001).

A diagnosis of depression is often accompanied by one or more additional psychiatric diagnoses, termed comorbidities. It is estimated that of children and adolescents diagnosed with depression, roughly half will have at least one other psychiatric diagnosis.

Anxiety disorders, oppositional disorders, attention deficit hyperactivity disorder (ADHD), and learning disorders are the most common comorbidities with depression (Ingersoll & Goldstein, 2001). All of these may seriously affect school performance, resulting in such problems as school phobia, poor-quality schoolwork, impulsive acting-out behavior, hopelessness, and unfulfilled educational potential. The combination of comorbid disorders may create significant ambiguity for the student, parents, and school staff who attempt to sort out which diagnosis is causing a particular problem. For one child, oppositional behavior may result in impaired learning. In another child, frustration from a specific learning disorder may be triggering oppositional behavior. The contribution of the school nurse in assessment and planning for these students is crucial, but a team approach that includes teachers, social workers, school psychologist, other school disciplines, parents, and the student is needed to provide a comprehensive view of the student's situation.

## Management

The therapeutic management of childhood depression begins with careful assessment and diagnosis. Assessment may take place in a primary care or mental health setting. It is important that it includes a multifactorial approach that considers psychosocial, genetic, educational, health, and other influences. Consideration of whether the depressive symptoms may be caused by a medical condition, for example, epilepsy or diabetes, must occur (Emslie et al., 2000). Recognition of the need for assessment may originate with parents, school staff, the child, the medical provider, or others associated with the child. The assessment findings will guide the types of interventions chosen to treat the depression. Treatment is most effective when it is part of a coordinated plan that spans the multiple settings of the child's life. Changes in family dynamics, modifications in a school schedule, psychotherapy to modify cognitive distortions and develop coping skills, and community referral to build a support network are all examples of a comprehensive approach for intervention (Saxhaug, Wolf, Sorum, & Moore, 2003; Ingersoll & Goldstein, 2001).

Psychotherapy is usually recommended for the depressed child and often for the parents and other family members as well. Of the various types of psychotherapy, cognitive behavioral therapy is viewed as being particularly effective for older children and for adolescents. Goals of therapy include modification of the cognitive distortions arising from depression and the development of coping skills. Younger children with more limited communication skills may benefit from play therapy, where play is used to express emotional difficulties and to demonstrate problem-solving skills. Family therapy seeks to correct disturbances in the way a family operates and works to improve communication and problem-solving skills (Ingersoll & Goldstein, 2001). There is no single agreed-upon approach to parenting, psychotherapy, educational method, or communication style that is used to successfully treat depression. Ongoing research is needed to help clarify which interventions for depression have shown the greatest efficacy.

The depressed child's school environment is viewed as having significant influence on the course of depression. When a child has a positive relationship with the teacher or with other key members of the staff, this becomes a protective factor that may diminish the negative impact of the depression. A classroom atmosphere that emphasizes cooperation over competition will enhance the child's sense of connectedness and support. When school expectations are clear that teasing, aggression, put-downs, and bullying are not tolerated, the depressed child is best able to feel secure (Ingersoll & Goldstein, 2001; MACMH, 2002). During a period of depression, it is common for a child's academic and behavioral performance to worsen. Self-esteem often deteriorates, relationships become strained, and social isolation may develop. Poor frustration tolerance, lethargy, decreased concentration, and other devastations of depression may contribute to school becoming an intolerable experience for the child. School interventions that are needed in order to address these problems may require a formal special education evaluation and plan as described in the Individuals with Disabilities Education Act (IDEA). Because mental health problems are often disabling, there is a potential that the student may meet criteria for special education services to be provided, if academic impairment has occurred. Depressed students may require accommodations in their school environment or academic requirements in order to be able to access their educational program. In this case, they may meet the requirements for services through section 504 of the Rehabilitation Act (Ingersoll & Goldstein, 2001; Saxhaug et al., 2002).

Psychotropic medication may also be indicated in the effective management of childhood depression. Research has pointed to the selective serotonin reuptake inhibitors (SSRIs) as the first line of medication treatment for childhood depression (Emslie et al., 2000). The use of psychotropic medication for children has remained controversial; however, the medication has not been around long enough to clearly indicate possible long-term effects. Medication use is of particular concern with children, because they are neurobiologically still developing. Even when the medication is helpful to the child and without side effects in the present, the medication's effect on developing brain cells is at this time an unknown. In the past, research studies on SSRI medication focused on an adult population. Application of this adult-oriented research to children has been necessary, because little other research has been available. Recently there has been a push for research specific to children. The U.S. Food and Drug Administration (FDA) has approved only fluoxetine (Prozac) for the treatment of childhood depression and obsessive-compulsive disorder. In addition, they have approved sertraline (Zoloft) and fluvoxamine (Luvox) for treatment of obsessive-compulsive disorder. All of the SSRIs, however, as well as several other antidepressants, have been prescribed for childhood depression and have been deemed effective. These medications lack FDA approval, however, until child-oriented research has taken place.

In March of 2004 the FDA issued a public health advisory about antidepressant medications, particularly the SSRIs. The advisory was given in response to research that raised concerns that these medications may trigger suicidal thoughts in certain individuals. Children were singled out for particular concern, and the FDA admonished that close monitoring of children taking these medications is important. Although close monitoring has always been recommended, the need for it has now been emphasized. Clearly, more research is needed to address these concerns, and the FDA has stated that an update is forthcoming (FDA, 2004). To put this advisory into perspective, however, it must be acknowledged that antidepressant medication has been shown to be effective for children with depression, while untreated depression is known to be a serious and sometimes life-threatening problem.

Suicide attempts are reported to occur at the peak of a depressive episode in up to 95% of cases (Suicide Awareness Voices of Education [SAVE], 2001). The cognitive distortions of depression influence thought processes such that the depressed child is unable to envision a way out of problems other than suicide. It is important for suicide prevention that the signs of suicidal risk are known and that help is sought when needed. An individual contemplating suicide may talk or even joke about suicide and death more frequently. Comments may be made that life seems hopeless and not worthwhile. A focus of interest might be guns, knives, or other lethal methods. Reckless and self-destructive behaviors may be evident, including substance abuse (SAVE, 2001).

Another self-destructive behavior associated with suicidal risk is self-mutilation, typically self-injurious cutting. Not as much a separate disorder as a symptom of other disorders, self-mutilation is associated with depression and suicidal behavior. The *DSM-IV-TR* lists it with the impulse control disorders, such as trichotillomania and gambling, for which an individual is unable to curtail actions that are known to be destructive. What drives the self-mutilator's desire to cut is often described as a perception that performing this action will release the individual's stress (Suyemoto & Kountz, 2000). Research has associated self-injurious cutting behaviors with individuals having low levels of the neurotransmitter serotonin. It is thus hypothesized that this is a disorder involving a dysregulation of neurotransmission. Psychologically, it seems to be a pathological coping mechanism. Self-injurious cutting is thought to be a physical expression of emotional pain, and may, at times, be done as a substitute for suicide. Although the intent of self-mutilation is said to not be suicidal, it remains that there is potential for it to inadvertently result in death. Self-mutilation is considered a risk factor for an individual becoming suicidal (Fong, 2003).

Assessment of the level of threat present in an individual's suicidal thinking, statement, or gesture is an important component of suicide prevention. A child or adolescent may think about suicide but lack a specific intent to act on this thought. Although the level of suicidal threat is lowered when there is no intent, all suicidal thinking must be taken seriously. The underlying problems that led to suicidal thoughts should be treated, with early interventions being shown to bring about the most successful outcomes. It is important that the suicidal child knows that key people in their life are listening to them and that problems are being taken seriously. The child needs to hear that suicide is not an acceptable option, with an emphasis that death is a permanent situation. All involved in the child's life need to receive education about suicide prevention. Suicidal risk factors, therapeutic communication methods, environmental structuring to remove weapons and other lethal methods, creating a support network, learning crisis numbers, and developing a crisis plan are all part of the essential learning needed by those involved with a suicidal child (Chlebus, 2004).

When a child or adolescent's suicidal thinking includes intent to act on the thoughts, urgent action is needed. Professional help must be sought, and a contract for safety made with the child. The contract is a formal agreement, usually written out and signed, that indicates that the suicidal individual commits to informing certain people if there is intent to act on a suicidal thought. If the individual will not agree to this contract, hospitalization is needed to ensure the child's safety. The school nurse and other staff involved with a suicidal child must be informed about suicide prevention plans and be ready to take urgent action when needed to ensure the child's safety (Chlebus, 2004).

## Individualized Healthcare Plan

### Assessment
*History*
- Developmental history
  - Prenatal history, including prenatal exposure to substances, complications of labor and delivery, gestational age
  - Developmental milestone achievement
- Medical history
  - General health in infancy and toddler years
  - Past medical conditions, surgeries, hospitalizations
  - Head injuries, other injuries
- Psychosocial history
  - Temperament in younger years
  - Temper tantrums
  - Incidents of abuse or neglect
  - Social development
  - Involvement with the legal system
- Family history
  - Medical and psychological history of extended family members
  - Chemical use/substance abuse in the family
  - Family functioning and stress level
  - Parental coping skills
  - Financial concerns
  - Presence of family violence
  - Parents' relationship
  - Family strengths

*Current Status and Management*
- Current medical status
  - Current general health, including sleep patterns, appetite, physical endurance/activity level
  - Height, weight, nutritional status
  - Current medical conditions
  - Current healthcare providers
  - Current management plan, including medication, therapy/counseling
- Current symptoms:
  - Anger management problems
  - Fears, phobias, worries
  - Presence of somatic complaints
  - Compulsive behaviors
  - Attentional difficulties
  - Low mood (suicidal behavior)
  - Chemical/substance use
  - Violence toward others or animals
  - Hallucinations or delusions

*Self-care*
- Student's knowledge of physical and mental health status
- Problem-solving, coping skills
- Availability of support network
- Ability to label and communicate emotional needs
- Level of independence in caring for hygiene needs
- Ability to ask for help when needed
- Ability to manage peer pressures
- Ability to follow through on tasks

*Psychosocial Status*
- Student's perception of physical and mental health status and impact on their life
- Temperament, adaptability
- Utilization of coping strategies: effective, ineffective
- Quality of social relationships: activities with peers, school-related and outside of school
- Parent's perception of physical and mental health status and impact on family life

*Academic*
- School performance, including academics and behavior, past and present
- Special education services: current services
- School health services needed: medications
- Speech/language issues
- Social interaction: relationships with staff and peers
- Attendance pattern: including reasons for absences
- School/classroom modifications needed: preferential seating, modified assignments, early release for counseling appointments, etc.

## Nursing Diagnoses (N.D.) (NANDA, 2003)

**N.D. 1** Chronic sorrow (NANDA 00137) related to emotional features of depressed mood
**N.D. 2** Hopelessness (NANDA 00124) related to emotional features of depressed mood
**N.D. 3** Powerlessness (NANDA 00125) related to emotional features of depressed mood
**N.D. 4** Chronic low self-esteem (NANDA 00119) related to altered self-view
**N.D. 5** Ineffective role performance (NANDA 00055) related to altered self-view
**N.D. 6** Social isolation (NANDA 00053) related to dysfunctional social relatedness
**N.D. 7** Impaired social interaction (NANDA 00052) related to dysfunctional social relatedness
**N.D. 8** Risk for loneliness (NANDA 00054) related to dysfunctional social relatedness
**N.D. 9** Decisional conflict (NANDA 00083) related to diminished decision-making and concentration skills
**N.D. 10** Ineffective coping (NANDA 00069) related to emotional stress

**N.D. 11** Defensive coping (NANDA 00071) related to emotional stress

**N.D. 12** Disturbed thought processes (NANDA 00130) related to emotional stress

**N.D.13** Risk for other directed violence (NANDA 000138) related to poor emotional and behavioral self-regulation

**N.D.14** Risk for self-directed violence (NANDA 000140) related to poor emotional and behavioral self-regulation

**N.D.15** Self-mutilation (NANDA 00139) related to:
- altered self-view and emotional stress
- poor emotional and behavioral self-regulation

**N.D.16** Risk for suicide (NANDA 00150) related to emotional stress

**N.D.17** Disturbed sleep pattern (NANDA 00095) related to emotional stress

**N.D.18** Fatigue (NANDA 00093) related to emotional stress

**N.D.19** Disturbed sensory perception (NANDA 00122) related to altered self-view

**N.D.20** Ineffective health maintenance (NANDA 00099) related to altered decision-making skills and altered self-view

**N.D.21** Risk for disproportionate growth (NANDA 00113) related to altered appetite and altered self-view

**N.D.22** Disturbed body image (NANDA 00118) related to altered self-view

**N.D.23** Sexual dysfunction (NANDA 0005) related to:
- altered self-view
- dysfunctional social relatedness

## Goals

The student will demonstrate developmentally appropriate mood and affect. (N.D. 1-4)

The student will develop and maintain social relationships with peers. (N.D. 6-8, 23)

The student will develop appropriate responses to stress. (N.D. 5, 10-12, 15-18)

The student will develop appropriate self-view and self-regulation skills. (N.D. 4, 5, 13-15, 19-23)

The student will develop sense of safety and respect from peers and staff. (N.D. 6-8)

The student will meet sleep needs to be well rested and alert in school. (N.D. 17, 18)

The student will learn developmentally appropriate hygiene and self-care skills. (N.D. 20-23)

The student will participate in school and classroom activities. (N.D. 5-8)

The student will maintain academic achievement and performance. (N.D. 5, 9)

## Nursing Interventions

- Assist student and parents/guardians in accessing mental health services. (N.D. 1-4)
- Assist student, staff and parents/guardians in monitoring student mood, stress level and self-regulation skills. (N.D. 1-5, 10, 11, 14-16)
- Assist the student to identify their strengths and abilities. (N.D. 1-7)
- Serve as resource for student, staff, and parents/guardians on mental health diagnoses, treatments, and the impact of mental health concerns on academic and social performance. (N.D. 1-4)
- Assist the student to learn and utilize effective coping strategies. (N.D. 9-11)
- Participate in school planning team to identify students at risk for depression and/or self-injury or suicide and to develop and implement an educational plan to address these concerns. (N.D. 1-4, 14)
- With student and parents/guardians, develop plan for nightly sleep needs and for monitoring alertness during school day (N.D. 17, 18)
- With student and parents/guardians, develop plan for monitoring student hygiene, growth, frequency of somatic complaints, visits to health office, and related health concerns. (N.D. 20-23)
- With student and parents/guardians, teachers, and administrators, identify student perceptions regarding sense of safety and respect in school and, if needed, work to develop plan to address these concerns (N.D. 6-8)
- If ordered, develop plan for psychotropic medication administration at school:
  -Obtain medication authorization from healthcare provider and parents/guardians
  -Assist student, parents/guardians, healthcare provider, and staff in monitoring medication benefits and side effects (N.D. 1-4)
- Participate on school crisis response team to develop plan for and provide physical and emotional care and safety for students who attempt or threaten suicide or other self-injury (N.D. 1-3, 12, 14-16)
- Assist teachers to provide needed instructional strategies and classroom accommodations. (N.D. 5, 12)
  -Provide acknowledgment for positive classroom contributions and performance, (e.g., acknowledge when one part is successfully completed and the student is ready to move on to the next part).

-Provide classroom accommodations: preferential seating, assistance needed with assignments, quiet or alternate work/study/test-taking area, breaking large projects into smaller parts.

-Assist student to get and complete assignments missed due to absences for health-related appointments or illness.

- Collaborate with student, parents/guardians, teachers, and other school staff to develop a plan for maintaining academic progress and achievement: (N.D. 5, 9, 12)

-Modification of course assignments or requirements, as needed

-School schedule modification, as needed

-Appropriate behavior reinforcement/reward system

-Task/assignment completion reinforcement/reward system

- Assist the student to identify school staff members he/she would feel comfortable talking with if he/she needed assistance coping with a problem or issue at school. (N.D. 1-10, 13-16, 22, 23)

- Assist the student to identify persons outside of school he/she feels comfortable talking with if he/she needed assistance coping with a problem or issue at home or in the community. (N.D. 1-20, 22, 23)

## Expected Student Outcomes

The student will:

- Demonstrate decrease in depressed mood. (N.D. 1-4)
- Demonstrate ability to create and maintain social relationships with peers and adults. (N.D. 6-8, 23)
- Demonstrate decrease in inappropriate responses to conflict [e.g., yelling, swearing, hitting, spitting]. (N.D. 9, 12, 15)
- Demonstrate increase in appropriate responses to conflict [e.g., calm voice, use conflict mediation skills, use problem-solving skills]. (N.D. 9, 12, 15)
- Demonstrate increase in effective response to stress [e.g., improved conflict mediation skills] talks with teacher/school counselor/school nurse when feeling stress at school]). (N.D. 5, 9-11, 14-17)
- Demonstrate an appropriate, realistic self-view [e.g., describes strengths and successes and limitations, accepts compliments from others, describes realistic goals]. (N.D. 4, 5)
- Demonstrate self-regulation skills [e.g., monitors his/her own behavior and chooses appropriate behavior in the classroom, identifies when he/she needs assistance from others and appropriately seeks it, identifies situations that make depressive symptoms worse, chooses healthy lifestyle behaviors that enhance feelings of well being, upholds contract not to harm him/herself]. (N.D. 13-15, 19-23)
- Report feeling safe and respected at school, to school staff and family members. (N.D. 6-8)
- Demonstrates respectful behavior toward peers in the school setting. (N.D. 5, 7
- Demonstrate alertness in classes (evidenced by paying attention to instruction, completing classroom assignments, not falling asleep in class, etc.) as reported by student and staff (N.D. 16, 17)
- Demonstrate age-appropriate personal hygiene patterns. (N.D. 20, 22)
- Demonstrate effective problem-solving skills [ e.g., breaking problem into smaller parts, responding less impulsively, identifying pros and cons of actions ](N.D. 9)
- Demonstrate effective coping strategies (asks for breaks when fatigued or stressed, uses hand-held manipulatives to relieve stress, etc.) (N.D. 10, 11)
- Complete classroom and homework assignments (on time, _____ %) of the time. (N.D. 5, 9)
- Actively participates in classroom activities with peers, as reported by teachers. (N.D. 5-7, 9, 18)
- Demonstrates a good school attendance pattern, (misses less than _____ days per year/quarter/semester). (N.D. 5, 6)
- Reports feeling (rested, less fatigue). (N.D. 18)

## Case Study

Willis is a 16-year-old student enrolled in a high school program for students with special education needs. He has the educational labels of emotional behavioral disorder (EBD) and specific learning disorder (SLD). He also has had a recent psychiatric and psychological evaluation completed at a local outpatient children's mental health clinic, which yielded the diagnoses of dysthymia and learning disorders in reading and math. His recommended treatment plan includes a psychotropic medication trial for the symptoms of depression, short-term cognitive behavioral therapy, and family therapy to help address social, academic, and self-regulation skill deficits. The treatment plan also recommended Willis's continued participation in special education services to address learning and social skill needs. Willis frequently states that he is "stupid" and "worthless." He often refuses to complete his work or attempt new tasks. Willis also frequently misinterprets comments and requests of others and will then respond in a verbally inappropriate manner.

Willis and his parents have requested that he receive his morning dose of Prozac at school on school days to address concerns that he may otherwise miss some doses of the medication because of forgetfulness and his tendency to oversleep. The school nurse will assist Willis and his parents in monitoring medication benefits and side effects. She will also provide information to his special education team on the impact of his mental health diagnosis on his academic performance, poor self-esteem, diminished ability to concentrate on schoolwork, significantly below-grade academic skills in reading and math, and threats of aggression to others when he was frustrated during challenging academic tasks.

# Depression

| Assessment Data | Nursing Diagnosis | Goals | Nursing Interventions | Expected Outcomes |
|---|---|---|---|---|
| Willis frequently states he is "stupid" and "worthless." | Chronic low self-esteem related to altered self-view. | Willis will develop appropriate realistic self-view. | Collaborate with student, parents, teachers, school psychologist, and other school staff to develop a plan to reframe student's comments about self and skills. Encourage Willis to ask for assistance when struggling with academic tasks. Assist Willis to identify his strengths and abilities. | Willis will demonstrate positive and appropriate self-esteem by: <br>• Identifying 4 personal strengths and abilities<br>• Identifying 3 recent successes<br>• Identifying 1 goal he is trying to achieve in school this year |
| Willis often refuses to complete classwork or to attempt new tasks. <br><br>Below-grade academic skills in reading and math. <br><br>Receives special education services in SLD and EBD. | Ineffective role performance related to altered self-view. | Willis will develop appropriate self-regulation skills related to academics. Willis will maintain academic achievement and performance. | Collaborate with student, parents, and teachers to develop plan for work completion:<br>• Modify assignments as needed<br>• Clear timelines and requirements<br>• Break large projects into smaller parts<br>• Opportunities for help with assignments during classes and before and after school<br><br>Assist parents and staff in providing motivations and rewards for completion of assignments and attempting new tasks. | Willis will complete assigned tasks, on time, 85% of the time. <br><br>Willis will demonstrate an increase in working on classroom assignments during work time in the classes. <br><br>Willis will increase completing and turning in homework assignments on time, 85% of the time. |

| Assessment Data | Nursing Diagnosis | Goals | Nursing Interventions | Expected Outcomes |
|---|---|---|---|---|
| Willis often demonstrates difficulty with task initiation, task completion, and appropriate verbal responses to staff. | Decisional conflict related to diminished decision-making and concentration skills. | Willis will develop appropriate responses to conflict.<br><br>Willis will increase problem-solving skills. | Collaborate with student, parents, teachers, and other school staff to develop plan to monitor task completion. With assistance of school counselor and teachers,<br>• Reward appropriate responses and practice appropriate social skills in class<br>• Assist Willis to identify and practice work skills that will help him be successful | Willis will demonstrate effective work skills, initiate tasks independently, work on class assignments during class work time.<br><br>Willis will demonstrate effective problem-solving skills.<br><br>Willis will demonstrate appropriate verbal responses to peers and staff.<br><br>Willis will decrease inappropriate responses to conflict, such as swearing and physical aggression. |
| Willis often overreacts to redirection, simple requests, peer comment due to misinterpretation of other's intent. | Risk for other directed violence related to poor emotional and behavioral self-regulation. | Willis will develop and maintain age-appropriate social relationships in the classroom.<br><br>Willis will increase appropriate peer interactions in the school setting. | Collaborate with student, parents, EBD case manager, school counselor, and other school staff to develop plan to improve self-regulation skills:<br>• ability to accurately interpret social interactions<br>• Assist Willis to identify inappropriate and appropriate responses to requests from others<br>• Assist Willis to identify when he is getting frustrated or angry and needs to remove himself from the situation (prearranged safe place where he may go with adult supervision to help calm down such as the EBD resource room) | Willis will demonstrate appropriate social interactions in the classroom.<br><br>Willis will not make threats to others when frustrated.<br><br>Willis will actively participate in classroom activities with peers.<br><br>Willis will identify when he is frustrated, inform the teacher, and go to the EBD resource room to talk with his case manager. |

| Assessment Data | Nursing Diagnosis | Goals | Nursing Interventions | Expected Outcomes |
|---|---|---|---|---|
| | | | • Assist Willis to learn strategies to deal with frustration or anger without hurting others or destroying property. | |
| Willis and his parents have requested that he receive his morning dose of Prozac at school on school days. Concerns that he may miss doses at home in the morning because of forgetfulness and tendency to oversleep. | Risk for noncompliance (with treatment plan medication) related to forgetfulness and tendency to oversleep. | Willis will be compliant with his health management plan. | Obtain authorization from parents and healthcare provider for administration of medication at school.

Assist parents to maintain a consistent supply of medication at home (for weekends and school breaks) and at school.

Assist Willis to take his medication every day upon arrival at school.
• Administer in a private space.
• Monitor for effects and side effects.

Assist Willis and his parents to attend any therapy sessions that are scheduled during school time.
• Excuse and release from class
• Getting missed work, notes, and assignments due to attending therapy appointments | Willis independently comes to the health office for medication daily upon arrival at school. |

## Rerences

American Psychiatric Association. (2000). *Diagnostic and statistical manual of mental disorders* (4th ed., text revision). Washington, DC: Author.

Biederman, J., Mick, E., Faraone, S. V., Spencer, T., Wilens, T. E., & Woznial, J. (2003). Current concepts in the validity diagnosis and treatment of paediatric bipolar disorder. *International Journal of Neuropsychopharmacology, 6,* 293–300.

Campo, J. V., Bridge, J., Ehmann, M., et al. (2003). Pediatric recurrent abdominal pain and emotional disorders in primary care. Program and abstracts of the American Academy of Child & Adolescent Psychiatry 50th Annual Meeting, October 14–19, 2003, Miami, FL. Retrieved March 16, 2004, from the World Wide Web: http://www.medscape.com.

Chlebus, P. M. (2004). Risk factors for adolescent suicide. *Advance for Nurse Practitioners, 12,* 49–56.

Emslie, G. J., Mayes, T. L., & Hughes, C. W. (2000). Depression: Recent developments and innovative treatments. *Psychiatric Clinics of North America, 23.* 813-835

Fong, T. ( 2003, February). Self-mutilation. *Current Psychiatry, 2,* 16–23.

Gelenberg, A. J. (2003). SSRIs for children. *Biological Therapies in Psychiatry, 26,* 33.

Ingersoll, B. D., & Goldstein, S. (2001). *Lonely, sad and angry.* Plantation, FL: Specialty Press.

Lott, D. (1999). Childhood trauma, CRF hypersecretion and depression. *Psychiatric Times, 16.* Retrieved January 10, 2001, from http://www.mhsource.com.

NANDA International. (2003). *Nursing diagnoses: Definitions & classification 2003-2004.* Philadelphia: Author.

National Institute of Mental Health. (2003, 2000 September). *Depression in children and adolescents.* A fact sheet for physicians (Publication No. 00-4744). Bethesda Maryland: Office of Communications and Public Liaison

Saxhaug, D., Wolf, L., Sorum, B., & Moore, C. (2003). *A teacher's guide to children's mental health.* St. Paul, MN: Minnesota Association for Children's Mental Health.

Suicide Awareness Voices of Education. (2001). *Depression awareness and suicide prevention.* Minneapolis, MN: Author.

Suyemoto, K. L., Kountz, X. (2000, November). Self-mutilation. *The Prevention Researcher, 7,* 1–11.

U.S. Food and Drug Administration. (2004, March). *Questions and answers on antidepressant use in children, adolescents, and adults.* Retrieved April 26, 2004, from http://www.fda.gov/cder/drug/antidepressants.htm

## Bibliographpy

Bergren, M. D. (2002). Child and adolescent mental health Web resources. *Journal of School Nursing, 18*(4), 226–228.

Delaney, K. R., Belmonte-Mann, F. (2001). Identifying the mental health needs of preschool children. *Journal of School Nursing, 17*(4), 222–226.

Denehy, J. (2002). The mental health needs of children and adolescents. *Journal of School Nursing, 18*(4), 189–190.

DeSocio, J., Hootman, J. (2004) Children's mental health and school success. *Journal of School Nursing, 20*(4), 189–196.

Frame, K. (2004). *Depression in school-age youth: The role of the school nurse* [Manual]. Scarborough, ME: National Association of School Nurses.

Hootman, J., Houck, G. M., King, M. C. (2002). A program to educate school nurses about mental health interventions. *Journal of School Nursing, 18*(4),191–195.

National Association of School Nurses. (n.d.). *Addressing the mental health needs of children and adolescence* [education program]. Retrieved November 7, 2004, from http://nasn.org/education/education.htm

National Association of School Nurses. (2000). *Issue Brief: Mental health and illness.* Scarborough, ME: Author.

National Association of School Nurses. (Revised 2000). *Position Statement: Mental health of students.* Scarborough, ME: Author.

Oria, J., Cureton, V. Y., Canham, D. (2001). Evaluation of the effectiveness of a youth leadership class in the prevention of depression in adolescents. *Journal of School Nursing, 17*(4), 204–209.

*Psychosocial screening* (Home Study Module Number 3). Scarborough, ME: National Association of School Nurses.

Riely, M. (2003). Facilitating children's grief. *Journal of School Nursing, 19*(4), 212–218.

# Resources

American Academy of Child and Adolescent
     Psychiatry (AACAP)
3615 Wisconsin Avenue, NW
Washington, DC 20016-3007
1-800-333-7636
www.aacap.org

Depression and Bipolar Support Alliance
730 North Franklin Street
Suite 501
Chicago, IL 60610-7224
1-800-826-3632
www.dbsalliance.org

National Alliance for the Mentally Ill (NAMI)
Colonial Place Three
2107 Wilson Boulevard
Suite 300
Arlington, VA 22201
1-800-950-6264
www.nami.org

National Information Center for Children and Youth
     With Disabilities
(NICHCY)
PO Box 1492
Washington, DC 20013
1-800-695-0285
www.nichcy.org

PACER Center (Parent Advocacy Coalition for
     Educational Rights)
8161 Normandale Boulevard
Bloomington, MN 55437-1044
1-800-537-2237
www.pacer.org

Suicide Awareness Voices of Education
7317 Cahill Road
Suite 207
Minneapolis, MN 55439-2080
952-946-7998
1-888-511-SAVE
www.save.org

U.S. Department of Education, Office of Special
     Education Programs (OSEP)
www.ed.gov/offices/OSERS/OSE/index.html

## Chapter Thirty-five

# Diabetes

### Tara S. Kaup and Jayne Chatterton

## Introduction

Diabetes in the school-aged population is on the rise. Approximately 206,000 people under the age of 20 have a diagnosis of either type 1 or type 2 diabetes (National Diabetes Information Clearinghouse, 2003). Along with an increase in the number of children diagnosed with type 1 diabetes, type 2 diabetes is becoming more common among specific ethnic groups and adolescents. Management of diabetes during the school day has dramatically changed over the last 10 years. Technological advances and new insulin analogs have been useful in the overall management of diabetes and prevention of both long-term and short-term complications. Along with these advances comes a need for expanded knowledge regarding new diabetes technologies in the school setting.

Management of a child with diabetes is a vital part of a student's academic experience. School nurses are important members of the management team for a student with diabetes. The nurse should develop the child's individualized healthcare plan (IHP) and then be involved in the coordination and implementation of the plan.

Diabetes and the classification of this disease have evolved over the past 10 years. Diabetes mellitus is a group of metabolic diseases characterized by hyperglycemia resulting from defects in insulin secretion, insulin action, or both (American Diabetes Association [ADA], 2003). Many different types of diabetes have been identified. The most common are type 1, type 2, and gestational diabetes. This chapter will focus on students who have type 1 or type 2 diabetes.

Gestational diabetes occurs in women who are pregnant. The school nurse may encounter a student who has a diagnosis of gestational diabetes, in which case the nurse should work with the student's healthcare provider to develop a plan of care for the school day. For most women, the diabetes resolves after the pregnancy. Some women may be reclassified as having either type 1 or type 2 diabetes (ADA, 2003).

## Type 1 Diabetes Mellitus

### Pathophysiology

Type 1 diabetes is characterized by autoimmune destruction of the beta cells, resulting in absolute insulin deficiency. Type 1 diabetes, or immune-mediated diabetes, accounts for approximately 10% of all people with a diabetes diagnosis. Type 1 diabetes previously encompassed the terms *insulin-dependent diabetes* and *juvenile onset diabetes* (ADA, 2004). Pathologic and biochemical changes may occur as long as 9 years before the clinical onset of type 1 diabetes (Ratner, 2003). Markers of immune destruction, including beta cell antibodies, are present in 85% to 90% of individuals with type 1 diabetes. One of the beta cell antibodies measured for diagnosis is islet cell antibody. The rate of beta cell destruction can be quite variable, ranging from rapid, mainly in infants and children, to slower in others, mainly older adolescents and adults.

Children and adults with type 1 diabetes are dependent on exogenous insulin to prevent ketoacidosis and sustain life. Common symptoms present at time of diagnosis include weight loss, polyuria, and polydypsia. When there is a deficiency of insulin, the body breaks down fat to create a fuel source, which explains the weight loss that often occurs prior to diagnosis of type 1 diabetes. Polyuria is the result of an attempt by the kidneys to eliminate excess blood glucose and polydypsia ensues to compensate for increased urine output. Other symptoms include increased hunger, vision changes, and fatigue.

Symptoms will progress rapidly, and if insulin therapy is not initiated, there is continued progression toward ketoacidosis. Whereas the clinical onset of symptoms may be abrupt, the pathophysiologic trigger that initiated the beta cell destruction is a slow, progressive phenomenon. Once insulin therapy is initiated, the beta cells may start to produce small amounts of insulin again. This phenomenon of remission is called the "honeymoon" phase. The pancreas begins producing variable amounts of insulin, often allowing for a decrease in the amount of exogenous insulin required. About 70% of children with type 1 diabetes move into the honeymoon phase, requiring decreased insulin doses (Drash, 1990). This period of remission can be quite variable, averaging 6 months; oftentimes this may be variable up to 1 to 2 years in older children (ADA, 2004).

### Etiology

Type 1 diabetes accounts for approximately 10% of individuals who have been diagnosed as having diabetes. Approximately one in every 400 to 500 children and adolescents has a diagnosis of type 1 diabetes (ADA, 2002b).

The incidence of type 1 diabetes increases with age and peaks at puberty, with the average age for girls around 10 to 12 years and the average age for boys around 12 to 14 (ADA, 2004). Currently there is no known cause for type 1 diabetes. Classification can be reliably made on the basis of clinical presentation and course of the disease. However, other tests, such as beta cell antibodies, C-peptide levels, and fasting insulin levels, may be required to clarify the diagnosis (ADA, 2003). People with a diagnosis of type 1 diabetes tend to have a higher risk of developing other autoimmune disorders, such as thyroid disease, Addison's disease, and celiac disease.

## Management
### Overview
There are four general goals in the management of type 1 diabetes for children and adolescents: (1) normal growth and development, (2) optimal glycemic control, (3) minimal acute (hypoglycemia/hyperglycemia) and chronic complications, and (4) positive social adjustment to diabetes.

Diabetes management strategies should focus on the balance of fluctuating food intake, insulin requirements, and exercise levels that are characteristic of the growing and developing child. Making frequent adjustments in insulin dosages to account for daily difference in food and activity is usually necessary (Betschart, 2001).

Management strategies discussed in this section reflect current trends in the general care of a child or adolescent with diabetes. Each child should have a care plan from the physician or diabetes care team that addresses the child's individual food, insulin, and activity needs; range of acceptable blood glucose levels; and action to be taken in the event of hypoglycemia or hyperglycemia.

All children who have type 1 diabetes must take insulin daily. The findings of the Diabetes Control and Complications Trial (DCCT) demonstrated the benefits of intensive therapy for the management of type 1 diabetes (Blum, 2002). Intensive therapy using multiple insulin injections or an insulin pump is the method used to mimic, as nearly as possible, the physiologic profile of insulin secretion. The advent of new insulin analogues has provided many more choices and greater flexibility in diabetes management strategies. Current methods of insulin delivery require the use of a syringe and needle, insulin pen, or insulin pump. Insulin therapy options have greatly expanded in the past few years.

### Meal Planning
A balance of food, insulin, and exercise is needed to achieve target blood glucose levels. The meal plan should not be a restriction of calories but is intended to ensure reasonable consistent food intake and a nutritionally balanced eating pattern. Insulin needs to be adjusted to cover the amount of food consumed (Franz, 2001).

In general, children need to focus on consuming sufficient calories for growth and development. Withholding food or having the child overeat in an effort to control should be discouraged. Withholding food can feel punitive to a child and eventually promote reluctance to honestly report extra food or high glucose levels (Betschart, 2001).

Meal plans must be individualized to meet individual food preferences, cultural influences, family eating patterns and schedules, age, weight, activity level, and insulin action peaks. Insulin therapy can be integrated into usual eating and exercise habits. In general, most children over 6 years of age require three meals per day as well as between-meal snacks. Meals and snacks are timed to correspond with the peak insulin action.

Meal planning is focused on carbohydrate content. A prescribed carbohydrate meal plan or a carbohydrate-counting meal plan may be used.

In the prescribed carbohydrate meal plan, the amount of carbohydrates (type can vary) is kept about the same for each meal and snacks for each day. Consistency is the key, with 15 grams of carbohydrate considered equal to one carbohydrate choice. More carbohydrates may be needed for increased activity.

### Meal Planning at School
To support children with diabetes in the school setting, the school nurse may need to include school nutrition services in the health plan for students. Issues related to food choice availability may be identified, and the nurse may need to advocate for students.

Access to nutritional information, primarily carbohydrate content of school menu items, is important. For all students, but particularly those students following a carbohydrate-counting meal plan, accurate carbohydrate information is essential to minimize "guessing" and ensure a proper insulin-carbohydrate ratio for dosing. Many prepared menu items combine different foods, and the support of school nutrition services staff will be required to provide the correct content information. The popularity of a-la-carte choices, offering a wide variety of food options, in many of the secondary schools provides an additional challenge because accurate carbohydrate information may not be readily available. Food labels are an option, but labels are often on the outside packaging of items and not on each individual item, so ready access to this information may be a problem for some students. The school nurse, in partnership with school nutrition services, can be helpful in obtaining this information for students.

### Class Parties
Class parties and special events are a very important aspect of the overall school experience, and children with diabetes should fully participate in these activities. Discussing these events at the time the health plan is devel-

oped is the best way to address these issues. Possible options to discuss include:

- Student will eat the treat
- Parents will provide a replacement alternative
- Treat will be placed in a bag and sent home to be eaten as part of a planned snack
- Other modifications

### Extended Field Trips

As students get older, there is often more opportunity for extended field trips. The student's safety is of paramount importance. The school nurse should facilitate communication involving the school staff, parents, and the student while overseeing preparations for the trip. Planning for extended field trips should include the following items:

- A copy of the student's IHP, including emergency information and phone numbers to be taken along on the trip
- Training of staff in the procedures for hypoglycemia recognition and treatment
- Assistance with and supplies for blood glucose monitoring
- Assistance with and supplies for insulin administration
- Provisions for proper storage of insulin
- Supply of meal/snack items (extra snacks may be needed for increased activity)
- For intensely active field trips, parents may elect to reduce the insulin dose to prevent hypoglycemia. This information should be addressed in the IHP.

### Exercise

Exercise is an important component in the treatment plan for diabetes management. The effect of exercise on blood glucose is very individual, but generally exercise will lower the blood glucose level. The blood glucose–lowering effect that occurs with exercise for an individual with diabetes can be attributed to a decreased need for, or better utilization of, insulin (Mullooly, 2001). Hypoglycemia is one of the main concerns with exercising, and it is important that blood glucose is tested before exercise. If the blood glucose level is not within a student's goal range, it needs be tested again while exercising. Generally, when the level is less than 100 mg/dl, an extra carbohydrate would be beneficial prior to exercising.

When blood glucose level is above 300 mg/dl and ketones are present in a student with type 1 diabetes, exercise is not encouraged. Exercising when ketones are present or blood glucose levels are severely high can lead to an even higher blood glucose level and more ketosis.

It is important for the school nurse to work with students, teachers, and parents to incorporate physical education classes into the student's IHP. This may mean that students with diabetes need extra snacks on days when they are more active, or they may need to adjust insulin to account for days where more activities like field trips and increased exercise are planned.

IHPs and emergency care plans (ECPs) should be in place for each student, and these should outline the appropriate plan of care for a specific student.

### Medications

Children generally require approximately 1 unit of insulin per kilogram of body weight per day (other than during remission). A range of 0.5 to 1.5 units/kg per day is acceptable and allows for individual differences based on age, activity, eating habits, and metabolic requirements. During puberty these dose ranges may increase according to the relative insulin resistance present during this time of growth and development. Approximately 50% of the total daily dose may be needed for basal or background insulin and is often given as intermediate-acting or long-acting insulin (Betschart, 2001). Site of the injection and exercise may influence insulin action (Chase, 2002). There may also be some variability from person to person and from one day to the next. **Table 1** shows the average times of insulin action.

### Insulin Storage Guidelines

- Insulin is affected by temperature extremes. Unopened vials should be stored in the refrigerator and are good through the manufacturer's expiration date.
- Opened vials may be stored at room temperature, between 59 and 86 °F, and used for 1 month.
- Storage guidelines for insulin pens and pen-fill cartridges vary.
- Insulin vials should be visually inspected for sediment before drawing an insulin dose.

### Insulin Dosing

Insulin is a medication obtained by prescription; therefore, physician authorization and parent authorization are required, as described in the school district's medication policy, for administration of prescription drugs in the school setting. The variability and individuality of diabetes add to the complexity of insulin dosing. From the time of diagnosis, patients and families are taught to recognize blood glucose trends and adjust insulin to balance blood glucose, food, and exercise. This philosophy leads to variable insulin doses. Insulin dose parameters at school need to outline these factors and allow the student and/or parents to adjust doses to balance blood glucose.

### Insulin Delivery Equipment

Depending upon the insulin regimen used, some students may require an insulin shot at school. In addition to the traditional method with vial and syringe, there are many new insulin pens available. Insulin pens are either

**Table 1. Insulin Actions**

| Type of Insulin | Onset of Action | Peak Action | Duration of Action | Visual Characteristics |
|---|---|---|---|---|
| *Rapid-acting*<br>Lispro or Aspart | 5-15 minutes | 60-90 minutes | 3-4 hours | Clear |
| *Fast-acting*<br>Regular | 30-60 minutes | 2-3 hours | 3-6 hours | Clear |
| *Intermediate-acting*<br>NPH | 1-2 hours | 4-8 hours | 10-16 hours | Cloudy |
| Lente | 3-4 hours | 6-12 hours | 12-18 hours | |
| *Long-acting*<br>Ultralente | 6-10 hours | 10-16 hours | 18-20 hours | Clear |
| Glargine | 1-2 hours | None | 24 hours | |
| *Combinations*<br>70/30 NPH/Regular | 30-60 minutes | Dual | 10-16 hours | Cloudy |
| 75/25<br>NPH/Humalog | 10-15 minutes | Dual | 10-16 hours | |

Adapted from: White, J.R., Campbell, R. K., (2003). Pharmacologic therapies for Glucose Management. In M. Franz, (Ed.), *A CORE curriculum for diabetes education* (5th ed., pp. 95-154). Chicago: American Association of Diabetes Educators.

prefilled or use an insulin cartridge. There are pens available that are able to dose in whole and half-unit doses. If it is available, an insulin pen should be used for insulin doses at school because there is less chance of error with insulin dosing.

### Insulin Pump Therapy

Insulin pump therapy, continuous subcutaneous insulin infusion, is a method for insulin delivery that uses a small mechanical pump to deliver a preset dose of short- or rapid-acting insulin. The insulin is delivered through small plastic tubing, which is connected to a subcutaneously placed catheter. This is called the *infusion set*. Insulin is dosed using a *basal* rate and a *bolus* dose. The basal insulin is the amount of insulin delivered in small amounts every few minutes, programmed to mimic pancreatic insulin release patterns. Bolus insulin doses are given to cover food intake or to correct a high blood glucose level.

### Insulin Pump Therapy at School

Most students using an insulin pump at school will be educated and proficient in the use of the pump. There may be times when, for a variety of reasons, a very young child may be using an insulin pump. Students who receive insulin via an insulin pump and are not able to manage the pump will require supervision and/or pump operation by or under the direction of a licensed school nurse. After completing an assessment of needs, the school nurse should develop an IHP that outlines the needs and interventions. The school must be notified prior to the student attending school so proper training and communication can occur. For students who are able to self-manage, school personnel training in how to suspend the pump at times of hypoglycemia should occur as part of a hypoglycemia emergency plan.

### Monitoring

The blood glucose levels measure the overall effects of balancing food, exercise, and medication for people with diabetes. Most people with type 1 diabetes monitor their blood glucose a minimum of four times a day. The technology for blood glucose monitoring is rapidly advancing. Blood glucose meters are compact, give fast results, and require a small sample of blood. Retractable lancets and wicking test strips have greatly minimized the risk of exposure to blood. Alternate-site (forearm) testing is also available with many of the new blood glucose meters. In the school setting, students who have demonstrated proper technique and understanding of results should be allowed to test their blood in multiple settings. Students requiring assistance with blood glucose testing or with interpreting the results should be provided assistance with testing.

Typically, blood glucose testing is done before a meal. However, postprandial testing may provide additional helpful information for evaluating the effectiveness of different insulin regimens or for persons with type 2 diabetes. If postprandial testing is required, the blood glucose reading should be obtained 2 to 3 hours after a meal or insulin dose.

Target blood glucose levels are individually determined and should be included in the student's IHP. Recording blood glucose results and regular communication of results to parents or healthcare providers are important aspects of the student's IHP.

The U.S. Food and Drug Administration (FDA) approved the continuous glucose monitoring system by MiniMed in 1999. This system involves the insertion of a small plastic catheter into the subcutaneous tissue. The catheter is attached to a small computer (sensor) that samples and reads the blood glucose every 10 seconds and provides an average reading every 5 minutes. When patients are wearing a sensor, they are required to keep accurate blood glucose, food, and insulin records. The sensor data is compared to patient records. Episodes of undetected hypoglycemia or hyperglycemia and blood glucose trends are identified by the sensor data. Patients often wear a sensor for 3 days and may be required to wear a sensor during the school day.

Ketone testing is an important aspect in the management of hyperglycemia and/or illness. Most students test ketones using urine ketone sticks. There is a blood glucose meter that also tests blood ketones. Access to equipment and tools for the monitoring of ketones should be incorporated into the student IHP.

## Diabetes Emergencies
### Hypoglycemia

All children who take insulin are at risk for hypoglycemia (low blood glucose). Hypoglycemia is one of the most immediate emergencies for a person with diabetes. With an emphasis on intensive management and a goal of near-normal blood glucose levels, the risk for hypoglycemia is greater (Hernandez, Bradish, Wilson, Rodger, & Rybansky, 1999; DCCT, 1996). Hypoglycemia is generally defined as a blood glucose level that is less than 70 mg/dl. However, with the evolution of glucose testing meters and for some children, 80 mg/dl or even 90 mg/dl may be considered low enough to treat the hypoglycemia. In the development of the school IHP and emergency plan, the school nurse will use the physician or diabetic treatment center's guidelines for the child. Children with diabetes are taught by their diabetes educators and physicians that if they experience any symptoms of low blood glucose (**Table 2**), they should treat these symptoms whether they have a specific blood glucose measurement or not. The three main causes of low blood glucose are too much insulin, meals and snacks that are delayed or missed, and extra exercise or activity.

Hypoglycemia can occur when a person with diabetes has an unusual amount of exercise, too much insulin, skipped or delayed meals or snacks, or an inadequate amount of food in the prescribed meal plan (Gonder-Frederick, 2001). Exercise helps the muscle utilize sugar in the blood (ADA, 2002a). If a student participates in more exercise than usual or forgets to eat a snack prior to exercise, his or her blood glucose level can get too low. Exercise can affect the blood glucose for up to 18 hours after exercising (ADA, 2002a). When a student has low blood glucose levels frequently after exercise or notices patterns of low blood glucose related to exercise, it is important to discuss a change in this student's diabetes regimen to prevent these low blood glucose occurrences. Examples include decreasing the rapid-acting insulin dose prior to a meal that is eaten before exercising, taking extra carbohydrates before and during exercise, and decreasing intermediate-acting insulin that may peak during exercise.

Taking more insulin than the body needs may cause low blood glucose. Students who calculate their insulin dose based on the carbohydrates they consume must follow through with their meal plan. Insulin-to-carbohydrate ratios can change for some students as they go through growth spurts or puberty or when they are ill. These incidences cause an increased secretion in specific growth and counterregulatory hormones that are related to insulin resistance, and therefore more insulin is required to metabolize carbohydrate intake. It is important to assess the student's ability to accurately calculate the amount of insulin based on his or her blood glucose level and carbohydrates as prescribed by the primary physician.

Missing a meal or taking in less food than the amount that was planned can cause low blood glucose levels. Students can be more flexible with meals and snacks with the newer rapid-acting insulin analogues available. With some of the short- and intermediate-acting insulin, a student may need to eat meals or snacks at a specific time to prevent a low blood glucose reaction. It is important for the school nurse to be knowledgeable about the type of insulin the student is taking and whether the student needs to strictly adhere to mealtimes or can be more flexible. When a student has difficulty following a strict meal schedule because of his or her insulin analogs, it may be beneficial to discuss changes in the insulin regimen with the student, parent or guardian, and physician so that low blood glucose reactions are prevented and a student has more flexibility.

Treatment for low blood glucose is very individualized, and it is important to know what symptoms, if any, a student has with low blood glucose reactions. The recommendation is to treat hypoglycemia at the first sign of symptoms, even if meter testing is unavailable to verify a low blood glucose (ADA, 2002b; Gonder-Frederick, 2001). The student and school nurse/health office should have fast-acting carbohydrates such as fruit juice, glucose tablets or gel, or regular soda pop available at all times in case of low blood glucose. It is important that the school nurse educates teachers and other school personnel about symptoms of low blood glucose and its treatment. Students who are having symptoms of low blood glucose should never be left unattended in case their blood glucose level goes too low and they lose consciousness.

Students should be encouraged to keep a supply of fast-acting carbohydrates in the classroom and in the nurse's office. During an episode of hypoglycemia, the student should consume 15 grams of carbohydrate. Examples of 15 grams of carbohydrate include the following:

- 4 oz of juice
- 8 oz of skim or 1% milk
- 5 or 6 hard candies (Lifesavers)
- 3 glucose tablets
- 1/2 cup of regular soda pop
- Cake icing (1 small tube)

When a student has a severe low blood glucose reaction, defined by loss of consciousness, seizure, or inability to swallow, the emergency medical services system should be called immediately and glucagon given according to the IHP. Turn the student on his or her side after the glucagon has been administered, because vomiting is a common side effect of this medication (Gonder-Frederick, 2001). The parent should always be contacted when a severe low blood glucose reaction occurs.

Students who have had mild to moderate low blood glucose reactions where the blood glucose result was lower than 50 mg/dl should wait at least 15 to 30 minutes before resuming normal activities (Gonder-Frederick, 2001). When blood glucose results are less than 40 mg/dl, mental and motor function may not return to normal for 1 hour or longer. Students who have had frequent episodes of mild hypoglycemia are at a greater risk for having a severe low blood glucose reaction.

Identifying each individual student's symptoms for hypoglycemia and the treatment they use is important. Hypoglycemia progresses through stages from mild to more severe, and if left untreated, it can progress to eventual loss of consciousness and seizures. Recognizing individual symptoms for hypoglycemia is very important for all school personnel who work with a child who has diabetes. A child with diabetes who has repeated episodes of hypoglycemia can start to lose the sensation to feel low blood glucose until it is dangerously low. This phenomenon is called *hypoglycemia unawareness*. In this situation, it is important to prevent episodes of hypoglycemia so that the child is eventually able to regain the sensation to feel low blood glucose at a safer level.

### Hyperglycemia

Hyperglycemia is generally considered a blood glucose level greater than 240 mg/dl. The physician's recommendations for a particular child may vary and will be used in developing the IHP for school. The benefit of blood glucose testing is the ability to monitor blood glucose to prevent dangerously high levels. Symptoms of high blood glucose are frequent urination, frequent thirst, blurred vision, fatigue, hunger, weight loss, abdominal pain, and numbness in extremities. Long periods of hyperglycemia can lead to damage of the blood vessels along with nerve endings and can affect major organs in the body, such as the circulatory system, eyes, kidneys, and nervous system (Andrus, Leggett-Frazier, & Pfeifer, 2001).

Most school-aged children are not concerned about the long-term effects of high blood glucose levels and often forget that this can be an emergency. When a person with type 1 diabetes does not take enough insulin, glucose

**Table 2. Reported Symptoms of Mild, Moderate, and Severe Hypoglycemia**

| Mild | Moderate | Severe |
|------|----------|--------|
| Hunger | Sleepiness | Inability to swallow |
| Irritability | Erratic behavior | Combativeness |
| Shakiness | Poor coordination | Unconsciousness |
| Weakness | Confusion | Seizures |
| Sweaty skin | Slurred speech | |
| Anxiety | Slow thinking | |
| Headache | Numbness | |
| Inability to concentrate | | |
| Not feeling well | | |
| "Feel funny" | | |
| Heart racing | | |
| Tingling in extremities | | |

Adapted from "Hypoglycemia," by L. Gonder-Frederick, in *A CORE Curriculum for Diabetes Education* (4th ed.) by M. Franz, et al., (Eds.), 2001, Chicago: American Association of Diabetes Educators. Copyright 2001 by AADE.

Diabetes

remains in the bloodstream and cannot be properly utilized for cellular energy. As the muscles need sugar for energy, the body responds by releasing stored fats and proteins for energy; ketones are formed, upsetting the pH balance and resulting in acidosis. This is a serious condition called diabetic ketoacidosis (DKA). Profound insulin deficiency is the main cause of DKA, but this condition is very complicated. If left untreated, DKA can progress to coma as the result of dehydration, electrolyte imbalance, and the acidosis (Davidson & Schwartz, 2001).

The insulin deficiency that occurs with DKA causes impaired protein degradation. The breakdown of stored fat and triglycerides is a result of severe insulin deficiency and increase in counterregulatory hormones that occur with DKA (Davidson & Schwartz, 2001).

Hyperglycemia can have many causes. Missed insulin doses or not taking enough insulin will lead to hyperglycemia. Eating more food than planned or foods that are high in carbohydrates and not taking enough insulin can also lead to hyperglycemia. Illness and growth may lead to hyperglycemia, along with some medications that may cause the blood glucose to become elevated. Some medications associated with hyperglycemia are corticosteroids, cyclosporine, diazide, diuretics, protease inhibitors, and thyroid products (White, Campbell, & Yarborough, 2001).

Guidelines for checking urine or blood ketones should be included in the IHP of students with type 1 diabetes. In most cases, when a student's blood glucose level is greater than 240 mg/dl or a student with type 1 diabetes is ill, the primary care provider may want to have urine or blood ketone level checked (ADA, 2002b). Some newer blood glucose meters on the market have a separate strip in the meter that can be used to test for blood ketones. It is important to remind students and parents that they need to have a supply of urine or blood ketone test strips at school at all times.

The student's IHP should describe steps to be taken if ketones are present when the blood glucose level is high. The student may need more insulin, may need more fluids for hydration, or may be sick and need to see his or her healthcare provider. Some students may have specific orders from their healthcare provider to take extra insulin to cover high blood glucose and/or ketones. When a student has ketones present, the parent and or physician should be contacted (Mullooly, 2001). A student should not participate in any physical activities, such as gym class, if ketones are present, because this may cause the blood glucose to increase and make ketosis worse.

When a student has a high blood glucose level and there are no ketones present, it may be helpful to determine what may have caused the high blood glucose level. Problem solving with a student regarding possible causes of high blood glucose may help keep levels within the goal range in the future. A student who has missed a dose of insulin may need to contact his or her parent regarding taking the insulin at school. Pattern management of blood glucose readings is an important aspect of diabetes self-management education. Students are instructed to look for patterns in variable blood glucose levels and make adjustments according to patterns rather than reacting to or "chasing" one high blood glucose episode.

Interventions for hyperglycemia when no ketones are present include drinking extra water, exercising moderately, and taking extra insulin, if this is part of the diabetes treatment plan. The student can return to the classroom if he or she is feeling better but should be encouraged to return to the health office if symptoms recur. Emergency care is needed for a student who is unable to tolerate fluids by mouth, has persistent vomiting or weakness, or has moderate or large ketones or a change in mental status.

### Blood Glucose Effects on Learning

The educational goal for children with a chronic condition is to provide a safe and supportive environment in school to ensure that students with chronic conditions have the same educational opportunities as other students (American Association of Diabetes Educators, 2000). Students with diabetes need to manage their illness to minimize the effect of diabetes symptoms on their learning capabilities. When the blood glucose level is high, they typically do not feel good and have symptoms of polyuria, polydipsia, fatigue, and hunger. They may have difficulty concentrating and may miss out on learning opportunities when they need to leave the classroom frequently.

Chronic hyperglycemia can be associated with reduced learning capacity (Northam et al., 2001). Some students with high blood glucose levels have symptoms of irritability and fatigue, leading to concentration difficulties and behavior issues. Students with diabetes should try to maintain their optimal blood glucose range while in school to maximize their learning potential. When a student is not succeeding in school, the student's blood glucose control should be reviewed to rule out fluctuations in blood glucose as a possible cause of poor performance.

Students who had low blood glucose levels, even mild low levels, showed impairment in regard to fine motor and motor speed activities or tasks (Hershey, Bhargava, Sadler, White, & Craft, 1999). Students who are having symptoms of mild hypoglycemia during the school day may not be able to comprehend instructions and may do poorly in testing situations. Consideration should be given to academic testing that follows a low blood glucose episode.

If the nurse notes that the child has had many blood glucose readings out of his or her target range, the parent or primary care provider should be consulted for a potential change in the insulin regimen. Frequent school absences may be an indicator of poor control. It is important to convey to the parents and student that school attendance is important and the school nurse can safely support the student in the classroom and school activities.

### Psychosocial Issues with Diabetes

School nurses understand the importance of assessing all students for issues related to psychosocial concerns. This assessment is significant for the student with diabetes because it has been shown that students with diabetes have more problems with self-esteem and depression (Grey, Davidson, Boland, & Tamborlane, 2001). Issues with poor self-esteem and depression can lead to other risk-taking behaviors. Eating disorders among females with type 1 diabetes have been a big concern. Girls with diabetes, more often than boys, misuse insulin for weight reduction, leading to higher blood glucose levels (Neumark-Sztainer et al., 2002). Studies have also shown that females who were more dissatisfied with their weight were more likely to use unhealthy weight control behaviors.

Family support is very important when assessing students' ability to manage their diabetes at school and when looking at psychosocial concerns. Studies have shown that continuing parental support and guidance appear to help adolescents achieve success in blood glucose control (Grey et al., 2001). The most significant predictor in this study of the impact of diabetes on quality of life was the youth's perception of the impact of diabetes on quality of life at diagnosis (Grey et al., 2001). This supports the need for school nurses to seek out and assist those students with type 1 diabetes who are depressed or withdrawn, along with those who have poor glucose control.

Compiled from "Diabetes During Childhood and Adolescence," by J. Betschart, in *A CORE Curriculum for Diabetes Education* (4th ed.), M. Franz, et al. (Eds.), 2001, Chicago: American Association of Diabetes Educators; *Pumper in the School: Insulin Pump Guide for School Nurses, School Personnel and Parents*, by L. Fredrickson and M. R. Griff, 2000, Sylmar, CA: MiniMed; and "School Nurse Tools," by M. Zombek, in *Pediatric Education for Diabetes in Schools: A Curriculum for Diabetes Care in the Schools*, 2001, Orange, CA: PADRE Foundation.

**Table 3. Age-Appropriate Diabetes Tasks With Educational Considerations**

| Age (years) | Developmental Issues | Diabetes Tasks | Educational Consideration |
|---|---|---|---|
| 4 to 5 | Knows likes and dislikes Identifies with "good" and "bad"<br><br>Fear of intrusive procedures<br><br>Magical thinking | Can pinch own skin<br><br>Collects urine for ketones Turns on glucose meter<br><br>Helps with recording<br><br>May begin to identify symptoms of hypoglycemia and alert an adult | Can use guided play, play therapy, artwork to express concerns and learn |
| 6 to 7 | Physically coordinated<br><br>Concrete reasoning<br><br>Able to share and cooperate | Can begin to identify carbohydrates in foods<br><br>Can help with injections<br><br>Can help with blood testing<br><br>Able to prick own finger<br><br>Able to activate bolus on pump with supervision<br><br>Able to connect and disconnect insulin pump with assistance | May need reminders and supervision |

**Table 3. Age-Appropriate Diabetes Tasks With Educational Considerations**

| Age (years) | Developmental Issues | Diabetes Tasks | Educational Consideration |
|---|---|---|---|
| 8 to 10 | Increased need for independence<br><br>Does not want to be different<br><br>Developing "scientific mind," intrigued by tests Feelings of sadness, anxiety, isolation, and friendlessness | Able to participate in meal planning<br><br>Correctly able to identify foods that fit into meal plan<br><br>Increased independence with injections, blood and urine testing<br><br>Able to keep records | Understands only immediate consequences of diabetes control, not long-term<br><br>Finds support groups, camps, individual counseling useful<br><br>Learns most effectively when information is presented in a fun and interesting way |
| 11 to 13 | Begins puberty; hormonal and physical changes may occur for females<br><br>Dependent versus independent struggles between parent and child<br><br>Aware of body image; concerned with not being different<br><br>More involved with peers than family | Can help plan meals and snacks along with starting carbohydrate counting<br><br>Able to recognize and treat hypoglycemia<br><br>Able to measure and inject own insulin<br><br>Able to recognize patterns in blood glucose levels<br><br>May need help in assessing urine tests<br><br>Able to connect and disconnect insulin pump<br><br>Able to calculate insulin to food intake | Peer pressure begins to influence decisions |
| 14+ | Begins puberty; hormonal and physical changes occur for males<br><br>Increased physical and social activities<br><br>Experimentation and risk-taking behaviors<br><br>Conflict in relationships with parents | Able to identify appropriate portion sizes<br><br>Able to alter food intake in relation to blood glucose level<br><br>Able to anticipate and prevent hypoglycemia<br><br>Able to calculate insulin dose based on blood glucose level | Still needs some parental supervision and review regarding insulin dosing<br><br>Knows consequences of poor diabetes control<br><br>More involved with risk taking and experimentation |

| Age (years) | Developmental Issues | Diabetes Tasks | Educational Consideration |
|---|---|---|---|
| | Strong peer pressure<br><br>Values independence and self-image | Can independently administer insulin<br><br>Able to understand role of exercise in calculating insulin needs | Finds assuming responsibility for self-management the most difficult task<br><br>At risk for eating disorders Learns best when educational content is pertinent to adolescent issues<br><br>Able to learn problem solving with adults and negotiate treatment<br><br>Likes discussion and support groups among peers. |

# Individualized Healthcare Plan

## Type 1 Diabetes

### Assessment
*History*
- Age at onset of diabetes
- Family history of diabetes, autoimmune disorders
- Other illness, current or chronic
- Range of hemoglobin $A_{1c}$
- History of severe hypoglycemia
- Support resources
- Management methods that have been successful

*Current Status and Management*
- Current diabetes management plan available from healthcare provider
- Blood glucose goal range
- Current insulin regimen
- Insulin delivery devices used (pump, pens, injection devices)
- Blood glucose monitoring schedule and equipment
- Current blood glucose testing and insulin administration techniques utilized
- Hypoglycemia action plan, including blood glucose range and carbohydrate replacement guideline, and glucagons availability
- Hyperglycemia action plan
- Current meal plan; nutritional preferences
- Plan for blood glucose management related to exercise and activity
- Current general health status

*Self-care*
- Diabetes self-management techniques the student performs independently and/or with supervision
- Parental supervision of diabetes care in the home setting

- Student's ability to verbalize the symptoms of hypoglycemia and state that action plan is in place
- The student carries a fast-acting carbohydrate food source
- The student states the plan for managing hyperglycemia, including ketone testing
- Student's independence in ability to perform blood glucose monitoring in the classroom or school setting
- Student ability to identify and follow the meal plan. Student's ability to appropriately count carbohydrates and follow the meal plan

### *Psychosocial Status*
- Family/student's perception of overall health
- Family/student's ability to cope with diagnosis of diabetes
- Student's ability to share the diagnosis with peer groups or expressed concern about peer groups' reactions
- Family and student's ability to identify a support group within their community
- Student's ability for age-appropriate reaction to the diagnosis of diabetes and ability to perform age-appropriate diabetes care tasks
- Student's ability to express concerns regarding depression or withdrawing from peers
- Community resources the family is currently using; identify what resources are available
- Student's involvement in support group for children with type 1 diabetes
- Student's attendance at camps for children/adolescents with type 1 diabetes
- Student's ability to exhibit a healthy level of self-esteem

### *Academic Issues*
- School attendance
- Academic performance patterns
- Special consideration of the impact of blood glucose control in relation to standardized testing accommodations
- Education resources past and present
- Determination if 504 plan is needed
- Regular education and special education issues as well as 504 plan
- School staff perceptions and education/training needs
- Healthcare needs during the school day: blood glucose testing, insulin and meal plan, consideration of exercise and activity levels
- School accommodations needed to ensure safety plan
- Field trip and extended school-day plans and alternate schedule in place
- School performance when blood glucose levels are in poor control

## Nursing Diagnosis (N.D.) (NANDA, 2003)

**N.D. 1** Risk for injury (NANDA 00035) related to development of acute complications of hypoglycemia or hyperglycemia

**N.D. 2** Deficient knowledge (NANDA 000126) related to:
- insulin administration
- blood glucose monitoring
- meal planning
- exercise effect on blood glucose

**N.D. 3** Ineffective coping (NANDA 00069) related to:
- knowledge deficit
- lack of resources
- normal developmental issues

**N.D. 4** Ineffective therapeutic regimen management (NANDA.00078)
related to:
- denial of chronic illness
- knowledge deficit
- not wanting to be different from peers

**N.D. 5** (Risk for) delayed growth and development (NANDA 00111) related to:
- poor nutritional choices
- poor glucose control
- knowledge deficit
- lack of resources

## Goals

The student will demonstrate increased knowledge regarding diabetes self-management. (N.D. 2, 3, 5)

The student will be able to verbalize symptoms of hypoglycemia/hyperglycemia and notify appropriate school personnel. (N.D. 1, 2)

The student will be able to follow meal plan while at school. (N.D. 2, 3, 4, 5)

The student will be able to administer medication independently or with the assistance of school personnel. (N.D. 1, 2, 3, 5)

The student will verbalize treatment for hypoglycemia/hyperglycemia. (N.D. 1, 2, 3, 5)

The student will identify exercise effect on blood glucose and identify action plan. (N.D. 1, 2, 3, 4, 5)

The student will actively participate in diabetes treatment plan in coordination with healthcare provider, family, and school personnel. (N.D. 1, 2, 3, 5)

## Nursing Interventions

Develop an individualized diabetes health plan. (N.D. 1–5)
- Include student, parent/guardian, healthcare provider, and teacher in the development process.
- Coordinate and incorporate the home diabetes health plan with parent/guardian and healthcare providers.
- Collaborate with student, family, and other school personnel to explore the need for 504 plan development and implementation.
- List and describe management measures to follow for high or low blood glucose.
- Include consideration for field trips and other extracurricular school activities.
- Establish guidelines for seeking assistance, including what to do with early warning signs, medications that may be used, how symptoms are after treatment, when to notify parent/guardian and/or healthcare provider, including phone numbers.

Obtain release of information for medical records and medical orders for blood glucose monitoring and medications or other interventions that will be needed at school. Work with parent/guardian and healthcare provider. (N.D. 1, 2, 4, 5.)
- For ongoing management of diabetes
- For management of hypoglycemia or hyperglycemia

Keep accurate records of diabetes management at school. (N.D. 1, 2, 4, 5)
- Time at onset of symptoms of hypoglycemia/hyperglycemia
- Describe presenting symptoms: shaky, sweaty, irritable, change in behavior or level of consciousness
- Action taken: treated with carbohydrate, testing of blood glucose, monitoring, fluids, ketone testing, or insulin administration per IHP
- Effectiveness of intervention used
- Name of person notified of the event, time of notification, who made the contact, and what the response was or further instructions

Provide in-service training for teachers and other appropriate school personnel. (N.D. 1–5)
- What is diabetes?
- What may attribute to changes in blood glucose control?
- What are the preventive measures needed at school?
- Note the importance of acknowledging and recognizing early warning symptoms.
- What to do in the event of a student having severe low or high blood glucose.
- Describe the importance of prompt management.
- Describe what may occur with no response to a student's symptoms.
- Describe effects of variable blood glucose levels on school performance.

Encourage and assist parent/guardians to talk with the student's teachers about the child and his/her diabetes by: (N.D. 1–5)
- Describing symptoms this child has had in the past when blood glucose levels were either too high or too low
- Identifying adult(s) for the child to seek out for the assistance with diabetes management
- Incorporating plans for parties into the child's meal plan
- Describing how symptoms are handled at home

Assist the student to administer prescribed medications and/or interventions appropriate for his/her knowledge and skills according to school district policy and legal mandates. (N.D. 2, 3, 4)

Facilitate arrangement that will encourage student to take responsibility and practice self-care. (N.D. 1, 2, 3)
- Fluids and restroom facilities will be easily accessible and unrestricted.
- Carbohydrate food sources will be easily accessible.

- Medications will be easily accessible and administered according to prescribed orders and school district policy and procedures. This includes self-administration of medications and blood glucose monitoring.
- Initiate plan for student to be escorted to health office when needed for assistance with treatment of low blood glucose.

Discuss with student: (N.D. 1–5)
- Importance of diabetes management and need to participate in school activities
- Goal to manage diabetes at school to promote school performance and prevent increased missed time from classroom
- Responsibility of self-management of diabetes and need to follow contract according to school district policy
- Symptoms that he/she should report to appropriate adult for further evaluation/intervention
- Responsibilities of notifying appropriate adult when symptoms first appear
- Responsibility to have adequate supplies at school for blood glucose monitoring, ketone testing, treatment of low blood glucose, and medication administration

Provide health education opportunities for individual instruction related to: (N.D. 1–5)
- Overview of diabetes disease process
- Signs and symptoms of diabetes
- Diabetes management strategies
- Treating symptoms of high or low blood glucose
- Psychosocial issues related to having a chronic illness
- Growth and development issues
- Self-management skills based on developmental abilities
- Reinforcement with self-management skills of blood glucose testing and medication administration

Assist the student to identify motivators and barriers to self-care. (N.D. 3)
- Acknowledge with students that diabetes can be overwhelming.
- Assist student to seek out other resources that may help with overcoming barriers or become motivators for a student to assume more self-care if appropriate.
- Acknowledge that many individuals with diabetes experience depression, and explore this with the student and family.

Assist the student to develop appropriate decision-making skills. (N.D. 2, 3)
- Encourage the student to actively participate in his/her diabetes management plan.
- Acknowledge changes that may affect decision making and pressures that may occur during adolescence.
- Discuss issues of compliance with diabetes management plan and academic performance in the school setting.

In collaboration with other school personnel, monitor attendance patterns and reasons for absences. (N.D. 3, 4)
In collaboration with teacher(s), monitor academic performance. (N.D. 2, 3, 4)
- Discuss with parent/guardian the relationship between academic performance and blood glucose control.
- Refer for evaluation as appropriate.
- Participate in 504 plan or individualized education plan (IEP) development as indicated. (Generally, the IHP can serve as the 504 plan. If accommodations for testing or other academic accommodations are needed, they would be addressed in the 504 plan.)

## Expected Student Outcomes

The student will:
- Participate in regular classroom activities, with modifications, such as in-classroom blood glucose testing and medication administration, if appropriate. (N.D. 1, 2, 3, 5)
- Define diabetes. (N.D. 2)
- List his/her medication treatment plan for home and school. (N.D. 1, 2, 3, 4)
- List his/her symptoms related to high or low blood glucose. (N.D. 1, 2, 4, 5)
- Recognize what symptoms of high or low blood glucose are and appropriate action to take. (N.D. 1, 2, 4, 5)
- Inform teacher when having symptoms of high or low blood glucose. (N.D. 1, 2, 3, 4)
- Demonstrate age-appropriate proper use of blood glucose testing equipment. (N.D. 2)
- Demonstrate age-appropriate proper use of medication administration (insulin-using pen, syringe, or pump). (N.D. 1, 2, 3)
- Describe how he/she participates in his/her diabetes management (dependent on demonstrated knowledge, skill, school district policy, and legal mandates). (N.D. 1, 2, 3, 4)
- List motivators and barriers to compliance with prescribed medications, blood glucose monitoring, and interventions. (N.D. 1, 2, 3)
- Demonstrate compliance with his/her diabetes management plan. (N.D. 1, 2, 3, 4)

• Have minimal disruptions in his/her educational program due to diabetes. (N.D. 1, 2, 3, 4, 5)

## Case Study

Eric, a 10-year-old boy, presented to his primary care physician's office with a 4-week history of polyuria, polydipsia, and an 8-lb weight loss. His parents noticed some bedwetting the past 3 nights. Eric was complaining of sore throat and headache. A throat culture was positive for *Streptococcus*. Based on his symptoms of polyuria and polydypsia, a urinalysis was done, revealing glucose in the urine and moderate urine ketoses. In the office Eric was found to have a blood glucose reading of 650 mg/dl. Eric was transferred to Children's Hospital and admitted with a new diagnosis of type 1 diabetes.

Admitting laboratory work includes hemoglobin $A_{1c}$, blood ketones, routine chemistry and insulin antibodies, celiac antibodies, thyroid-stimulating hormone (TSH), and thyroxine (T4). An insulin regimen was prescribed, consisting of NPH and NovoLog insulin, with three injections per day: a mixed dose of NovoLog and NPH insulin in the morning, NovoLog insulin at the evening meal, and NPH insulin at bedtime. After 3 days Eric was discharged to home and is returning to school today.

The diabetes management plan that was sent from Eric's healthcare provider outlines a plan for aspects of diabetes management at school. Blood glucose monitoring before lunch each day and as needed for symptoms of hypoglycemia or hyperglycemia, a meal plan with specific carbohydrate amounts at specific times of day, an action plan for hypoglycemia including glucagon administration, and an action plan for management of hyperglycemia.

Eric has expressed to his parents that he is afraid his friends will treat him differently now that he has diabetes.

# Type 1 Diabetes

| Assessment Data | Nursing Diagnosis | Goals | Nursing Interventions | Expected Outcomes |
|---|---|---|---|---|
| New diagnosis of type 1 diabetes. | Ineffective therapeutic regimen management related to new diagnosis. | Student will be able to learn and practice self-management skills. | Reinforce education regarding appropriate technique with blood glucose monitoring. | Student will demonstrate correct technique with use of blood glucose meter. |
| Diabetes management involves care at school. | Ineffective coping related to normal adolescent development issues and change in diabetes management regimen. | Student will demonstrate competence with blood glucose testing. | Observe technique; assist with skill and problem solving. | Student will demonstrate accurate documentation and follow action plan for blood glucose results. |
| Student at risk for hypoglycemic episodes | | Student will verbalize understanding of hypoglycemia signs/symptoms treatment and prevention. | Assist with interpretation of blood glucose results and appropriate action to take. Educate student regarding purpose, mechanism of action of insulin. | Student will verbalize and demonstrate appropriate response to blood glucose results. |
| Parents report student is feeling overwhelmed with diabetes self-management care and is concerned about being different from peers. | | Student will have an IHP and ECP in place to include student, staff, and parental roles in preventing and managing diabetes care needs. | Educate school staff on the early signs of hypoglycemia and the appropriate steps to take for treatment. | School staff is informed of potential for hypoglycemia and signs and symptoms and action steps to take. |
| | | Student will be able to correctly demonstrate technique with new diabetes management regimen (medications, blood glucose monitoring, carbohydrate counting). | Reinforce correct technique with blood glucose monitoring. | Student will be independent in diabetes blood glucose monitoring. |
| | | | Provide positive reinforcement regarding follow-through on diabetes management regimen. | Student will verbalize confidence in self-management of diabetes. |
| | | Student will be able to verbalize feelings regarding having a chronic illness and how this affects peer relationships. | Reinforce education promoting diabetes self-management. | Student will be able to verbalize rationale in diabetes medication and management regimen. |
| | | | Provide opportunities for student to verbalize feelings regarding diabetes. | Student will be able to verbalize feelings about new diabetes diagnosis. |
| | | | Provide student and family with support groups for children with diabetes or other chronic illnesses. | Student will be able to identify community and school resources that will be a support. |

# Emergency Care Plan
## Diabetes

Student Name: _____          Date: _____

Birth date:_____          Grade/Room: _____

ID #: _____

Parent/Guardian Name: _____          Phone: (_____)_____

Emergency Contact: _____          Phone: (_____)_____

Emergency Contact: _____          Phone: (_____)_____

Healthcare Provider: _____          Phone: (_____)_____

Hospital in Case of Emergency: _____

**Emergency supplies located:**_____

\* Never send a child with suspected low blood glucose anywhere alone.

## Symptoms*
### Low Blood Sugar

| **Mild** | **Moderate** | **Severe** |
|---|---|---|
| Hunger   Pallor   Dizziness<br>Irritability   Crying   Shakiness<br>Weakness   Sweating   Anxiety<br>Drowsiness   Headache<br><br>Irritability to concentrate<br><br>Other: _____ | Sleepiness<br>Erratic behavior<br>Confusion<br>Slurred speech<br>Poor coordination | Irritability to swallow<br>Combativeness<br>Unconsciousness<br>Seizures |

## Action

Treat symptoms as listed below
• Check Blood Sugar      • Notify School Nurse:

Name: _____

Pager: _____

| **Mild** | **Moderate** | **Severe** |
|---|---|---|
| Provide sugar source:<br>• 2–3 glucose tabs<br>• 4 oz juice<br>• 4 oz regular soda or glucose gel<br><br>Wait 10 to 15 minutes<br><br>Retest glucose if less than _____mg/dl retreat with sugar source.<br><br>If blood sugar within target range: _____mg/dl student may return to class. | Provide sugar source:<br>• 2–3 glucose tabs<br>• 4 oz juice<br>• 4 oz regular soda or glucose gel<br><br>Wait 10 to 15 minutes<br><br>Retest glucose if less than _____mg/dl retreat with sugar source.<br><br>Notify parent or guardian<br><br>Provide snack if no meal for more than 1 hour<br><br>If blood sugar within target range: _____mg/dl student may return to class. | Call 911<br><br>Give glucagon, if ordered<br><br>Position on side<br><br>Contact parent/guardian & school nurse |

S.N. Signature: _____ Date_____

Copy given to: _____ Date_____

Adapted from *Pediatric Education for Diabetes in School (PEDS), National Version* (p. 173), 2003, Castle Rock, CO: PADRE Foundation, National Association of School Nurses. Copyright 2003 by PADRE Foundation and National Association of School Nurses.

# Type 2 Diabetes Mellitus

## Pathophysiology

Type 2 diabetes is characterized by diminished liver, muscle, and adipose tissue sensitivity to insulin, also known as insulin resistance, and impaired beta cell function (ADA, 1998). As with adults, it is speculated that in children the development of type 2 diabetes is a result of both genetic and environmental factors (Libman & Arslanian, 1999). Although genetic susceptibility is present with type 2 diabetes, it is thought that environmental factors such as obesity, physical inactivity, and diet high in fat and refined carbohydrates are the main factors contributing to the development of this disease (Libman & Arslanian).

With type 2 diabetes, basal insulin concentration is normal or increased until late in the disease course. The impaired insulin sensitivity that occurs with type 2 diabetes is believed to be related to obesity and hyperinsulinemia and may be genetically determined (ADA, 2003). Beta cell deficiency in individuals with type 2 diabetes is not entirely known, but unlike type 1 diabetes, autoimmune destruction of the beta cells does not occur (ADA, 2003). It is believed that in children with type 2 diabetes, the initial abnormality is impaired insulin action, and a later development is beta cell failure (ADA, 2000).

Epidemiologic data support higher hyperinsulinemia or insulin resistance in African American and other ethnic groups, along with lower insulin sensitivity, compared with Caucasian youth (Libman & Arslanian, 1999). Diagnosis of type 2 diabetes tends to occur at a higher rate in midpuberty, most likely related to temporary evolution of insulin resistance during this developmental phase, which accounts for approximately a 30% reduction in insulin action compared with prepubertal children or adults (Libman & Arslanian).

## Etiology

Type 2 diabetes is defined by the ADA (2003) as a type of diabetes that is primarily due to insulin resistance along with some insulin deficiency. Eighty percent to 90% of all individuals with diabetes are considered to have type 2 diabetes (ADA, 2002b). Children account for 2% to 3% of the total number of individuals with diabetes (Libman & Arslanian, 1999). Studies indicate that there has been a 30% increase in type 2 diabetes diagnosed in youth over the last 20 years (Rosenbloom, Joe, Young, & Winter, 1999). The increase in type 2 diabetes among children may be occurring because of increased obesity in children, along with inactivity. Most people who are diagnosed with type 2 diabetes are overweight and have some family history of diabetes. The incidence tends to be higher in females and occurs more often during pubertal and postpubertal development, with an average age of 13 years, due to the stress of obesity and increased demand for insulin during this growth phase (Rosenbloom et al., 1999; Brosnan, Upchurch, & Schreiner, 2001).

The prevalence of type 2 diabetes varies among different populations and in different areas of the world. It has been reported that 8% to 45% of new cases of type 2 diabetes are among the pediatric population in urban areas (Kaufman, 2002). The above variance in this statistic speaks to the fact that type 2 diabetes in children, while on the rise, has not been well researched and documented up to this time. The TODAY study, 2004, will look closely at development and trends in type 2 diabetes in youth. Type 2 diabetes tends to be higher in certain ethnic populations, such as African American, Hispanic, Asian, and Native American (Ruiz, Robertson, & Boyd, 2001). Acanthosis nigricans, a thickening and hyperpigmentation of the skin at the neck and flexural areas, typically signifies insulin resistance and can be a marker for type 2 diabetes. Up to 60% to 90% of youth who develop acanthosis nigricans develop type 2 diabetes (Kaufman, 2002).

Studies also support that poor nutrition in fetal and early infant life could put individuals at risk for developing diabetes during adolescence related to the thrifty phenotype hypothesis. This hypothesis claims that defective insulin action in utero results in decreased fetal growth as a conservation mechanism, but at the cost of obesity-induced diabetes later in childhood or adulthood (Rosenbloom et al., 1999).

## Management

Type 2 diabetes in youth is challenging for many reasons. It is difficult for this group to adhere to lifestyle modifications and medical treatment because of socioeconomic conditions and availability of resources for management. The challenge also lies in adolescents' perceptions regarding health along with their lack of concern for the long-term complications of this disease. Type 2 diabetes tends to occur in specific ethnic groups that may also come from lower socioeconomic backgrounds. Obesity, peer pressure, and lack of resources are factors that can prohibit students from participating in activities and following through on the prescribed plan of care (Rosenbloom et al., 1999).

Diabetes management requires an individual approach; achieving blood glucose control is important as well as facilitating a normal life for persons with diabetes. The goal for diabetes management and treatment is to decrease the risk of acute and chronic complications associated with diabetes (ADA, 2000). The components of blood glucose balance are nutrition (meal planning), medication, and exercise.

## Meal Planning

Meal planning and nutrition are vital in the control of type 2 diabetes. The goal for children with type 2 diabetes is similar to goals in type 1 diabetes in that normal growth and development are essential. Concerns related to obesity, hypertension, and hyperlipidemia also need to be considered. For youth with type 2 diabetes, achieving and maintaining a healthy weight through healthy eating habits and exercise can help control blood glucose levels, contribute to management of other health concerns, and delay the progression of the chronic complications of diabetes (Franz, 2001). An individualized meal plan should address personal preferences, cultural aspects, and the need or willingness to change one's lifestyle or adapt to a meal plan. The plan should be made available to the school personnel working with the student.

### Exercise

Exercise is an important component in the treatment plan for diabetes management. Typically, exercise will lower blood glucose levels, but this effect is very individualized. The effects of exercise on blood glucose can be attributed to a decreased need for or better utilization of insulin (Mullooly, 2001). Many individuals with type 2 diabetes are able to maintain good blood glucose control with meal planning and exercise and may not need the use of medications for diabetes. Exercise can be as simple as a student being more active, or as challenging as a student being involved in numerous extracurricular activities. Collaborating with student, family, and the healthcare team to maximize a student's exercise will have beneficial effects on blood glucose.

When a student is taking a medication that will lower blood glucose levels, hypoglycemia may occur with exercise. Utilizing an IHP, monitoring patterns of blood glucose, testing before exercise, and coordinating with student, family, and healthcare provider will help to minimize occurrences of low blood glucose levels related to exercise. Some students may require different doses of medication on the days when they know they will be exercising. Generally, it is not recommended that students with type 2 diabetes take extra snacks before exercising. Parents and/or healthcare providers should be contacted to determine if changes in medications are warranted if a student with type 2 diabetes has repeated episodes of low blood glucose with exercise. The school nurse should address this in a student's IHP.

### Medications

Children who have type 2 diabetes may be treated with oral medications, insulin, or both. Use of insulin is addressed in the previous section on type 1 diabetes. The following section will discuss different oral medications that are available for management of type 2 diabetes. Students may take their medications at home or at school. It is important to keep in mind that a student who is taking insulin will always be at risk for hypoglycemia, even though the student may take the insulin at home and not at school. Knowing specific medication that a student is taking either at home or at school is important when developing a student's IHP.

When type 2 diabetes cannot be controlled by diet and exercise, medication should be added. Some children with type 2 diabetes may have insulin only or oral medication only, whereas others may have insulin in combination with oral medication. Metformin (glucophage) is the oral medication typically used to treat children and adolescents with type 2 diabetes (Ruiz et al., 2001). This medication's main effect in controlling blood glucose is to decrease glucose production by the liver, and it also helps with insulin sensitivity. Metformin is the only oral diabetes medication approved by the FDA for the treatment of type 2 diabetes in children. **Table 4** compares oral diabetes medications. For information on insulin, refer to the discussion in the section on type 1 diabetes.

## Diabetes Emergencies

### Hypoglycemia

Children with type 2 diabetes are at less risk for severe hypoglycemia than children with type 1 diabetes. Hypoglycemia is defined as a blood glucose level that is less than 70 mg/dl (Gonder-Frederick, 2001). Symptoms identified can vary as well as the blood glucose level at which individuals feel these symptoms (Hernandez et al., 1999; Ryan, Dulay, Suprasongsin, & Becker, 2002). Identifying each individual student's symptoms for hypoglycemia and the treatment they use is important.

Only those students with type 2 diabetes who are taking medications such as insulin and sulfonylureas are at a risk for low blood glucose. Treatment for low blood glucose levels with type 2 diabetes may be different from that for type 1 diabetes. Use of 10 to 15 grams of carbohydrate is typically all that is needed to treat low blood glucose in students with type 2 diabetes. Students should be encouraged to keep a supply of fast-acting carbohydrates in the classroom and in the nurse's office.

Examples of snacks that contain 15 grams of carbohydrate include the following:
- 4 oz of juice
- 1/2 cup of regular soda pop
- 5 or 6 hard candies (Lifesavers)
- 3 glucose tablets
- 8 oz of skim or 1% milk
- Cake icing (1 small tube)

### Hyperglycemia

High blood glucose is defined by the ADA (2003) as a blood glucose level that is greater than 240 mg/dl. Many children with diabetes have different blood glucose goal ranges and may have guidelines that define high blood glucose at a level that is closer to 300 mg/dl. When a student comes into the office with a blood glucose reading that is above his or her goal range, it is important to determine what may have caused the elevated level. In managing diabetes, it is important not to react to one blood glucose result but to look at patterns of blood glucose to determine possible causes and treatment.

Many things can cause blood glucose levels to become elevated. Missed insulin doses or not taking enough insulin will lead to hyperglycemia. Eating more food than planned or foods that are high in carbohydrates and not taking enough insulin can also lead to hyperglycemia.

**Table 4. Oral Diabetes Medications by Classification and Action**

| Drug Name | Drug Classification | Dose Range | Side Effects | Comments |
|---|---|---|---|---|
| Glucophage (Metformin)  Biguanides (insulin sensitizer) | Biguanides (insulin sensitizer) | 500-850 mg tid or 1,000 mg bid  Doses start low and titrate up | Gastrointestinal (GI) side effects, sweating, headache | Used alone is not associated with hypoglycemia |
| Glipizide (Glucotrol, Glucotrol XL), glimepiride (Amaryl) | Sulfonylurea(insulin secretagogue) | Glucotrol, 2.5-20 mg, single or divided doses; Amaryl 1-4 mg, single dose | Hypoglycemia, weight gain, skin rash | Is associated with hypoglycemia |
| Pioglitazone (Actos), rosiglitazone maleate (Avandia) | Thiazolidinediones (TZDs) (insulin sensitizer) | Actos, 15-, 30-, 45-mg doses; Avandia 2-, 4-, 8-mg doses | Elevated hepatic enzymes, edema | Reduce insulin resistance  Used alone will not cause hypoglycemia  Not approved for children |
| Acrabose (Precose) | Alpha-glucosidase inhibitor; blocks gut absorption of complex sugars | 25 mg/day; may increase to maximum split dose of 300 mg (150 mg for weight <60kg) | Gas and bloating | Should not be used if GI disorders |
| Repaglinide (Prandin)  Nateglinide (Starlix) | Meglitinide  Phenylalanine derivative; increases insulin release from pancreas | 0.5-2 mg before meals  120 mg, or 60 mg 3 times a day | Hypoglycemia, weight gain, hyperinsulinemia | Should medicate 30 minutes before meals |

Adapted from "Pharmacologic Therapies," by J. R. White, R. K. Campbell, and P. C. Yarborough, in *A CORE Curriculum for Diabetes Education* (4th ed.), M. Franz, et al. (Eds.), 2001, Chicago: American Association of Diabetes Educators

Illness and growth may cause hyperglycemia, along with some medications. (For further information on hyperglycemia, refer to the discussion in the section on type 1 diabetes management.)

Interventions for hyperglycemia include drinking extra water, exercising moderately, and taking extra insulin if this is part of the student's diabetes treatment plan. The student can return to the classroom if he or she is feeling better but should be encouraged to return to health office if symptoms recur. Ketones are generally not checked in a student with type 2 diabetes unless specified by the healthcare provider and noted in the student's IHP. For information on blood glucose effects on learning, psychosocial issues, and age-appropriate diabetes tasks with educational considerations, refer to the discussions in the section on type 1 diabetes.

# Individualized Healthcare Plan

## Type 2 Diabetes

### Assessment
*History*
- Age at onset of diabetes
- Family history of diabetes, hypertension, hyperlipidemia
- Other illness, current or chronic
- Presence of acanthosis nigricans
- Level of diabetes control currently and in the past
- Previous diabetes education, camps
- Previous difficulties in management of diabetes

*Current Status and Management*
- Current diabetes management plan available from physician
- Blood glucose goal range and treatment plan available
- Current medication
- Current blood glucose testing and insulin administration techniques utilized
- Current ability to perform self-management tasks
- Frequency of hypoglycemia/hyperglycemia and treatment plan
- Nutritional status and current meal plan
- Exercise plan
- Current health status

*Self-care*
- Ability of student to perform diabetes self-management techniques independently or with supervision
- Student's independence in self-care management of diabetes at home or need for supervision from parent or guardians
- Student's ability to identify symptoms of hypoglycemia and hyperglycemia and treat appropriately
- Student's ability to do blood glucose testing in classroom independently
- Student's ability to identify and follow meal plan as well as ability to appropriately count carbohydrates

*Psychosocial Status*
- Family/student's perception of overall health
- Family/student's ability to cope with diagnosis of diabetes
- Student's ability to share diagnosis with peer groups or expressed concerns about peer groups' reactions
- Family and student's ability to identify a support group within their community
- Student's ability for age-appropriate reaction to the diagnosis of diabetes and ability to perform age-appropriate diabetes care tasks
- Student's ability to express concerns regarding depression or withdrawing from peers
- Community resources the family is currently using along with other resources that are available
- Student's involvement in any support group for children with type 2 diabetes
- Level of self-esteem

*Academic Issues*
- School attendance
- Academic performance patterns
- Regular education and special education issues
- School staff perceptions
- Healthcare needs during the school day: medications, blood glucose testing
- School performance when blood glucose levels are in poor control

**Nursing Diagnoses (N.D.)** (NANDA, 2003)

**N.D. 1** Risk for injury (NANDA 00035) related to development of acute complications to hypoglycemia or hyperglycemia.

**N.D. 2** Deficient knowledge (NANDA 00126) related to:
- meal planning
- insulin administration
- blood glucose monitoring
- oral hyperglycemic medications
- exercise plan

**N.D. 3** Ineffective coping (NANDA 00069) related to:
- knowledge deficit
- lack of resources
- normal developmental issues

**N.D. 4** Ineffective therapeutic regimen management (NANDA. 00078) related to:
- denial of chronic illness
- knowledge deficit
- not wanting to be different from peers

**N.D. 5** Imbalanced nutrition: More than body requirements (NANDA 00001) related to:
- excessive intake in relation to body needs
- inactivity

## Goals

The student will demonstrate increased knowledge regarding diabetes self-management. (N.D. 2, 3, 5).

The student will be able to verbalize symptoms of hypoglycemia/hyperglycemia and notify appropriate school personnel. (N.D. 1, 2).

The student will be able to follow meal plan while at school. (N.D. 2, 3 4, 6).

The student will demonstrate skill in blood glucose monitoring. (N.D. 1,2,3,4).

The student will be able to administer medication independently or with the assistance of school personnel. (N.D. 1, 2, 3, 5).

The student will verbalize treatment for hypoglycemia/hyperglycemia. (N.D. 1, 2, 3, 6).

The student will identify exercise plan. (N.D. 2, 3, 4, 5, 6).

The student will actively participate in diabetes treatment plan in coordination with healthcare provider, family, and school personnel. (N.D. 2, 3, 5, 6).

## Nursing Interventions

Develop an individualized diabetes health plan. (N.D. 1–5)
- Include student, parent/guardian, healthcare provider, teacher in the development process.
- Coordinate and incorporate the home diabetes health plan with parent/guardian and healthcare providers.
- Collaborate with student, family, and other school personnel to explore need for 504 plan development and implementation. (Generally your IHP/ECP can serve as the 504 plan. If a student needs accommodations for testing or other academic accommodations, then those would be addressed in the 504 plan.)
- List and describe management measures to follow for high or low blood glucose.
- Include consideration for field trips and other extracurricular school activities.
- Establish guidelines for seeking assistance, including what to do with early warning signs, medications that may be used, how symptoms are after treatment, when to notify parent/guardian and/or healthcare provider, including phone numbers.

Obtain release of information for medical records and medical orders for blood glucose monitoring and medications or other interventions that will be needed at school. Work with parent/guardian and healthcare provider. (N.D. 1, 2, 4, 5.)
- For ongoing management of diabetes
- For management of hypoglycemia or hyperglycemia

Keep accurate records of diabetes management at school. ( N.D.1, 2, 4, 5)
- Time at onset of symptoms of hypoglycemia/hyperglycemia
- Describe presenting symptoms: shaky, sweaty, irritable, change in behavior or level of consciousness

- Action taken: treated with carbohydrate, testing of blood glucose, monitoring, fluids, ketone testing, or insulin administration per IHP
- Effectiveness of intervention used
- Name of person notified of the event, time of notification, who made the contact, and what the response was or further instructions

Provide in-service training to teachers and other appropriate school personnel. (N.D. 1–5)
- What is diabetes?
- What may attribute to changes in blood glucose control?
- What are the preventive measures needed at school?
- Note the importance of acknowledging and recognizing early warning symptoms.
- What to do in the event of a student having severe low or high blood glucose.
- Describe the importance of prompt management.
- Describe what may occur with no response to a student's symptoms.
- Describe effects of variable blood glucose levels on school performance.

Encourage and assist parent/guardians to talk with the student's teachers about the child and his/her diabetes. (N.D. 1–5)
- What previous symptoms has this child had in the past when blood glucose levels were either too high or too low?
- When would this child seek out the assistance of another adult for help with diabetes management?
- How do you usually plan for parties and incorporate this into your child's meal plan?
- How do you handle symptoms at home?

Assist the student to administer prescribed medications and/or interventions appropriate for his/her knowledge and skills according to school district policy and legal mandates. (N.D. 2, 3, 4)

Facilitate arrangement that will encourage student to take responsibility and practice self care.
- Fluids and restroom facilities will be easily accessible
- Carbohydrate food sources will be easily accessible
- Medications will be easily accessible and administered according to prescribed orders and school district policy and procedures. This includes self-administration of medications and blood glucose monitoring.
- Student should always be escorted to health office when needing assistance with treatment of low blood glucose.

Discuss with student: (N.D. 1–5)
- Importance of diabetes management and need to participate in school activities
- Goal to manage diabetes at school to promote school performance and prevent increased missed time from classroom
- Responsibility of self-management of diabetes and need to follow contract according to school district policy
- Symptoms that he/she should report to appropriate adult for further evaluation/intervention
- Responsibilities of notifying appropriate adult when symptoms first appear
- Responsibility to have adequate supplies at school for blood glucose monitoring, ketone testing, treatment of low blood glucose, and medication administration

Provide health education opportunities for individual instruction related to: (N.D. 1–5)
- What diabetes is
- What are signs and symptoms of diabetes
- What can be done to manage diabetes
- What to do for symptoms of high or low blood glucose
- Psychosocial issues related to having a chronic illness
- Growth and development issues
- How to learn self-management skills based on developmental abilities
- Reinforcement with self-management skills of blood glucose testing and medication administration

Assist the student to identify motivators and barriers to self-care. (N.D. 3).
- Acknowledge with students that diabetes can be overwhelming.
- Assist student to seek out other resources that may help with overcoming barriers or become motivators for a student to assume more self-care if appropriate.
- Acknowledge that many individuals with diabetes experience depression, and explore this with the student and family.

Assist the student to develop appropriate decision-making skills. (N.D. 2, 3)
- Encourage the student to actively participate in his or her diabetes management plan.
- Acknowledge changes that may affect decision making and pressures that may occur during adolescence.
- Discuss issues of compliance with diabetes management plan and academic performance in the school setting.

Monitor attendance patterns and reasons for absences. (N.D. 3, 4) Monitor academic performance. (N.D. 2, 3, 4)

- Discuss with parent/guardian the relationship between academic performance and blood glucose control.
- Refer for evaluation as appropriate.
- Participate in IEP development as indicated.

## Expected Student Outcomes

The student will:

- Participate in regular classroom activities, with modifications, such as in classroom blood glucose testing and medication administration, if appropriate. (N.D. 1, 2, 3, 4).
- Define diabetes and effects on the body. (N.D. 1, 2).
- List his/her medication treatment plan for home and school. (N.D. 1, 2, 3, 4).
- List his/her symptoms related to high or low blood glucose. (N.D. 1, 2, 3, 4).
- Recognize what symptoms of high or low blood glucose are and appropriate action to take. (N.D. 1, 2, 3, 4).
- Inform student's teacher when having symptoms of high or low blood glucose. (N.D. 1, 2, 3, 4)
- Demonstrate age-appropriate proper use of blood glucose testing equipment. (N.D. 1, 2, 3, 4)
- Demonstrate age-appropriate proper use of medication administration (insulin-using pen, syringe, or pump). (N.D. 1, 2, 3, 4)
- Describe how he/she participates in his/her diabetes management (dependent on demonstrated knowledge, skill, school district policy, and legal mandates). (N.D. 1, 2, 3, 4)
- Describe the benefits of specific interventions. (N.D. 1, 2, 3, 4, 5)
- Describe the consequences of not using specific interventions. (N.D. 1, 2, 3, 4, 5)
- List motivators and barriers to compliance with prescribed medications, blood glucose monitoring, and interventions. (N.D. 1, 2, 3, 4)
- Demonstrate compliance with his/her diabetes management plan. (N.D. 1, 2, 3, 4, 5)
- Have minimal disruptions in his/her educational program due to diabetes. (N.D. 1, 2, 3, 4)

## Case Study

Maria Garcia, a 13-year-old Hispanic girl who was diagnosed with type 2 diabetes at the age of 12, is currently enrolled in 8th grade. She is 60 inches tall and weighs 185 lb, which gives her a body mass index of 36. Her blood pressure is 148/90, which is above the normal limits. Recent laboratory results from the primary provider show an elevated lipid panel with total cholesterol of 250, HDL of 35, LDL of 120, and a triglyceride level of 300. Her most recent hemoglobin $A_{1c}$ is 11.0, which gives her an average blood glucose level over the last 3 months of 310 mg/dl. Maria's immunizations are up to date. She currently has a primary provider, Dr. Health, and also sees Dr. Sharp at the Children's Diabetes Center. She recently saw her diabetes specialist and is coming to school with medication orders and orders for blood glucose testing.

Maria's mother states that Mary had been controlling her diabetes by watching what she eats and by walking. Maria was walking every day in her previous home, but she has recently moved to a new town and school and her mother is concerned that her activity may decrease because of the change in weather. Her mother states that Maria has seemed more tired lately, and she attributes this to her being up at night going to the bathroom. Maria is now supposed to start medication for her diabetes and test her blood glucose at school; in the past she did not test blood glucose at school.

Orders received from the physician state that Maria is to take her Metformin (glucophage) with breakfast (she eats breakfast at school) and with supper. She is to test her blood glucose at school, 1 hour after she has eaten lunch or when symptoms of high blood glucose occur.

Maria had recently been missing more school because she has felt so tired. Her teachers are concerned because she was falling asleep in class. Maria has been withdrawn, has not been interacting with her peers, and has not been participating in school activities that she had previously participated in. Maria has stated to her mother that she does not want to have diabetes, take medicine, check her blood glucose, or eat differently from her friends. Maria does not have any special education services, and teachers feel that she can be successful in school if she is awake and alert.

## Type 2 Diabetes

| Assessment Data | Nursing Diagnosis | Goals | Nursing Interventions | Expected Outcomes |
|---|---|---|---|---|
| Mother reports diagnosis of type 2 diabetes with recent addition of medications. | Ineffective therapeutic regimen management related to change in diabetes management plan. | Student will demonstrate increased knowledge regarding diabetes self-management.<br><br>Student will administer medication independently or with assistance of school personnel. | Develop IHP that includes education on skills like blood glucose self-monitoring and medication administration.<br><br>Observe technique and assist with skill.<br><br>Keep accurate records of diabetes management at school.<br><br>Discuss with student symptoms that she should report to appropriate adult for further evaluation/intervention.<br><br>Assist the student to administer prescribed medications appropriate for her knowledge and skills according to school district policy and legal mandates. | Student will demonstrate skill in blood glucose monitoring.<br><br>Student will demonstrate age-appropriate proper use of blood glucose testing equipment.<br><br>Student will recognize what symptoms of high or low blood glucose are and appropriate action to take.<br><br>Student will inform teacher or adult when having symptoms of high or low blood glucose.<br><br>Student will list his/her medication plan at home and school.<br><br>Student will participate in regular classroom activities, with modifications made as necessary.<br><br>Student will demonstrate age-appropriate proper use of medication administration. |

| Assessment Data | Nursing Diagnosis | Goals | Nursing Interventions | Expected Outcomes |
|---|---|---|---|---|
| Mother reports student feeling overwhelmed with diabetes self-management cares and is concerned about being different from her peers. | Ineffective coping related to normal adolescent development issues and change in diabetes management regimen. | Student will actively participate in diabetes treatment plan in coordination with healthcare provider, family, and school personnel.<br><br>Student will identify motivators and barriers to self-care. | Provide health education opportunities for individual instruction related to growth and development issues along with psychosocial issues related to having a chronic illness.<br><br>Assist student to identify motivators and barriers to self-care.<br><br>Assist student to develop appropriate decision-making skills. | Student will describe how she participates in her diabetes management.<br><br>Student will participate in regular classroom activities, with modifications made as necessary.<br><br>Student will list motivators and barriers to compliance with prescribed mediations, blood glucose monitoring, and interventions.<br><br>Student will verbalize benefits of specific interventions as well as consequences of not using specific interventions. |

# References

American Association of Diabetes Educators. (2000). Position statement: Management of children with diabetes in the school setting. *Diabetes Educator, 26*(1), 32–34.

American Diabetes Association. (1998). *Medical management of type 2 diabetes* (4th ed., pp. 21–33). Canada: American Diabetes Association.

American Diabetes Association. (2000). Type 2 diabetes in children and adolescents. *Diabetes Care, 23,* 381–389.

American Diabetes Association. (2002a). Position statement: Diabetes and exercise. *Diabetes* Care, *25* (Suppl.1), 64S.

American Diabetes Association. (2002b). Standards of medical care for patients with diabetes mellitus. *Diabetes Care, 25*(1), 213–229.

American Diabetes Association. (2003). Report of the expert committee on the diagnosis and classification of diabetes mellitus. *Diabetes Care, 26,* S5–S20.

American Diabetes Association. (2004). Report of the expert committee on the diagnosis and classification of diabetes mellitus. *Diabetes Care, 27,* S5–10.

Andrus, M., Leggett-Frazier, N., & Pfeifer, M. (2001). Chronic complications of diabetes: An overview. In M. Franz, K. Kulkarni, W. Polonsky, P. Yarborough, & V. Zamudio (Eds.), *A CORE curriculum for diabetes education* (4th ed., pp. 45–61). Chicago: American Association of Diabetes Educators.

Betschart, J. (2001). Diabetes during childhood and adolescence. In M. Franz, K. Kulkarni, W., Polonsky, P. Yarborough, & V. Zamudio (Eds.), *A CORE curriculum for diabetes education* (4th ed., pp. 3–25). Chicago: American Association of Diabetes Educators.

Blum, M. (2002). Are school nurses using the recommendations of the diabetes control and complications trial in the care of students with diabetes? *Journal of School Nursing, 18,* 138–143.

Brosnan, C. A., Upchurch, S., & Schreiner, B. (2001). Type 2 diabetes in children and adolescents: An emerging disease. *Journal of Pediatric Health Care, 15,* 187–193.

Chase, H. P. (2002). *Understanding diabetes* (10th ed.). Denver, CO: Children's Diabetes Foundation at Denver. Retrieved January, 5, 2005, from http://www.childrensdiabetesfdn.org/publ.htm

Davidson, M., & Schwartz, S. (2001). Hyperglycemia. In M. Franz, K. Kulkarni, W. Polonsky, P. Yarborough, & V. Zamudio (Eds.), *A CORE curriculum for diabetes education* (4th ed., pp. 21–39). Chicago: American Association of Diabetes Educators.

Diabetes Control and Complications Trial Research Group. (1996). Epidemiology of severe hypoglycemia in the diabetes control and complications trial. *Journal of American Medical Association, 90,* 450–459.

Drash, A. (1990). Management of the child with diabetes mellitus: Clinical course, therapeutic strategies and monitoring techniques. In F. Lifshitz (Ed.), *Pediatric endocrinology: A clinical guide* (2nd ed., pp. 681–700). New York: Marcel Dekker.

Franz, M. J. (2001). Medical nutrition therapy for diabetes. In M. Franz, K. Kulkarni, W. Polonsky, P. Yarborough, & V. Zamudio (Eds.), *A CORE curriculum for diabetes education* (4th ed., pp. 203–231). Chicago: American Association of Diabetes Educators.

Fredrickson, L., & Griff, M. R. (2000). *Pumper in the school: Insulin pump guide for school nurses, school personnel and parents.* Sylmar, CA: MiniMed Inc.

Gonder-Frederick, L. (2001). Hypoglycemia. In M. Franz, K. Kulkarni, W. Polonsky, P. Yarborough, & V. Zamudio (Eds.), *A CORE curriculum for diabetes education* (4th ed., pp. 231–257). Chicago: American Association of Diabetes Educators.

Grey, M., Davidson, M., Boland, E., & Tamborlane, W. (2001). Clinical and psychosocial factors associated with achievement of treatment goals in adolescents with diabetes mellitus. *Journal of Adolescent Health, 25,* 377–385.

Hernandez, C., Bradish, G., Wilson Rodger, N., & Rybansky, S. (1999). Self-awareness in diabetes: Using body cues, circumstances, and strategies. *Diabetes Educator, 25,* 576–584.

Hershey, T., Bhargava, N., Sadler, M., White, N., & Craft, S. (1999). Conventional versus intensive diabetes therapy in children with type 1 diabetes. *Diabetes Care, 22,* 1318–1325.

Kaufman, F. (2002). Type 2 diabetes in children and young adults: A "new epidemic." *Clinical Diabetes, 20,* 217–218.

Libman, I., & Arslanian, S. (1999). Type II diabetes mellitus: No longer just adults. *Pediatric Annals, 28*(9), 589–593.

Mullooly, C. (2001). Exercise. In M. Franz, K. Kulkarni, W. Polonsky, P. Yarborough, & V. Zamudio (Eds.), *A CORE curriculum for diabetes education* (4th ed., pp. 55–88). Chicago: American Association of Diabetes Educators.

National Diabetes Information Clearinghouse. (2003). *National diabetes statistics.* Retrieved February 2, 2005, from http://diabetes.niddk.nih.gov/

Neumark-Sztainer, D., Patterson, J., Mellin, A., Ackard, D., Utter, J., & Story, M., et al. (2002). Weight control practices and disordered eating behaviors among adolescent females and males with type 1 diabetes. *Diabetes Care, 25*, 1289–1297.

Northam, E., Anderson, P., Jacobs, R., Hughes, M., Warne, G., & Werther, G. (2001). Neuropsychological profiles of children with type 1 diabetes 6 years after disease onset. *Diabetes Care, 24*, 1541–1546.

NANDA International. (NANDA). (2003). *Nursing diagnoses: Definitions & classification 2003-2004.* Philadelphia: Author.

P.E.D.S. (Pediatric Education for Diabetes in Schools, National Version). (2003). PADRE Foundation. Castle Rock, CO: National Association of School Nurses.

Ratner, R. (2003). Pathophysiology of the diabetes state. In M. Franz (Ed.), *A CORE curriculum for diabetes education* (5th ed., pp. 1–18). Chicago: American Association of Diabetes Educators

Rosenbloom, A., Joe, J., Young, R., & Winter, W. (1999). Emerging epidemic of type 2 diabetes in youth. *Diabetes Care, 22*, 345–354.

Ryan, C., Dulay, D., Suprasongsin, C., & Becker, D. (2002). Detection of symptoms by adolescents and young adults with type 1 diabetes during experimental induction of mild hypoglycemia. *Diabetes Care, 21*, 852–858.

Ruiz, E., Robertson, C., & Boyd, L. (2001). Type 2 diabetes in children. *RN, 64*, 44–51.

National Institute of diabetes and Digestive and Kidney Diseases. (2004). TODAY study: Treatment options for type 2 diabetes in adolescents and youth. Retrieved November, 18, 2004, from http://www.todaystudy.org/index.cgi

White, J.R., Campbell, R. K., & Yarborough, P. C. (2001). Pharmacologic therapies. In M. Franz, K. Kulkarni, W. Polonsky, P. Yarborough, & V. Zamudio (Eds.), *A CORE curriculum for diabetes education* (4th ed., pp. 91–147). Chicago: American Association of Diabetes Educators.

Zombek, M. (2001). Section 3: School nurse tools. In *Pediatric education for diabetes in schools: A curriculum for diabetes care in the schools* (pp. 47–48). Orange, CA: PADRE Foundation.

## Bibliography

Barrett, J. C., Goodwin, D. K., & Kendrick, O. (2002). Nursing, food service, and the child with diabetes. *Journal of School Nursing, 18*(3), 150–156.

Boland, E. A., & Grey, M. (2004). Diabetes mellitus (types 1 and 2). In P. J. Allen & J. A. Vessey (Eds.). *Primary care of the child with a chronic condition* (4th ed., pp. 426–444). St. Louis, MO: Mosby.

Hockenberry, M. J., Wilson, D., Windkelstein, M. L., & Kline, N. E. (2003). *Wong's nursing care of infants and children* (7th ed., pp. 1732–1756). St. Louis, MO: Mosby.

Lewis, K. D., & Bear, B. J. (2002). *Manual of school health* 2nd ed., St. Louis, MO: Saunders.

National Association of School Nurses. (Adopted 2001). *Position Statement: Blood sugar monitoring in the school setting.* Scarborough, ME: Author.

National Association of School Nurses. (Adopted 2001). *Position Statement: School nurse role in care and management of the child with diabetes in the school setting.* Scarborough, ME: Author.

National Association of School Nurses. (Revised 2004). *Position Statement: Emergency care plans for students with special health care needs.* Scarborough, ME: Author.

National Association of School Nurses. (n.d.). *Pediatric education for diabetes in schools (PEDS)* [education program]. Retrieved November 7, 2004, from http://nasn.org/education/education.htm

Quarry-Horn, J. L., Evans, B. J., & Kerrigan, J. R. (2003). Type 2 diabetes mellitus in youth. *Journal of School Nursing, 19*(4), 195–203.

## Resources

American Association of Diabetes Educators
100 West Monroe Street
Suite 400
Chicago, IL 60603
1-800-338-3633
312-424-2427 (fax)
www.aadenet.org

American Council on Exercise
4851 Paramount Drive
San Diego, CA 92123
858-279-8227
1-800-825-3636
858-279-8064 (fax)
www.acefitness.org

American Diabetes Association
Attn: National Call Center
1701 North Beauregard Street
Alexandria, VA 22311
1-800-342-2383
www.diabetes.org

Diabetes

American Dietetic Association
120 South Riverside Plaza
Suite 2000
Chicago, IL 60606-6995
1-800-877-1600
www.eatright.org

American School Health
    Association
7263 State Route 43
PO Box 708
Kent, OH 44240
330-678-1601
www.ashaweb.org

Centers for Disease Control and
    Prevention
Clifton Road
Atlanta, GA 30333
404-639-3311
404-639-3534 (public inquiries)
1-800-311-3435
www.cdc.gov
Division of Diabetes Translation:
www.cdc.gov/diabetes
Division of Nutrition and Physical
    Activity:
www.cdc.gov/nccdphp/dnpa
Division of Adolescent and School
    Health:
www.cdc.gov/nccdphp/dash

Children With Diabetes
www.childrenwithdiabetes.com
The on-line community for kids,
    families and adults with dia-
    betes.

Diabetes Exercise and Sports
    Association
8001 Montcastle Drive
Nashville, TN 37221
1-800-898-4322
615-673-2077 (fax)
www.diabetes-exercise.org

Disability Rights Education and
    Defense Fund
Main Office
2212 Sixth Street
Berkeley, CA 94710
510-644-2555 (V/TTY)
510-841-8645 (fax)
www.dredf.org

Indian Health Service HIS
    National Diabetes Program
Indian Health Service (HQ)
The Reyes Building
801 Thompson Avenue
Suite 400
Rockville, MD 20852-1627
http://www.ihs.gov/MedicalProgra
    ms/Diabetes/index.asp

Joslin Diabetes Center
617 732 2400
www.joslin.harvard.edu

Juvenile Diabetes Research
    International
1400 K Street, NW
Suite 1212
Washington, DC 20005
202-371-9746
1-800-533-1868
202-371-2760 (fax)
www.jdrf.org

National Association of School
    Nurses
Western Office:
1416 Park Street
Suite A
Castle Rock, CO 80109
303-663-2329
1-866-627-6767
303-663-0403 (fax)
Eastern Office:
PO Box 1300 (163. U.S. Route 1)
Scarborough, ME 04070
207-883-2117
1-877-627-6476
207-883-2683 (fax)
www.nasn.org

National Diabetes Education
    Program
One Diabetes Way
Bethesda, MD 20814-9692
301-496-3583
www.ndep.nih.gov

National Diabetes Information
    Clearinghouse
http://diabetes.niddk.nih.gov/

National Institute of Diabetes and
    Digestive and Kidney Diseases
Building 31, Room 9A04
31 Center Drive, MSC 2560
Bethesda, MD 20892-2560
www.niddk.nih.gov

Pediatric Adolescent Diabetes
    Research Education (PADRE
    Foundation)
455 South Main Street
Orange, CA 92868
714-532-8330
www.peds.ws

Pediatric Endocrinology Nursing
    Society
7794 Graw Drive
Pensacola, FL 32514
850-475-5223
1-877-936-7367
www.pens.org

*Federal Laws Related to the
Education of Students With
Disabilities:*
Individuals with Disabilities
    Education Act
www.ed.gov/offices/OSERS/OSEP
Section 504 of the Rehabilitation
    Act of 1973
www.ed.gov/ocr/disability.html
Title II of the Americans with
    Disabilities Act of 1990
www.ed.gov/ocr.disability.html

# Chapter Thirty-six

# Down Syndrome

## Roxanne Truen

## Introduction

Down syndrome is the most common chromosomal cause of mental retardation, occurring in approximately 1 in 800 to 1,000 live births (Allen & Vessey, 2004). Down syndrome results when extra chromosome 21 material is present (Trisomy 21). Three genetic mechanisms can allow Down syndrome to occur. The first and most common is nondisjunction. Nondisjunction (uneven chromosome division) occurs when an entire extra chromosome 21 is present in all cells. The second type, mosaicism, occurs when some but not all cells have the trisomy 21 defect. Individuals with mosaic Down syndrome may have fewer phenotypic features of the syndrome and be more mildly affected. Translocation is the third form of Down syndrome and is the least common, occurring in 3% to 5% of total cases. In these individuals, part or all of an extra chromosome 21 attaches to another chromosome. Down syndrome caused by translocation can be hereditary, and parents may be encouraged to seek genetic testing to determine their carrier status and risk of recurrence in future pregnancies (Allen & Vessey, 2004; Benke, Carver, & Donahue, 1995; Roizen, 1997).

The likelihood of having a child with Down syndrome increases with advancing maternal age. At age 25, the risk of Down syndrome is approximately 1:1,500, increasing to approximately 1:20 by age 45 (Allen & Vessey, 2004). Down syndrome is often diagnosed at birth as a result of its distinctive clinical features. Many physical characteristics of Down syndrome may be evident at birth; some of the most common of these include generalized hypotonia, single transverse palmar creases (most individuals have two transverse flexion creases on their palms), small, low-set ears, large tongue, epicanthal folds (skinfold covering inner corner of the eye, creating the appearance of slanted eyes), incurved fifth finger, flattened nasal bridge, excess nuchal (neck) skin, and widely spaced first and second toes (Allen & Vessey, 2004; Bosch, 2003).

## Pathophysiology

A variety of associated physical problems may occur with Down syndrome:

### Mental Retardation

Intellectual abilities may be greatly varied. Most people with Down syndrome fall into the range of moderate impairment; others may be either mildly or severely impaired (Allen & Vessey, 2004). Factors shown to correlate with the child's intelligence and adaptive behavior skills include the physical condition of the child, individualized early intervention, and home environment (Allen & Vessey, 2004).

Individuals with mental retardation may also be affected by behavior disorders, such as inattention, noncompliance, social withdrawal, and depression. Autistic-type behaviors and psychotic episodes have been reported (Allen & Vessey, 2004; Bosch, 2003).

### Cardiac Defects

Cardiac defects occur in up to 60% of children with Down syndrome (Roizen, 1997; Van Riper & Cohen, 2001; Allen & Vessey, 2004). The most commonly occurring cardiac anomalies include atrioventricular canal, ventricular septal defect, atrial septal defect, tetralogy of Fallot, and patent ductus arteriosus (Allen & Vessey, 2004; Azra & Seward, 2000; Roizen, 1997). In addition, these conditions may be associated with pulmonary vascular obstructive disease, a significant complication that can lead to congestive heart failure. It has also been noted that even individuals with Down syndrome who do not have a congenital heart defect are at risk of developing mitral valve prolapse. This condition, which can cause deterioration of cardiac function, may be present in up to 50% of individuals by the end of adolescence. Regular monitoring by healthcare providers is important for early diagnosis and management (Allen & Vessey, 2004).

### Endocrine Abnormalities/Growth Issues

Velocity of linear growth is slower in children with Down syndrome, especially during infancy and adolescence. Multiple causes for decreased growth may be considered, including hypothalamic dysfunction, congenital heart disease, nutrition/feeding problems, and thyroid disease (Allen & Vessey, 2004; Castiglia, 1998). Congenital hypothyroidism is more prevalent in children with Down syndrome, affecting 1 in 141 infants, a rate 28 times that of the general population (Fort et. al., 1984, as cited in Roizen, 1997). Any suspected growth problem should be thoroughly evaluated.

Although slow weight gain and growth may occur initially, by the second year of life, children with Down syndrome often develop a tendency to be overweight. This trend continues and results in 30% to 60% of children and adolescents with Down syndrome being overweight (Allen & Vessey, 2004; Roizen, 1997; Van Riper & Cohen, 2001). In addition, persons with Down syndrome are of shorter stature than those unaffected, thus illustrating the importance of utilizing growth charts specific to individuals with Down syndrome.

The onset of puberty in children with Down syndrome may or may not occur earlier than in unaffected children. Although males with Down syndrome are virtually always sterile, females are capable of reproduction (Allen & Vessey, 2004).

### Sensory impairments
#### Vision

Several types of vision disorders tend to occur with Down syndrome. The most common are refractive errors, strabismus, nystagmus, blepharitis (inflammation of eyelids), cataract, tear duct obstruction, and ptosis (drooping of eyelids) (Allen & Vessey, 2004; Pueschel, S.M., 1992, as cited in Texas Deafblind Outreach, 1998). Because some of these conditions may go undetected initially and may result in loss of acuity, it is crucial for children with Down syndrome to receive screening in school and regular ophthalmologic examinations.

#### Hearing

Sixty percent to 80% of children with Down syndrome have some type of hearing loss (Allen & Vessey, 2004; Roizen, 1997; TSBVI, 1998). These losses may be due to structural abnormalities of the skull, middle and inner ears, external auditory canal, and/or throat, and are often complicated by eustachian tube dysfunction (Allen & Vessey, 2004). The hearing loss can be conductive or sensorineural, congenital or acquired. It may be bilateral or unilateral. Decreased immunity affecting many individuals with Down syndrome may increase susceptibility to chronic otitis media and other upper respiratory infections that can ultimately impact hearing (Allen & Vessey, 2004). In addition, because individuals with Down syndrome often have small ear canals, performing otoscopic examinations may prove difficult. Identification of ear infections and possible hearing loss is crucial, however, as they may greatly impact cognitive development and speech.

### Musculoskeletal and Motor Abilities

Orthopedic problems are quite common in Down syndrome. Hyperflexibility and hypotonia occur in nearly all children with Down syndrome (Allen & Vessey, 2004; Bosch, 2003). Among the possible orthopedic conditions that may be seen are patellar subluxation, scoliosis, dislocated hips, atlantoaxial subluxation, joint and muscle pain, and muscle fatigue (Allen & Vessey, 2004). Of these, atlantoaxial subluxation may be the most potentially serious. Atlantoaxial instability results when a "loose joint" occurs between the C1 and C2 vertebrae, causing increased space between the atlas and the odontoid process (Allen & Vessey, 2004, p. 450). The vast majority, 98% to 99% of children affected, are asymptomatic (Allen & Vessey, 2004). However, the condition has potential to progress to subluxation or dislocation, which can lead to compression of the spinal cord. Symptoms of subluxation may include neck pain, head tilt, torticollis, deterioration of gait, changes in bowel and bladder function, and decreased hand function due to weakness or paralysis (Allen & Vessey, 2004; Leshin, 2000; Roizen, 1997; Van Riper & Cohen, 2001). Because of this potential for serious sequelae, it is recommended that children with Down syndrome have a cervical x-ray to rule out atlantoaxial subluxation prior to engaging in activities that can cause the head to jerk back and potentially result in subluxation (Allen & Vessey, 2004).

### Gastrointestinal Tract Abnormalities

Gastrointestinal anomalies commonly occurring in Down syndrome include tracheoesophageal fistula, duodenal atresia/stenosis, imperforate anus, Hirschsprung's disease, and pyloric stenosis (Allen & Vessey, 2004; Bosch, 2003; Roizen, 1997). Most of these anomalies require surgical intervention and long-term monitoring.

### Immune System Deficits

Children with Down syndrome have diminished immune function. This can contribute to an increased incidence of other disorders, such as respiratory illness, diabetes mellitus, adrenal dysfunction, periodontal disease, thyroid disorders, leukemia, and joint problems (Allen & Vessey, 2004). Immunizations are important in the prevention of disease; the addition of the pneumococcal and influenza vaccines should be considered as well (Bosch, 2003). The incidence of insulin-dependent diabetes mellitus is more than twice the rate in the general population, occurring in 1 in 250 children with Down syndrome (Pueschel et al, 1999, as cited in Allen & Vessey, 2004).

### Seizure Disorders

Approximately 5% to 10% of children with Down syndrome are diagnosed as having seizure disorders. The onset of seizures peaks prior to 3 years of age, then again in adults in their 30s (Allen & Vessey, 2004; Roizen, 1997).

### Leukemia

Children with Down syndrome are 18 to 20 times more likely to be diagnosed with leukemia than children without Down syndrome (Tolmie, 2002, as cited in Allen & Vessey, 2004). The reasons for this predisposition are not clear.

### Dental Issues

Due to the anatomic anomalies present in the face and oral cavity, various dental problems (malocclusion, microdontia, periodontal disease) are more prevalent in children with Down syndrome (Allen & Vessey, 2004; Hennequin, Faulks, Veyrune & Bourdiol, 1999). Of these, the most serious is periodontal disease, which affects the tissues that support the teeth. This condition is likely related to diminished immune function, abnormal chewing, and difficulty with oral hygiene. Juvenile periodontitis is characterized by periods of swelling, inflammation, and pain. If it progresses, it may be associated with loss of supporting tissues of the teeth and eventual tooth loss. The incidence of periodontal disease in the Down syndrome population is high, affecting approximately 94% to 100% of individuals (Allen & Vessey, 2004; Hannequin et al., 1999). Periodontal disease is cause for additional concern for those children with congenital heart disease, as any dental infection can potentially cause endocarditis. It is crucial that children with Down syndrome receive regular dental care.

### Respiratory Problems

Because of diminished immunity, children with Down syndrome tend to experience more respiratory and upper airway infections than the unaffected population (Allen & Vessey, 2004).

### Sleep Apnea

The anatomic anomalies associated with Down syndrome (large tongue, midfacial hypoplasia) may predispose children with Down syndrome to sleep apnea (Allen & Vessey, 2004; Bosch, 2003). This may result in fatigue and difficulty attending to schoolwork and should be considered if a child appears unusually sleepy or tired during the day. Surgical intervention (tonsillectomy, adenoidectomy, partial reduction of tongue) and/or other treatments such as use of a continuous positive airway pressure (CPAP) device may prove helpful in reducing sleep apnea (Allen & Vessey, 2004; Bosch, 2003).

### Behavior Concerns

Children with Down syndrome may be affected by behavior problems similar to other children, such as conduct disorders, depression, attention deficit hyperactivity disorder (ADHD), obsessive compulsive disorder (OCD), and self-injurious behaviors (Bosch, 2003). These disorders may be difficult to identify and manage owing to lower cognitive functioning.

### Mental Illness

Individuals with Down syndrome and mental retardation may be more isolated and experience rejection, which can lead to feelings of loss and depression. Depression and other mental illnesses may not be readily recognized in persons with Down syndrome because of their cognitive disabilities. This may lead to ineffective treatment or lack of treatment (Hurley, 1996).

## Management

The child with Down syndrome will require a multidisciplinary team of individuals to provide a comprehensive approach to management. Depending on the level of physical needs and mental retardation, the child may receive services from multiple medical specialists, such as developmental pediatrician, cardiologist, endocrinologist, ophthalmologist, ears, nose, and throat (ENT) specialist, orthopedist, gastrointestinal specialist, neurologist, hematologist, nutritionist, and psychologist. In addition, many require occupational, physical, and/or speech therapy. In the school setting, the child will require services based on individual needs. These services may include a special education teacher, school nurse, physical therapist, occupational therapist, speech therapist, adaptive physical education teacher, school psychologist, and paraprofessionals (Vessey & Swanson, 1993) The child may also require adaptations to the school environment for safety and school success.

# Individualized Healthcare Plan

**Assessment**

*History*
- Down syndrome diagnosis (prenatal, postnatal)
- Neonatal history:
  - cardiac
  - gastrointestinal
  - ENT
  - respiratory
  - feeding problems
  - thyroid dysfunction
  - vision and hearing problems (testing done)
  - length of stay in hospital
- Surgeries
- Procedures
- Growth: percentiles, growth concerns, obesity
- Development: age when milestones reached, early intervention
- Orthopedic: atlantoaxial testing done, results; activity restrictions
- Sleep concerns, apnea
- History of frequent infections, type
- Behavior concerns
- Student/family perceptions

*Current Status and Management*
Health concerns in the following areas:
- Cardiac: taking medication, symptoms, activity restrictions, need future surgeries, procedures
- Gastrointestinal: symptoms, medications, food restrictions/allergies
- Orthopedic: atlantoaxial subluxation results (if positive, what activities restricted); joint pain, hip problems
- Neurologic: seizures, cognitive level
- Respiratory: frequency of infections, asthma, medications
- ENT: frequency of ear infections, hearing loss, pressure equalization tubes, sleep apnea
- Dental: evidence of periodontal disease (bleeding gums, loose teeth), oral hygiene habits, frequency of dental care, need for prophylaxis antibiotics
- Vision: receiving regular care, vision problems, acuity, need for glasses
- Thyroid: thyroid screen done, symptoms
- Growth: height, weight, percentiles on Down syndrome and standard growth charts, obesity concerns
- Toileting: status of toilet training, concerns
- Current medications, treatments, etc.
- Current providers: name, name of clinic, phone numbers
- Current therapies: occupational therapy, physical therapy, speech, etc.
- Outside agencies: home care nursing, equipment/supply company, etc.
- Receiving waivered services, respite, etc.
- Family/social: household members, any changes or concerns, support system perception of disorder and delays

*Self-care*
- Level of independence with activities of daily living (feeding, dressing, toileting, ambulating, etc.)
- Communication: abilities, methods, augmentative devices
- Community activities: participation, level of independence
- Knowledge of own health status, needs

*Psychosocial Status*
- Interaction with peers, family, adults
- Participation in activities in community, with family, with peers
- Behavior concerns
- Mental health concerns
- Sexuality education, concerns related to vulnerability and exploitation

- Participation in school activities
- Potential for vulnerability to exploitation

*Academic Issues*
- School health services needed: procedures, medications, monitoring/assessments needed during school day, case management needs
- Inclusion in regular education
- Need for adaptations/modifications to environment (adaptive seating, accessible bathroom, etc.)
- Curriculum adaptations
- Need for emergency evacuation
- Transportation issues: busing
- Special education services needed
- Adaptive physical education
- Need for aide in classroom
- Attendance: past, current, reasons for absences
- Transition issues
- Additional support services

## Nursing Diagnoses (N.D.) (NANDA, 2003)

**N.D. 1** Risk for activity intolerance (NANDA 00094) related to:
- decreased cardiac output
- increased weight.

**N.D. 2** Risk for decreased cardiac output (NANDA 00029) related to congenital heart defect.

**N.D. 3** Risk for impaired verbal communication (NANDA 00051) related to:
- hearing loss
- oral-facial structure anomalies.

**N.D. 4** Risk for impaired verbal communication (NANDA 00051) related to speech delay/mental retardation.

**N.D. 5** Risk for constipation (NANDA 00015) related to decreased motility of gastrointestinal tract.

**N.D. 6** Risk for infection (NANDA 00004) related to alteration in immune response.

**N.D. 7** Risk for infection (NANDA 00004) related to exposure to pathogens.

**N.D. 8** Risk for imbalanced nutrition: more than body requirements (NANDA 00003) related to decreased metabolism.

**N.D. 9** Risk for injury (NANDA 00035) related to:
- decreased muscle tone
- cognitive delays

**N.D. 10** Risk for injury (NANDA 0035) to spinal cord due to atlantoaxial subluxation.

**N.D. 11** Risk for disturbed sensory perception: visual (NANDA 00122) related to vision deficit.

**N.D. 12** Risk for disturbed sensory perception: auditory (NANDA 00122) related to hearing loss.

**N.D. 13** Risk for impaired skin integrity (NANDA 00047) related to orthotics.

**N.D. 14** Risk for delayed development related to Down syndrome.

**N.D. 15** Risk for impaired oral mucous membranes and dentition (NANDA 00045) related to periodontal disease.

## Goals

The student will participate in appropriate physical activities. (N.D.1, 2, 10)
The student will decrease energy expenditure based on activity tolerance level. (N.D. 1, 2)
The student will maintain adequate nutrition. (N.D. 5, 8)
The student will communicate effectively. (N.D. 3, 4)
The student will have optimal visual acuity. (N.D. 11)
The student will have optimal hearing acuity. (N.D. 3, 12)
The student will increase independence. (N.D. 14)
The student will be free from injuries. (N.D. 9, 13)
The student will be free from infections. (N.D. 6, 7)
The student will have optimal oral health. (N.D. 15)

## Nursing Interventions

Monitor activity tolerance, level of fatigue, and any contributing factors. (N.D. 1, 2)

Inform teachers and staff working with the student on signs and symptoms of activity intolerance and fatigue. (N.D. 1, 2)

Allow for rest periods in classroom or in health office as needed. (N.D.1)

With physical education teacher, plan for modifications in physical education curriculum if needed. (N.D. 1, 2, 9, 10, 14)

Obtain results of cervical x-rays for atlantoaxial instability. Inform staff about restrictions if appropriate. (N.D. 10)

Monitor student's cardiac status, obtain and document baseline pulse rate, rhythm, and blood pressure (N.D. 2)

Monitor skin for signs of redness, pressure, and/or breakdown under orthotics. Consult with physical therapist or health care provider as needed. (N.D. 13)

Monitor student's height and weight; record on both standardized growth chart and Down syndrome growth chart. (N.D. 8)

Assess nutritional intake. (N.D. 8)

Encourage intake of high-fiber foods. (N.D. 5)

Team with parents/guardians, healthcare provider, and school nutrition services to provide reduced calorie meals if needed. (N.D. 8)

Provide yearly vision screening. (N.D. 11)

Monitor wearing of glasses if prescribed. (N.D. 11)

Inform teachers and classroom staff of student's possible visual needs (preferential seating near board, large-print formats, etc.). (N.D. 11)

Provide yearly hearing screening. (N.D. 3, 12)

Monitor wearing of hearing aids if prescribed; consult with school audiologist as needed. (N.D. 3, 12)

Encourage referral for speech evaluation and therapy. (N.D. 4)

Inform teachers and classroom staff of student's possible hearing needs (seating near speaker, minimizing background noise, etc.). (N.D. 3, 12)

Assess for otitis media using otoscopic examination as needed. (N.D. 6, 7,12)

Encourage routine dental visits with prophylactic antibiotics administered before dental work if student has cardiac involvement. (N.D. 6, 7, 15)

Assess mouth for evidence of periodontal disease regularly. (N.D. 15)

Encourage staff and student to use good hand-washing techniques. (N.D. 6, 7)

Encourage following recommended schedule of vaccinations. Provide information to family about additional vaccines available, such as flu and pneumococcal vaccines. (N.D. 6, 7)

Assist family in obtaining outside therapies if needed. (N.D. 14)

## Expected Student Outcomes

The student will:
- Participate in physical education activities as appropriate with modifications made as needed. (N.D. 1, 2, 9, 10, 14)
- Communicate the need to rest if necessary. (N.D. 1)
- Wear glasses as prescribed during the school day. (N.D. 11)
- Participate in speech therapy as recommended. (N.D. 3, 4)
- Wear hearing aids as prescribed during the school day. (N.D. 3, 12)
- Eat a well-balanced diet. (N.D. 5, 8)
- Maintain stable and appropriate weight. (N.D. 8)
- Maintain regular bowel-elimination patterns. (N.D. 5)
- Wear orthotic devices if prescribed. (N.D. 9)
- Demonstrate progress in acquiring self-care skills. (N.D. 14)
- Remain free from skin breakdown under orthotics. (N.D. 13)
- Wear glasses as prescribed during the school day. (N.D. 11)
- Maintain prescribed use of orthotics. (N.D. 9, 13)
- Demonstrate a regular attendance pattern. (N.D. 6, 7)
- Maintain a routine of oral health that includes cleaning teeth after meals in school. (N.D. 15)

# Case Study

Michael is a 7-year-old boy who was diagnosed as having Down syndrome shortly after birth. He was hospitalized for 6 weeks on account of multiple complications. He was found to have a large ventricular septal defect and underwent repair at 1 month of age. He recovered well. A hearing test (BAER) done in the neonatal intensive care unit found moderate hearing loss on the left side. He was discharged home and followed by the Down syndrome clinic at the children's hospital. His parents were connected with early intervention through their school district prior to Michael's second birthday.

Currently, Michael is in the 2nd grade in a special education classroom. He is mainstreamed with his peers for part of the school day in his resource room and spends the remainder of the day in his special education classroom. Michael has friends in both of his classrooms. Due to his hearing loss, he wears a hearing aide on the left side. He has had occasional ear infections (one or two a year), but they have responded well to antibiotic treatment. Michael was recently found to have myopia, and glasses were prescribed. Michael ambulates independently with a slightly shuffling gait. He has low muscle tone and wears bilateral ankle-foot orthoses to improve his alignment and function. His atlantoaxial subluxation x-ray was normal, and he has no activity restrictions. He does, however, tend to become fatigued at times after prolonged physical activity or sometimes at the end of a busy school day. Michael has no long-term sequelae from his congenital heart defect and takes no medications. He is followed yearly by his cardiologist.

Michael's current weight of 70 pounds is at the 95th percentile on the Down syndrome growth chart. His height of 44 inches is at the 75th percentile. Michael's mom verbalizes concern about his weight and states that he tends to snack often and doesn't like many vegetables.

Michael has no other current health concerns. He is a social, interactive child. Parents state that he can be stubborn at times but has no significant behavior concerns.

## Down Syndrome

| Assessment Data | Nursing Diagnosis | Goals | Nursing Interventions | Expected Outcomes |
|---|---|---|---|---|
| Fatigue after high level of activity, or at end of school day. | Risk for activity intolerance related to lack of muscle strength. | Student will participate in daily school activities and physical education (PE) without excessive fatigue. | 1. Monitor activity tolerance and level of fatigue.<br>2. Allow for rest periods as needed.<br>3. With PE teacher, plan for modifications in physical education curriculum as needed. | Student will participate in PE activities as appropriate with modifications as needed.<br><br>Student will communicate the need to rest before becoming overly fatigued. |
| Low muscle tone, walks with slightly shuffling gait. Wears bilateral ankle-foot orthoses (AFOs) to improve alignment and function. | Risk for injury related to decreased muscle tone. | Student will be free from injuries. | 1. Encourage student to wear AFOs as prescribed<br>2. Assess environment for factors that may contribute to injury.<br>3. Allow for rest if needed. | Student will maintain independence without experiencing injuries. |
| Weight at 95th percentile on Down syndrome chart; height at 75th percentile. Parents report he is a picky eater, doesn't like vegetables. Likes to snack. | Risk for imbalanced nutrition: more than body requirements related to decreased metabolism | Michael will maintain a stable and appropriate weight. | 1. Monitor height and weight. Record on Down syndrome growth chart and standardized chart.<br>2. With parents and school nutrition services, provide reduced-calorie meals if necessary.<br>3. Assist parents with referral to nutritionist if desired. | Michael will eat a well-balanced diet.<br><br>He will maintain an appropriate and stable weight. |
| Michael wears bilateral AFOs. | Risk for impaired skin integrity related to orthotics. | Michael will maintain prescribed use of AFOs. | 1. Monitor for signs of redness, pressure, and/or skin breakdown under AFOs.<br>2. Consult with school physical therapist or Michael's healthcare provider with concerns regarding AFOs. | Michael's skin will remain free from skin breakdown under AFOs. |

| Assessment Data | Nursing Diagnosis | Goals | Nursing Interventions | Expected Outcomes |
|---|---|---|---|---|
| Michael has moderate-to-severe hearing loss on the left side. A hearing aid is prescribed for the affected side. | Disturbed sensory perception: auditory related to hearing loss. | Michael will maximize his hearing potential. | 1. Encourage Michael to wear his hearing aid as prescribed during the school day.<br>2. Consult with audiologist as needed for concerns regarding the hearing aid. Seating with right ear (good ear) toward speaker. | Michael will wear his hearing aid as prescribed during the school day. |
| Michael has a diagnosis of myopia. Glasses have been prescribed. | Disturbed sensory perception: visual related to vision deficit. | Michael will maximize his visual potential. | 1. Encourage Michael to wear his glasses as prescribed.<br>2. Preferential seating in front of class if glasses not available. | Michael will wear his glasses as prescribed during the school day. |

## References

Allen, P. J., & Vessey, J. A. (2004). Down syndrome. In *Primary care of the child with a chronic condition* (4th ed., (pp. 445–468). St. Louis, MO: Mosby.

Azra, A., & Seward, J. B. ( 2000). Echocardiographic features of genetic diseases: Part 6. Complex cardiovascular defects. *Journal of the American Society of Echocardiography, 13*(6), 637–643.

Benke, M. J., carver, V. & Donahue, R. (1995). Risk and recurrence risk of Down syndrome. Retrieved July 29, 2004, from http://www.nas.com/downsyn/benke.html.

Bosch, J. J. (2003). Health maintenance throughout the life span for individuals with Down syndrome. *Journal of the American Academy of Nurse Practitioners, 15*(1), 5–17.

Castiglia, P.T. (1998). Trisomy 21 syndrome: Is there anything new? *Journal of Pediatric Health Care, 12*(1), 35–37.

Hennequin, M., Faulks, D., Veyrune, J-L., Bourdiol, P. (1999). Significance of oral health in persons with Down syndrome: A literature review. *Developmental Medicine & Child Neurology, 41*(4), 275–283.

Hurley, A.D. (1996). Identifying psychiatric disorders in persons with mental retardation: A model illustrated by depression in down syndrome. *Journal of Rehabilitation, 62*(1), 27–33.

Leshin, L. (2000). Atlantoaxial instability in Down syndrome: Controversy and commentary. Retrieved February 24, 2004, from http://www.ds-health.com/aai.htm

NANDA International. (2003). *Nursing diagnoses: Definitions & classification 2003-2004.* Philadelphia: Author.

Roizen, N. J. (1997) Down syndrome. In M. L. Batshaw (Ed.), *Children with disabilities* (4th ed., pp. 361–376). Baltimore: Paul H. Brooks.

Texas Deafblind Outreach (TSBVI). (1998). Hearing and vision loss associated with Down syndrome. Retrieved March 30, 2004, from http://www.tsbvi.edu/Outreach/seehear/summer98/downsynd.htm

Van Riper, M., & Cohen, M.I. (2001). Caring for children with Down syndrome and their families. *Journal of Pediatric Health Care, 15*(3), 123–131.

Vessey, J.A., & Swanson, M. N. (1993). Caring for the child with Down syndrome. *Journal of School Nursing, 9*(1), 20–36.

## Bibliography

American Academy of Pediatrics. (2001). Health supervision for children with Down syndrome. *Pediatrics, 107*(2), 442–449.

Batshaw, M.L. (1997). *Children with disabilities* (4th ed.). Baltimore: Paul H. Brooks.

Hahn, J.E. (2003). Addressing the need for education: Curriculum development for nurses about intellectual and developmental disabilities. *Nursing Clinics of North America, 38*(2), 185–204.

Hill, J.L. (1999). *Meeting the needs of students with special physical and health care needs.* Columbus, OH; Prentice Hall.

Jain, R., Thomasma, D. C., & Ragas, R. (2002). Down syndrome: Still a social stigma. *American Journal of Perinatology, 19*(2), 99–107.

National Institute of Child Health & Human Development. (2002). Facts about Down syndrome. Retrieved February 24, 2004, from http://www.nichd.nig.gov/publications/pubs/downsyndrome/down.htm

Roizen, N. J. (1997). New advancements in medical treatment of young children with Down syndrome: Implications for early intervention. *Infants and Young Children, 9*(4), 36–42.

# Resources

## National Organizations:

The Arc of the United States
1010 Wayne Avenue
Suite 650
Silver Spring, MD 20910
http://www.thearc.org
301-565-3842

Canadian Down Syndrome Society
811-14 Street NW
Calgary, Alberta T2N 2A4
http://www.cdss.ca
403-270-8500

Learning Disabilities Association of America
4156 Library Road
Pittsburgh, PA 15234-1349
1-888-300-6710
http://wwwldanatl.org

March of Dimes
1275 Mamaroneck Avenue
White Plains, NY 10605
1-888-MODIMES
http://www.modimes.org

National Association for Down Syndrome
PO Box 206
Wilmetter, IL 60091
http://www.nads.org

National Down Syndrome Congress
1370 Center Drive
Suite 102
Atlanta, GA 30338
1-800-232-6372
http://www.ndsccenter.org

National Down Syndrome Society
666 Broadway
8th Floor
New York, NY 10012
1-800-221-4602
http://www.ndss.org

National Information Center for Children and Youth
With Disabilities
PO Box 1492
Washington, DC 20013
1-800-884-8200
http://www.nichcy.org

## Other resources

*Down Syndrome Quarterly*
Denison University
Granville, Ohio
http://www.denison.edu/org

Dr. Len Leshim's comprehensive Web site
http://www.ds-health.com

## Chapter Thirty-seven

# Duchenne Muscular Dystrophy

### Judith F. Harrigan

## Introduction

Muscular dystrophies are the largest and most important group of muscle diseases affecting children. *Muscular dystrophy* refers to a group of inherited diseases marked by progressive weakness and degeneration of the skeletal muscles. The muscular dystrophies constitute the largest group of muscle diseases that affect children. In all forms of muscular dystrophy there is insidious loss of strength, but in each there is a difference in muscle groups affected, age at onset, rate of progression, and inheritance patterns. The etiology of the muscular dystrophies is unknown, although it is probable that the basic defect is caused by a metabolic disturbance that is unrelated to the nervous system. Recent theory supports the belief that the muscle itself is the site of the primary defect.

## Pathophysiology

Duchenne (pseudohypertrophic) muscular dystrophy (DMD), first recognized in 1861, is the most common and severe form of muscular dystrophy affecting children and is characterized by progressive, symmetric weakness and wasting of skeletal muscles, with increasing disability and deformity. Duchenne muscular dystrophy is X-linked and therefore affects males almost exclusively with an incidence of approximately 1 in 3,500 male births. Major complications of DMD include contractures, muscle atrophy, respiratory infections, obesity, and cardiopulmonary problems.

Although there is laboratory evidence that the disease is present from birth and there may be an early history of motor delay, the onset of muscle weakness is generally not exhibited until the child is between 3 and 5 years of age. The child generally achieves early developmental milestones such as raising his head while lying prone, rolling, and sitting upright. The disability becomes apparent when the child begins to stand and walk. Developmental symptoms include delay in walking, unsteady gait, and a tendency to walk on tiptoes. At this point the child may be described as clumsy with a slightly waddling gait, frequently falling and exhibiting a characteristic method of rising from a sitting position on the floor by "walking" his hands up his legs (Gowers' sign). **Table 1** charts the progression of DMD. Unless there is suspicion of DMD related to family history, these signs may be attributed to the normal clumsiness of a developing child. The diagnosis may not be made until the late preschool years, when the child's inability to physically keep up with his peers becomes significant. (Emery & Muntoni, 2003)

The boy with DMD often seems to be particularly well developed muscularly because of the bilateral hypertrophied muscles characteristic of the disease. The name pseudohypertrophy is applied to DMD because muscles, especially in the calves and upper arms, become enlarged from fatty infiltrates and are often described as "firm" or "woody" (Emery & Muntoni, 2003). Leg pain, lordosis, progressive muscle weakness, and more frequent falls become problematic as the child enters school. Stair climbing, running, and jumping become difficult or impossible for the child with DMD. Mild mental retardation may be associated with muscular dystrophy. Anxiety and depression are also common, first as the child begins to realize that he is not able to keep up with peers, and later when he becomes confined to a wheelchair.

Significant muscle atrophy, contractures, and deformities involving many joints occur in later stages of the disease. Ambulation usually becomes impossible by the time the child approaches his second decade of life. A progressive kyphoscoliosis develops, interfering with an already weakened respiratory system. In its terminal stages, the disease process involves the facial, oropharyngeal, and respiratory muscles, with death resulting from pneumonia and respiratory failure and cardiomyopathy (Pourmand, 2001). Evidence of limb girdle weakness, elevated serum creatine kinasa levels, characteristic muscle biopsy, and DNA testing confirm the diagnosis (Emery & Muntoni, 2003).

**Table 1. Insulin Actions**

| Age | Signs |
|---|---|
| <2 years | No symptoms; normal developmental milestones |
| 2 years | Clumsiness, frequent falls, unsteady gait, walks on tiptoes |
| 2 – 3 years | Bilateral hypertrophy of calf muscles; Gower's sign upon standing from floor |
| 3 – 4 years | Beginning lordosis; waddling gait |
| 5 – 6 years | Increasing difficulty running, jumping, climbing stairs |
| 7 – 8 years | Decreasing respiratory status; winging of scapula, increased lordosis; contractures may develop; walking becomes difficult |
| 8 – 9 years | Unable to stand from floor; progressive gait deterioration; contractures limit or prevent ambulation; bracing and surgical interventions may prolong ambulation |
| 10 – 12 years | Begin use of wheelchair, progressing to full-time use |
| >12 years | Increasing respiratory problems with increased severity of respiratory infections; scoliosis; death, usually by late teens or early 20s |

From *Neuromuscular diseases: Expert clinicians' view*, by R. Pourmand, 2001, Boston: Butterworth Heinemann. Copyright 2001 by Butterworth Heinmann.

## Management

Although many studies are currently under way, there is no effective treatment for DMD; at present it is an incurable disease. Maintaining function of muscles for as long as possible is the primary goal of treatment. Passive stretching of heel cords and the application of nighttime splints may impede foot and ankle deformities. Maintenance of function often includes surgery to release contractures, bracing, and assistance with activities of daily living. Despite best preventive efforts, most patients eventually become confined to a wheelchair, and contractures accelerate to include knee, hip, and arm joints. Stretching exercises should include these joints. As kyphoscoliosis begins to develop, a body jacket or wheelchair insert may be used to impede progression.

Progression of scoliosis is often related to failure to comply with the body jacket regimen. Patients must use the brace in order for it to be effective. Ancillary assistive devices may benefit the child who has difficulty performing activities of daily living. Consultation with physical and occupational therapists will be helpful in determining aids that will enable the child to participate as much as possible in all aspects of his life (Emery & Muntoni, 2003). Medications that may affect the progression of the disease include steroids (improve muscle strength and slow progression), creatine (improve muscle strength), and dantrolene (decrease pain, contractures, and creatine kinase levels). Gene therapy also proves to be promising. (Pourmand, 2001; Karpoti, Hilton-Jones, & Griggs, 2001)

# Individualized Healthcare Plan

## Assessment
### History
- When the diagnosis was made
- Degree and pattern of progression of physical disability related to DMD
- Past hospitalizations, surgeries, medications—respiratory complications, tendon release, scoliosis, tracheostomy
- Previous physical, occupational, and respiratory therapy
- Assistive devices (braces, splints, feeding equipment, computers, etc.) that have been used previously
- Other illnesses and/or complications related to DMD
- Family genogram—including history of others with muscular dystrophy
- Family history in relation to management of cares, stresses, finances, and the demands of having a physically disabled child with a terminal illness

### Current Status and Management
- Severity of the student's DMD
- Prognosis
- Compliance with DMD plan of care
- Effectiveness of DMD plan of care
- Growth pattern—current height and weight
- Daily nutritional pattern
- Daily activity schedule—including DMD management measures
- Bowel elimination pattern
- Respiratory status—past and present
- Description and general knowledge about DMD—student and family
- Involvement of support persons/systems
- Heathcare providers involved in management of DMD and routine health maintenance
- Participation in regular exercise program—school-related or non-school-related

### Self-care
- Knowledge about DMD—student, family, and school personnel
- Knowledge about skin care, use of assistive devices, respiratory health, prevention of constipation, etc.—student, family, and school personnel
- Student's participation in development and implementation of DMD plan of care
- Assistive devices needed for daily activities
- Ability to manage activities of daily living
- Motivation to do self-care
- Barriers to self-care
- Experience with self-care at home

### Psychosocial Status
- Current developmental stage of the student
- Current developmental stage of the family
- Communication skills—student and family
- Student's self-concept
- Student's feelings about having DMD
- Student's fears, anxieties, and concerns
- Student's perception of his health and DMD
- Student's perception of his abilities and disabilities
- Family's perception of student's health and DMD
- Decision-making skills and problem-solving skills
- Coping skills—student and family
- Student's locus of control—health, school, family, and activities of daily living
- Ability to interact with peers and adults
- Support systems—student and family
- Family values

*Academic Issues*
- Level of cognitive functioning—learning problems
- Academic, developmental, and social strengths and weaknesses
- Patterns of academic performance—grades, progress, changes in academic performance
- School attendance patterns—current and past, absences related to DMD
- Accommodations needed: accessibility to school building, classrooms, field trips, emergency evacuation plan
- Special education services needed: academic, related services
- Transportation services needed: lift bus
- School health services needed
- Student's perceptions about school—his own strengths and weaknesses
- Teacher's perception of student's academic performance and classroom functioning
- Comparison of student's behavior, social skills, and academic performance to peers
- Participation in school activities: regular and adapted

## Nursing Diagnoses (N.D.) (NANDA 2003)

**N.D. 1** Impaired physical mobility (NANDA 00085) related to:
- muscle weakness
- contractures

**N.D. 2** Self-care deficit: feeding (NANDA 00102), bathing/hygiene (NANDA 00108), dressing/grooming (NANDA 00109), toileting (NANDA 00110) related to:
- mobility limitations
- muscle weakness
- contractures

**N.D. 3** Chronic low self-esteem (NANDA 00119) related to:
- physical limitations
- grieving
- embarrassment
- feelings of being different/physical changes
- loss of control
- intimacy concerns
- perception of stigma

**N.D. 4** Risk for injury (NANDA 00035) related to:
- poor balance and coordination
- falls

**N.D. 5** Ineffective airway clearance (NANDA 00031) related to weakness of muscles in diaphragm

**N.D. 6** Constipation (NANDA 00011) related to immobility

**N.D. 7** Risk for impaired skin integrity (NANDA 00046) related to:
- pressure from braces and wheelchair
- immobility

**N.D. 8** Powerlessness (NANDA 00125) related to:
- deteriorating physical condition
- terminal prognosis

**N.D. 9** Risk for imbalanced nutrition: more than body requirements (NANDA 00001) related to immobility

**N.D. 10** Delayed development (cognitive, gross motor, fine motor, social) (NANDA 00111) related to:
- muscle weakness
- absences from school

## Goals

The student will develop and maintain range of motion in joints to prevent/minimize joint deformity. (N.D. 1)

The student will maintain mobility throughout the school using a wheelchair and/or other assistive devices. (N.D. 1)

The student will maintain maximum independence in school and classroom and activities of daily living. (N.D. 2)

The student will maintain and/or improve self-management skills. (N.D. 2)

The student will be actively participate in making decisions about managing his/her health condition. (N.D. 2, 3, 8)

The student will maintain positive self-image and self-esteem. (N.D. 3)

The student will safe in the school environment and remain free from physical injury. (N.D. 4)

The student will assist in preventing respiratory infections. (N.D. 5)

The student will maintain regular, soft bowel movements. (N.D. 6)

The student will assist in maintaining good skin integrity. (N.D. 7)

The student will express feelings regarding his/her health conditions to others, concerns, and optimism about the present. (N.D. 8)

The student will increase his/her knowledge about his/her health condition. (N.D. 8)

The student will increase his/her locus of control over aspects of his/her life and functioning at school. (N.D. 8)

The student will develop and maintain positive, healthy relationships with peers. (N.D. 8)

The student will maintain appropriate weight for height. (N.D. 9)

The student will choose low-fat, healthy foods in appropriate portions. (N.D. 9)

The student will maintain an optimal level of exercise, with modifications as necessary. (N.D. 9)

The student will maintain a good school attendance pattern. (N.D. 5, 10)

The student will achieve and maintain academic success and progress (appropriate to age and cognitive abilities). (N.D. 10)

## Nursing Interventions

Observe and monitor student's ability to perform self-management skills. (N.D. 1, 2)

Collaborate with occupational therapy (OT)/physical therapy (PT) staff to instruct student in methods to improve/maintain physical abilities and maximize potential. (N.D. 1, 2)

Collaborate with OT/PT staff in providing appropriate assistive devices to increase independence in self-care and classroom activities and mobility around the school setting and on field trips and monitor their use. (N.D. 1, 2)

Collaborate with PT to encourage student and parent/guardian to maintain use of splints and standing table at home according to medical management plan to prevent/reduce contractures. (N.D. 1)

Collaborate with social worker to assist family to obtain assistive devices for use at home. (N.D. 1)

Assist parent/guardian and school administrators in making arrangements for appropriate transportation to and from school. (N.D. 1)

Instruct classroom staff and assistive personnel in performance of and provide supervision of: (N.D. 1, 4)
- stretching exercises
- application of braces
- transfer to and from wheelchair

Assist administrator and school staff in determining and providing the student with assistance for daily school activities, as needed. (N.D. 1)

Monitor student's ability to perform self-management skills. (N.D. 2)

Provide educational opportunities for the student to improve his self-care skills and maximize potential. (N.D. 2)

Maintain regular communication with student and parent/guardian about healthcare plan. (N.D. 2)

Encourage student to share feelings about his condition, its management requirements, limits, the stigma it imposes, and the prognosis. (N.D. 3)

Asssist student to identify his own strengths and weaknesses. (N.D. 3)

Assist student in developing strategies to handle teasing and discrimination. (N.D. 3)

Encourage age-appropriate, positive peer interactions and relationships. (N.D. 3)

Refer student and parent/guardian to support groups, counseling, family therapy, and/or clergy, as indicated. (N.D. 3, 8, 10)

Assess school environment for accessibility and safety: (N. D. 4)
- Facilitate installation of equipment such as ramps, railings, etc. to allow safe access.
- Collaborate with school staff and emergency personnel to establish an evacuation plan in case of fire or other emergency. (N.D. 4)

Monitor student's health and the school population for the presence of infectious diseases, especially respiratory infections, such as pneumonia, influenza. and pertussis. (N.D. 5)

Inform parent/guardian and student when infectious diseases (especially respiratory infections such as influenza, pneumonia, pertussis) are present in the school population and the student's possible exposure or not.

Assist student to use prevention methods to minimize/decrease exposure to infectious diseases. (N.D. 5)

Assist student to cough and clear airway effectively. (N.D. 5)

Assist student to maintain adequate hydration (to thin secretions) during the school day. (N.D. 5)

Provide in-service training for school staff working with the student:
- proper technique for airway clearance (N.D. 5)
- need for adequate hydration during the school day. (N.D. 5, 6)
- detection of early skin breakdown (N.D. 7)
- safety issues in the school environment and on field trips (N.D. 4)

Arrange for private space and time for toileting at school. (N.D. 6)

Collaborate with parent/guardian and classroom and food services personnel to provide appropriate foods and fluids to decrease constipation. (N.D. 6)

Assist student and parent/guardian to learn and observe for signs of early skin breakdown. (N.D. 7)

Instruct student and parent/guardian in management of skin care, as indicated (N.D. 7)

Encourage student to shift his weight in his wheelchair approximately every 15 minutes to prevent skin breakdown. (N.D. 7)

Assist student to identify activities he enjoys (at school, at home, in the community, with family members, with peers, etc.). (N.D. 8)

Reinforce student's positive abilities, interactions, etc. (N.D. 8)

Listen to student and family and encourage expressions of concern, grief, fear, and anxiety. (N.D. 8)

Assist staff to identify opportunities for the student to make choices and decisions. (N.D. 3, 8)

Provide opportunities for the student to problem solve and make decisions regarding his/her healthcare at school. (N.D. 8)

Monitor student's growth with height and weight measurements twice a year. (N.D. 9)

Assist student and parent/guardian in planning nutritional diet for school that is low in calories and fat and high in protein and fiber. (N.D. 9)

Collaborate with school food services director on inclusion of appropriate food choices. (N.D. 9)

Promote wellness for student and family with teaching and support. (N.D. 8)

Refer to special education team or 504 team for evaluation of academic program needs, as needed. (N.D. 10)

Participate as a member of the special education interdisciplinary team. (N.D. 10)

Encourage parent/guardian and other family members to play a supportive role in assisting the student to manage his/her care in the school setting and at home. (N.D. 8)

## Expected Student Outcomes

The student will:
- Demonstrate mobility around the school building and in classrooms (with assistance from adults, as needed). (N.D. 1)
- Actively participate in classroom and school activities, with assistance from adults as needed. (N.D. 2)
- Participate in classroom and school activities, with assistance from adults as needed. (N.D. 2)
- Consistently wear braces, as prescribed by medical management plan. (N.D. 1)
- Actively participate in daily stretching activities at school. (N.D. 1)
- Utilize standing table daily at school, as prescribed in medical management plan. (N.D. 1)
- Actively participate in range-of-motion activities for ankles, knees, and hips. (N.D. 1)
- Use his braces at home for increasing times, as determined by tolerance of the activity, as reported by parent/guardian. (N.D. 1)
- Demonstrate use of assistive devices at (school, home) to (achieve, maintain) an optimal (level of independence, participation) in self-care. (N.D. 1, 2)
- Student will demonstrate safe and appropriate technique in
  – toileting, during the school day (N.D. 2)
  – transferring in and out of the wheelchair during the school day (N.D. 1, 2)
  – medication administration (N.D. 2)
  – skin care (N.D. 7)
- Report early symptoms indicating problems to (teacher, health office personnel). (N.D. 2, 4, 6, 7)
- Demonstrate positive interactions with peers (in the classroom, during lunch, during recess). (N.D. 10)
- Demonstrate effective problem-solving skills regarding (specific: classroom issues, peer issues) (N.D. 2, 3, 8)
- Demonstrate effective decision-making skills regarding (specific: care, school work, other. (N.D. 2, 3, 8)
- Verbalize feelings to appropriate adults about his/her concerns, grief, anger, anxiety, fear, and limitations and others' reactions to his/her disability. (N.D. 3, 8)
- Verbalize positive feelings about himself and identify his/her strengths. (N.D. 3)
- Develop answers to questions others (peer, adults) ask him and will use them to explain about his disability and limitations. (N.D. 3)
- Demonstrate activities (hand washing, covering a cough, etc) that assist in preventing the spread of diseases to others. (N.D. 5)
- Identify signs and symptoms of respiratory infections. (N.D. 5)
- Report signs or symptoms of infections to (school staff, parent/guardian) when they occur. (N.D. 5)

- Demonstrate a good school attendance pattern (specific criteria). (N.D. 5, 10)
- Demonstrate effective airway clearing. (N.D. 5)
- Drink 3 to 4 glasses of water or juice each day in school. (N.D. 5, 6)
- Have regular bowel movements, as reported by student and parent. (N.D. 6)
- Demonstrate appropriate food choices to maintain regular bowel activity. (N.D. 6)
- Identify (number of signs) and symptoms of skin breakdown. (N.D. 7)
- Demonstrate preventive skin care techniques. (N.D. 7)
- Demonstrate weight shifts in wheelchair (number of times per class period) to prevent skin breakdown, as reported by student and classroom teachers/paras. (N.D. 7)
- Actively participate in activities and functions that he enjoys. (N.D. 8)
- Participate in counseling, if appropriate. (N.D. 8)
- Maintain weight that is appropriate for height, as plotted on growth chart. (N.D. 9)
- Consistently choose appropriate, nutritional foods. (N.D. 9)
- Actively participate in physical education and physical therapy programs and in games played in class, with modifications as necessary. (N.D. 9)
- Describe his roles and responsibilities in the family and the roles and responsibilities of other family members. (N.D. 8)
- Demonstrate academic success and achievement. (N.D. 10)

## Evacuation Plan

Discussion must take place with parents, teachers, administrators and local emergency personnel to plan for evacuation of physically disabled students in case of emergencies that require vacating the school building.

The plan should include how the student would evacuate the school building for each class on his/her schedule, as well as from the media center, cafeteria, auditorium, and other common areas of the building. It should also include a designation of staff persons who would stay and assist in evacuating the student from the building. Elevators should not be used during an emergency evacuation.

Evacuation plans should be developed with consideration to building construction, district finances, advice from emergency personnel, and the student's personal needs.

## Case Study

Jason is an 11-year-old boy who was diagnosed at the age of 4 years as having Duchenne muscular dystrophy after his parents began to recognize symptoms of falling and progressive weakness that they had previously seen in young cousins in both the mother's and father's families. Jason did not begin to walk until he was almost 2 years old and has never been able to run or jump. He started school 1 year later than his peers and is described by his teachers as being immature and unable to accomplish many routine activities in the classroom without assistance. Psychological tests reveal him to be mildly mentally impaired. He is reported to be highly distractible with poor academic interest and problems with short-term and rote memory. He currently attends is in special education and has an individualized education program (IEP). He receives speech, physical therapy, occupational therapy, and developmental adapted physical education (DAPE) services. He has assistance from paras in his mainstream classes. He has had many absences from school because of frequent respiratory infections and has been hospitalized twice in the past 2 years with pneumonia.

During the last year Jason has begun to rapidly lose function. He is no longer able to ambulate, and his parents have stopped using his long leg braces at home. He is developing contractures in his ankles, knees, and hips. Jason spends most of each day in his wheelchair and is becoming more proficient in maneuvering his wheelchair. His doctor has just written a prescription for him to resume use of his braces and to stand in his braces at a standing table. The physical therapist will be monitoring this process. He has gained 12 pounds in the past 6 months. He takes prednisone, 12.5 mg per day. His mother reports that he has problems with constipation.

The school nurse met with Jason and his mother in her office to discuss Jason's rapidly changing physical status and to develop a healthcare plan that would accommodate his needs in school. He arrived in his wheelchair, which was pushed by his mother. His mother repeatedly answered questions that were directed to Jason and assured the nurse that he was unable to accomplish dressing, bathing, and toileting without assistance. Jason was silly and immature during the meeting and did not seem to be interested in the discussion about his care plan. When asked what he likes best about school, he stated that he did not like school.

In a private discussion with the nurse, his mother expressed guilt that "We knew this ran in the family. It's our fault that he has muscular dystrophy." She also stated that she feels so bad when he has difficulty with activities of daily living that she helps him, even though she knows she should let him do things for himself.

# Duchene Muscular Dystrophy

| Assessment Data | Nursing Diagnosis | Goals | Nursing Interventions | Expected Outcomes |
|---|---|---|---|---|
| Diagnosed at age 4. Recently has had rapid loss of functioning.<br><br>No longer able to ambulate.<br><br>Uses wheelchair for mobility.<br><br>Developing contractures in his ankles, knees and hips.<br><br>Physician order for use of long leg braces and standing table.<br><br>Teachers report that Jason is unable to accomplish many routine activities in the classroom setting without assistance. | Impaired physical mobility related to muscle weakness and contractures. | Jason will maintain mobility in the school setting using his wheelchair, with assistive devices and adult assistance as needed.<br><br>Jason will assist in preventing increase in contractures by wearing braces in school as prescribed by physician. | Collaborate with PT staff for assisting Jason with:<br>• Increasing independence and proficiency in using and maneuvering his wheelchair<br>• Maintaining physical abilities<br>• Use of leg braces and standing table during the school day<br>• Use of appropriate assistive devices in the classroom<br>• Daily stretching exercises<br>• Transferring to and from his wheelchair<br><br>Encourage student and parents to utilize leg braces at home according to medical management plan.<br><br>Assist parent/guardian and administrators in making arrangements for transportation to and from school.<br><br>Develop Emergency Evacuation Plan (EEP) for evacuating Jason from the building safely and quickly, if needed. | Jason will demonstrate effective mobility around the school environment, with assistance from adults as needed.<br><br>Jason will independently use and maneuver his wheelchair in the classroom and school setting.<br><br>Jason demonstrates compliance with wearing leg braces and using standing table, as prescribed.<br><br>Jason will actively participate in physical therapy activities in the school setting.<br><br>Jason will actively participate in a drill of his EEP.<br><br>Jason will evacuate the building quickly. and safely, as needed. |
| Jason is unable to accomplish dressing, bathing, and toileting without assistance.<br><br>Psychological testing indicates that Jason is mildly mentally impaired. | Self-care deficit related to muscle weakness, contractures resulting in need for adult assistance with dressing, toileting, hygiene needs. | Jason will improve self-management skills.<br><br>Jason will participate in daily self-care activities, (dressing, hygiene, feeding, and toileting) | Observe and monitor Jason's ability to perform self-care skills. | Jason will demonstrate active participation in self-care activities, with assistance from adults as needed.<br>• dressing and undressing<br>• hygiene<br>• toileting |

| Assessment Data | Nursing Diagnosis | Goals | Nursing Interventions | Expected Outcomes |
|---|---|---|---|---|
| Jason acts silly and immature during meeting.<br><br>Unsure of Jason's ability to make decisions or choices regarding his care at school.<br><br>Parent states that she sometimes helps Jason when she knows she should let him do things for himself. | | Jason will actively participate in making decisions about managing his health condition. | Assist Jason and school staff to identify things Jason can do independently and things he needs assistance with:<br>• dressing and undressing<br>• hygiene<br>• toileting<br><br>Collaborate with OT, PT, and parents to find and utilize assistive devices that allow Jason to develop and/or maintain independence in self-care.<br><br>Assist in providing staffing to meet Jason's need for assistance with dressing, hygiene, feeding, and toileting during the school day.<br><br>Assist school staff working with Jason to maintain safety for Jason and themselves during self-care activities.<br><br>Assist school staff to identify opportunities at school when Jason can make choices and decisions to assist him in developing and maintaining a sense of control and independence.<br><br>Encourage parents to allow Jason to make decisions and choices to assist him in developing and maintaining a sense of control and independence. | Jason will utilize assistive devices to improve and maintain his ability to participate in self-care activities.<br>Jason asks for assistance from adults and peers if he feels he needs it.<br><br>Jason will demonstrate effective decision-making skills regarding his health care at school.<br>Jason will make choices daily regarding his care at school.<br><br>Jason will make decisions and choices at home regarding his care, as reported by Jason and his parents. |

## Duchenne Muscular Dystrophy

| Assessment Data | Nursing Diagnosis | Goals | Nursing Interventions | Expected Outcomes |
|---|---|---|---|---|
| Frequent respiratory infections Hospitalized twice in the past 2 years for pneumonia. | Risk for infection related to muscle weakness resulting in ineffective airway clearance. | Jason will assist in preventing respiratory infections by maintaining effective airway clearance. | Assist Jason to cough and clear airway effectively. | Jason will demonstrate effective airway clearing. |
| | | | Assist student to maintain adequate hydration during the school day to keep secretions thin. | Jason will drink 3 glasses of water or juice at school each day. |
| | | | In-service staff working with Jason about: <br> • need for adequate hydration <br> • proper coughing technique <br> • signs and symptoms of respiratory infections. | Jason will report signs and symptoms of respiratory infection to school staff and parents if they occur. |
| | | | Assist staff working with Jason to monitor for signs of respiratory and other infections. | |
| | | | Monitor school population for evidence of respiratory illnesses, especially influenza, pneumonia, and pertussis. | |
| | | | Inform parents when respiratory infections (especially influenza, pneumonia, and pertussis) are present in the school population and th student's possible exposure or not. | |
| Started school 2 year later than peers. | Delayed development (cognitive, gross and fine motor, and social) related to neuromuscular disease. | Jason will achieve and maintain academic success and progress. | Participate with special education team in developing and providing an individualized education program (IEP) for Jason. | Jason will actively participate in activities in the classroom. |

| Assessment Data | Nursing Diagnosis | Goals | Nursing Interventions | Expected Outcomes |
|---|---|---|---|---|
| Mildly mentally impaired. Highly distractable, poor academic interest, problems with short-term and rote memory Teachers report he is unable to accomplish many routine activities in the classroom without assistance.<br><br>Special education classes, speech, OT, PT, and DAPE services.<br><br>Assistance from paras in mainstream classes.<br><br>Many absences from school. When asked what he likes best about school, Jason stated he hated school. | | Jason will develop and maintain positive, healthy relationships with peers. | Assist Jason to identify things he is good at in classes at school.<br><br>Provide positive reinforcement to Jason for actively participating and interacting with peers in classroom activities.<br><br>Collaborate with OT and PT staff in providing appropriate assistive devices that allow Jason to maintain independence in classroom activities.<br><br>Assist teachers and paras to provide opportunities that allow Jason to interact and participate with peers in the classroom setting, without direct adult assistance or supervision.<br><br>Encourage parents to provide opportunities for Jason to play with his peers, especially classmates from school. | Jason will meet IEP goals and objectives.<br><br>Jason will demonstrate positive interactions with peers during classroom activities.<br><br>Jason will demonstrate positive interactions with peers during lunch. |

## References

Emery, A. E. H., & Muntoni, F. (2003). *Duchenne muscular dystrophy* (3rd ed.). Oxford, England: Oxford University Press.

Karpati, G., Hilton-Jones, D., & Griggs, R. C. (Eds.). (2001). *Disorders of voluntary muscle* (7th ed). Cambridge, England: Cambridge University Press.

NANDA International. (2003). *NANDA nursing diagnoses: Definitions & classification 2003–2004.* Philadelphia: Author.

Pourmand, R. (Ed.). (2001). *Neuromuscular diseases: Expert clinicians' view.* Boston: Butterworth Heinemann.

## Bibliography

Hockenberry, M. J. (2003). *Wong's nursing care of infants and children* (7th ed.). St. Louis, MO: Mosby.

Muscular Dystrophy Association. (1998). *Journey of love: A parent's guide to Duchenne muscular dystrophy.* Tucson, AZ: Author.

Porter, P. B., Hall, C. D. & Williams, F. (1999). *A teacher's guide to Duchenne muscular dystrophy.* Retrieved March, 12, 2005. from http://mdausa.org/publications/tchrdmd/

## Resources

Muscular Dystrophy Association
National Headquarters
3300 East Sunrise Drive
Tucson, AZ 85718
1-800-572-1777
http://www.mdausa.org/disease.cfm

## Chapter Thirty-eight

# Eating Disorders

Tona L. Leiker and Elaine Level

## Introduction

Disordered eating has been recorded throughout history and throughout the world. However, the prevalence of eating-related disorders is increasing at staggering rates in the United States. Our obsessions with fast food, busy lifestyles, dieting, and allowing the media images to define our self-worth places our school-aged children at high risk for food-related health conditions.

The United States has recorded a rise in the prevalence of anorexia nervosa, bulimia, and obesity over the last 20 years. The school nurse is in a position to effectively intervene with students experiencing potentially negative consequences of food choices. Physical problems begin when body weight is below or above ideal body weights.

It is estimated that 7.5% to 11% of adolescent females and 2.0% to 4.5% of adolescent males have eating disorders, with a 5% death rate of anorexia patients, 50% of which are suicides (Jellinek, Patel, & Froehle, 2002). Caucasian, upper/middle class adolescent females are at greatest risk of developing an eating disorder (Cochrane, 1998).

Primary years of onset are 13 to 20 years; however, elementary school children are not immune from these problems. Bulimia nervosa occurs in 2% to 4% of the population in which the patient's weight is usually normal. Among high school and college-aged females, bulimia may occur in up to 15% of the population. Urban areas have a higher incidence of disordered eating, anorexia, and bulimia than the rural areas (Cochrane).

## Pathophysiology

Pathologically, studies indicate there is a deregulation of feeding/satiety related to altered serotonin and amino acid levels in the brain, with biologic, psychological, environmental, and sociocultural influences. Research is not clear as to which comes first, the deregulation of feeding/satiety or other influences that result in altered brain chemicals (Antai-Ontong, 2003; Cochrane, 1998).

Students with eating disorders may experience a perceived loss of control or perceived excessive caloric intake or have a history of food restrictions, fasting patterns, or use of laxatives, diet pills, diuretics or following excessive periods of exercise. Symptomatically, the student may present with:
- Altered vital signs
- Abnormal height/weight ratios
- Dry, scaly skin, possibly with lanugo
- Cardiovascular complaints, such as fainting or tachycardia
- Dental problems
- Delayed puberty and sexual development
- History of substance and/or sexual abuse
- Family history of eating disorders
- Comorbid psychological disorders, such as anxiety disorder or depression (Cochrane, 1998; Green, 2002; Jellinek, et al., 2002).

Cochrane (1998) suggests the use of two questions as brief screening for potential eating disorders: (1) Are you satisfied with your eating patterns? and (2) Do you ever eat in secret?

It is important for the school nurse to be aware of the diagnostic criteria for eating disorders described in the American Psychiatric Association's *Diagnosis and Statistical Manual of Mental Disorders (DSM- IV-TR)* (2000). There are two primary diagnoses for eating disorders: (1) anorexia nervosa with restricting type or binge eating/purging type and (2) bulimia nervosa with purging or nonpurging type. The four primary criteria for anorexia nervosa include refusal to maintain body weight at or above minimally normal weight for age and height, intense fear of weight gain, body image disturbance, and amenorrhea of at least three consecutive menstrual cycles. Primary criteria for bulimia nervosa include binge eating, lack of control over eating, recurrent inappropriate compensatory behavior at least twice a week for 3 months, and critical self-evaluation. (DSM IV-TR).

While obesity is not specifically listed as an eating disorder in the *DSM-IV-TR* (2000), the health complications of obesity are escalating healthcare costs at an alarming rate. Secondary health problems related to obesity include hypertension, elevated cholesterol and triglyceride levels, strokes, other cardiovascular diseases, and type 2 diabetes. These illnesses can result from mild obesity. Risk increases as body mass index (BMI) increases. Younger children with cardiovascular changes and type 2 diabetes are presenting in school health offices in growing numbers.

Obesity occurs on a continuum, as do all the eating disorders, from healthy nutrition and body weight to death, secondary to health related-disease states. Obesity may be defined as overweight, obese, and morbid obesity. BMIs greater than 25th to 26th percentile begin the definition of overweight. Cultural/genetic variations may alter the BMI for overweight slightly; for example, persons Asian descent may be considered overweight with a slightly lower BMI, and persons of Polynesian descent may be considered overweight with a slightly higher BMI. Government nutrition Web sites, found in the Resource section at the end of this chapter, provide current and specific charts on BMIs related to obesity. Healthy eating may be reinforced from a perspective of balanced food choices, no forbidden foods, not promoting food fads personally or with other school staff, and providing concrete examples of accurate food serving sizes, not our large and super-sized meal portions. Teaching the importance of balanced food choices, including a variety of proteins, carbohydrates, and fats, is a key role of the school nurse in every decision related to food choices in the academic setting.

The brain is the primary consumer of calories, and research is clarifying the importance of essential fatty acids, vitamins, and minerals for optimal brain function. The United States' distorted vision of female body sizes and types may contribute to the prevalence of adolescent altered body images. With a few gains in promoting models of all body types and sizes, a focused review of print and video materials will increase one's awareness of our society's obsession with diets and weights and the popular waif-like appearance of models today.

The school nurse may serve as an information source in communicating to adolescents that their physical maturation in puberty is a normal, healthy, and an expected life event. The average healthy female adolescent will increase her body fat from 8% to 22 % during adolescence (Green, 2002). Teaching students about normal growth and development and the role genetics plays in our body shapes and sizes, while promoting positive self-image, is of great importance.

Eating disorders are closely correlated with other psychiatric diagnoses, especially depression and anxiety. A comprehensive evaluation is critical to determine correct diagnoses and interventions and plan for school expectations.

## Management

The school nurse is in a key position to promote nutrition education in a variety of school arenas: in health and physical education classes, in family and consumer science courses, through collaborative efforts with the school's athletic trainer/coaches, in special education programs, and in school food service programs (Green, 2002).

Early identification and successful intervention improve the outcomes of disordered eating patterns. Students, faculty, and staff who had intervention within the first months of disordered eating patterns have significantly higher rates of recovery than those ignored or unidentified for more than 1 year (Green, 2002).

Students experiencing difficulties with anorexia may present with headaches, fatigue, rapid heart rate, fainting episode during activity, diaphoresis, clamminess, and/or hypoglycemic episodes (Cochrane, 1998; Green, 2002; Jellinek, et al., 2002; Krupnick, & Wade, 1999).

Students experiencing binging and purging may present with sore throats, vomiting, diarrhea, stomachaches, mouth sores, and/or sores on fingers and hands (Cochrane, 1998; Green, 2002; Jellinek, et al., 2002; Krupnick, & Wade, 1999).

The school nurse's role in promoting healthy behaviors, healthy food choices, and the view that food consumption is like fuel to keep our bodies functioning optimally or like medicine for the anorexic client will assist in removing the psychological incongruence associated with eating and current emotional state. Managing eating disorders in the school environment begins first with comprehensive health education programs that address mental health issues, including eating disorders of anorexia nervosa, bulimia nervosa, and obesity. The school nurse's involvement in health education allows for preventative services to be provided while establishing a trusting relationship between the students and the school nurse.

Effective planning of an intervention process with the student and parents is essential when an eating disorder is suspected. Denial of a problem with anger as the initial response is not uncommon when the student or parent is approached about a possible eating disorder. Before the problem can be successfully addressed, the student and the parents must acknowledge that there is a potential problem. To assist the student in the recovery process, the school nurse may be instrumental in making appropriate referrals, providing support during the treatment process, and facilitating reentry into the school environment. The school nurse's awareness of eating disorders is critical to prevent endemic episodes of disordered eating within peer groups.

Appropriate school management strategies include:
- Positive reinforcement, as defined by the student and in compliance with the treatment plan; for example, time with friends or extra privileges in the home environment
- Modification of the educational environment to decrease stressors. Consider need for 504 accommodation plan to assist with management.
- Consensus regarding participation in extracurricular activities during active treatment process, especially if weight or nutritional intake is such that it places student at risk for sudden death.
- Immediate referral to parents/physician/therapist if suicidal ideation/attempts identified by school personnel.

The school nurse should be an advocate and facilitator of appropriate parental interventions that should include:
- Parental support and family education regarding specific eating issues
- Counseling services to enhance family function
- Ongoing assessment to identify sabotage, control issues, treatment barriers

# Individualized Healthcare Plan

## Assessment

### History
- Student's complete health history, including any major illness or injury
- Date of last physical examination or visit to primary healthcare provider or sports physical
- Date of last mental health examination
- History of any major illness, injury, or chronic health issue with immediate family member
- Student's past response to stress
- History of use of laxatives, diuretics, enemas, self-induced vomiting, binging, fasting, exercise
- Relationship with parents over time, noting recent changes
- Any major changes in the student's home life or school activities
- Onset and duration of eating issues at hand, including recent weight changes
- History of substance abuse (Cochrane, 1998; Green, 2002; Jellinek, et al., 2002; Krupnick, & Wade, 1999)

### Current Status and Management
- Current treatment plan for disordered eating issues
- Medications to be taken at home or administered during school hours
- Activities outside the school setting
- Parental response, including participation in treatment process with student
- Key physical assessment findings include:
  - Altered vital signs
  - Abnormal height/weight ratios
  - Dry, scaly skin, possibly with lanugo
  - Cardiovascular complaints, such as fainting or tachycardia
  - Dental problems
  - Delayed puberty and sexual development
  - Sore throats
  - Vomiting
  - Constipation or diarrhea
  - Stomachaches
  - Mouth sores
  - Sores on fingers, knuckles
  - Dental problems
  - Hair loss, development of lanugo
  - Poor concentration
  - Preoccupation with food
  - Obsession with body image and size
  - Amenorrhea
  - Lack of breast tissue development
  - Anemia
  - Cyanosis of extremities
  - Hypertension
  - Electrolyte imbalances
  - Aspiration pneumonia
  - Bleeding gums
  - Esophagitis
  - Gastric rupture
  - Muscle weakness
  - Dizziness or fainting (Cochrane, 1998; Green, 2002; Jellinek, et al., 2002; Krupnick, & Wade, 1999)
- Student's ability to verbalize and identify the source of anxiety or fear
- Student's ability to utilize relaxation methods to decrease urgency to refuse food, binge, or purge

### Self-care
- Student's ability to recognize the sources of anxiety and fears that precede disordered eating episodes
- Student's ability to verbalize positive statements to improve self-esteem
- Use of school and community resources for increasing effective coping skills
- Student's ability to terminate disordered eating patterns of starvation, binging, purging

*Psychosocial Status*
- Student's opinion of academic achievement
- Student's perception of parental expectations
- Student's perception of body image

*Academic Issues*
- Current academic standing
- Classroom modifications to decrease stress and anxiety, especially around eating issues
- Need for 504 plan

## Nursing Diagnoses (N.D.) (NANDA, 2003)

**N.D. 1** Anxiety (NANDA 00146) related to:
- eating and discovery of eating behaviors
- eating rituals resulting in disordered eating patterns

**N.D. 2** Activity intolerance (NANDA 00092) related to pain or fatigue when engaged in physical activity

**N.D. 3** Imbalanced nutrition, less than body requirements, (NANDA 00002) related to:
- self-imposed starvation
- self-induced vomiting

**N.D. 4** Imbalanced nutrition, more than body requirements, (NANDA 00001) related to excessive caloric intake.

**N.D. 5** Disturbed body image (NANDA 00118) related to an unrealistic ideal of thinness.

**N.D. 6** Fatigue (NANDA 00093) related to:
- low caloric intake
- excessive caloric intake
- increased physical exercise.

**N.D. 7** Risk for injury (NANDA 00035) related to:
malnourished condition
- obesity
- dental damage
- aspiration of vomitus
- esophageal erosion and/or rupture.

**N.D. 8** Delayed growth and development (NANDA 00111) related to low caloric intake.

**N.D. 9** Readiness for enhanced nutrition (NANDA 00163) related to willingness to learn healthy eating patterns and make educated food choices.

**N.D. 10** Disturbed thought processes (NANDA 00130) related to:
- malnourished state
- low self-esteem
- unrealistic body image.

**N.D. 11** Deficient knowledge (NANDA 00126) of healthy eating habits, proper nutrition, and treatment for disordered eating.

**N.D. 12** Situational low self-esteem (NANDA 00120) related to:
- disturbed body image
- feelings of worthlessness and/or shame.

## Goals

The student will recognize the sources of anxiety and fears. (N.D. 1, 10, 12)

The student will employ relaxation methods to decrease anxiety. (N.D. 1, 10, 12)

The student will verbalize improved self-esteem. (N.D. 5, 12)

The student will verbalize a more realistic self-perception of body size. (N.D. 4, 5)

The student will identify stressors that increase disordered eating episodes. (N.D. 1, 2, 3, 4)

The student will request assistance with and make use of school and community resources for increasing effective coping skills. (N.D. 4, 5, 9, 10, 11, 12)

The student will learn healthy eating patterns and make educated food choices. (N.D. 4, 5, 6, 11)

The student will engage in appropriate levels of regular, healthy activity. (N.D. 2, 3, 4, 8)

The student will terminate disordered eating patterns of starvation, binging, purging. (N.D. 3, 4, 5, 6, 7, 8, 9)

The student will develop flexible thought patterns, with decreased concrete, black-and-white thinking. (N.D. 10)

The student will decrease episodes of obsessive thoughts. (N.D. 10)
The student will decrease hypersensitivity to environmental stimuli. (N.D. 1, 5, 10, 12)

## Nursing Interventions

- Treat food consumption as a medication order. (N.D. 2, 3)
- Provide a safe environment in which the student may eat snacks or meals. (N.D. 1, 3, 9)
- Allow the student to visit the health office when feeling overwhelmed. (N.D. 1, 2, 6, 10, 12)
- Provide diversional activities that are calming to the student. (N.D. 1, 10, 12)
- Provide active listening to assist student in expressing anxieties regarding food. (N.D. 1)
- Supervise release for participation in physical education, sports, and other school activities. (N.D. 2, 7)
- Facilitate and educate school staff on the need to adjust activity levels per physician/therapist orders. (N.D. 2, 7)
- Monitor student participation, observing for signs and symptoms of intolerance. (N.D. 2, 7)
- Discretely monitor food intake, without student awareness. (N.D. 1, 3, 4, 6, 8)
- Enlist counseling staff or trusted cafeteria employee to monitor food intake if school nurse is unable. (N.D. 1, 3, 4, 6, 8)
- Communicate with therapist or parent as directed by treatment plan. (N.D.1–12)
- Support healthy food choices, balanced meal and snack choices. (N.D. 3, 4, 6, 8, 9, 11)
- Provide education and support healthy food choices. (N.D. 3, 4, 6, 8, 9, 11)
- Offer a safe environment. (N.D. 1-4, 6, 7, 9-12)
- Provide diversional activities that are calming to the student, such as drawing, reading, or craft activities (N.D 1, 10, 12).
- Provide emotional support and active listening for the student to express concerns about body image. (N.D. 1, 5, 10, 12)
- Do not feed into distorted images or perceptions. (N.D. 1, 5, 10, 12)
- Provide education and awareness to students of media distortion of body image. (N.D. 1, 5, 10, 12)
- Provide education regarding genetics as indicator of body size and type. (N.D. 5, 10, 11, 12)
- Report disturbed statements to therapist/parent as agreed upon in team meetings. (N.D. 1–12)
- Encourage healthy hydration. (N.D. 2-4, 6, 7)
- Allow short rest periods, if needed and supported by therapist, being careful that rest periods are not used to avoid appropriate emotional and/or physical activity. (N.D. 6)
- Monitor and assess for signs and symptoms of suicide using standardized assessment tools. (N.D. 7, 10)
- Monitor for signs of purging behavior. (N.D. 7)
- Coordinate with physical education and/or athletic coaches for safe participation in class and activities. (N.D. 2, 7)
- Monitor onset of menses in females and report amenorrhea to parents as agreed to in planning meeting. (N.D. 8)
- Provide education regarding the consequences of anorexia, bulimia, and obesity. (N.D. 9, 11)
- Provide education and resources to food services teams to promote healthy food choices in school cafeterias and vending machines. (N.D. 9, 11)
- Provide materials and/or provide age-appropriate education about eating disorders in the classroom setting. (N.D. 9, 11)
- Provide rational feedback to the student in a safe and supportive environment. (N.D. 1-7, 9-12)
- Provide ongoing communication to parents and the treatment team regarding thought processes and behavior, with appropriate privacy compliance. (N.D. 1-12)
- Facilitate and educate the student regarding:
  – appropriate activity
  – serving sizes
  – healthy food choices
  – realistic perception of body image. (N.D. 1-7, 9, 11, 12)
- Facilitate and provide staff education regarding disordered eating, eating behaviors, and treatment modalities. (N.D. 11)
- Collaborate with student, family, and other school personnel to:
  – explore need for 504 plan
  – participate in development of 504 plan
  – implement 504 plan (N.D. 1-5, 7)
- Facilitate and provide peer education regarding the dangers of disordered eating. (N.D. 11)

- Monitor for compliance if any medications are taken at school (N.D. 7, 11)
- Educate school personnel regarding healthy lifestyle, including healthy food choices and appropriate exercise, rather than current fad diets (N.D 3-6, 9, 10).
- Provide support and awareness of hypersensitivity of persons with eating disorders, especially emotions surrounding eating and eating behaviors. (N.D. 12)
- Identify and encourage positive qualities, traits, and abilities of the student to help build self-esteem. (N.D. 12)
- Educate faculty members regarding the role of stressors in the classroom and impact of disordered eating. (N.D. 12)

## Expected Student Outcomes

The student will:
- Verbalize importance of frequent small meals and snacks as an important intervention toward health within __ weeks. (N.D. 1, 5, 8, 9).
- Eat at least 50% of prescribed food for meals and snacks during the school day within __ weeks. (N.D. 1, 5, 8, 9)
- Make educated food choices in the school cafeteria or sack lunches within 3 weeks. N.D. 9, 11)
- Make three positive statements regarding her talents and abilities within 2 weeks. (N.D. 12)
- Verbalize and identify the source(s) of anxiety and fears. (N.D. 1, 10, 12)
- Differentiate between effective and ineffective methods of coping with anxiety. (N.D. 1, 10, 12)
- Report a decrease in anxiety at school over a __ week period (N.D. 1, 10-12)
- Describe physiologic responses to anxiety and fear. (N.D.1, 10, 12)
- Employ relaxation methods to decrease anxiety. (N.D. 1, 10, 12)
- Verbalize improved self-esteem. (N.D. 5, 12)
- Verbalize a more realistic self-perception of body size. (N.D. 4, 5)
- Identify stressors that increase disordered eating episodes. (N.D. 1-4)
- Request assistance with and make use of school and community resources for increasing effective coping skills. (N.D. 4, 5, 8-12)
- Describe healthy eating patterns and make educated food choices. (N.D. 4, 5, 6, 8, 9, 11)
- Engage in appropriate levels of regular, healthy activity. (N.D. 2-4, 7)
- Terminate disordered eating patterns of starvation, binging, purging. (N.D. 3-7)
- Develop flexible thought patterns, with decreased concrete, black-and-white thinking. (N.D. 1, 2, 5, 10)
- Not harm self in the school setting. (N.D. 7)
- Report episodes of suicidal or other self-harming thoughts to trusted adult in school setting. (N.D. 7, 10,12)
- Decrease episodes of obsessive thoughts. (N.D. 1, 10)
- Verbalize fewer statements reflective of disturbed thoughts within ___ weeks. (N.D. 10)
- Decrease hypersensitivity to environmental stimuli. (N.D. 1, 5, 10, 12)

To support student's academic success, the parent(s) will:
- Accept that an eating disorder does exist. (N.D. 4, 6)
- Maintain communication with the school nurse. (N.D. 4, 6)
- Identify the impact of disordered eating patterns on the family. (N.D. 4)
- Verbalize their feelings regarding their child's eating disorder or obesity. (N.D. 4)
- Attend follow-up meetings and conferences regarding their child. (N.D. 4)
- Access appropriate healthcare resources to support, treat, and care for their child and themselves. (N.D. 4)
- Request assistance with and make use of school and community resources for increasing effective coping skills. (N.D. 4, 6, 7)

# Case Study

Susan is a 16-year-old student in high school this year. She is in the accelerated-learning program, Scholar's Bowl, drama club, cheerleading, basketball, and track. Susan was mildly obese in elementary school and middle school. Susan entered puberty as a freshman in high school, growing 8 inches and gaining 20 lbs. Susan is the youngest child in her family, and her older siblings are attending colleges on scholarships and continuing to achieve academically.

Susan places a lot of pressure on herself to excel in school and school activities. Her mother is a model for the local department store and expects Susan to always look her best and pursue her drama interests in hopes of a modeling career. Her father is a business manager and expects academic excellence and varsity starting positions in basketball and track; he sees Susan as a potential athletic and academic scholarship recipient at a Division 1 private school. Susan's mother is supportive, yet demanding, and Susan's father perceives the world and its events from a very self-centered perspective.

Susan has returned to school this fall, and in reviewing the athletic physical, the school nurse noticed that she has lost 30 pounds since her previous athletic physical in the spring. On the spring physical, Susan noted that she wanted to weigh less than her current weight at 140 lb. She is 5 feet 8 inches tall.

As Susan's school nurse, you note her food choices at lunch in the cafeteria. Susan has a paper sack lunch from home, which has six grapes, three saltines, and a diet soda.

Susan's cheerleading coach and her accelerated-program teacher came to you separately, each providing additional information indicating a possible eating disorder, anorexia nervosa. You have met with Susan and her parents. Susan believes that she is fat and that her classmates are talking about this during cheerleading practices. Susan begins obsessing about going to cafeteria for lunch by 10 a.m. each school day. Susan's teacher is letting her skip lunch and stay in the classroom.

Although reluctant, the parents agreed to have Susan be seen by their family physician, who astutely referred Susan to specialists in eating disorders. Susan has returned to school and continues in outpatient therapy with medications for anorexia nervosa, anxiety, and depression. Susan was agreeable, and her parents signed the Release of Information forms so the school nurse could exchange information with the therapist. The therapist reports that Susan doesn't feel good about herself or her body; verbalized to the therapist suicidal thoughts 6 months prior to beginning therapy; described elaborate rituals regarding food preparation, cleaning, moving, and not consuming; and continues to verbalize feelings of fullness and overeating, but verbalized desire to learn more about healthy eating patterns so she can return to sports and regular routine. Her therapist is addressing this issue in therapy. According to the discharge planning papers, Susan's body weight is 75% of target weight for young adult females.

Susan is not allowed to begin participation in school activities until released from her physician. Susan's father and coaches want to begin participation next week. The therapist is providing education regarding anorexia nervosa and provided complimentary brochures to the school nurse for education and consistency with interventions and terminology of care.

# Eating Disorders

| Assessment Data | Nursing Diagnosis | Goals | Nursing Interventions | Expected Outcomes |
|---|---|---|---|---|
| Susan reports elaborate rituals regarding food preparation, cleaning, moving, and not consuming. | Anxiety related to eating and discovery of eating rituals resulting in disordered eating patterns. | Susan will recognize the sources of anxiety and fears. | Allow the student to visit the health office when feeling overwhelmed. Provide active listening to assist Susan in expressing anxieties regarding food. Report disturbing statements to therapist/parent as agreed upon in team meetings. Provide rational feedback to Susan in a safe and supportive environment. | The student will verbalize and identify the source(s) of anxiety and fears. The student will describe physiologic responses to anxiety and fear. Susan reports a decrease in anxiety at school over a 4-week period. |
| Susan's body weight is 75% of target weight for young adult female, according to discharge planning papers. | Imbalanced nutrition, less than body requirements, related to self-imposed starvation. | Susan will identify stressors that increase disordered eating episodes. | Treat food consumption as a medication order. Discretely monitor food intake, without Susan's awareness. Enlist counseling staff or trusted cafeteria employee to monitor food intake if school nurse is unable. | Susan will identify stressors that increase disordered eating episodes. |
| Susan's therapist is providing education regarding anorexia nervosa and provided complimentary brochures to the school nurse for education and consistency with interventions and terminology of care. | Disturbed body image related to an unrealistic ideal of thinness. | Susan will verbalize a more realistic self-perception of body size. | Provide emotional support and active listening for Susan to express concerns about body image without validating distorted perceptions. Provide education and awareness to Susan of media distortion of body image. Provide education regarding genetics as indicator of body size and type. | Susan will verbalize a more realistic self-perception of body size. |

| Assessment Data | Nursing Diagnosis | Goals | Nursing Interventions | Expected Outcomes |
|---|---|---|---|---|
| Susan is not allowed to begin participation in school activities until released from physician. Susan verbalized to therapist suicidal thoughts 6 months prior to beginning therapy. Susan's father and coaches want to begin participation next week. | Risk for injury related to malnourished condition. | Susan will request assistance with and make use of school and community resources for increasing effective coping skills. | Monitor and assess for signs and symptoms of suicide using standardized assessment tools.<br><br>Supervise release for participation in physical education, sports, and other school activities.<br><br>Facilitate and educate school staff on the need to adjust activity levels per physician/therapist orders.<br><br>Monitor Susan's participation, observing for signs and symptoms of intolerance.<br><br>Communicate with therapist or parent as directed by treatment plan.<br><br>Encourage healthy hydration. | Susan will not harm herself in the school setting.<br><br>She will seek out school nurse or other trusted adult if she experiences thoughts of suicide or other types of self-harm. |
| Susan continues to verbalize feelings of fullness and overeating, but verbalized desire to learn more about healthy eating patterns so she can return to sports and regular routine. | Readiness for enhanced nutrition related to willingness to learn healthy eating patterns and make educated food choices. | Susan will terminate disordered eating patterns of starvation. | Provide a safe environment in which Susan may eat snacks or meals.<br><br>Support healthy food choices, balanced meal and snack choices. | Susan will verbalize importance of frequent small meals and snacks as an important intervention toward health within 2 weeks.<br><br>Susan will eat at least 50% of prescribed food for meals and snacks during the school day, within 2 weeks. |

| Assessment Data | Nursing Diagnosis | Goals | Nursing Interventions | Expected Outcomes |
|---|---|---|---|---|
| Susan believes she is fat and that her classmates are talking about this during cheer-leading practices.<br><br>Susan begins obsessing about going to cafeteria for lunch by 10 a.m. each school day. Susan's teacher is letting her skip lunch and stay in the classroom | Disturbed thought processes related to malnourished state, low self-esteem, and unrealistic body image. | Susan will develop flexible thought patterns.<br><br>Susan will decrease episodes of obsessive thoughts. | Provide diversional activities that are calming to Susan, such as drawing, reading, or craft activities.<br><br>Educate school personnel regarding healthy lifestyle, including healthy food choices and appropriate exercise, rather than current fad diets. | Susan will verbalize fewer statements reflective of disturbed thoughts within 4 weeks. |
| Susan is not yet eating at school, and her therapist is addressing this issue in therapy. Susan is taking medication daily as well, for anxiety, depression, and disordered eating patterns. | Deficient knowledge of healthy eating habits, proper nutrition, and treatment for disordered eating. | Susan will learn healthy eating patterns and make educated food choices. | Facilitate and provide staff education regarding disordered eating, eating behaviors, and treatment modalities.<br><br>Provide education and support healthy food choices.<br><br>Create a safe environment for learning.<br><br>Monitor for compliance if any medications are taken at school. | Susan will make educated food choices in the school cafeteria or sack lunches within 3 weeks. |
| Susan doesn't feel good about herself or her body, as indicated in her discharge summary and in meeting with school nurse and therapist. | Situational low self-esteem related to disturbed body image and feelings of worthlessness. | Susan will verbalize improved self-esteem. | Provide support and awareness of hypersensitivity of persons with eating disorders, especially emotions surrounding eating and eating behaviors.<br><br>Identify and encourage positive qualities, traits, and abilities of Susan to help build self-esteem.<br><br>Elevate faculty members' awareness of the role of stressors in the classroom and impact on disordered eating. | Susan will make 3 positive statements regarding her talents and abilities within 2 weeks. |

# References

American Psychiatric Association. (2000). *Diagnosis and statistical manual of mental disorders* (4th ed., text revision) (DSM-IV-TR) [CD ROM]. Washington, DC: Author.

Antai-Otong, D. (2003). *Psychiatric nursing: Biological & behavioral concepts.* Clifton Park, NY: Delmar Learning.

Cochrane, C. E. (1998). Eating regulation responses and eating disorders. In G. Stuart, & M. Laraia (Eds.), (6th ed.). *Stuart & Sundeen's principles and practice of psychiatric nursing* (pp. 523–543). St. Louis, MO: Mosby.

Green, M. (2002). *Beneath the surface of eating disorders: An overview of anorexia, bulimia, and binge eating disorders.* Castle Rock, CO: National Association of School Nurses.

Jellinek, M., Patel, B. P., & Froehle, M. C. (Eds.), (2002). *Bright futures in practice: Mental health.* Arlington, VA: National Center for Education in Maternal and Child Health.

Krupnick, S. L. W., & Wade, A. (1999). *Psychiatric care planning* (2nd ed). Springhouse, PA: Springhouse.

NANDA International. (2003). *Nursing diagnoses: Definitions & classification 2003-2004.* Philadelphia: Author.

# Bibliography

*Body mass index (BMI) wheel.* Scarborough, ME: National Association of School Nurses.

Denehy, J. (2002). Taking action to address the problem of obesity. *Journal of School Nursing, 18*(2), 65–67.

Fox, J. A. (1997). *Primary health care of children.* St. Louis, MO: Mosby.

Green, M. (2002). *Beneath the surface of eating disorders* [Manual]. Scarborough, ME: National Association of School Nurses.

National Association of School Nurses. (2002). *Issue Brief: Eating disorders.* Scarborough, ME: Author.

National Association of School Nurses. (Adopted 2002). *Position Statement: Overweight children and adolescents.* Scarborough, ME: Author.

Mosca, N. (2005). *Overweight children: Making a difference—the school nurse role* [Manual]. Scarborough, ME: National Association of School Nurses.

Seidel, H. M. (1999). *Mosby's guide to physical examination* (4th ed.). St. Louis, MO: Mosby.

Skybo, T., Ryan-Wenger, N. (2003). Measures of overweight status in school-age children. *Journal of School Nursing, 19*(3). 172–180.

Zive, M. M., & Pelletier, R. (1997-2000). *Nursing assessment of school age youth. Nutritional status.* (Home Study Module Number 8). Scarborough, ME: National Association of School Nurses.

# Resources

American Academy of Pediatrics
141 Northwest Point Boulevard
Elk Grove Village, IL 60007-1098
847-434-4000
847-434-8000 (fax)
www.aap.org

American Dietetic Association
120 South Riverside Plaza
Suite 2000
Chicago, IL 60606-6995
1-800-877-1600
www.eatright.org

Bright Futures Project
Georgetown University
Box 571272
Washington, DC 20057-1272
202-784-9556
202-784-9777 (fax)
www.brightfutures.org

Food and Nutrition Information Center
Agricultural Research Service, USDA
National Agricultural Library, Room 105
10301 Baltimore Avenue
Beltsville, MD 20705-2351
301-504-5719
www.nal.usda.gov/fnic

National Association of Anorexia Nervosa and
Associated Disorders (ANAS)
PO Box 7
Highland Park, IL 60035
847-831-3438
www.anad.org

National Association of School Nurses
PO Box 1300
Scarborough, ME 04070
1-877-627-6476
www.nasn.org

National Center for Education in Maternal and Child
Health
Georgetown University
Box 571272
Washington, DC 20057-1272
202-784-9770
www.ncemch.org

NHLBI Health Information Center
PO Box 30105
Bethesda, MD 20824-0105
301-592-8573
http://www.nhlbisupport.com/bmi/bmicalc.htm

Screening for Mental Health
One Washington Street
Suite 304
Wellesley Hills, MA 02481
781-239-0071
781-431-7447 (fax)
http://www.mentalhealthscreening.org/eat.htm

# Chapter Thirty-nine

# Encopresis

## Nancy W. Mosca and Kella Haren

## Introduction

Encopresis is defined as stool incontinence after an age when a child should be able to control his or her bowel movements, usually 4 years of age. Primary encopresis occurs when a child has never established fecal continence; secondary encopresis is when the incontinence develops after a period of established fecal continence. The central characteristic of encopresis is repeated passage of feces into inappropriate places such as one's clothing. Most often this is involuntary, but in rare instances it may be intentional (Schmitt, 2001).

## Pathophysiology

DiLorenzo and Benninga (2004) classify fecal incontinence into four categories, each with a distinct pathophysiology: functional fecal retention with overflow soiling, functional nonretentive fecal soiling, anorectal malformations, and spinal defects. Surgical interventions are typical treatment for congenital anorectal and spinal defects and are beyond the scope of this chapter. Medical literature uses the term *encopresis* interchangeably to describe the first two categories (American Psychiatric Association [APA], 2000).

Encopresis most often is involuntary and associated with constipation and stool retention. Most children with encopresis have a history of constipation or a history of passing large and/or painful bowel movements. Because of painful bowel movements and constipation, children may not completely empty themselves when they go to the bathroom. Over a period of time, the large intestine fills with stool and stretches out of shape. With this overextension and stretching, liquid stool from the small intestine begins to leak around the formed stool in the colon. Leakage is usually in small amounts at first. As time goes on, and the intestine stretches further, the amount of leakage increases to a point where a child will pass whole bowel movements in their underwear. The child does not typically feel an urge to defecate when the accident occurs. Since the rectum almost always contains stool, and the nerves that signal the brain to empty are continually being stimulated, the child's brain learns to ignore the signal, tuning out the signal to pass a bowel movement. With the chronic stretching and expanding of the large intestine

(megacolon), the colon's muscles and nerves become damaged. Sensations of impending bowel movements get suppressed and confused, resulting in fecal soiling or encopresis (DiLorenzo & Benninga, 2004). What usually begins as a functional voluntary withholding progresses to a decreased urge to defecate because of rectal enlargement and loss of sensation of a full rectum.

On occasion, encopresis can be voluntary. When this is the case, there is no evidence of constipation by history or physical examination. The child's bowel movements are typically of normal form and consistency, and soiling is intermittent. Stool may be deposited in a prominent location. Historically, this uncommon type of encopresis has been considered a symptom of an emotional disturbance in children, representing an impulsive action triggered by unconscious anger (DiLorenzo & Benninga, 2004). Differential diagnoses associated with this uncommon type of encopresis include child abuse, depression, autism, and attention deficit disorder (University of Michigan Health System [UMHS], 2003). The *Diagnostic and Statistical Manual of Mental Disorders (DSM-IV-TR)* (APA, 2000) associates this type of nonretentive encopresis with the presence of oppositional defiant disorder or conduct disorder. However, this theory is being disputed in newer studies, where serious psychological disorders have not been observed with encopretic children, and psychotherapy treatment alone is often unsuccessful (DiLorenzo & Benninga, 2004; Cox, Morris, Borowitz, & Sutphen, 2002; McGrath, Mellon, & Murphy, 2000). Recent trends suggest a greater appreciation by pediatricians of encopresis as primarily a physical condition rather than psychological in nature (Fishman, Rappaport, Schonwald, & Nurko, 2003).

Physical complications of encopresis can include anal fissures from passing large hard formed stools; urinary incontinence; and bladder infection due to the large full colon pressing on the bladder and preventing it from emptying completely (DiLorenzo & Benninga, 2004).

Psychological complications resulting from encopresis center around self-esteem issues related to embarrassment about the condition and treatment of peers or family members. Isolation for children with encopresis is common (Fishman et al., 2003).

## Management

Treatment for encopresis typically includes three phases: catharsis, maintenance, and follow-up. Education is a key component to success. The importance of explaining the physiologic basis of constipation and soiling to both the child and family helps to alleviate blame and enlists cooperation. Along with personal face-to-face opportunities to educate the family, Internet instruction for both parent and child has been demonstrated to provide a comfortable source for education and actually improve treatment outcome in some instances (Borowitz et al., 2003).

### Catharsis Phase

The goal of this phase is to empty the bowel. A 3-day regimen of enema (day 1), rectal suppository (day 2), and laxative (day 3), repeated for four cycles, is common management practice. A child may need to be hospitalized for catharsis if the retention is severe, home compliance is poor, or parents should not administer enemas for psychological reasons (Dunn, 2000).

### Maintenance Phase

The goal of the second phase is to establish regular soft bowel movements, increase the child's ability to sense the urge to defecate, and eliminate soiling. This phase involves medication, behavior, and dietary components (Mikkelsen, 2001; UMHS, 2003). Stool softeners such as mineral oil are often used in combination or alternatively with laxatives. One laxative that has demonstrated success with encopresis is polyethylene glycol 3350 (PEG), also known by its trade name, Miralax (Loening-Baucke, 2002; Pashankar, Bishop, & Loening-Baucke, 2003). A significant advantage of this drug is its odorless and tasteless characteristics. As a powder, PEG can be added to other fluids without altering the taste.

Behavior training includes maintaining a toileting diary, instituting toileting routines, providing positive reinforcement for the child's accomplishments, and maintaining neutral to positive attitudes around toileting by caregivers. Toileting diaries should document time, amount, and location of bowel movements, to include soiling episodes. Stool frequency of once or twice a day and no soiling indicates no impaction. Stool frequency of less than every 3 days and/or an increase in soiling suggests impaction. The toileting diary will help to determine the times of day that toilet sitting will be most successful (UMHS, 2003).

Toilet sitting should be at regular times, usually after meals and at bedtime for about 5 to 10 minutes. Scheduling after a meal is eaten takes advantage of the gastrocolic reflex, where consuming a meal stimulates evacuation of the colon and rectum. Use of a timer is helpful. Children should be shown the proper positioning on the toilet, with their upper body flexed forward slightly at the hips and use of foot support (UMHS, 2003). Fun reading material, music, or other enjoyable activity can be arranged to occur with a toilet sit. Child should be praised for cooperation with the various components of treatment. Caregivers should maintain positive attitude around the child's progress with toileting. Punitive approaches and embarrassment should be avoided at all cost. A standard clean-up procedure, carried out matter-of-factly and emotionally neutral, should be protocol.

High-fiber foods are included as part of the child's daily intake. The American Heart Association's recommended fiber intake for children over 2 years of age is their age in years plus 5 g (http://www.americanheart.org, 2004). For example, a 10-year-old child should have a dietary fiber intake of 15 g per day (10 + 5). Some recommendations for children with functional constipation and soiling include increasing daily fiber intake to 10 g plus the

**Table 1. Sample High-Fiber Food Choices**

| Food Item | Serving Size | Fiber Content (grams) | Calories (kcal) |
|---|---|---|---|
| Wheat bran raisin muffin | 1 muffin | 2.8 | 106 |
| Whole-grain/mixed-grain/7-grain bread | 0.92-ounce slice | 1.7 | 65 |
| Oat bran bread | 1.1-ounce slice | 1.4 | 71 |
| Oatmeal cooked, quick/regular | 1 cup | 4.0 | 145 |
| Oatmeal, instant dry, apples & cinnamon, Malt-O-Meal | 1.8-ounce packet | 5.0 | 190 |
| Cheerios, General Mills | 1 cup (1.1 ounces) | 2.7 | 111 |
| Cracklin' Oat Bran, Kellogg's | 3/4 cup (1.9 ounces) | 6.4 | 225 |
| Bran, 100% , Post | 1/3 cup (1 ounce) | 8.3 | 83 |

**Table 1. Sample High-Fiber Food Choices**

| Food Item | Serving Size | Fiber Content (grams) | Calories (kcal) |
|---|---|---|---|
| Fiber One , General Mills | 1/2 cup (1.1 ounce) | 14.4 | 59 |
| Frosted Mini Wheats, bite size, Kellogg's | 1 cup (1.9 ounces) | 5.5 | 189 |
| Brown Rice, long grain, cooked | 1 cup | 3.5 | 216 |
| Rye wafer cracker | One triple cracker | 5.7 | 84 |
| Whole wheat cracker | 0.5 ounce (~ 3.5 crackers) | 1.5 | 63 |
| Broccoli | 1 medium stalk | 5.2 | 50 |
| Brussels sprouts | 1/2 cup | 2.0 | 30 |
| Collards, chopped, boiled | 1 cup | 5.3 | 49 |
| Peas, green, boiled | 1 cup | 8.8 | 134 |
| Corn, fresh yellow, boiled | 1 cup | 4.6 | 177 |
| Sweet potato, boiled, without skin, mashed | 1 cup | 5.9 | 344 |
| Apple, raw, with skin | 1 medium, (2 3/4" diameter) | 3.7 | 81 |
| Blueberries, raw | 1 cup | 3.9 | 81 |
| Apricots, dried | 1 cup, halves | 9.5 | 313 |
| Fig, dried | 1 fig | 2.3 | 48 |
| Orange, raw | 1 medium, (2 5/8" diameter) | 3.1 | 62 |
| Pear, raw | 1 medium | 4.0 | 98 |
| Raisins | 1/4 cup | 2.0 | 130 |
| Strawberries, raw | 1 cup, whole | 3.3 | 43 |
| Baked beans, Bush's homestyle | 1/2 cup | 8.0 | 150 |
| Chickpeas (garbanzo beans), canned | 1/2 cup | 5.3 | 143 |
| Kidney beans, canned | 1/2 cup | 4.5 | 104 |
| Refried beans, canned | 1/2 cup | 6.7 | 119 |
| Popcorn, plain, air-popped | 1 ounce (3.5 cups) | 4.3 | 108 |
| Sunflower seeds, whole, roasted and toasted | 1 ounce | 4.0 | 160 |
| Peanuts, dry roasted | 1 ounce (28 nuts) | 2.3 | 166 |
| Walnuts | 1 ounce (14 halves) | 1.9 | 185 |

Adapted from Bowes and Church's Food Values of Portions Commonly Used (18th ed.), by J. A. Pennington and J. S. Douglass, 2005, Philadelphia: Lippincott Williams & Wilkins. Copyright 2005 by Lippincott William & Wilkins.

child's age in years (UMHS, 2003). High-fiber foods include bran muffins, whole-grain breads and cereals, brown rice, raw vegetables, cooked vegetables, dried fruits such as raisins and plums, raw fruits (especially those with seeds or skins), legumes (beans), popcorn, nuts, seeds, and high-fiber snack bars. Refer to **Table 1** for examples of high-fiber food. Fiber retains water for softer stool consistency and adds bulk to the stool, facilitating propulsion through the intestinal tract.

Adequate fluid intake is also essential to prevent constipation from recurring. In general, 2 ounces of nondairy fluids are recommended for each gram of fiber intake (UMHS, 2003). Frequent opportunities for extra fluid intake should be provided. Sorbitol-based juices such as prune, pear, and apple increase the water content of stools.

*Follow-up Phase*

The goal of normal defecation without constipation is long-range and can have setbacks. In general, 4 to 6 weeks of consistent treatment may be required before substantial and consistent improvement in symptoms is achieved. Typical follow-up appointments are every 2 weeks in this phase, reviewing success and problems with the treatment regimen. Once maintenance therapy is well established, follow-up intervals can be from 1 to 3 months until medication is weaned (UMHS, 2003). Recurrences are common if the family stops the diet regimen, there is an interruption in routine (holidays, vacation), or the child has an illness causing a gastric disruption (Christopherson & Mortsweet, 2005). For complex cases, referral to a child psychologist is beneficial for long-term success.

## Individualized Healthcare Plan

### Assessment

*History* (from parent interview, regarding child of concern)
- Child's history of toilet training: age at onset, techniques used, persons responsible, age when bladder training completed, age when bowel training completed
- Child's bowel patterns since toilet training: description of frequency, consistency and amount, past episodes of constipation, and methods used to treat, crying or distress during bowel movements, blood in stool, unusual position used to defecate.
- Child's bowel patterns since soiling began: precipitated by constipation, frequency of soiling, amount of soiling (smears versus whole stool), timing and circumstances surrounding soiling episodes (time of day, activities engaged in at the time of, and/or precipitating, the soiling event)
- Child's diet history: Describe child's typical daily diet, amount of fiber and fluids in typical day, describe child's appetite, recent weight loss or gain, any refusal to eat

*History* (from interview with child)
- Child's perception: what is causing the soiling, child's feelings about the issue.

*Current Status and Management* (from parent interview, medical records)
- Diagnostic/treatment regimen: examinations and tests done, physician orders and recommendations
- Medication use: all medicines taken regularly or as needed, doses and frequencies
- Diet: 24-hour recall, noting amount of fiber (fruits, vegetables, and whole grain servings). Amount of fiber servings recommended by physician.
- Fluid intake: amount of fluid ingested per day. Amount recommended by physician. Use of water bottle in school.
- GI: any vomiting, complaints of nausea, stomach pain or discomfort, gas
- Bowel elimination: last bowel movement: time of day, stool consistency, color, amount, pain or strain with evacuation, blood present. Body position used when on toilet to defecate. Ability to contract sphincter muscles at will. When catharsis phase of treatment was completed, describe regimen, and where student currently is in treatment protocol. Does child feel the urge to defecate? If so, what do they do when it occurs?
- Exercise: amount and type of physical activity engaged in daily

*Self-care* (from parent/child interview)
- Words used for bowel movement, urination
- Assistance needed to handle soiling clean-up
- Ability to use school restroom, both psychomotor coordination and comfort level, fears
- Willing to stop playing at recess to go to the bathroom; having time after school dismissal to use bathroom before getting on the bus
- Willing to ask teacher to use the bathroom

*Psychosocial Status* (from parent/child interview)
- Age, developmental age, intellectual age
- Affect, general attitude toward condition, description of typical mood
- Relationships with peers, any teasing or bullying behavior
- Participation in social activities during or after school
- Relationship with family members, any crisis at home
- Description of typical school day, condition student is in when arrives home
- Any reluctance to attend school
- Description of typical day off from school

*Academic Issues* (from teacher interview)
- Attendance record: number of absences in current school year, and reasons. Number of days sent home for soiling, number of days missed for doctor appointments. Frequency of leaving classroom for bathroom breaks.
- Academic performance: past and current achievement, changes in grades
- Classroom behavior: behavior problems in the classroom, withdrawn behavior, posturing (i.e., stiffening, standing in a corner, straight-legged, flushed face, wiggling, doing "a little dance," rocking); victim of teasing, bullying, classroom relationships with classmates
- Need for modifications in school day routine: Inclusion of extra fluids and fiber foods during school day, access to private bathroom, frequent bathroom breaks, modified lunch time
- Determine need for 504 plan or individualized education program (IEP) evaluation.

## Nursing Diagnoses (N.D.) (NANDA, 2003)

N.D. 1 Bowel incontinence (NANDA 00014) related to:
- environmental factors (i.e., inaccessible bathroom)
- incomplete emptying of bowel
- impaction
- dietary habits
- toileting self-care deficit

N.D. 2 Constipation (NANDA 00011) related to:
- environmental changes
- habitual denial/ignoring of urge to defecate
- insufficient physical activity
- irregular defecation habits
- inadequate toileting (i.e., timeliness, positioning, privacy)
- poor eating habits
- insufficient fiber intake
- insufficient fluid intake
- change in usual foods and eating pattern

N.D. 3 Bathing/hygiene self-care deficit (NANDA 00108) related to:
- decreased or lack of motivation
- severe anxiety
- perceptual or cognitive impairment
- pain
- environmental barriers

N.D. 4 Toileting self-care deficit (NANDA 00110) related to:
- environmental barriers
- decreased or lack of motivation
- severe anxiety
- pain

N.D.5 Situational low self-esteem (NANDA 00120) related to:
- developmental changes
- disturbed body image
- functional impairment (soiling)
- failures/rejections

**N.D.6** Risk for situational low self-esteem (NANDA 00153) related to:
- developmental changes
- disturbed body image
- functional impairment (soiling)
- failures/rejections

**N.D.7** Delayed growth and development (NANDA 00111) related to:
- indifference
- effects of physical disability
- inadequate caretaking

**N.D.8** Impaired social interaction (NANDA 00052) related to:
- environmental barriers
- self-concept disturbance

## Goals

The student will establish a normal pattern of bowel functioning. (N.D. 1, 2)

The student will be continent of stool with no soiling episodes. (N.D. 1)

The student will recognize the urge to move bowels. (N.D. 1, 4)

The student will perform needed hygiene activity with soiling episode. (N.D. 3)

The student will use toilet facility at school when recognizing urge to defecate, or during scheduled timed attempts. (N.D. 1, 4)

The student will follow diet and medication regimen as prescribed. (N.D. 2)

The student will keep a daily toileting diary. (N.D. 1, 2, 4)

The student will display behaviors of positive self-esteem. (N.D. 5, 6)

The student will participate in developmentally appropriate peer group social activities. (N.D. 7, 8)

## Nursing Interventions

Meet with parents/guardian to assess their understanding and obtain the prescribed treatment regimen. (N.D 1, 2)

Establish a plan for monitoring bowel patterns with student while at school. (N.D. 1, 2)

Maintain daily toileting diary with student. (N.D. 1, 2)

Arrange for student to come to nurse's office after lunch every day for a toilet sit and, if necessary, at the beginning of each school day if student unable to toilet-sit at home before school. (N.D. 1, 2, 4)

Assist student to learn to bear down using technique of blowing on a balloon while sitting on toilet and using foot support. (N.D. 1, 2, 4)

Oversee diet regimen as prescribed. Arrange for fiber foods to be available at school. (N.D. 1, 2)

Encourage generous amounts of fluid intake throughout the day. (N.D. 1, 2)

Arrange for permission for student to use the bathroom any time student requests. (N.D. 1, 4)

Arrange for privacy while child is in bathroom and provide elevated foot support, if appropriate. (N.D. 3, 4, 5, 6)

Develop a standard clean-up procedure, carried out matter-of-factly and emotionally neutral. (N.D. 1, 3, 4 )

Reward with praise. Tie other rewards or incentives offered to passage of stool in the toilet, rather than for "not soiling" underwear. (N.D 1, 5, 6)

Communicate with parents/guardian regularly regarding progress. (N.D. 1, 7)

Refer to school counselor for individual supportive counseling surrounding esteem and social interactions with peer group issues. (N.D. 5, 6, 7, 8)

Monitor for signs and symptoms of constipation. (N.D. 1, 2)

Monitor bowel movements through use of diary. (N.D. 1, 2)

Encourage fluids throughout the school day. (N.D. 1, 2)

Instruct student on high-fiber food choices. (N.D. 1, 2)

Institute a toileting schedule at school. (N.D. 1, 2)

Ensure that student performs daily toilet-sits using proper positioning as scheduled. (N.D. 1,3)

Provide privacy during scheduled toilet-sits. (N.D.1, 3)

Keep change of clothes available in health office. (N.D. 3, 4)

Provide soap, towels, cleansing wipes as needed in a private, accessible place, maintaining student's privacy. (N.D. 3, 7)

Establish student's food preferences. (N.D. 2)

Instruct student on high-fiber food choices. (N.D. 1, 2)

*Chapter Thirty-nine: Encopresis*

Incorporate fiber into student's food preferences. (N.D. 2)

Review fiber and diet intake with student during each visit to the health office. (N.D.2, 7)

Instruct student on needed 2 ounces of nondairy fluids per each gram of fiber intake (N.D. 2)

Provide access to fluids throughout the school day. (N.D. 2)

Arrange for use of water bottle in the classroom. (N.D. 2)

Review fluid intake with student during each visit to health office. (N.D. 2, 7)

Encourage student to identify strengths. (N.D. 5, 6, 7)

Reinforce personal strengths student identifies. (N.D. 5, 6)

Convey confidence in student's ability to handle situation. (N.D. 5, 6, 7)

Provide privacy in the nurse's office for discussions, toileting, or cleaning activities. (N.D. 5, 6 )

Consult with teacher to provide activities in classroom that allow for success. (N.D. 5, 6, 7, 8)

Consult with teacher to monitor for signs of teasing or bullying by peers (N.D. 5, 6, 7, 8)

Encourage teacher to incorporate lessons on tolerance of differences, understanding physical disabilities, and/or value of empathy toward students faced with challenges. (N.D. 5, 6, 7, 8)

Refer to school counselor for individual supportive counseling surrounding esteem and social interactions with peer group issues. (N.D. 5, 6, 7, 8)

Build trusting relationship with student. (N.D. 5, 6, 7)

Build trusting relationship with parents/guardians. (N.D. 5, 6, 7)

Encourage student to be independent in performing toileting and hygiene care. (N.D. 3, 4, 7)

Encourage participation in school activities. (N.D. 5, 6, 7, 8)

Comfort student when upset or after incontinence episode. (N.D. 5, 6, 7)

Encourage independence in maintaining daily toileting diary. (N.D. 7)

Consult with teacher for ways to include student in group activities. (N.D. 8 )

Give student feedback in improvement of personal appearance. (N.D. 8 )

## Expected Student Outcomes

The student will:
- Attend school each day. (N.D. 7)
- Report to the health office for daily toilet-sitting at prescribed time. (N.D. 1)
- Return to class promptly, within 3 minutes, after daily visit to health office. (N.D. 1, 7)
- Participate in curricular school activities. (N.D. 5, 6, 7, 8)
- Recognize the urge to defecate. (N.D. 1)
- Control stool passage. (N.D. 1)
- Evacuate stool at least every 2 days. (N.D. 1, 2)
- Respond to urge in a timely manner. (N.D. 1, 2)
- Drink an adequate amount of fluid each school day. (N.D. 2)
- Eat at least two high-fiber foods each school day. (N.D. 2)
- Maintain toileting diary. (N.D. 1, 2)
- Toilet independently. (N.D. 4)
- Stay soil-free throughout the school day. (N.D. 1, 4, 6, 7, 8)
- Include high-fiber foods in diet daily to prevent constipation. (N.D. 2)
- Drink adequate amount of fluid during school day to prevent constipation. (N.D. 2)
- Use toileting diary to monitor constipation symptoms over time. (N.D. 1, 2)
- Clean perineal area after soiling incident. (N.D. 3)
- Wash hands following cleaning up after soiling incident. (N.D. 3)
- Keep clean change of clothing at school for hygiene needs. (N.D. 3)
- Clean up bathroom area once performing self-care after soiling incident. (N.D. 3)
- Respond to urge to have a bowel movement in timely manner. (N.D. 4)
- Get to and from toilet. (N.D. 4)
- Position self on toilet to facilitate bowel movement. (N.D. 4)
- Empty bowel in toilet. (N.D. 4)
- Wipe self after bowel movement. (N.D. 4)
- Wash hands after toileting complete. (N.D. 4)
- Stand erect with head raised. (N.D. 5, 6)
- Maintain eye contact. (N.D. 5, 6)

- Openly engage in conversation. (N.D. 5, 6)
- Exhibit pleasant, bright facial expression, smiles. (N.D. 5, 6)
- Describe successes in school work. (N.D. 5, 6, 7)
- Describe successes with friends. (N.D. 5, 6, 7,8)
- Express feelings of self-worth. (N.D. 5, 6)
- Practice good health habits regarding diet. (N.D. 7)
- Develop close friendships. (N.D. 5, 6, 7, 8)
- Use effective social interaction skills. (N.D. 7, 8)
- Display self-confidence. (N.D. 5, 6, 7)
- Assume responsibility for following treatment regimen. (N.D. 7)
- Perform in school to level of ability. (N.D. 7)
- Interact with close friends. (N.D. 7, 8)
- Participate as a member of a group at school. (N.D. 7, 8)
- Interact with family members. (N.D. 7, 8)
- Cooperate with others. (N.D. 7, 8)
- Exhibit warmth. (N.D. 5, 6, 7, 8)
- Appear relaxed. (N.D. 5, 6, 8)

## Case Study

Eleven-year-old Daniel Winslow is a sixth-grade boy, new to the middle school this school year. This fall he was sent to the school nurse's office several times by his math teacher because of foul-smelling fecal odor. Students in math class make comments about the odor and complain to the teacher about Daniel stinking. Each time, Daniel comes into the school nurse's office with his head down, eyes gazed at the floor. He offers no explanation, saying he can't help it, answering in a soft voice with a flat affect.

After the first incident, the school nurse phoned Daniel's mother, and she agreed to take him to the pediatrician to be evaluated. Several more incidents occurred between that conversation and Mrs. Winslow reporting back to the school nurse that the pediatrician diagnosed Daniel with encopresis and started him on a treatment schedule to resolve the problem. Daniel received enemas and mineral oil treatment over the first weekend and is now on a daily stool softener. According to his mother, the doctor wants Daniel to drink "extra" fluids and increase fiber in his diet. Also, he is supposed to have regular toilet sitting time 15 minutes after eating lunch. Daniel is refusing to do this in the students' bathroom, saying kids will bother him.

The school nurse meets with Daniel and works out a plan to help him stay continent at school. Daniel agrees to come to the nurse's office after lunch and sit on the toilet in the single bathroom in her office for 10 minutes each day. The school nurse promises Daniel privacy and no interruptions during that time. In addition, Daniel and the school nurse discuss the diet/toileting diary the pediatrician wants Daniel to keep for 2 months. Daniel agrees to bring it every Friday to review his progress with her. They will also go over the school lunch menu for the following week at that time to identify food choices high in fiber. Arrangements are made for Daniel to be able to have a water bottle in class to support his increased fluid intake needs.

# Encopresis

| Assessment Data | Nursing Diagnosis | Goals | Nursing Interventions | Expected Outcomes |
|---|---|---|---|---|
| Soiling incidents occurring 2 to 3 times a week.<br><br>Reports "doesn't feel like he has to go." | Does not like to use the student bathroom in school.<br><br>Bowel incontinence related to environmental factors (i.e., Inaccessible bathroom), incomplete emptying of bowel, impaction, dietary habits, toileting self-care deficit. | Daniel will be continent of stool with no soiling incidents during school within 1 month.<br><br>Daniel will establish a normal pattern of bowel functioning by the end of 2 months. | Meet with parents to assess their understanding and review the prescribed treatment regimen.<br><br>Assist Daniel to maintain toileting diary.<br><br>Arrange permission for Daniel to use the bathroom any time during the school day he requests.<br><br>Arrange for Daniel to have privacy in health office bathroom for daily toilet sits after lunch.<br><br>Communicate with parents regularly regarding Daniel's progress. | Daniel will recognize urge to defecate.<br><br>Daniel will come to the health office daily for toilet sits after lunch<br><br>Daniel will have a bowel movement at least every 2 days.<br><br>Daniel will maintain his diet/toileting diary each day.<br><br>Daniel will stay soil-free throughout the school day. |
| History of 4 days or more without bowel movement.<br><br>History of diet including no or very little fiber.<br><br>History of pain and discomfort when passing stool.<br><br>Stool reported in past to often be of hard consistency.<br><br>Currently diagnosed with retentive encopresis, and under medical management. | Constipation related to environmental changes, habitual denial/ ignoring of urge to defecate, insufficient physical activity, irregular defecation habits, inadequate toileting (i.e., timeliness, positioning, privacy), poor eating habits, insufficient fiber intake, insufficient fluid intake, change in usual foods and eating pattern. | Daniel will establish a pattern of bowel functioning with no reports of hard, painful stools by the end of 1 month. | Establish Daniel's food preferences, exploring ways to incorporate fiber.<br><br>Work with Daniel to recognize high-fiber food choices on school lunch menus.<br><br>Keep high-fiber snack in health office for Daniel when school lunch is limited in fiber options.<br><br>Monitor for signs and symptoms of constipation. | Daniel includes high-fiber foods in every lunch meal.<br><br>Daniel drinks at least 2 ounces of fluid for every gram of fiber ingested.<br><br>Daniel uses diet/toileting diary to monitor constipation symptoms. |

| Assessment Data | Nursing Diagnosis | Goals | Nursing Interventions | Expected Outcomes |
|---|---|---|---|---|
| Frequently smells of feces in school.<br><br>Soiling incidents in school. | Bathing/hygiene self-care deficit related to decreased or lack of motivation, severe anxiety, perceptual or cognitive impairment, pain, environmental barriers. | Daniel will independently manage hygiene clean-up after soiling incident within 1 week. | Monitor Daniel's fluid and fiber intake during school day, for compliance with treatment regimen.<br><br>Encourage Daniel to drink at least 2 ounces for every gram of fiber ingested.<br><br>Obtain permission for Daniel to have a water bottle in the classroom.<br><br>Review diet/toileting diary with Daniel weekly, assisting him to recognize relationship of diet and activity to constipation symptoms.<br><br>Provide privacy for clean-up.<br><br>Keep change of clothes available in health office.<br><br>Provide soap, towels, cleansing wipes, plastic bag for soiled clothes in a place where Daniel can always access, with some privacy, or with minimal attention of others.<br><br>Maintain an emotionally neutral, matter-of-fact approach with Daniel during soiling and clean-up episodes. | Daniel will clean perineal area after soiling incident using soap, cleansing wipes, towels.<br><br>Daniel will wash hands following clean-up from soiling incident.<br><br>Daniel will bring in a replacement set of clean clothes from home when using extra set at school. |

| Assessment Data | Nursing Diagnosis | Goals | Nursing Interventions | Expected Outcomes |
|---|---|---|---|---|
| Soiling episodes occurring at school.<br><br>Classmates complaining of smell, not wanting Daniel in group activities.<br><br>Slouching posture, head down, rarely making eye contact with others. | Risk for situational low self-esteem related to developmental changes, disturbed body image, functional impairment (soiling), failures/rejections. | Daniel will display behaviors of positive self-esteem within 1 month of treatment regimen commencing. | Engage Daniel in discussion of issues other than his bowel movements and soiling.<br><br>Encourage Daniel to identify his strengths.<br><br>Reinforce Daniel's identified personal strengths.<br><br>Reward with praise.<br><br>Convey confidence in Daniel to manage the situation.<br><br>Provide privacy for Daniel during discussions, toileting, or cleaning activities. | Daniel will maintain eye contact when engaged with another in conversation.<br><br>Daniel will initiate and openly engage in conversation with teacher, school nurse, classmates.<br><br>Daniel's facial expression will be pleasant, bright, with smiles noted.<br><br>Daniel will describe successes in school or at home.<br><br>Daniel will describe successes with peers. |
| | | | Consult with teacher to provide activities in the classroom that allow for success.<br><br>Encourage teacher to incorporate lessons on tolerance of differences, understanding physical disabilities, and empathy toward students faced with challenges.<br><br>Refer to school counselor or child psychologist for individual supportive counseling surrounding esteem. Daniel will stand erect with head raised. | |

| Assessment Data | Nursing Diagnosis | Goals | Nursing Interventions | Expected Outcomes |
|---|---|---|---|---|
| Frequently observed alone in lunch room. | Teacher reports classmates not including Daniel in conversations, activities<br><br>Impaired social interaction related environmental barriers, self-concept disturbance. | Daniel will participate in developmentally appropriate peer group social activities (i.e., attending lunch-time intramural boys basketball, joining science club, sit with peers at the lunch table) by end of first grading period. | Consult with teacher for ways to include Daniel in group activities.<br><br>Discuss with Daniel his interests and willingness to join a group or activity.<br><br>Encourage Daniel to join one new activity.<br><br>Provide Daniel positive feedback with any personal appearance improvement.<br><br>Compliment Daniel when he is observed engaging in conversation with another student. | Daniel interacts with close friends.<br><br>Daniel participates as a member of a group at school.<br><br>Daniel interacts with family members.<br><br>Daniel displays warmth and cooperation in his interaction with others.<br><br>Daniel displays a relaxed appearance when in group settings with his peers. |

# References

American Psychiatric Association. (2000). *Diagnostic and statistical manual of mental disorders* (4th ed., text revision) *(DSM-IV-TR)*. Washington DC: Author.

Borowitz, S., Cox, D. J., Kovatchev, B., McKnight, L., Ritterband, L. M., & Sutphen, J. (2003). An internet intervention as adjunctive therapy for pediatric encopresis. *Journal of Consulting and Clinical Psychology, 71*(5), 910–917.

Christopherson, E., & Mortsweet, S. L. (2005). Soiling problems (encopresis). In L. M. Osborn, T. G. DeWitt, L. R. First, & J. A. Zenel (Eds.). *Pediatrics* (pp. 1614-1619). Philadelphia: Mosby.

Cox, D. J., Morris, J., Borowitz, S. M., & Sutphen, J. L. (2002). Psychological differences of children with and without chronic encopresis. *Journal of Pediatric Psychology, 27*, 585–591.

DiLorenzo, C., & Benninga, M. A. (2004). Pathophysiology of pediatric fecal incontinence. *Gastroenterology, 126*(1 Suppl. 1), 533–540.

Dunn, A. M. (2000). Elimination patterns. In C.E. Burns, M.A. Brady, A.M. Dunn, & N.B. Starr (Eds.). *Pediatric Primary Care: A Handbook for Nurse Practitioners* (2nd ed., pp. 327-342). Philadelphia: Saunders.

Fishman, L., Rappaport, L., Schonwald, A., & Nurko, S. (2003). Trends in referral to a single encopresis clinic over 20 years. *Pediatrics, 111*(5), e604–607.

Loening-Baucke, V. (2002). Encopresis. *Current Opinion in Pediatrics, 14*, 570–575.

Loening-Baucke, V., Miele, E., & Staiano, A. (2004). Fiber (glucomannan) is beneficial in the treatment of childhood constipation. *Pediatrics, 113*(3), e259–264.

McGrath, M. L., Mellon, M. W., & Murphy, L. (2000). Empirically supported treatments in pediatric psychology: Constipation and encopresis. *Journal of Pediatric Psychology, 25*, 225–254.

Mikkelsen, E. J. (2001). Enuresis and encopresis: Ten years of progress. *Journal of American Academy of Child and Adolescent Psychiatry, 40*(10), 1146–1158.

NANDA International (2003). *Nursing diagnoses: definitions & classification 2003-2004*. Philadelphia: Author.

Pashankar, D. S., Bishop, W. P., & Loening-Baucke, V. (2003). Long-term efficacy of polyethylene glycol 3350 for the treatment of chronic constipation in children with and without encopresis. *Clinical Pediatrics, 42*(9), 815–819.

Pennington, J. A., & Douglass, J. S. (2005). *Bowes & Church's food values of portions commonly* used (18th ed.). Philadelphia: Lippincott Williams & Wilkins.

Schmitt, B. D. (2001). Encopresis. In Hoekelman, et al., (Eds.), *Primary pediatric care*, (4th ed.). St. Louis, MO: Mosby.

University of Michigan Health System. (2003). *Functional constipation and soiling in children: Guidelines for clinical care*. Retrieved November, 17, 2004, from http://cme.med.umich.edu/iCME/constipation03/guideline.asp

Galvin M. (1989). *Clouds and clocks: A story for children who soil*. Washington, DC: Magination Press.

# Resources

Your Child and Encopresis
http://www.medicine.uiowa.edu/uhs/enco.cfm

Ucanpooptoo Program
http://www.ucanpooptoo.com
A controlled intervention program to be used by students ideally between 6 and 12 years of age. Developed by researchers at the University of Virginia.

Encopresis
http://www.healthsystem.virginia.edu/uvahealth/peds_digest/encopres.cfm

UMHS Your Child: Development and Behavior Resources
http://www.med.umich.edu/1libr/yourchild/encopre.htm

# Chapter Forty

# Fragile X Syndrome

Mary Jo Martin

## Introduction

Fragile X syndrome knows no boundaries. It appears in children of all ethnic, racial, and socioeconomic backgrounds. Fragile X, or Martin-Bell, syndrome is a sex-linked genetic disorder and is the most common form of inherited mental retardation (Fast, 2003). In recent years, more has been learned about fragile X syndrome. Adults and children with no known cause for their mental impairment are being tested and correctly diagnosed. Multidisciplinary school programs must be provided to meet the educational and health needs of these special individuals.

## Pathophysiology

The fragile X syndrome is caused by an abnormal gene on the lower end of the long arm of the X chromosome. This fragile site has been determined to be caused by a gene mutation that results in excessive repeats of nucleotide in a specific deoxyribonucleic acid (DNA) segment on the chromosome (Wong, 2001).

Like other sex-linked disorders, fragile X syndrome primarily affects males. Approximately four times as many males as females have the disorder. Because females have two X chromosomes and males have one X and one Y chromosome, men with the fragile X gene pass it on to all of their daughters and none of their sons. Mothers have a 50-50 chance of passing it on to either their son or their daughter (Warren & Nelson, 1994).

The physical characteristics of fragile X may be quite subtle or pronounced. Features can include a long, narrow face, large ears, high palate, mitral valve prolapse, and enlarged testicles (macroorchidism) in males. Connective tissue and muscle abnormalities along with poor muscle tone can cause motor delays, double-jointed fingers, curvature of the back, flat feet, strabismus, and slack facial features, especially in younger children (Warren & Nelson, 1994).

Boys are typically more severely affected than girls. Whereas most boys have mental retardation, only one third to one half of girls have significant intellectual impairment. Short attention span, hyperactivity, anxiety, and unstable mood are common in both sexes. Behavior is usually socially engaging, but individuals tend to avoid direct eye contact during conversation. Hand flapping, hand bit-

ing, and fascination with spinning objects are common. Sensory skills are often poor, and those with fragile X can be easily overwhelmed by crowds, noises, textures, and so on. They may not like being touched or held (Wong, 2001; Warren & Nelson, 1994; FRAXA Research Foundation, 2003; Hagerman & Hagerman, 2002).

Speech and language development are often delayed. Studies have shown that the specific communication problems associated with fragile X cannot be attributed just to mental retardation. Compared to males with Down syndrome, males with fragile X have more jargon (unintelligible strings of syllables), perseveration (frequent and inappropriate repetition of words, phrases, or a specific topic), and echolalia (repetition of verbalizations of a previous speaker, which usually indicates a lack of understanding) (Wong, 2001).

A DNA-based blood test was developed in 1992 to diagnose fragile X syndrome. It is an accurate test and can detect both carriers and fully affected individuals. A blood sample is collected and sent to a laboratory that offers the test. It usually takes several weeks to receive the results (FRAXA Research Foundation, 2003). Families are advised to seek genetic counseling to understand the inheritable nature of fragile X syndrome and discuss the likelihood of other family members or future offspring having the disorder. A positive diagnosis often produces grief over the loss of the normal child the parents had hoped and expected to have. Seeking support from family, friends, and professionals is essential in coping with theses intense feelings.

## Management

Currently no cure exists for fragile X syndrome, but there are treatments that have been shown to be extremely effective. Medical treatment may include the use of serotonin agents such as carbamazepine (Tegretol) or fluoxetine (Prozac) to control violent tempers and outbursts and the use of central nervous system (CNS) stimulants or clonidine (Catapres) to improve attention span and decrease hyperactivity. The use of folic acid, which affects the metabolism of CNS transmitters, is controversial (Wong, 2001).

The significant sensory processing, cognitive, and regulation problems that children with fragile X have makes learning in the typical classroom challenging. These challenges require early intervention; without it, children with fragile X can experience a progressive decline in IQ (Hagerman & Hagerman, 2002). The intervention of multiple professions promotes optimal learning. Health, occupational, physical, and speech therapies should be included in the child's individualized education program (IEP) (National Institute of Child Health and Human Development, 2003).

## Individualized Healthcare Plan

### Assessment

*History*
- Family (genetic) factors that predispose to fragile X syndrome
- Review of any medical (including genetic) and/or educational testing
- Age that diagnosis was made
- Developmental milestones
- Medication history
- Other health/medical issues
- Review of any previous special education assessment or interventions
- History from family:
  - Family knowledge base of fragile X syndrome
  - Any other family member affected?
  - Family's concerns and needs
  - Family's coping abilities

*Current Status and Management*
- Results of special education assessment, including developmental (motor and cognitive), behavioral and psychological assessments
- Results of speech and language assessment
- Vision and hearing assessment
- Ability to function in school environment (interview teachers)

*Self-care*
- Self-care skill level (toilet training, dressing, eating skills)
- Barriers to self-care
- Willingness and desire to participate in self-care

*Psychosocial Status*
- Ability to communicate with others
- Ability to interact with peers
- Sources of emotional stress
- Development of play skills
- Development of social skills (e.g., turn-taking, eye contact)
- Ability to deal with transition and tolerate change
- Reaction to different environments (home, school, community settings)
- Effective motivators of appropriate behavior (home, school)

*Academic Issues*
- Ability to stay on task
- Ability to follow directions
- Review IEP or individual family service plan
- Consult with teacher, special education teacher, speech therapist, occupational therapist, and any others on IEP multidisciplinary team

## Nursing Diagnoses (N.D.) (NANDA 2003)

**N.D. 1** Impaired verbal communication (NANDA 00051) related to speech and language delays

**N.D. 2** Impaired social interaction (NANDA 00052) related to communication barriers, anxiety, and altered thought processes

**N.D. 3** Disturbed thought processes (NANDA 00130) related to:
- impaired attention span
- impaired ability to recall information
- impaired perception
- impaired judgment
- impaired decision-making skills
- impaired conceptual reasoning ability
- sensory integration difficulties

**N.D. 4** Risk for injury (NANDA 00035) related to perceptual and cognitive impairment

**N.D. 5** Ineffective health maintenance: bathing/hygiene, dressing/grooming, toileting (NANDA 00099) related to perceptual and cognitive impairment

**N.D. 6** Chronic low self-esteem (NANDA 00119) related to impaired cognitive, perceptual, verbal communication and social interaction

## Goals

The student will develop abilities to communicate needs. (N.D. 1)

The student will engage in healthy social interaction. (N.D. 2)

The student will participate in an environment that encourages the student to learn. (N.D.3)

The student will be free from injury. (N.D. 4)

The student will increase participation in activities of daily living within cognitive/emotional/physical limits. (N.D. 5)

The student will develop and/or maintain effective family communication patterns. (N.D. 6)

The student will seek and obtain community support for self and his/her family. (N.D. 6)

## Nursing Interventions

### Referral

Refer to special education team for assessment if not already involved. (N.D. 1–5)

Participate in child study team meetings to monitor student's needs in the classroom. (N.D. 1–5)

Determine differences in chronologic age and mastery of developmental milestones. (N.D. 1–6)

### Communication Enhancement

Interact with student on appropriate cognitive level. (N.D. 1–5)

Consult with speech therapists about methods/strategies to enhance communication. (N.D. 1)

Provide alternative ways of communication when needed (signing or using pictures). (N.D. 1)

Encourage activities that involve communication with others, especially peers: describing wants and needs, making choices, explaining experiences (home, school, friends, etc.). (N.D. 1)

### Socialization Enhancement

Encourage student interaction with peers in the classroom, lunchroom, etc. (N.D. 2)

### Environmental Management

Provide the student with a calm atmosphere when external stimuli are overwhelming. (N.D. 3)

Provide consistent approach in care: same teacher, same routine. (N.D. 3)

Prepare the child for anticipated changes, such as having a substitute teacher tomorrow. (N.D. 3)

Allow for ample rest periods, which are important for optimal cognitive/perceptual functioning. (N.D. 3)

Provide a safe physical environment, including supervision in classroom, hallways, lunchroom, gym, bus, and so on, as necessary. (N.D. 4)

Encourage staff to select and provide toys and supplies appropriate to cognitive age. (N.D. 3, 4)

*Self-care Assistance*
Teach appropriate skills necessary for self-care with sensitivity to the student's cognitive and developmental needs for repetition, practice, and encouragement. (N.D. 5)
Encourage continued development of self-help skills. (N.D. 5)
Encourage continued health maintenance. (N.D. 5)
Provide opportunities to enhance the student's confidence in performing self-care. (N.D. 5)

*Family Mobilization*
Encourage family to utilize alternative methods/strategies of communication when needed. (N.D. 1)
Establish a caring atmosphere to keep communication open. (N.D. 6)
Involve family in case management. (N.D. 6)
Encourage parents and family members to discuss their fears and feelings. (N.D. 6)

*Caregiver Support*
Assist in referral for respite care for family, if indicated. (N.D. 6)
Refer to genetic counseling services and other community resources as needed. (N.D. 6)

## Expected Student Outcomes

The student will:
*Communication: Expressive*
- Demonstrate effective communication abilities (verbal, signing, augmentative assistive). (N.D. 1)
- Communicate his/her needs (using alternative forms of communication if necessary). (N.D. 1)

*Social Interaction*
- Interact with peers (at home, in school, in the community) (N.D. 2)

*Social Involvement*
- Participate in classroom activities, with modifications made as necessary (N.D. 1–3)

*Self-care: Instrumental Activities of Daily Living*
- Perform (or participate in) (specific) activities of daily living skill (N.D. 5)

*Safe Environment*
- Not experience injury (N.D. 4)

*Social Support*
- Identify family and others that provide care and support (N.D. 6)

## Case Study

Carl is 4 years and 9 months old. His history was obtained from Carl's mother at his IEP conference on November 26, 2003, and from a review of health records.

Carl was delivered at full-term vaginally after a normal pregnancy. He experienced mild difficulties with sucking initially, but weight gain progressed typically. Developmental milestones included sitting at 9 months, crawling at 11 months, and walking at 18 months. Carl continued to be nonverbal and had poor eye contact. His parents became concerned and sought help through a variety of doctors. In May 2001, genetic testing was conducted, and Carl was diagnosed with fragile X syndrome. There is a family history of the disorder: the mother's brother is affected, as is a maternal uncle and a child of a maternal aunt (all diagnoses late in life). Further testing was conducted in November 2002, and Carl was also diagnosed with autism.

Carl suffered from recurrent otitis media infections beginning in his first year and tympanostomy tubes were placed at 18 months. Currently, Carl's mom states that the tubes are in place and he has a resolving infection. Carl's immunizations are up to date.

# Fragile X Syndrome

| Assessment Data | Nursing Diagnosis | Goals | Nursing Interventions | Expected Outcomes |
|---|---|---|---|---|
| Carl has impaired verbal communication. | Impaired verbal communication related to speech and language delays. | Carl will learn to communicate needs using words or signs by pointing to pictures. | Consult with special education teacher and speech therapist about modes to enhance communications. Look directly at Carl and speak slowly. Encourage use of visual aids for reinforcement. Discuss communications strategies at team meetings. | Carl will communicate his needs effectively. |
| Carl is unable to toilet, dress, or bathe independently. | Ineffective health maintenance: toileting, bathing, dressing related to perceptual and cognitive impairment. | Carl will perform activities of daily living within his developmental capabilities. | Consult with parents and staff and develop a toileting plan to be followed at home and school. Staff will teach the appropriate skills for self-care in Carl's terms with sensitivity to developmental needs. Provide opportunities to enhance Carl's confidence in performing self-care. | Carl will demonstrate an increase in self-care skills. |
| Carl has poor family functioning. | Compromised family coping: related to having a child with fragile X syndrome. | Provide support to Carl and his family. | Encourage verbalization of feelings regarding student's special needs. Use a notebook to facilitate communication between parents and the numerous professionals working with him. Refer family to ECSE Parent Support Group. Refer family to community agencies and resources as needed. | Carl will give and receive support within the family systems. |

# References

Fast, D. (2003). Summary of fragile X syndrome. In *What is fragile X?* Retrieved September 20, 2003, from http://www.fragilex.org

FRAXA Research Foundation. (2003). About fragile X. In *What is fragile X?* Retrieved September 20, 2003, from http://www.fraxa.org

Hagerman, R.J., & Hagerman, P.J. (2002). *Fragile X syndrome: Diagnosis, treatment, and research.* Baltimore: Johns Hopkins University Press.

NANDA International. (2003). *Nursing diagnoses: Definitions & classification, 2003-2004.* Philadelphia: Author.

National Institute of Child Health and Human Development. (2003). *Families and fragile X syndrome* (NICHD Publication No. 96-3402). Rockville, MD: U.S. Government Printing Office. (pp. 61–132). New York: Oxford University Press.

Warren, S. T., & Nelson, D. T. (1994). Advances in molecular analysis of fragile X syndrome. *Journal of the American Medical Association, 271*(7), 536–542.

Wong D. L. (2001). *Wong's essentials of pediatric nursing,* St. Louis, MO: Mosby.

# Bibliography

Braden, M. L. (2000). *Fragile X, handle with care: More about fragile X syndrome—adolescents and adults.* Dillon, CO: Spectra Publishing.

Dykens E., Hodapp R., & Leckman J. (1994). *Behavior and development in fragile X syndrome.* Thousand Oaks, CA: Sage Publications.

Hagerman, R. J. (1999). Fragile X syndrome. In *Neurodevelopmental disorders: Diagnosis and treatment* (pp. 61–132). New York: Oxford University Press.

Schopmeyer, B., & Lowe, F. (1992). *The fragile X child.* San Diego, CA: Singular Publishing Group.

Wilson, P., Stackhouse, T., O'Connor, R., Scharfenaker, S., & Hagerman, R. (1994). *Issues and strategies for educating children with fragile X syndrome: A monograph.* Dillon, CO: Spectra Publishing.

# Resources

FRAXA Research Foundation
45 Pleasant Street
Newburyport, MA 01950
978-462-1866
978-463-9985 (fax)
http://www.fraxa.org
info@fraxa.org

The National Fragile X Foundation
PO Box 190488
San Francisco, CA 94119
925-938-9300
1-800-688-8765
925-938-9315 (fax)
http://www.nfxf.org
NATLFX@FragileX.org

*Chapter Forty-one*

# Gastroesophageal Reflux Disease

Penny J. Makuchal

## Introduction

Gastroesophageal reflux is the backward flow of gastric contents into the esophagus. The most common symptom of reflux is typically chronic heartburn or acid indigestion, which is described as a burning sensation just beneath the lower end of the sternum. Dysphagia, which is difficulty swallowing, is another common symptom (Kahrilas, 1998). Although reflux is most common in infants, women during pregnancy, and the elderly, reflux can be experienced at any age. It is estimated that approximately 15 million Americans experience acid indigestion on a daily basis (American College of Gastroenterology, 2004).

Causes of gastroesophageal reflux vary with age, and there can be multiple causes. An immature digestive system is the most common cause of reflux in infants; however, laryngomalacia (prolapse of supraglottic structures during inspiration) and tracheomalacia (narrowing of the trachea) are also associated with reflux in infants (Rayhorn, Argel, & Demchak, 2003). In children and adults, reflux is commonly linked to diet selections, medications, obesity, and increases in intra-abdominal pressure. The incidence of reflux in children is also associated with developmental problems and asthma (Rayhorn et al., 2003). Pregnancy, alcohol use, excessive stress, and smoking are also contributing factors among young adults. When occasional episodes of reflux, such as heartburn, begin to occur more frequently and become severe, the condition may progress to the disease stage. Gastroesophageal reflux disease (GERD) is a chronic condition that requires medical management.

## Pathophysiology

The superior gastrointestinal tract includes the mouth, esophagus, and the stomach. Food is broken down in the mouth and then passes through the esophagus into the stomach. The stomach has sphincters at each end that allow food to enter and exit respectfully. The esophageal sphincter connects the esophagus and the stomach. If this sphincter becomes weakened or loosened, gastric contents can leak or reflux back into the esophagus. This condition is most common in children and adults. The pyloric sphincter, located at the end of the stomach, can be too tight and cause a narrowing known as pyloric stenosis. This condition is most common in newborns and infants.

## Management

School nurses are more likely to care for children with episodic reflux, who need symptom management, rather than chronic cases that require implementing medical management recommendations. Medical management of GERD involves identifying triggers and decreasing stomach acid. In its milder forms, GERD can be managed by avoiding problem foods and beverages, avoiding increases in intra-abdominal pressure, decreasing stress, ceasing smoking, losing weight, and maintaining an upright body position following meals. Over-the-counter antacids and acid-blocking medications known as $H_2$ receptor antagonists, such as Axid, Pepcid, Tagamet, and Zantac, may be useful. Severe cases of GERD may require prescription-strength proton pump inhibitors, such as Aciphex, Nexium, Prevacid, Prilosec, and Protonix, which decrease gastric acid. If treatment with medication is unsuccessful, tests and possible surgical interventions may be required. Fundoplication is one such surgical procedure that helps to strengthen the sphincter. If left untreated, premalignant conditions such as Barrett's esophagus could develop.

# Individualized Healthcare Plan

## Assessment
### History
- Diagnosis. Date of diagnosis
- Identified cause of the condition
- Student health history, including medical and surgical history
- Family history of gastrointestinal disorders
- Known allergies to foods, medications, insects, dust
- Developmental problems
- Identification of asthma

### Current Status and Management
- Height and weight
- Healthcare providers caring for this student
- Current treatment plan (medications, diet modifications, activity limitations)
- Current experience of discomfort or pain related to GERD, including frequency and severity, precipitating factors, home management of pain
- Activity restrictions

### Self-care
- Medication administration or treatments done independently by student
- Identification of trigger foods
- Adult-supervised or self-planned appropriate diet
- Student's feelings regarding diet modifications and/or activity restrictions
- Barriers preventing the student from participating in self-care

### Psychosocial Status
- Student's perception of health condition
- Family's perception of the student's health condition
- Student's support system—family, friends, classmates
- Extracurricular activity involvement—sports, clubs, community
- Student's family structure (nuclear, extended, etc.)
- Student's perception of current stress level

### Academic Issues
- Student's school attendance record, prior to diagnosis and current
- Students' academic history
- Accommodations such as 504 plan or individualized education plan
- Modifications needed during the school day (pain management, dietary changes, etc.)
- Health services needed during the school day

## Nursing Diagnoses (N.D.) (NANDA, 2003).

**N.D. 1** (Risk for) Acute pain (NANDA 00132) related to reflux symptoms:
- burning sensation in chest

**N.D. 2** (Risk for) Imbalanced nutrition: less than body requirements (NANDA 00002) related to:
- inadequate intake
- lack of knowledge regarding appropriate diet
- abdominal pain associated with eating

**N.D. 3** Deficient knowledge (NANDA 00126) related to:
- recent diagnosis of GERD
- treatment regimen and management of GERD

**N.D. 4** (Risk for) Noncompliance of management plan (NANDA 00079) related to:
- denial of condition

- knowledge deficit
- cultural and religious dietary influences

**N.D. 5** (Risk for) Ineffective role performance (NANDA 00055) related to:
- absences
- abdominal discomfort/pain
- barriers to learning

**N.D. 6** Activity intolerance (NANDA 00094) related to:
- abdominal discomfort
- medication side effects
- frequency and severity of symptoms

**N.D. 7** (Risk for) Situational low self-esteem (NANDA 00153) related to:
- altered role performance
- frequency and severity of symptoms
- activity intolerance

## Goals

The student will experience an increased level of comfort after interventions. (N.D. 1)

The student will demonstrate an improvement in nutritional choices at school. (N.D. 2, 3, 4)

The student will demonstrate increased knowledge of GERD and the management plan. (N.D. 3)

The student will seek treatment for symptoms of GERD when they first appear. (N.D. 1, 5, 6)

The student will comply with prescribed GERD management plan. (N.D. 3, 4)

The student will attend school daily and participate fully in student role activities with modifications as prescribed. (N.D. 5, 6, 7)

The student will demonstrate improved self-esteem. (N.D. 7)

## Nursing Interventions

Observe student for signs and symptoms of GERD. (N.D. 1, 4, 5)

Obtain a signed physician's order for medications/treatments to manage pain during school. (N.D. 1, 3)

Assist student in rating pain on a pain scale. (N.D. 1, 4, 6)

Administer pain medication per physician's order and monitor effectiveness. (N.D. 1)

Observe for medication side effects. (N.D. 1, 4, 6)

Teach student to observe for signs and symptoms of GERD and actions to take if they occur. (N.D. 1, 3)

Collaborate with student's medical care team to increase student's understanding in the use of over-the-counter and prescription medications. (N.D. 1).

Observe student's body position and explain importance of avoiding lying down 2 to 3 hours after a meal and several hours before bedtime. (N.D. 1, 4)

Encourage student to sleep in reverse Trendelenburg position and discuss with parents how to elevate the head of the bed 4 to 6 inches using blocks, if recommend by physician. (N.D. 1)

Discuss techniques to avoid increases in intra-abdominal pressure: avoiding wearing tight clothing, avoid straining, and avoid cigarette smoking. (N.D. 1)

Provide nutritional counseling: (N.D. 2, 3)
- Select bland foods by avoiding fatty, greasy, acidic food (such as tomato-based or citric products), acidic beverages (such as carbonated drinks, fruit juices, alcohol).
- Eat several small meals daily.

Collaborate with dietary staff and assist in planning for dietary restrictions and substitutions. (N.D. 2)

Provide student, family, and designated school staff with educational materials and counseling about GERD. (N.D. 3, 5)

Monitor student's compliance with treatment plan. (N.D. 4)

Assist student in removing barriers to treatment compliance. (N.D. 4, 5)

Collaborate with other school personnel to monitor student's daily attendance. (N.D. 5, 6)

Collaborate with student, family, and other school personnel to: (N.D. 5)
- Explore need for 504 plan
- Develop 504 plan
- Implement 504 plan

Discuss goal setting with student, physical education teacher, and sports coaches (N.D. 5, 6, 7)

Assist school staff in modifying current activities to accommodate physician's order for physical limitations/restrictions (N.D. 5, 6, 7)

Discuss appropriate school activities with healthcare provider and parents (N.D. 6)
Arrange for modifications in physical education and other activities as indicated. (N.D. 6)
Obtain physician's orders for physical education and sports limitations/restrictions. (N.D. 6)
Promote self-esteem enhancement by: (N.D. 7)
- Providing support and encouragement
- Assisting student in planning ahead for activities and events that require a diet or activity modification
- Monitoring for signs and symptoms of withdrawal
- Encouraging school attendance and participation by assisting school staff in modifications

## Expected Student Outcomes

The student will:
- Utilize knowledge of pain management to make appropriate health-related decisions. (N.D. 1).
- Experience a decrease in the incidence of pain associated with reflux symptoms. (N.D. 1, 3, 4)
- Rate pain on the pain scale and identify pain management needed. (N.D. 1, 3)
- Utilize knowledge of pain management to make appropriate health-related decisions (N.D. 1, 3, 6).
- Identify and avoid foods that trigger reflux symptoms. (N.D. 2, 3)
- Select and eat GERD-friendly foods. (N.D. 2, 4)
- Recognize the signs and symptoms of GERD and inform parents, teachers, and school nurse when symptoms occur. (N.D. 1, 3, 5, 6)
- State ways to decrease the pain associated with signs and symptoms, both pharmacologic and nonpharmacologic. (N.D. 3)
- Attend school daily. (N.D. 5)
- Work cooperatively with teachers, coaches, and school nurse to modify activities to allow for sports and physical education participation. (N.D. 5, 6, 7)
- Identify activities that trigger reflux symptoms and will modify lifestyle to accommodate adjustments. (N.D. 3, 6)
- Complete the school day participating in all activities with modifications (N.D. 5, 6, 7)
- Show evidence of improved self-esteem by participating in physical education class with modifications, in after-school activities with friends, and in extracurricular activities and sports. (N.D. 7)

## Case Study

Maranda is a 16-year-old girl who is a junior in high school. Although she has experienced numerous episodes of "indigestion" and "upset stomachs," she only recently sought medical treatment after experiencing a severe burning sensation in the epigastric area following a pizza dinner to celebrate her field hockey team's championship win and her scoring the winning goal. Throughout her high school career, Maranda has received annual perfect attendance awards; however, she has been absent 10 days this school year for health-related reasons. Lately she has complained about abdominal pain during physical activity. Maranda has decided to quit her gymnastics team because of "pain" during exercise.

She is an academic honors student who is involved in numerous extracurricular sports and clubs. Maranda has no other chronic illnesses or conditions and no known allergies, and prior to her diagnosis she did not take any medications. Her current weight is100 lbs, and height is 5 feet 3 inches. She has lost 8 lbs in the last 2 months.

During her appointment with a gastroentrologist yesterday, she was diagnosed with GERD. She and her parents have brought a management plan to school. To control her symptoms, the gastroenterologist prescribed Nexium, bid, and Gaviscon, 1 tablespoon orally every 3 to 4 hours, as needed, if pain is rated "6" or higher on pain scale of 1 to 10. She is to follow a bland diet for 2 weeks and avoid acid-producing foods for the next month. She was given a note by her physician to modify exercise to avoid activities involving bending at the waist. The doctor recommends that she sleep in reverse Trendelenburg position by elevating the head of the bed using 4- to 6-inch blocks.

Maranda's family is very concerned about her absences, inability to participate in activities, and modifications needed in the school setting. The parents are very supportive and involved in all aspects of Maranda's management plan. They report that Maranda has stopped after-school food-related activities with friends. They ask about the school dietary staff's understanding of GERD and if GERD-friendly foods are available. Maranda has not had experience in using a pain rating scale.

# Gastroesophageal Reflux Disease

| Assessment Data | Nursing Diagnosis | Goals | Nursing Interventions | Expected Outcomes |
|---|---|---|---|---|
| Gastroenterologist appointment yesterday, diagnosed with GERD.<br><br>Healthcare provider's management plan received today.<br><br>Medications:<br>• Nexium bid.<br>• Gaviscon, 1 Tbsp PO q3-4h as needed if pain is rated "6" or higher on pain rating scale of 1 to 10.<br><br>Maranda has complained of "pain" during physical education classes and when participating in gymnastics.<br><br>Maranda does not currently use a pain rating scale, although she was given a copy of one by her physician at yesterday's visit. | Risk for acute pain related to reflux symptoms<br>• burning sensation in chest | Maranda will seek treatment for signs and symptoms of GERD when they first appear.<br><br>Maranda will experience an increased level of comfort after interventions. | 1. Observe Maranda for signs and symptoms of GERD.<br><br>2. Obtain a signed physician's order for medications/treatments to manage pain during the school day.<br><br>3. Assist Maranda in rating her pain on a pain scale of 1 to 10.<br><br>4. Administer pain medication(s) per physician's orders.<br><br>5. Monitor effectiveness of medication(s) and observe for side effects.<br><br>6. Collaborate with student's medical care team to increase student's understanding in using over-the-counter and prescription medications.<br><br>7. Observe student's body position and discuss importance of avoiding lying down 2 to 3 hours after a meal and several hours before bedtime.<br><br>8. Encourage student to sleep in reverse Trendelenburg position by elevating the head of the bed using 4- to 6-inch blocks. | Maranda will experience a decreased incidence of pain associated with reflux symptoms.<br><br>Maranda will rate her pain on the pain scale and identify pain management needed.<br><br>Maranda will utilize her knowledge of pain management to make appropriate health-related decisions. |

| Assessment Data | Nursing Diagnosis | Goals | Nursing Interventions | Expected Outcomes |
|---|---|---|---|---|
| | | | 9. Discuss techniques to avoid increases in intra-abdominal pressure:<br>• Avoid wearing tight clothing, especially around waist.<br>• Avoid cigarette smoking.<br>• Avoid straining (constipation). | |
| Current weight: 100 lbs.<br><br>Current height: 5 feet, 3 inches.<br><br>Weight loss of 8 lbs in last 2 months.<br><br>Physician-ordered bland diet for 2 weeks followed by avoidance of acid-producing foods for 1 month. | Risk for imbalanced nutrition: less than body requirements related to weight loss, inappropriate menu selections. | Maranda will demonstrate an improved nutritional status. | 1. Provide nutritional counseling:<br>• Select bland foods.<br>• Eat several small meals daily.<br><br>2. Collaborate with dietary staff and assist in planning for dietary restrictions and substitutions. | Maranda will identify and avoid foods that trigger her reflux symptoms.<br><br>Maranda will select and eat GERD-friendly foods. |
| Newly diagnosed with GERD. | Student unfamiliar with food choices that contribute to condition, unaware of treatment regimen. | Deficient knowledge related to recent diagnosis, and treatment and management of GERD<br><br>Maranda will demonstrate an increased knowledge of GERD and the management plan. | 1. Teach Maranda the signs and symptoms of GERD and actions to take if they occur.<br><br>2. Obtain a signed physician's order for GERD management.<br><br>3. Provide student, family, and designated school staff with educational materials and counseling about GERD. | Maranda recognizes the signs and symptoms of GERD and informs teachers and school nurse if symptoms occur at school.<br><br>Maranda will state ways to decrease the pain associated with signs and symptoms, both pharmacologic and non-pharmacologic. |

| Assessment Data | Nursing Diagnosis | Goals | Nursing Interventions | Expected Outcomes |
|---|---|---|---|---|
| Student unaware of GERD-friendly foods. Parents concerned student will continue to make personal food selections that are not listed on her bland diet checklist. Prior to diagnosis, Maranda has been seen participating in activities that increase intra-abdominal pressure (i.e., sports). | Risk for noncompliance of management plan related to knowledge deficit. | Maranda will comply with the prescribed GERD management plan. | 1. Assist student in removing barriers to treatment compliance by counseling, discussing importance of treatment management plan, reteach, instruct, help student identify why she is not in compliance. | Maranda will show evidence of compliance as evidenced by: • making GERD-friendly food selections • working cooperatively with coaches to modify activities to allow for participation |
| Maranda has been absent 10 days this school year. Maranda has decided to quit her gymnastics team because of "pain" during exercise. | Risk for ineffective role performance related to absences and abdominal pain. | Maranda will attend school daily and participate fully with modifications as prescribed. | 1. Collaborate with other school personnel to monitor Maranda's daily attendance. 2. Discuss realistic goal setting with Maranda and her physical education teacher and sports coaches. 3. Assist school staff in modifying current activities to accommodate physician's order for physical limitation/restrictions. | Maranda will attend school daily. Maranda will work cooperatively with teachers and coaches to modify activities to allow for sports and physical education participation. |
| Maranda has complained of pain during exercise and when participating in sports activities. Maranda has decided to quit her gymnastics team because of "pain" during exercise. | Activity intolerance related to abdominal discomfort. | Maranda will participate fully in school and extracurricular activities with modifications as prescribed. | 1. Collaborate with other school personnel to monitor Maranda's daily attendance. 2. Discuss appropriate activities with healthcare provider and parents. | Maranda will identify activities that trigger reflux symptoms and will modify lifestyle to accommodate adjustments. Maranda will be able to complete the school day participating in all activities with modifications. |

| Assessment Data | Nursing Diagnosis | Goals | Nursing Interventions | Expected Outcomes |
|---|---|---|---|---|
| | | | 3. Arrange for modifications in physical education and other activities as indicated.<br><br>4. Obtain physician's orders for physical education and sports limitations/restrictions. | |
| Parents report Maranda has stopped after-school time with friends in activities that are food-related.<br><br>Maranda has decided to quit her gymnastics team because of "pain" during exercise. | Risk for situational low self-esteem related to inability to eat the same foods as friends, lack of participating in activities. | Maranda will demonstrate improved self-esteem. | 1. Promote self-esteem enhancement by:<br>• providing support and encouragement<br>• assisting Maranda in planning ahead for activities and events that require a diet or activity modification<br>• monitoring for signs and symptoms of withdrawal<br>• encouraging school attendance and participation by assisting school staff in modifications | Maranda will show evidence of improved self-esteem by participating in physical education class with modifications, in after-school activities with friends, and in extracurricular activities and sports. |

# References

American College of Gastroenterology. (2004). *Patient information: Common GI problems* (Vol. 1). Retrieved 03/01/04 from http://www.acg.gi.org/patientinfo/cgp/cgpvol1.html

Kahrilas, P. J. (1998). Gastroesophageal reflux disease and its compliance. In *Sleisenger & Fordtran's gastrointestinal and liver disease* (6th ed.). Philadelphia: Saunders.

NANDA International. (2003). *Nursing diagnoses: Definitions and classifications 2003-2004.* Philadelphia: Author.

Rayhorn, N., Argel, N., & Demchak, K. (2003). Gastroesophageal reflux disease. *Nursing 2003, 33*(10), 36–41.

# Resources

American College of Gastroenterology
4900 B South 31st Street
Arlington, VA 22206
703-820-7400
1-800-HRT-BURN
http://www.acg.gi.org/patientinfo/frame gerd.asp

American Gastroenterological Association
4930 Del Ray Avenue
Bethesda, MD 20814
301-654-2055
http://www.gastro.org

National Digestive Diseases Information Clearinghouse
2 Information Way
Bethesda, MD 20892
301-654-3810
http://www.niddk.nih.gov

National Institute of Diabetes and Digestive and Kidney Diseases
National Institutes of Health
31 Center Drive
Bethesda, MD 20892
http://www.niddk.nih.gov

North American Society for Pediatric Gastroenterology, Hepatology, and Nutrition
PO Box 6
Flourtown, PA 19031
215-233-0808
http://www.naspghan.org

Pediatric/Adolescent Gastroesophageal Reflux Association, Inc.
PO Box 1153
Germantown, MD 20875
301-601-9541
http://www.reflux.org

# Chapter Forty-two

# Hearing Deficit

Elisabeth Barclay

## Introduction

Hearing is defined as the ability to sense or perceive sounds. Humans use our sense of hearing as a primary means of communication (Northern & Downs, 2002). Hearing deficits occur when there is a decrease in the ability to hear sounds.

Approximately 30 million Americans are affected by hearing deficits (National Association of School Nurses [NASN], 2003), and nearly 14% of school-aged children present with hearing deficits (American Academy of Pediatrics [AAP], 2002). The ability to hear provides the communication skills needed to have a positive impact on the social, emotional, and educational development and self-esteem of the student (NASN, 2003). Therefore, early detection and treatment of hearing deficits is vital for a student to be successful in both school and community settings.

## Pathophysiology

### The Ear and Hearing

The sensory organ for hearing is the ear. The ear has three parts: the external (auricle or pinna), middle, and inner ear (**Figure 1**). The shape of the external ear allows sound waves to travel into its opening (Jarvis, 2004). Sound waves travel through the external auditory canal to the tympanic membrane (eardrum), causing the tympanic membrane to vibrate. The sound vibrations then enter the middle ear.

The middle ear serves three functions: (1) It transmits sound vibrations from the tympanic membrane of the external ear into the inner ear, (2) it protects the inner ear by reducing the amplitude of loud sounds, and (3) its eustachian tube allows equalization of air pressure on each side of the tympanic membrane so that the membrane does not rupture (e.g., during altitude changes in an airplane) (Jarvis, 2004, p. 343). The sound vibrations then enter the inner ear. The inner ear is composed of several complex structures used for hearing and balance. Within the structures of the inner ear lies the auditory nerve (cranial nerve VIII), where the ability to sense or perceive sound is formed.

**Figure 1. Diagram of the external, middle, and inner ear.**

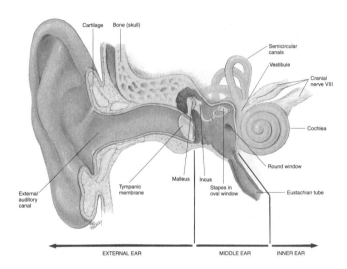

From *Physical Examination and Health Assessment* (4th ed.), by C. Jarvis, 2004, St. Louis, MO: Saunders. Copyright 2004 by Saunders. Reprinted with permission.

### Hearing Deficit

As noted above, hearing deficits occur when there is a decrease in the ability to hear sounds. There are several different types and also varying degrees of hearing deficits. Some hearing deficits can be medically treated, whereas others cannot. Hearing deficits can be classified into three categories: conductive, sensorineural, or mixed (a combination of conductive and sensorineural losses in the same ear) (Jarvis, 2004). Presbycusis is considered normal hearing deficit due to the aging process.

Another form of hearing deficit is called central auditory dysfunction. This deficit occurs when the components of the ear function within normal limits yet there is a decrease in the ability to recognize or interpret speech, "which may lead to learning disabilities" (Northern & Downs, 2002, p. 10). A complete discussion of central auditory dysfunction is beyond the scope of this chapter.

### Conductive

In conductive hearing deficits there is an interference of sound from the external or middle ear to the inner ear. The inner ear has the ability to function within normal limits; the dysfunction is in the external or middle ear (Lewis & Bear, 2002). Causes of conductive hearing deficits in the external ear include cerumen buildup, external otitis (inflammation or infection of the auricle or auditory canal), a foreign body lodged in the ear canal, and a perforation or scarring of the tympanic membrane. Causes of conductive hearing deficits in the middle ear include otitis media (inflammation or infection of the middle ear), fluid buildup, tumors, and otosclerosis. Conductive hearing deficits involve a disturbance in the loudness of sounds (Wong, 2003).

### Sensorineural

Sensorineural hearing deficits are caused by a dysfunction of the inner ear, auditory nerve (cranial nerve VIII), or damaged auditory areas in the brain. Sensorineural hearing deficits are either congenital defects

**Table 1. Classification of Hearing Deficit and Implications**

| Hearing Deficit | Effects/Educational Implications |
|---|---|
| Mild (26-40 dB) | Soft or distant speech may be difficult. |
| | At 30-dB loss, child can miss up to 10% of conversations. |
| | At 35 to 40-dB loss, child can miss 50% of conversations. |
| | Preferential seating indicated. |
| | May experience fatigue due to effort needed to listen. |
| | Amplification or assistive hearing device beneficial. |
| | Face-to-face conversation understood at 3 to 5 feet. |
| Moderate (41 to 55 dB) | At 50-dB loss, child can miss 80% to 100% of conversations. |
| | Vocabulary and articulation may be difficult. |
| | Preferential seating indicated. |
| | Amplification or assistive hearing device indicated. |
| | Speech therapy indicated. |
| | Usually cannot understand speech by hearing alone. |
| Moderately severe (56 to 70 dB) | Others must speak loudly to be understood. |
| | Difficulty participating in classroom discussions. |
| | Preferential seating and speech therapy indicated. |
| | Full-time use of amplification/assistive hearing device indicated. |
| | May require teacher assistant in classroom and school setting. |
| Severe (71 to 90 dB) | May hear voices within 1 foot of ear. |
| | May discriminate environmental sounds. |
| | Language may not develop spontaneously. |
| | Amplification device necessary. |
| | Requires special services at regular education school. |
| | Services to focus on speech, language, and auditory training. |
| | Teacher assistant needed in regular classroom and school setting. |
| Profound (91+ dB) | Some loud noises may be audible. |
| | Vision is primary method for communication and learning. |
| | Language may not develop spontaneously. |
| | Requires special services at regular education school. |
| | Possibly requires school for hearing impaired. |
| | May be considered for cochlear implant. |

From *The Manual of School Health* (2nd ed.), by K. Lewis and B. J. Bear, 2002, Philadelphia, PA: Elsevier, and *Wong's Nursing Care of Infants and Children* (7th ed.), by D. L. Wong, M. J. Hockenberry, D. Wilson, M. L. Winkelstein, and N. E. Kline, 2003, Philadelphia, PA: Elsevier. Adapted with permission.

(hereditary or genetic) or nonhereditary (acquired at some point after birth) (Lewis & Bear, 2002). Causes of sensorineural deficits include noise-induced (loud music, machinery, gunfire), trauma-induced, ototoxic drug–related, tumors, viral diseases, and perinatal infections. Sensorineural hearing deficits involve a distortion in sounds. Although a student with a sensorineural hearing deficit will hear most sounds and conversations, the sounds will be distorted and will negatively affect sound discrimination and comprehension (Wong, 2003).

*Mixed*

A mixed hearing deficit refers to a combination of both conductive and sensorineural deficits in the same ear.

*Classification of Degree and Severity of Hearing Deficit*

Hearing deficits are also classified by the degree of hearing loss (Table 1). Common categories include: mild hearing loss (26 to 40 dB), moderate hearing loss (41 to 55 dB), moderately severe (56 to 70 dB), severe hearing loss (71 to 90 dB), profound hearing loss (91+ dB), and total hearing loss (Lewis & Bear, 2002).

## Management
### Screening Tools

Early detection of hearing deficits is valuable. The child with a hearing deficit has a greater chance to develop appropriate speech and language skills if the deficit is identified early and interventions are started as soon as possible. Several screening tools can be used. Many newborns are routinely screened for hearing deficits prior to being sent home from the hospital. One of the screening tools used is the auditory brain-stem response. This response determines how the "brain stem (the part of the nerve that carries sound from the ear to the brain) and the brain respond to sound" by simply placing headphones over the ears and electrodes on the head and ears (National Institute on Deafness and Other Communication Disorders [NIDCD], 2001, p.2). This tool is fast, effective, and easy to use, and it alerts the screener when further medical attention is needed.

Another reliable screening tool is the otoacoustic emission response screening. This tool is used in the hospital setting and can be used in the school setting for early detection of hearing deficits. The otoacoustic emission "is a measurement of the inner ear (cochlear) response to a sound introduced into the external ear" (Lewis & Bear, 2002, p.94). In a person with normal hearing, an "echo" of the sound is measured; if there is no "echo," a hearing deficit may be indicated (NIDCD, 2001). This screening tool is able to detect both conductive hearing deficits and sensorineural deficits. Again, this tool is fast, effective, easy to use, and alerts the screener when further medical attention is needed.

Ideally, hearing deficits would be recognized and diagnosed at an early age. However, some hearing deficits may not develop or may go undiscovered until later in life.

Because of this, many states require annual hearing screenings for children in any public or private school setting. The school screening guidelines are usually regulated by the Department of Public Health in each state. Typically, the screening process includes introducing different levels of tones (hertz [Hz]) at a particular level loudness or intensity (decibel [dB]) (**Figure 2**). If the student fails the screening, then a medical referral must be made for further evaluation.

**Figure 2. Diagram of audiogram showing typical sounds heard at various decibels and frequencies.**

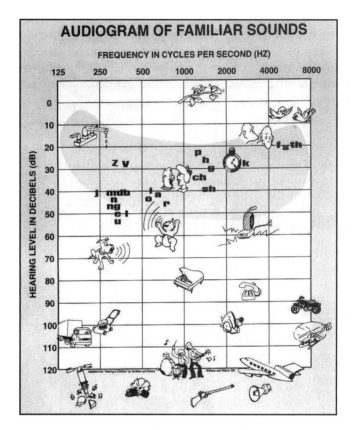

From *Audiogram of Familiar Sounds*, 1978, Reston, VA: American Academy of Audiology. Copyright 1978 by American Academy of Audiology. Reprinted with permission.

## Medical Interventions

There are several medical interventions for each type of hearing deficit. Proper care will directly affect the student's success in the community and the school setting. Such care may include treatment provided by a pediatrician or family physician, an ear, nose and throat specialist, an audiologist, or an otologist.

*Conductive*

Treatment options for conductive hearing deficit include removing wax buildup by irrigation or using a wax softener, medications (antibiotics, antifungals, or possibly oral steroids), surgery, hearing aids, speech therapy, and otoplasty (plastic surgery) (Lewis & Bear, 2002).

## Sensorineural

Treatment options for sensorineural hearing deficit include hearing aids or other amplification option, early diagnosis and treatment of ear infections, speech and language therapy, and auditory training; also, because vision is greatly relied on, it is important to offer an annual vision screening to rule out any vision deficits (Lewis & Bear, 2002).

## Mixed

Treatment options for mixed hearing deficit include hearing aids, prompt and appropriate treatment of the conductive hearing deficit, preferential classroom seating as needed (typically center of second row so student can also use visual cues from other students), and using a classroom partner to alert the student of important information; also, because vision is greatly relied on, it is important to offer an annual vision screening to rule out any vision deficits (Lewis & Bear, 2002).

## Amplification Options

The use of an amplification or an assistive listening device is an important intervention that will strengthen the relationship between hearing, speech, and language development. An amplification device increases the loudness of a sound (i.e., hearing aids, personal FM system that has a transmitter and receiver and functions similar to a radio, and cochlear implants). An assistive listening device promotes more independent functioning in daily communication situations (American Speech-Language-Hearing Association, 2004) (i.e., text telephones, alerting devices, and closed-captioned TV). These examples are several options available for students with hearing deficits to improve their communication skills.

## Educational Interventions

The school nurse should provide health-related recommendations and services, including yearly audiometer screenings; referrals for speech, language, and academic development; and referral to a physician if medical treatment is needed. In addition, classroom teachers may provide accommodations for students with hearing deficits. Several accommodations include gaining the student's attention before speaking, using familiar vocabulary, rephrasing misunderstood statements and not just repeating them, using visual supplements, preferential seating, and minimizing noise interference (Northern & Downs, 2002).

# Individualized Healthcare Plan

## Assessment

### History
- History of earaches or ear infections
- History of ear tubes
- Discharge from ear(s)
- History of any hearing deficit
- Exposure to any extreme environmental noise
- Complaints of tinnitus (ringing or buzzing in the ears)
- Complaints of vertigo (feeling as though the room is spinning)
- Complaints of not being able to hear or ears feeling plugged
- Most recent hearing screening
- Successful management strategies

There are many possible behaviors that may indicate a hearing deficit. Compare the child's behaviors to this list. The behaviors include, but are not limited to:
- Inattentiveness or daydreaming
- Asking to have questions or directions repeated
- Watching others' faces when they talk (attempting to lip-read)
- Watching for visual cues from others before starting a task
- Turning ear toward the speaker
- Inappropriate answers or statements related to class discussion
- Difficult time taking written notes in class while listening to a lecture or watching a video
- Inappropriate speech volume (too loud or too soft)
- Mispronunciation of common words
- No response to loud sounds located next to or behind the student
- Concerned or teased about their speech
- Has trouble getting words out; hesitates, stops, and starts over
- Talks too fast or too slow
- Seldom seeks help from teacher and may not ask for clarification

*Current Status and Management*
- Current performance level
- Current management strategies
- Ability to function in the mainstream classroom
- Current medical treatment; any procedures to be completed at school

*Self-care*
- Knowledge level and understanding of hearing deficit
- Willingness to actively participate in decisions related to the hearing deficit
- Ability to care for own hearing aid device(s)
- Ability to communicate own needs to teachers and students

*Psychosocial Status*
- Perception of self compared to peers in the same environment
- Ability to communicate with others
- Involvement in school and community activities

*Academic Issues*
- Current and past academic achievement levels
- School services needed based on speech and language evaluation
- Preferential seating
- Use of hearing amplification device: hearing aids or personal listening device
- Printed copies of lectures, other verbal communication, or additional information
- Need to modify assignments
- Need for personal teacher assistant
- School health services needed throughout the school day

## Nursing Diagnoses (N.D.) (NANDA 2003)

**N.D. 1** (Risk for) ineffective therapeutic regimen management (NANDA 00078) related to inadequate information regarding hearing deficit treatment options

**N.D. 2** (Risk for) ineffective health maintenance (NANDA 00099) related to:
- inadequate information regarding hearing deficit
- ineffective individual coping regarding hearing deficit

**N.D. 3** (Risk for) fatigue (NANDA 00093) related to amount of energy being used to hear everyday conversations

**N.D. 4** Disturbed sensory perception (auditory) (NANDA 00122) related to specific hearing deficit

**N.D. 5** (Risk for) deficient knowledge (NANDA 00126) related to:
- hearing deficit type
- management
- treatment options

**N.D. 6** (Risk for) impaired verbal communication (NANDA 00051) related to hearing deficit

**N.D. 7** Risk for situational low self-esteem (NANDA 00153) related to perception of hearing deficit

**N.D. 8** (Risk for) disturbed body image (NANDA 00118) related to perception of hearing deficit

**N.D. 9** (Risk for) noncompliance (NANDA 00079) related to beliefs regarding hearing deficit

**N.D. 10** (Risk for) social isolation (NANDA 00053) related to hearing deficit

**N.D. 11** Risk for delayed development (NANDA 00112) related to hearing deficit

## Goals

The student will reach and sustain highest level of hearing. (N.D. 1, 2)

The student will reduce or remove factors that may cause or contribute to the hearing deficit. (N.D. 3, 4, 6–8)

The student will reduce or remove barriers to communication and learning in the classroom and school setting. (N.D. 3, 4, 6, 9)

The student will communicate effectively with teachers, staff, students, and family members. (N.D. 2, 3, 6, 10, 11)

The student will seek situations that support and maintain the ability to learn. (N.D. 4, 6, 11)

The student will gain knowledge and skills in the use and care of amplification or assistive devices. (N.D. 1, 2, 5, 9)

The student will effectively interact in social settings at school, at home, and in the community. (N.D. 7, 8, 10)

The student will assist in an age-appropriate decision-making process regarding health management. (N.D. 1, 2, 7)

The student will identify abilities, disabilities, and appearance in a realistic manner. (N.D. 7, 8, 10)

## Nursing Interventions

Perform annual threshold screenings on students with known hearing deficits. (N.D. 1, 2)

Collaborate with audiologist or otologist to receive current level of hearing with and without amplification or assistive devices. (N.D. 1, 2)

Explain to adults working with the student, the student's hearing deficit diagnosis, use of amplification or assistive hearing devices, and the impact on the student's ability to communicate and learn. (N.D. 1, 2, 5, 9)

Provide opportunities to reduce or remove factors that may cause or contribute to the hearing deficit in the school setting. (N.D. 2, 3, 4, 6, 9)

Provide in-service opportunities for school personnel that teach ways to promote communication and learning for the student with a hearing deficit. (N.D. 1, 2, 4, 6, 9, 10, 11)

Collaborate with student, family, and other school personnel to determine need for accommodations, 504 plan, or individualized education plan (IEP) related services. If needed, develop and implement the accommodations, 504 plan, or IEP-related services in the classroom and school setting. (N.D. 1, 2, 9)

Collaborate with teachers and assist in a referral process for further academic, speech and language, hearing, and vision assessment if academic abilities or learning needs are not progressing or being met as expected. (N.D. 1, 2, 9)

Provide educational opportunities regarding hearing deficits, management, and treatment options for the student. (N.D. 1, 2, 5, 7, 8, 9)

Provide space for extra batteries or other supplies to be stored at school. (N.D. 1, 2, 9)

In collaboration with the teacher, make accommodations to improve student's ability to communicate and learn by (list accommodations to be made). (N.D. 4–6)

Monitor the effectiveness of using the amplification or assistive hearing device. (N.D. 1, 2, 4, 5, 9)

Encourage student to tell an adult when the amplification or assistive hearing device is not working properly. (N.D. 2, 6, 7–9)

Assist the student in maintaining open communication with school personnel and family members. (N.D. 6, 10)

Provide opportunities to learn and use appropriate social skills. (N.D. 10, 11)

Encourage the student to actively participate in at least one extracurricular activity in school or the community. (N.D. 7, 8, 10, 11)

Support the student in expressing emotional needs to adults. (N.D. 6–9)

Provide opportunities where the student can make decisions regarding hearing deficit management in the school setting. (N.D. 6–9)

Encourage the student to problem-solve and to approach teachers with appropriate solutions to issues related to hearing deficit. (N.D. 2, 3, 6, 7, 9, 10)

Stress importance of the student's strengths and abilities. (N.D.7, 8)

## Expected Student Outcomes

The student will:

- Understand and describe type, cause, and severity of hearing deficit. (N.D. 1, 2, 4, 5)
- Understand and describe how the hearing deficit affects communication and learning ability. (N.D. 2, 4, 5, 6, 11)
- Follow through on medication regimens for prevention and treatment of ear infections. (N.D. 1, 5, 9)
- List and identify the names of teachers and other school personnel who can provide communication and learning assistance. (N.D. 6, 10)
- Describe (and apply) options to improve communication with others in the school and community setting. (N.D. 2–4, 6–8)
- Describe (and apply) options to reduce or remove background noise in the school and community setting. (N.D. 2, 3, 6)
- Tell others when communication efforts are ineffective. (N.D. 2, 3, 6, 7)
- Communicate appropriately and effectively with others in the school and community setting. (N.D. 2, 3, 6)
- Name the hearing amplification or assistive hearing device being used. (N.D. 1, 2, 6)
- Understand and describe how a hearing amplification or assistive device will improve the hearing and communication process. (N.D. 1–6, 9)

- Understand and describe why a hearing amplification or assistive device will positively influence educational and social situations. (N.D. 1–10)
- Demonstrate appropriate use and care of amplification or assistive hearing device. (N.D. 1, 2, 4, 5, 9)
- Wear amplification or assistive hearing device as prescribed. (N.D. 1, 2, 9).
- Know when to seek assistance if device is not working properly. (N.D. 1, 2, 6, 7, 9)
- Provide the names of friends at school and other community settings. (N.D. 7, 8, 10, 11)
- Gather a list of extracurricular activities they may be interested in participating in from the office staff, counselor, physical education teachers, and/or coaches. (N.D. 7, 8, 10, 11)
- Actively participate in at least one extracurricular activity in the school or community. (N.D. 7, 8, 10, 11)
- Demonstrate appropriate social skills in the school and community settings. (N.D. 10, 11)

## Case Study

Addison is an 11-year-old girl who will begin at TJ Middle School this fall. She is a gifted, outgoing girl who has a moderate sensorineural hearing deficit. Addison's sensorineural hearing deficit is caused by a congenital defect. She wears a hearing aid for amplification of sounds.

Addison will be placed on a mainstream sixth-grade team. Due to Addison's high level of functioning at this time, she does not require any direct assistance.

During a meeting with Addison and her parents, Addison told the school nurse that she doesn't like to call attention to herself by asking to be excused from class to change her hearing aid batteries. The father said that in the past, teachers have accused Addison of not paying attention or not following directions. Addison's mother is hopeful that her daughter will socialize with a wider group of friends. She is concerned that making friends beyond the ones from elementary school will be difficult. After the meeting with Addison and her parents, several recommendations were discussed:

1. Addison may need an emergency evacuation plan in place.
2. Addison will need time and space to install extra hearing aid batteries if needed. She will carry these in her binder and is capable of knowing when and how to change the batteries.
3. Because of Addison's hearing deficit, her parents would like to request preferential seating in all of her classrooms. Preferential seating refers to the center of the second row so she can also use visual cues from the other students.
4. In small-group situations and laboratory sessions, handouts provided prior to explaining the assignment and instruction would be beneficial.

### Emergency Evacuation Plan

**Student's Name:** Addison
**Grade:** 6
**School Building:** TJ Middle School
**Deficit Area:** Hearing deficit

**Concerned Personnel:** Teachers, Teacher's Assistant, Administrators, Support Personnel (i.e., Nurse, Counselor, Case Manager, Social Worker, Custodian, Bus Driver)

**Concern:** Addison has a hearing deficit and may not be aware when an emergency situation occurs in the school setting. Although she currently wears a hearing aid, additional assistance may be required in the event of an emergency situation in the school setting.

**Plan:** Addison may or may not be able to hear the audible emergency alarm. For this reason, it may be necessary to gain her attention by the use of visual cues. If a visual (flashing light) alarm system is not available in the building, gain Addison's attention by flickering the lights, using hand gestures, or writing a note explaining the emergency situation and the evacuation route (i.e., "Fire drill. Go out the front door to the sidewalk."). Addison will be paired with an able hearing person to assist her in the evacuation process when in the building or on the bus.

## Hearing Deficit

| Assessment Data | Nursing Diagnosis | Goals | Nursing Interventions | Expected Outcomes |
|---|---|---|---|---|
| Addison's parents worry that she is socializing with the same group of friends from her elementary school and does not seem to be making any new friends this school year. | Addison was reluctant to ask for permission to change her hearing aid batteries during third period. She waited until her fifth period lunch hour. | Risk for ineffective health maintenance related to ineffective coping by not installing new hearing aid batteries when needed. | Addison will communicate effectively with teachers and school staff.<br><br>Addison will gain knowledge and skills in the use and proper care of her hearing aid. | Explain to the adults working with Addison her hearing deficit diagnosis<br>1. use of hearing aids<br>2. the impact of hearing deficit on her ability to communicate and learn.<br><br>Provide opportunities to reduce factors that may cause or contribute to the hearing deficit in school by<br>1. explaining to the teachers the needed classroom modifications<br>2. requesting appropriate seating in the classroom.<br><br>Provide a space in the nurse's office for Addison to store and replace batteries. Encourage Addison to tell her teacher when she needs to change her hearing aid battery. |
| Occasionally Addison is accused of not paying attention or following directions during science lab. When this occurs, her comments seem inappropriate. | Disturbed sensory perception (auditory) and risk for impaired verbal communication related to moderate sensorineural hearing deficit. | Addison will reduce or remove barriers to communication and learning in the classroom and school setting by<br>1. wearing her hearing aids at all times and<br>2. asking for handouts prior to lab demonstrations and discussions. | In collaboration with the teacher, make accommodations to improve Addison's ability to communicate and learn by<br>1. seating Addison in the middle second row of the classroom<br>2. providing handouts prior to lab sessions.<br><br>Assist Addison in maintaining open communication with school personnel and parents. | Addison will understand and describe how her hearing deficit affects communication and learning abilities.<br><br>Addison will describe and apply options to improve communication with others in the school and community setting. |

| Assessment Data | Nursing Diagnosis | Goals | Nursing Interventions | Expected Outcomes |
|---|---|---|---|---|
| Addison's parents worry that she is socializing with the same group of friends from her elementary school and does not seem to be making any new friends this school year. | Risk for situational low self-esteem and social isolation related to hearing deficit in the new school environment and to other people's perception of hearing deficits. | Addison will communicate effectively with peers in the school setting. Addison will effectively interact in at least one extracurricular activity this school year. Addison will identify her abilities, disabilities, and appearance in a realistic manner. | Provide opportunities for Addison to make decisions regarding hearing deficit management in the school setting. Encourage Addison to problem-solve and approach teachers with appropriate solutions | Addison will describe and apply ways to reduce or remove background noise in the school and community setting. Addison will know what type of hearing aid she wears. Addison will understand and describe why wearing her hearing aid will positively influence educational and social situations. Addison will demonstrate appropriate use and care of her hearing aid. Addison will wear her hearing aid as prescribed. Addison will know when to seek assistance if her hearing aid is not working properly. |
| | | | Encourage Addison to actively participate in at least one extracurricular activity in school or the community. Assist Addison in maintaining open communication with school personnel and family members, talking about her social activities and level of involvement. | Addison will list and identify the names of teachers and other school personnel who can provide communication and learning assistance. Addison will know how and practice options to improve communications with others in the school and community settings. |

| Assessment Data | Nursing Diagnosis | Goals | Nursing Interventions | Expected Outcomes |
|---|---|---|---|---|
| | | | Provide opportunities to learn and use appropriate social skills by introducing Addison to other students with interests similar to hers. | Addison will tell others when she realizes communication efforts are ineffective. |
| | | | | Addison will provide the names of friends at school and other community settings. |
| | | | | Addison will provide a list of extracurricular activities to participate in. |
| | | | | Addison will actively participate in at least one extracurricular activity in the school or community. |
| | | | | Addison will demonstrate appropriate social skills in the school and community settings. |

# References

American Academy of Audiology. (1978.). *Audiogram of familiar sounds*. Reston, VA: American Academy of Audiology.

American Academy of Pediatrics (AAP). (2002). *Pediatric academic societies* [abstract]. Retrieved January 26, 2005, from http://www.aap.org/research/abstracts/02abstract17.htm

American Speech-Language-Hearing Association (ASHA). *Assistive technology*. Retrieved April 22, 2004, from http://www.asha.org/public/hearing/treatment/assist_tech.htm

Jarvis, C. (2004). *Physical examination & health assessment* (4th ed.). St. Louis, MO: Saunders.

Lewis, K. & Bear, B.J . (2002). *Manual of school health* (2nd ed.). St. Louis, MO: Saunders.

NANDA International. (2003). *Nursing diagnoses: Definitions & classification 2003-2004*. Philadelphia: Author.

National Association of School Nurses (NASN), (2003). *Position statement: Noise induced hearing loss*. Scarborough, ME: Author.

National Institute of Deafness and Other Communication Disorders (NIDCD). (2001). *Has your baby's hearing been screened?* Retrieved November 4, 2004, from www.nidcd.nih.gov/health/hearing/screened.asp

Northern, J. L.& Downs, M. P. (2002). *Hearing in children* (5th ed.). Philadelphia: Lippincott, Williams & Wilkins.

Wong, D. L., Hockenberry, M. J., Wilson, D., Winkelstein, M. L., & Kline, N. E. (2003).The child with cognitive, sensory, and communication impairment. In *Wong's nursing care of infants and children* (7th ed., pp. 994–1000). St. Louis, MO: Mosby.

# Bibliography

Gregory, E. K. (1998). *The ear & hearing: A guide for school nurses* [Manual]. Scarborough, ME: National Association of School Nurses.

Yockel, N. J. (2002). A comparison of audiometry and audiometry with tympanometry to determine middle ear status in school-age children. *Journal of School Nursing, 18*(5), 287–292.

# Resources

American Academy of Audiology
11730 Plaza America Drive
Suite 300
Reston, VA 20190
1-800-AAA-2336
www.audiology.org

American Academy of Pediatrics
141 Northwest Point Boulevard
Elk Grove Village, IL 60007-1098
847-434-4000
www.aap.org

American Speech-Language-Hearing Association
10801 Rockville Pike
Rockville, MD 20852
1-800-498-2071
www.asha.org

Cochlear Implant Association, Inc.
5335 Wisconsin Avenue, NW
Suite 440
Washington, DC 20015-2052
202-895-2781
www.cici.org

National Association of School Nurses
*Western Office:*
1416 Park Street
Suite A
Castle Rock, CO 80109
303-663-2329
 1-866-627-6767
303-663-0403 (fax)
nasn@nasn.org
*Eastern Office:*
PO Box 1300 (163 US Route 1)
Scarborough, ME 04070
207-883-2117
1-877-627-6476
207-883-2683 (fax)
nasn@nasn.org

National Institute on Deafness and Other Communication Disorders
National Institutes of Health
31 Center Drive
MSC 2320
Bethesda, MD 20892-2320
www.nidcd.nih.gov

## Chapter Forty-three

# Hemophilia

Clara J. Richardson and Lindsey W. Minchella

## Introduction

Hemophilia is the term used for a group of bleeding disorders characterized by the congenital deficiency of a specific plasma protein required for coagulation. The most common forms of hemophilia are hemophilia A and B. The combined prevalence of these two forms is 13 cases per 10,000 male births, or approximately 17,000 cases in the United States (Soucie, Rickles & Evatt, 2000).

Hemophilia A (classic hemophilia) is the deficiency of clotting factor VIII and accounts for about 80% of all cases. Its incidence is 1 in 10,000 male births (Soucie et al., 2000). Hemophilia B (Christmas disease) is less common than hemophilia A, with an incidence of 1 in 40,000 male births (Soucie et al., 2000). Factor IX is the deficient clotting factor in hemophilia B.

Hemophilia is a sex-linked recessive disorder with the defective gene located on the X chromosome, meaning that hemophilia usually affects males. Females are usually carriers of the trait. In rare cases, females can have hemophilia if their father is affected and their mother is a carrier. Up to one third of cases are due to a gene mutation and have no identified family history (Hemophilia A, n.d.).

### Pathophysiology

Hemophilia involves the impaired clotting ability of the blood resulting in prolonged bleeding. Children with hemophilia bleed longer, not faster. Bleeding into joints and muscles is most common, but bleeding into tissues can occur anywhere. Bleeding of the mouth, neck, and thorax can lead to difficulty breathing or even airway obstruction. Intracranial bleeds may result in chronic neurologic impairment or even death. Early signs include headache, nausea, vomiting, decreased level of consciousness, or changes in vision. These symptoms can occur several days after trauma. Bleeding in the gastrointestinal tract may result in anemia and may be indicated by nausea, pain, or blood in stool or vomitus. Pain in the lower abdomen or groin, limited hip extension, and numbness over the anterior quadriceps are signs of iliopsoas muscle bleeding. Testicular injury with resulting fertility or urinary tract compromise is possible. Spinal cord bleeds may cause paralysis. Other problems include nosebleeds, spontaneous hematuria, and anemia. (Hockenberry, 2003).

Hemarthrosis, bleeding into joints, is the most frequent type of internal bleeding. Initial signs are stiffness, tingling, swelling, pain, decreased range of motion, warmth, and redness. Recurrent episodes can cause synovial hypertrophy with progressive damage of cartilage and subchondral bone. Individuals with inadequate treatment of bleeding episodes may suffer from severe joint pathology, including fixed flexion, joint deformity, and muscle-wasting resulting in impaired mobility and pain (Bolton-Maggs & Pasi, 2003).

The severity of hemophilia varies greatly and is classified as mild, moderate, or severe. Approximately 60% to 70% of children with hemophilia have the severe form (Hockenberry, 2003).

- Mild: Clotting factor activity level between 5% and 50% of normal. Prolonged bleeding episode only with severe trauma or surgery.
- Moderate: Clotting factor activity level between 1% and 5% of normal. Prolonged bleeding with trauma.
- Severe: Clotting factor activity level less than or equal to 1% of normal. Spontaneous bleeding without trauma.

Laboratory tests confirm the diagnosis of hemophilia in a child who has a history of prolonged bleeding episodes. Tests of platelet function are normal, whereas tests of blood clotting mechanisms may be abnormal (Hockenberry, 2003; Cavanaugh, 2003).

- Platelet function
  - Bleeding time: normal
  - Clot retraction test: normal
- Blood clotting mechanisms
  - Whole blood clotting time: prolonged with severe hemophilia, but may be normal with mild or moderate forms
  - Prothrombin time (PT): normal
  - Partial thromboplastin time (PTT): prolonged
  - Prothrombin consumption time test: shortened
- Coagulation factor assays identify the specific clotting factor deficiency, as well as the severity of the disease.

### Management

The National Hemophilia Foundation has a prevention program called "Do the 5!"

(National Prevention Program, n.d.) The program's goal is to prevent or reduce the complications of bleeding disorders by following their five strategies for healthy living:

1. Annual comprehensive checkup at a hemophilia treatment center
2. Early and adequate treatment of bleeds
3. Hepatitis A and B vaccinations
4. Exercise to protect joints
5. Regular testing for blood-borne infections

Federal funding for hemophilia treatment centers became available in 1975, and there are approximately 140 centers in the United States (Catlin, 1999). Healthcare teams of hematology specialists staff these centers and offer comprehensive care emphasizing self-management and home care rather than repeated hospitalizations.

Treatment of hemophilia depends on the type and severity of the disease as well as the type of injury. Bleeding from minor cuts, scrapes, or abrasions may be managed as noted in **Table 1**. More severe bleeding or internal bleeding is treated primarily by the replacement of the missing clotting factor along with the nursing interventions noted in the chart.

Desmopressin (DDAVP) is recommended for the treatment of mild hemophilia A (Medical and Scientific Advisory Council [MASAC], 2003). This synthetic agent that causes the release of factor VIII may be administered intravenously or as a nasal spray.

More severe forms of hemophilia A require replacement with recombinant or plasma-derived factor VIII concentrates via intravenous infusion. Genetically engineered recombinants have been available since 1992. The third-generation forms are not derived from animal or human plasma proteins at all and should eliminate the risk of viral contamination; therefore, these recombinants are considered the treatment of choice (MASAC, 2003).

Technologically advanced viral-depleting processes and improved donor screening practices have greatly lowered, but not eliminated, the risk of viral transmission by plasma-derived factor concentrates.

Cryoprecipitate, derived from human plasma, is no longer recommended for the treatment of hemophilia because it carries a slightly higher risk of viral contamination.

The treatment of choice for hemophilia B is recombinant factor IX concentrate. Plasma-derived factor IX concentrate is also available. These agents have the same advantages and carry the same risks as recombinant factor VIII (MASAC, 2003).

The amount of factor concentrate administered is determined by the child's size as well as the site and severity of the bleed. Families trained to do intravenous infusions can provide factor replacement in the home at the first signs of bleeding. Early home management serves to prevent complications and to decrease the number of hospitalizations. Administration by a family member is rec-

## Table 1. Treatment of Hemophilia

| Site of Bleeding | Nursing Interventions |
|---|---|
| Minor cuts, scrapes, skin abrasions | Clean with soap and water<br>Sterile dressing<br>Firm pressure until bleeding stops<br>Ice pack |
| Tooth, mouth | Ice pack to face for 20 minutes<br>Have child bite on cold pack |
| Nosebleed | Pressure to nares for 20 minutes<br>Nasal pack may be necessary |
| Joint | RICE: rest area, ice pack, compression with Ace wrap, elevate affected area<br>Avoid weight bearing if hip, knee, or ankle |
| Soft tissue, muscle | RICE<br>Complete bedrest if iliopsoas muscle |

Adapted from "Hypoglycemia," by L. Gonder-Frederick, in *A CORE Curriculum for Diabetes Education* (4th ed.) by M. Franz, et al., (Eds.), 2001, Chicago: American Association of Diabetes Educators. Copyright 2001 by AADE.

Hemophilia

ommended for children over 2 years of age, and self-administration is possible by age 8 to 12 years (Hockenberry, 2003)

Prophylactic management is also an option for children with hemophilia. Primary prophylaxis, or regular administration of factor concentrate two to three times each week, has been shown to decrease long-term joint problems (Hockenberry, 2003). Due to its often prohibitive cost and potential complications, this option is reserved for individuals with severe hemophilia (Butler, McClure & Wulfe, 2003, Prophylaxis, n.d.). Secondary prophylaxis involves regular administration for a limited period of time after a bleeding episode to prevent repeated bleeding into the same area.

Other medications may be included in a child's management plan (Hockenberry, 2003). Acetaminophen is usually recommended for pain during a bleeding episode. Corticosteriods may be used for hematuria, acute hemarthrosis, or chronic synovitis. Nonsteroidal anti-inflammatory drugs (NSAIDs) may be used to treat synovitis pain but are used cautiously because they can inhibit platelet function. Oral epsilon aminocaproic acid (EACA, Amicar) may be prescribed to maintain clots before oral surgery or after mouth trauma.

In addition to avoiding situations that might cause bleeding, additional measures may prevent bleeding episodes (Hemophilia A, n.d.). Prophylactic factor administration or DDAVP may be given before dental extractions or surgeries. Drugs to be avoided include aspirin, heparin, and coumadin. Practicing good dental care, including regular brushing, flossing, and checkups, will decrease tissue trauma during cleaning by the hygienist and prevent the need for tooth extractions.

Vaccination for hepatitis A and B is strongly recommended to prevent transmission of the disease from plasma-derived factor concentrates. Improved methods of viral inactivation have greatly decreased, but not eliminated, the risk of transmission. Hepatitis B can be killed, but hepatitis A is resistant to these methods (Hepatitis, n.d.).

Regular exercise will strengthen the muscles surrounding joints providing protection for the joints and hopefully decreasing the occurrence of spontaneous bleeds. Contact sports with a high risk for injury should be avoided, but activities such as walking, biking, swimming, and golfing are very effective forms of exercise. Weight control is also necessary to avoid excess stress on joints. Adequate calcium and protein intake is helpful to promote healthy bones and joints.

Regular testing for blood-borne infections will allow early identification and treatment. Although vaccines are available to prevent hepatitis A and B, there is no vaccine for hepatitis C. Without annual testing, hepatitis C might go undiagnosed, because it can be mild or without obvious symptoms. Transmission of human immunodeficiency virus (HIV) has been a major concern for individuals with hemophilia. In the early 1980s, about 60% of those treated with plasma-derived factor concentrates were infected with HIV (hemophilia A, n.d.). After considerable technological innovation in viral inactivation methods and advanced donor screening techniques, the risk of becoming infected with HIV via currently used products has been virtually eliminated (HIV/AIDS FAQs, n.d.).

Another concern for those with hemophilia is the possibility of developing inhibitors, or antibodies that develop after replacement therapy. Inhibitors occur in 15% to 30% of people with hemophilia A and 2% to 5% of those with hemophilia B (Disorder Overview, n.d.). Inhibitor titers are measured in Bethesda units (BU) and determine the type of replacement therapy that can be used to treat bleeding episodes. Individuals with titers <10 BU are considered to be low responders who can receive the usual factor replacement products in higher doses. High responders have titers >10 BU and are only given the usual products for life- or limb-threatening bleeding complications. In other situations, they receive prothrombin complex concentration, activated prothrombin complex concentration, or recombinant factor VIIa. These products may cause adverse reactions and are less effective than factor VIII or IX concentrates. Other interventions, such as plasmapheresis, porcine factor VIII, and immune tolerance therapy, are extremely costly and of limited usefulness in treating inhibitors (Disorder Overview, n.d.).

Gene therapy, involving the introduction of a working copy of the defective factor into people with hemophilia, is in the research stage and may become a management strategy in the future. In the meantime, following the steps of "Do the 5!" can maximize the quality of life for children with hemophilia.

## Individualized Healthcare Plan

### Assessment
*History*
- Developmental history and health history prior to diagnosis of hemophilia
- Date of initial hemophilia diagnosis
- Type of hemophilia; severity of factor deficiency
- Tests for HIV, hepatitis (family may choose not to share results, but advise to have these done)
- History of immunizations (including hepatitis A and B)
- Family history, including genetic testing for hemophilia
- Injuries, surgeries, and related bleeding episodes
- Signs and symptoms of past bleeding episodes

- History of bleeding episode treatment and response to treatment
- Frequency of hospitalizations, emergency department visits, physical therapy treatments
- History of school attendance patterns
- Activity restrictions advised; past participation in activities, sports, physical education

### Current Status and Management
- Primary physician
- Hemophilia treatment center/phone numbers/frequency of contacts
- Medical provider contact numbers (doctors, nurses, physical therapists)
- Personal contact numbers (family, work numbers, emergency contacts)
- Access to medical care (transportation, insurance)
- Recent contacts with primary physician and with hemophilia treatment center
- Medications
- Factor replacement (products used, guidelines for administration, prophylaxis)
- Pain management plan
- Allergies
- Height and weight (recent changes)
- General health status
- Nutritional status (diet history focusing on fiber, calcium, protein, texture, fluid intake)
- Dental care status
- Present problems related to hemophilia (anemia, joint or muscle problems, bruising, other bleeding)
- Posture, gait, coordination, balance
- Activities (e.g., sports involvement, hobbies)
- Activity restrictions; guidelines for physical education; safety equipment advised
- Current therapy (physical, occupational)
- Current management plan for minor injuries and major injuries
- Medical alert identification?

### Self-care
- Student's knowledge about current health status and about hemophilia
- Student's perception of his/her abilities or restrictions
- Parent's perceptions of student's abilities or restrictions
- Student's decision-making skills
- Student's ability to recognize signs of bleeding
- Student's ability to self-administer Factor
- Student's motivation to follow up with hemophilia care
- Family's knowledge about disease and treatment
- Family's sources for information about hemophilia
- Student's barriers to participation in self-care

### Psychosocial Status
- Student's contact and interactions with family
- Student's contact and interactions with peers and adults
- Student's locus of control
- Student's involvement with support persons, groups, and community services
- Student's participation in family, peer, school, and community activities
- Student's strengths, concerns, and needs (peer and teacher relationships, feelings of fairness)
- Family's strengths, concerns, and needs (relationships, finances, genetic counseling)

### Academic Issues
- Past academic achievement
- Current academic achievement; strengths and concerns
- Number and type of schools student has attended
- Special educational services: past services, current needs
- Teacher/staff knowledge about disease and treatment
- Participation in school activities, physical education, and extracurricular activities
- School and classroom modifications needed (elevator pass, extended passing period, and alternate activities during bleeding episodes)

- Specialized healthcare procedures required during the school day
- Emergency evacuation and information to emergency personnel

## Nursing Diagnoses (N.D.) (NANDA 2003)

**N.D. 1** Risk for acute injury (NANDA, 00035) related to deficiency of clotting factor.
**N.D. 2** Risk for acute pain (NANDA, 00132) related to:
- bleeding episode
- swelling

**N.D. 3** Risk for impaired physical mobility (NANDA, 00085) related to:
- bleeding episode
- swelling
- discomfort

**N.D. 4** Risk for chronic injury (NANDA, 00035) related to:
- repeated bleeding into joint
- musculoskeletal deformity

**N.D. 5** Deficient knowledge (NANDA, 00126) related to:
- lack of exposure to information about hemophilia
- unfamiliarity with information resources about hemophilia

**N.D. 6** Risk for noncompliance with healthcare plan (NANDA, 00079) related to:
- deficient knowledge
- complexity of healthcare plan
- health beliefs about diagnosis

**N.D. 7** Risk for ineffective student role performance (NANDA, 00055) related to:
- absences from school due to bleeding episodes
- restriction of participation in activities due to risk for injury, recuperation period after bleeding episode

**N.D. 8** Risk for chronic pain (NANDA, 00133) related to:
- altered mobility
- musculoskeletal deformity

**N.D. 9** Risk for disturbed body image (NANDA, 00118) related to:
- perceived difference from peers
- restriction of participation in activities due to risk for injury, recuperation period after bleeding episode

**N.D. 10** Risk for powerlessness (NANDA, 00125) related to:
- deficient knowledge
- complexity of healthcare plan
- body image

## Goals

The student will identify and respond to bleeding episodes promptly and adequately. (N.D 1, 3, 4, 6, 10)
The student will evaluate effectiveness of pain management techniques. (N.D. 2, 8, 10)
The student will participate in an exercise plan to strengthen muscles, protect joints, and minimize risk of bleeding episodes. (N.D. 1–4, 10)
The student will increase his/her knowledge about hemophilia. (N.D. 5, 10)
The student will utilize information resources about hemophilia. (N.D. 5, 10)
The student will comply with safety measures to prevent bleeding episodes. (N.D. 1, 4, 6, 10)
The student will comply with treatment measures. (N.D. 1–3, 6, 10)
The student will comply with school policies for absences and make up assignments. (N.D. 6, 7)
The student will maximize participation in school activities. (N.D. 4, 7, 9, 10)

## Nursing Interventions

*Environmental management: safety*
With the student, family, and teacher, identify potential sources of injury: (N.D. 1, 4, 10)
- classroom
- playground
- hallways
- physical education class

- sports activities
- school field trips

With the student, family, and teacher, implement safety measures to prevent acute injuries and bleeding episodes. (N.D. 1, 2, 3, 10)

### Bleeding precautions

With the student and school staff, implement safety measures to prevent injury: (N.D. 1, 4, 10)
- enforcement of school safety policies
- educate peers, teachers, staff about injury prevention
- use protective padding and equipment according to activity
- annual update of medical ID bracelet, including diagnosis, treatment product, and blood type

### Emergency care

With student, family, and healthcare providers, design emergency care plan (ECP), including: (N.D. 1–4)
- assessment of injury
- treatment guidelines for minor injuries and suspected internal bleeding
- contact numbers and guidelines for contacting family members, healthcare providers, emergency management system
- guidelines for fieldtrips
- authorization for medications to be administered by school staff

With student, family, and healthcare providers, implement ECP to treat bleeding episodes promptly and adequately. (N.D. 1-4, 10)

### Supply management

Obtain medications, equipment, and supplies to be utilized in implementation of the ECP. (N.D. 1–3)

### Bleeding reduction

With student, implement ECP: (N.D. 1–4, 8, 10)
- immobilize area of bleed when student has pain
- apply ice to area of bleeding
- apply gentle compression to area of bleeding
- elevate affected area
- active range of motion as pain subsides (avoid passive range of motion to avoid further injury)
- soft diet for mouth bleeding

### Pain management

With student, assess and treat acute pain during a bleeding episode: (N.D. 2, 10)
- use a pain scale (FACES, 1–10) to assess need for and to evaluate effectiveness of medication
- administer pain medication according to ECP guidelines
- evaluate effectiveness of pain management techniques

### Medication management

With student, assess and treat chronic pain: (N.D. 8, 10)
- discuss student's perception of comfort level
- evaluate effectiveness of medication regimen
- monitor for adverse reactions to medication

### Documentation

Document implementation steps and effectiveness of ECP during a bleeding episode. (N.D. 1–4)

### Staff development

Provide in-service education for school staff (teachers, principal, aides, lunchroom supervisor, playground supervisor, secretary) including: (N.D. 1–4, 7)
- definition of hemophilia
- type and severity of student's hemophilia
- potential sources of injury
- measures to prevent injury

Hemophilia

- activity restrictions
- assessment of injury
- signs of bleeding
- treatment of minor injuries
- treatment of suspected bleeding
- pain management techniques
- prevention of joint bleeding
- information resources about hemophilia

Discuss with school staff the potential for intracranial bleeding which might result in learning problems. (N.D. 1, 4, 7)

Acknowledge school staff members' possible fear of HIV infection and provide information regarding transmission and current safety of treatment. (N.D. 9)

### Sports-injury prevention: youth
Discuss with student, family, and school staff, strategies to prevent bleeding into joints: (N.D. 1, 4, 8, 10)
- regular exercise to strengthen muscles surrounding joints
- avoidance of contact sports that have a high risk for injury
- maintenance of weight and good nutrition
- adherence to safety rules
- use of protective padding and equipment
- early recognition and treatment of bleeding episodes

### Consultation
Refer to physical and/or occupational therapist for evaluation. (N.D. 3, 4)
Refer to special education team for evaluation. (N.D. 7)

### Teaching: disease process
Assess student's and family's knowledge about hemophilia, including: (N.D. 5–10)
- pathophysiology
- genetic implications
- potential complications
- classification of severity
- measures to prevent bleeding
- signs of bleeding
- treatment measures
- administration of medications and factor products
- self-administration of factor products
- implications of treatment choices (risks and benefits of various factor products, prophylaxis)
- importance of good nutrition and avoidance of obesity
- importance of exercise and physical activities with decreased risk of injury
- importance of dental hygiene and regular dental care
- hepatitis immunizations
- regular testing for blood-borne infections, anemia, and microscopic hematuria
- possible development of inhibitors

### Teaching: prescribed activity/exercise
Discuss activity restrictions to: (N.D. 1, 4, 6–10)
- prevent injury
- allow recuperation after a bleeding episode
- maximize participation in school and extracurricular activities

### Health education
Assess student's and family's awareness of and use of information resources about hemophilia, including: (N.D. 5, 6, 10)
- nearest hemophilia treatment center
- National Hemophilia Foundation
- Hemophilia and AIDS/HIV Network for Dissemination of Information (HANDI)
- Canadian Hemophilia Society

*Self-responsibility facilitation*
Discuss barriers to compliance with student and family including: (N.D. 5, 6, 7, 9, 10)
- knowledge about hemophilia
- concerns about emergency treatment plan
- barriers to self-care
- student concerns (peer and teacher relationships, potential complications)
- family concerns (potential complications, finances, eligibility for medical insurance, genetic and cultural implications)
- relationships with healthcare providers (especially during transition from adolescence to adulthood)

*Health system guidance*
Refer to available community resources as indicated by identified barriers. (N. D. 6, 10)

*Role enhancement*
Discuss school policies and special adaptations needed for absence and make up assignments with student, family, and teacher. (N.D. 7)

*Self-esteem enhancement*
Refer to school counselor as indicated. (N.D. 6, 9, 10)
Refer to available hemophilia support groups. (N.D. 6, 9, 10)

## Expected Student Outcomes

The student will:
*Personal safety behavior*
- Identify potential sources of injury within the school environment. (N.D. 1, 4, 10)
- Identify safety measures to prevent injury. (N.D. 1, 4, 10)
- Follow school safety policies. (N.D. 1, 4, 6, 10)
- Discuss injury prevention with peers, teachers, staff. (N.D. 1, 4, 10)
- Use protective padding and equipment to prevent injury. (N.D. 1, 4, 6, 10)
- Wear medical ID bracelet. (N.D. 1, 4, 6, 10)
- Avoid contact sports that have a high risk of injury. (N.D. 1, 4, 5, 6, 10)
- Evaluate risks of chosen school activities. (N.D. 1, 4, 5, 7, 10)

*Health-seeking behavior*
- Report injuries promptly to school staff. (N.D. 1–4, 5, 6, 10)
- Report injuries to parent after school. (N.D. 1–4, 5, 6, 10)
- Seek additional information about hemophilia and its treatment from school nurse, parent, healthcare providers. (N.D. 5, 6, 9, 10)

*Health-promoting behavior*
- Discuss importance of weight and health maintenance with school nurse, parent, healthcare providers. (N.D. 1, 4, 5, 6, 10)
- Discuss importance of nutrition and special dietary needs, which might include soft diet, high fiber, protein, calcium, fluid intake. (N.D. 1,5,6,10)
- Discuss importance of regular vision, hearing, blood pressure, urine, and blood screening. (N.D. 1, 5, 6, 10)

*Oral hygiene*
- Practice good dental hygiene. (N.D. 1, 5, 6, 10)
- Discuss the importance of regular dental care. (N.D. 1, 5, 6, 10)

*Compliance behavior*
- Report suspected bleeding promptly. (N.D. 1–4, 5, 6, 10)
- Comply with steps of emergency management plan. (N.D. 1–4, 6,10)
- Comply with immobilization, ice, compression, and elevation techniques. (N.D. 1–4, 5, 6, 10)
- Comply with regular dental checkups. (N.D. 1, 5, 6, 10)
- Comply with scheduled visits to healthcare providers and hemophilia treatment center. (N.D. 5, 6, 10)
- Comply with activity restrictions as recommended. (N.D. 3–6, 9 ,10)

*Participation in healthcare decisions*
- Participate in design of ECP. (N.D. 1–4,10)
- Participate in development and implementation of exercise plan. (N.D. 1, 4, 5, 6, 10)

*Blood loss severity*
- Recognize signs of bleeding. (N.D. 1–5)
- Report signs of bleeding promptly to initiate ECP. (N.D. 1–6, 10)

*Mobility*
- Institute active range of motion as pain subsides. (N.D. 1–4, 5, 6, 8, 10)

*Knowledge: treatment regimen*
- Increase knowledge about hemophilia and its treatment. (N.D. 5, 6, 9, 10)
- Increase knowledge about self-administration of medications and factor products. (N.D. 1–5, 10)

*Self-care: parenteral medication*
- Increase self-management of hemophilia. (N.D. 1–6,10)

*Role performance*
- Follow school policies on absences and make-up assignments. (N.D. 7)

*Social involvement*
- Identify areas of interest in school activities. (N.D. 7, 9)
- Participate in a variety of school activities. (N.D. 7, 9, 10)

*Body image*
- Relate concerns about how hemophilia affects life to parent, school nurse, healthcare providers. (N.D. 6, 7, 9)
- Discuss the importance of safe-sex practices (N.D. 5)

## Case Study

Matt, aged 13, is a new student at Superstar Middle School. Matt and his mother moved to the area from a neighboring state because Matt's mother found work in the area. They do not have a support system in the area, and they have not yet established a primary healthcare provider. Matt is socially inclined and enjoys sports. He is proud to be a member of his school's 7th-grade basketball team.

### Past Health History

Matt was diagnosed with hemophilia when he had a tonsillectomy at age 5. During the procedure, he had persistent bleeding. When the bleeding was reported to Matt's mother, she revealed that her brother had hemophilia. Matt was found to have moderate hemophilia A with 4% factor VIII deficiency. Matt required cauterization and received factor VIII with good response. Matt and his mother were referred to and followed up with a hemophilia treatment center after diagnosis. He received hepatitis A and B immunizations.

Matt had two episodes of joint swelling after falls when he was 8 and 10. He was treated with factor VIII. Matt has always bruised easily and has had frequent but manageable nosebleeds. He had not had significant bleeding since the joint bleed when he was 10. Matt has no other health concerns.

Matt's mother worries about Matt's sport activity and recalls that the hemophilia treatment center had advised against playing contact sports. She is not sure if basketball is a contact sport. Matt assured his mother that he will stop playing basketball if it is dangerous.

Matt has never been to the school nurse, and on account of Matt's request, he and his mother have not yet shared his hemophilia diagnosis with anyone at Superstar Middle School.

### Current Injury

Matt injured his right ankle during basketball practice after school. The ankle did not appear swollen at the time of injury. The coach advised Matt to rest, ice his ankle, and elevate it, and to tell his mother about the injury. Matt followed the advice but did not tell his mother about the injury, hoping that it would improve quickly. His ankle swelled significantly overnight. Matt's mother went to work before he awoke. Matt's homeroom teacher noted that Matt had trouble walking and sent Matt to see the school nurse.

Matt told the nurse, "I came down on my ankle while I was practicing basketball. I iced it and elevated it like Coach said." The right ankle is spongy, warm, and tender, with dark bluish-red discoloration. There is limited range of motion of the right ankle, and Matt does not bear full weight on it. Matt's blood pressure is 108/64, pulse 84, and respirations 24. Matt appears anxious and in pain. The right ankle appears to be fluid-filled, possibly with blood. There is possible bleeding into joint and possible sprain or fracture. The nurse contacts Matt's mother to seek medical evaluation. The nurse will follow-up after evaluation to determine diagnosis and will discuss care of ankle and prevention of future injuries with student.

## Interventions

The nurse called Matt's mother at work and advised her to take Matt for medical care. Mother reported Matt's history of hemophilia. While waiting for Matt's mother, the nurse revealed to Matt that his mother reported his diagnosis of hemophilia. While affirming Matt's desire to avoid standing out as having a special need with his peers, the nurse imparted the safety aspect of communicating his diagnosis and providing prompt attention to injuries. Matt's mother talked with the nurse about the lack of a medical provider. She reported that she had worked at her job just long enough to receive insurance coverage. The nurse referred her to a local emergency care facility and gave information about pediatricians and the closest hemophilia treatment center. The nurse asked Matt's mother to keep her updated about Matt's status. The nurse noted that an individualized healthcare plan (IHP) and an ECP would be developed with input from Matt, his mother, and their healthcare provider.

Mother took Matt to the emergency facility. An x-ray showed no fractures. Factor VIII was given to control bleeding. Appropriate pain medication and crutches were prescribed. An appointment was made for 3 days later at the closest hemophilia treatment center.

## Follow-up

The nurse asked Matt's mother to sign consents to obtain information and doctor's orders/guidelines from the hemophilia treatment center. A health-planning meeting was held for the purpose of gathering information to develop an IHP and an ECP. Alternatives to basketball were considered because the new doctor restricted Matt from playing contact sports, including competitive basketball. Matt became a manager for the basketball team and was allowed to shoot free throws with the team. He thought he might consider trying swimming or bowling teams in the future.

School staff met with Matt, his mother, and the nurse to develop a school plan incorporating health and educational accommodations. The school nurse discussed safety with Matt, and they decided to give a presentation to Matt's health class about hemophilia. The school nurse met with appropriate staff to teach about Matt's IHP and ECP.

# Hemophilia

| Assessment Data | Nursing Diagnosis | Goals | Nursing Interventions | Expected Outcomes |
|---|---|---|---|---|
| Student with moderate hemophilia A with 4% factor VIII deficiency.<br><br>Student has had four past bleeding episodes:<br>1. during surgery when 5 years old<br>2. joint bleed from fall when 8 years old<br>3. joint bleed from fall when 10 years old<br>4. joint bleed from ankle injury when 13 years old (present time)<br><br>Student bruises easily and has had nosebleeds, which have been manageable. | Risk for injury causing prolonged bleeding related to deficiency of clotting factor. | Matt will participate in implementation of safety measures to prevent acute injuries/bleeding episodes.<br><br>Matt will participate in planning peer education/safety measures.<br><br>Matt will participate in development and implementation of ECP for bleeding episodes.<br><br>Matt will participate in identifying and treating bleeding episodes promptly and adequately. | Coordinate with physical therapist to obtain doctor's activity/PT orders, and with Matt, develop mobility safety plan for prevention of injuries in the school environment.<br><br>Meet with appropriate school staff to teach about safety plan (include PE teacher, classroom teachers, bus driver).<br><br>Discuss with Matt about educating peers about hemophilia and safety measures to avoid injury.<br><br>Contact hemophilia treatment center outreach nurse; plan and coordinate peer education program with Matt, who has expressed interest in participating in a presentation on hemophilia in health class.<br><br>Educate Matt and his mother about medical ID bracelet for student, as a way to inform public about care needed in an emergency.<br><br>Develop an ECP with Matt and mother.<br><br>Meet to discuss ECP with appropriate school staff to teach about ECP. | School safety plan will be developed and incorporated in IHP/504 plan by Date:<br><br>Meet with staff by Date: ___<br><br>Matt will verbalize understanding of safety measures to prevent injury when among peers by Date: ___<br><br>Matt will participate in planning and giving program about hemophilia for health class by Date: ___<br><br>Matt will wear medical ID bracelet by Date: ___<br><br>Develop ECP by Date: ___ (See attached ECP).<br><br>Meet with staff by Date: ___<br><br>Matt will verbalize signs and symptoms of potential bleeding episodes, including the most common episodes (joint and muscle) and the nonobvious episodes (internal bleeding episodes) as listed in the ECP, by Date: ___<br><br>Matt will verbalize his signs and symptoms of a bleeding episode. |

**Hemophilia**

| Assessment Data | Nursing Diagnosis | Goals | Nursing Interventions | Expected Outcomes |
|---|---|---|---|---|
| | | | Discuss with Matt the signs and symptoms of bleeding episodes noted in ECP.<br><br>Discuss with Matt how to seek prompt treatment for bleeding episodes. | Matt will verbalize what he will do when a bleeding episode occurs at school, during after-school activities, and on field trips by Date: ____.<br><br>Matt will follow the ECP when an episode occurs.<br><br>Matt will effectively manage bleeding, pain, and swelling at school.<br><br>Matt will comply with hemophilia treatment measures.<br><br>Discuss with Matt ECP and management of bleeding episodes, pain, and swelling.<br><br>Discuss with Matt the prescribed hemophilia treatment following injury or bleeding episode.<br><br>Matt will verbalize 2 reasons for prompt treatment following injuries (to decrease swelling and pain, to prevent long-term complications) by Date: ____. |

| Assessment Data | Nursing Diagnosis | Goals | Nursing Interventions | Expected Outcomes |
|---|---|---|---|---|
| Adolescent who enjoys typical peer activities and active lifestyle may have repeated injuries involving pain and swelling. | Risk for acute pain associated with bleeding and swelling. | Matt will report pain and discomfort as they occur. | Discuss pain/swelling management plan with Matt and mother to ensure comfort and ease of mobility. | Matt will verbalize 2 reasons for exercise plan (to strengthen muscles and to protect joints to minimize risk of bleeding episodes) by Date: |
| Adolescent who enjoys typical adolescent peer activities and active lifestyle may have repeated injuries involving pain and swelling which may impair mobility. | Risk for impaired physical mobility related to joint/muscle bleeding episodes causing swelling and discomfort. | Matt will participate in an exercise plan to strengthen muscles, protect joints, and minimize risk of bleeding episodes. | Discuss with Matt need to follow up with his doctor and physical therapists' plan to strengthen muscles and protect joints to minimize risk of bleeding episodes. | Matt will comply with activity restriction plan during bleeding episodes. |
| | | Matt will participate in a plan for alternative activity, according to physical therapist and doctor's orders, during episodes of impaired mobility. | Coordinate with school physical therapist re: exercise program for Matt to maintain joint and muscle strength at school. | |
| | | | Discuss activity plan, such as elevator use or lengthened passing period, with Mat and staff during injury episodes when altered activity is necessary. | |
| Student and parent are new in area and had limited access with hemophilia treatment center since diagnosis of hemophilia. | Deficient knowledge related to lack of exposure to information about hemophilia and unfamiliarity with information resources about hemophilia. | Matt will increase his knowledge about hemophilia.<br><br>Matt will have access to utilize information resources about hemophilia. | Coordinate with hemophilia treatment center nurse to assess Matt's knowledge about hemophilia, including its treatment, complications, prevention of complications, and long-term implications.<br><br>Coordinate with hemophilia treatment center nurse to reinforce teaching of information with Matt about above listed implications of hemophilia. | Matt will verbalize current understanding about hemophilia, its treatment, complications that can occur, prevention of complications, and long-term implications, by Date:<br><br>Matt will follow up with hemophilia treatment center treatment and education program with school nurse for reinforcement of information. |

| Assessment Data | Nursing Diagnosis | Goals | Nursing Interventions | Expected Outcomes |
|---|---|---|---|---|
| | | | Provide information resources about National Hemophilia Foundation, support groups, and useful Web sites.<br><br>Discuss with Matt importance of following up with hemophilia treatment center.<br><br>Coordinate with treatment center nurse, Matt, and Matt's mother to develop a resource notebook to keep information about hemophilia. | Matt will maintain resource and reference notebook to keep useful information about hemophilia (including information about factor, diary of bleeding episodes, and immunization records) by Date: _____. |
| Adolescent student, who desires to be like peers, be active in sports, socially active.<br><br>Student and parent unclear of definition of contact sports.<br><br>Had not established health-care provider. | Risk for noncompliance with healthcare plan related to deficient knowledge. | Matt will comply with health-care plan, including activity restrictions to prevent injury and activity restrictions after bleeding episodes to allow healing. | Coordinate with hemophilia treatment center nurse to have Matt discuss barriers to compliance with student and family (including concerns about long-term implications, peer perceptions, wearing of ID bracelet, activity restrictions, peer relationships).<br><br>Refer to school counselor if needed.<br><br>Coordinate with hemophilia treatment center about referring Matt to support groups or chat rooms for adolescents with hemophilia.<br><br>Encourage Matt to keep diary to express his feelings.<br><br>Refer mother/Matt to community agencies as needed. | Matt will verbalize his perceptions of his/his family's barriers to compliance by Date: _____.<br><br>Matt will verbalize plan to increase compliance in one specific area, such as activity restriction, by Date: _____.<br><br>Matt will have access to adolescent and family support systems when needed. |

| Assessment Data | Nursing Diagnosis | Goals | Nursing Interventions | Expected Outcomes |
|---|---|---|---|---|
| Student playing contact sport. Student not telling anyone at school about diagnosis. | Disturbed body image related to restriction of physical activity. | Matt will comply with activity restrictions and safety measures. Matt will maximize participation in school activities. Matt will discuss diagnosis with school staff. | Discuss sports injury prevention with Matt, mother, and school staff. Discuss noncontact sports alternatives with Matt. Discuss need for school staff to have knowledge about diagnosis with Matt and mother. Refer to school counselor regarding body image issues. | Matt will evaluate risks of chosen activities by Date: ____. Matt will identify areas of interest and participate in noncontact sports by Date: ____. Matt will participate in a variety of school activities throughout school year. Matt will relate concerns about diagnosis to school staff. |
| Restriction of basketball participation. Student not telling mother about injury. Referral to school nurse by teacher. | Sense of powerlessness related to deficient knowledge and disturbance of body image. | Matt will actively participate in development of IHP and ECP. Matt will increase his knowledge about hemophilia. Matt will comply with treatment measures prescribed by doctor. Matt will verbalize pain and discomfort to school nurse when they occur. Matt will utilize available community resources. Matt will verbalize increased sense of control. Matt will participate in presentation about hemophilia to health class. Matt will promptly identify and respond to bleeding episodes and injuries to initiate ECP. | Include Matt in all healthcare-planning meetings. Assess Matt's knowledge about hemophilia. Provide Matt with information resources. Provide Matt with contact to local hemophilia support group. Discuss with Matt any concerns about coping with diagnosis. Assist Matt in planning and implementing presentation on hemophilia to health class. | Matt will actively participate in development of Individual Healthcare Plan and Emergency Care Plan by Date: ____. Matt will seek information about hemophilia as needed. Matt will contact local hemophilia support group as needed. Matt will verbalize concerns to school staff. Matt will design presentation about hemophilia for health class by Date: ____. Matt will promptly report bleeding and injuries to school staff, school nurse, and mother. |

# Emergency Care Plan
# Hemophilia

Date: _____  Parent(s)/Guardian(s): _____

Student: _____  _____

Date of birth: _____

Parent(s)/Guardian(s): _____  Home telephone: _____

_____  Work: _____

_____  Cell: _____

Emergency/Contacts: _____  Telephone: _____

_____  Telephone: _____

Primary Doctor/

Care Center: _____  Telephone: _____

Telephone: _____

**General information about student with Hemophilia** - Hemophilia is an inherited blood disorder in which blood does not clot properly. People with hemophilia bleed longer, not faster. Severity can be mild, moderate, or severe. Internal bleeds in joints or muscles are most common. Minor injuries, such as small cuts or abrasions, nosebleeds, and mouth bleeds are usually not serious but must be assessed promptly and monitored to ensure bleeding has stopped. If possible, a school nurse should assess injuries. If there is no school nurse in the school or for field trips, designated staff should be trained by a school nurse in first aid for the student. A responsible person should accompany students to the health clinic. Parent should be notified of injuries. A blow to the head, neck, abdomen, or groin may cause internal bleeding and should be assessed promptly by medical personnel. **Use Universal Precautions in all cases of First Aid.**

| If this happens | Actions to take |
|---|---|
| **1. Nosebleed** | a. Position sitting with the head upright, slightly forward.<br>b. Apply firm continuous pressure to the nose by pinching the nose for 20 minutes (have student do this if possible).<br>c. Apply a cold pack if needed.<br>d. Call parent to come if bleeding has not stopped after 20 minutes. |
| **2. Mouth bleed** | a. Apply cold compress with firm continuous pressure 20 minutes.<br>b. Call parent to come if bleeding has not stopped after 20 minutes |

Hemophilia

| If this happens | Actions to take |
|---|---|
| **3. Bleeding from a cut, scrape, or laceration** | a. Clean the wound with soap and water.<br>b. Apply firm pressure and elevate the body part until bleeding stops.<br>c. Apply bandage or dressing.<br>d. Apply an ice pack to the area over the dressing if needed.<br>e. Observe wound for 20 minutes.<br>f. Call parent to come if bleeding continues or if laceration may require sutures.<br>g. Call 911 if bleeding is severe and if parent cannot be reached. |
| **4. Joint or muscle injury or possible fracture**<br><br>*Signs/symptoms of bleeding into a joint*<br>• Bubbling, prickly, or tingling feeling in the joint<br>• Feeling of warmth or swelling in a joint<br>• Decreased range of motion, stiffness, pain, or tenderness<br>• Blueness or discoloration of surrounding skin<br><br>*Signs/symptoms of bleeding into a muscle*<br>• Gradually intensifying pain, tightness, swelling<br>• Limitation of movement in surrounding joints<br>• Numbness or loss of sensation in the limb<br>• Blueness or discoloration of surrounding skin<br>• Pain in lower abdomen & groin if iliopsoas muscle bleed<br><br>*Student may say "I am having a bleeding episode"* | a. Notify parent of need for evaluation for possible fracture or hemophilia treatment.<br>b. Immobilize the area of injury/Rest<br>c. Apply ice<br>d. Elevate area of injury<br>e. Follow doctor's orders regarding compression bandage, supports to immobilize area, medication, and exercise after injury<br>f. Call 911 if possible fracture or severe joint bleed and parent cannot be reached.<br>g. Call 911 if bleed suspected in iliopsoas muscle. |
| **5. Blow injury or fall affecting head, neck, abdomen, groin; possibly causing internal bleeding**<br><br>**Signs and symptoms of internal bleeding:**<br>• Bruising/discoloration/swelling/pain of injured area<br>• Blood in urine (urine may be pink, red, or cola colored)<br>• Vomit or respiratory secretions with red or brown material<br>• Severe headache, irritability, confusion, drowsiness<br>• Trouble swallowing or breathing<br>• Blurred or double vision, vision changes, unequal pupils<br>• Blood in stools (tarry or bloody)<br><br>*Note: slow bleed after trauma may delay symptoms for days* | a. Call parent immediately.<br>b. Call doctor or Hemophilia Treatment Center if the parent cannot be reached.<br>c. Call 911 if parent cannot be reached and there has been a blow to the head, neck or abdomen.<br>d. Have student rest and keep student calm.<br>e. Evaluate blood pressure, pulse, respirations, level of consciousness, orientation, color<br>f. Be prepared to treat for shock if needed. |

This emergency healthcare plan was developed to provide school staff with information about caring for this student at school. Staff and parents, please keep the School Nurse updated about significant health information for this student.

**Signatures:**

School Nurse_____ Phone_____ Date_____

Parent/guardian (if required)_____ Date_____

# References

Bolton-Maggs, P., & Pasi, K. J. (2003). Haemophilias A and B [Electronic version]. *Lancet, 361,* 1801–1809.

Butler, R. B., McClure, W., & Wulfe, K. (2003). Practice patterns in haemophilia A therapy: A survey of treatment centers in the United States [Electronic version]. *Haemophilia, 9,* 549–554.

Catlin, A. J., & Schaefer, J. (1999). Ethical dilemmas in the pediatric community ?Electronic version?. *Pediatric Nursing, 5,* 537–539.

Cavanaugh, B. M. (2003). *Nurse's manual of laboratory and diagnostic tests* (4th ed.). Philadelphia: Davis.

Disorder overview. (n.d.). Retrieved March 1, 2004, from National Hemophilia Foundation Web site: http://www.hemophilia.org/inhibitors/providers.html

Hemophilia A. (n.d.). Retrieved January 22, 2004, from National Hemophilia Foundation Web site: http://www.hemophilia.org/bdi/bdi_types1.htm

HIV/AIDS FAQs. (n.d.). Retrieved February 23, 2004, from National Hemophilia Foundation Web site: http://www.hemophilia.org/bdi/bdi_safety3b.htm

Hockenberry, M. J. (2003). *Wong's nursing care of infants and children* (7th ed.). St. Louis, MO: Mosby.

NANDA International. (2003). *NANDA nursing diagnoses: Definitions & classification 2003-2004.* Philadelphia: Author.

Medical and scientific advisory council recommendations concerning the treatment of hemophilia and other bleeding disorders document 151. (2003, November 9). Retrieved January 22, 2004, from National Hemophilia Foundation Web site: http://www.hemophilia.org/research/masac/masac.151.htm.

National prevention program. (n.d.). Retrieved January 22, 2004, from National Hemophilia Foundation Web site: http://www.hemophilia.org/programs/npp/npp.htm

Prophylaxis: A fact sheet for parents. Retrieved November 29, 2004, from National Hemophilia Foundation Web site: http://www.hemophilia.org/resources/prophylaxis.htm

Soucie, J. M., Rickles, F., & Evatt, B. L. (2000). Surveillance for hemophilia and inherited hematologic disorders. In Khoury, M. J., Burke, W., & Thomson, E. J. (Eds,), *Genetics and public health in the 21st century.* New York: Oxford University Press. Retrieved August 31, 2004, from Centers for Disease Control and Prevention Web site: http://www.cdc.gov/genomics/oldWeb01_16_04/info/book/21stcentury.htm

# Bibliography

Allen, P. J., & Vessey, J. A. (2004). Bleeding disorders. In *Primary care of the child with a chronic condition* (4th ed., pp. 239–257). St. Louis, MO: Mosby.

Betz, C. L., & Sowden, L. A. (2000). Hemophilia. In *Mosby's pediatric nursing reference* (4th ed., pp. 184–188). St. Louis, MO: Mosby.

Bleeding disorders: Pathways and processes in the school setting. (n.d.). Retrieved August 31, 2004, from National Association of School Nurses Web site: http://www.nasn.org/profession/nasne.htm

Bolton-Maggs, P., & Pasi, K. J. (2003). Haemophilias A and B [Electronic version]. *Lancet,* 1801–1809.

Butler, R. B., McClure, W., & Wulfe, K. (2003). Practice patterns in haemophilia A therapy: A survey of treatment centers in the United States [Electronic version]. *Haemophilia, 9,* 549–554.

Catlin, A. J., & Schaefer, J. (1999). Ethical dilemmas in the pediatric hemophilia community ?Electronic version?. *Pediatric Nursing, 5,* 537–539.

Cavanaugh, B. M. (2003). *Nurse's manual of laboratory and diagnostic tests* (4th ed.). Philadelphia: Davis.

Disorder overview. (n.d.). Retrieved March 1, 2004, from National Hemophilia Foundation Web site: http://www.hemophilia.org/inhibitors/providers.html

Dochterman, J., & Bulechek, G. (2004). *Nursing interventions classification (NIC)* (4th ed.). St. Louis: Mosby.

Fahrenkrug, M. A. (2003). Development of a nursing data set for school nursing. *Journal of School Nursing, 19,* 238–248.

Hemophilia A. (n.d.). Retrieved January 22, 2004, from National Hemophilia Foundation Web site: http://www.hemophilia.org/bdi/bdi_types1.htm

Hemophilia B. (n.d.). Retrieved January 22, 2004, from National Hemophilia Foundation Web site: http://www.hemophilia.org/bdi/bdi_types2.htm

Hepatitis. (n.d.). Retrieved February 16, 2004, from National Hemophilia Foundation Web site: http://www.hemophilia.org/bdi/bdi_safety2.htm

HIV/AIDS FAQs. (n.d.). Retrieved February 23, 2004, from National Hemophilia Foundation Web site: http://www.hemophilia.org/bdi/bdi_safety3b.htm

Hockenberry, M. J., (2003). *Wong's nursing care of infants and children* (7th ed.). St. Louis, MO: Mosby.

Hemophilia

Information for teachers & childcare providers. (n.d.). Retrieved January 22, 2004, from National Hemophilia Foundation Web site: http://www.hemophilia.org/bdi/bdi_providers.htm

Lusher, J. M. (2002, May 19–24). *Highlights from the XXV International Congress of the World Federation of Hemophilia.* Retrieved January 20, 2004, from Medscape Web site: http://www.medscape.com/viewarticle/436527_print

Medical and scientific advisory council guidelines for emergency department Management of individuals with hemophilia document 155. (2003, November 9). Retrieved January 22, 2004, from National Hemophilia Foundation Web site: http://www.hemophilia.org/research/masac/masac155.htm

Medical and scientific advisory council recommendations concerning the treatment of hemophilia and other bleeding disorders document 151. (2003, November 9). Retrieved January 22, 2004, from National Hemophilia Foundation Web site: http://www.hemophilia.org/research/masac/masac151.htm

Morehead, S., Johnson, M., & Maas, M. (2004). *Nursing outcomes classification (NOC)* (3rd ed.). St. Louis, MO: Mosby.

National Association of School Nurses. (n.d.). *Bleeding disorders: Pathways and processes in the school setting* [Online Continuing Education Module]. Retrieved November 7, 2004, from http://nasn.org/education/nasnce.htm

National prevention program. (n.d.). Retrieved January 22, 2004, from National Hemophilia Foundation Web site: http://www.hemophilia.org/programs/npp/npp.htm

Prophylaxis: A fact sheet for parents. Retrieved November 29, 2004, from National Hemophilia Foundation Web site: http://www.hemophilia.org/resources/prophylaxis.htm

Recombinant factor. In *Hemophilia encyclopedia.* Retrieved January 22, 2004, from Hemophilia Galaxy Web site: http://www.hemophiliagalaxy.com/1_PATIENTS/ENCYCLOPEDIA/index.html

Silkworth, C. K. (1993). IHP: Hemophilia. In Hass, M. K. (Ed.), *The school nurse's source book of individualized healthcare plans* (Vol. 1, pp. 299–308). North Branch, MN: Sunrise River Press.

Soucie, J. M., Rickles, F., & Evatt, B. L. (2000). Surveillance for hemophilia and inherited hematologic disorders. In Khoury, M. J., Burke, W., & Thomson, E. J. (Ed.), *Genetics and public health in the 21st century.* New York: Oxford University Press. Retrieved August 31, 2004, from Centers for Disease Control and Prevention Web site: http://www.cdc.gov/genomics/oldWeb01_16_04/info/book/21stcentury.htm

## Resources

Ask Noah About Hemophilia and Bleeding
   Disorders
(New York Online Access to Health)
www.noah-health.org/english/illness/genetic_diseases/hemophilia.html

Canadian Hemophilia Society
625 President Kennedy Avenue
Suite 505
Montreal, Quebec H3A 1K2
514-848-0503
1-800-668-2686
514-848-9661 (fax)
www.hemophilia.ca

Centers for Disease Control and Prevention
1600 Clifton Road
Atlanta, GA 30333
404-639-3311
1-800-311-3435
www.cdc.gov/ncidod/dastlr/Hematology/aboutHDB.htm

HANDI (Hemophilia and AIDS/HIV Network for
   the Disseminating of Information)
The Information Center for NHF

1-800-42-HANDI
www.hemophilia.org/resources/handi.htm
HANDI provides free single copies of the following
   brochures (and others) on request: "Caring for
   Your Child and Hemophilia," "The Child With a
   Bleeding Disorder: First Aid for School
   Personnel," "Hemophilia, Sports and Exercise,"
   and "What You Should Know About Bleeding
   Disorders." Hemophilia Treatment Centers
   (HTCs) are located throughout the United States
   and Canada. They offer comprehensive medical
   services, risk reduction information, counseling,
   HIV education, and referrals. The National
   Hemophilia Foundation can refer you to the
   nearest HTC.

National Hemophilia Foundation
116 West 32nd St
11th Floor
New York, NY 10001
212-328-3700
1-800-42-HANDI
212-328-3777 (fax)
www.hemophilia.org

# Chapter Forty-four

# Hepatitis, Viral

Sharon D. Martin and Marcia S. Mullen

## Introduction

Viral hepatitis is not a single disease but a group of diseases caused by different viruses, all attacking the liver. Worldwide, eight distinct hepatitis viruses have been identified, hepatitis A (HAV), B (HBV), C (HCV), D (HDV or delta virus), E (HEV), G (HGV), TT (TTV), and SEN (SENV) (Poovorawan, Chatchatee, & Chongsrisawat, 2002). Hepatitis F was tentatively identified in 1994 but not confirmed; therefore, there is currently no recognized hepatitis F virus (Johns Hopkins University, n.d., Hepatitis F fact sheet.).

Of the eight recognized hepatitis viruses, the Centers for Disease Control and Prevention (CDC) in Atlanta, Georgia, lists hepatitis A, B, C, D, and E as most likely to be found in the United States. Therefore, this chapter will focus on hepatitis A through E. There are more than 50,000 new cases of viral hepatitis reported yearly (versus the *actual* number of cases, which would be much higher). Of reported cases in the United States, 32% are HAV, 43% HBV, 21% HCV, and 4% unidentified (Holcomb, 2002).

## Pathophysiology

The hepatitis viruses are divided into two major groups:
- Those transmitted via the fecal-oral route (enteric) that cause acute illness without chronic carrier state (hepatitis A and E)
- Those that are parenterally transmitted, major causes of chronic liver disease (hepatitis B, C, and D). Hepatitis D is actually a virusoid that requires HBV to replicate. Thus, it appears as either a coinfection or superinfection of people with HBV rather than a stand-alone disease (Poovorawan et al., 2002; CDC, National Center for Infectious Diseases [NCID], n.d., Hepatitis A–E slide set).

### Acute, Enteric Hepatitis A and E

Hepatitis A, one of the most frequently reported vaccine-preventable diseases in the United States, gained notoriety in extensive news coverage in 2003 when hundreds of patrons of a Pennsylvania restaurant were sickened and several died after eating raw green onions in salsa (Morbidity and Mortality Weekly Report, 2003). According to the National Center for Health Statistics, in

2001 (the latest year for which we have data) there were 10,609 new cases of HAV *reported* to the CDC with a rate of 3.8 cases per 100,000 U.S. citizens (CDC, National Center for Health Statistics, n.d., Fast stats A to Z, Viral hepatitis). However, the CDC estimates the *actual* number of new infections in 2001 was 93,000, with about half showing symptoms. The burden is more evident when one notes that about 31% of Americans show antibodies to HAV (CDC, NCID, Division of Viral Hepatitis, n.d., Disease burden from viral hepatitis A, B, and C in the United States). The number of cases within the school-aged population is not available.

Transmission of HAV is usually fecal-oral, either food/water-borne or person-to-person. The highest rates exist where food and water are fecal-contaminated or from person to person transmission by putting something contaminated with HAV in the mouth (often contaminated hands). "Most infections result from contact with a household member or sex partner who has hepatitis A. Casual contact, as in the usual office, factory, or school setting, does not spread the virus" (CDC, NCID, n.d., Viral hepatitis A, Frequently asked questions).

Hepatitis A incubates for 10 to 50 days, depending upon the number of infectious particles consumed. "The period of communicability extends from early in the incubation period to about a week after the development of jaundice. The greatest danger of spreading the disease to others occurs during the middle of the incubation period, well before the first presentation of symptoms. Many infections with HAV do not result in clinical disease, especially in children. When disease does occur, it is usually mild and recovery is complete in 1-2 weeks" (US Food & Drug Administration [FDA], Center for Food Safety & Applied Nutrition, n.d., Foodborne pathogenic microorganisms and natural toxins handbook, Hepatitis A virus).

Only half of infected persons, *children less likely than adults*, will show symptoms. If present, symptoms, which usually last less than 2 months, occur abruptly and often require hospitalization but rarely result in death; these include:
- jaundice,
- fatigue, tiredness,
- abdominal pain or discomfort,
- loss of appetite,

- nausea,
- diarrhea,
- fever,
- dark urine, and
- flulike symptoms (CDC, NCID, n.d., Viral hepatitis A, Frequently asked questions).

Though there is no chronic carrier state and a natural HAV infection provides lifetime immunity, "about 15% of people infected with HAV will have prolonged or relapsing symptoms over a 6-9 month period" (CDC, NCID, n.d., Viral hepatitis A, Fact sheet).

- Those at greatest risk of infection are:
- household contacts or sex contacts of infected persons,
- people, especially children, living in areas or traveling to countries with increased rates of HAV,
- men who have sex with men,
- injecting and noninjecting drug users,
- children and employees in child-care centers,
- residents and staff of institutions for developmentally disabled persons,
- workers who handle HAV-infected animals, and
- persons with clotting disorders who receive factor concentrates (Minnesota Department of Health, 1999).

Prevention is twofold. First, there is effective long-term protection with HAV vaccine (see "HAV Vaccine Considerations"). Also, some short-term protection is available from immune globulin if given before or within 2 weeks after exposure. The second part of prevention is controlling transmission by thorough hand washing with soap and water after using the bathroom, changing diapers, engaging in any activity that causes contact with human feces, and before preparing and eating food (CDC, NCID, n.d., Viral hepatitis A, Fact sheet).

Hepatitis E, sometimes called enterically transmitted non-A, non-B hepatitis (ET-NANBH), is clinically indistinguishable from HAV, and no serologic test to diagnose HEV is available in the United States. Therefore, the diagnosis is made based upon the characteristics of the outbreak and the exclusion of HAV and HBV by serologic test. Because HEV is so similar to HAV, we note the *differences* rather than the similarities here. Hepatitis E, unlike hepatitis A, is:

- uncommon and not currently endemic in the United States. All cases, except one, have occurred among travelers returning from HEV-endemic areas, which includes most developing countries.
- most likely to cause symptoms in people aged 15 to 40 years. As with HAV, younger people are less likely to have symptoms.
- commonly transmitted via fecally contaminated drinking water rather than food-borne; person-to-person transmission is uncommon.
- serious among pregnant women with a fatality rate close to 20%. Like HAV, the disease is mild and usually resolves in 2 weeks in most other people.

- of unknown period of infectivity, but virus has been found in the stool up to 14 days after illness onset.
- of unknown risk factors.
- without a vaccine, and immune globulin from donors in Western countries does not prevent infection.
- prevented by use of clean water when traveling in HEV endemic areas (CDC, NCID, n.d., Hepatitis E virus; U.S. FDA, Center for Food Safety & Applied Nutrition, n.d., Foodborne pathogenic microorganisms and natural toxins handbook, Hepatitis E virus; Johns Hopkins University, n.d., Hepatitis E fact sheet).

### Blood and Body Fluid–Borne Hepatitis B, C, and D

According to the National Center for Health Statistics, in 2001 there were 7,844 new cases of HBV reported to the CDC, with a rate of 2.8 cases per 100,000 U.S. citizens (CDC, National Center for Health Statistics, n.d., Fast stats A to Z, Viral hepatitis). However, the CDC estimates the *actual* number of new infections in 2001 at 78,000, with about 30% showing no acute symptoms. About 5% of Americans show antibodies to HBV, 1.25 million have chronic HBV infection, and an estimated 5,000 die each year of related liver disease (CDC, NCID, Division of Viral Hepatitis, n.d., Disease burden from viral hepatitis A, B, and C in the United States). In the United States, hepatitis D rates are estimated at less than 10% among asymptomatic HBV carriers and less than 25% among people with chronic HBV-related liver disease (CDC, NCID, n.d., Hepatitis D virus). School-age-related data are not available.

In comparison, the number of hepatitis C cases was not reported to the CDC in 2001; therefore, the agency *estimates* the actual number of new infections in 2001 at 25,000, with 80% showing no acute symptoms. About 2% of Americans show antibodies to HCV, 2.7 million have chronic HCV infection (note that this is significantly higher than the estimated number of chronic HBV infections), and an estimated 8,000 to 10,000 die each year of related liver disease (slightly higher than the estimated deaths from HBV) (CDC, NCID, Division of Viral Hepatitis, n.d., Disease burden from viral hepatitis A, B, and C in the United States). School-age-related data are not available.

The signs and symptoms of hepatitis B, C, and D are the same as those of HAV (discussed earlier), though HBV occasionally causes skin rashes, arthralgias, and arthritis (Finelli & Alter, 2002). As with HAV, children are less likely to show symptoms of infection than adults. Long-term effects of chronic HBV include hepatic necrosis, chronic hepatitis, liver cancer, and cirrhosis. Chronic infection occurs in 90% of infants infected at birth, 30% of children infected at age 1 through 5, and 6% of persons infected after age 5. Fifteen to 25% of chronically infected persons will die of liver disease. In HCV, 75% to 85% of persons infected will suffer chronic infection and 70% will develop liver disease. HCV has become the leading cause for liver transplant in the United States.

Transmission of HBV, HCV, and HDV all occur through blood and body fluids. HBV is considered more likely to be spread by sexual contact than HCV. Sharing needles in IV drug use or tattooing or exposure of an infant to the blood of an infected mother during birth can also lead to infection.

Primary prevention differs between HBV/HDV and HCV because an effective vaccine exists for HBV (which then protects against HDV), but no vaccine exists for HCV (see "HBV Vaccine Considerations"). The vaccine, which is considered the best protection against HBV, will not cure an existing infection. Recently, the vaccination of U.S. infants at birth has been initiated, so the rates of HBV/HDV disease should drop over time. The following general recommendations help prevent spread of HBV, HDV, and HCV:

- Do not share needles, syringes, razors, toothbrushes, dental appliances, nail-grooming equipment, or any items contaminated with blood (even if the blood is not visible).
- Cover skin cuts, sores, and rashes.
- Consider the risks of tattoos and body piercing; tools or artist/piercer may be infected.
- Use condoms if sexually active with more than one steady partner whose hepatitis and HIV status is negative.
- If you have hepatitis, do not donate blood, organs, or tissue.
- Follow universal precautions to avoid contact with the blood and body fluids of others.

## Management

HBV and HCV are treated with various antivirals, which can significantly decrease or rid the body of the virus in some people, though complete cure is not currently possible. Unfortunately, antivirals are not licensed for children under age 18, so children with hepatitis should be referred to a specialist in childhood liver disease. People should be advised to take these drugs exactly as prescribed and to avoid discontinuing use without physician advice. Also, pregnant women should not take them. People with hepatitis should avoid drinking alcohol (CDC, NCID, n.d., Viral hepatitis B, Fact sheet; CDC, NCID, n.d., Viral hepatitis B, Frequently asked questions; CDC, NCID, n.d., Viral hepatitis C, Fact sheet; CDC, NCID, n.d., Viral hepatitis C, Frequently asked questions).

Management of the child with hepatitis in the school involves the nurse, healthcare provider, teacher, staff, and family. According to the CDC (Hepatitis Information Line, 1-888-4-HEP-CDC, personal communication, March 11, 2004), assuming the child is well enough to attend, there is no need to exclude a child from school for acute or chronic hepatitis A through E. Of course, local, state, and school policies may differ from CDC recommendations; therefore these should be checked and adhered to.

The nurse should identify the type of hepatitis diagnosed in order to understand the modes of transmission and prevention requirements. Local, state, and school policies are followed regarding the potential exclusion of children with active disease, but recall that *most children will show no symptoms of hepatitis*. It is quite possible that there are or have been children with hepatitis in the school without the knowledge of school personnel. Therefore staff should be taught and encouraged to treat all students (and others) as though they are infectious.

- Management measures include the following:
- *Analysis of the need for immune globulin* for those exposed should be done based upon consultation with the school medical director, student's own healthcare provider, state or local public health department, or the CDC.
- *Education* of the student, the student's family, teachers, and staff regarding universal precautions and/or enteric precautions as applicable. School personnel should be knowledgeable and follow these guidelines every day with all students, so there should be little different about the interactions with the child with hepatitis. Education regarding the disease and primary, secondary, and tertiary prevention should be offered to all in a language and at a level that they can understand. Specific attention to hand washing is crucial with enteric hepatitis, and attention to the avoidance of blood, body fluids, and proper disposal of needles and sharps is crucial with blood-borne hepatitis. Decontamination after direct human contact or contact with contaminated surfaces or inanimate objects should be covered.
- *Medication administered* as ordered for the infected student.
- *Adequate equipment* must be available to school personnel to protect themselves and others from infection, e.g., gloves, cleaning solutions.
- *Privacy* of the student must be maintained while others are educated and protected from infection.
- *Psychological support* may be needed because the student may have fears about having hepatitis, especially if it is a chronic condition or the student is experiencing troubling symptoms. Adults and children who have come into contact with the infected student may be fearful of contracting the disease.

# Individualized Healthcare Plan

## Assessment

*History*

- Student age, development, behavior, and health prior to infection
- Date of diagnosis, prognosis, name and contact information of healthcare provider(s)
- Family considerations, such as siblings in the school system, parents or others living in the home who may be infected or at risk of infection
- Home characteristics that impact care, e.g., absence of clean running water
- Possible source of infection
- If required, date infection was reported to state
- Medication history
- Care to date and most recent evaluation
- Teaching student, family, school personnel have received to date and from whom

*Current Status and Management*

- Vital signs, growth, height and weight
- Presence of jaundice, fatigue, tiredness, abdominal pain or discomfort, loss of appetite, nausea, diarrhea, fever, dark urine, flulike symptoms, skin cuts, sores, or rashes
- Medications at home and during school hours
- Impact of any signs and symptoms on school functioning
- Nutrition requirements
- Symptom control

*Self-care*

- Knowledge of disease and prevention techniques
- Student's willingness, motivation, and ability to follow appropriate prevention instructions, e.g., frequent hand washing, especially after using the bathroom and before eating, and to participate in prescribed medication plan
- Barriers to participation in self-care

*Psychosocial Status*

- Student, parent, and school perception of and concerns about the disease or its symptoms

*Academic Issues*

- Past and current academic achievement and services
- Time lost from school due to infection
- Potential impact of fatigue/tiredness on academic schedule
- Ability to participate in-age appropriate activities with peers

## Nursing Diagnoses (N.D.) (NANDA 2003)

N.D. 1 Fatigue (NANDA 00093) related to disease process.
N.D. 2 Risk for activity intolerance (00094) related to disease process.
N.D. 3 Hyperthermia (00007) related to disease process.
N.D. 4 Nausea (00134) related to disease process.
N.D. 5 Imbalanced nutrition: Less than body requirements (00002) related to:
- loss of appetite
- vomiting

N.D. 6 Disturbed body image (00118) related to:
- yellow eyes or skin
- dark urine

N.D. 7 Acute pain (00132) related to muscle, abdominal, stomach, or joint aches.
N.D. 8 Diarrhea (00013) related to disease process.
N.D. 9 Impaired skin integrity (00046) related to rash.
N.D. 10 Knowledge deficit (00126) related to:
- disease process
- symptoms

- transmission
- prescribed medications
- laboratory tests
- prognosis

## Goals

The student will demonstrate behaviors consistent with prevention of transmission of hepatitis. (N.D. 10)
The student will participate in prescribed medication and laboratory regimen, and attend scheduled healthcare visits. (N.D. 10)
The student will maintain optimal body temperature. (N.D. 3)
The student will maintain adequate dietary and fluid intake. (N.D. 4, 5, 8)
The student will demonstrate knowledge of disease process. (N.D. 1, 3, 4, 6–10)
The student will cope successfully with altered body image. (N.D. 6)
The student will remain pain-free. (N.D. 7)
The student will maintain intact skin integrity. (N.D. 9)
The student will participate in usual school activities. (N.D. 1, 2)

## Nursing Interventions

After determining the causative virus (A through E), ensure that the student is able and willing to follow instructions to prevent disease transmission by providing education, reinforcement, and monitoring of behavior. (N.D. 10)
Identify anyone living in close contact with the student who may also be enrolled in or working/volunteering in the school to determine the need for testing/treatment and to make referrals as needed. (N.D. 10)
Ensure that the school medical director, primary healthcare provider, principal, and any agencies (local or state public health departments) are notified according to school policy and local or state law. (N.D. 10)
Participate in the investigation of the source of the infection as may be conducted by local, state, or federal public health officials. (N.D. 10)
Observe for and report additional cases of hepatitis or students/staff who may be symptomatic within the school population. (N.D. 10)
Establish an IHP with input from the healthcare provider, student, and family. (N.D. 1–10)
Establish contact with the child's healthcare provider(s), especially those responsible for the treatment of the hepatitis. (N.D. 10)
Establish contact with the child's parent(s) or legal guardians. (N.D. 10)
Educate student, teachers, and staff about the disease process, symptoms, transmission prevention, and universal precautions. (N.D. 10)
Ensure confidentiality. (N.D. 1–10)
Ensure that all members of the school community have access to adequate resources (i.e., gloves, cleaning solutions) to prevent transmission. (N.D. 10)
Educate student about prescribed medications, laboratory tests, and prognosis. (N.D. 10)
Anticipate future needs and provide education about sexuality. (N.D. 10)
Assist student to identify activity tolerance and, in conjunction with teachers, to develop a plan for appropriate school activities, rest breaks if needed. (N.D. 1, 2)
Assess temperature and vital signs during the first week after returning to school and as needed thereafter. (N.D. 3)
Assess child daily during the first week after returning to school and as needed thereafter for symptoms that may interfere with school activities, such as:
- nausea
- vomiting
- loss of appetite
- jaundice
- dark urine
- pain or discomfort in abdomen, stomach, joints, or muscles
- diarrhea
- skin rash (N.D. 4, 6–9)

Encourage and monitor nutrition and fluid intake if student has nausea, vomiting, loss of appetite, or diarrhea. (N.D. 4, 5, 8)
Provide emotional support as needed, especially if child suffers visible symptoms (i.e., jaundice). (N.D. 6)

Provide emotional support as needed to other students, staff, and faculty who may be fearful of contracting the disease while maintaining student confidentiality. (N.D. 6)

Keep infected student's skin lesions covered. (N.D. 9)

Encourage frequent hand washing. (N.D. 10)

Assist child to notify parent(s) if any symptoms require the student leave school. (N.D 1–5, 7, 8)

## Expected Student Outcomes

The student will:

- Demonstrate understanding, willingness, and behavior of necessary activities to prevent disease transmission before returning to school, such as:
  – hand washing
  – covering open wounds
  – blood-borne precautions
  – sexual precautions (N.D. 10)
- Demonstrate knowledge of and compliance with established medical regimen, including reporting signs and symptoms, taking medications, and attending appointments for laboratory work or healthcare visits on the first school day after diagnosis and ongoing thereafter. (N.D. 10)
- Take rest breaks as needed or planned by the end of the first week of school after diagnosis. (N.D. 1, 2)
- Maintain optimum body temperature upon return to school and ongoing. (N.D. 3)
- Maintain adequate dietary and fluid intake upon return to school and ongoing. (N.D. 4, 5, 8)
- Demonstrate knowledge of disease process, signs and symptoms, and willingness to report to the nurse as they occur by the end of the first week of school after diagnosis. (N.D. 1, 3, 4, 6–10)
- Demonstrate effective coping with altered body image by the end of the first week of school after diagnosis. (N.D. 6)
- Be pain-free upon return to school and ongoing. (N.D. 7)
- Maintain intact skin or keep skin lesions covered upon return to school and ongoing. (N.D. 9)
- Participate in the usual school activities as soon as physically able. (N.D. 1, 2)

## Case Study

Sarah, an 8-year-old third grader, has been absent from school for 7 days. After a brief period of fever and nausea, Sarah became jaundiced. Her primary care provider diagnosed hepatitis A after IgM anti-HAV was detected in her blood. The state bureau of health was contacted. The infectious source could not be determined, but the school lunch program was eliminated as a possible source. Her mother called to inform the school nurse that Sarah would be back to school on Monday because she is now feeling well enough to be in school. There are no limitations to her activity, although she continues to fatigue easily and some jaundice remains.

Considerations for the individualized healthcare plan include:

1. The effect of Sarah's absence from school and present fatigue and its effect on her academic performance
2. Education of staff working with Sarah
3. Sarah's participation in frequent hand washing
4. Cooperation with the bureau of health, parent, and healthcare provider related to the public health of the community
5. Confidentiality

# Viral Hepatitis

| Assessment Data | Nursing Diagnosis | Goals | Nursing Interventions | Expected Outcomes |
|---|---|---|---|---|
| Tires easily with normal daily activity during convalescent stage of HAV. | Fatigue related to disease process. | Sarah will be able to participate in the school program to her level of tolerance. | Meet with parent and Sarah's teachers to develop a modified school program that may include shortened day or frequent rest breaks.<br><br>Monitor activity tolerance, encouraging return to normal program, as she is able.<br><br>Consider the need for a 504 Accommodation Plan if the recovery is delayed and it impacts Sarah's participation or attendance. | Plan for modified school day is developed.<br><br>Sarah is gradually able to participate in normal school day. |
| Sarah forgets to wash her hands after toileting. | Knowledge deficit related to disease process, symptoms, transmission, and prognosis. | Sarah will practice appropriate hand washing without reminders. | Observe Sarah's hand washing technique and provide education and reinforcement.<br><br>Meet with teachers and staff who work with Sarah to reinforce the need for universal precautions.<br><br>Educate teachers and staff about disease process, transmission and prevention. | Sarah will demonstrate appropriate hand washing behavior. |
| Sarah is uncomfortable returning to school because she is concerned students will be afraid of her or will tease her. | Disturbed body image related to yellow eyes and skin (NANDA 00118) | Sarah will cope successfully with altered body image by the end of the first week of school. | Provide emotional support for Sarah as she copes with the illness by allowing her to express her feelings.<br><br>Discuss with Sarah and her parent the information appropriate to be shared with Sarah's peers. | Sarah will feel comfortable with her body image as she recovers. |

| Assessment Data | Nursing Diagnosis | Goals | Nursing Interventions | Expected Outcomes |
|---|---|---|---|---|
| | | | Encourage teachers, staff and peers to be sensitive to Sarah's discomfort.<br><br>Protect Sarah's privacy by providing necessary information to only those individuals with a need to know. | |

# References

Centers for Disease Control and Prevention. (2000). Notice to readers: Alternate two-dose hepatitis B vaccination schedule for adolescents aged 11-15 years. *Morbidity and Mortality Weekly Report, 49*(12), 261.

Centers for Disease Control and Prevention, National Center for Health Statistics. (n.d.). *Fast stats A to Z: Viral hepatitis.* Retrieved March 8, 2004, from http://www.cdc.gov/nchs/fastats/hepatits.htm

Centers for Disease Control and Prevention, National Center for Infectious Diseases, Division of Viral Hepatitis. (n.d.). *Disease burden from viral hepatitis A, B, and C in the United States.* Retrieved March 8, 2004, from http://www.cdc.gov/ncidod/diseases/hepatitis/resource/PDFs/disease_burden2002.pdf

Centers for Disease Control and Prevention, National Center for Infectious Diseases. (n.d.). *Hepatitis A–E slide set.* Retrieved March 8, 2004, from http://www.cdc.gov/ncidod/diseases/hepatitis/slideset/hep_d/slide_2.htm

Centers for Disease Control and Prevention, National Center for Infectious Diseases. (n.d.). *Viral hepatitis A: Fact sheet.* Retrieved March 8, 2004, from http://www.cdc.gov/ncidod/diseases/hepatitis/a/fact.htm

Centers for Disease Control and Prevention, National Center for Infectious Diseases. (n.d.). *Viral hepatitis A: Frequently asked questions.* Retrieved March 8 and 9, 2004, from http://www.cdc.gov/ncidod/diseases/hepatitis/a/faqa.htm

Centers for Disease Control and Prevention, National Center for Infectious Diseases. (n.d.). *Viral Hepatitis B: Fact sheet.* Retrieved March 8, 2004, from http://www.cdc.gov/ncidod/diseases/hepatitis/b/fact.htm

Centers for Disease Control and Prevention, National Center for Infectious Diseases. (n.d.). *Viral hepatitis B: Frequently asked questions.* Retrieved March 8, 2004, from http://www.cdc.gov/ncidod/diseases/hepatitis/b/faqb.htm

Centers for Disease Control and Prevention, National Center for Infectious Diseases. (n.d.). *Viral hepatitis C: Fact sheet.* Retrieved March 8, 2004, from http://www.cdc.gov/ncidod/diseases/hepatitis/c/fact.htm

Centers for Disease Control and Prevention, National Center for Infectious Diseases. (n.d.). *Viral hepatitis C, Frequently asked questions.* Retrieved March 8, 2004, from http://www.cdc.gov/ncidod/diseases/hepatitis/c/faq.htm

Centers for Disease Control and Prevention, National Center for Infectious Diseases. (n.d.). *Hepatitis D virus.* Retrieved March 10, 2004, from http://www.cdc.gov/ncidod/diseases/hepatitis/slideset/hep_d/slide_6.htm

Centers for Disease Control and Prevention, National Center for Infectious Diseases. (n.d.). *Hepatitis E virus.* Retrieved March 9, 2004, from http://www.cdc.gov/ncidod/diseases/hepatitis/slideset/hep_e/slide_1.htm

Centers for Disease Control and Prevention, National Immunization Program. (1998 August 25). *Hepatitis A vaccine: Vaccine information statement.* Retrieved March 8, 2004, from http://www.cdc.gov/nip/publications/VIS/vis-hep-a.pdf

Centers for Disease Control and Prevention, National Immunization Program. (2001 July 11). *Hepatitis B vaccine: Vaccine information statement.* Retrieved March 26, 2004, from http://www.cdc.gov/nip/publications/VIS/vis-hep-b.pdf

Finelli, L. & Alter, M. (2002). Hepatitis B. In Centers for Disease Control and Prevention, National Immunization Program, *VPD surveillance manual* (3rd ed.), Chapter 4. Retrieved March 11, 2004, from http://www.cdc.gov/nip/publications/surv-manual/chpt04_hepb.pdf

GlaxoSmithKline Biologicals. (2003). *ENGERIX-B Prescribing information.* Retrieved March 10, 2004, from http://us.gsk.com/products/assets/us_engerixb.pdf

Holcomb, S. (2002). An update on hepatitis. *Dimensions of Critical Care Nursing, 21*(5), 1700–1791.

Johns Hopkins University. (n.d.). *Hepatitis E fact sheet.* Retrieved March 9, 2004, from http://hopkins-id.edu/diseases/hepatitis/hev_faq.html

Johns Hopkins University. (n.d.). *Hepatitis F fact sheet.* Retrieved March 8, 2004, from http://hopkins-id.edu/diseases/hepatitis/hfv_faq.html

Minnesota Department of Health. (1999). Hepatitis A Prevention. *Morbidity and Mortality Weekly Report.* (2003). *Hepatitis A outbreak associated with green onions at a restaurant—Monaca, Pennsylvania.* November 21, 52 dispatch;1-3. Retrieved March 8, 2004 from http://www.cdc.gov/mmwr/preview/mmwrhtml/mm52d1121a1.htm

NANDA International. (2003). *Nursing diagnoses: Definitions & classification 2003-2004.* Philadelphia: Author.

Poovorawan, Y., Chatchatee, P., & Chongsrisawat, V. (2002). Epidemiology and prophylaxis of viral hepatitis: A global perspective. *Journal of Gastroenterology and Hepatology, 17*(Suppl.), S155–S166.

U.S. Food & Drug Administration, Center for Food Safety & Applied Nutrition. (n.d.). *Foodborne pathogenic microorganisms and natural toxins handbook, Hepatitis A virus.* Retrieved March 9, 2004, from http://vm.cfsan.fda.gov/~mow/chap31.html

U.S. Food & Drug Administration, Center for Food Safety & Applied Nutrition. (n.d.). *Foodborne pathogenic microorganisms and natural toxins handbook, Hepatitis E virus.* Retrieved March 9, 2004 from http://vm.cfsan.fda.gov/~mow/chap32.html

## Bibliography

Champion, C. (1999). *Occupational exposure to blood-borne pathogens* [Manual]. Scarborough, ME: National Association of School Nurses.

Chin, J. (2000). *Control of communicable diseases manual* (17th ed.). Washington, DC: American Public Health Association

National Association of School Nurses. (n.d.). *Managing infectious diseases in the school setting* [Online Continuing Education Module]. Retrieved November 7, 2004, from http://nasn.org/education/nasnceinfectdis.htm

National Association of School Nurses. (Revised 2003). *Position Statement: Bloodborne pathogens in the school setting, Regulations on.* Scarborough, ME: Author.

National Association of School Nurses. (Revised 2001). *Position Statement: Infectious diseases.* Scarborough, ME: Author.

## Resources

Centers for Disease Control and Prevention
1600 Clifton Road
Atlanta, GA 30333
1-800-311-3435
National Center for Infectious Diseases
Division of Viral Hepatitis
1-888-4-HEP-CDC
http://www.cdc.gov/ncidod/diseases/hepatitis/

Hepatitis B Foundation
700 East Butler Avenue
Doylestown, PA 18901-2697
215-489-4900
http://www.hepb.org

Hepatitis Foundation International
504 Blick Drive
Silver Spring, MD 20904-2901
301-622-4200
1-800-891-0707
http://www.hepfi.org/

Immunization Action Coalition
1573 Selby Avenue
Suite 234
St. Paul, MN 55104
651-647-9009
http://www.immunize.org/hepa/index.htm (hepatitis A information)
http://www.immunize.org/hepb/index.htm (hepatitis B information)

MedlinePlus, Hepatitis
National Library of Medicine
National Institute of Health
http://www.nlm.nih.gov/medlineplus/hepatitis.html

Parents of Kids with Infectious Diseases
PO Box 5666
Vancouver, WA 98668
1-877-55-PKIDS
http://pkids.org

# HAV Vaccine Considerations

Two HAV vaccines (HAVRIX, manufactured by GlaxoSmithKline, and VAQTA, manufactured by Merck & Co., Inc) are currently licensed in the United States for use with persons aged 2 years and older with any of the following characteristics:

- Traveling in areas with increased rates of HAV, such as Mexico, some South and Central American countries, many African countries, and many Asian countries (except Japan), the Caribbean, and southern or eastern Europe. The vaccine series must be started at least 1 month before traveling.
- Suffering from clotting-factor disorders (e.g., hemophilia) or chronic liver disease
- Men who have sex with men, and injecting or noninjecting drug users
- People living in communities with high rates of HAV (e.g., American Indian, Alaska Native, Pacific Islander)
- Children living in areas with increased rates of HAV during the baseline period of 1987 to 1997. Generally, in the United States the western states have higher rates of HAV, although it is important to determine an area's rate of HAV by contacting the local or state public health division. "Children living in states, counties, and communities where rates of hepatitis A are at least twice the national average (≥20 cases/100,000) in baseline period should be routinely vaccinated beginning at 2 years of age. High rates of hepatitis A have been found in these populations, both in urban and rural settings. In addition, to effectively prevent epidemics of hepatitis A, vaccination of previously unvaccinated older children is recommended within 5 years of initiation of routine childhood vaccination programs. Although rates differ among areas, available data indicate that a reasonable cutoff age in many areas is 10 to 15 years of age, because older persons have often already had hepatitis A. Vaccination of children before they enter school should receive highest priority, followed by vaccination of older children who have not been vaccinated" (Centers for Disease Control and Prevention, National Center for Infectious Diseases, n.d., Viral hepatitis A: Frequently asked questions; Centers for Disease Control and Prevention, National Immunization Program, (1998, August 25), Hepatitis A vaccine: Vaccine information statement).

*Dosages and schedules for hepatitis A vaccines*

## Recommended Dosages of HAVRIX*

| Vaccinee's age (years) | Dose (ELU)† | Volume (mL) | No. doses | Schedule (mo) |
|---|---|---|---|---|
| 2-18 | 720 | 0.5 | 2 | 0,6-12 |
| >18 | 1,440 | 1.0 | 2 | 0,6-12 |

ELU = Elisa units.
*Hepatitis A vaccine, inactivated, GlaxoSmithKline.
†0 months represents timing of the initial dose; subsequent numbers represent months after the initial dose.

## Recommended Dosages of VAQTA*

| Vaccinee's age (years) | Dose (ELU)† | Volume (mL) | No. doses | Schedule (mo) |
|---|---|---|---|---|
| 2-18 | 25 | 0.5 | 2 | 0,6-18 |
| >18 | 50 | 1.0 | 2 | 0,6-12 |

*Hepatitis A vaccine, inactivated, Merck & Co., Inc.
†0 months represents timing of the initial dose; subsequent numbers represent months after the initial dose.

Tables adapted from *Viral hepatitis A: Frequently asked questions.* Centers for Disease Control and Prevention, National Center for Infectious Diseases, n.d., available at: http://www.cdc.gov/ncidod/diseases/hepatitis/a/faqa.htm.

# HAV Vaccine Considerations

## Other Considerations

Hepatitis A vaccine can be given at the same time as hepatitis B, diphtheria, poliovirus (oral and inactivated), tetanus, oral typhoid, cholera, Japanese encephalitis, rabies, yellow fever vaccine, or immune globulin, but at a different injection site. The vaccine is very safe with no serious adverse events attributed definitively to it. Soreness at the injection site, headache, loss of appetite, and tiredness are the most frequently reported side effects. In addition:

- There is no live virus in hepatitis A vaccine, so there is less risk of a systemic reaction, the vaccine cannot cause a hepatitis infection, and it is safer to use with those who are immune compromised.
- It is estimated that vaccine protection will last for at least 20 years.
- Protection against hepatitis A begins 4 weeks after the first dose of the vaccine.
- Hepatitis A vaccine is not licensed for use *after exposure* to the virus. Immune globulin should be used instead.
- Prevaccination testing is done only in specific instances to control cost with persons who were likely to have had hepatitis A in the past (e.g., people born in countries with high levels of HAV, the elderly, those who have clotting factor disorders and may have received factor concentrates in the past).
- Postvaccination testing is not recommended.
- It is unclear whether the vaccine is safe in pregnancy; therefore check with the healthcare provider regarding administration.
- The vaccine can be given to immunocompromised persons (e.g., those receiving hemodialysis or persons with AIDS).
- Twinrix is a combined hepatitis A and hepatitis B vaccine for use in persons aged 18 years and older.

(Information adapted from *Viral hepatitis A: Frequently asked questions.* Centers for Disease Control and Prevention, National Center for Infectious Diseases, n.d., available at: http://www.cdc.gov/ncidod/diseases/hepatitis/a/faqa.htm)

# HBV Vaccine Considerations

Two HBV vaccines (ENGERIX-B, manufactured by GlaxoSmithKline, and Recombivax HB, manufactured by Merck & Co., Inc) are currently licensed in the United States in pediatric/adolescent and adult formulations. In addition, Twinrix is a combined hepatitis A and hepatitis B vaccine for use in persons aged 18 years and older.

Because a vaccination strategy limited to high-risk individuals has failed to substantially lower the overall incidence of hepatitis B infection, the Advisory Committee on Immunization Practices recommends vaccination of all persons from birth to age 18. The Committee on Infectious diseases of the American Academy of Pediatrics (AAP) has also endorsed universal infant immunization as part of a comprehensive strategy for the control of hepatitis B infection. The AAP, American Academy of Family Physicians, and American Medical Association also recommend routine vaccination of adolescents 11 to 12 years of age who have not been vaccinated previously. The AAP further recommends that providers administer hepatitis B vaccine to all previously unvaccinated adolescents (GlaxoSmithKline Biologicals, 2003, p. 2).

Children, adolescents, or adults should get three doses of hepatitis B vaccine as follows:

- First dose: any time
- Second dose: 1 to 2 months after first dose
- Third dose: 4 to 6 months after first dose

Adolescents 11 to 15 years old may need only two doses of vaccine, separated by 4 to 6 months (CDC, 2000). A blood titer may be ordered after the last dose to ensure immune status. This vaccine may be given at the same time as other vaccines. Common problems with the vaccine are soreness at the injection site and fever (CDC, National Immunization Program, 2001 July 11).

*Chapter Forty-five*

# HIV/AIDS

Mary E. Newell

## Introduction

The history of the human immunodeficiency virus (HIV) epidemic in the United States is relatively short. AIDS (acquired immunodeficiency syndrome) was first documented by physicians and public health officials beginning in 1981. In the two decades since the first reports of the disease, AIDS has become a major worldwide epidemic. HIV is most commonly spread through sexual contact with an infected partner. It can be transmitted through contact with infected blood or by sharing needles or syringes contaminated with the virus. Untreated women with HIV can also pass the infection to their babies during pregnancy or through their breast milk.

By 1985, the causative agent—HIV—had been identified, and AIDS was determined to be the end stage of a chronic infection with HIV. In addition, an antibody test was developed, and routes of transmission were determined. Drug therapy for the infection became available in 1987 with the release of zidovudine (ZDV, AZT, Retrovir), and treatment has since expanded (Wilson, 1997). Since 1994 several important advances have been made, including the development of laboratory tests to assess viral levels in the blood, the production of new groups of antiretroviral agents, multidrug therapy, and treatment to decrease the risk of perinatal transmission. These advances have made it possible to improve both the quality and quantity of life for someone with HIV. Although great medical advances have been made, the HIV epidemic is far from being over, and nursing care remains a critical component in improving the life of someone diagnosed with HIV.

### Pathophysiology
#### Significance of the Problem

More that 830,000 cases of AIDS have been diagnosed in the United States since 1981 (NIAID, 2003), and over 501,700 AIDS-related deaths have been reported (CDC, 2002). Of equal concern is the fact that an estimated 950,000 Americans may be infected with HIV, one quarter of whom are unaware of their infection. The epidemic is growing most rapidly among whites, Hispanics, and Asians/Pacific Islanders and has remained consistently level among blacks see **Table 1.** (CDC, 2002).

**Table 1. Estimated Numbers of Diagnoses of HIV/AIDS, by Year of Diagnosis and Selected Characteristics of Persons, 1999-2002**

| Race/Ethnicity | Year of Diagnosis | | | | Cumulative through 2002 |
|---|---|---|---|---|---|
| | **1999** | **2000** | **2001** | **2002** | |
| White, not Hispanic | 7,718 | 7,985 | 8,040 | 8,347 | 115,134 |
| Black, not Hispanic | 14,398 | 14,129 | 14,090 | 14,398 | 162,950 |
| Hispanic | 2,631 | 2,920 | 3,012 | 3,321 | 29,315 |
| Asian/Pacific Islander | 123 | 150 | 140 | 149 | 1,262 |
| American Indian, Alaskan Native | 153 | 147 | 142 | 168 | 1,795 |

Adapted from the Centers for Disease Control and Prevention. *HIV/AIDS Surveillance Report 2002.*

## Structure of HIV

HIV is an RNA virus that was discovered in 1983. RNA viruses are known as retroviruses because they replicate in a reverse or backward fashion. Like all viruses, HIV cannot replicate until it has entered a living cell. HIV enters a cell by binding to a receptor site on the cell's surface. CD4 is an antigen on the surface of T helper cells that acts as the primary receptor for HIV. Once bound, the genetic material of the virus enters the cell. Through the use of a viral enzyme, reverse transcriptase, the viral RNA is converted to DNA and inserted into the infected cell's genetic material. If the cell is activated, viral proliferation may occur, resulting in lysis and death of the infected cell. If the cell remains dormant, the viral material continues to replicate and is integrated into the cell's DNA. It may then remain dormant for years.

The HIV virus infects primarily CD4$^+$ T cells (also known as T helper cells, or lymphocytes). Once activated, the virus causes the destruction of CD4$^+$ cells. CD4$^+$ cell destruction and eventual depletion have a profound effect on the immune system. The major concern related to immune suppression is the potential development of infections and cancers, which can cause morbidity and result in mortality (Lisanti, 1997).

## Transmission of HIV

HIV is a fragile virus that can be transmitted only under specific conditions which allow contact with infected body fluids, including blood, semen, vaginal secretions, and breast milk (Lisanti, 1997). Transmission of HIV can occur through sexual intercourse with an infected partner, by internalized exposure to HIV-infected blood or blood products, or by perinatal transmission during pregnancy, or at the time of delivery or through breast-feeding (Lisanti).

HIV is not spread casually. The virus cannot be transmitted through hugging, dry kissing, shaking hands, sharing eating utensils, or attending school or working with an HIV-infected person. It is not transmitted through tears, saliva, urine, emesis, sputum, feces, or sweat. In addition, there is no evidence that the virus can be transmitted by insects or fomites.

HIV can infect anyone who practices risky behaviors, such as:

- Sharing drug needles or syringes
- Having unprotected sexual contact with an infected person
- Having sexual contact with someone whose HIV status is unknown
- Having another sexually transmitted disease such as syphilis, genital herpes, chlamydial infection, gonorrhea, or bacterial vaginosis appears to leave individuals more susceptible to HIV infection as a result of sexual contact with infected partners.

## Stages of HIV/AIDS

The typical course of HIV infection follows the pattern shown in Figure 1. It is important to remember that HIV is very individualized. The information depicted in **Figure 1** represents data from a large group of people and should not be used to predict any one individual's life span after HIV infection.

---

**Figure 1. Timeline for the Spectrum of HIV Infection\***

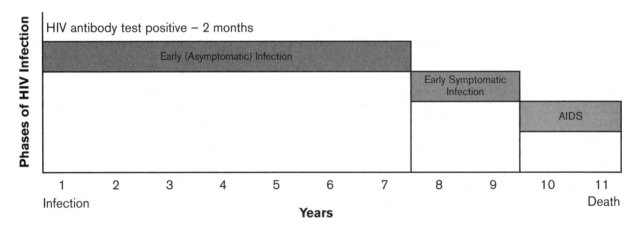

Figure 1. Timeline for the spectrum of HIV infection. The timeline represents the course of the illness from the time of infection to clinical manifestations of disease. Reprinted with permission

From *Medical Surgical Nursing* (5th ed.) (p.244), by S. Lewis, M. Heitkemper, and S. Dirksen, (Eds.), 2000, St. Louis, MO: Elsevier. Copyright 2000 by Elsevier.

At the time of diagnosis the HIV-infected individual may manifest one of four conditions: serologically negative, serologically positive but asymptomatic, early stage of HIV disease, or AIDS.

Many people do not have symptoms when they first become infected with HIV. The symptoms of HIV and AIDS vary depending on the phase of infection. Some people do experience a brief flulike illness within 2 to 6 weeks after exposure to the virus. This illness may include:

- Fever
- Headache
- Fatigue
- Enlarged lymph nodes

These symptoms of an initial infection usually disappear within a week to a month and are often mistaken for those of another viral infection. During this period, even if symptoms are not present, individuals are very infectious and HIV is present in large quantities in their genital fluids.

An individual may remain symptom-free for 8 to 10 years. During this time the virus continues to multiply and destroy immune cells. Tests are likely to show a sharp decline in the number of these cells in the body.

Eventually, mild infections or chronic symptoms develop, such as:

- Swollen lymph nodes, often one of the first signs of HIV infection
- Diarrhea
- Weight loss
- Fever
- Cough
- Shortness of breath

More persistent or severe symptoms may not appear for 10 years or more after HIV first enters the body in adults, or within 2 years for children born with HIV infection.

The term *AIDS* applies to the most advanced stages of HIV infection. CDC's definition of AIDS includes all HIV-infected people who have fewer than 200 CD4$^+$ T cells per cubic millimeter of blood. Additional diagnostic criteria (**Table 2**) are more likely to occur when the immune system becomes severely compromised as the disease progresses and the CD4$^+$ T-cell count decreases. Therefore, the amount of HIV that can be detected in the blood is increased.

---

**Table 2. Diagnostic Criteria for AIDS**

AIDS is diagnosed when an individual with HIV has at least one of the following additional conditions:

1. CD4$^+$ T-cell count drops below 200/$\mu$L.

2. Development of one of the following opportunistic infections:
   - *Fungal:* candidiasis of bronchi, trachea, lungs, or esophagus; *Pneumocystis carinii* pneumonia; disseminated or extrapulmonary histoplasmosis
   - *Viral:* cytomegalovirus (CMV) disease other than the liver, spleen, or nodes; CMV retinitis (with loss of vision); herpes simplex with chronic ulcer(s) or bronchitis, pneumonitis, or esophagitis; progressive multifocal leukoencephalopathy; extrapulmonary cryptococcosis
   - *Protozoal:* disseminated or extrapulmonary coccidioidomycosis, toxoplasmosis of the brain, chronic intestinal isosporiasis; chronic intestinal cryptosporidiosis

   - *Bacterial: Mycobacterium tuberculosis* (any site; any disseminated or extrapulmonary mycobacterium, including M. avium complex or M. kansasii; recurrent pneumonia or recurrent Salmonella septicemia

3. Development of one of the following opportunistic cancers:
   - invasive cervical cancer, Kaposi's sarcoma, Burkitt's lymphoma, immunoblastic lymphoma, or primary lymphoma of the brain

4. Wasting syndrome occurs. Wasting syndrome is defined as a loss of 10% or more of ideal body mass.

5. Dementia develops.

Modified from "1993 revised classification system for HIV infection and expanded surveillance case definition for AIDS among adolescents and adults," 1992, *MMWR , 41*(RR-17), p. 1.

Children who are HIV-positive often fail to gain weight or grow at the expected pace. As the disease progresses, they can have difficulty walking or delayed mental development and they may develop cerebral palsy. Children are also susceptible to the same opportunistic infections as adults are and may have severe forms of common childhood illnesses, such as otitis media, pneumonia, and tonsillitis.

The median time for survival after a diagnosis of AIDS is 2 years, but this time varies greatly. Some people with AIDS live for 6 or more years, whereas others survive for only a few months. There is also a wide variation in morbidity. Some people with AIDS are severely ill, yet others are able to continue usual routines with lifestyle adjustments to obtain healthcare and cope with symptoms, such as fatigue. Advances in the treatment and diagnosis of HIV infection, opportunistic diseases, and constitutional symptoms have increased survival times, but AIDS fatality rates remain high.

### Opportunistic Disease

Opportunistic diseases, commonly a reactivation of a previous infection, generally do not occur in the presence of a functioning immune system. Numerous infections, a variety of malignancies, wasting, and dementia can result from HIV-related immune impairment. Children with AIDS may develop the same opportunistic infections as adults with the disease. In addition, they may also acquire severe forms of the bacterial infections that commonly occur among all children, such as conjunctivitis (pink eye), ear infections, and tonsillitis. Organisms that are nonvirulent or cause limited or localized disease in immunocompetent individuals can cause severe debilitating and life-threatening opportunistic infections in AIDS patients. Unfortunately, multiple opportunistic diseases tend to occur at the same time, further complicating the difficulties of diagnosis and treatment.

### Diagnosis

The most useful screening tests for HIV are those that can detect HIV-specific antibodies. The major problem with these tests is that there is a median delay of 2 months after infection, before detectable antibodies are produced. This creates a window period, during which an infected individual will not test positive for HIV-antibody. HIV-antibody screening is generally done in the sequence outlined in **Table 3**.

Most healthcare providers can perform HIV testing and will usually offer counseling to the patient at the same time. Of course, individuals can be tested anonymously at many clinic sites if they are concerned about confidentiality.

Healthcare providers diagnose HIV infection by

---

**Table 2. Diagnostic Criteria for AIDS**

The following steps are used in the process of testing blood for antibodies to HIV:

1. A highly sensitive enzyme immunoassay (EIA, ELISA) is done to detect serum antibodies that bind to HIV antigens on test plates. Blood samples that are negative on this test are reported as negative.

2. If the blood is EIA-reactive, the test is repeated.

3. If the blood is repeatedly EIA-reactive, a more specific confirming test, such as the Western blot (WB) or immunofluorescence assay (IFA), is done.
   • WB testing uses purified HIV antigens electrophoresed on gels. These are incubated with serum samples. If antibody in the serum is present, it can be detected.
   • IFA is used to identify HIV in infected cells. Blood is treated with a fluorescent antibody against p17 or p24 antigen and then examined using a fluorescent microscope.

4. Blood that is reactive in all of the first three steps is reported as HIV-antibody positive.

5. If the results are indeterminant, testing should be repeated within 6 months. Consistently indeterminant test results require the use of polymerase chain reaction (PCR), viral culture, and other diagnostic measures.
   • PCR analyzes DNA extracted from lymphocytes and/or HIV from serum using an in vitro amplification procedure.
   • A cell culture system can be used to grow viruses from infected lymphocytes.

Because these tests are expensive and difficult to do, they are usually not used for screening purposes, but may be done in situations where the index of suspicion is high and antibody tests are negative.

---

Modified from "1993 revised classification system for HIV infection and expanded surveillance case definition for AIDS among adolescents and adults," 1992, *MMWR*, *41* (RR-17), p. 1.

using two different types of antibody tests: ELISA and Western blot. If a person is highly likely to be infected with HIV and yet both tests are negative, the healthcare provider may request additional tests. The individual may also be told to repeat antibody testing at a later date, when antibodies to HIV are more likely to have developed.

Diagnosis of HIV in newborns can be problematic. All infants born to HIV-infected mothers will test positive for HIV antibodies because maternal antibodies cross the placental barrier and these antibodies remain present in the infant for up to 18 months. For that reason, early detection of HIV infection in infants depends on testing for HIV antigen through the use of polymerase chain reaction (PCR) or viral culture. These tests can definitely diagnose HIV in infected infants, by age 4 weeks (CDC, 2004).

### Course of Disease in Children

The pediatric and adolescent course of HIV infection and AIDS differs from that of adults in the following ways:

- Pediatric infection is usually intergenerational, meaning that an HIV-positive mother while pregnant transfers the virus to the unborn child
- Blood transfusion, an HIV-positive mother while pregnant transfers the virus to the unborn child via mixing of maternal and fetal blood.

The first priority for an infant is to correctly identify antibody status. Due to maternal antibody transfer and an immature immune system, an accurate diagnosis may not be possible until the child is at least 15 months old. The majority of infants with perinatally acquired HIV infection are clinically normal during infancy, developing symptoms by 18 to 24 months (Wong, Hockenberry, Wilson, Winkelstein, Kline, 2003). Clinical signs and symptoms of AIDS are usually present within months after birth.

Children also respond differently to anti-HIV medications. They have larger increases in T-cell counts and more diverse T cells. They also seem to recover more of their immune response than adults.

Infants' bodies contain more fat and water. Because of this, fewer medications are available for them. Children have a very high rate of metabolism. This gradually slows as they mature. The liver processes drugs and removes them from the body. It takes several years for a child's liver to mature. As it matures, drug levels in children can change dramatically. Therefore, correct medication doses are not always easy to determine. Children's doses are sometimes based on their weight. Another method is to determine body surface area, which considers both height and weight. Dosing may have to be adjusted several times as the child grows and develops.

The course of the disease varies in adolescents and is complicated by factors such as sexually transmitted diseases, chemical use/abuse, denial, depression, problems with compliance with medical regimes, and the vulnerability of the adolescent. Adherence to their treatment regimen is a major challenge. Many adolescents do not understand why they should put up with the medication's side effects.

The impact on the families of children with HIV/AIDS is significant. The parents are usually HIV-positive. They may have their own difficulties with HIV/AIDS to deal with while they are also trying to provide nurturing care to their own infected child. For the adolescent, the problems may include exclusion from the family. Parents may have difficulty accepting their child's risky behavior and/or sexual orientation. Expected responses could include grief and mourning for the loss of the healthy as well as shame and guilt if the parent transmitted HIV to the child.

## Management

When HIV was first identified in the early 1980s, there were no medications to combat the underlying immune deficiency and few treatments existed for the resulting opportunistic diseases. A number of medications have since been developed to treat both HIV/AIDS and opportunistic infections. For both adults and children, newer treatments have extended and improved the quality of life. Unfortunately, none of these drugs can cure HIV/AIDS, many have side effects that can be quite severe, and treatment is often expensive.

According to current guidelines, treatment should focus on achieving the maximum suppression of symptoms for as long as possible. This aggressive approach is known as highly active antiretroviral therapy (HAART). The aim of HAART is to reduce the amount of virus in the individual's blood to a very low level, although this does not mean the virus is completely gone. Eradication of the virus is usually accomplished with a combination of three or more drugs (CDC, 2004).

The U.S. Food and Drug Administration (FDA) has approved a number of drugs for treating HIV infection. The first group of drugs used to treat HIV infection, called nucleoside analogue reverse transcriptase (NRT) inhibitors, interrupt an early stage of the virus, when it is making copies of itself. Included in this class of drugs (called nucleoside analogs) are AZT (zidovudine), ddC (zalcitabine), ddl (dideoxyinosine), d4T (stavudine), 3TC (lamivudine), abacavir (Ziagen), and tenofovir (Viread). These drugs may slow the spread of HIV in the body and delay the start of opportunistic infections.

Healthcare providers can prescribe nonnucleoside reverse transcriptase inhibitors (NNRTIs), such as delavardine (Rescriptor), nevirapine (Viramune), and efravirenz (Sustiva), in combination with other antiretroviral drugs. These drugs bind directly to the enzyme, reverse transcriptase.

The FDA has also approved a second class of drugs for treating HIV infection. These drugs, called protease inhibitors, interrupt virus replication at a later step in its life cycle by interfering with an enzyme known as HIV protease. They include:

- Ritonavir (Norvir)
- Saquinivir (Fortovase)
- Indinavir (Crixivan)
- Amprenivir (Agenerase)

- Nelfinavir (Viracept)
- Lopinavir (Kaletra)

In addition to antiretroviral therapy, healthcare providers treat adults with HIV, whose CD4$^+$ T-cell counts drop below 200, to prevent the occurrence of Pneumocystis carinii pneumonia (PCP). PCP is one of the most common and deadly opportunistic infections associated with HIV. They administer PCP to children as preventive therapy, when their CD4$^+$ T-cell counts drop to levels considered below normal for their age group. Regardless of their CD4+ T-cell counts, HIV-infected children and adults who have survived an episode of PCP take drugs for the rest of their lives to prevent a recurrence of pneumonia. Treatment guidelines also emphasize the importance of quality of life. Thus, the major goal of AIDS treatment is to find not only the most effective regimen but also the one that is the least complicated and has the fewest side effects.

### School Considerations

All children have the constitutional right to a free appropriate educational program of experiences in the least restrictive environment. It is well established that the risk of HIV transmission in school settings is virtually nonexistent.

**Table 4. Managing HIV/AIDS Infections in School**

The following public health recommendations address the management of persons infected with HIV/AIDS who are attending school. These recommendations follow guidelines developed by the U.S. Public Health Service.

1. Risk of transmission of HIV infection is virtually non-existent in the normal unrestricted school setting because the primary pathways of HIV infection do not exist in school activities. For this reason, children with AIDS or HIV infection should be allowed to attend school and after-school day care without restriction, except when medical or behavioral impairments exist that are severe enough to be a hazard to the infected child or to his/her classmates. (See 2 and 3 below.)

2. Infected children who may be neurologically impaired, lack control of body functions, bite, or have uncoverable oozing lesions should be educated in restricted settings until their medical or behavioral problems improve. Educational settings should minimize exposure of other children to blood or body fluids.

3. The decision to limit the educational setting for any particular child because of medical or behavioral reasons should be made jointly by the child's physician, child's parents and guardians, school nurse, and school administrator. Decisions should be made on an individual case-by-case basis after weighing risks and benefits to the infected child as well as to others in the school or day care setting.

4. Teachers or other employees, including food handlers, who may have AIDS or HIV infection should be under no work restrictions. They present no appreciable risk of infection to school children or other employees under normal school work conditions.

5. Persons providing care and education for children with AIDS or HIV infection should respect each child's right to privacy, including maintaining confidentiality. The number of personnel aware of the child's condition should be kept to a minimum, according to state laws.

6. School officials should notify parents of children known to have AIDS or HIV infection when illnesses that may represent a threat to immunosuppressed children are occurring in the school. These include chickenpox, measles, whooping cough, meningitis, and influenza.

7. Guidelines for cleaning up blood or body fluid spills should be followed at all times, regardless of the presence of HIV-infected individuals in the school. These provisions will prevent infection with HIV, hepatitis B, herpes virus, and other infectious agents.

8. School personnel should receive training about HIV/AIDS and other infectious diseases, including information about how these disease are acquired, how transmission can be prevented, and how to handle body fluids in schools.

From *JLCD Student Health: Students with HIV/AIDS. Guidelines for the Education and Care of Preschool and School-Age Children Who Have Diagnosed AIDS,* by Maine School Administrative District 40, 2000. Retrieved January 26, 2004, from http://msad40.org/POLICY/jled.html. Adapted with permission.

Decisions regarding the most appropriate educational setting for a child with AIDS should be based upon the child's behavior, neurologic development, physical condition, and anticipated interaction with others. These decisions are best made on a case-by-case basis by a team representative of school personnel, including the school nurse, child's physician, parents and guardians, and the school administrator. In each case, the risks and benefits to both the infected child and others within the educational setting must be carefully considered.

For most AIDS-infected school-aged children, the benefit of an unrestricted setting would outweigh the risk of their acquiring potentially harmful infections and the apparent nonexistent risk of transmitting AIDS. The nurse's role in the care of the child with HIV is multifaceted. The nurse serves as an educator, direct care provider, case manager, and advocate. **Table 4** outlines how to manage HIV/AIDS infections in a school setting.

The school should respect the right-to-privacy of the individual; therefore, knowledge that a child has AIDS should be confined to those persons with a direct need to know (e.g., school administrator, school nurse, teacher). Confidentiality is a major issue in school attendance. Parents and legal guardians have a right to decide whether they inform a school of their child's HIV diagnosis.

## Individualized Healthcare Plan

### Assessment
*History*
- Health prior to diagnosis
- Date of diagnosis and age of student
- Prognosis
- Growth and developmental stage
- Stage of illness
- Treatment regimen
- Support system(s)
- Recurrent infections
- Most recent reevaluation
- Housing status: home/homeless/shelter
- Use of intravenous drugs
- Homosexual or bisexual preference
- Engagement in unsafe sexual practices

*Current Status and Management*
- Overall appearance/hygiene
- Immune system status: lymph nodes
- Pattern of recurring infections: bacterial, viral
- Cardiovascular system: cardiopathy, vasculitis
- Skin disorders
- Neoplasms: lymphoma
- Nutritional status: diarrhea, appetite pattern, signs of malnutrition/malabsorption and dehydration, nutritional supplements
- Neurological status: neuropathy, mental/cognition, socio-emotional state, fatigue
- Growth: height and weight
- Daily activity schedule: energy use, need for rest
- Sleep pattern
- Current therapy: medications, physical, recreational, spiritual

*Self-care*
- Knowledge about current health status, treatment regimen and risk for infection
- Health beliefs
- Parent/guardian's perception of student's knowledge of health status and disease progress
- Student's decision-making skills
- Level of independence/dependence; self-control
- Participation in routine health maintenance
- Participation in treatment plan: medication, specialized healthcare procedures

*Psychosocial Status*
- Student's contact and interaction with family, peers, and adult
- Student's locus of control
- Previous losses (real/perceived)
- Decision-making skills
- Involvement with support persons, groups, and community services
- Availability of parent/guardian, or other family members for support

*Academic Issues*
- Past and current academic achievement
- Attendance patterns: reasons for absences
- Schools the student has attended, including hospital-based and homebound instruction
- Transportation to and from school
- School health services needs: medications, rest periods, monitoring infectious disease in the school environment
- Education program needs: individualized education program (IEP): modified school schedule, modified school day
- 504 plan
- Confidentiality issues surrounding student disclosure and "need to know" status for others involved in daily care

## Nursing Diagnoses (NANDA, 2003)

**N.D. 1** Imbalanced nutrition: less than body requirements (NANDA 00002) related to:
- recurrent illness
- diarrhea losses
- loss of appetite
- wasting syndrome

**N.D. 2** Risk for infection (NANDA 00004) related to:
- impaired body defenses
- presence of infectious organisms

**N.D. 3** Impaired social interaction (NANDA 00052) related to:
- physical limitations, hospitalizations
- social stigma toward HIV/AIDS
- inability to engage in satisfactory peer relationships

**N.D. 4** Powerlessness (NANDA 00125) related to:
- nature of the disease
- social isolation

**N.D. 5** Ineffective sexuality patterns (NANDA 00065) related to:
- risk of HIV disease transmission to others

**N.D. 6** Deficient knowledge (educational) (NANDA 00126) related to:
- existing disease condition
- interruption of education
- frequent absences

**N.D. 7** Risk for activity intolerance (NANDA 00094) related to:
- active infectious process
- fatigue

**N.D. 8** Anxiety (NANDA 00146) related to:
- uncertainty of health status
- role change
- stigma associated with HIV/AIDS

**N.D. 9** Disturbed body image (NANDA 00118) related to:
- advanced disease process
- wasting syndrome
- activity intolerance

**N.D. 10** Ineffective health maintenance (NANDA 00099) related to:
- ineffective individual coping
- change in health status

**N.D. 11** Risk for noncompliance (NANDA 00079) related to:
- inability to perform task

- nontherapeutic environment
- knowledge deficit
- complex treatment regimen

**N.D. 12** Ineffective therapeutic regimen management (NANDA 00078) related to:
- family conflict
- complexity of therapeutic regimen
- powerlessness

**N.D. 13** Fatigue (NANDA 00093) related to:
- malnutrition
- wasting syndrome

**N.D. 14** Pain; acute pain (NANDA 00136) or chronic pain (NANDA 00133) related to:
- disease process

**N.D. 15** Anticipatory grieving (NANDA 00136) related to:
- deteriorating physical condition
- terminal prognosis

**N.D. 16** Hopelessness (NANDA 00124) related to:
- deteriorating physical condition
- terminal process

**N.D. 17** Delayed growth and development (NANDA 00111) related to:
- disease process
- recurring infections
- malnutrition

## Goals

The student will maintain weight and optimal nutrition. (N.D. 1, 2, 13, 17)
The student will minimize risk for infection. (N.D. 2, 7)
The student will learn and utilize measures to prevent the spread of the disease to others. (N.D. 2, 5, 7)
The student will participate in peer-group, community, school, and family activities. (N.D. 3, 4, 8, 9)
The student will identify current problems, concerns, and stressors. (N.D. 4, 8, 10, 16)
The student will actively participate in identifying and implementing coping skills and strategies to assist in addressing and managing problems, concerns, and stressors. (N.D. 4, 8, 10-12, 16)
The student will identify sexuality issues regarding his/her health condition and demonstrate positive sexual decisions. (N.D. 5)
The student will increase knowledge of health condition. (N.D. 6, 11)
The student will consistently attend classes and complete all assigned projects. (N.D. 6)
The student will achieve optimal activity level. (N.D. 7, 13)
The student will develop positive coping skills. (N.D. 8, 12, 15, 16)
The student will demonstrate improved body image. (N.D. 9, 12)
The student will participate in self-management of personal healthcare. (N.D. 10-12)
The student will decrease episodes of pain or irritability. (N.D. 11, 12, 14)
The student will utilize family members, community resources, and school staff to assist in meeting their health and educational needs. (N.D. 15)

## Nursing Interventions

Assess understanding of nutritional principles and teach as needed. (N.D. 1, 2, 12, 17)
Assess understanding of need for adequate nutrition intake and teach as needed. (N.D. 1, 2, 12, 17)
Assist the parent/guardian and student to:
- Provide high-calorie, high-protein meals and snacks to meet body requirements for metabolism and weight maintenance. (N.D. 1, 2, 12, 17)
- Fortify foods with nutritional supplements to maximize quality of intake. (N.D. 1, 2, 12, 17)
- Monitor student's weight and growth so that additional nutritional interventions can be implemented if weight drops. (N.D. 1, 2, 12, 17)

Encourage all students and staff to utilize proper hand-washing technique to minimize exposure to infectious organisms. (N.D. 2, 5, 7)
Develop and implement standard precautions to prevent spread of viruses. (N.D. 2, 5, 7)
Provide in-service education opportunities for school staff:

- appropriate precautions (N.D. 1, 2, 6)
- clarify any misconceptions about communicability of the virus (N.D. 2, 5, 6, 7, 9)
- injury prevention strategies, including environment: classroom, P.E., bus, and playground (N.D. 2, 5, 7)
- proper procedures for cleaning and bandaging minor wounds, disposal of wound-care products, reinforce as well (N.D. 2, 5, 7)
- ways to prevent social isolation (N.D. 3, 4, 8, 9)

Assist student in identifying personal strengths to facilitate coping. (N.D. 3, 4, 8, 9, 12)

Provide opportunities for student to develop and maintain peer relationships. (N.D. 3-5, 8, 9)

Encourage active participation in school and extracurricular activities. (N.D. 3, 4, 8, 9)

Assist student in identifying problems, concerns, and/or stressors. (N.D. 4, 8-10)

Assist school staff to provide a supportive environment that encourages the student to express feelings and concerns. (N.D. 4, 8-10)

Assist student in identifying and utilizing support systems. (N.D. 4, 8-12)

Assist student in identifying and utilizing coping strategies. (N.D. 4, 8-12)

Educate the student about:
- sexual transmission (N.D. 2,5)
- risk of infection (N.D. 2)
- abstinence (N.D. 5)
- use of condoms (N.D. 5)
- dangers of promiscuity (N.D. 5)

Assist student to identify physical and psychosocial aspects of sexual growth and development. (N.D. 5)

Encourage the student to talk about feelings and concerns related to sexuality. (N.D. 5, 10)

Assist student in building effective relationships. (N.D. 5, 9, 10)

Assist student in building effective decision-making skills. (N.D. 5, 9, 10)

In collaboration with teachers, develop and implement 504 plan that addresses:
- absences (N.D. 6)
- assignment completion as needed (N.D. 6)

Provide a supportive environment for the student to ask questions. (N.D. 6, 10-12)

Assist student in identifying supportive community resources. (N.D. 6, 10-12)

Monitor activity level and tolerance weekly. (N.D. 7)

With teaching staff, assist in developing adaptive activities based on current activity tolerance level. (N.D. 7, 13)

Teach student about signs and symptoms that indicate appropriate activity level, activity tolerance level, and overexertion. (N.D. 7, 13)

Provide positive feedback to the student with honesty and sincerity. (N.D. 9, 10)

Teach student correct administration of medication or other healthcare procedures, including rationale, correct steps, and documentation. (N.D. 10-12, 14)

Monitor medications/healthcare procedures when student self-administers care. (N.D. 10-12)

Teach student self-assessment of pain/discomfort. (N.D. 10-12, 14)

Teach comfort measures to help decrease the pain/discomfort. (N.D. 10-12, 14)

Teach stress management/relaxation techniques and medication methods for pain control. (N.D. 10-12, 14)

Convey an attitude of caring for the student and family. (N.D. 15)

Involve parent/guardian and student in decision making about healthcare and educational programming at school. (N.D. 15)

Maintain privacy and confidentiality. (N.D. 15)

Review school district's policies and guidelines regarding: (N.D. 2, 3, 5, 6, 8)
- confidentiality
- self-disclosure
- data privacy
- attendance for student/ faculty member diagnosed with communicable diseases, including HIV/AIDS
- HIV/AIDS curriculum
- substance abuse curriculum
- sexual health curriculum

Design an educational program to support staff, faculty, and students that will help to increase their knowledge base regarding HIV/AIDS. (N.D. 3, 6)

## Expected Student Outcomes

The student will:
- List nutritional principles that are important to maintain optimal nutrition and weight. (N.D. 1, 2, 12, 17)
- Choose well-balanced meals and healthy snacks. (N.D. 1, 2, 12, 17)
- Demonstrate intake of sufficient number of nutrients and calories (specific nutrients/specific calorie amount) to maintain weight. (N.D. 1, 2, 12, 17)
- Decrease contact with persons with infectious diseases or contaminated articles. (N.D. 2, 7)
- Demonstrate good health practices: hand washing, covering mouth with tissue when coughing/sneezing. (N.D. 2, 5, 7)
- Exhibit no signs or symptoms of opportunistic infections. (N.D. 2, 7)
- Demonstrate and utilize infection-control practices to not transmit the disease to others. (N.D. 2, 5, 7)
- Actively participate in (peer, community, school, family) activities. (N.D. 3, 4, 8, 9)
- Demonstrate effective coping skills to deal with (identify specific problems, concerns, or stressors). (N.D. 4, 8, 10)
- Utilize effective coping skills to effectively resolve/manage an identified problem/concern. (N.D. 4, 8, 10)
- Demonstrate a healthy sexual behavior. (N.D. 5)
- Verbally describe HIV/AIDS:
  – how it is transmitted
  – how to prevent transmission
  – how to seek and access information (N.D. 6, 11, 12)
- Actively participate in healthcare procedures and administration of medications. (N.D. 10, 11, 12)
- Demonstrate good school and classroom attendance, (fewer than ____ missed days/classes, per year/quarter/semester). (N.D. 6)
- Complete assigned work. (N.D. 6)
- Maintain activity level with intolerance level by modifying or substituting activities when required by physical condition, with assistance from (parent/guardian, teachers, school nurse), as needed. (N.D. 7, 13)
- Identify and describe fears and concerns to school nurse/staff member. (N.D. 8)
- Describe self in positive terms (what they can do, what they do know, how they are functioning, what they have accomplished). (N.D. 9)
- Utilize effective measures to decrease/manage pain. (N.D. 11, 12, 14)
- Utilize effective measure to decrease/manage irritability. (N.D. 8)
- Student will discuss feelings. (N.D. 15)

## Case Study

Peter is a 9-year-old boy who has started third grade at Pine Lake Elementary School. Peter is an articulate child who is small for his age. He was diagnosed with HIV at 26 months of age. He did not have any of the childhood vaccinations. Peter's mother was a known IV-drug user, and he was put into foster care following the initial diagnosis. Peter's foster parents have two other physically disabled children who are older than Peter, and they attend the same school. His foster siblings are not HIV-positive. Peter eats about one third of his meals and is 15% below his ideal body weight. He is very shy, and it is difficult for him to interact with other students. He is also not physically active because of a decrease in his energy level. He usually stands alone at recess and during physical education class.

Two days into the new school year, Peter was involved in a playground fight. Three classmates were picking on "the new small guy." On the following morning, parents of the three students who started the fight called the principal concerned that other students had shared information that Peter was HIV-positive. The principal called Peter's foster parents to share this information, and his foster parents confirmed the HIV-positive diagnosis. They asked the principal to keep this information confidential. He agreed that he would but needed to share the information with the school nurse. The foster parents agreed that sharing the information with the school nurse was acceptable.

In talking with Peter about his health condition, you determine that he has little knowledge or understanding of HIV infection and the disease process. His foster mother also reports that he seems to know little about his health condition.

# HIV/AIDS

| Assessment Data | Nursing Diagnosis | Goals | Nursing Interventions | Expected Outcomes |
|---|---|---|---|---|
| Peter is a new student.<br><br>Peter stands alone at recess and during P.E. class. Not physically active due to decreased energy level.<br><br>Other students reported to their parents that Peter has HIV. | Impaired social interaction related to stigma toward HIV/AIDS, inability to engage in satisfactory peer interaction. | Peter will participate in peer-group and school activities. | Implement and carry out standard precautions to prevent spread of virus.<br><br>With teachers and school counselor, provide opportunities for Peter to develop and maintain peer relationships. | Peter will actively participate in peer and school activities. |
| Peter eats about one third of his lunch. He is 15% below his ideal body weight. | Imbalanced nutrition: less than body requirements related to loss of appetite. | Peter will maintain optimal nutrition for weight gain. | Assess Peter's knowledge of nutrition and provide instruction, as needed.<br><br>In collaboration with Peter's foster parents and physician, assist in fortifying Peter's foods with nutritional supplements to maximize quality of food intake.<br><br>Monitor Peter's weight and growth.<br><br>Implement additional nutritional interventions, as prescribed, if weight continues to drop. | Peter will list two nutritional principles that are important to maintain optimal nutrition and weight gain.<br><br>Peter will choose well-balanced meals and healthy snacks.<br><br>Peter's weight will demonstrate increase in weight, (closer to normal range for his height). |
| Peter's knowledge and understanding of his health condition and HIV/AIDS disease process is poor. | Deficient knowledge, education related to existing disease condition. | Peter will increase knowledge of his health condition. | Instruct teaching staff:<br>• about HIV infection and AIDS<br>• in appropriate precautions<br>• clarify any misconceptions about communicability of the virus | Peter will describe<br>• HIV/AIDS (age appropriate)<br>• how it is transmitted (age appropriate)<br>• how to prevent transmission<br>• how to seek and access information |

| Assessment Data | Nursing Diagnosis | Goals | Nursing Interventions | Expected Outcomes |
|---|---|---|---|---|
| | | | Provide Peter with educational opportunities to learn about his health condition in collaboration with his foster parents, physician, and teachers.<br><br>Teach prevention strategies:<br>• hand washing<br>• universal precautions | Peter will demonstrate proper hand-washing technique.<br><br>Peter will demonstrate covering his mouth when he sneezes or coughs. |
| Peter is immunocompromised.<br><br>Peter is not immunized against childhood diseases. | Risk for infection related to impaired body defenses and not being immunized. | Peter will decrease his risk of infection in the school setting. | Assist Peter to learn about precautions to prevent the spread of diseases:<br>• hand washing<br>• cover mouth when sneeze/cough<br><br>Monitor school environment for current potential infections.<br><br>Notify Peter's foster parents when there is an infectious disease present in the classroom:<br>• influenza<br>• pneumonia<br>• chickenpox<br><br>Encourage Peter's foster parents to discuss getting influenza and pneumococcal and other immunizations with healthcare providers. | Peter will minimize contact with other students with known infectious diseases at school.<br><br>Peter will exhibit no signs or symptoms of an infectious disease. |

# References

Centers for Disease Control and Prevention (CDC), Division of HIV/AIDS Prevention. (2002). *Basic statistics.* Retrieved January 12, 2004, from http://www.cdc/gov/hiv/stats.htm

Centers for Disease Control and Prevention (CDC). (2002). *HIV/AIDS surveillance report.* Retrieved January 12, 2004, from http://www.cdc.gov/hiv.htm

Centers for Disease Control and Prevention (CDC). (2004). Treating opportunistic infections among HIV infected children. *Morbidity and Mortality Weekly Report (MMRW).* Retrieved December 2, 2004, from http://www.cdc.gov/mmwr/preview/mmwrhtml/rr5314a1.htm

Lewis, S., Heitkemper, M., & Dirksen, S. (2000). Nursing management of human immunodeficiency virus infection. In *Medical surgical nursing* (5th ed.). St. Louis, MO: Mosby.

Lisanti, P., & Zwolski, K. (1997). Understanding the devastation of AIDS. *American Journal of Nursing, 97,* 26.

Maine School Administrative District 40. (2000). *JLCD student health: Students with HIV/AIDS. Guidelines for the education and care of preschool and school-age children who have diagnosed AIDS.* Retrieved January 26, 2004, from http://msad40.org/POLICY/jled.html

NANDA International. (2003). *Nursing diagnoses: Definitions & classification 2003-2004.* Philadelphia: Author.

National Institute of Allergy and Infectious Diseases (NIAID). (2003). *HIV infection and AIDS: An overview.* Retrieved January 12, 2004, from http://www.niais.nih.gov/factsheets/hivinf.htm

Wilson, B. A. (1997). Understanding strategies for treating HIV. *MEDSURG Nursing, 6,* 109.

Wong, D. L., Hockenberry, M.J ., Wilson, D., Winkelstein, M. L., & Kline, N. E. (2003). The child with hematologic or immunologic dysfunction. In *Nursing care of infants and children* (7th ed.). St. Louis, MO: Mosby.

# Bibliography

Advocates for Youth. (2003). *Guide to implementing TAP (Teens for AIDS Prevention): A peer education program to prevent HIV and STI.* Retrieved January 15, 2004, from http://www.advocatesforyouth.org/publications/tap.htm

American Foundation for AIDS Research (amfAR). (2003). *New reports show increase in infections and AIDS deaths.* Retrieved January 27, 2004, from http://www.amfar.org/cgi-bin/iowa/news/record.html

Casey, K. M. (1996). *ANAC's core curriculum for HIV/AIDS nursing.* Philadelphia: Nursecom

Centers for Disease Control and Prevention (CDC). (2004). Heterosexual transmission of HIV–29 states, 1999-2002. *Morbidity and Mortality Weekly Report (MMWR).* Retrieved February 23, 2004, from http://www.cdc.gov/mmwr/preview/mmwrhtml/mm5306a3.htm

Centers for Disease Control and Prevention (CDC), Division of HIV/AIDS Prevention. (n.d.). *Human immunodeficiency virus type 2.* Retrieved January 12, 2004, from http://www.cdc.gov/hiv/pubs/facts/hiv2.htm

Centers for Disease Control and Prevention (CDC), Division of HIV/AIDS Prevention. (2002). *Living with HIV/AIDS.* Retrieved January 12, 2004, from http://www.cdc.gov/hiv/pubs/brochure/livingwithhiv.htm

Centers for Disease Control and Prevention (CDC), Division of HIV/AIDS Prevention. (2003). *HIV causes AIDS.* Retrieved January 12, 2004, from http://www.cdc.gov/hiv/hivinfo/overview.htm

Centers for Disease Control and Prevention (CDC), Office of Communication. (2003). *New study shows overall increase in HIV diagnoses.* Retrieved February 3, 2004, from http://www.cdc.gov/od/oc/media/pressrel/r031126,htm

Champion, C. (1999). *Occupational exposure to blood-borne pathogens* [Manual]. Scarborough, ME: National Association of School Nurses.

Facente, A. C. (2001). Adolescents and HIV: Knowledge, behaviors, influences, and risk perceptions. *Journal of School Nursing, 17*(4), 198–203.

Iowa Intervention Project. (1996). *Nursing interventions classifications (NIC).* St. Louis, MO: Mosby

Kaiser Family Foundation, State Health Facts Online. (2003). *State health facts online. 50 state comparisons: state requirements.* Retrieved January 15, 2004, from http://www.statehealthfacts.kff.org/cgi-bin/healthfacts.cgi?action=compare&category=HIV

Lewis, K. D., & Bear B. J. (2002). *Manual of school health* (2nd ed.). St. Louis, MO: Saunders.

Marick, J. (2002). HIV/AIDS peer education: A rural health project. *Journal of School Nursing, 18*(1), 41–47.

Mayo Foundation for Medical Education and Research (MFMER). (2004). *HIV/AIDS.* Retrieved February 3, 2004, from http://www,mayoclinic.com

McCane, K. L., & Huether, S. E. (1998). Infection and alternations in Immunity and inflammation. In *Pathophysiology: The biologic basis for disease in adults and children* (3rd ed.). St. Louis, MO: Mosby.

National Association of School Nurses. (n.d.). *Managing infectious diseases in the school setting* [Online Continuing Education Module]. Retrieved November 7, 2004, from http://nasn.org/education/nasnceinfectdis.htm

National Association of School Nurses. (Revised 2001). *Position Statement: Infections diseases.* Scarborough, ME: Author.

National Association of School Nurses. (Revised 2003). *Position Statement: Regulations on bloodborne pathogens in the school setting.* Scarborough, ME: Author.

National Association of State Boards of Education (NASBE). (2002). *The continuing role of schools in HIV prevention and education.* Retrieved January 12, 2004, from http://www.nasbe.org/Educational_Issues/Policy_Updates/8_18p.html

National Center for Education in Maternal and Child Health and Georgetown University (2004). *AIDS/HIV: Annotated lists of organizations on key topics in maternal and child health.* Retrieved January 12, 2004, from http://www.mchlibrary.info/databases/action.lasso?-database=Organizations&-layout=Web

National Institute of Allergy and Infectious Diseases (NIAID). (2001). *How HIV causes AIDS.* Retrieved January 12, 2004, from http://www.niaid.nih.gov/factsheets/howhiv.htm

National Institute of Allergy and Infectious Diseases (NIAID). (2002). *Basic information about HIV disease and AIDS, AIDS 101.* Retrieved January 12, 2004, from http://www.aegis.com/topics/basics/whataidsis.html

New Mexico AIDS Education and Training Center, University of New Mexico Health Sciences Center. (2003). *Children and HIV.* Retrieved January 26, 2004, from http://www.aidsinfonet.org/articles.php?articleID=612

New Mexico AIDS InfoNet. (2003). *New Mexico AIDS InfoNet fact sheet number 101. What is AIDS?* Retrieved January 27, 2004, from http://www.thebody.com/nmai/whaisaids.htm

University of Chicago Student Care Center. (2001). *HIV infection and AIDS.* Retrieved January 29, 2004, from http://scc.uchicago.edu/hivaids.htm

Windal, C. (1997). HIV/AIDS education isn't only for health class—it's for English, math science, Spanish ... *Education World.* Retrieved January 26, 2004, from http://www.education-world.com/a_curr/curr013.shtml

## Resources

AIDS Alliance for Children, Youth and Families
1600 K Street, NW
Suite 300
Washington, DC 20006
202-785-3564
1-888-917-AIDS
info@aids-alliance.org
http://www.aids-alliance.org

AIDSinfo
PO Box 6303
Rockville, MD 20849-6303
1-800-448-0440
ContactUs@aidsinfo.nih.gov
http://aidsinfo.nih.gov

CDC National STD and AIDS Hotlines
PO Box 13827
Research Triangle Park, NC 27709
1-800-342-2437
std-hivnet@ashastd.org
http://www.ashastd.org

Health Initiatives for Youth
235 Montgomery Street
Suite 430
San Francisco, CA 94102-2902
415-274-1970
dolan@hify.com

Mother, Child & Adolescent HIV Program
University of California at San Diego
150 West Washington Street
Suite 100

San Diego, CA 92103
616-543-8080
mcaffery@uscd.edu

National AIDS Fund
1030 15th Street, NW
Suite 860
Washington, DC 20005
202-408-4848
info@aidsfund.org
http://www.aidsfund.org

National Association of People with AIDS
1413 K Street, NW
Seventh Floor
Washington, DC 20005
202-898-0414
napwa@napwa.org
http://www.napwa.org

National Center for HIV, STD, and TB Prevention
1600 Clifton Road, NE
Mailstop E-07
Atlanta, GA 30333
1-800-311-3435
nchstp@cdc.gov
http://www.cdc.gov/nchstp/od/nchstp.html

National Foundation for Infectious Diseases
4733 Bethesda Avenue
Suite 750
Bethesda, MD 20814
1-800-851-3420
http://www.nfid.org

National Institute of Allergy and Infectious Diseases
MSC 2520
31 Center Drive
Bethesda, MD 20892-2520
310-496-5717
ocpostoffice@niaid.nih.gov
http://www.niaid.nih.gov

National Pediatric and Family HIV Resource Center
30 Bergen Street
ADMC No. 4
Newark, NJ 07103
1-800-362-0071
questions@pedhivaids.org
http://pedhivaids.org

*Chapter Forty-six*

# Immune Thrombocytopenic Purpura

### Mary A. Swanson

## Introduction

Immune thrombocytopenic purpura (ITP), also called idiopathic thrombocytopenic purpura and autoimmune thrombocytopenic purpura, is usually an acute self-limited disease in young children. It is classified as an autoimmune disorder in that the person produces antiplatelet autoantibodies, which results in the destruction of platelets (Blanchette & Carcao, 2000).

The incidence of ITP is estimated at 1 in 25,000 children (Bolton-Maggs, 2003). Acute ITP occurs most often in children after a viral illness, lasts 1 to 2 months, and rarely persists longer than 6 months. Both sexes are affected equally in acute ITP. Chronic ITP is most often seen in adults and may last for years or indefinitely. Acute ITP is considered a milder disorder with a better prognosis than the chronic form of the disorder. About 20% to 30% of children with acute disease (mostly older children) develop chronic ITP, defined as exhibiting thrombocytopenia with a platelet count of less that 150,000 per microliter beyond 6 months. The mortality rate is extremely low (Blanchette &Carcao, 2000, Medeiros & Buchanan, 2000, Tarantino, 2002).

The school-aged and adolescent child with ITP may have activity and/or sports restrictions, extremely cautious or anxious parents, multiple laboratory tests, and treatments with severe or chronic symptoms. The child lives with the threat of a minor or major bleeding episode but needs to experience activity and peer relationships as near to normal as possible.

## Pathophysiology

In this autoimmune disorder, the person produces autoantibody (primarily IgG type), which binds to circulating platelets resulting in phagocytic destruction of these cells, primarily in the spleen. What triggers this production of autoantibody is not entirely understood, but it often follows a viral illness. The balance between the antibody-mediated platelet destruction and the increased platelet production from megakaryocytes in the bone marrow determines the severity of the individual's thrombocytopenia. This thrombocytopenia induces purpura and

hemorrhage if the platelet count reaches a critical level (usually <30,000/microliter). The bleeding is predominantly seen in the skin and mucous membranes. Petechiae are noticed in dependent areas of the body. Common areas for bleeding are the mucous membranes of the nose, mouth, gastrointestinal tract, and uterus. Conjunctival and retinal hemorrhages can also occur but are rare. There is often a case history of easy bruising in absence of trauma, frequent nosebleeds, gum bleeding, prolonged menses, and hematuria. The most serious, but rare, complication is bleeding into the central nervous system (CNS), or intercranial hemorrhage, which can be fatal and must be rapidly and vigorously treated. The risk of hemorrhage varies and probably depends on such factors as platelet age, mean platelet volume and surface coverage, and capillary integrity (Blanchette & Carcao, 2000; Buchanan, 2003; Medeiros & Buchanan, 2000).

In 1996, the American Society of Hematology published guidelines for the diagnosis and treatment of ITP (George, Woolf, & Raskob, 1998). As a result of controversies over the guideline limitations, an intercontinental childhood ITP study group was established to collect data, network, and share results regarding the diagnosis and treatment of childhood ITP (Kumne, 2003). The criteria (Blanchette & Carcao, 2000; Buchanan, 2003; Medeiros & Buchanan, 2000) for diagnosis of ITP are based principally on the child's age, history, physical examination, complete blood cell count, and examination of the peripheral blood smear that are compatible with a diagnosis of acute ITP and also exclude other causes of thrombocytopenia. The child with acute ITP:

- Is usually healthy and presents with sudden onset of bruising, petechiae, and occasionally epistaxis
- May have a history of recent viral infection or, rarely, a recent live virus immunization
- Has no evidence of other disorders, such as systemic lupus erythematosus, HIV infection, or drug-induced thrombocytopenia
- May have hemorrhage of mucous membranes, such as menorrhagia, gastrointestinal bleeding, or oral blood blisters

The peripheral blood smear data consistent with a diagnosis of ITP include:

- Thrombocytopenia. Platelets are normal in size or may appear larger than normal, but consistently giant platelets should be absent.
- Normal red blood cell morphology
- Normal white blood cell morphology

The need for an initial bone marrow aspiration in children with typical acute ITP is controversial, but often recommended before starting corticosteroid therapy (Blanchette & Carcao, 2000).

## Management

Numerous therapeutic modalities for ITP have been suggested and tried over the years, but none has been uniformly curative. Treatments are aimed at maintaining the platelet count at a level that enables the child to lead a normal life, usually a count above 30,000 per microliter. Many children are able to recover spontaneously without treatment. This is the preferred option if they do not have an excessively low platelet count and they lack severe symptoms, such as frequent nosebleeds or heavy bruising. The parent and child need to be informed about the risk of bleeding and management of bleeding episodes, medications that impair platelet functioning, need for platelet monitoring, and treatment options. Platelet counts are monitored intermittently, and the child's activities and lifestyle may be restricted if the platelet levels fall below 30,000 cells per microliter to reduce the risk of internal injury and bleeding (Blanchette, 2002, Bolton-Maggs, Dickerhoff & Vora, 2001, George, et al. 1998, Medeiros & Buchanan, 2000).

The American Society of Hematology practice guidelines recommend that children with acute ITP and platelet counts less than 20,000 microliters plus significant mucous membrane bleeding or those with platelet counts less than 10,000 and minor purpura be treated with specific regimens of immune globulin or oral corticosteroids. The goal is to rapidly increase the circulating platelet counts to a safe level until the autoimmune reaction subsides. Other medical therapies have included methyl prednisolone, dexamethasone, anti-D, and immunosuppressive drugs. Steroids such as prednisone or dexamethasone have been used to impair antibody production and/or binding to platelets. These have been given in high dosages for a short time with good responses for both acute and chronic ITP. Immunoglobins or anti-D have been given intravenously over a number of days and with further single doses and may be given in combination with steroids. Intravenous gamma globulin blocks the destruction of antibody-coated platelets by the reticuloendothelial system. Immunosuppressive drugs such as vincristine, azathioprine (Imuran), danazol, cyclophosphamide, and cyclosporine have many side effects and are prescribed for

patients only in severe cases when other treatments have failed (Blanchette & Price, 2003; Blanchette, 2002; Bolton-Maggs et al., 2001; George et al., 1998; Tarantino, 2000).

Splenectomy may be performed in cases of chronic ITP or in the case of acute ITP when severe or life-threatening bleeding occurs. A splenectomy removes the potential site for destruction of damaged platelets and a significant source of antiplatelet antibody production. In children with chronic ITP, splenectomy improves the platelet count in approximately 70% of the cases. Following a splenectomy, the child will be monitored closely for infections and treated with antibiotics prophylactically (Blanchette & Price, 2003; Blanchette, 2002; Bolton-Maggs, 2003; Tarantino, 2000).

If a child has extensive hemorrhage and there is evidence of imminent or existing CNS bleeding (platelet count below 10,000/microliter), emergency treatment is required. This emergency treatment may include intravenous gammaglobulin, high-dose intravenous corticosteroids, and platelet transfusions (Blanchette & Price, 2003; Blanchette, 2002; Tarantino, 2000).

The child and parents must be educated about ITP so that they promptly report bleeding problems and injuries that could lead to hemorrhage. Parents are often frightened to see their previously healthy child with a sudden onset of petechiae, bruises, and perhaps bleeding from their nose or mouth. The day-to-day uncertainty of the platelet count places the prescription for restriction of physical activity at the discretion of the physician, which may increase the anxiety of the parents. Most contact sports are restricted until the platelet count is consistently above 100,000 per microliter. Most noncontact sports can be safely enjoyed by children with a platelet count greater than 30,000 per microliter. It is important that parents and the child understand ITP, the significance of the platelet counts, safety issues, emergency treatment, activity restrictions, and side effects of medications and treatments. In a study designed to develop quality-of-life instruments for children with ITP and their parents, Barnard et al. (2003) reported that parents experienced stress or felt a burden from the impact on their own lives and on the lives of their family, and they also felt stress from the burden they perceived that their child endured. Areas of greatest concern for parents included wanting to understand more about ITP, feeling the need to check the child frequently and to protect the child from injury, worrying about complications of ITP, and concern about potential complications of treatment. The areas of concern identified by young children with ITP included worrying about their platelet count and receiving treatment through an intravenous infusion. Resource organizations for patient and family education, support, and networking are available, including the ITP Foundation and the Platelet Disorder Support Association (see Resources listed at the end of this chapter).

Immune Thrombocytopenic Purpura

# Individualized Healthcare Plan

## Assessment

### History
- Date of initial diagnosis
- Symptoms experienced (bruising, petechia, nosebleeds, menorrhagia)
- Platelet count history

### Current Status and Management
- Healthcare providers: Frequency of visits
- Current health status
- Current management plan
- Current medications: Other medications used
- Current platelet count: Frequency of platelet counts
- Physical activity restrictions
- Plan for emergency management (i.e., head injury, trauma, unconsciousness)

### Self-care
- Parent knowledge of disease and treatment
- Student knowledge of disease and treatment
- Student wears Medic Alert bracelet
- Student's involvement in planning/implementation of treatment plan, including school emergency care plan (ECP)
- Student's willingness and ability to follow treatment plan
- Motivators to compliance with plan
- Barriers to compliance with plan

### Psychosocial Status
- Involvement of family/ support persons
- Activities with friends, peers
- Usual school and community activities
- Usual physical activity (sports, etc.)
- Student's perception of his/her condition and possible outcomes
- Student's perceptions and feelings about being different

### Academic Issues
- Physical education limitations (i.e., contact sports): Physical education requirements
- School attendance patterns: Current and prior to ITP diagnosis, related to diagnosis, other reasons
- Academic performance
- Modifications needed in academic program: course requirements, exemption from specific activities
- Need for academic support: 504 plan, referral for special education assessment

## Nursing Diagnoses (N.D.) (NANDA 2003)

**N.D. 1** Risk for injury (NANDA 00035) related to thrombocytopenia

**N.D. 2** Social isolation (NANDA 00052) related to altered state of wellness affecting activity with peers

**N.D. 3** Ineffective student role performance (NANDA 00055) related to health alterations affecting:
- activity
- school attendance

**N.D. 4** Noncompliance (NANDA 00079) related to:
- complexity of healthcare plan and unpredictability of ITP
- motivation
- knowledge and skill relevant to care regimen

**N.D. 5** Knowledge deficit about ITP and its management (NANDA 00126) related to:
- lack of information
- no experience with using the information

## Goals

The student will be safe in the school environment and remain free from physical injury. (N.D. 1)

The student will maintain peer relationships and activities. (N.D. 2, 3)

The student will participate in classroom and school activities with modifications made as needed. (N.D. 3)

The student will participate in the development and implementation of an action plan to manage bleeding episodes promptly (including an emergency care plan). (N.D. 1, 5)

The student will maintain a good school attendance pattern. (N.D. 3)

The student will comply with medical treatment measures. (N.D. 4)

The student will demonstrate increased knowledge about ITP and its management. (N.D. 5)

The student will demonstrate increased independence in implementing his management plan. (N.D. 5)

## Nursing Interventions

Develop ECP with student and parents/guardians for care of injuries and bleeding episodes. (N.D.1) Include:
- Specific directions for observations and bleeding, head injuries, abdominal trauma, and unconsciousness
- Plan for transportation
- Plan for notification of parent

Assist in modifying educational program as needed. (N.D. 1, 3)
- Modify physical education requirements, identify alternative activities
- Modify classroom assignments, especially those that may increase potential for injury
- Plan for make-up work for school days absent
- Homebound instruction if platelets are dangerously low

Monitor playground activities; set limits on activities as necessary. (N.D. 1, 3)
- Inform student
- Inform teachers and playground supervisor

Provide in-service training for teachers and staff on ITP and ECP. (N.D. 1, 3)

Assist physical education teachers and classroom teachers in modifying activities as needed. (N.D. 3)

Discuss with student: (N.D. 1, 2, 3, 4, 5)
- What ITP is and how it can be managed
- Symptoms of lowered platelet count that need medical attention
- How platelet counts affect his or her activity and lifestyle to reduce risk of injury
- Importance of having a plan to treat injury or bleeding
- Alternatives for peer activities when platelet counts are low
- Use of Medic Alert bracelet
- Use of over-the-counter medications that contain aspirin or affect platelet formation/functioning

Monitor school attendance and academic performance. (N.D. 3)

Request note from physician to document need for activity limitations/restrictions. (N.D. 1, 3)

Discuss possible ways to continue to be part of a sports team with student, parents, and coach (if physical activities are restricted). (N.D. 2)

Assist student to notify parents if he/she has signs/symptoms of infections. (N.D. 4, 5)

Request parent notify the school if there is a change in status, especially if a decrease in platelet count occurs. (N.D. 1, 3, 5)

Provide resources, including Web sites of ITP Foundation and Platelet Disorder Support Association to parents and student for educational and networking support. (N.D. 2, 5)

## Expected Student Outcomes

The student will:
- Describe symptoms that need medical attention. (N.D. 1, 5)
- Wear a Medic Alert bracelet. (N.D. 1, 5)
- Describe risks of injury when platelet counts are decreased. (N.D. 4, 5)
- Modify his/her activities when platelet counts are low. (N.D. 3, 4, 5)
- Maintain good school attendance pattern. (N.D. 2, 3)
- Report results of each platelet count to the school nurse and identify its implications for safety and activities. (N.D. 1, 4, 5)
- Participate in physical activities (regular or modified, appropriate to platelet count). (N.D. 2, 3)

Immune Thrombocytopenic Purpura

- Participate in activities with friends and peers (appropriate to platelet counts). (N.D. 2)
- Identify appropriate use and safety of over-the-counter medications. (N.D. 5)
- Utilize resource organizations (i.e., via Web sites) for education and networking. (N.D. 2, 5)

## Case Study

Christopher T., age 15, was taken to the doctor by his parents in November when they noticed bruising on his legs and he had several lengthy nosebleeds. He was diagnosed with ITP following several laboratory blood studies and a bone marrow examination. His platelet count was initially 23,000 per microliter. He was treated with corticosteroid bursts over several months with his platelet count responding to 80,000 to 120,000 initially each time, but falling again to less than 30,000 per microliter. His doctor recommended that he not attend school when his platelet count was below 20,000 per microliter because of the potential of injury-related or spontaneous bleeding. He also advised him not to participate in gym or contact sports when his platelet levels were below 80,000 per microliter. Christopher had platelet counts done one to two times per week over several months and attended school when his platelet count was above 20,000 per microliter. His parents requested homework and homebound instruction so that he could keep up with his coursework. At the beginning of second semester, Christopher was placed on a 504 plan to provide an alternative for his physical education class and continued on homebound instruction when his platelet checked went below 20,000 per microliter. It was hoped that he could spontaneously recover and return to school and his normal activities.

Christopher was completing his coursework successfully at home with a homebound teacher. His mother arranged for him to complete a daily exercise program with an athletic trainer at the family's athletic club. Christopher logged his activities and physical education skills to submit to school for the physical education requirement. Christopher was able to attend school for part of the second semester because his platelet count continued to fluctuate between 18,000 and 123,000 per microliter. His physician diagnosed chronic ITP in May and planned a splenectomy for July. When Christopher, following splenectomy, returned to school in September, he had platelet counts between 150,000 and 200,000 per microliter and no activity restrictions. He is participating in mainstream classes and is participating in his tenth-grade physical education class. His physician continues to monitor his platelet count every 3 months and wants him to seek medical attention when signs of infection and fever occur.

# Emergency Care Plan
## Immune Thrombocytopenic Purpura

Date: 12-12-03

Student: Christopher T.

Date of birth: 6-2-88

School: HHS

Grade: 9

Parent(s)/Guardian(s): Marie T.

Dave T.

Home telephone: 456-3333

Father's work: 456-8828

Mother's work: _____

Emergency Contact: Bill and Sue R.

Telephone: 456-7877

Healthcare Provider: Dr. G. Seal

Telephone: 456-6756

Emergency plan written by: M. Swanson, LS

Medical Diagnosis: _____

Persons Authorized to Administer Treatment: _____

Parent/Student Signature: _____

**Health Condition:** Christopher was diagnosed with immune thrombocytopenic purpura (ITP) in November 2003. His platelet count has been fluctuating between 18,000 and 120,000 per microliter. He has been treated with corticosteroid bursts and responds with a higher platelet count initially, but it gradually falls over two to three weeks. The physician will be monitoring his platelet count one to two times per week and plans to continue with corticosteroids until Christopher's platelets stabilize at 100,000 per microliter or higher. There is a risk for uncontrolled bleeding if Christopher has an injury (internally or externally) because he has fewer platelets that normally clot his blood. Prevention of injuries is important, but should an accident occur, it is an emergency and Christopher will need prompt medical attention for his injuries.

| Signs of Emergency | Actions to Take |
|---|---|
| If Christopher sustains a cut or bruise that bleeds slowly | Apply pressure to wound and escort Christopher to the nurse's office or call school nurse to come to you (extension 8809). |
| If Christopher has a large injury with large amount of visible bleeding | Apply pressure to wound if possible.<br><br>Call 911.<br><br>Stay with student, and direct someone else to call the operator (dial 0) to obtain help from the principal and the school nurse.<br><br>Notify parents of emergency.<br><br>Call 911. |
| If Christopher complains of sudden headache and/or has a change in consciousness or orientation to his environment:<br><br>**Christopher wears a Medic Alert bracelet.** | Stay with student, and direct someone to call the operator (dial 0) to obtain help from the principal and school nurse.<br><br>Notify parents of emergency.<br><br>**Provide the information on this plan to the paramedics.** |

# Section 504 Student Accomodatin Plan

Name: <u>Christopher T. 12-12-03</u>          Date: <u>12-12-03</u>

School: <u>Hamilton High School</u>          Grade: <u>9</u>

Birth date: <u>6-2-88</u>

1. **Describe the nature of the concern:**
   Christopher was diagnosed with ITP (immune thrombocytopenic purpura) in November 2003. When his platelet count is below normal, he has a higher risk for hemorrhage/bleeding with injury, trauma, or spontaneously.

2. **Describe the basis for the determination of handicap (if any):**
   Christopher cannot attend school when his platelet count is below 20,000/microliter because he is at high risk for hemorrhage/bleeding. He is taking corticosteroids (treatment), which can affect his attention span and mental stability.

3. **Describe how the handicap affects a major life activity:**
   - Christopher cannot attend school when platelets are below 20,000 per microliter.
   - Christopher cannot participate in gym/contact sports when platelets are below 80,000 per microliter.
   - Christopher is taking corticosteroids, sometimes at high doses, which may affect his attention span and mood.

4. **Describe the reasonable accommodations that are necessary:**
   - Homebound instruction (1 hour/week/class of school missed) will be available to Christopher as needed for absence from school related to his ITP.
   - Christopher will discuss with teachers his need for extra time for assignments/projects/tests, as needed when he misses school.
   - Christopher will provide an activity log (physical education skills) to counselor/assistant principal for one physical education credit consideration.
   - Christopher will wear his Medic Alert bracelet and keep the school nurse informed of his platelet count and ITP status.

Review/Reassessment Date: 3/17/04

Participants (Name and title)

| | | | |
|---|---|---|---|
| Sue T. | (Parent) | Bob B. | (Math teacher) |
| Christopher T. | (Student) | Mary S. | (School nurse) |
| Mark K. | (Spanish teacher) | Paula A. | (English teacher) |
| Tom P. | (Academic counselor) | Judy M. | (Assistant principal) |
| Dan H. | (Science teacher) | Marla P. | (Physical education teacher) |

cc. Student's Cumulative File

Attachment: Information regarding Section 504 of the Rehabilitation Act of 1973

Immune Thrombocytopenic Purpura

# Immune Thrombocytopenic Purpura

| Assessment Data | Nursing Diagnosis | Goals | Nursing Interventions | Expected Outcomes |
|---|---|---|---|---|
| Platelets fluctuate between 18,000 and 110,000/micro-liters. | Risk for injury related to thrombocytopenia. | Christopher will be safe in school and remain free from physical injury.<br><br>Christopher will participate in the development and implementation of an action plan to manage bleeding episodes promptly. | Modify phy ed requirements (see 504 plan). Develop emergency care plan with Christopher and family.<br><br>Discuss ITP with and distribute emergency plan to teachers/staff. | Christopher will wear a Medic Alert bracelet.<br><br>Christopher will describe his symptoms that need medical attention.<br><br>Christopher will report his platelet count to the school nurse weekly. |
| Christopher can attend school if platelets >20,000/microliters. | Ineffective student role performance related to activity restrictions and absence from school. | Christopher will participate in school activities with modifications.<br><br>Christopher will maintain a good school attendance pattern. | Classroom assignments modified.<br><br>Homebound instruction if platelets <20,000/microliters (see 504 plan).<br><br>Monitor school attendance. | Christopher will maintain a good school attendance pattern. Christopher will participate in school and physical activities (appropriate to platelet count). |
| Christopher diagnosed with ITP in November 2003. | Knowledge deficit about ITP and its management related to lack of exposure and unfamiliarity. | Christopher will demonstrate increased knowledge of ITP and its management.<br><br>Christopher will demonstrate increased independence in implementing his plan. | Discuss with student:<br>1. ITP and management<br>2. relationship of platelet count to bleeding risk<br>3. alternatives for peer activities<br>4. use of over-the-counter medications<br><br>Provide ITP-related Web sites for educational and networking support. | Christopher will describe activities with friends and peers (appropriate to platelet counts).<br><br>Christopher will identify the implications of his platelet counts.<br><br>Christopher will modify his activities when platelet counts are low.<br><br>Christopher will identify appropriate use of OTC medications. |

# References

Barnard, D., Woloski, M., Feeny, D., McCuster, P., Wu, J., & David, M., et al. (2003). Development of disease-specific health-related quality-of-life instruments for children with immune thrombocytopenic purpura and their parents. *Journal of Pediatric Hematology/Oncology, 25*, 56–62.

Blanchette, F. S., & Price, V. (2003). Childhood chronic immune thrombocytopenic purpura: Unresolved issues. *Journal of Pediatric Hematology/Oncology, 25*(Suppl.1), 28–33.

Blanchette, V. (2002). Childhood chronic immune thrombocytopenic purpura (ITP). *Blood Reviews, 16*, 23–26.

Blanchette, V., & Carcao, M. Approach to the investigation and management of immune thrombocytopenic purpura in children. *Seminars in Hematology, 37*, 299–314.

Bolton-Maggs, P. (2003). Severe bleeding in idiopathic thrombocytopenic purpura. *Journal of Pediatric Hematology/Oncology, 25*(Suppl. 3), 47–51.

Bolton-Maggs, P., Dickerhoff, R., & Vora, A. (2001). The nontreatment of childhood ITP (or "the art of medicine consists of amusing the patient until nature cures the disease"). *Seminars in Thrombosis and Hemostasis, 27*, 269–275.

Buchanan, G. R. (2003). Bleeding signs in children with idiopathic thrombocytopenic purpura. *Journal of Hematology/Oncology, 25*(Suppl. 3), 42–46.

George, J. N., Woolf, S. H., & Raskob, G. F. (1998). Idiopathic thrombocytopenic purpura: A guideline for diagnosis and management of children and adults. *Annuals of Medicine, 30*, 38–44.

Kumne, T. (2003). Investigation and management of newly diagnosed childhood idiopathic thrombocytopenic purpura: Problems and proposed solutions. *Journal of Pediatric Hematology/Oncology, 25*(Suppl. 3), 24–27.

Medeiros, D., & Buchanan, G. R. (2000). Idiopathic thrombocytopenic purpura: Beyond consensus. *Current Opinions in Pediatrics, 12*, 4–9.

NANDA International. (2003). *Nursing diagnosis: Definitions & classification, 2003-2004*. Philadelphia: Author.

Tarantino, M. D. (2000). Treatment options for chronic immune (idiopathic) thrombocytopenia purpura in children. *Seminars in Hematology, 37*(Suppl. 1): 35–41.

Tarantino, M. D. (2002). Acute immune (idiopathic) thrombocytopenic purpura in childhood. *Blood Reviews, 16*, 19–21.

# Bibliography

George, J. N., Woolf, S. H., Raskob, G. E., Wasser. J. S., Aledort, L. M., Ballern, P. J., et al. (1996). Idiopathic thrombocytopenic purpura: A practice guideline developed by explicit methods for the american society of hematology. *Blood 88*(1), 3–40.

Handlin, R. I. (1998). Disorders of the platelet and vessel wall. In A. S. Fauci, J. D. Wilson, & E. Braunwald, et al. (Eds.), *Harrison's principles of internal medicine* (14th ed., pp. 730–735). New York: McGraw-Hill.

Homas, A. (1999). Disorders of platelet quantity and function. In S. S. Gellis & B. M. Kagen (Eds.), *Current pediatric therapy* (Vol. 16, pp. 705–708). Philadelphia: Saunders.

*Idiopathic thrombocytopenic purpura.* Accessed April 17, 2004, from http://rarediseases.about.com

Radin, A. & Radin, B. (1996). *What's it called again?* New York: ITP Society of The Children's Blood Foundation.

# Resources

ITP Foundation
381 Post Road
Darien, CT 06820
203-655-6954
203-655-7997 (fax)
info@itpfoundation.org
http://www.itpfoundation.org

Platelet Disorder Support Association
PO Box 61533
Potomac, MD 20859
301-770-6638
1-877-528-3538
301-770-6638 (fax)
pdsa@pdsa.org
http://www.pdsa.org

*Chapter Forty-seven*

# Immunodeficiency Diseases

## Lacy E. Scott

## Introduction

Immunodeficiency diseases occur when part of the body's immune system is missing or not functioning properly (Immune Deficiency Foundation, 2004). Immunodeficiency diseases can be primary (inherited or congenital) or acquired. Both can lead to autoimmune disorders. Refer to the HIV/AIDs chapter in this book for further discussion of this disease.

### Primary Immunodeficiency

There are over 100 identified primary immunodeficiency diseases (Buckley, 2004). Primary immunodeficiency affects approximately 1 in 10,000 individuals (Cunningham-Rundles, 2002). The severity of a primary immunodeficiency varies greatly and is dependent on the particular immune response affected. Primary immunodeficiency diseases are classified in terms of the disrupted immunologic mechanism. There are three main groups of primary immunodeficiency diseases: antibody deficiencies, cellular deficiencies, and combined B-cell and T-cell deficiencies. There are also classifications for defects in phagocyte function and complement deficiency.

In childhood, primary immunodeficiency can be recognized by symptoms associated with immunologic abnormalities but usually presents as recurrent, severe, or unusual infections or symptomatic infections of low pathogenicity. Common features of primary immunodeficiency are recurrent infections, chronic inflammation, and autoimmunity. A complete blood cell count and quantitative immunoglobulins will detect most primary immunodeficiencies. Early diagnosis is vital to ensure the best prognosis, reduce morbidity, improve long-term quality of life, and prevent rapid deterioration of the immune system (Bonilla & Geha, 2003; Champi, 2002; Gennery, Spencer & Cant, 2004; Peake & Roberton, 2001; Simonte & Cunningham-Rundles, 2003).

Antibody deficiencies make up 50% of all congenital immunodeficiencies. Their prevalence is 4 to 5 persons per 100,000. It is evidenced by low serum levels of one or more Ig classes and/or relative impairment of antibody responses. The body essentially does not produce neutralizing antibodies or B-cell memory. Typically, an individual has recurrent bacterial infections of upper or lower respiratory tract, pyogenic skin infections, osteomyelitis, meningitis, and sepsis. Predominant organisms responsible for infections are encapsulated bacteria, *Streptococcus pneumoniae, Haemophilus influenzae, Staphylococcus aureus, and Neisseria meningitidis.* Treatment consists of antimicrobial agents per infectious event, antibiotic prophylaxis, and intravenous immunoglobulin (IVIG) therapy approximately every 2 to 4 weeks. Antibiotic doses are not necessarily adjusted for individuals based on their history of primary immunodeficiency; however, duration of antibiotic course may be lengthened (Geha, Leung, Sampson, & Szefler, 2003; Glauser, 2000; Patrick, 2001).

Cellular deficiencies occur in 1 in every 50,000 to 100,000 live births. T-lymphocytes are a component of adaptive immunity and mediate resistance to intracellualar pathogens. Impaired T-cell function ultimately results in autoimmunity. All T-cell immunodeficiency diseases have significant morbidity and some high early-onset mortality (Geha et al., 2003).

The 10 warning signs of primary immunodeficiency are:

1. Eight or more new ear infections within a year
2. Two or more serious sinus infections within a year
3. Two or more months on antibiotics with little effect
4. Two or more pneumonias within a year
5. Failure for an infant to gain weight or grow normally
6. Recurrent deep skin or organ abscesses
7. Persistent thrush in mouth or elsewhere on skin, after age of 1 year
8. Need for intravenous antibiotics to clear infections
9. Two or more deep-seated infections, such as meningitis, osteomyelitis, cellulitis, or sepsis
10. A family history of primary immunodeficiency (National Primary Immunodeficiency Resource Center, 2004)

### Acquired Immunodeficiency

These are complications of other conditions and diseases, such as malnutrition, chickenpox, cytomegalovirus, German measles, measles, tuberculosis, infectious mononucleosis (Epstein-Barr virus), human immunodeficiency virus, chronic hepatitis, and lupus. Chemotherapy and antirejection medications for organ transplant can also cause acquired immunodeficiency (Lohr, 2004).

## Pathophysiology

### B-lymphocyte Humoral Deficiencies

#### X-Linked Agammaglobulinemia

This is a genetic disorder due to mutation on X chromosome affecting B-cell maturation.

- Affects males only
- Occurs in 1 in 100,000 live births
- Half of those affected will have a family history of affected males on maternal side
- Clinical illness presents at 4 to 18 months of age as maternal antibodies wane
- Characterized by absence or marked deficiency of immunoglobulins
- Presence of tonsils rare and notably reduced lymphoid tissue, spleen, lymph nodes, and adenoids
- Normal T-cell numbers and function
- Signs and symptoms include chronic enteroviral meningoencephalitis, viral infections, meningitis, septic arthritis, failure to thrive, and chronic diarrhea
- Opportunistic infections rare
- Complications include bronchiectasis
- Specific medical management includes immunoglobulin therapy

(Ballow, 2002; Geha et al., 2003; National Institute of Health, National Institute of Child Health & Human Development, 1999; Patrick, 2001; Spickett, 1999)

### Selective IgA Deficiency

There is no evidence of immune defects in selective IgA deficiency; however, familial occurrence is prevalent. IgA immunoglobulins are found in secretions and mucous membranes.

- Most common form of primary immunodeficiency
- Affects 1 in 200 to 700 individuals
- Characterized by serum IgA level of less than 10 mg/dL
- Typically asymptomatic, but chronic sinopulmonary infections occur, as well as allergic disorders
- Complications include atopic diseases, celiac disease, immune thrombocytopenia, rheumatoid arthritis, systemic lupus erythematosus, hepatitis, Sjogren's syndrome, insulin-dependent diabetes mellitus, Crohn's disease, lymphoid/gastrointestinal malignancies, asthma, pulmonary hemosiderosis, endocrinopathy
- Special considerations include cases of acquired IgA deficiency from anticonvulsant use, association with some chromosomal abnormalities, possible severe allergic reaction after exposure to blood products containing IgA
- Specific medical management targets treatments of diseases associated with selective IgA deficiency

(Geha et al., 2003; National Institute of Health, National Institute of Child Health & Human Development, 1999; National Primary Immunodeficiency Resource Center, 2004; Patrick, 2001)

### IgG Subclass Deficiency

This condition is not a result of genetic lesions. IgG immunoglobulins are composed of four subtypes of IgG molecules.

- Normal total levels of IgG, IgA, and IgM
- Poor responses to diphtheria, tetanus toxoid, and pneumococcal immunizations
- Characterized by lack of or low levels of one or more IgG subclasses
- Signs and symptoms include recurrent sinopulmonary infections, frequent viral infections, chronic diarrhea
- Complications include rheumatologic disorders, vasculitis, impaired lung function, asthma, chronic rhinitis, and hearing loss
- Specific medical management includes prophylactic antibiotics, gamma globulin replacement therapy

(Geha et al., 2003; Reisman & Slavin, 1999)

### Common Variable Immunodeficiency (CVID)

No well-defined molecular defect has been identified in this condition.

- Commonly reported in the second and third decades of life
- Characterized by lack of serum IgG, IgA, and IgM
- 40% of affected individuals also have disrupted T-cell function
- Signs and symptoms include recurrent sinopulmonary diseases, chronic rhinitis, meningitis, infectious arthritis, exudative enteropathy, giardiasis, arthropathy, and enteroviral infections
- Complications include autoimmune disorders, lymphoid and gastrointestinal malignancies, lymphoma, malabsorption, inflammatory bowel syndrome, cytopenias, pernicious anemia, and lymphoproliferation may cause splenomegaly, adenopathy, and/or intestinal lymphonodular hyperplasia
- Specific medical management includes gamma globulin therapy

(Bonilla & Geha, 2003; Geha et al., 2003; Patrick, 2001)

## T-Lymphocyte Cellular Deficiencies

### DiGeorge Syndrome

DiGeorge syndrome is not inherited; it is a developmental anomaly occurring during fetal development.

- Presents within days of birth due to heart disease and/or hypocalcemia
- All tissues affected by viral illnesses
- Characterized by an underdeveloped thymus or absent thymus
- Signs and symptoms include hypoparathyroidism, dysmorphic features, hypocalcemic seizures
- T-lymphocyte production improves over time
- Complications include autoimmune manifestations due to dysregulation of thymic function
- Special considerations include no live vaccines

- Specific medical management includes *Pneumocystis carinii* pneumonia prophylaxis, bone marrow transplant, thymic transplantation, supplementation of calcium and vitamin D, surgical repair of heart defect

(Geha et al., 2003; Lohr, 2004)

### Wiskott-Aldrich Syndrome

- X-linked disorder
- Prevalence is 4 per one million male births
- Characterized by reduced numbers and size of platelets, congenital thrombocytopenia
- Signs and symptoms include increased tendency to bleed, eczema, food allergies, and recurrent bacterial, viral, and fungal infections
- Complications include autoimmune manifestations, tumors, leukemia, lymphoma, cerebral hemorrhage
- Special considerations include no live vaccines
- Specific medical management includes platelet transfusions, splenectomy, bone marrow transplant, cordblood stem-cell transplant, prophylactic antibiotics

(Geha et al., 2003; National Primary Immunodeficiency Resource Center, 2004)

### X-linked Hyper-IgM

- Characterized by no IgA, low levels of IgG, high levels of IgM, and possibly a low neutrophil count
- Poor prognosis due to liver disease
- Signs and symptoms include opportunistic bacterial infections, especially pneumocystis pneumonia, otitis media, sinusitis
- Complications include liver/biliary disease, autoimmune diseases, chronic diarrhea, anemia, increased occurrence of liver tumors
- Special considerations include drinking sterile/filtered water, nonmyeloablative regimens
- Specific medical management includes G-CSF protein to produce granulocytes, routine intravenous immunoglobulin

(Geha et al., 2003; National Institute of Health, National Institute of Child Health & Human Development, 1999)

### Chronic Granulomatous Disease (CGD)

- This inherited group of four types of immunodeficiency diseases is caused by faulty phagocytes, identified by a different gene defect. One is on the X chromosome, and the remaining three are recessive genes on autosomes.
- Affects males four times more than females
- Clinical presentation as early as 3 months of age and diagnosis usually by age 1
- Characterized by inability of phagocytes to produce oxygen by-products necessary to kill certain bacteria and fungi
- Normal antibody function, T-cell function, and complement system

- Signs and symptoms include skin infections, rashes, lung disease, pneumonia, liver and lung abscesses, and osteomyelitis
- Complications include chronic inflammatory conditions, gum disease, inflammatory bowel disease, enlarged lymph glands, development of granulomas in the skin, lungs, lymph nodes, liver, or bone
- Special considerations include avoiding swimming in salt water and fresh water lakes due to increased possible exposure to organisms, abstention from smoking marijuana due to likelihood of *Aspergillus* contamination, avoidance of environments with dusty conditions or containing moldy grass, hay, or compost
- Specific medical management includes granulocyte transfusions for life-threatening infections after failed aggressive antibiotic treatment, surgical drainage of abscesses, prophylactic antibiotics, steroids, gamma interferon

(National Institute of Health, National Institute of Child Health & Human Development, 1999; National Primary Immunodeficiency Resource Center, 2004; Rosenzweig & Holland, 2004 )

## Combined B-cell and T-cell Deficiencies

### Ataxia Telangiectasia (AT)

Autosomal recessive disorder

- Clinical presentation noted between 12 and 18 months of age
- Poor prognosis, progressive disorder
- Affects several body systems
- Characterized by decreased B-cell response, decreased maturity and numbers of T-cells, and immature thymus gland
- Signs and symptoms include neurologic sequelae, ataxia, telangiectasia, poor quality of gross motor skills, oculomotor apraxia, dystharia, susceptibility of bacterial or viral sinopulmonary infections
- Do not develop opportunistic infections
- Complications include increased occurrence of leukemia, lymphoma, dysgerminoma, gonadoblastoma
- Special considerations include limiting diagnostic x-rays, routine monitoring of swallow function
- Specific medical management includes prophylactic antibiotic, chest physiotherapy, IVIG

(Geha et al., 2003; National Institute of Health, National Institute of Child Health & Human Development, 1999; National Primary Immunodeficiency Resource Center, 2004)

### Severe Combined Immunodeficiency (SCID)

This heterogenous group of inherited disorders is caused by mutations of different genes. Only one form is X-linked; all others are autosomal recessive.

- Most severe primary immunodeficiency
- Prevalence of one in every one million persons
- Presents at 4 to 6 months of age

- Opportunistic infections can be bacterial, viral, and fungal
- Characterized by severe abnormalities in both B-cell and T-cell function
- Signs and symptoms include failure to thrive, protracted diarrhea, high frequency of *Pneumocystis carinii* pneumonia, severe respiratory infections, persistent candidiasis (oral thrush), skin rash, erythrodermia, alopecia
- Complications include blindness, sensorineural hearing loss, bronchiolitis obliterans, chronic hepatitis
- Special considerations include no live vaccines and eradication of blood products prior to transfusion
- Specific medical management includes bone marrow transplant

(Geha et al., 2003; National Institute of Health, National Institute of Child Health & Human Development, 1999)

## Management

Early diagnosis is essential to determine an appropriate therapeutic regimen and medical intervention to minimize long-term sequelae in patients with primary immunodeficiency diseases.

Self-management includes gaining education about the condition, finding resources needed for medical care and lifestyle changes, and implementation of knowledge into daily lifestyle by:

- Maintaining a healthy diet; malnutrition aggravates immunodeficiencies
- Practicing good personal hygiene, including dental care
- Avoiding eating undercooked food, a potential source of bacteria

- Avoiding unnecessary exposure to communicable disease

Medical management includes determining the correct diagnosis and developing a treatment plan that includes medications, various therapies, education, resource support, and continuing evaluation and follow-up. Elements of medical management include:

- Baseline laboratory tests
- Avoid contact with persons with communicable disease
- Prophylactic antibiotic treatment
- Antibiotic treatment for specific infectious agents
- IVIG (intravenous Immunoglobulin)
- Bone marrow transplant
- Enzyme replacement therapy
- Gene therapy
- No live vaccines
- Routine vaccinations and boosters: Pneumovax, Hib, meningococcal boosters every 2 to 3 years
- Assess pulmonary status with high-resolution computed tomography and spirometry at baseline and every 12 to 24 months
- Splenectomy
- Postural drainage
- Passive immunity
- Stem-cell transplant
- Growth factor injections
- Cytokine injections
- Gamma interferon

(Glauser, 2000; Immune Deficiency Foundation, 2004; National Institute of Health, National Institute of Child Health & Human Development, 1999; Reisman & Slavin, 1999)

# Individualized Healthcare Plan

## Assessment

*History*
- Specific immunodeficiency disease
- Severity of disease
- Date of diagnosis
- Contributing medical conditions
- Prognosis

Family history of autoimmune diseases and/or immunodeficiency disease
- Past infections
- Past hospitalizations
- Past treatments and responses to treatments
- Previous height and weight
- Immunizations

*Current Status and Management*
- Healthcare providers, primary and specialists
- Current treatment plan, including alternative or naturopathic therapies
- Current medications and side effects
- Oxygen requirement, gastric tube, and/or MediPort
- Specific nutritional needs

- Skin care
- Oral hygiene
- Current developmental assessment
- Physical examination
  – Normal linear growth
  – Dysmorphic features
  – Skin lesions: eczema, scars, wound healing, pigment changes
  – Nutritional status
  – Tonsils: present or absent
  – Mucosal abnormalities: dental/periodontal disease, ulcerations, candidiasis, aphthous lesions
  – Visceral or perianal abnormalities
  – Muscular/joint pain
  – Neurologic signs: vision, hearing loss, tactile sensibility, cerebellar or motor function
  – Structural damage: lungs, sinuses, ears
  – Autoimmune features
  – Height and weight: failure to thrive
  – Respiratory: asthma, oxygen requirement
  – Gastrointestinal: malabsorption, gastric tube

(Glauser, 2000; Spickett, 1999)

*Self-care*
- Parent's knowledge of specific immunodeficiency disease
- Student's knowledge of specific immunodeficiency disease
- Student's hygiene practices
- Family's food-preparation skills
- Student's level of involvement in disease management
- Barriers to self-care; financial resources, transportation

*Psychosocial Status*
- Family participation in disease-specific support group
- Student's participation in disease-specific support group
- Family/student's involvement in community, church
- Student's participation in sports, recreation, and/or school activities
- Student's peer group

*Academic Issues*
- Developmental delays
- School attendance record
- Individualized education plan (IEP) or 504 plan
- Effect of health on academic progress
- Modifications or accommodations during school day

## Nursing Diagnoses (N.D.) (NANDA, 2003)

**N.D. 1** Risk for infection (NANDA 00004) related to: specific immunodeficiency disease
- inadequate acquired immunity
- chronic disease
- increased environmental exposure to pathogens

**N.D. 2** Ineffective (student) role performance (NANDA 00055) related to:
- inadequate role socialization
- inadequate support system
- physical illness
- health alterations
- frequent absences

**N.D. 3** Risk for delayed development (NANDA 00112) related to:
- chronic illness
- possible vision impairment
- possible hearing impairment
- social isolation

**N.D. 4** Imbalanced nutrition: less than body requirements (NANDA 00002) related to:
- malabsorption
- specific immunodeficiency disease

**N.D. 5** Social isolation (NANDA 00053) related to:
- chronic illness
- frequent absences

**N.D. 6** Ineffective health maintenance (NANDA 00099) related to:
- lack of resources
- lack of knowledge regarding basic health practices
- developmental age; desire to fit in with peers

**N.D. 7** Risk for activity intolerance (NANDA 0094) related to:
- fatigue
- frequent infections

**N.D. 8** Risk for impaired skin integrity (NANDA 00047) related to:
- gastric tube placement
- MediPort/catheter placement
- eczema

**N.D. 9** Ineffective coping (NANDA 00069) related to:
- school attendance pattern
- chronic illness
- inability to meet role expectation
- fear of future sequelae

**N.D. 10** Deficient knowledge (NANDA 00126) related to lack of knowledge of:
- specific immunodeficiency disease
- signs and symptoms of illness
- signs and symptoms of infection of MediPort and/or gastric tube
- health promotion lifestyle, hygiene practices, proper nutrition, hydration, adequate sleep patterns and appropriately accessing resources as warranted by present health status

## Goals

The student will be free of infection. (N.D. 1, 7)

The student will recognize and verbalize signs and symptoms of infection to promote early intervention and treatment. (N.D. 1, 7)

The student will utilize health office for substantiated signs and symptoms of illness and/or infection. (N.D. 1, 2, 6, 9, 10)

The student will practice good hygiene as reported/observed by classroom staff and student. (N.D. 1, 6, 8, 10)

The student will prevent physical injuries. (N.D. 1, 6)

The student will maintain good attendance pattern as evidenced by school records. (N.D. 2, 9)

The student will maintain academic progress as appropriate for developmental and cognitive abilities as reported by teacher. (N.D. 2, 3)

The student will eat and maintain a balanced diet as reported by parents/student and observed by school personnel. (N.D. 4, 6, 10)

The student will develop/maintain meaningful relationships with peer group as evidenced by participation in at least one extracurricular activity. (N.D. 5, 9)

The student will communicate with peers during periods of school absences. (N.D. 5)

The student will achieve and maintain developmental standardized norms as evidenced by: _____ (N.D. 2, 5)

## Nursing Intervention

Modify individualized healthcare plan (IHP) as student's health status and needs change. (N.D. 1)

Monitor and observe student for:

- signs and symptoms of infection (N.D. 1)
- respiratory status (N.D. 1, 6, 7)
- skin for breakdown, warmth, redness, and/or drainage (N.D. 8)

Instruct student on signs and symptoms of illness/infection and periodically review teaching as child's cognitive abilities change. (N.D. 1, 8, 10)

Establish guidelines with student for visiting health office. (N.D. 1, 2, 6, 9, 10)

Administer school treatment plan as prescribed by physician (such as): (N.D 1, 2, 6)
- Medications and other treatments needed during school hours
- Scheduling changes related to field trips, class parties, etc
- Perform chest physiotherapy and postural drainage as indicated and prescribed

Collaborate with school personnel to avoid placing student in classroom with any students with known communicable diseases. (N.D. 1)

Monitor school environment for communicable diseases. (N.D. 1)

Maintain communication with classroom teacher to identify infectious diseases in classroom. (N.D. 1)

Notify parent/guardian of student's exposure to communicable diseases. (N.D. 1)

Review universal precautions with student, parent, and teachers. (N.D. 1)

Instruct student on good hygiene practices. (N.D. 1)

Teach proper hand-washing technique; periodically review teaching as child's cognitive abilities change. (N.D. 1)

Notify teachers of student's potential adverse reaction to medication and/or treatment plan. (N.D. 1-3, 5, 9)

Facilitate classroom communication with student during absences. (N.D. 1, 2, 5, 9)

Evaluate cleaning practices and chemicals used by janitorial/custodial staff and make recommendations. (N.D. 1)

Obtain signed release of information from parent/guardian in order to facilitate communication and collaboration with student's healthcare providers regarding student's health status and needs in the school setting. (N.D. 1)

Obtain medical exemption for contraindicated immunizations. (N.D. 1)

Educate staff on specific immunodeficiency disease. (N.D. 1-3, 5, 10)

Recommend student wear Medic Alert bracelet (i.e., blood transfusions). (N.D. 1, 6)

Encourage parent/student to consult healthcare providers regarding vaccination boosters every 2 to 3 years. (N.D. 1, 6, 10)

Collaborate with student to develop plan for making up missed assignments. (N.D. 2, 9)

Arrange for/facilitate homebound instruction for extended periods of absences. (N.D. 2, 9)

Advocate for student to have additional textbooks and materials to utilize during absences. (N.D. 2)

Encourage medical management and scheduling of medical appointments outside school hours and during school breaks. (N.D. 2, 5, 10)

Collaborate with staff to facilitate regular assessments of academic achievement in all areas of development. (N.D. 3)

In cooperation with student, parents, and other school personnel, consider the need for 504 plan or more complete educational evaluation. (N.D. 1-3, 6, 7, 9)

Participate in development of student's IEP or 504 as indicated. (N.D. 1-3, 6, 7, 9)

Collaborate with staff to facilitate regular assessments of academic achievement in all areas of development. (N.D. 3)

Discuss healthy eating habits with student and parents. (N.D. 4, 10)

Consult cafeteria staff regarding any necessary modifications. (N.D. 4)

Encourage student participation in social activities; specify activity . (N.D. 5, 9)

Discuss strategies to minimize social isolation during school absences; specific strategies. (N.D. 5, 9)

Assist student in educating classmates regarding specific disease. (N.D. 5, 9, 10)

Assist parents in locating community resources for financial assistance, support groups, and respite care. (N.D. 6, 10)

Provide parent anticipatory guidance and information regarding illness. (N.D. 6, 10)

Notify local fire department and emergency medical services of student with special requirement/conditions: oxygen, latex allergy, high risk for infection. (N.D. 6)

Ascertain student's ability to participate in physical activity. (N.D. 7)

In cooperation with physical education staff, establish accommodations in physical education consistent with present health status and endurance. (N.D. 7)

Adjust school hours to achieve maximum participation in academic setting. (N.D. 7)

Rehearse techniques with student necessary to cope with chronic illness, social isolation, and future sequelae. (N.D. 9)

Coordinate referrals to relevant community resources and healthcare providers as indicated by present health status. (N.D. 10)

## Expected Student Outcomes

The student will:
- Be free of infection until next annual review of IHP. (N.D. 1)
- Promptly report any sign or symptom of an illness and/or infection of MediPort and/or gastric tube to the school nurse and parents. (N.D. 1, 6, 8, 10)
- Describe signs and symptoms of infection in a pretest and posttest during first week of school. (N.D. 1, 6, 8, 10)
- Limit visits to health office in accordance with established guidelines. (N.D. 1, 2, 6, 9, 10)
- Seek medical attention if exhibiting signs and symptoms of illness/infection as evidenced by documentation from healthcare provider. (N.D. 1, 6, 10)
- Practice hand washing 100% of the time before lunch/snacks and after recess and toileting. (N.D. 1, 2, 6, 8, 10)
- Demonstrate proper hand washing technique. (N.D. 1, 6)
- Practice good hygiene. (N.D. 1, 6, 8, 10)
- Identify strategies for making up missed assignments. (N.D. 2, 9)
- Exhibit a decline in number of reported absences quarterly as evidenced by school records. (N.D. 2)
- Schedule appointments outside school hours when possible. (N.D. 2)
- Demonstrate academic performance/achievement consistent with ability. (N.D. 2, 3)
- Not miss lunch or recess for treatment plan during the school year. (N.D. 2, 5)
- Eat a balanced diet and snacks as reported by student and observed by school staff. (N.D. 4, 6)
- Keep a log of dietary intake. (N.D. 4, 6)
- Maintain contact with classroom peers during absences through letters, telephone, or visits. (N.D. 5, 9)
- Regularly participate in at least one school-related extracurricular interest with peer group or developmentally appropriate social/recreational activity outside of school setting; specify activity. (N.D. 5, 9)
- Identify at least one meaningful relationship within peer group. (N.D. 5)
- Attend disease-specific or chronic illness camp during summer break. (N.D. 5, 9)

## Case Study

Jessica is an 11-year-old attending fourth grade. Jessica was diagnosed with IgG subclass 2 deficiency at age 7. During infancy, Jessica suffered chronic sinus infections, otitis media, upper respiratory tract infections, and pneumonia. She underwent an adenoidectomy, tonsillectomy, and placement of seven sets of pressure equalization tubes. At age 3, she was diagnosed with acute lymphocytic leukemia, requiring chemotherapy for 2 years. After ending chemotherapy treatment, she experienced an additional two bouts of pneumonia. Subsequent computed tomographic scans revealed packed sinuses, prompting four sinus surgeries, including drainage of sinuses and placing of windows.

Jessica's pneumonia infection at age 7 hospitalized her for 6 weeks, and she did not respond to any antibiotic treatment. At that time, an immunologist collaborated with her medical management and she received intravenous immunoglobulin (IVIG) while awaiting results of her immunologic studies. She recovered dramatically after receiving the IVIG therapy. Her antibody profile indicated an IgG subclass 2 serum level of zero. Her initial treatment plan began with IVIG therapy once a week for 1 year and every other week for 6 months. She has had two Broviac catheters, three peripherally inserted central catheter lines, and five MediPorts over the past 5 years.

She currently receives IVIG every 3 weeks and has a physical examination prior to infusion. Infusions last approximately 5 hours, and she is also given intravenous Benadryl and hydrocortisone. She usually spikes a fever after treatment and is tired and lethargic. Typically, she misses a day of school afterwards.

Jessica has a MediPort, which is replaced every 3 to 5 years or sooner if deemed medically necessary due to blockage or infection. She also takes Septra prophylactically. Once a year she has blood cell counts done. She has recently been diagnosed with Hashimoto's disease, and Synthroid has been prescribed.

Jessica's parents are concerned about the possible shortage of IVIG, because Jessica will need treatment for the rest of her life unless she undergoes a bone marrow transplant.

The nurse and other school personnel met with Jessica and her parents. On the basis of the discussion, the nurse developed this list of health concerns to be addressed in the school setting:
- Risk for infection needs to be minimized related to placement in a classroom, monitoring for communicable diseases, Jessica's self-care. Monitoring by the nurse will be ongoing.
- Need for absence from school for treatments and other absences or visits to the health room that impair doing assignments or benefiting from classroom activities.
- Socialization with peers is limited. Best friend since first grade recently moved away. Jessica's feelings of isolation due to risk of infection, absence from school, feeling she doesn't fit in. The family lives on an acreage, so there are no houses close by, limiting neighborhood friendships.

# Immunodeficiency Diseases

| Assessment Data | Nursing Diagnosis | Goals | Nursing Interventions | Expected Outcomes |
|---|---|---|---|---|
| IgG subclass 2 deficiency, risk of infection, monitor school environment and limit exposure to communicable disease.<br><br>Inconsistencies in Jessica's routine use of good hygiene practices, such as hand washing at school. | Risk for infection related to IgG subclass deficiency, inadequate acquired immunity, chronic disease, and increased environmental exposure to pathogens in school setting. | Jessica will recognize and verbalize primary signs and symptoms of an illness and infection of MediPort to promote early intervention and treatment.<br><br>Jessica will wash her hands before lunch/snack, and after recess and toileting. | Monitor and observe Jessica for signs of infection.<br><br>Review signs and symptoms of illness and infection of MediPort.<br><br>Teach hand-washing technique.<br><br>Review universal precautions with Jessica, student peers, and classroom staff.<br><br>Monitor school environment for communicable diseases.<br><br>Notify parents of any exposure to communicable diseases in school setting. | Jessica will describe four signs and symptoms of illness and infection of her MediPort in a pretest/posttest during the first week of school and periodically throughout the school year.<br><br>Jessica will promptly report any signs and symptoms of an illness and/or infection of MediPort to school nurse and parents.<br><br>Jessica will practice good hygiene (hand washing) 100% of the time before lunch/snacks and after recess and toileting. |
| Jessica misses at least 2 days of school every 3 weeks for medical treatment, sometimes misses other days or parts of days because she is tired and doesn't feel well. She doesn't routinely complete missed assignments, ultimately affecting her grades. She frequents the health room several times a week, complaining of vague symptoms. | Ineffective (student) role performance related to frequent absences, inadequate role socialization, health alterations, and physical illness. | Jessica will maintain academic progress consistent with developmental and cognitive abilities.<br><br>Jessica will utilize health office for substantiated signs and symptoms of illness and/or infection. | Collaborate with Jessica to develop a plan for making up missed assignments.<br><br>Encourage medical management and scheduling of medical appointments outside of school hours.<br><br>Establish guidelines with Jessica for visiting health office.<br><br>In cooperation with student, parents, and other school personnel, consider the need for 504 plan. | Jessica will demonstrate academic performance/achievement consistent with ability.<br><br>Jessica will identify strategies for making up missed assignments.<br><br>Jessica will limit visits to health office in accordance with established guidelines.<br><br>Jessica will exhibit a decline in number of reported absences quarterly as evidenced by school attendance record. |

| Assessment Data | Nursing Diagnosis | Goals | Nursing Interventions | Expected Outcomes |
|---|---|---|---|---|
| Excessive absences noted for routine medical care and frequent sequelae of her immunodeficiency disease.<br><br>Jessica's reluctance to develop friendships, feelings of dissimilarity, or feelings of rejection by others, best friend recently moved away, fear of socialization related to risk of infection. | Social isolation related to chronic illness and frequent absences. | Jessica will develop meaningful relationships with peer group.<br><br>Jessica will communicate with peers during periods of school absences. | Encourage Jessica's participation in social activities: role play, introduce her to preselected peer for an activity.<br><br>Discuss strategies to decrease social isolation from absences; play "what if," to help her prepare for situations.<br><br>Assist Jessica in educating classmates regarding her IgG subclass 2 deficiency, risk for infection, and need for medical treatments.<br><br>Jessica will regularly participate in her school's chess club. | Jessica will maintain contact with classmates by exchanging letters via traveling journal.<br><br>Jessica will cooperatively participate in educating classmates about her condition; active participation will depend on her comfort level. |

*Chapter Forty-seven: Immunodeficiency Diseases*

# References

Ballow, M. (2002). Primary immunodeficiency disorders: Antibody deficiency. *Journal of Allergy and Clinical Immunology, 109*(4), 581–591.

Bonilla, F. A., & Geha, R. S. (2003). Primary immunodeficiency diseases. *Journal of Allergy and Clinical Immunology, 111*(2, part 2), 571–581.

Buckley, R. H. (2004). Pulmonary complications of primary immunodeficiencies. *Paediatric Respiratory Reviews, 5*(1), S225–S233.

Champi, C. (2002). Primary immunodeficiency disorders in children: Prompt diagnosis can lead to lifesaving treatment. *Journal of Pediatric Health Care, 16*(1), 16–21.

Cunningham-Rundles, C. (2002). Hematological complications of primary immune deficiencies. *Blood Reviews, 16*(1), 61–64.

Geha, R. S., Leung, D. Y., Sampson, H. A., & Szefler, S. J. (2003). *Pediatric allergy: Principles and practice.* St. Louis, MO: Mosby.

Gennery, A. R., Spencer, D. A., & Cant, A. J. (2004). Immune deficiency and the lung. *Current Paediatrics, 14*(2), 115–121.

Glauser, M. P. (2000). *Management of infections in immunocompromised patients.* London: Saunders Harcourt.

Immune Deficiency Foundation. (2004). *About primary immunodeficiencies.* Retrieved February 6, 2004, from http://www.primaryimmune.org/pid/whatis_pid.htm

Lohr, J. T. (2004). *Immunodeficiency.* Retrieved March 22, 2004, from http://ehendrick.com/healthy

NANDA International (2003). *Nursing diagnoses: Definitions & classifications 2003-2004.* Philadelphia: Author.

National Institutes of Health, National Institute of Child Health & Human Development. (1999). *Primary immunodeficiency.* Retrieved February 6, 2004, from http://www.nich.nih.gov/publications/pubs/primaryimmuno-booklet.htm

National Primary Immunodeficiency Resource Center. (2004). *NPI interactive FAQ's.* Retrieved March 22, 2004, from http://npi.jmfworld.org/faq/index.cfm?section=faq&CFID=2813523&CFTOKEN=39718732

National Primary Immunodeficiency Resource Center. (2004). *10 warning signs of primary immunodeficiency.* Retrieved March 22, 2004, from http://npi.jmfworld.org/patienttopatient/index.cfm?section=patienttopatient&content=warningsigns

Patrick, C. C. (2001). *Clinical management of infections in immunocompromised infants and children.* Philadelphia: Lippincott Williams & Wilkins.

Peake, J., & Roberton, D. (2001). Advances in the diagnosis of primary immunodeficiency disorders in childhood. *Current Paediatrics, 11*(2), 149–157.

Reisman, R. E., & Slavin, R. G. (1999). *Expert guide to allergy & immunology.* Philadelphia: American College of Physicians.

Rosenzweig, S. D., & Holland, S. M. (2004). Phagocyte immunodeficiency and their infections. *Journal of Allergy & Clinical Immunology, 113*(4), 620–626.

Simonte, S. J., & Cunningham-Rundles, C. (2003). Update on primary immunodeficiency: defects of lymphocytes. *Clinical immunology, 109*(3), 249.

Spickett, G. (1999). *Oxford handbook of clinical immunology.* New York: Oxford University Press.

# Bibliography

Ashwill, J. W., Droske, S. C., & James, S. R. (2002). *Nursing care of children: Principles and practice* (2nd ed.). Philadelphia: Saunders.

Brown, R. T. (1999). *Cognitive aspects of chronic illness in children.* New York: Guilford Press.

Buckley, R. H. (2002). Primary cellular immunodeficiencies. *Journal of Allergy and Clinical Immunology, 109*(5), 747–757.

Wong, D. L., Hockenberry, M. J., Wilson, D., Winkelson, M. L., & Kline, N. E. (2003). The child with hematologic or immunologic dysfunction. *Nursing care of infants and children* (pp. 1570–1580). St. Louis, MO: Mosby.

# Resources

American Academy of Allergy, Asthma & Immunology
611 East Wells Street
Milwaukee, WI 53202
1-800-822-2762
www.aaaai.org

Children's Immune Deficiency Foundation
5666 La Jolla Boulevard
La Jolla, CA 92037
www.healingkids.net

Immune Deficiency Foundation
40 West Chesapeake Avenue
Suite 308
Towson, MD 21204
1-800-296-4433
www.primaryimmune.org

Jeffrey Modell Foundation
747 Third Avenue
New York, NY 10017
1-866-INFO-4-PI
www.info4pi.org

National Institute of Child Health and Human
Development
NIH Public Information and Communications Branch
31 Center Drive
Room 2A32
Bethesda, MD 20892-2425
301-496-5133
www.nichd.nih.gov

Pediatric Primary Immune Deficiency
www.pedpid.com

*Chapter Forty-eight*

# Infectious Mononucleosis

## Sally Zenter Schoessler

## Introduction

Infectious mononucleosis is a relatively common disease with fairly nonspecific symptoms. This viral infection impacts the school-aged child and adolescent not as a severe illness with dramatic complications, but as a somewhat long-term infection that creates a need to modify both the student's and family's lifestyle until the course of the illness is over.

Although infectious mononucleosis can occur in any child or adolescent, children in lower socioeconomic groups have a higher incidence of mononucleosis (Behrmann & Klingman, 2004). Adolescents from lower socioeconomic levels can have up to 60% to 80% of their peers test seropositive for the virus (Behrmann & Klingman, 2004).

Because of the prolonged nature of the symptoms of the infection, mononucleosis can be a difficult illness for the student and family to cope with. The school nurse is in a unique position to assist the student and parents in coordinating efforts to address the child's physical and academic needs during recuperation, as well the family's ability to cope with the child.

## Pathophysiology

The infection is caused by the Epstein-Barr virus, which is a DNA virus (KidsHealth, 2004). It is spread by salivary exchange, contact with contaminated objects, or, less commonly, by blood transfusions (NY Dept. of Health, 2003). The illness is mildly contagious, and because the most common mode of transmission is that of salivary exchange, "mono" is often referred to as "the kissing disease."

Infectious mononucleosis is often diagnosed well into the course of the illness on account of the nonspecific nature of the symptoms. After an incubation period of 4 to 6 weeks (NY Dept. of Health, 2003), an initial period of the infection with symptoms of malaise, fatigue, headache, nausea, and/or abdominal pain is often mistaken for influenza or many other viral infections. As the infection progresses, the symptoms become more pronounced. The student presents with severe pharyngitis (often with enlarged tonsils and a membranous exudate), high fever, lymphadenopathy (in the neck and throughout the body), and upper abdominal pain, indicative of an enlarged spleen.

Occasionally, the child will experience a rash that appears most prominently on the trunk of the body (Wong, Hockenbery-Eaton, Wilson, Winkelstein, & Kline, 2003).

The symptoms usually disappear in 1 to 3 weeks (the fatigue may persist for up to several months). It is not known how long the child remains infectious (Family Doctor.org, 2003).

Blood tests are important in the diagnosis of infectious mononucleosis because of the nonspecific nature of the symptoms. Blood work should be done to check for elevated lymphocytes. The other important test to be done is the "monospot," which screens for heterophil antibodies. However, these antibodies show a decline after the individual has reached the fourth week of illness, and the mono test will become negative as the infection resolves (Lab Tests Online, 2001).

Infants and young children tend to experience a milder case of infectious mononucleosis or remain asymptomatic. They often experience what appears to be a mild case of tonsillitis or an upper respiratory tract infection with an accompanying low-grade fever, because they tend to contract the virus by hand-to-hand contact or by an encounter with a contaminated object. Adolescents and college-aged students, who tend to spread the disease by intimate salivary contact, are disposed toward a more significant case of the disease because their exposure tends to be more intimate (Behrmann & Klingman, 2004).

Complications are not common but can include neurologic problems, pneumonitis, myocarditis, hemolytic anemia, thrombocytopenia, and rupturing of the spleen (Wong et al., 2003).

## Management

Treatment is very simple. The child should be limited to bed rest during the more acute phase of the illness, followed by the addition of activities based on the child's activity tolerance level. There is no need to isolate the student.

Because of the viral nature of infectious mononucleosis, treatment is mainly supportive and aimed at relieving the child's symptoms. Over-the-counter analgesics can be used to relieve the pain of headache and discomfort of malaise. Penicillin is prescribed to treat the accompanying tonsillitis if B strep is present. In severe cases, prednisone is used to lessen some of the symptoms of mononucleosis (Family Doctor.org, 2003).

Soft foods, with attention to caloric and nutritional content, should be encouraged if the child is experiencing pharyngitis (Wong et al., 2003).

If spleen enlargement is present, the child should be instructed to avoid activities that may result in an injury, such as contact sports.

## Individualized Healthcare Plan

### Assessment

*History*

- Symptoms that led to the diagnosis of infectious mononucleosis
- Diagnosis confirmed by a healthcare provider—Date: _____
- Friends or family members diagnosed with infectious mononucleosis in the past 6 weeks
- Treatment that has been effective
- Complications:
  – hepatitis
  – encephalitis
  – ruptured spleen
  – pneumonia
- Course of the illness

*Current Status and Management*

- Current management plan
- Fatigue and malaise affecting activities of daily living
- Accommodations that have been made
- Student's activity tolerance
- Symptoms the student is currently experiencing
  – fever
  – streptococcal infection
  – enlarged lymph nodes
  – enlarged spleen or tenderness
  – rash
  – fatigue
- Sleep/rest pattern
- Nutritional and hydration status

*Self-care*

- Ability to self-monitor tolerance of activity
- Ability to modify activities to accommodate limitations due to fatigue and malaise
- Ability to engage in activities of daily living

*Psychosocial Status*

- Maintenance of peer relationships throughout prolonged absence from school and other activities
- Feelings about alteration in student role are altered due to illness or related symptoms
- Student's and family's coping strategies for management of symptoms and treatment

*Academic Issues*

- School attendance pattern
- Total days the student has been absent this school year for any reason
- Accommodations needed to facilitate attendance in partial or full days of school
- Anticipated date the student may resume participation in physical education or sports activities
- Academic achievement/progress
- Plan for picking up/dropping off homework on days absent from school
- Plan is in place to make up missed work at a manageable pace
- Modification of assignments/requirements/grading
- Plan for teacher contact (e-mail, phone); arrange communication time

## Nursing Diagnoses (N.D.) (NANDA 2003)

**N.D. 1** Activity intolerance (NANDA 00092) related to:
- symptoms of malaise
- symptoms of fatigue

**N.D. 2** Ineffective role performance (student) (NANDA 00055) related to:
- prolonged absences from school
- fatigue

**N.D. 3** Risk for infection (NANDA 00004) related to increased susceptibility to other infections

**N.D. 4** Compromised individual/family coping (NANDA 00074) related to prolonged illness of self/child

**N.D. 5** Altered health maintenance (NANDA 00132) related to prolonged symptoms associated with infectious mononucleosis

**N.D. 6** Acute pain (NANDA 00132) related to infection (sore throat, headache, malaise, enlarged spleen)

**N.D. 7** Imbalanced nutrition, less than body requirements (NANDA 00002), related to symptoms making swallowing difficult and painful (sore throat, swollen glands)

**N.D. 8** Deficient knowledge (NANDA 00126) related to:
- infectious mononucleosis
- infection management

**N.D. 9** Fatigue (NANDA 00093) related to viral infection.

**N.D. 10** Risk for situational low self-esteem (NANDA 00193) related to:
- activity intolerance
- inability to attend to full school days with peers

## Goals

The student will increase school attendance pattern beginning with half days and moving to full days over 1 to 2 weeks. (N.D. 1, 2)

The student will rest as needed at school and home. (N.D. 1)

The student will contract with teachers to complete class work missed in small, manageable amounts. (N.D. 2)

The student will participate in extracurricular activities as activity tolerance allows. (N.D. 2)

The student will participate in physical education and sports activities as directed by his/her healthcare provider and as activity tolerance allows. (N.D. 2)

The student will increase his/her knowledge of signs and symptoms of infections to promote early intervention and treatment. (N.D. 3)

The student will verbalize concerns/issues experienced by family due to prolonged illness. (N.D. 4)

The student will assist in developing a management plan for symptoms. (N.D. 5, 6)

The student will participate in management of discomfort. (N.D. 6)

The student will maintain good fluid and nutritional intake. (N.D. 7)

The student will increase knowledge to adequately manage infection and recovery. (N.D. 8)

The student will maximize energy and deal appropriately with periods of fatigue at school. (N.D. 9)

The student will have intact self-esteem as he/she deals with absences and alteration in activity tolerance. (N.D. 10)

## Nursing Interventions

Monitor student's attendance on a daily basis. (N.D. 1)

Encourage and assist student to recognize signs of fatigue and rest appropriately. (N.D. 1, 6, 9)

Provide student with an opportunity to rest as needed. (N.D. 1, 6, 9)

Obtain written documentation from healthcare provider regarding physical activity and sports limitations. (N.D. 1)

Collaborate with physical education staff to modify physical education activities as needed. (N.D. 1, 9)

Arrange for use of elevator if needed. (N.D. 1, 9)

Meet with student, parent, and teachers to plan for school reentry. (N.D. 1)

Discuss appropriate activity level with student and parents to ensure consistent approach between home and school. (N.D. 1, 9)

Discuss appropriate time for student to rejoin extracurricular activities. (N.D. 1)

Notify the student's teachers and other staff working directly with the student (with parent permission) as to student's health status. (N.D. 2)

Collaborate with the student and staff in setting realistic goals and modifying assignments for missed days or partial days during student's recovery period. (N.D. 2)

Discuss activity limitations with athletic department coaches. Find alternate role for student (i.e., timekeeper or statistician) during recuperation so that he/she can remain a member of his/her team. (N.D. 2)

Observe for signs and symptoms of infections and/or potential complications. (N.D. 3)
- fever/chills
- sore throat
- rash
- swollen glands
- fatigue
- malaise
- abdominal pain

Discuss with student and parents which signs and symptoms should be reported to their healthcare provider. (N.D. 3)

Discuss strategies to manage symptoms of malaise and fatigue in the school setting. (N.D. 5, 9)

Instruct student in strategies to avoid spread of communicable diseases (hand washing, not sharing cups or utensils, etc.). (N.D. 3)

Monitor possible exposure to communicable diseases such as streptococcal sore throat, chickenpox, influenza, pneumonia, etc. (N.D. 3)

Family will identify and employ positive coping strategies in dealing with student's illness. (N.D. 4)

Discuss with parents and student how the family is coping with the student's illness. (N.D. 4, 6)

Allow parent an opportunity to express personal issues or concerns in regard to the student's illness (large block of time missed at work while caring for child, lack of patience with symptoms of fatigue, impact on siblings, etc.). (N.D. 4)

Allow student an opportunity to express feelings about being ill. (N.D. 4, 10)

Assist parents and school administration in arranging for homebound instruction if absenteeism becomes a long-term necessity. (N.D. 5)

Assist parents in accessing healthcare provider as needed for support of illness. (N.D. 5)

Discuss techniques for management of discomfort related to symptoms (lozenges for sore throat, medication as needed at school for headache, etc.). (N.D. 6)

Offer student small, frequent meals of soft, cool foods to provide for nutritional intake while experiencing throat pain. (N.D. 7)

Encourage good hydration and nutritional pattern for student. (N.D. 7)

Provide refrigeration of foods brought from home for lunch or snack. (N.D. 7)

Provide student with information related to disease process and recovery to facilitate self-care. (N.D. 8)

Permit water bottle in classes. (N.D. 7)

Provide time for snacks if needed. (N.D. 7)

Monitor self-care practices and provide education as needed. (N.D. 8)

Student will receive needed academic modifications or supports as needed to complete schoolwork during periods of fatigue. (N.D. 9)

Encourage half-day attendance at school to begin with, moving to full day over 1- to 2-week period when student is ready to return to school. (N.D. 9)

Allow the student time to verbalize feelings about the limitations that his/her illness places on activities of daily living. (N.D. 10)

Provide student with opportunities to relate with peers in relaxed atmosphere to facilitate maintenance of peer relationships during period of illness. (N.D. 10)

Encourage peers to write cards and letters to student during absences from school. (N.D. 10)

## Expected Student Outcomes

The student will:
- Attend school (half days for 1 week, then increasing to full days over the next 2 weeks). (N.D. 1, 2)
- Identify periods of fatigue and rest in health office as needed. (N.D. 1)
- Participate in physical education activities (as appropriate) with modifications made as needed. (N.D. 1, 2)
- Arrange to complete missed course work with his/her teachers. (N.D. 2)
- Collaborate with faculty and staff to modify school activities as needed. (N.D. 2)
- Identify symptoms of infection. (N.D. 3)
- Report any symptoms to the school nurse and parent. (N.D. 3)
- Practice good hygiene behaviors. (N.D. 3)
- Express feelings about having an illness and the impact it has on him/her and his/her family. (N.D. 4, 10)
- Identify positive coping strategies that can be used to cope with child's illness. (N.D. 4, 5)

- Demonstrate positive coping strategies in dealing with issues of illness. (N.D. 5)
- Identify and demonstrate strategies for managing discomfort from symptoms. (N.D. 6)
- Eat several small meals a day and drink appropriate fluids to support nutritional needs. (N.D. 7)
- Demonstrate understanding of infection management to facilitate recovery. (N.D. 8)
- Cope well with periods of fatigue at school. (N.D. 9)
- Have a positive self-esteem throughout the duration of the illness. (N.D. 10)

## Case Study

Ann Capen is a 16-year-old girl who was diagnosed with infectious mononucleosis 14 days ago. Prior to diagnosis, she had complained of nonspecific symptoms and stated she felt "lousy." She had a temperature of 102°F (oral) and presented with a sore throat, swollen glands, and upper abdominal discomfort. She was diagnosed with a case of strep throat and was placed on an antibiotic. Ann's symptoms were not relieved during treatment with the antibiotic, and she continued to experience a worsening sore throat and extreme fatigue. After 5 days of treatment, Ann's mother returned to her healthcare provider, Dr. Louise Clarke, and a monospot test was performed. The test came back positive, and Ann's mother called the school to inform the health office of the diagnosis of infectious mononucleosis. The sore throat continued, and Ann was not able to take solid food or rest due to throat swelling and pain. Her spleen became enlarged as a part of the viral process. Ann was placed on prednisone following the completion of the antibiotic, and experienced relief from the throat pain. She began to eat a soft diet and take in adequate fluids.

Ann has missed 10 full days of school and is now attending half days. She has a physician's note excusing her from physical education and sports until further evaluation. She has obtained homework assignments but is having trouble completing them and managing her current homework load. She states, "It's so hard to make it through the time that I'm at school, and then I'm so exhausted that all I can do when I get home is sleep." She reports feeling overwhelmed by the amount of course work that remains incomplete. She is also the starting goalie for the varsity soccer team and reports feeling that she is letting her team down by not being able to play. She commented, "I've always defined myself as a soccer player; now I feel lost not being with the team."

During the acute phase of Ann's mononucleosis, her mother felt the need to be at home with her, because she remained febrile for more than 7 days. Her mother has been feeling pressured by her employer to be at work as much as possible and feels frustrated at needing and wanting to care for Ann and also fulfilling her responsibilities at work. She feels additional stress because Ann's younger brother, aged 3, has regressed to the point that, although he had been "toilet trained" for 8 months, he is soiling his underwear instead of using the toilet. Ann's mother feels that this is directly related to the amount of attention that she has needed to direct toward Ann and her illness.

# Infectious Mononucleosis

| Assessment Data | Nursing Diagnosis | Goals | Nursing Interventions | Expected Outcomes |
|---|---|---|---|---|
| Ann is often tired and complains of "feeling sick." Ann should not be participating in contact sports. | Activity intolerance related to symptoms of malaise and fatigue. | Ann will increase school attendance pattern beginning with half days and moving to full days over 1 to 2 weeks. Ann will rest as needed at school and home. | Monitor Ann's attendance on a daily basis. Encourage and assist Ann to recognize signs of fatigue and rest appropriately. Provide Ann with an opportunity to rest as needed. Obtain written documentation from healthcare provider regarding physical activity and sports limitations. Collaborate with physical education staff to modify physical education activities as needed. Discuss appropriate activity level with Ann and parents to ensure consistent approach between home and school. | Ann will attend school (half days for 1 week, then increasing to full days over the next 2 weeks). Ann will identify periods of fatigue and rest in health office as needed. Ann will participate in physical education activities (as appropriate) with modifications made as needed. |
| Ann was absent for 10 full days of school and is now attending only half days. Ann is unable to compete although she is a member of the varsity soccer team. | Ineffective role performance (student) related to prolonged absences from school and fatigue. | Ann will contract with teachers to complete class work missed in small, manageable amounts. Ann will participate in physical education and sports activities as directed by her healthcare provider and as activity tolerance allows. | Notify Ann's teachers and other staff working directly with Ann (with parent permission) as to Ann's health status. Collaborate with Ann and staff in setting realistic goals and modifying assignments for missed days or partial days during Ann's recovery period. Discuss activity limitations with athletic department coaches. Find alternate role for Ann (e.g., timekeeper or statistician) during recuperation so that she can remain a member of her team. | Ann will arrange to complete missed course work with her teachers. Ann will participate in physical education activities (as appropriate) with modifications made as needed. Ann will collaborate with faculty and staff to modify school activities as needed. |

| Assessment Data | Nursing Diagnosis | Goals | Nursing Interventions | Expected Outcomes |
|---|---|---|---|---|
| Ann is at increased risk for infections. | Risk for infection related to increased susceptibility to other infections. | Ann will increase her knowledge of signs and symptoms of infections to promote early intervention and treatment. | Observe for signs and symptoms of infections and/or potential complications.<br><br>Instruct Ann in strategies to avoid spread of communicable diseases (hand washing, not sharing cups or utensils, etc.)<br><br>Monitor possible exposure to communicable diseases such as streptococcal sore throat, chickenpox, influenza, pneumonia, etc. | Ann will identify symptoms of infection.<br><br>Ann will report any symptoms to the school nurse and parent.<br><br>Ann will practice good hygiene behaviors. |
| Ann's mother has missed many days of work to care for Ann. Ann expresses frustration with the length of time that she has been ill.<br><br>Ann's younger brother is exhibiting regression due to attention given to sister's illness. | Compromised individual coping related to prolonged illness. | Ann will verbalize concerns/issues experienced by family due to prolonged illness. | Discuss with parents and Ann how the family is coping with Ann's illness.<br><br>Allow parent an opportunity to express personal issues or concerns in regard to Ann's illness (large block of time missed at work while caring for child, lack of patience with symptoms of fatigue, impact on siblings, etc.)<br><br>Allow Ann an opportunity to express feelings about being ill. | Ann will express feelings about having an illness and the impact it has on her and her family.<br><br>Ann will identify positive coping strategies that can be used to cope with this illness. |

## References

Behrmann, R. E., & Klingman, R. M. (2004) *Nelson essentials of pediatrics* (17th ed.). Philadelphia: Saunders.

KidsHealth. *Infectious mononucleosis* (2004) Retrieved June 6, 2004, from http://www.kidshealth.org/parent/infections/bacterial_viral/mononucleosis_p2.html

New York State Department of Health. (2003). *Infectious mononucleosis.* Retrieved June 6, 2004, from http://www.health.state.ny.us/nysdoh/communicable_diseases/en/infect.htm

Wong, D. L., Hockenbery-Eaton, M., Wilson, D., Winkelstein, M. L., & Kline, N. E. (2003). *Whaley and Wong's nursing care of infants and children* (6th ed.). St. Louis, MO: Mosby.

Family Doctor.org. (2003). *Mononucleosis.* Retrieved June 6, 2004, from http://familydoctor.org/handouts/077.html

Lab Tests Online. (2001) *Mono test.* Retrieved June 6, 2004, from http://www.labtestsonline.org/understanding/analytes/mono/test.html

North American Nursing Diagnosis Association. (2003). *NANDA nursing diagnoses: Definitions & classification 2003-2004.* Philadelphia: Author.

## Bibliography

Beers, M. (2003). *Merck manual of medical information* (2nd home ed.). Whitehouse Station, NY: Merck & Co.

Centers for Disease Control (2002). *Epstein-Barr virus and infectious mononucleosis.* Retrieved August 29, 2004, from http://www.cdc.gov/ncidod/diseases/ebv.htm

Chin, J. (2000). Control of communicable diseases manual (17th ed.). Washington, DC: American Public Health Association.

Litin, S. (2003). *Mayo Clinic family health book* (3rd ed.). New York: Harper.

Mayo Clinic.com. (2004). *Mononucleosis.* Retrieved August 29, 2004, from http://www.mayoclinic.com/invoke.cfm?id=DS00352

MedlinePlus. (2004) *Mononucleosis.* Retrieved August 29, 2004, from http://www.nlm.nih.gov/medlineplus/ency/article/000591.htm

Nettina, S. (2001). *Lippincott manual of nursing practice* (7th ed.). Philadelphia: Lippincott, Williams & Wilkins.

*Professional guide to signs and symptoms* (4th ed.). (2003). Philadelphia: Lippincott, Williams & Wilkins.

## Resources

KidsHealth.org
Parent's information: www.kidshealth.org/infections/bacterial_viral/mononucleosis.html
Teen information: www.kidshealth.org/teen/infections/common/mononucleosis.html

FamilyDoctor.org
www.familydoctor.org (click on Health Topics, then search on the term "mononucleosis")

MedicineNet.com http://www.medicinenet.com/Infectious_Mononucleosis/article.htm

Infectious Mononucleosis

## Chapter Forty-nine

# Inflammatory Bowel Disease

### MaryAnn Tapper Strawhacker

## Introduction

*Inflammatory bowel disease* (IBD) is a term used to describe the two most common types of gastrointestinal conditions: Crohn's disease and ulcerative colitis. Because both diseases share many of the same symptoms, as well as diagnostic tests and treatments, they are often referred to collectively as IBD. IBD is a chronic condition that persists throughout life with periods of exacerbation and remission. The peak age at onset is 15 to 35 years. IBD is more common among Caucasians, especially those of Jewish European descent, and those who have a family history of the disease. It occurs equally in males and females (Crohn's & Colitis Foundation of America [CCFA], 2003c, 2003d; Mayo Clinic, 2002).

## Pathophysiology

The exact causes of IBD are not known. Research has proven that the immune system within the intestinal wall does not function properly in IBD. Current research focuses on examining immune response, environmental effects, and heredity. The link between heredity and trigger mechanisms is unknown (CCFA, 2003c, 2003d; Mayo Clinic, 2002). It is now known, however, that IBD is a medical disorder and is not caused by food, stress, or anxiety. Stress can, however, exacerbate the illness (CCFA, 2003a, 2003c, 2003d; Mayo Clinic, 2002).

The student with IBD usually presents with one or more of the following symptoms: abdominal pain, diarrhea, fever, fatigue, blood in the stool, and weight loss (Kirschner & Black, 2002). Growth and sexual maturation may also be delayed. Although somewhat less common, IBD may also present with symptoms outside the gastrointestinal tract, such as arthritis, skin conditions, and eye, liver, and joint complications (CCFA, 2003b; Rayhorn & Rayhorn, 2002). Multiple tests are used to diagnosis IBD. After a complete medical history and physical examination, blood is drawn. The student with active IBD often shows anemia due to blood loss, a high white blood cell count, and an elevated erythrocyte sedimentation rate, due to inflammation. Additional blood tests may be done to check for the nutritional imbalances caused by poor absorption of nutrients. A stool sample is tested to detect bleeding and/or infection. Upper and lower gastrointestinal barium x-rays may be taken. The x-rays look for areas of inflammation that may be seen as a narrowing or swelling on the film. Upper and lower endoscopy may also be done to examine tissue and collect a biopsy sample to confirm diagnosis. Collective data helps the physician distinguish whether the student has Crohn's disease, ulcerative colitis, or another type of inflammatory bowel disorder (National Digestive Diseases Information Clearinghouse [NDDIC], 2003a, 2003b; Mayo Clinic, 2002).

## Crohn's Disease

Although many similarities exist with ulcerative colitis, Crohn's disease does have some unique features. Crohn's disease may be found in any part of the gastrointestinal tract but is most common in the lower part of the small intestine and beginning of the large intestine. All layers of the intestinal wall are involved. Diseased areas can be segmental with disease-free areas in between. Abdominal pain is most common in the right lower quadrant. Weight loss and malnutrition are related to anorexia as well as malabsorption. Anal and perianal skin tags, fissures, and fistulas are common. Intestinal obstruction is the most common complication (NDDIC, 2003a; CCFA, 2003c). Approximately 75% of the children with Crohn's disease require surgery at some point in the course of the disease. Emergency surgery is indicated for excessive bleeding, bowel perforation, intestinal obstruction, abscess formation, or toxic megacolon, a severe colonic dilatation and loss of muscle tone that may cause perforation. Elective surgery is performed when medical treatments fail to control symptoms or side effects of treatments are intolerable. Even though diseased segments have been removed, Crohn's disease may reoccur at the surgical site (CCFA, 2003e).

## Ulcerative Colitis

Ulcerative colitis involves only the innermost lining of the colon causing inflammation and ulceration. The area of disease is continuous with no areas of healthy bowel in between, as with Crohn's disease. Crampy urgent lower bowel pain is usually followed by frequent loose, often bloody stools. During an acute episode the student often experiences tenesmus, which is the persistent urge to empty the bowel caused by inflammation (CCFA, 2003d; NDDIC, 2003b).

Surgery may be required at some point in 25% to 40% of children with the disease. Emergency surgery may be necessary for colon perforation, sudden severe episodes, and toxic megacolon (CCFA, 2003f). Starting 10 years after diagnosis, those with ulcerative colitis are at an increased risk for colon cancer, which continues to grow with each decade of life (Sondheimer, 2001). Elective surgery may be performed when medical treatments fail to control symptoms, when side effects of treatments are intolerable, or to treat premalignant cell changes. The most common procedure is removal of the colon and rectum. This requires that either an illeostomy or a proctocolectomy be performed. A proctocolectomy attaches the remaining ileum, which has been fashioned into a reservoir, to the anus. This procedure is preferred because it preserves continence. After this procedure, students will average six soft bowel movements per day. Bowel obstruction due to adhesion scar tissue is a potential complication, as is pouchitis, a condition that occurs in 30% of recipients. Symptoms are variable and may include diarrhea, abdominal pain, fever, dehydration, and joint pain. Antibiotics are used to treat pouchitis. Unlike in Crohn's disease, surgical removal of the colon will cure ulcerative colitis (CFFA, 2003f).

## Management

Dietary modifications are not usually necessary with IBD. Overall, it is important to eat a well-balanced healthy diet. Because of the associated anorexia and weight loss, the student should be encouraged to select preferred foods high in nutritional value. Sometimes vitamin and mineral deficiencies occur and supplementation will be required. When the ileum is severely inflamed, producing a narrow lumen, some may report certain foods cause digestive symptoms. Avoidance is the best treatment until symptoms subside. For children with severe disease in need of calories, the physician may order oral liquid supplements during the day or continuous drip feedings at night through a feeding tube (CCFA, 2003a). Complete elemental diet through formula has been tried successfully in severe cases of IBD to induce remission, obtain catch-up growth, and allow for bowel rest (Rayhorn & Rayhorn, 2002). It is important to note that with active disease or malabsorption, use of oral contraception is not effective. Parenteral hormone routes or barrier methods are recommended. In teens with stable or quiescent IBD, oral contraception may be used cautiously (Neinstein, 2002).

Inflammatory bowel disease does not necessarily limit activity. During acute episodes, abdominal pain, fever, anemia, and diarrhea will affect tolerance and stamina. If the disease is under control, the student should be able to participate in sports. If strenuous sports cause fatigue or aggravate symptoms, such as abdominal or joint pain, some activity restrictions may be needed (Rayhorn & Rayhorn, 2002).

Research continues to produce new drugs and improved treatment options for children diagnosed with IBD. The most common drugs prescribed are aminosalicylates (5-ASA agents), which help control inflammation in the colon. These drugs may be administered either orally or rectally. Side effects may include headaches, gastrointestinal upset, and impaired folate absorption. Allergic reaction, leukopenia, and worsening of symptoms may also occur. A newer medication, mesalamine, is similar to sulfasalazine in its local anti-inflammatory action, but is better tolerated and has less potential to cause allergic reactions. Rare but serious complications of mesalamine treatment include nephritis and blood dyscrasias (CCFA, 2003g).

Corticosteroids are useful to control moderate to severe symptoms and during acute exacerbations. For disease limited to the distal colon, medication can be delivered in enemas or suppositories. When IBD involves the other areas of the gastrointestinal tract, oral or intravenous medication is necessary. Side effects of corticosteroids include weight gain, acne, facial hair, hypertension, mood swings, and increased risk of infection (NDDIC, 2003a, 2003b; CFFA, 2003c, 2003d, 2003g). Prednisone is the oral drug of choice, and when used in combination with a 5-ASA agent, it is often effective in achieving remission. Once therapeutic results are achieved, the dose of prednisone can be gradually tapered while monitoring the student's symptoms and laboratory values. If successful, the student will be maintained on a 5-ASA agent alone. If symptoms resume or intensify, the dose of prednisone may be continued or an immunomodulatory medication may be added

Immunomodulatory medications, including azathioprine, 6-mercaptopurine, methotrexate, and cyclosporine, are used to alter how immune cells participate in the inflammatory process. These medications are prescribed when routine drugs have been ineffective. Immunomodulatory medications have been shown in some individuals to reduce dependence on corticosteroids and to be useful in maintaining remissions. Complications may include pancreatitis, hepatitis, reduced white blood cell count, and lowered resistance to infection (NDDIC, 2003a, 2003b).

Because of side effects, noncompliance with treatment continues to be a concern. In a study of adults in remission from ulcerative colitis, nonadherence with medication had greater than a fivefold risk of symptom recurrence (Kane, Huo, Aikens, & Hanauer, 2003). Newer treatments aim to reduce symptoms with fewer side effects. Budesonide has been found effective for treating symptoms of mild to moderate Crohn's disease in children aged 8 to 18 years. Remission rates were similar to those with prednisone treatment; however, budesonide had significantly fewer cosmetic side effects, an important consideration for children and adolescents (Levine et al., 2003). Another promising area of research focuses on use of biologic agents, molecules made by living organisms (NDDIC, 2003b). Incidence of complementary and alternative medicine use is also on the rise among those with IBD (Hilsden, Verhoef, Best, & Pocobelli, 2003).

Students with IBD must cope with the psychosocial implications of both disease symptoms and medication side effects. Symptoms such as urgent bowel movements, abdominal pain, fatigue, and weight loss can affect the desire to participate in social interactions. Altered appearance due to corticosteroid use and delayed puberty can impact self-confidence (Pediatric Crohn's & Colitis Association, n.d.). A study conducted with adolescents looked at the effects of chronic digestive disease on social position. IBD was negatively associated with social position in the following areas: education, leisure activities, labor participation, financial situation, partnership, and sexuality (Calsbeek et al., 2002).

## Individualized Healthcare Plan

### Assessment
*History*
- Medical diagnosis and age at diagnosis
- Hospitalizations and surgical treatment related to IBD
- Student's disease course, include exacerbations and remissions
- Other health concerns
- Prognosis
- Date of last physical examination

*Current Status and Management*
- Areas of the bowel affected
- Healthcare providers involved in the student's care (primary care physicians, specialists, practitioners)
- Current medical treatment regimen (medications, dietary supplements, treatments)
- Student's tolerance of treatment, including medication side effects
- Supplies/medications/equipment needed during the school day
- Notification method preferred by family when additional supplies are needed at school
- Student's nutritional status, including need for supplements/snacks
- Recommended fluid requirements
- Need for dietary restrictions
- Experience with extraintestinal symptoms
- Experience with IBD-associated discomfort
- Use of over-the-counter medications or herbal remedies
- Change in the student's activity level or tolerance noticed by family
- Activity restrictions or limitations

*Self-care*
- Medications/treatments/procedures student administers independently at home and with supervision
- Self-care skills currently taught and reinforced at home
- Incidence of soiling and need for assistance with personal hygiene during acute exacerbations
- Experiences with food intolerances and self-monitoring of offending foods
- Ability to self-regulate activity level when fatigued and need for adult supervision

*Psychosocial Status*
- Family and student perception of overall health status
- Student and family coping strategies utilized
- Experience with disruption of usual activities
- Degree of disclosure of IBD diagnosis with peers and peer response
- Concerns expressed either by parents or student regarding peer reactions
- Degree of participation in extracurricular activities with peers
- Problems with teasing at school or in the community
- Family members' perception of changes in dress or behavior since IBD diagnosis
- Availability of social support within extended family or community
- Use of community resources and need for additional resources

*Academic Issues*
- School attendance record, including recent or past pattern of absences and reason for absences
- Note academic history and any observable trends since diagnosis
- Modifications, adaptations, and accommodations made during the school day to date

- Need for additional modifications during the school day, including recess, physical education, and extracurricular activities
- Need for unlimited or private bathroom privileges, snack breaks, rest periods, or modified class schedule
- Existence of a 504 plan or an individualized educational program to address health and educational accommodations, modifications, and adaptations
- School staff training needs
- Provisions for pain management and symptom management at school

## Nursing Diagnoses (N.D.) (NANDA 2003)

**N.D. 1** (Risk for) diarrhea (NANDA 00013)
**N.D. 2** Risk for acute pain (NANDA 0132) related to exacerbation of IBD symptoms
**N.D. 3** (Risk for) imbalanced nutrition: less than body requirements (NANDA 00002) related to:
- inadequate intake
- impaired intestinal absorption

**N.D. 4** Activity intolerance (NANDA 00092) related to:
- joint pain
- fatigue
- anemia
- fever
- medication side effects

**N.D. 5** Disturbed body image (NANDA 00118) related to:
- exacerbation of IBD symptoms
- weight loss
- medication side effects
- surgical interventions
- pain
- fatigue

**N.D. 6** Situational low self-esteem (NANDA 00120) related to:
- exacerbation of IBD symptoms
- fatigue
- impaired body image
- altered role performance

**N.D. 7** Ineffective role performance (NANDA 00055) related to:
- absence from school/class due to exacerbation of symptoms
- fatigue
- inadequate coping
- depressed mood
- impaired body image

**N.D. 8** Deficient knowledge (NANDA 0126) related to:
- recent diagnosis of IBD
- complicated management of IBD
- recent change in IBD therapeutic regimen

**N.D. 9** (Risk for) noncompliance with prescribed medications (NANDA 00079) related to:
- denial of need for medication
- recent change in therapeutic regimen
- perceived ineffectiveness of medication
- undesirable side effects of medication
- knowledge deficit

## Goals

The student will attend school/class and participate with modifications made as needed. (N.D. 1, 2, 4, 7)
The student will experience an increased level of comfort, allowing active participation in school activities. (N.D. 2)
The student will perform self-care skills with assistance as needed. (N.D. 1, 6–9)
The student will show improved nutritional status. (N.D. 3, 5)
The student will demonstrate improved physical activity tolerance. (N.D. 4)
The student will progress toward adapting to living with a chronic illness. (N.D. 4–9)

The student will demonstrate improved self-esteem. (N.D. 5–7)

The student will be involved in planning and implementation of his/her IBD treatment plan at school. (N.D. 6–9)

The student will demonstrate increased knowledge of IBD. (N.D. 8, 9)

The student will comply with prescribed IBD treatment plan. (N.D. 8, 9)

## Nursing Interventions

Obtain a signed release of information to obtain pertinent medical records and to share information with the medical provider. (N.D. 1–9)

Obtain parental and student permission to share relevant medical information with school personnel. (N.D. 1–9)

Provide IBD educational materials to designated school personnel and allow time for questions. (N.D. 1–9)

Provide emotional support to the student and family. (N.D. 1–9)

- Provide support and encouragement to student.
- Develop trusting, open communication with the student and encourage verbalization of feelings of anger, frustration, depression, concerns, and fears.
- Establish a preferred mode of scheduled communication with parents/guardians to facilitate coordination of medical treatment and to monitor the student's social and emotional adjustment.
- Refer family to counseling resources as needed to facilitate student's adaptation to living with a chronic illness.

Obtain medical orders for IBD management in the school setting. (N.D. 1-4)

In collaboration with medical provider, determine when 911 will be called and to which medical facility the student should be transported. (N.D. 1, 2)

Instruct staff when to notify the school nurse for provision of additional assessment and possible emergency intervention. (N.D. 1, 2)

Refer to building student assistance team or 504 coordinator, if not already involved. (N.D. 1-9)

Outline for school staff possible student medical accommodations, such as: (N.D. 1–7)

- Unrestricted restroom pass
- Access to private restroom with a vent.
- Modified physical education class for joint pain and fatigue
- Rest periods scheduled into the school day
- Need for nutritious snacks during the school day
- Access to private shower time after physical education class or team sports if student has body image concerns
- Modified work load if health deteriorates, or if hospitalization or surgery is required
- Shortened school day during severe acute exacerbations
- Assign seating next to classroom exit

Provide pain management. (N.D. 2, 4, 6, 7, 9)

- Observe student for signs of discomfort.
- Encourage student to monitor level of discomfort and intervene as needed.
- Determine impact of discomfort on student's school performance.
- In association with the student, family, and medical team, evaluate effectiveness of present comfort measures.
- Modify environmental factors that may contribute to the student's discomfort.
- In association with the family, assemble a list of comfort measures and help the student to select appropriate choices based on level of discomfort.

Provide medication management. (N.D. 1, 2, 6–9)

- Facilitate self-medication administration when appropriate and in accordance with district policy.
- Monitor student's medication/treatment compliance and assist in removing existing barriers. (N.D. 9)
- Identify the type and quantity of over-the-counter analgesics used.
- Instruct student/family to seek information from pharmacist when adding new medications.
- Review with the student/family appropriate use of over-the-counter as well as prescription medications.
- Discuss use of herbals and alternative therapies that may interact with over-the-counter or prescription medication.
- Review medication actions and side effects.
- Instruct student to report any unusual side effects to the school nurse.
- Instruct student when to consult physician regarding medication management.

Provide nutritional counseling. (N.D. 3–5)

- Determine student's knowledge of nutritional guidelines in making healthy food choices.
- Determine quantity and quality of food intake and general eating habits.
- Discuss nutritional requirements.
- Discuss food intolerances and suggest nutritional alternatives.

- Discuss student's food preferences.
- Discuss ways to modify and/or supplement school lunches to provide adequate intake.
- Discuss ways to increase fluid intake during the school day.

Promote nutritional therapy in collaboration with the student's medical team: (N.D. 3, 9)
- Monitor food and fluid intake per physician request.
- Facilitate consumption of nutritious snacks.
- Ensure availability of well-tolerated foods in the school lunch program.
- Encourage family to send nutritious snacks.

Assist student with energy management. (N.D. 4–7)
- Determine causes of fatigue.
- Encourage rest alternating with periods of activity.
- Educate teacher(s) as to the need to monitor student's activity tolerance and to make adjustments in scheduling as needed.

Provide opportunities for student/family/nurse to educate classmates about IBD. (N.D. 4–9)

Promote body image enhancement (N.D. 5–7)
- Encourage discussion of body changes since diagnosis of IBD.
- Monitor self-critical statements made by the student.
- Determine student's perceptions of body image alteration and compare with reality.
- Discuss ways of minimizing outward signs of illness through clothing styles or cosmetics.
- Identify coping strategies used by the student.
- Monitor student for signs of social isolation.
- Assist student to separate physical appearance from feelings of self-worth.
- Identify support groups available locally to the student.

Promote self-esteem enhancement. (N.D. 5–7)
- Facilitate an environment that encourages positive self-esteem.
- Provide experiences that increase the student's autonomy as appropriate for developmental age.
- Assist student to examine negative self-perceptions and reasons for self-criticism.
- Assist student to problem-solve social situations made difficult because of IBD.
- Encourage increased level of self-care and responsibility.
- Encourage student to discuss impact of peer group on feelings of self-worth.
- Assist student to identify strengths and reinforce examples of those strengths when observed.
- Convey confidence in the student's abilities.
- Monitor levels of self-esteem over the course of the semester.

Promote knowledge enhancement. (N.D. 8)
- Obtain release of information to determine content of education while hospitalized and during follow-up visits.
- Assess student's knowledge of IBD.
- Determine the readiness and ability of the student to learn the necessary skills to manage IBD.
- Begin instruction after the student shows readiness to learn the necessary skills.
- Provide an environment that is conducive to learning.
- Encourage student's active participation in learning.
- Review the known pathophysiologic processes with the student at a developmentally appropriate level.
- Review prescribed treatment strategies.
- Reinforce IBD education completed while hospitalized and during clinic visits.
- Provide current IBD resources as needed.
- Reinforce teaching with the student and her primary caregiver on an ongoing basis.

Monitor student's medication/treatment compliance and assist in removing existing barriers.

## Expected Student Outcomes

The student will:
- Participate in classroom, physical education, and selected extracurricular activities with accommodations as needed. (N.D. 1–7)
- Have access to collaboratively planned IBD treatment. (N.D. 1–9)
- Report an improved level of comfort after interventions. (N.D. 2)
- Progress toward self-monitoring of comfort interventions. (N.D. 2, 6)
- Make healthy selections from the school lunch menu. (N.D. 3)
- Maintain current weight without further loss. (N.D. 3)
- Progress toward self-monitoring of activity level and seek assistance as needed from school staff. (N.D. 4, 6)
- Show evidence of improved personal appearance. (N.D. 5, 6)
- Demonstrate a reduction in self-critical comments. (N.D. 5–7)
- Obtain counseling as needed. (N.D. 5–7)
- Identify and utilize existing community IBD resources as needed. (N.D. 6–8)
- Attend his/her school health planning meetings. (N.D. 6–9)
- Self-administer medications in compliance with prescribed orders and district policy/procedures. (N.D. 6–9)
- Actively participate in making IBD management/treatment choices. (N.D. 6–9)
- Demonstrate an understanding of the IBD disease process and begin to use that knowledge to make health management decisions. (N.D. 8)
- Comply with the medically prescribed treatment. (N.D. 9)

## Case Study

Nicole Birch is a 14-year-old female recently diagnosed with IBD. She sought treatment after experiencing difficulties with low-grade fever, abdominal pain, ankle swelling, joint pain, weight loss, and anemia. She had also experienced several bouts of diarrhea that she had blamed on the "flu" and had missed several school days due to abdominal pain. Nicole has no previous family history of IBD. After the lower gastrointestinal series showed two areas of acute inflammation, one in the proximal duodenum and one in the lower colon, the diagnosis of Crohn's disease was made. The gastroenterologist placed Nicole on oral prednisone (bid) and Pentasa (tid) to help control her symptoms. She was told by her physician to limit strenuous physical activity until her ankle swelling resolved. The physician also suspected that Nicole might have a milk intolerance. She is to limit her milk intake to 1 cup per day. The family is very supportive of Nicole but is unsure of what accommodations are needed in the school setting. Nicole has no other chronic health conditions and takes no other medications except calcium and iron supplements. Tylenol is ordered for menstrual discomfort.

# Inflammatory Bowel Disease

| Assessment Data | Nursing Diagnosis | Goals | Nursing Interventions | Expected Outcomes |
|---|---|---|---|---|
| • Parents report Nicole has had several days this summer spent in bed due to abdominal cramping and leg pain.<br><br>• Visible edema of the lower extremities with +2 pitting noted on physical assessment<br><br>• Nicole expressed concern over walking and climbing stairs in the old high school building.<br><br>• Tylenol and elevation used to relieve leg discomfort at home | Acute pain related to exacerbation of IBD symptoms. | Nicole will perform self-care skills with assistance as needed. | 1. Obtain medical orders for IBD medication management at school.<br>2. Facilitate self-medication administration in accordance with district policy.<br>3. Monitor Nicole's medication/treatment compliance and assist in removing existing barriers.<br>4. Identify the type and quantity of over-the-counter analgesics used.<br>5. Instruct Nicole/family to seek information from pharmacist when adding new medications.<br>6. Review with the Nicole/family appropriate use of over-the-counter as well as prescription medications.<br>7. Discuss use of herbals and alternative therapies that may interact with over-the-counter or prescription medication.<br>8. Review medication actions and side effects.<br>9. Instruct Nicole to report any unusual side effects to the school nurse.<br>10. Instruct Nicole when to consult physician regarding medication management. | Nicole will self-administer medications in compliance with prescribed orders and district policy/procedures. |

| Assessment Data | Nursing Diagnosis | Goals | Nursing Interventions | Expected Outcomes |
|---|---|---|---|---|
| | | Nicole will experience an increased level of comfort, allowing active participation in school activities. | 1. Observe Nicole for signs of discomfort.<br>2. Encourage Nicole to monitor level of discomfort and intervene as needed.<br>3. Determine impact of discomfort on Nicole's school performance.<br>4. In association with Nicole, her family, and medical team, evaluate effectiveness of present comfort measures.<br>5. Modify environmental factors that may contribute to Nicole's discomfort.<br>6. In association with the family, assemble a list of comfort measures and help Nicole to select appropriate choices based on level of discomfort. | Nicole will actively participate in making IBD management/treatment choices. |
| • Diagnosed with IBD at start of school year<br><br>• History of low-grade fever, abdominal pain, ankle swelling, joint pain, and anemia<br><br>• Four episodes of loose stools lasting 2 to 3 weeks<br><br>• Lower GI series showed two areas of inflammation; diagnosed with Crohn's end of first quarter | Knowledge deficit related to recent diagnosis of IBD. | Nicole will demonstrate an increased knowledge of IBD. | 1. Obtain release of information to determine content of education while hospitalized and during follow-up visits.<br>2. Assess Nicole's knowledge of IBD.<br>3. Determine the readiness and ability of Nicole to learn the necessary skills to manage her IBD.<br>4. Begin instruction after Nicole shows readiness to learn the necessary skills. | Nicole will demonstrate an understanding of the IBD disease process and begin to use that knowledge to make health management decisions. |

| Assessment Data | Nursing Diagnosis | Goals | Nursing Interventions | Expected Outcomes |
|---|---|---|---|---|
| • No other chronic illnesses or conditions<br><br>• No hospitalizations since birth<br><br>• Pentasa and Tylenol are the only medications to be given at school; takes her medications independently at home, including oral prednisone.<br><br>• Rectal fissures may need topical medication during the school day which she self-administers<br><br>• Parents request high school staff be trained in IBD symptoms and necessary accommodations | | | 5. Provide an environment that is conducive to learning.<br>6. Encourage Nicole's active participation in learning.<br>7. Review the known pathophysiologic processes with Nicole at a developmentally appropriate level.<br>8. Review prescribed treatment strategies.<br>9. Reinforce IBD education completed while hospitalized.<br>10. Provide current IBD resources as needed.<br>11. Reinforce teaching with Nicole and her primary caregiver on an ongoing basis. | |
| • Weight loss of 15 lbs in last 3 months. Current weight 100 lbs, height 5 feet 4 inches<br><br>• Milk intolerance diagnosed<br><br>• Family will review school menu and send sack lunch as needed.<br><br>• Parents request that dietary department assist them to make menu selections | Imbalanced nutrition: less than body requirements related to inadequate intake | Nicole will show improved nutritional status. | 1. Determine quantity and quality of food intake and general eating habits.<br>2. Review fluid requirements.<br>3. Monitor food and fluid intake per physician request.<br>4. Discuss nutritional requirements.<br>5. Discuss Nicole's knowledge of the food pyramid in making healthy food choices.<br>6. Facilitate consumption of nutritious snacks. | Nicole will make healthy selections from the school lunch menu. |

| Assessment Data | Nursing Diagnosis | Goals | Nursing Interventions | Expected Outcomes |
|---|---|---|---|---|
| • Calcium and iron supplements prescribed for home use<br><br>• Has complained of decreased energy and stamina<br><br>• Reports "not feeling hungry" and skipping meals<br><br>• Last hemoglobin was 8.4 g/dl<br><br>• Suggested fluid intake of 64 oz per day | | | 7. Ensure availability of well-tolerated foods in the school lunch program.<br>8. Provide lunch menu to parents to assist with planning lunches.<br>9. Discuss food intolerances and suggest alternatives.<br>10. Discuss Nicole's food preferences and suggest nutritious combinations.<br>11. Discuss ways to modify and/or supplement school lunches to provide adequate intake.<br>12. Refer for nutritional consult as needed.<br>13. Contact the physician quarterly and as needed for follow-up/coordination of prescribed nutritional treatment regimen. | |
| • Has dropped out of the swim team because she "can't keep up" with the practices<br><br>• Has complained of decreased energy and stamina.<br><br>• Parents report Nicole sleeps an average of 12 to 14 hours per night yet still complains of being tired.<br><br>• Nicole's grade point for last semester was 3.00, down from 3.25. | Activity intolerance related to fatigue. | Nicole will demonstrate improved physical activity tolerance. | 1. Determine causes of fatigue during the school day and at home.<br>2. Encourage rest to alternate with periods of activity while at school.<br>3. Educate teacher(s) as to the need to monitor Nicole's activity tolerance and make adjustments in scheduling as needed.<br>4. Refer to building student assistance team.<br>5. Outline for staff any required medical accommodations. | Nicole will progress toward self-monitoring of activity level and seek assistance as needed from school staff. |

| Assessment Data | Nursing Diagnosis | Goals | Nursing Interventions | Expected Outcomes |
|---|---|---|---|---|
| • Nicole missed 40 days last school year. She missed 8 days the previous year.<br><br>• Parents report Nicole is wearing nothing but baggy clothes, has stopped wearing make-up, and seems to care less about her physical appearance. Also report she refuses to wear a swimsuit.<br><br>• Ankle swelling continues to be a problem along with pain, per Nicole.<br><br>• Teachers report observing older teens tease Nicole about being "skinny" and looking sick.<br><br>• Refuses to discuss Crohn's disease with her peers.<br><br>• Refuses to go to the school counselor. Parents are willing to pay for a private therapist. | Situational low self-esteem related to impaired body image. | Nicole will demonstrate improved self-esteem. | 1. Facilitate an environment that encourages self-esteem.<br>2. Assist Nicole to examine negative self-perceptions and reasons for self-criticism.<br>3. Encourage discussion of body changes since diagnosis of IBD.<br>4. Assist Nicole to problem-solve social situations made difficult because of IBD.<br>5. Encourage increased level of self-care and responsibility.<br>6. Encourage Nicole to discuss impact of peer group on feelings of self-worth.<br>7. Assist Nicole to identify strengths and reinforce examples of those strengths when observed.<br>8. Convey confidence in Nicole's abilities and strengths<br>9. Provide experiences that increase Nicole's autonomy as appropriate for her developmental age.<br>10. Identify support groups available locally. | Nicole will show evidence of improved personal appearance.<br><br>Nicole will demonstrate a reduction in self-critical comments. |

| Assessment Data | Nursing Diagnosis | Goals | Nursing Interventions | Expected Outcomes |
|---|---|---|---|---|
| | | | 11. Refer family to counseling resources as needed to facilitate student's adaptation to living with a chronic illness.<br>12. Monitor levels of self-esteem over the course of the semester. | |

# References

Calsbeek, H., Rijken, M., Bekkers, M. J., Kerssens, J. J., Dekker, J., & van Berge Henegouwen, G. P. (2002). Social position of adolescents with chronic digestive disorders. *European Journal of Gastroenterology and Hepatology* *14*(5), 543–549.

Crohn's & Colitis Foundation of America. (2003a). *Diet and nutrition.* Retrieved September 29, 2003, from http://www.ccfa.org/medinfo/medinfo/diet.html

Crohn's & Colitis Foundation of America. (2003b). *Extraintestinal complications of IBD.* Retrieved September 12, 2003, from http://www.ccfa.org/medinfo/medinfo/complications.html

Crohn's & Colitis Foundation of America. (2003c). *Introduction to Crohn's disease.* Retrieved September 29, 2003, from http://www.ccfa.org/medinfo/medinfo/aboutcd.html

Crohn's & Colitis Foundation of America. (2003d). *Introduction to ulcerative colitis.* Retrieved September 29, 2003, from http://www.ccfa.org/medinfo/medinfo/aboutuc.html

Crohn's & Colitis Foundation of America. (2003e). *Surgery for Crohn's disease.* Retrieved September 12, 2003, from http://www.ccfa.org/medinfo/medinfo/surgerycd.html

Crohn's & Colitis Foundation of America. (2003f). *Surgery for ulcerative colitis.* Retrieved September 12, 2003, from http://www.ccfa.org/medinfo/medinfo/surgeryuc.html

Crohn's & Colitis Foundation of America. (2003g). *Treating children and adolescents.* Retrieved September 12, 2003, from http://www.ccfa.org/medinfo/medinfo/kidsmeds.html

Hilsden, R. J., Verhoef, M. J., Best, A., & Pocobelli, G. (2003). Complementary and alternative medicine use by Canadian patients with inflammatory bowel disease: Results from a national survey. *The American Journal of Gastroenterology* *98*(7), 1563–1568.

Kane, S., Huo, D., Aikens, J., & Hanauer, S. (2003). Medication nonadherence and the outcomes of patients with quiescent ulcerative colitis. *The American Journal of Medicine* *114*(1), 39–43.

Kirschner, B. S., & Black, D. D. (2002). The gastrointestinal tract. In R. E. Behrman & R. M. Kliegman (Eds.), *Nelson essentials of pediatrics* (4th ed., pp. 497–499). Philadelphia: Saunders.

Levine A., Weizman, Z., Broide, E., Shamir, R., Shaoul, R., & Pacht, A., et al. (2003). A comparison of budesonide and prednisone for the treatment of active pediatric Crohn disease. *Journal of Pediatric Gastroenterology and Nutrition* *36*, 248–252.

Mayo Clinic. (2002). *Inflammatory bowel disease.* Retrieved September 12, 2003, from http://www.Mayoclinic.com/invoke.cfm?objected=908EOEEE-98DF-4A18-8E426B22F7133

National Digestive Diseases Information Clearinghouse. (2003a). *Crohn's disease.* Publication NIH 03-3410. Retrieved September 12, 2003, from http://digestive.niddk.nih.gov/ddiseases/ pubs/chrohns/index.htm

National Digestive Diseases Information Clearinghouse. (2003b). *Ulcerative colitis.* Publication NIH 03-1597. Retrieved September 24, 2003, from http://digestive.niddk.nih.gov/ddiseases/pubs/colitis/index.htm

Neinstein, L. S. (2002). Contraception. In L. S. Neinstein (Ed.), *Adolescent health care: A practical guide.* Philadelphia: Lippincott Williams & Wilkins.

NANDA International. (2003). *Nursing diagnosis: Definitions & classification 2003-2004.* Philadelphia: Author.

Pediatric Crohn's & Colitis Association. (n.d.). *The ABC's of pediatric IBD.* Retrieved September 12, 2003, from http://pcca.hypermart.net/abcs.html

Rayhorn, N. & Rayhorn, D. (2002). Inflammatory bowel disease: Symptoms in the bowel and beyond. *The Nurse Practitioner* *27*(11), 13–27.

Sondheimer, J. M. (2001). Gastrointestinal tract. In W. W. Hay, A. R. Hayward, M J. Levin, & J. M. Sondheimer (Eds.), *Current pediatric diagnosis & treatment* (15th ed., pp. 565–568). New York: McGraw-Hill.

# Bibliography

Beers, M. H., & Berkow, R. (Eds.). (1999). *The Merck Manual* (17th ed., pp. 302–315). Whitehouse Station, NJ: Merck Research Laboratories.

Corkins, M. R., Gohil, A. D., & Fitzgerald, J. F. (2003). The insulin-like growth factor axis in children with inflammatory bowel disease. *Journal of Pediatric Gastroenterology and Nutrition* *36*, 228–224.

Kundhal, P. S., Critch, J. N., Zachos, M., Otley, A. R., Stephens, D., & Griffiths, A. M. (2003). Pediatric Crohn disease activity index: Responsive to short-term change. *Journal of Pediatric Gastroenterology and Nutrition* *36*, 83–89.

McCloskey, J. C., & Bulechek, G. M. (Eds.).(2000*). Nursing interventions classification (NIC)* (3rd ed.). St. Louis, MO: Mosby Yearbook.

Morpurgo, E., Petras, R., Kimberling, J., Ziegler, C., & Galandiuk, L. (2002). Characterization and clinical behavior of Crohn's disease initially presenting predominantly as colitis. *Diseases of the Colon and Rectum 46*, 918–924.

Pediatric Crohn's & Colitis Association. (n.d.). *Growth problems associated with GI disorders.* Retrieved September 12, 2003, from http://pcca.hypermart.net/growth.html

Ramaswamy, K., Jacobson, K., Jevon, G., & Israel, D. (2003). Esophageal Crohn disease in children: A clinical spectrum. *Journal of Pediatric Gastroenterology and Nutrition 36*, 454–458.

## Resources

Crohn's & Colitis Foundation of America Inc.
386 Park Avenue South
17th Floor
New York, NY 10016-8804
212-685-3440
1-800-932-2423
212-779-4098 (fax)
info@ccfa.org
http://www.ccfa.org (PDF brochures for teachers, parents, and students)

National Digestive Diseases Information Clearinghouse
2 Information Way
Bethesda, MD 20892-3570
nddic@info.niddk.nih.gov
http://digestive.niddk.nih.gov/

Pediatric Crohn's & Colitis Association Inc.
PO Box 188
Newton, MA 02468
617-489-5854
http://www.pcca.hypermart.net

Reach Out for Youth With Ileitis and Colitis Inc.
84 Northgate Circle
Melville, NY 11747
631-293-3102
631-293-3103 (fax)
reachoutforyouth@reachoutforyouth.org
http://www.reachoutforyouth.org

United Ostomy Association Inc.
19772 MacArthur Boulevard
Suite 200
Irvine, CA 92612-2405
949-660-8624
1-800-826-0826
949-660-9262 (fax)
info@uoa.org
http://www.uoa.org

## Chapter Fifty

# Latex Allergy

Constance M. Cotter and Mariann Smith

## Introduction

The school environment can be a source of allergens to some students. Allergic reactions to food, insect stings, chalk dust, and more are well known in schools. An allergy less commonly known, but potentially life-threatening in the school environment, is the allergy to latex (Cotter et al., 1996). Allergic reactions to latex can range from annoying to life-threatening. The school environment has many sources of latex; therefore, it is important for school personnel to be aware of procedures for identification and treatment of potentially serious allergic reactions to latex products.

Students with spina bifida and those who have undergone multiple surgical procedures, especially from infancy, are at risk for latex allergy. The Spina Bifida Association of America reports 18% to 73% of children and adolescents with spina bifida are sensitive to latex. However, any student with a history of respiratory symptoms or skin problems when in contact with latex/rubber products (e.g., balloons, condoms, gloves) should be considered at risk for latex allergy. Other students who should be considered at risk are those who have had conditions associated with continuous or intermittent bowel/bladder management programs, students who are allergic to bananas, avocados, kiwis, and chestnuts, and students with a history of other allergies (Evangelisto, 1997). Students with a known latex allergy should wear a medical alert bracelet or necklace indicating an allergy to latex.

The student's school environment should be examined for latex products. Examples of sources of latex in the school are erasers, paints, glue, rubber bands, lab and gym supplies, flooring, and latex gloves. A complete list of latex in the community can be found in Appendix A. (*Latex in the Home and Community*, published by the Spina Bifida Association, 2002). This list includes latex-free alternatives. The individualized healthcare plan (IHP) should include information about the student's history of allergic reaction and causes, management of the latex response, environmental controls, the emergency care plan (ECP) for reactions that occur at school, and identification of the student's ability to participate in the school health plan and activities.

## Pathophysiology

Latex is described as a raw material (milky sap) derived from the tropical rubber tree, *Hevea brasiliensis*, used to make many medical and consumer products (e.g., surgical gloves, balloons, rubber additives). People who are repeatedly exposed to latex (e.g., through multiple surgical and treatment procedures) become sensitized to the latex antigen and are at risk for developing an allergic reaction. The antigen that triggers the allergic response is believed to be a water-soluble protein that occurs naturally in the latex. Reactions can include watery and itchy eyes, nasal congestion, rhinorrhea, sneezing and coughing, urticaria (hives), as well as swelling of mucosal tissues (lips, tongue, uvula, and/or throat). Other reactions can include shortness of breath, tightness in the chest, wheezing, and nausea and/or abdominal cramping. There are also reactions that have delayed onset that present as contact dermatitis and can be seen several days after contact (Blaylock, 1997). More serious reactions can include bronchospasm leading to respiratory arrest and/or life-threatening changes in blood pressure and circulation (anaphylactic shock).

## Management

Management of the student who has a latex allergy consists of two steps: (1) modifying the school environment to remove as many latex sources as possible and (2) treating any allergic reaction that occurs. The school environment constantly changes (class location, field trips, transportation, etc.); therefore school personnel should receive periodic in-service training about sources of latex, latex-free alternatives, and necessary modifications to the environment. Nonlatex gloves should be used throughout the school. Barriers need to be provided between the skin and any latex product if no alternative is available (e.g., gym floors). Use of latex balloons should be discouraged. Parents should be notified about any party, dance, or other activity where balloons will be used for decoration. Parents will then be able to decide if the student can attend the function. Health service and first-aid supplies should be latex-free for all students. Additionally, emergency medical service (EMS) personnel should be aware of the student with latex allergy so they will also have appropriate supplies.

Treating an allergic reaction involves teaching school personnel about symptoms of the allergic reaction and appropriate management. School personnel need to know that a latex allergy can be a potential medical emergency. The ECP needs to specify treatment protocol as well as who is trained and responsible for carrying out the plan. It is critical that a source of epinephrine (usually an EpiPen) and antihistamines is readily available. School personnel will need to inform EMS personnel (if called) that the student has a latex allergy and what treatment has already been given at school.

## Individualized Healthcare Plan

### Assessment
*History*
- Student's medical diagnosis
- Student's medical and surgical history
- Past healthcare records
- Number of reactions to latex
- Student's signs and symptoms of an allergic reaction (mild to severe)
- Date of the last allergic reaction
- Previous allergic reactions other than to latex
- Family knowledge base in relation to treatment (e.g., medications) and environmental sources of latex
- Past history of episodes at school
- Past school environmental modifications and how well they worked to prevent reactions

*Current Status and Management*
- Current treatment plan for the allergic reaction(s), including prescribed medications
- Knowledge about condition (student, parent, guardian, teacher, para, etc.)
- Knowledge about early warning signs (student, school staff)
- Identification of potential sources of latex in school environment
- Healthcare provider involved in assessment and treatment
- Assistance needed to implement management plan (e.g., parent, sibling, teacher, nurse)

*Self-care*
- Physical and cognitive ability to self-administer medications
- Self-awareness of early signs and symptoms of an allergic reaction
- Knowledge and ability to inform appropriate personnel when experiencing allergic symptoms and assist with treatment
- Physical and/or cognitive ability to explain his/her needs during an allergic reaction
- Knowledge and ability to avoid latex products

*Psychosocial Status*
- Effect of the latex allergy on student's daily living activities
- Student's perception of what school staff and peers think and feel about student having latex allergy
- Student's affect, outlook, and general attitude toward the condition
- Student's age, developmental level, and intellectual level
- Student's ability to participate in normal activities of community, church, school clubs, or athletic activities
- Student's support system: family, friends, other

*Academic Issues*
- School environment: latex allergen sources
- Alternative products and procedures needed to minimize latex in the school environment
- Faculty awareness and knowledge of condition and potential problems
- School environment modifications needed so student may safely participate in school and classroom activities
- Activity restrictions that are necessary due to possible latex exposure

### Nursing Diagnoses (N.D.) (NANDA, 2003)

N.D. 1. Latex allergy response (NANDA 00041) related to:
- type and characteristics of allergic reaction(s)

**N.D. 2.** Risk for latex allergy response (NANDA 00042) related to:
- history of exposure, reactions, and/or environmental conditions

**N.D. 3.** Deficient knowledge (NANDA 00126) related to:
- latex sources
- signs and symptoms of an allergic reaction

**N.D. 4.** Effective therapeutic regimen management (NANDA 00082) related to:
- student's physical and/or cognitive ability to self-medicate
- student's ability to alert staff of needs
- emergency care plan

**N.D. 5.** Powerlessness (NANDA 00125) related to:
- the uncertainty of an allergic reaction and its outcome in the school environment

## Goals

The student will increase knowledge about symptoms of an allergic reaction/anaphylaxis. (N.D. 1, 2, 3)

The student will increase knowledge about sources of latex and latex-free alternatives. (N.D. 3, 4, 5)

The student will participate in developing and implementing healthcare plans at school in order to effectively prevent and manage a reaction to latex. (N.D. 1–5)

The student will identify possible products or conditions in the school environment that may cause an allergic response. (N.D. 2, 3)

The student will remain in the least restrictive educational environment. (N.D. 5)

The student will feel safe in the school environment. (N.D. 5)

## Nursing Interventions

In-service school staff and bus staff (as needed) about allergic reaction/anaphylaxis. (N.D. 1, 2, 3) Discuss:
- Significance of latex allergy
- Symptoms of mild to severe allergic reactions, including anaphylaxis
- Importance of early warning signs and prompt treatment
- Specific guidelines for treatment from mild to severe (ECP)
- Documentation of reactions that occur

Provide in-service training for school staff and bus staff (as needed) about common sources of latex and latex-free alternatives. (N.D. 2, 3)
- List items containing latex that are commonly found in the school environment.
- Provide list of latex-free alternative items.
- Discuss ways to minimize student's exposure to latex.
- Explain classroom modifications that may be needed.
- Discuss transportation modifications that may be needed.
- Outline field trip modifications that may be needed.
- Provide modifications for extracurricular activity (dances, carnivals, etc.) that may be needed.

Monitor school and bus environment at regular intervals for new sources of latex. (N.D. 2, 3, 5)
- Discourage use of latex balloons in school environment, especially in classrooms with students with known latex allergy (Mylar balloons should be used as an alternative.)

Inform staff of students who have a latex allergy. (N.D. 1, 2, 5)
- Encourage parents to have the student wear an allergy alert bracelet indicating a severe latex allergy.

Develop and implement a latex allergy ECP. (N.D. 1–5)
- List and describe measures to follow if reaction occurs.
- Include student, parent/guardian, appropriate school personnel, and healthcare provider, and coordinate school plan with home plan.
- Include student and parent on tour of student's school environment to identify latex sources.
- Allow for modifications to plan(s) as needed.
- Assist parents to supply (and resupply, as needed) a source of epinephrine (EpiPen, Anakit, etc.) to always be available in school and on field trips.
- Assist parents to obtain physician authorization for use of epinephrine and other needed medications in school.

Provide counseling for student regarding concerns. (N.D. 5)
- Safety in the school environment
- Relationship with peers regarding need to eliminate latex sources from the school environment

Encourage parent and student to keep school personnel informed. (N.D. 4, 5)
- Changes in health status
- Changes in health management plan

Have latex-free first-aid supplies available. (N.D. 2–5)
- Assist parents in obtaining and supplying latex-free health procedure supplies (catheters, gloves, etc.).
- Supply health office with latex-free supplies (Band-Aids, gloves, etc.).

Provide necessary health education for student to participate in self-care (depending on the student's cognitive and/or physical ability). (N.D. 1–5)
- Review symptoms of allergic reaction.
- Review sources of latex.
- Review treatment methods, including how/when to report allergic symptoms to school personnel and parents/guardians.
- Teach proper technique for self-administration of epinephrine and other medications prescribed for an allergic reaction.

## Expected Student Outcomes

The student will:
- Avoid sources of potential allergens. (N.D. 2–5)
- Participate in school and classroom activities with modifications, as necessary. (N.D. 3, 4, 5)
- Describe his/her symptoms of an allergic reaction (from mild to severe). (N.D. 1, 3, 4)
- Identify common sources of latex in school environment. (N.D. 3)
- Inform school staff of products at school that might contain latex and that might cause allergic symptoms. (N.D. 2, 3)
- Inform school staff when experiencing allergic symptoms. (N.D. 4)
- Demonstrate proper technique of self-medication if appropriate. (N.D. 4)
- Identify location of EpiPen. (N.D. 4)
- Wear latex allergy alert bracelet/necklace. (N.D.1, 2, 5)
- Follow steps in ECP if a reaction occurs. (N.D. 4)
- Identify school personnel that can assist him/her if a reaction occurs. (N.D. 4, 5)
- Participate in counseling, addressing issues of school safety and peer knowledge of his latex allergy. (N.D. 5)

## Case Study

J. D. is a 13-year-old student at Wecare Middle School. He was born with spina bifida. He lives with his mother, father, brother, and sister. This past summer, J. D. had a serious allergic reaction to latex while hospitalized for orthopedic problems. He has had a long history of exposure to latex through numerous surgeries, treatments, bowel-management programs, and intermittent catheterization procedures. Initially, his mother plans to transport him to school this year because she is unsure of the latex sources on the school bus.

J. D. is unable to walk and will spend his school day in a wheelchair. The school is easily accessible for him, but the environment needs to be examined for latex sources on account of his recent diagnosis of "severe reaction to latex." The bus will also need to be evaluated for sources of latex that he might be exposed to on his ride to and from school. J. D.'s physician has ordered that EpiPen be available at school. Mom has also requested that we speak with the local EMS personnel, who might be called for emergency problems with J. D. Because of a learning deficit, if J. D. would inadvertently be exposed to latex in the school (balloon bouquet, balls, etc.), he may not be able to advise school staff of his allergic symptoms and his need for medication or emergency treatment.

# Emergency Care Plan
# Latex Allergy

School: _____     Phone: _____

Date: _____     FAX : _____


Pupil's Name: _____     Physician's Name: _____

I.D.#: _____     Address: _____

Birth date: _____     Phone: _____

Address: _____     FAX: _____

Phone: _____     Hospital: _____


Parents:

Mother: _____     Day Phone: _____

Father: _____     Day Phone: _____


Parent Designee: _____     Day Phone: _____


**Medical Condition:** Latex Allergy—severe reactions in past


**Location of medication and other supplies:** _____


**Persons authorized to administer treatment:**

    School Nurse: _____

    Nurse Designee: _____


**Signs of emergency:** urticaria (hives) and itching, swelling of mucosal tissues (tonsils, throat, tongue), wheezing, shortness of breath, itching eyes, feeling faint, nausea/vomiting, diarrhea, abdominal cramps


**Treatment for Severe Allergic Reaction:**

1. Administer epinephrine injection or assist with self-administration
2. Call 911, informing EMS of severe latex allergy reaction and that epinephrine injection has been given
3. Call parent or parent designee
4. Call student's physician to inform of emergency situation
5. Record administration or self-administration of medication in student's health record (include date, time, source of exposure, treatment, if EMS was called, and signature)
6. EMS to transport to (hospital reference) or nearest emergency department

# Latex Allergy

| Assessment Data | Nursing Diagnosis | Goals | Nursing Interventions | Expected Outcomes | |
|---|---|---|---|---|---|
| J.D. has had a history of allergic response to natural latex rubber products.<br><br>J.D. had serious allergic reaction to latex last summer. | Latex allergy response related to type and characteristics of allergic reaction(s). | J.D. will increase knowledge about symptoms of an allergic reaction. | Educate school and bus personnel on significance of latex allergy and allergic signs and symptoms (mild to severe).<br><br>Provide necessary health education for J.D. to be able to identify his symptoms of allergic reaction.<br><br>Inform staff that J.D. has a latex allergy.<br><br>Encourage parent to obtain medical alert bracelet/necklace for student. | J.D. will describe his symptoms of allergic reaction (mild and severe).<br><br>J.D. will inform school staff when experiencing allergic symptoms.<br><br>J.D. will wear medical alert bracelet/necklace at all times. | |
| J.D. is at risk for allergic response to natural latex rubber products in the school and bus environment.<br><br>Parent unsure of all potential sources of latex in school environment as well as on school bus. | Risk for latex allergy response related to history of exposure, reactions, and/or environmental conditions. | J.D. will identify possible products and conditions in the school environment that can cause allergic response. | J.D. and parent will accompany school nurse on tour of student's school environment to identify latex sources and discuss ways to minimize student's exposure to latex.<br><br>J.D., parent, and school nurse will be notified in advance of field trips and other extracurricular activities so possible sources of latex can be identified and modified as needed.<br><br>J.D., parent, school nurse, and bus personnel will discuss bus modifications that may be needed. | J.D. will inform staff of products at school that might contain latex and cause allergic symptoms (including field trips and transportation).<br><br>J.D. will avoid potential allergens. | |

| Assessment Data | Nursing Diagnosis | Goals | Nursing Interventions | Expected Outcomes |
|---|---|---|---|---|
| J.D. has a learning deficit, which will affect his ability to alert staff to symptoms of latex allergy. | Deficient knowledge related to latex sources and signs and symptoms of an allergic reaction. | J.D. will increase knowledge of potential allergens, allergic reactions, and latex-free sources. | Provide list and suggestions for latex-free alternative products, barriers, or modifications to school personnel. | J.D. will identify common latex sources and potential allergic reactions. |
| J.D. has physical and cognitive deficits, which will affect his ability to alert staff of treatment needs and his ability to self-medicate. | Effective therapeutic regimen management related to student's physical and/or cognitive ability to self-medicate, ability to alert staff of needs, and ECP. | J.D. will participate in development and implementation of health care plans in school in order to effectively prevent and manage a reaction to latex. | Develop ECP with signs and symptoms, treatment protocols, location of emergency supplies, persons trained to administer medications, and proper documentation of reaction that occurs. | J.D. will identify school personnel who can assist him if a reaction occurs as well as location of emergency medications. |
| J.D.'s physician ordered EpiPen to be available at school. | | | Coordinate ECP with home plan, including student, parent/guardian, appropriate school personnel, and health-care provider. | J.D. will follow steps in ECP if a reaction occurs. |
| | | | Modify ECP when needed. | J.D. will demonstrate proper technique of self-administration of EpiPen with staff supervision. |
| | | | Assist parent to obtain and supply latex-free health procedure supplies. | J.D. will participate in school and classroom activities, with modification as needed. |
| J.D. is concerned about his ability to make his needs known and receive proper treatment. | Powerlessness related to uncertainty of allergic reaction and the outcome in school environment. | J.D. will remain in least restrictive educational environment.

J.D. will feel safe at school. | Evaluate J.D. and provide necessary health education for student to participate in self-care and treatment protocol. | J.D. will participate in counseling, addressing issues of school safety and peer knowledge of his latex allergy. |
| J.D. is concerned about the changing school environment and unknown sources of latex. | | | Provide ongoing monitoring and education about latex allergy and student's medical condition. | |
| J.D. is concerned about peer's awareness of his latex allergy. | | | Provide ongoing health counseling to J.D. to increase his confidence that school is safe.

Provide ongoing health counseling to peers with regard to safety and health concerns of student with latex allergy. | |

## References

Blaylock, B. (1997). Latex allergies: Overview, prevention and implications for nursing care. *Ostomy/Wound Management, 43*(3), 46–53.

Cotter, C., Burbach, C., Boyer, M., Engelhardt, M., Smith, M., & Hubka, K. (1996). Latex allergy and the student with spina bifida. *Journal of School Nursing, 12,* 14–18.

Evangelisto, N. (1997). Handle with care: Identifying and treating patients with latex allergy. *Today's Surgical Nurse, 19*(6), 30–35.

National Association of School Nurses. (Adopted 2000). *Position Statement: Natural rubber latex allergy.* Scarborough, ME: Author.

Spina Bifida Association of America (2002). *Latex in the home and community.* Washington, DC: Author.

## Bibliography

American Academy of Pediatrics (AAP). (2001). *Policy statement: Guidelines for emergency care in school.* Retrieved August 12, 2003, from http://www.aap.org/policy/re9954.html

Barton, E. C. (1993). Latex allergy: Recognition and management of a modern problem. *Nurse Practitioner, 18*(11), 54–59.

Degenhardt, P., Golla, S., Wahn, F., & Niggemann, B. (2001). Latex allergy in pediatric surgery is dependent on repeated operations in the first year of life. *Journal of Pediatric Surgery, 36*(8), 1535–1539.

Gold J. (1994). Ask about latex. *RN,* June, 32–34.

Lewis, K. D., & Bear, B. J. (2002). *Manual of school health* (2nd ed). Philadelphia: Saunders.

Meropol, E. (1997). *Alert: Latex allergy in children and youth assisted by medical technology educational settings: Guidelines for care.* Baltimore: Paul H. Brooks.

Meeropol, E. V. (1998). The R.U.B.B.E.R. tool: Screening children for latex allergy. *Pediatric Health Care, 12*(1), 320–323.

NANDA International. (2003). *Nursing diagnoses: Definitions & classification 2003-2004.* Philadelphia: Author.

National Association of School Nurses (NASN). (2001). *Position Statement: Natural rubber latex allergy.* Retrieved August 12, 2003, from http://www.nasn.org/positions/allergy.htm

National Association of School Nurses (NASN). (2001). Position *Statement: The role of the school nurse in allergy/anaphylaxis Management.* Retrieved August 12, 2003, from http://www.nasn.org/positions/allergy.htm

Wynn, S. R. (1993). Anaphylaxis at school. *Journal of School Nursing, 9,* 5–11.

Young, M. A, Meyers, M. (1997). Latex allergy: Considerations for the care of pediatric patients and employee safety. *Nursing Clinics of North America, 32,* 169–182.

Young, M. A, Meyers M., McCulloch, L. D, & Brown, L. J. (1997). Latex allergy. *AORN J, 56,* 488–501.

## Resources

Alternative Resource Catalog
135 Walnut Drive
 No. 214C
Saint Charles, IL 60174-1551
1-800-618-3129
niccirn@aol.com

American Academy of Allergy, Asthma & Immunology
611 East Wells Street
Milwaukee, WI 53202
414-272-6071
1-800-822-2742
http://www.aaaai.org

American Academy of Pediatrics
141 Northwest Point Boulevard
Elk Grove Village, IL 60007-1098
847-434-4000
1-800-842-7777
http://www.aap.org

American College of Allergy, Asthma & Immunology
85 West Algonquin Road
Suite 550
Arlington Heights, IL 60005
847-427-1200
http://www.allergy.mcg.edu/physicians/ltxhome.html

Latex Allergy Information Service
176 Roosevelt Avenue
Torrington, CT 06790
http://www.latexallergyhelp.com

Myloons (self-sealing balloon)
Marketing Innovation Enterprises
200 East 94th Street
Suite 603
New York, NY 10128

National Association of School Nurses (NASN)
Western office:
1416 Park Street
Suite A
Castle Rock, CO 80109
1-866-627-6767
Eastern office:
PO Box 1300
Scarborough, ME 04070-1300
1-877-627-6476
www.nasn.org

Spina Bifida Association of America
4590 MacArthur Boulevard, NW
Suite 250
Washington, DC 20007-4226
1-800-621-3141
http://www.sbaa.org

# Appendix A: Latex in the Home and Community

| Products That May Contain Latex | Latex-Safe Alternatives |
|---|---|
| Art supplies, paints, glue, erasers, fabric paints | Elmer's, Faber-Castell erasers, Liquitex paints, acrylic paints, soap erasers, Crayola (except stamps, erasers), Play-Doh |
| Balloons | Mylar balloons, self-sealing Myloons |
| Balls: Koosh, tennis, bowling, ball pits | PVC (Hedstrom), Nerf foam balls |
| Carpet backing, gym floor, basement sealants | Provide barrier cloth or mat |
| Chewing gum | Wrigley gums, Bubblicious, Trident (Warner-Lambert) |
| Clothes: liquid appliqués on tee shirts, elastic on socks, underwear, sneakers, sandals | Cloth-covered elastic, neoprene, Buster Brown elastic-free socks |
| Condoms, diaphragms, contraceptive sponges | Polyurethane wideseal silicone diaphragms, Trojan Supra condom, others |
| Crutch tips, hand grips, axillary pads | Cover with cloth or tape |
| Diapers, rubber pants, incontinence pads | Huggies, Gold Seal, some Attends, Drypers, Always, Pampers, Luvs, others |
| Food handled with latex gloves | Synthnetic gloves for food handling |
| Handles on rackets, tools, bicycles | Vinyl, leather handles or cover with cloth or tape |
| Kitchen cleaning gloves | PVC, cotton liners |
| Latex paint | There is no natural rubber in latex paint |
| Newsprint, ads, coupons | Provide barrier such as gloves |
| Toys, such as old Barbies, Stretch Armstrong | 1992 Barbie, Mattell dolls, Kenner figures, toys by Fisher Price, Playschool, others |
| Rubber bands | String, plastic bands |
| Water toys, swimming equipment, bathing suits | Plastic, PVC, nylon, SuitsMe swimwear |
| Wheelchair cushions, tires | Jay, ROHO, cover seat, use gloves |
| Zippered plastic storage bags | Waxed paper, plain plastic bags, Ziploc bags |

Adapted from *Latex in the Home and Community*, 2002, Washington, DC: Spina Bifida Association of America.

*Chapter Fifty-one*

# Lyme Disease

Heidi M. Toth

## Introduction

Lyme disease is the most common and rapidly emerging vector-borne infectious disease in the United States. The Centers for Disease Control and Prevention (CDC) initiated Lyme disease surveillance in 1982, and since that time, more than 157,000 cases have been reported. There were 23,763 cases reported in 2002 (CDC, 2003). The national incidence rate is approximately 7 per 100,000 population. Cases of Lyme disease have been reported in 49 states and the District of Columbia. A geographic pattern exists in which the majority of Lyme disease cases are found in the northeastern, mid-Atlantic and North Central regions; several states exceed an incidence of 20 per 100,000, including Connecticut, Delaware, New Jersey, New York, Pennsylvania, and Rhode Island. The highest reported incidence according to age was among children aged 5 through 9 years. From 1991 through 2000, the incidence of Lyme disease nearly doubled, making it a public health threat for the school-aged population (CDC, 2002; CDC, *Lyme Disease Epidemiology*).

Dr. Steere first described Lyme disease in the United States in 1975 when he described an epidemic of juvenile arthritis in Old Lyme, Connecticut. However, reports of the clinical manifestations have been available for more than 100 years (Nachman & Pontrelli, 2003). Lyme disease is a zoonosis and is acquired by the transmission of the spirochete *Borrelia burgdorferi* from infected ticks to humans. It is a multisystem infection with numerous manifestations similar to the disease presentation of syphilis, which is known as the "great imitator." Lyme disease has been called the "new great imitator" because of its tendency to be acute, subacute, chronic, symptomatic, or asymptomatic (Pachner, 1989).

The vector is the deer tick, or *Ixodes scapularis,* which is responsible for most Lyme disease cases in the United States. These ticks have a 2-year three-stage life cycle: larva, nymph, and adult. The larvae hatch usually uninfected in the summer and become infected with *B. burgdorferi* by feeding on an infected host such as a mouse or other small mammal. The larvae then emerge in the spring in the nymphal stage, which is considered the most likely time for the tick to transmit the infection. This is possibly due to the minute size of the nymph, which makes it difficult to detect and remove in a timely manner

(Shapiro & Gerber, 2000). The risk of transmission of *B. burgdorferi* from infected ticks also appears to be dependent on the length of feeding. Nymphs normally need to feed on a human for 40 or more hours before *B. burgdorferi* is transferred. They are at the peak of their feeding frenzy in the late spring and early summer (Rawlings, 1999). People who have exposure to tick-infested woods or fields near woods in endemic areas are at higher risk of acquiring Lyme disease (Shapiro & Gerber). Thus, children who spend more time outdoors are at greatest risk for contracting Lyme disease.

## Pathophysiology

After a tick injects *B. burgdorferi* and the incubation period of 3 to 32 days passes, the spirochete multiplies locally and the characteristic "bull's-eye" rash, or erythema migrans, may appear at the site of tick attachment (Steere, 1989). Erythema migrans begins as a red macule or papule that typically enlarges over several days or weeks to become an annular red lesion, which may have variable degrees of central clearing. The lesion can differ greatly from person to person; it may be itchy and painful or asymptomatic. There may be nonspecific symptoms such as fever, malaise, headaches, muscle aches, or joint aches (Shapiro & Gerber, 2000). This stage is considered early localized, and if the characteristic erythema migrans is not present, diagnosis may be extremely difficult.

The next stage is early disseminated disease, which occurs 3 to 12 weeks after the tick bite and includes multiple annular erythematous lesions, aseptic meningitis, cranial nerve palsies, and, rarely, radiculopathy and encephalitis. Cardiac abnormalities, such as atrioventricular heart block, rarely occur in children (Nachmann & Pontrelli, 2003). Eye involvement, such as iritis, optic neuritis, and uveitis, has also been reported (Shapiro & Gerber, 2000). The most frequent neurologic sign in the pediatric population is cranial neuropathy. The most common nerve affected is the facial nerve, reported in as many as 73% of children with central nervous system (CNS) Lyme disease; however, abnormalities of all cranial nerves have been described (Nachman & Pontrelli). Facial palsy typically occurs anywhere from 40 to 170 days after the occurrence of the rash. In endemic areas, facial nerve palsy may be a marker for meningitis; therefore, the cerebrospinal fluid should be examined (Belman et al.,1997).

Lyme meningitis occurs in 10% to 40% of Lyme disease cases. The most common symptoms include headache, neck discomfort, papilledema (inflammation of the optic nerve) and irritation of the brain and spinal cord (Nachman & Pontrelli). The long-term neuropsychological effects in children with facial nerve palsy attributable to Lyme disease were comparable to normal children according to a recent study done at the Yale Child Study Center (Vazquez, Sparrow, & Shapiro, 2003).

Late Lyme disease, evidenced by arthritis and/or chronic CNS involvement, can occur if early symptoms are untreated or undiagnosed. When untreated, the symptoms may emerge anywhere from 1 month to 14 years after infection, with remissions and recurrences (Fallon, Kochevar, Gaito, & Nields, 1998). Arthritis is the most common, affecting the large joints, especially the knee, within weeks to months after the initial infection. The joint might be swollen and tender intermittently; however, severe pain is usually not present as compared to septic arthritis (Shapiro & Gerber, 2000). Less frequent are the CNS involvements that consist of mild to severe encephalopathy, polyneuropathy, and severe fatigue (Fallon et al., 1992). Typical reported symptoms of chronic Lyme disease include difficulty with concentration and memory, disturbances in mood and sleep, and severe fatigue (Nachmann & Pontrelli, 2003). There is also concern of subtle cognitive impairments. Lyme encephalopathy can affect short-term memory, verbal fluency, reaction time, and attention. According to Fallon et al. (1998), some of these patients are so distractible that they may appear to have attention deficit disorder (ADD). Impulsivity and hyperactivity might also be seen; however, Lyme-induced attention deficit disorder usually meets the criteria for the inattention type (Fallon et al.,1998). The onset of the illness is not dramatic and is gradual in the child and adolescent. Children may have difficulty keeping up with their peers academically and might label themselves as incompetent. A study by Tager et al. (2001) suggests that children with Lyme disease had significantly more cognitive and psychiatric disturbances, resulting in psychosocial and academic difficulties. A study by Bloom, Wyckoff, Meissner, & Steere (1998) revealed evidence of behavioral changes, forgetfulness, decreased school performance, and mild to moderate deficits in visual or auditory processing in children after infection with Lyme disease. Nonetheless, there are also experts who question whether chronic CNS infection actually exists as a disease entity. Currently, there are randomized controlled studies in progress of patients who remain ill after standard courses of antibiotic therapy for Lyme disease. At this time, "chronic Lyme disease" is not a separate diagnostic entity (Wormser et al., 2000).

Lyme disease may be difficult to diagnose due to the nonspecific manifestations and poor standardization of diagnostic tests. Attempts have been made to develop antigen-based diagnostic tests; however, they should be considered experimental until additional studies are done. The confirmation of Lyme disease is based on IgM and IgG antibodies (which usually appear 6 to 8 weeks after infection) to *B. burgdorferi* in the patient's blood through the enzyme-linked immunsorbent assay (ELISA). This test is sensitive; however, it lacks specificity, leading to false positives due to cross-reactive antibodies from other spirochetal infections, viral infections, and autoimmune diseases. If the ELISA is positive or equivocal, a Western blot, which is an immunoblot for serum antibodies to *B. burgdorferi,* should be done for confirmation (Shapiro & Gerber, 2000).

## Management

Early Lyme disease or early localized disease may be treated with oral antibiotics (doxycycline for patients over age 8, or amoxicillin) for 14 to 21 days (**Table 1**). Doxycycline is contraindicated for children under age 8 because of the potential for dental staining; however, it has been used for up to 2 weeks safely without staining. If these antibiotics cannot be used on account of allergies, the more expensive cefuroxime axetil may be used. The child should be observed for any side effects. Disadvantages of doxycycline therapy include photosensitivity reactions (which may be significant, because early Lyme disease in usually treated in the warmer months) and esophageal ulcerations (Eppes, 2003). Encouraging the administration of antibiotics with food will lessen the gastrointestinal effects. Flulike symptoms such as myalgia, arthralgia, fever, headache, or fatigue may also occur during the early localized stage. The child should be encouraged to report any of these symptoms so that appropriate comfort measures may be used.

In early disseminated disease or with CNS symptoms, intravenous antibiotics ceftriaxone or penicillin G are indicated for 14 to 28 days. Lyme arthritis requires 28 days of doxycycline or amoxicillin (Wormser et al., 2003). Children who have both arthritis and CNS symptoms may benefit from intravenous therapy (Nachman & Pontrelli, 2003). The child might have intravenous access, typically with a peripherally inserted central catheter (PICC). The child with a PICC should be monitored for any fever, chills, or feelings of malaise, oozing from around the line, cracks or leaks from the line, dislodgement, or pain, redness, or swelling around the site or in the neck or arm.

Lyme Disease

**Table 1. Recommended Therapy for Lyme Disease**

| Disease Type | Type Treatment |
|---|---|
| Early localized disease:<br>Erythema migrans, fever, malaise, headache, muscle ache, joint ache | Children less than 8 years:<br>Amoxicillin, 14-21 days<br>Children over 8 years:<br>Doxycycline or amoxicillin, 14-21 days<br>Alternative:<br>Cefuroxime axetil |
| Early disseminated disease:<br>Multiple erythema migrans<br>Cardiac symptoms<br>1st or 2nd degree heart block<br>3rd degree heart block<br>Cranial nerve palsy<br>Meningitis/CNS involvement | Same as early localized disease<br><br>Same as early localized disease<br>Same as meningitis<br>Same as early localized disease<br>Ceftriaxone IV, 14-28 days<br>Alternative:<br>Penicillin G IV |
| Late disease:<br>Arthritis<br><br>CNS involvement | Same as early localized disease, but for 28 days<br><br>Same as meningitis |

Lyme disease may cause discomfort in various body systems, and the pain should be adequately assessed. Pain is now considered to be the "fifth vital sign," according to the American Pain Society (as cited in Wong, Hockenberry, Wilson, Winkelstein, & Kline, 2003).

One assessment strategy is using the technique QUESTT:

Question the child.

Use pain rating scales.

Evaluate behavior and physiologic changes.

Secure parents' involvement.

Take cause of pain into account.

Take action and evaluate results (Baker & Wong, 1987, as cited in Wong et al., 2003, p. 1049).

Several pain rating scales exist; one example is the FACES pain rating scale, which consists of six cartoon faces ranging from smiling for no pain to a crying face for "worst pain" (Wong et al., 2003).

The child with late stage Lyme disease will benefit from a collaborative approach in managing the disease. Physical effects may include pain, visual disturbances, joint swelling, headaches, cardiac changes, and fatigue. Adaptation for physical education should be considered due to the pain and fatigue. Cognitive function such as short-term memory issues and visual and auditory processing difficulties may affect school performance and require modifications in the classroom setting. Mood changes, irritability, lifestyle changes, and depression will affect the child's emotional state. Addressing these issues with effective nursing interventions will support the student in achieving academic success.

Educational materials for children and parents focusing on preventing exposure to Lyme disease should also address the possibility of reinfection with continued exposure.

The best available method for preventing Lyme disease is to avoid tick-infected areas, particularly in the spring and summer, when nymphal ticks are feeding. Ticks prefer a moist, shaded location with leaf litter and low-lying vegetation in wooded or overgrown grassy areas. A single application of pesticides to tick-infested habitats may reduce the tick population but may be harmful to other wildlife and people. Landscape the yard to reduce ticks by removing leaf litter and laying down wood chips where lawns abut the woods. Reducing deer and rodent hosts will also decrease the tick population. Using fences to exclude deer from yards and keeping your pets free of ticks will lessen your exposure (Hayes & Piesman, 2003; CDC, *Lyme Disease Prevention and Control*).

If exposure to tick habitats is unavoidable, some additional measures are recommended to decrease the risk of acquiring Lyme disease. Protective clothing such as a hat, long-sleeved shirt tight at the wrists and tucked into pants, and pants tucked into socks should be worn. Light-colored clothing allows better visibility of ticks and increases the probability of removing the tick before it can attach (Wormser et al., 2000). Insect repellents containing DEET (N,N-diethylmetatoluamide) may be applied to clothes and exposed skin, providing additional protection. DEET should not be applied to a child's hands, face, or irritated skin because of potential neurotoxicity. It should be applied sparingly to other exposed skin. The skin should be washed after the child returns indoors. Permethrin, (a synthetic pyrethroid repellent), which kills ticks on contact, can be applied to clothing only (Shapiro & Gerber, 2000). The package directions should be followed when using over-the-counter protection products.

Promote daily tick checks by inspecting the child's body and clothing after possible exposure to ticks. Studies indicate a prolonged duration of attachment is necessary to cause transmission; consequently, prompt removal of any ticks is important. Embedded ticks should be grasped with tweezers as close to the skin as possible and the tick should be gently pulled straight out. Any mouth parts that remain embedded should be left alone, because they eventually extrude. Repeated attempts to remove them cause tissue damage and may increase the risk of bacterial infection (Shapiro & Gerber, 2000). The area should be cleansed with an antiseptic or soap and water. Analysis of ticks for *B. burgdorferi* is not recommended except for research studies. Routine use of prophylactic antimicrobials after a tick bite is not recommended according to the Infectious Diseases Society of America Guidelines (Wormser et al., 2000). However, a recent study indicated that a single dose of doxycycline given within 72 hours after a tick bite may prevent the development of Lyme disease in adults and might be indicated, depending on the degree of engorgement and the prevalence of tick-transmitted diseases in the area (Nadelman et al., 2001). Dosing and efficacy of prophylactic treatment have not been studied in children. Monitor closely anyone affected by a tick bite for signs and symptoms of Lyme disease for 30 days, and monitor specifically for any skin lesion at the site of the bite. Anyone with symptoms or a skin lesion should seek medical attention.

The United States Food and Drug Administration had licensed LYMErix vaccine in 1998 to prevent Lyme disease; however, it was removed from the market in February 2002 because of poor sales (Nachman & Pontrelli, 2003).

## Individualized Healthcare Plan

### Assessment
*History*
- Diagnosis and medical testing
- Onset of signs and symptoms
- Past hospitalizations, medications, or treatments
- Course of the disease
- Other health concerns or illnesses
- Family and student knowledge base
- Body system involvement: cardiac, musculoskeletal, neurologic
- Sleep disturbances

*Current Status and Management*
- Level of function, physical restrictions due to pain or fatigue
- Medications, at home and school
- Level of pain
- Daily activity level: energy use, rest period as needed
- PICC or intravenous line present
- Current stage of Lyme disease and prognosis
- Cardiac manifestations (assess apical rate and blood pressure as indicated)
- Neurologic manifestations, such as headaches, memory loss, visual or auditory processing difficulties; need for referral to outside health personnel and learning consultant for evaluation
- Current management of sleep disturbances
- Management plan

*Self-care*
- Knowledge about current health status and management plan
- Perception of the illness and its effect
- Ability to manage activities and self-impose restrictions or rest periods
- Decision-making and problem-solving skills

*Psychosocial Status*
- Perception of self
- Support system: family, peers, other
- Ability to participate in extracurricular activities
- Student's feelings related to his/her role due to the illness
- Student's ability to cope with the illness

*Academic Issues*
- Student or teacher report regarding difficulty concentrating, memory loss, unusual sensations, irritability, and difficulty with directions or recalling information
- Past and current academic achievement, strengths, and weaknesses
- School health services needed and/or medications required during the school day
- School, curriculum, and classroom modifications; what plan is available to make up missed work
- School staff and peer perceptions, information they need to know
- Teacher's and student's perception of academic performance and limitations
- Need for a 504 plan or individualized education program (IEP)
- Days the student has been absent from class due to Lyme disease compared to student's attendance before infected with Lyme disease

## Nursing Diagnosis (N.D.) (NANDA, 2003)

**N.D. 1** Risk for deficient diversional activity (NANDA 00097) related to difficulty participating in usual activities
**N.D. 2** Risk for ineffective health maintenance (NANDA 00099) related to:
- perceived ineffectiveness of interventions
- information misinterpretation

**N.D. 3** Impaired physical mobility (NANDA 00085) related to:
- pain
- swelling
- musculoskeletal impairment

**N.D. 4** Fatigue (NANDA 00093) related to:
- inability to maintain usual routines
- decreased performance
- musculoskeletal impairments
- sleep disturbances

**N.D. 5** Risk for activity intolerance (NANDA 00092) related to:
- impaired mobility
- musculoskeletal impairment
- generalized weakness or fatigue

**N.D. 6** Risk for impaired memory (NANDA 00131) related to:
- neurologic manifestations
- concentration difficulty secondary to pain and sleep disturbances

**N.D. 7** Risk for injury (NANDA 00035) related to:
- impaired mobility secondary to musculoskeletal impairments
- fatigue

**N.D. 8** Chronic pain (NANDA 00133) related to:
- musculoskeletal symptoms
- gastrointestinal symptoms, e.g., nausea

**N.D. 9** Knowledge deficit (NANDA 00126) related to:
- impaired auditory or visual processing
- inaccurate perception of health status or plan
- lack of or misinformation of Lyme disease

**N.D. 10** Risk for ineffective coping (NANDA 00069) related to:
- inability to meet role expectations
- inability to conserve adaptive energies

**N.D. 11** Risk for powerlessness (NANDA 00152) related to;
- prolonged symptoms
- inability to participate in normal activities
- inability to control situation

**N.D. 12** Risk for situational low self-esteem (NANDA 00120) related to;
- functional impairment
- academic difficulties

**N.D. 13** Risk for infection (NANDA 00004) related to:
- presence of invasive lines
- exposure to ticks

**N.D. 14** Risk for ineffective therapeutic regimen management (NANDA 00078) related to:
- barriers to comprehension secondary to memory problems and fatigue
- lack of or misinformation of Lyme disease or treatment
- risk of infection

## Goals

The student will participate in classroom and school activities with modifications as needed. (N.D. 1, 3, 5)

The student will participate in extracurricular activities as tolerance allows or substitute new activities as indicated. (N.D. 1, 3, 5)

The student will demonstrate knowledge of medications and treatment modalities. (N.D. 2, 9, 14)

The student will be involved in the management of his/her condition and improve self-management skills. (N.D. 2, 9, 14)

The student will increase activity as tolerated with adequate musculoskeletal function. (N.D. 3, 5, 7)

The student will maintain adequate energy level during the school day. (N.D. 3, 4, 7)

The student will be safe in the school environment and remain free from physical injury. (N.D. 3, 7)

The student will maintain skin integrity and prevent infection at the invasive line. (N.D. 13, 14)

The student will exhibit signs of reduced joint inflammation. (N.D. 3, 5, 8)

The student will exhibit no pain or reduction of pain to a tolerable level. (N.D. 3, 8)

The student will express feelings and concerns. (N.D. 10, 11, 12, 14)

The student will maintain normal sleep pattern. (N.D. 4, 6, 7, 10,)

The student will utilize healthy adaptation and coping skills. (N.D. 10, 11, 12, 14)

The student will make decisions regarding health management, school, and peer activities. (N.D. 1, 9, 11, 12, 14)

The student will receive assistance in managing medications in school setting. (N.D. 2, 8, 9, 14)

The student will demonstrate increased adaptation to and psychological comfort with body changes and lifestyle requirements. (N.D. 1, 5, 10, 11, 12)

The student will increase knowledge of Lyme disease and prevention of further tick-related diseases. (N.D. 2, 9, 13, 14)

The student will utilize adaptive coping methods. (N.D. 10, 11, 12)

## Nursing Interventions

Monitor the student's response to activities based on pain, fatigue, or weakness. (N.D. 1, 5)

Encourage student to: (N.D. 1, 10, 11, 12)
- Identify activities available in and outside of school
- Plan schedule and find alternate activities if limitations are present (e.g., manager of team, school newspaper, drama club)
- Verbalize fears and concerns about participating in activities
- Socialize with peers; social development is as important as cognitive development
- Challenge himself/herself by learning a new skill or pursuing a new interest
- Join a support group either in or out of school, which can boost self-esteem and self-worth and provide a sense of belonging.

Examine student's health and cultural beliefs and past experiences related to illness and assess their impact on his/her desire to learn. (N.D. 2, 9, 14)

Assess for barriers to learning, have student explain effective intervention and treatment plan, adapt teaching to student's physical and psychological status (e.g., comfort, fatigue, cognitive). (N.D. 2, 9, 14)

Consult with parents and healthcare provider in regard to limitations of physical activity or a modified program. (N.D. 3, 4, 5)

Encourage student's natural tendency to be physically active and in a way that does not excessively strain affected joints (e.g., swimming, isometric exercises). (N.D. 3, 5)

Allow the application of heat or cold to affected joints (dependent on physician recommendation) to reduce or prevent pain and inflammation. (N.D. 3, 5, 8)

Notify staff of student's health status after parental permission is obtained. (N.D. 10, 12, 14)

Schedule regular periods for rest, especially during acute phase, to conserve energy; include the teachers and student in planning for needed rest during the day to have the minimal effect on academic needs. (N.D. 4, 7, 8, 12)

Discuss with the guidance department the possibility of schedule changes (e.g., specials in the morning, study hall and lunch together to facilitate a midday rest, academics in the afternoon). (N.D. 4, 5, 12)

Help the student to identify activities that are difficult and encourage him/her to verbalize how fatigue may cause frustration. (N.D. 4, 5, 7, 10, 12)

Emphasize student's past accomplishments and help develop goals with the student based on this information. (N.D. 1, 10, 11, 12)

Teach the student to maximize pleasant experiences and to anticipate what he/she enjoys each day. (N.D. 8, 10, 11, 12)

Consult with student and parents regarding sleep patterns and assist with exploring strategies for dealing with the problem (medication-related, calming techniques, soft music, white noise, caffeine avoidance, bedtime snack of foods high in L-tyrptophan. (N.D. 4, 6, 10)

Collaborate with the physical education staff to: (N.D. 3, 4, 5, 7)
- Increase the student's tolerance for activity by performing it more slowly or for a shorter period of time with rest periods.
- Provide a modified physical education program as needed.
- Encourage muscle-strengthening exercises.

Help student identify the progress made; do not underestimate the value of praise and encouragement as an effective motivational technique. (N.D. 10, 11, 12)

Discuss with student factors that increase risk of injury and ways to prevent injuries. (N.D. 7)

Assist student in managing their pain by: (N.D. 8, 9, 11)
- Utilizing a developmentally appropriate and consistent pain scale, such as FACES or a 0-10 scale with 0 being no pain and 10 being the worst pain
- Obtaining medical orders and administering pharmacologic interventions as indicated
- Assessing the response to pain, rate the severity before and after interventions to evaluate their effectiveness
- Using nonpharmacologic interventions to supplement, not replace, pharmacologic interventions, such as heat/cold therapy, distractions, relaxation exercises, guided imagery, positive self-talk, thought stopping, cutaneous stimulation, and behavioral contracting

Reduce or eliminate other factors, such as fatigue, which may increase the pain experience. Explain that pain contributes to stress, which increases fatigue. (N.D. 4, 8, 9, 11)

Provide instruction at student's level of understanding when giving health information; repeat information as necessary; check for accurate feedback. (N.D. 2, 9, 14)

Provide medication instruction at student's level of understanding, including purpose, adverse effects, and dosage. Discuss interventions to lessen adverse effects. (N.D. 2, 8, 9, 14)
- Take deep breaths and swallow voluntarily to decrease vomiting reflex if nausea occurs.
- Take medications with meals if indicated to lessen gastrointestinal side effects.
- Avoid sun and use sunscreen if taking medications that cause photosensitivity (doxycycline).

Discuss the benefit of regular medical supervision, nutritious eating, and regular exercise for health maintenance. (N.D. 2, 9, 14)

Review student's understanding of diagnosis and prescribed treatment, clarify any misconceptions student has in regard to his/her care and education. (N.D. 2, 9, 14)

Encourage student to promote personal achievement, self-esteem, and externalize anxieties. (N.D. 10, 11, 12)
- Establish rapport with the student and provide a supportive environment.
- Convey honesty and empathy.
- Identify alternate support persons in the school setting.
- Reinforce use of self-esteem-building exercises, such as self-affirmations, meditation, relaxation, or humor.
- Help to identify negative thoughts and unrealistic expectations.
- Encourage to verbalize concerns and feelings.

Have student describe previous encounters with conflict and stressors and how he/she managed to resolve them.

Encourage the student to look at his/her own behavior. Reinforce adaptive coping mechanisms. (N.D. 10, 11, 12)

Explore options to assist student in coping with anxieties and concerns: (N.D. 10, 11, 12, 14)
- Relaxation techniques for stress control (guided imagery, positive self-talk, thought stopping, music therapy)
- Referral to counseling/support resources in school and community
- Use of distractions
- Identification of problems that are out of his/her control

Discuss alternatives to problems (e.g., doing nothing, talking over the problem, or trying to change the situations). What will be the consequences? Practice self-talk about the change and consequences. (N.D. 10, 11, 12)

If the student has an invasive line (N.D. 9, 13, 14)
- Instruct student and family on appropriate practices to prevent infection: assess every 24 hours for redness, inflammation, drainage, or tenderness.
- Monitor temperature every 24 hours, and notify the physician if febrile.
- Maintain aseptic technique.
- Have available an additional dressing kit, spare clamps, heparin, saline, and syringes with prescribed dosage of flush.
- Determine when and under what conditions the tubing or the dressing should be handled.

Determine current knowledge about Lyme disease and educate the student and family about: (N. D. 2, 9, 13, 14)
- Mode of tick transmission
- Body checks after being in tick-infested areas
- The use of repellents and protective clothing
- Prompt and proper removal of ticks from people and animals

Reinforce positive efforts taken by student who follows through with treatment plan. (N.D. 2, 11)

Allow student to make choices, and encourage student to assume responsibility for self-care and health management whenever possible. (N.D. 2, 11, 14)

Collaborate with student, family, and other school personnel to: (N.D. 6, 9, 10, 12)
- Explore the need for a 504 plan or IEP referral.
- Participate in development of 504 plan or IEP.
- Implement aspects of 504 plan or IEP.

## Expected Student Outcomes

The student will:
- Rate on a scale of 1 to 10 how satisfied he/she is with current activity level (1 = not at all satisfied and 10+ very satisfied). (N.D. 1, 5, 10, 11)
- Identify one enjoyable activity each day. (N.D. 1, 10, 11)
- Verbalize understanding of the disease, treatment plan, and interventions. (N.D. 2, 9, 14)
- Participate in classroom activities with modifications as needed. (N.D. 1, 3–8, 10–12)
- Participate in physical education and sports with appropriate modifications. (N.D. 3, 5, 7)
- Report an increase in strength, endurance, and overall improved physical activity tolerance. (N.D. 3, 5, 7)
- Demonstrate measures to increase mobility and describe rationale for the interventions. (N. D. 3, 5, 7)
- Identify any symptoms of infection and report to nurse and parent. (N.D. 2, 13, 14)
- Share feelings regarding the effect of fatigue on his/her life and describe interventions that assist him/her with normal sleep patterns. (N.D. 4, 6, 10, 12)
- Gradually reduce rest periods as energy and stamina increase. (N.D. 3, 4, 5, 7)
- Complete activities despite fatigue. (N.D. 4, 5)
- Progress to activity status prior to disease onset and identify methods to reduce activity intolerance. (N.D. 3, 4, 5, 9, 14)
- Report acceptable control of pain and use relief measures as indicated. (N.D. 8, 9, 14)
- Identify and demonstrate the use of nonpharmacologic approaches to pain. (N.D. 2, 8, 9, 14)
- Identify any side effects of medications and describe factors to eliminate. (N.D. 8, 9, 14)
- Make decisions and follow through with appropriate actions. (N.D. 10, 11, 12)
- Verbalize feelings related to emotional state, and identify their personal strengths in dealing with adversity. (N.D. 10, 11, 12)
- Express a positive outlook for the future. (N.D. 10, 11, 12)
- Practice health behaviors to recover from his/her illness and prevent reinfection. (N.D. 2, 14)
- Verbalize satisfaction in balancing treatment, school, leisure, rest, and nutrition. (N.D. 1, 2, 4, 10, 14)
- Demonstrate the use of adaptive coping skills. (N.D. 10, 11, 12)

# Case Study

Brittany is a 13-year-old eighth grader with a recent diagnosis of Lyme disease. Her initial symptoms appeared to start in mid-summer with frequent complaints of headaches and fatigue. She also developed left-sided knee tenderness and swelling for approximately 2 weeks that was attributed to her competitive field hockey schedule. In late September, Brittany developed photophobia, dizziness, and difficulty sleeping, even though she felt extremely fatigued. Her right knee then became tender and swollen. Brittany's blood work included an ELISA with highly reactive IgG antibody response to *Borrelia burgdorferi*, which is consistent with late-stage Lyme disease. The laboratory result was confirmed with Western blot testing. After a PICC line was inserted and intravenous ceftriaxone therapy initiated, she was discharged from the hospital to her home. Her doctor allowed her to return to school; however, she is excused from physical education and sports until further notice.

Brittany still has a PICC line, which is managed at home, and she will receive a total of 28 days of intravenous antibiotics. Brittany is to take ibuprofen as needed for discomfort. Brittany has returned to school but has had to leave early several days on account of fatigue and headaches. She reports feeling "left out" of her social circle because she has not been able to return to field hockey, nor has she been able to attend her student council meetings and chorus practices before school. She is finding it too hard to get up that early. Brittany missed 9 full days of school and several half days. She is having trouble making up the work and managing the current work assignments. She has always been on the high honor roll; however, this school year she reports, "I do not know what is the matter with me, I feel so dumb all of a sudden!" Brittany is unaware of when she acquired Lyme disease. She lives in New Jersey, an endemic area for Lyme disease, and she spends a lot of times outdoors. She does not do regular body checks for ticks. She did say she finds occasional ticks on her two dogs at home.

# Lyme Disease

| Assessment Data | Nursing Diagnosis | Goals | Nursing Interventions | Expected Outcomes |
|---|---|---|---|---|
| Brittany is experiencing headaches and joint pain. | Chronic pain related to physical symptoms. | Brittany will have a reduction of pain to a tolerable level. | Allow Brittany to use ice packs as necessary to reduce her knee pain and inflammation. | Brittany will report adequate pain control (less than 3 out of 10). |
| | | | Assess Brittany's pain level by utilizing a 0-10 scale to assess the intensity of the pain. (0 being no pain and 10 being the worst pain). | Brittany will use relief measures. |
| | | | Administer pain medications as ordered: assess Brittany's response to pain medication and its effectiveness. | Brittany will identify two non-pharmacologic approaches to manage pain. |
| | | | Incorporate nonpharmacologic approaches to supplement pain medication (e.g., music therapy, guided imagery, and relaxation exercises). | Brittany will demonstrate the use of relaxation exercises to assist with pain control. |
| | | | Reduce or eliminate other factors, such as fatigue, that may increase the pain experience. | |
| Brittany was recently diagnosed with late-stage Lyme disease.<br><br>Symptoms started several months prior to diagnosis.<br><br>Brittany does not practice health behaviors to prevent Lyme disease. | Knowledge deficit and ineffective therapeutic regimen management related to lack of information about the disease and treatment plan and barrier to comprehension secondary to fatigue. | Brittany will demonstrate knowledge of medications and treatment modalities.<br><br>Brittany will increase her knowledge of Lyme disease and prevention of tick-related diseases. | Examine Brittany's health and cultural beliefs and past experiences related to illness and assess their impact on her desire to learn.<br><br>Assess for barriers to learning, adapt teaching time to when Brittany is less fatigued and not in pain. | Brittany will verbalize adequate and correct knowledge in regard to her disease and treatment plan.<br><br>Brittany will practice health behaviors to recover from her illness and prevent reinfection with Lyme disease. |

| Assessment Data | Nursing Diagnosis | Goals | Nursing Interventions | Expected Outcomes |
|---|---|---|---|---|
| | | | Provide instruction at Brittany's level of understanding, repeat information as necessary, and check for accurate feedback. | |
| | | | Review Brittany's understanding of diagnosis and prescribed treatment, clarify any misconceptions. | |
| | | | Determine current knowledge about Lyme disease and educate Brittany and her family: mode of transmission, body checks after being in tick-infested areas, use of repellents and protective clothing, prompt and proper removal of ticks from people and her dogs. | |
| Brittany has complained of extreme fatigue and difficulty sleeping. | Fatigue related to decreased performance, inability to maintain usual routines, and sleep disturbances. | Brittany will maintain an adequate energy level and a normal sleep pattern. | Discuss with the guidance department to change schedule to provide regular rest periods during the school day (lunch and study hall) to help conserve energy and minimize the impact on academic classes. | Brittany will be able to complete her school day despite her fatigue. |
| Brittany is unable to maintain her normal school activities. | | | Help Brittany to identify which activities or times of day cause the most fatigue. | Brittany will gradually reduce her rest periods as her energy and stamina increase. |
| | | | Consult with Brittany and her parents regarding her sleep patterns. | Brittany will describe interventions to assist with normal sleep patterns. |

| Assessment Data | Nursing Diagnosis | Goals | Nursing Interventions | Expected Outcomes |
|---|---|---|---|---|
| | | | Explore strategies to help improve sleep patterns (e.g., calming techniques, soft music, white noise, bedtime snack of foods high in ʟ-tyrptophan. | |
| Brittany is unable to participate in sports or physical education classes.<br><br>Brittany is experiencing knee swelling and pain. | Activity intolerance related to fatigue and musculoskeletal impairment. | Brittany will increase her activity as tolerated with adequate musculoskeletal function. | Consult with Brittany's health care provider in regard to physical education restrictions and the possibility of a modified program.<br><br>Encourage Brittany's natural tendency to be physically active in a less strenuous way, such as isometric exercises or swimming.<br><br>Collaborate with physical education staff to provide a modified physical education program with muscle-strengthening exercise when Brittany is ready to increase her activity and increase tolerance for activity by performing it more slowly or for a shorter period of time with rest periods. | Brittany will progress to activity status prior to disease onset.<br><br>Brittany will identify methods to reduce activity intolerance.<br><br>Brittany will participate in physical education and sports when appropriate and with appropriate modifications.<br><br>Brittany will report an increase in strength, endurance, and overall physical activity tolerance. |
| Brittany states, "I feel so dumb."<br><br>Brittany is having trouble making up the work and managing her current work assignment. | Risk for situational low self-esteem related to her academic difficulties. | Brittany will participate in classroom and school activities with modifications as needed. | Emphasize Brittany's past accomplishments and help her to develop goals based on her success in the past.<br><br>Educate Brittany's teachers on assistive measures that are needed in the classroom. | Brittany will participate in all classroom activities with modifications as needed. |

| Assessment Data | Nursing Diagnosis | Goals | Nursing Interventions | Expected Outcomes |
|---|---|---|---|---|
| Her grades have made her ineligible for high honor roll, which she accomplished in the past. | | | Collaborate with Brittany's teachers to assist in setting realistic goals.<br><br>Encourage Brittany to promote her personal achievements and self-esteem: establish rapport and provide a supportive environment; convey honesty and empathy; reinforce use of self-esteem-building exercises such as self-affirmations, meditation, relaxation, and humor; help to identify negative thoughts and unrealistic expectations. | |
| Brittany has a PICC line. | Risk for infection related to presence of invasive line. | Brittany will maintain skin integrity and prevent infection at invasive line. | Instruct student and family on appropriate practices to prevent infection: inspect her PICC line every 24 hours for redness, inflammation, drainage, or tenderness.<br><br>Monitor temperature every 24 hours and notify the physician if febrile.<br><br>Maintain aseptic technique.<br><br>Brittany's family will provide an additional dressing kit, spare clamp, heparin, saline, and syringes for school as necessary. | Brittany will identify any symptoms of infection and report to nurse and parent. |

| Assessment Data | Nursing Diagnosis | Goals | Nursing Interventions | Expected Outcomes |
|---|---|---|---|---|
| | | | Consult with Brittany's physician, and obtain orders to determine when and under what conditions the tubing or the dressing should be handled, prescribed dosage of flush with use of correct syringe size, and correct amount of flush. | |
| Brittany is unable to participate in extracurricular and school activities due to Lyme disease. | Deficient diversional activity related to inability to participate in field hockey, chorus, and student council. | Brittany will participate in extracurricular activities as tolerated or substitute new activities. | Monitor Brittany's response to her current activities.<br><br>Identify activities available in and outside of school.<br><br>Encourage Brittany to find alternate ways to stay involved in her current activities (e.g., become the manager for her field hockey team, discuss with student council alternate to share role, attend half the chorus practices until stronger).<br><br>Encourage Brittany to look at alternate activities that are less physically demanding (e.g., newspaper club). | Brittany will report satisfaction with her extracurricular activity level by rating on a scale of 1-10 (1 = not at all satisfied and 10 = very satisfied).<br><br>Brittany will identify an enjoyable activity she participates in each day. |
| Brittany reports feeling " left out" of her social circle.<br><br>Brittany missed 9 days of school and has had to leave school early several times. She continues to feel fatigued. | Ineffective coping related to inability to meet role expectations and fatigue. | Brittany will express feelings and concerns.<br><br>Brittany will demonstrate increased adaptation to and psychological comfort with body changes and lifestyle requirements. | Encourage Brittany to verbalize fears and concerns about participating in activities.<br><br>Help Brittany to identify activities that are difficult, and encourage her to verbalize how her fatigue may increase frustration. | Brittany will verbalize feelings related to emotional state and identify her personal strengths in dealing with adversity. |

| Assessment Data | Nursing Diagnosis | Goals | Nursing Interventions | Expected Outcomes |
|---|---|---|---|---|
| Brittany stated, "I feel so dumb all of a sudden" and is having difficulty keeping up with her schoolwork. | | Brittany will utilize healthy adaptive coping methods. | Explore options to assist Brittany in coping with anxieties and concerns: relaxation techniques such as guided imagery and positive self-talk, identifying problems that are out of her control, and referral to the guidance counselor as an additional support person.<br><br>Help Brittany describe previous encounters with stress and conflict and how she managed to resolve them. Reinforce her adaptive coping mechanism.<br><br>Have Brittany identify the progress made; do not underestimate the value of praise and encouragement as an effective motivational technique. | Brittany will verbalize satisfaction in balancing her treatment, school, leisure, rest, and nutrition.<br><br>Brittany will demonstrate the use of adaptive coping skills. |

# References

Belman, A. L., Reynolds, L., Preston, T., Postels, D., Grimson, R., & Coyle, P. K. (1997). Cerebrospinal fluid findings in children with Lyme disease-associated facial nerve palsy. *Archives of Pediatric Adolescent Medicine, 151*(12), 1224–1228.

Bloom, B. J., Wyckoff, P. M., Meissner, H. C., & Steere, A. C. (1998). Neurocognitive abnormalities in children after classic manifestations of Lyme disease. *Pediatric Infectious Diseases, 17*(3), 189–196.

Carpenito, L. J. (2002). *Nursing diagnosis: Application to clinical practice.* Philadelphia: Lippincott.

Centers for Disease Control and Prevention. (2003 August 8). Notice to readers: Final 2002 reports of notifiable diseases. *MMWR Morbidity and Mortality Weekly Report, 52*(31), 741–750.

Centers for Disease Control and Prevention. (2002, January 18). Lyme disease—United States, 2000. *MMWR Morbidity and Mortality Weekly, 51*(02), 29–31.

Centers for Disease Control and Prevention. (n.d.). *Lyme disease epidemiology—CDC divison of vector-borne infectious disease.* Retrieved January 30, 2004, from http://www.cdc.gov/ncidod/dvbid/lyme/epi.htm

Centers for Disease Control and Prevention. (n.d.). *Lyme disease prevention and control—CDC division of vector-borne infectious diseases.* Retrieved February 20, 2004, from http://www.cdc.gov/ncidod/dvbid/lyme/prevent.htm

Eppes, S. C. (2003). Diagnosis, treatment, and prevention of Lyme disease in children. *Pediatric Drugs, 5*(6), 363–372.

Fallon, B. A., Kochevar, J. M., Gaito, A., & Nields, J. A. (1998). The underdiagnosis of neuropsychiatric Lyme disease in children and adults. *Psychiatric Clinics of North America, 21*(3), 693–703

Fallon, B. A., Nields, J., Burrascano, J. J., Liegner, K., DelBene, D., & Liebowitz, M. R. (1992). The neuropsychiatric manifestations of Lyme borreliosis, *Psychiatric Quarterly 63*(1), Retrieved January 30, 2004, from http://library.lymenet.org

Hayes, E.B., & Piesman, J. (2003). How can we prevent Lyme diseases? *New England Journal of Medicine 348*(24), 2424–2430.

Nachman, S. A., & Pontrelli, L. (2003). Central nervous system Lyme disease. *Seminars in Pediatric Infectious Diseases, 14*(2), 123–130.

Nadelman, R. B., Nowakowski, J., Fish, D., Falco, R. C., Freeman, K., McKenna, D., et al. (2001). Prophylaxis with single-dose doxycycline for the prevention of Lyme disease after an *Ixodes scapularis* tick bite. *New England Journal of Medicine, 345*(2), 79–84.

NANDA International. (2003). *NANDA nursing diagnosis: Definitions & classification 2003-2004.* Philadelphia: Author.

Pachner, A. R. (1989). Neurologic manifestations of Lyme disease, the new "great imitator." *Reviews of Infectious Diseases , 11*(6), 1482–1486.

Rawlings, J. (1999). The epizootiology and prevention and control of selected tick-borne diseases. *12th international conference on Lyme disease and other spirochetal and tick-borne disorders,* Retrieved February 2, 2004, from http://www.medscape.com/viewprogram/1689_pnt

Shapiro, E. D., & Gerber, M. A. (2000). *Clinical infectious diseases, 31,* 533–542.

Steere, A. C. (1989). Lyme disease. *New England Journal of Medicine, 321,* 586–596.

Tager, F .A., Fallon, B. A., Keilp, J., Rissenberg, M., Jones, C.R., & Liebowitz, M. R. (2001). A controlled study of cognitive deficits in children with Lyme disease. *Journal of Neuropsychiatry and Clinical Neurosciences, 13*(4), 500–507.

Vazquez, M., Sparrow, S., & Shapiro, E. D. (2003). Long-term neuropsychologic and health outcomes of children with facial nerve palsy attributable to Lyme disease. *Pediatrics, 112*(2), e93–e97.

Wong, D. L., Hockenberry, M. J., Wilson, D., Winkelstein, M. L., & Kline, N. E. (2003). Chapter 26: Family centered care of the child during illness and hospitalization. *Nursing Care of Infants and Children* (pp. 1031–1100). St. Louis, MO: Mosby.

Wormser, G. P., Nadelman, R. B., Dattwyler, R. J., Dennis, D. T., Shapiro, E. D., & Steere, A. C., et al. (2000). Practice guidelines for the treatment of Lyme disease. *Clinical Infectious Diseases, 31*(Supp 1), S1–14.

Lyme Disease

## Bibliography

*Atlas of Dermatology*
http://www.dermis.net/doia/diagnose.asp?zugr=d&lang=e&diagnr=88810&topic=t
Photographs of erythema migrans.

Centers for Disease Control and Prevention (CDC)
http://www.cdc.gov/ncidod/dvbid/lyme/index.htm
CDC's Lyme disease home page.

*Lyme Disease: The Facts The Challenge*
http://www.niaid.nih.gov/publications/lyme/niaid%20lymedisbookf2.pdf
Booklet published by National Institutes of Health.

National Institute of Allergy and Infectious Diseases, National Institutes of Health
http://www.niaid.nih.gov/dmid/lyme
Information about Lyme disease.

## Resources

American Lyme Disease Foundation
Mill Pond Offices
293 Route 100
Somers, NY 10589
914-277-6970
http://www.aldf.com

Columbia University Lyme Disease Research
Columbia Presbyterian Medical Center
New York State Psychiatric Institute
1051 Riverside Drive
Room 3200
New York, NY 10032
http://www.columbia-lyme.org

Lyme Disease Association
PO Box 1438
Jackson, NJ 08527
1-888-366-6611
http://www.lymediseaseassociation.org/index.htm

Lyme Disease Network of New Jersey
43 Winton Road
East Brunswick, NJ, 08816
http://www.lymenet.org

## Chapter Fifty-two

# Marfan Syndrome

Deborah Kotlas Ilardi

## Introduction

In 1986, Flo Hyman, an Olympic silver medalist in volleyball, died suddenly during a championship match. In 1996, Jonathan Larson, a Broadway composer, died following his last trip to the emergency department, where clinicians improperly diagnosed gastroenteritis. Both of these people died of an aortic rupture secondary to undiagnosed Marfan syndrome, a somewhat rare connective tissue disorder in which cardiac and other complications can cause sudden death (especially from physical exertion) or greatly impair quality of life (Ryan-Krause, 2002).

Marfan syndrome is an inheritable condition that affects the connective tissue. The primary purpose of connective tissue is to hold the body together and provide a framework for growth and development. In Marfan syndrome, the connective tissue is defective and does not act as it should. Because connective tissue is found throughout the body, Marfan syndrome can affect many body systems, including the skeleton, eyes, heart and blood vessels, nervous system, skin, and lungs. Marfan syndrome affects men, women, and children and has been found among people of all races and ethnic backgrounds. It is estimated that at least 1 in 5,000 people in the United States have the disorder (National Marfan Foundation, 2004a).

Students with Marfan syndrome will each present to the school nurse with a unique set of needs based on the body systems affected, their age, and their progression in the illness itself. This creates a unique challenge for the school nurse in preparing the plan for their care. Most of these students will require frequent assessment and modification of their plan. Explaining this changing picture to the school staff with whom the student spends most of the day presents a second set of challenges, both complex and time-consuming. Because outwardly the student may appear healthy, the job is even more difficult. Students with Marfan syndrome rarely need to be home-schooled because of their illness, even when potential life-threatening risks are present.

## Pathophysiology

Marfan syndrome is caused by a defect (mutation) in the gene that determines the structure of fibrillin, a protein that is an important part of connective tissue. A person with Marfan syndrome is born with the disorder, even though it may not be diagnosed until later in life (National

Marfan Foundation, 2004a). Interestingly, each person with the disease will experience unique body system involvement. This is called variable expression, and it means basically that each person's body and other genetics will determine to what degree the weakened fibrillin affects the person. This expression of the syndrome is something that is beyond scientific understanding at this time. Whether mild or severe, in most cases the disease progresses as the person ages.

The defective gene can be inherited: The child of a person who had Marfan syndrome has a 50% chance of inheriting the disease. But even without family history, sometimes a gene defect occurs during the formation of sperm or egg cells. Still, two unaffected parents have only a 1 in 10,000 chance of having a child with Marfan syndrome. Possibly 25% of the cases are due to a spontaneous mutation at the time of conception (National Marfan Foundation, 2004a).

Characteristics of body systems most often affected are as follows:

- *Skeleton:* affected persons typically are very tall, slender, and loose jointed; affects long bones such that arms, legs, fingers, and toes may be disproportionate in relation to the rest of the body; long, narrow face; arched, high palate causing teeth to be crowded; indented or protruding sternum; scoliosis; flat feet
- *Eyes:* more than half experience dislocation of the lenses of one or both eyes, either minimally or pronounced and obvious to the skilled ophthalmologist; retinal detachment is a serious complication of the disorder; often nearsighted (myopic); some develop glaucoma or cataracts
- *Cardiovascular:* heart murmur, mitral valve prolapse; tachycardic arrythmias; aortic dilatation, dissection, or rupture is possible, causing sudden death
- *Nervous system:* dural ectasia, a weakened and stretched dura in the spinal column, can cause symptoms of mild discomfort or radiating pain in the abdomen, or pain, numbness, or weakness of the legs
- *Skin:* stretch marks without weight change that can occur at any age; abdominal or inguinal hernia
- *Lungs:* there is a risk of pneumothorax if the alveoli become stretched and swollen; sleep-related disorders such as snoring or sleep apnea

(Marfan Syndrome Fact Book, 2004)

## Management

There is no cure for Marfan syndrome. The range of treatment options can minimize and sometimes prevent complications. Individual specialists will need to individualize care, depending upon which body systems have been affected. While it is a lifelong disorder, early diagnosis and advances in medical technology have improved the quality of life for people with Marfan syndrome and lengthened their lifespan. Advances being made by researchers provide hope for the future. With early diagnosis and appropriate management, the life expectancy for someone with Marfan syndrome is similar to that of the average person (Marfan Syndrome Fact Book, 2004). With the increasing emphasis on physical fitness and sports participation, ensuring that all children can safely engage in vigorous activity is crucial. Timely diagnosis and appropriate interdisciplinary management of Marfan syndrome are vital in preventing early deaths, unnecessary disabilities, and poor adjustment to this chronic condition (Ryan-Krause, 2002).

Management includes the following:
- *Skeletal:* Annual evaluations are needed to detect change in the spine and the sternum, particularly during times of rapid growth, such as adolescence. Serious deformity can cause disfigurement and also prevent the heart and lungs from functioning properly. Bracing and surgery are possible interventions.
- *Eyes:* Regular eye examinations are crucial. Corrective lenses, either glasses or contact lenses, can correct acuity; surgery may be needed for lens displacement or detached retina.
- *Cardiovascular:* Regular examinations and echocardiograms evaluate the size of the heart and aorta and the way the heart functions. Awareness of the signs of difficulty, including chest, back, or abdominal pain, is crucial prevention. Beta-blockers may be required to decrease the stress on the aorta; surgery to repair or replace a valve or to repair the aorta may be needed. Endocarditis is a complication of heart surgery, and premedicating for dental work will be required prophylaxis afterward [emergency identification is prudent.]
- *Nervous system:* Medication may minimize pain if dural ectasia develops. This condition is best identified through magnetic resonance imaging (MRI); myelogram, computed tomography (CT) scan, or spinal x-rays may also be helpful.
- *Lungs:* Discourage smoking; manage other respiratory symptoms as needed; emergency care is needed for spontaneous pneumothorax.

Pregnancy should not be lightly undertaken. Specialists should monitor the high-risk status of a pregnant woman with Marfan syndrome (Marfan Syndrome Fact Book, 2004).

Those providing care should always consider the emotional and psychosocial effects of living with chronic disease. Marfan syndrome affects the family system, and the appropriate professionals on an ongoing basis should address everyone's needs.

Exercise is important for students with Marfan syndrome. It instills a sense of physical and psychological well-being, improves exercise endurance, lowers blood pressure, reduces weight, regulates metabolism and gastrointestinal function, increases bone density and physical strength, and often leads to beneficial lifestyle changes such as smoking cessation, moderation of alcohol consumption, and improved nutrition. People with Marfan syndrome and their families, as well as physical educators and healthcare professionals charged with overseeing the physical activity of students, should be aware of the impact different forms of exercise have on their bodies and basic guidelines for participating safely in physical activities (**Table 1**). Because most exercise and athletic activities involve combinations of isokinetic and isometric muscle work and aerobic and anaerobic energy use, and because the proportion of work and energy is determined by the nature of the activity, decisions about how strenuously a person participates and sometimes even the position played in a team sport require significant discussion. Students with Marfan syndrome should always avoid contact sports. The risk of damage to the aorta and the eyes is too great.

The school nurse can be a welcomed link in the care of students with Marfan syndrome. There are several areas in which to excel:

Share knowledge of Marfan syndrome with students, families, and school staff. Explain what it is and how it appears in those affected.

Provide emotional support. Students diagnosed may go through a "why me?" phase as they learn about the potential complications.

Encourage frequent checkups and genetic counseling to maximize health. Emphasize the importance of prescribed medications (beta-blockers), following activity restrictions and avoiding smoking (Delong, 2004).

Encourage evaluation for possible Marfan syndrome when suspicious symptoms are noted during nursing assessment of a child or adolescent.

# Individualized Healthcare Plan

## Assessment

### History

- Family health history
- Growth, development, and health prior to diagnosis
- Age at diagnosis
- Circumstances prompting evaluation and diagnosis
- Initial care and lifestyle changes
- Systems currently affected, severity
- Immediate and long-term prognosis
- Program of medical and surgical care
- Frequency of evaluations
- Results of last evaluation
- Family development of acceptance
- Student's development of acceptance
- Past supportive persons, support group involvement
- Past professional eye-examination reports

### Current Status and Management

- Height and weight
- Deformity of the sternum and spinal curves
- Appearance of limbs, fingers, and toes
- Arm span
- Current vision, interval screening for vision complaints
- Emergency care plans (ECPs) for aortic dilation and dissection or rupture, lens dislocation and retinal detachment, sudden shortness of breath and pain associated with breathing
- Current circulatory status: blood pressure, apical and radial pulse
- Stretch marks and abdominal, inguinal, or umbilical bulges or weaknesses
- Current respiratory status: bilateral lung sounds, respiratory rate and effort initially and if symptomatic
- Current medications
- Current therapies
- Nervous system function of lower extremities (weakness, numbness, pain)
- Current management plan
- Student's and family's understanding of management plan
- Spinal bracing
- Current activity tolerance: getting to and from school, traveling around both inside and outside the campus, recreational play, and physical education classes

### Self-care

- Student's knowledge of health-care needs and management plan
- Ability to self-monitor: activity tolerance, vision, skin, breathing
- Student's ability to advocate for self with staff
- Decision-making skills

### Psychosocial Status

- Student's acceptance of family interventions
- Student's utilization of coping strategies to deal with health condition: effective, ineffective
- Family's utilization of coping strategies to deal with health condition: effective, ineffective
- Behavioral issues: risk-taking behaviors, fear of performance
- Feelings about visible deformity and activity limitations
- Participation in school activities, community activities, family activities
- Supportive persons he/she is comfortable talking to (parents, physicians, school staff, psychologist, etc.)

- Academic achievement: past and current
- School attendance pattern: reasons for absences
- Physical education and other activity restrictions
- Modifications needed in curriculum or course requirements: alternative assignments due to physical education restrictions, extended timelines for completion of assignments, and process to obtain missed assignments due to absences for appointments or illness
- ECPs needed
- School reentry plan following surgery

## Nursing Diagnoses (N.D.) (NANDA, 2003)

**N.D. 1** Chronic self-esteem disturbance (NANDA 00119) related to diagnosis of chronic illness with multiple unknowns

**N.D. 2** Risk for activity intolerance (NANDA 00094 or 00092) related to:
- joint laxity, respiratory problems
- cardiac problems

**N.D. 3** Imbalanced nutrition: less than body requirements (NANDA 00002) related to: loss of balance between nutritional intake and exercise

**N.D. 4** Risk for disproportionate growth (NANDA 00113) related to: (potential for) abnormal bone development (progressive spinal deformity, sternal protrusion or concavity, long bone development)

**N.D. 5** Risk for impaired skin integrity (NANDA 00044 or 00047) related to: altered fibrillin efficiency

**N.D. 6** Ineffective breathing pattern (NANDA 00032) related to: loss of elasticity of alveoli and potential for pneumothorax

**N.D. 7** Risk for powerlessness (NANDA 00152 or 00125) related to: current (or potential for) life-threatening health complications

**N.D. 8** Impaired physical mobility (NANDA 00085) related to: potential for spinal deformity

**N.D. 9** Disturbance in body image (NANDA 00118) related to (perception of physical disability):
- scoliosis
- limb length
- joint laxity
- surgical scars

**N.D. 10** Risk for injury (NANDA 00035) related to aortic dilation, dissection or rupture

## Goals

The student will participate in development and implementation of ECP. (N.D. 6, 10)

The student will participate in development and implementation of emergency evacuation plan. (N.D. 2, 10)

The student will be independent in school setting. (N.D. 1, 2)

The student will increase self-acceptance and positive self-esteem. (N.D. 1, 7, 9)

The student will increase his/her knowledge of the disease process (N.D. 1, 5, 7)

The student will assist in identifying and implementing modifications to plan of care. (N.D. 7)

The student will share personal health information appropriately with staff and peers. (N.D. 4, 7)

The student will maintain adequate dietary and fluid intake. (N.D. 3)

The student will utilize healthy adaptation and coping skills. (N.D. 1, 4, 7, 10)

The student will prevent predictable physical injury. (N.D. 4)

The student will manage his/her pain effectively. (N.D. 4, 8)

The student will communicate effectively with parents/guardians and school staff about school-day health needs (N.D. 1, 9, 10).

## Nursing Interventions

Periodically update health information with parent/guardian and student. (N.D. 3, 4, 10)

Assist the student to manage episodes of pain during the school day (ice-packing joints, medication, rest, etc.). (N.D. 2, 6, 8, 10)

Obtain parent and physician authorization for administration of medication. (N.D. 2, 4-6, 8, 10)

Develop ECPs and revise as needed. (N.D. 10)

Decide when and how information will be shared with education staff. Review and update regularly. (N.D. 7, 10)

Establish plan with parents/guardians and student to obtain health updates and share information. Review regularly. (N.D. 7, 10)

Educate school staff on student's individual needs and review emergency plans (N.D. 10)

Assist teachers to modify physical education activities and requirements, as needed. (N.D. 8)

Review playground safety rules with student. (N.D. 8)

Encourage student to report changes in skin, vision, breathing, leg pain, activity intolerance, getting through halls, stairs, on and off bus, etc. (N.D. 7)

Encourage independence and activity that does not put the student at risk for injury. (N.D. 1, 7, 8, 10)

Screen vision, height, weight, spine as needed or as agreed upon with parents and physician. (N.D. 3, 5, 6)

Encourage student to verbalize feelings about chronic illness. (N.D. 1)

Provide positive feedback to student, parents/guardians, and staff regarding effective management of symptoms. (N.D. 1, 7)

Provide age-appropriate information on Marfan syndrome to the student. (N.D. 1)

If surgery is required, assist in planning for homebound instruction and reintegration back into school. (N.D. 2)

Provide student with opportunities to take on responsibilities for his/her care and control situations when appropriate (i.e., talking to primary care provider office for appointments with parent permission). (N.D. 1)

Clarify misconceptions the student has about self-care. (N.D. 1)

Provide assessment of student's subjective concerns as they occur, such as respiratory difficulty, irregular heart rate, or activity intolerance. (N.D. 2, 3, 4, 5)

Teach student how to report abnormal symptoms to the teacher, health office, and parents/guardians. (N.D. 5, 6, 10)

Teach students how to advocate responsibly for self (N.D. 9)

Encourage student to express how he/she feels about or views himself/herself. (N.D. 1, 9)

Encourage student to ask questions at home and at school to assist in making good decisions or problem solving. (N.D. 1, 7, 9)

Assist teachers to organize school day to minimize:
- pain and discomfort (N.D. 2)
- energy expenditure, if activity tolerance is occurring. (N.D. 2, 8)

Assist the student and parents/guardians to obtain medical emergency identification bracelet or necklace. (N.D. 6, 10)

Encourage the student to wear medical emergency identification bracelet or necklace. (N.D. 6, 10)

## Expected Student Outcomes

The student will:
- Effectively communicate health concerns and needs to parents/guardians and school staff. (N.D. 1, 7)
- Identify and describe potential health problems. (N.D. 3, 5, 6, 7)
- Demonstrate avoidance of risk activities that could cause injury. (N.D. 10)
- Follow ECP(s) and evacuation plan when required. (N.D. 8, 10)
- Demonstrate adequate nutritional and fluid intake during the school day. (N.D. 3)
- Describe what Marfan syndrome is and how it affects his/her body (age-appropriate). (N.D. 2, 4, 5, 6, 8, 10)
- Participate in classroom activities, with specific activity limitations as needed. (N.D. 1, 2, 6, 8, 10)
- Demonstrate compliance with activity limitations. (N.D. 2, 10)
- Demonstrate effective coping and adaptation skills. (N.D. 1, 7, 9)
- Demonstrate independent mobility in the school environments. (N.D. 8)
- Utilize measures to minimize pain and discomfort during the school day. (N.D. 2, 4, 5, 6, 8)
- Consistently wear medical emergency information bracelet or necklace. (N.D. 6, 10)

# Case Study

Andrew James is a 16-year-old who attends St. Joseph's High School. He was diagnosed with Marfan syndrome at age 2. His mother and sister also have Marfan syndrome. His mother is 42 years old and has been in a wheelchair as long as Andy can remember. He has seen a video of his mother walking when she was younger and he was an infant. The family does not share the specifics of her illness with the school. Andy just knows that her back is curved and she doesn't walk. Andy's sister's illness is manifest in her physical appearance, but she does not have cardiac involvement at this time.

Andy's symptoms are physical appearance, skeletal and cardiac. He is tall and slender. His sternum curves inward (pectus excavatum). He has long fingers and toes, a wide arm span, mild scoliosis, and a 4.8-cm aortic aneurysm. He is scheduled for surgical repair in 2 weeks, during a school vacation. Then he will be on homebound status for approximately 4 weeks. He will receive homebound instruction. When he returns to school, he will require modifications in activities and in his plan of care.

Andy has two close friends that he has known since elementary school, Kim and Matt . They also know his family. They feel they know how to keep Andy safe. They have proven to be trustworthy, and Andy shares his health information with them openly. They also try to help him maintain some privacy by not discussing his information with others. Andy and his friends have visited the school nurse together. They know they can share concerns with her.

Each fall the school nurse meets with Andy to review and revise his plan. The school nurse keeps in touch with his mother by phone. Plans typically include:

1. Cardiac precautions
- ECP
- Notification of teachers and staff
- Emergency medical identification
- Activity tolerance and modifications for physical education and recess
- Evacuation plan
2. School health screenings
- Height and weight twice yearly
- Vision twice yearly
- Hearing once yearly
- Spinal screening twice yearly
- Results documented and shared with parent, primary care provider, eye care professional, orthopedic care provider, cardiac care provider
- Release of information signed each fall with names and numbers of above
3. Activity tolerance
- School has three floors, walk stairs as tolerated; however, Andy also is given a pass to use the elevator as needed for low-tolerance days; pass also excuses lateness of up to 5 minutes during hall passing time
- Andy does not want to be excused from physical education requirements whenever possible. However, activity limitations from his physician and parents require Andy to walk during running activities and no participation in contact sports. Because each physical education session of 5 weeks offers at least one noncontact activity, Andy will be given priority to choose the appropriate one for his level of activity tolerance. If there are any problems, he will talk with his physical education teacher or come to the nurse for assistance. He will not put himself at risk by participating.

# Marfan Syndrome

| Assessment Data | Nursing Diagnosis | Goals | Nursing Interventions | Expected Outcomes |
|---|---|---|---|---|
| Physician order received for no physical education activities until after surgery and recovery. Homebound instruction for approximately 4 weeks following surgery. | Activity intolerance related to cardiac complications. | Andy will participate in physical education classes, without participating in physical activities. Andy will actively participate in homebound instruction. | Inform physical education teacher of activity limitations. Educate school staff about student's individual needs. Explain excuse policy to Andy and parents. He can still participate in class without doing activities (learning rules, learning how the sport is played, scored, etc., and still get credit). | Andy will comply with activity limitations. Andy will participate in classroom activities with physical limitations. |
| Andy expresses concern over earning credit and graduating on time (he will miss 4 weeks of school and midterm exams). | Self-esteem disturbance related to chronic illness resulting in need to miss 4 weeks of school. | Andy will effectively communicate his academic needs and concerns to parents and teachers. | Inform Andy's teachers of his need to be out of the classroom for 4 weeks and discuss the possible need for modified assignments or course requirements. Collaborate with Andy's guidance counselor, teachers, and parents to assist Andy to maintain academic achievement. Contact parents by phone to review plan after he is home from the hospital and ready for homebound instruction. Encourage Andy to advocate for himself with teachers. | Andy will successfully complete coursework with modifications as needed. Andy will maintain successful academic progress. |
| Andy has a 4.8-cm aortic aneurysm. Surgery is planned in 2 weeks. | Risk for injury related to aortic aneurysm. | Andy will assist in preventing and managing predictable physical injury. | Encourage Andy and his parents to communicate with teachers by phone or e-mail. Develop ECP with parent, Andy, and physician regarding what to do if a rupture of the aneurysm occurs. | Andy will demonstrate avoidance of risk activities that could cause his aneurysm to dissect or rupture. Andy informs school staff immediately if signs or symptoms develop. |

# Emergency Care Plan
# St. Joseph's High School

Date: _____  HR: 912 _____

Student: Andrew James _____  Grade: 10 _____

Date of birth: 1-1-87 _____

Parent(s)/Guardian(s): Michael & _____  Home telephone: 567-1199 _____

Marie James _____  Father's work: 646-5542 _____

Address: 7406 Ventura Circle, Brightsville  Mother's work: 67-8642 _____

Mother's cell: 236-3814 _____

Primary Care Provider: Dr. Mary Dillard _____  Telephone: 567-2987 _____

Hospital Preferance: St. Joseph's Hospital, Brightsville _____

Ambulance Preferance: none _____

Health Insurance: BCBS (father primary – family coverage) _____

Health Condition: Marfan syndrome—aortic aneurysm, vision problems _____

## Cardiac:

1. **General:** Do not go anywhere in the building or on the grounds alone; sit on the ground or lay down if dizziness develops, send friend for adult help, take own pulse if possible; tell friends about health problems, wear medical emergency ID or carry emergency card at all times.

2. **Aortic aneurysm (severe pain in the chest or loss of consciousness):** Friend to call "O" from nearest phone or get nearest adult to do it and page the nurse, give your name, Andy's name, your location; if asked to call 911 be prepared to provide answers to same questions above until someone else arrives; locate the nearest AED and bring it to the site.

3. **Abnormal symptoms (uneasiness, rapid heart rate, respiratory difficulty):** Same as "2" above, but relay that Andy is conscious, ask nurse's office to bring a wheelchair.

## Vision:

**For sudden changes in visual field, spots, floaters, or loss of vision in one or both eyes:** Cup hand over affected eye for protection, tell the nearest adult you are having an eye-related emergency, come to the nurse with another student or have someone call the nurse to come to you.

Signatures:

Reviewed by _____ Date_____

Student _____ Date_____

School Nurse_____ Date_____

Parent/guardian (if required)_____ Date_____

# Emergency Evacuation Plan
# St. Joseph's High School

Date: _____     HR: 912 _____

Student: Andrew James _____     Grade: 10 _____

Date of birth: 1-1-87 _____

Parent(s)/Guardian(s): Michael & _____     Home telephone: 567-1199 _____

Marie James _____     Father's work: 646-5542 _____

Address: 7406 Ventura Circle, Brightsville     Mother's work: 67-8642 _____

Mother's cell: 236-3814 _____

Health Condition: Marfan syndrome—aortic aneurysm, vision problems _____

## Emergency Evacuation From the School Building:

**If feeling well:**
1. Exit, with class, to first floor
2. Exit with friend through front doors to flagpole meeting area and wait for the school nurse's instruction.
3. If exit is blocked, go to the closest administrator with a walkie-talkie, have them notify the school nurse of your location.
4. Follow school nurse's instructions.

**If not feeling well:**
1. Report to the area of refuge (Rooms 116, 216, or 316) and wait for adult assistance and/or direction.
2. Once outside, have an administrator advise the nurse of your location.
3. If students are placed on buses, report the number of the bus you are on. (This may have to be done by radio, through the transportation office and back to the school, depending on the nature of the emergency.)
4. If none of this is possible, make sure the adult you are with knows that you have special, potentially life-threatening health concerns.

**Table 1. Physical Education and Activity Guidelines**

Prepared by the National Marfan Foundation Professional Advisory Board

Exercise is important for people with Marfan syndrome. It instills a sense of physical and psychological well-being, improves exercise endurance, lowers blood pressure, reduces weight, regulates metabolism and gastrointestinal function, increases bone density and physical strength, and often leads to beneficial lifestyle changes, such as smoking cessation, moderation of alcohol consumption, and improved nutrition.

## Classification of Sports and Activities
(Modified from a classification devised by the American Academy of Pediatrics, 2001)

Before you apply this chart to your specific situation, it is important to realize that many sports can fall within several categories, depending on the intensity of your participation. It is essential to talk to your doctor about the sports and activities that are safe for you, and how to monitor your exertion level so that exercise remains safe throughout your involvement.

| | |
|---|---|
| **Contact/collision high potential:** strenuous | Boxing, field hockey, football, ice hockey, lacrosse, martial arts, rodeo, skiing (water), soccer, wrestling |
| **Limited contact:** strenuous | Baseball, bicycling (intense), gymnastics, horseback riding, skating (ice and roller), skiing (downhill and cross-country), softball, squash, volleyball |
| **Noncontact:** strenuous | Aerobic dancing (high-impact), crew, running (fast), weight lifting |
| **Noncontact:** moderately strenuous | Aerobic dancing (low-impact), badminton, bicycling (leisurely), jogging, swimming (leisurely), table tennis, tennis |
| **Noncontact:** nonstrenuous | Golf, bowling, riflery, walking |

People with Marfan syndrome should always avoid contact sports because of the risk of damaging the aorta and injuring the eyes. Strenuous activities also should be avoided because of the stress placed on the aorta. Every activity has graduations, and no recommendations hold in all circumstances. For example, shooting baskets in the driveway is different from full-court basketball, and bicycling 10 miles in 1 hour on a level course is different from competing in a triathlon. To maximize safety of low-intensity, noncontact activities, it is important to take necessary precautions, such as not carrying a heavy bag of golf clubs, and to avoid intense competitive efforts. In short, it is essential for each individual with Marfan syndrome to discuss physical activities, and specific activity levels, with his/her healthcare provider(s) so that exercise can be incorporated safely into the regular healthcare routine.

# References

American Academy of Pediatrics, Committee on Sports Medicine and Fitness. (2001). Medical conditions affecting sports participation. *Pediatrics, 107*(5), 1205–1209.

Delong, M. F. (2004). NurseWeek: *Marfan syndrome.* Retrieved March 1, 2004, from http://www.nurseweek.com/ce/ce1102a.html

Health Newsflash. (2004). *Marfan syndrome fact book.* Retrieved February 26, 2004, from http://www.healthnewsflash.com/conditions/marfan_syndrome.

National Marfan Foundation. (2004a). *About Marfan syndrome: What is Marfan syndrome?* Retrieved February 26, 2004, from http://www.marfan.org/nmf

National Marfan Foundation. (2004b). *Physical education and activity guidelines: National Marfan Foundation.* Retrieved February 26, 2004, from http://www.marfan.org/nmf/GetSubContentRequestHandler.do?type=print&sub_menu_item_co

NANDA International. (2003). *Nursing diagnoses: Definitions & classification 2003-2004.* Philadelphia: Author

Ryan-Krause, P. (2002). Identify and manage Marfan syndrome in children. *Nurse Practitioner: American Journal of Primary Health Care, 27*(10), 26–36.

# Bibliography

American Academy of Pediatrics. (1998). Health supervision of children with Marfan syndrome. *Pediatrics, 98*(5), 978–982.

American Academy of Pediatrics. (2002). AAP guidelines for pediatricians: Sudden cardiac death (SCD). Retrieved January 16, 2005, from http://www.aap.org/family/sportsshorts

Behrmann, R. E., & Klingman, R. M. (2001). *Nelson's essentials of pediatrics* (4th ed.). Philadelphia: Saunders.

Connecticut Department of Education. (1992). *Serving students with special care needs.* Hartford, CT: State of Connecticut DOE.

Pyeritz, R. E., & Gasner, C. (2001). *Marfan syndrome* (5th ed.). Port Washington, NY: National Marfan Foundation.

Rubenstein, A.., & Korf, F. B. (1990). *A Handbook for Patients, Families, and Health Care Professionals.* New York: Thieme Medical.

Wong, D. L. (1996). *Clinical manual of pediatric nursing* (4th ed.). St. Louis, MO: Mosby-Year Book.

Wong, D. L., Hockenberry, M. J., Wilson, D., Winkelstein, M. L., & Kline, N. E. (2003). *Wong's nursing care of infants and children* (7th ed.). St. Louis, MO: Mosby.

# Resources

American Academy of Pediatrics
141 Northwest Point Boulevard
Elk Grove Village, IL 60007-1098
847-434-4000
847-434-8000 (fax)
http://www.aap.org

American Heart Association
National Center
7272 Greenville Avenue
Dallas, TX 75231
1-800-242-8721
http://www.americanheart.org/children

National Institute of Arthritis and Musculoskeletal and Skin Diseases
National Institutes of Health
1 AMS Circle
Bethesda, MD 20892-3675
301-495-4484

301-565-2966 (TTY)
1-877-226-NIAMS (4267)
301-718-6366 (fax)
http:// www.niams.nih.gov

National Human Genome Research Institute
National Institutes of Health
9000 Rockville Pike
Bethesda, MD 20892
1- 800-411-1222 (information about entering a clinical study)
http://genom.gov

National Marfan Foundation
22 Manhasset Avenue
Port Washington, NY 11050
516-883-8712
1-800-8-MARFAN
http://www.marfan.org

## Chapter Fifty-three

# Metachromatic Leukodystrophy

Jeanette H. Williams

## Introduction

Metachromatic leukodystrophy (MLD) is an inherited, progressive disorder that affects the central nervous system and peripheral nerves. Because of absence of the enzyme arysulfatase A, a material called cerebroside sulfate accumulates and is toxic to cells, especially neurons (MedlinePlus, 2003). It is derived from the Greek word *leuko* (white) because it affects the white matter of the nervous system and *dystrophy*, meaning imperfect growth (United Leukodystrophy Foundation, 2003). Some of the other forms of leukodystrophies are adrenoleukodystrophy (ALD)/adrenomyeloneuropathy (AMN), Aicardi-Goiutieres syndrome, Alexander's disease, CACH (childhood ataxia with central nervous system hypomyelination or vanishing white matter disease), CADASIL (cerebral autosomal dominant arteriopathy with subcortical infarcts and leukoencephalopathy), Canavan's disease, cerebrotendinous xanthomatosis (CTX), Krabbe's disease, neonatal adrenoleukodystrophy, Pelizaeus-Merzbacher disease, Refsum's disease, van der Knaap syndrome, and Zellweger syndrome (United Leukodystrophy Foundation).

The incidence of MLD is about 1 in 40,000 to 100,000 (MLD Foundation, 2003), although a high incidence of the disease occurs in the Habbanite Jewish community, with 1 in 75 births (Zlotogora et al., 1995).

MLD is devastating to families. It takes a severe emotional, financial, and physical toll on them. The constant and total care required over an extended period of time is extremely difficult. Families need nursing and respite care in order to cope with caring for a child with this serious illness. There is also a sense of guilt in having passed on this horrible disease to their child. Because the disease is inherited, families usually do not have additional children once a diagnosis has been made. Counseling and extended family support will help the parents to remain stable during this trying period of their lives.

## Pathophysiology

MLD, the most common form of leukodystrophy (National Organization for Rare Diseases [NORD], 2003), is an inherited neurometabolic disorder that involves primarily the white matter of the brain and central nervous system (MLD Foundation, 2003). MLD is an autosomal recessive degenerative disease, which means both parents must be carriers. Offspring have a 25% chance of having the disease and a 50% chance of being carriers. The MLD defect is found on chromosome 22 (Ouvrier, McLeod, & Pollard, 1999).

MLD is a disorder caused by a buildup of sulfatides in the central nervous system and also in various organs of the body, including the kidney, liver, and gallbladder. This accumulation of sulfatides is due to a missing enzyme or deficit in the activity of the enzyme arylsulfatase A (Tylki-Szymanska, Czartoryska, & Lugowska, 1998; MLD Foundation, 2003). Biochemically, it is characterized by accumulation of sulfatide in certain tissues, brain, peripheral nerves, kidney, liver, gallbladder, and possibly spleen. It causes a lack of growth and severe loss of the myelin sheath (fatty covering), which acts as an insulator on nerve fibers (National Institutes of Health, 1997). Demyelinization is diffuse, and accumulation of metachromatic granules occurs in the central and peripheral nervous system as well as other organs (kidney, liver, and gallbladder). A severe loss of myelin occurs, especially in the late infantile form of MLD (Tylki-Szymanska et al., 1998). The early signs and symptoms may be vague and gradual in onset.

Most experts speak of three types of MLD: (1) late infantile, with symptoms appearing between age 6 months and 2 years; (2) juvenile, with onset between early childhood and late adolescence; and (3) adult, with onset after age 16 (Kaye, 2001; MLD Foundation, 2003, Gieselmann, Kreysing, & vonFigura, 1994). Ouvrier et al. (1999) also include a fourth type, multiple sulfatase deficiency, and a fifth type, the AB variant.

In type 1, the late infantile form, the child has normal development until 6 months to 2 years of age. Clinical features include blindness, loss of motor function, rigidity, loss of mental abilities, seizures, and impaired swallowing ability. Seizures are common (Balslev, Cortex, Blaser, & Haslam, 1997; National Institutes of Health, 1997; McDonald, 1999). Gastrointestinal reflux is also associated with the disorder (Malde, Naik, Pantvaidya, & Oak, 1997). The child quickly regresses and becomes totally dependent as the disease progresses. If the child has reached the stage of crawling or walking, this ability is soon lost. Loss of the swallow reflex occurs, and the child must be tube-fed. Because of poor swallowing ability, aspiration frequently occurs and pneumonia and respiratory infections are common. The child will be floppy, and mental development will halt. The child's arms and legs will later become spastic (Kaye, 2001). Death normally occurs within 3 to 6 years, although there are exceptions because of outstanding parental and medical provider care.

Onset of type 2, the juvenile form, may vary greatly, ranging from early childhood to late adolescence. If the child develops symptoms at a later age, school problems and behavior problems are key features (Kaye, 2001). In many cases, normal development occurs from 4 to 12 years of age, with loss of developmental milestones usually by age 10. Symptoms are gait disturbances, behavioral and cognitive problems, slurred speech, seizures, urinary incontinence, and optic atrophy, including blindness. Death usually occurs 4 to 6 years after diagnosis (National Institute of Neurological Disorders and Stroke [NINDS], 2003).

Symptoms of the adult form, type 3, include normal development until around puberty, and then cognitive and behavioral abnormalities are seen. Progressive clumsiness and slowing occur. Seizures, peripheral neuropathy, urinary incontinence, nystagmus, optic atrophy, and blindness may also occur. Death usually occurs within 5 to 10 years of diagnosis (Malde et al., 1997).

## Management

There is no cure for MLD. Therapy is generally symptomatic. Bone marrow transplants have been used and have delayed the progression of the disease in some cases (Landrien et al., 1998; NINDS, 2001; Malm et al., 1996; Shapiro et al., 1995; Peters & Steward, 2003). In some cases, the progression of the disease has been halted (United Leukodystrophy Foundation, 2003).

Gene therapy and immunosuppressant therapy are being investigated (Landrien et al.,1998). There is a report of some increase in strength in a child treated with immunotherapy for 2 years (Nevo, Pestronk, Lopate, & Carroll, 1996; Ohashi et al., 1996).

Management of MLD is supportive and treats the symptoms as they occur.

- Nutritional support is necessary through gastrostomy tube feedings.
- Suctioning and appropriate drugs are used to enhance breathing and to minimize respiratory difficulties.
- Good infection control should be practiced in the child's environment to minimize infection, particularly respiratory infection.
- Medications are used to control respiratory infections and seizures.
- Counseling and extended family support are necessary to help the parents cope with the physical and emotional impacts of the disease.
- Respite and nursing care should be available to families to ensure that the family may continue the child's care in the home.
- Occupational and physical therapy services help minimize contractures, rigidity, and loss of bone strength related to neuromuscular disease and lack of weight bearing.
- Good skin care is necessary to prevent bedsores and skin breakdown around gastrostomy stoma site and genital area.

## Individualized Healthcare Plan

### Assessment
*History*
- Present age and developmental level of the student
- Age diagnosis was made
- Healthcare providers involved in the management and care of the student
- Student's history of growth and weight gain
- Student's medical management plan (past and current)
- Medications the student takes
- Respiratory status
  - Tracheostomy
  - Suctioning
- Nutritional management
- Method by which student is fed (orally or tube feeding).
- Age gastrostomy was done
- Oral nutrition
- Nutritional supplements
- Episodes of skin breakdown
- Medication used to prevent or treat skin breakdown
- Family understanding of the disease process
- Family counseling support and utilization

- Family functioning
- Modifications to the home/family environment
- Effectiveness of family care for child and coping with disease process
- Support persons/systems available and involvement
- Respiratory symptoms related to respiratory dysfunction:
  - Respiratory episodes/infection requiring emergency department visits and/or hospitalization
  - Experience with respiratory episodes at school
    - Medications used and effectiveness
    - Length of time and frequency of time that student has required suctioning
    - Past school attendance pattern, including number of days missed
    - Plan for calling emergency medical team and order for resuscitation or "Do not resuscitate" (DNR)
- Seizures
  - Age when seizures began
  - Types of seizures that have been observed and how often they occur
  - Seizures lasting longer than 5 minutes, intervention needed
  - Medications used to control seizures

### Current Status and Management
- Gross and fine motor functioning
- Mobility: walk, crawl, or move by self
  - Use of wheelchair or other assistive device
  - Need for range-of-motion or other exercises
- Cognitive status
- Current nutritional and pattern, including:
  - Placement on growth chart (height and weight)
  - Gastrostomy feedings
  - Equipment and feeding formula, how much and how often
  - Bowel elimination patterns
  - Stoma care
- Skin integrity
- Any skin breakdown
  - At pressure points
  - At stoma site
  - In genital area
- Use of any medication to treat or prevent skin breakdown
- Current respiratory status, including:
  - Rate, rhythm, depth
  - Ability to cough
  - Breath sounds
- Current procedures used to maintain respiratory function, including:
  - Positioning
  - Suctioning
  - Medications and side effects
- Current status of seizure activity, including:
  - Frequency
  - Duration
  - Behavior observed
  - Change in level of consciousness
  - Incidence of status epilepticus
  - Medication used to control seizures and side effects
- Hearing and visual status

### Self-care
- Student's ability to participate in personal care, assistance needed

### Psychosocial Status
- Family members involved with the student
- Parents' perception of student's health and condition

- Extended family members who help with the child's care
- Connection with a respite care agency and/or family access to nursing care part of every day
- Family grieving, functional manner
- DNR order

*Academic Issues*
- Cognitive level of student: academic performance
  – Individualized education program (IEP) related services (physical therapy [PT], occupational therapy [OT], and Developmentally Appropriate Physical Education [DAPE], health services)
  – Assistance needed for academic issues
- Health services needed at school:
  – Assistance needed for health conditions
  – Feeding-equipment cleaning procedures and guidelines
  – Emergency care plan for seizures, gastrostomy tube dislodgement
  – Health procedures needed: gastrostomy tube feedings, skin care
- Staff in-service needs regarding
  – Metachromatic leukodystrophy
  – Gastrostomy and feedings
  – Potential for exposure to infection in school setting
  – Infection control procedures needed
  – Early warning signs of respiratory difficulty
  – Seizure disorders
- Medications needed at school
- Transportation needs

## Nursing Diagnoses (N.D.) (NANDA, 2003)

**N.D. 1** Deficient knowledge related to cognitive limitation and neuromuscular disease (NANDA 00126)

**N.D. 2** Risk for injury related to developmental age and altered mobility and neuromuscular impairment (NANDA 00035)

**N.D. 3** Self-care deficit related to developmental age and neuromuscular dysfunction:
- bathing/hygiene. (NANDA 00108)
- dressing/grooming (NANDA 00109)
- toileting (NANDA 00110)

**N.D. 4** Risk for imbalanced nutrition—less than body requirements related to inability to swallow (NANDA 00002)

**N.D. 5** Risk for disproportionate, altered growth related to inability to consume adequate nutrition (NANDA 00113)

**N.D. 6** Risk for diarrhea related to tube feeding (NANDA 00113)

**N.D. 7** Risk for impaired skin integrity related to gastrostomy stoma, incontinence, and immobility (NANDA 00047)

**N.D. 8** Risk for aspiration related to: (NANDA 00039)
- increased intragastric pressure secondary to tube feeding
- impaired swallowing
- seizures

**N.D. 9** Ineffective breathing pattern related to neuromuscular dysfunction (NANDA 00032)

**N.D. 10** Ineffective airway clearance related to retained oral secretions caused by neuromuscular dysfunction (NANDA 00031)

**N.D. 11** Impaired gas exchange related to increased mucus production and/or inability to clear oral secretions (NANDA 00030)

**N.D. 12** Risk for infection related to inability to clear secretions or aspiration (NANDA 00004)

**N.D. 13** Risk for injury related to seizures (NANDA 00035)

**N.D. 14** Impaired physical mobility use of assistive devices, related to decreased strength and endurance related to neuromuscular disease (NANDA 00085)

## Goals

The student will maintain the maximum cognitive function possible. (N.D. 1)

The student will remain safe in school environment (classroom, bus, etc.). Student will be evacuated from building in a timely and safe manner in an emergency situation. (N.D. 2)

The student will maintain good hygiene and grooming. (N.D. 3)

The student will maintain adequate nutrition and hydration and facilitate weight gain as measured by growth chart. (N.D. 4–5)

The student will maintain normal bowel consistency. (N.D. 6)

The student will maintain skin integrity at stoma site and pressure areas. (N.D. 7)

The student will not have skin breakdown from incontinence. (N.D. 7)

The student will not aspirate during feedings or seizures. (N.D. 8)

The student will maintain optimal breathing pattern and pulmonary function. (N.D. 9–12)

The student will breathe without difficulty. (N.D. 9–12)

The student will have minimal respiratory infections as measured by number of respiratory infections this school year as compared to last year. (N.D. 12)

The student will remain safe from injury during seizure activity. (N.D. 13)

The student's muscles will remain flexible and maintain strength to the extent possible. (N.D. 14)

The student will utilize appropriate assistive devices. (N.D. 14)

## Nursing Interventions

Assist administrators, teachers, and parents to determine the specific healthcare needs of the student and healthcare services needed during the school day. (N.D. 1–14)

Work with staff to stimulate student with appropriate devices/equipment to prevent/delay further losses in cognitive skills. (N.D. 1)

Develop plan for evacuation of student in case of emergency. (N.D. 2, 14)

Collaborate with transportation staff to develop plan to meet student's needs in possible emergency on bus. (N.D. 2, 8-11, 13, 14)

Collaborate with other staff in identifying safety issues and providing for safe environment at school. (N.D. 2, 8-14).

Provide in-service opportunities for staff working with student to increase their skills and knowledge to care for student's needs, including:
- information about the condition, medication administration
- oral suctioning
- Gastrostomy tube feeding
- seizure care
- infection control with emphasis on hand washing
- positioning
- range-of-motion exercises
- signs of respiration difficulty or possible infection (N.D. 2–14)

Provide cardiopulmonary resuscitation (CPR)–trained staff coverage for the building (at least two staff members) (N.D. 2, 8-10, 13).

Assist staff in developing procedures and providing care for the student: (N.D. 3):
- toileting
- diapering
- dressing
- mobility
- grooming (hands, face, hair)

Administer tube feeding as ordered by physician. (N.D. 4, 5)
- Develop procedure in collaboration with parents, physician.
- If delegated, train, observe, and supervise staff.
- Position properly and feed through gastrostomy tube at recommended rate of flow and recommended amount as prescribed by physician.
- Document each tube feeding given.

Monitor weight (in collaboration with physician and parents) to ascertain maintenance of weight and appropriate gain. (N.D. 4, 5)

Monitor stools for diarrhea, and contact parent if necessary. (N.D. 6)

Change diapers frequently:
- Clean well.
- Give skin care as needed to maintain skin integrity in genital area. (N.D. 7)

Keep gastrostomy stoma site clean and dry:
- Observe for redness or irritation.
- Report any abnormalities to parents and/or physician. (N.D. 7)

Reposition student frequently to prevent pressure sores. (N.D. 7)

Position on side during seizure. (N.D. 8)

Suction as necessary to maintain airway. (N.D. 8–12)

Position student to drain secretions to prevent aspiration at all times. (N.D.8–12)

Develop emergency care plan (ECP) for incidences of breathing difficulty. (N.D. 9–12)

Monitor respiratory secretions for color, amount, and consistency. (N.D. 12)

Use good infection-control practices and prevent transmission of infection to student. (N.D. 12)

Obtain physician orders for procedures (feeding, suctioning, stoma care) that will be done at school. (N.D. 2–13)

Obtain physician order for medications given at school. (N.D. 4–13)

Administer medications as prescribed and according to school district policies and procedures. (N.D. 8–13)

Document all seizure activity. (N.D. 13)
- Protect student from injury during seizure activity.
- Remove all sharp objects from area of student.
- Loosen clothing if possible. (N.D. 13)

Develop ECP for seizures lasting longer than 5 minutes. (N.D. 13).

Consult with OT and PT for appropriate mobility equipment, interventions, and positioning. (N.D. 14)

Consult with district administration regarding district policy with regard to DNR and assist in informing parents of the policy. (N.D. 8–13)

If DNR orders are allowed by district policy and if DNR order exists, obtain necessary documents so that parents' wishes may be honored if it becomes necessary to utilize emergency medical personnel. (N.D. 8–12)

Provide support to the family:
- Encourage counseling.
- Provide information about support groups for parents of terminal children.
- Encourage use of respite and/or available nursing care. (N.D. 1-14)

Encourage use of extended family support and community resources. (N.D 1–14)

Encourage expression of feelings. (N.D. 1–14)

Assist family in developing and utilizing effective coping skills to deal with their child's terminal illness and the child's care. (N.D. 1–14)

## Expected Student Outcomes

The student will:
- Function at maximum cognitive potential as measured by goals on IEP. (N.D. 1)
- Remain safe in educational environment. (N.D. 2)
- Be evacuated from building in a timely and safe manner in an emergency situation.(N.D. 2–14)
- Participate in grooming, hygiene, dressing, toileting with assistance from staff as needed. (N.D. 3)
- Maintain good hygiene and grooming. (N.D. 3)
- Maintain adequate nutrition/hydration. (N.D. 4, 5)
- Maintain physical growth as measured by height and weight done at beginning, middle, and end of school year. (N.D. 4, 5)
- Remain free of diarrhea. (N.D. 6)
- Have gastrostomy stoma site that remains intact and uninfected. (N.D. 7)
- Remain free of pressure sores. (N.D. 7)
- Not have skin breakdown due to incontinence. (N.D. 7)
- Not aspirate during tube feedings. (N.D. 8)
- Remain free of infection. (N.D. 9–12 )
- Have good school attendance pattern as measured by number of days absent because of illness as compared to previous year. (N.D. 12)

- Breathe comfortably as measured by normal breathing pattern. (N.D. 9–12)
- Maintain good airway clearance with staff assistance as needed. (N.D. 2–13)
- Remain safe during seizure. (N.D. 12)
- Not aspirate during seizures. (N.D. 13)
- Maintain flexibility and maintain muscle strength, with staff assistance. (N.D. 14)
- Utilize assistive equipment and devices. (N.D. 14)

## Case Study

Justin is a 4-year-old early childhood special education student at West Elementary. He was diagnosed with MLD at age 18 months. He lives with his mother, father, and brother, Alex, who is 8 years old. Alex is in the second grade and doing well.

Justin was the product of a 9-month nonremarkable pregnancy with no history of maternal drug use, alcohol abuse, or nicotine use. He was delivered by a normal vaginal delivery, and his condition was listed as good. Justin weighed 8 pounds 11 ounces and was discharged from the hospital with his mother.

Justin was an easygoing baby as an infant and fed well. He responded to his mother's voice and touch and smiled and cooed in response to pleasurable stimuli. He cried and showed displeasure and discomfort in appropriate circumstances. He gained head control and rolled over at age expectancy.

At about 9 months of age, Justin's mother became worried because she felt he had not made any motor progress. He was not scooting or trying to crawl and was unable to sit up alone. He began coughing while feeding and became resistant to eating. He was hospitalized at 11 months on account of pneumonia. Soon Justin was unable to swallow well and was losing weight. A swallow study showed he was aspirating. Justin had stopped his verbal communication and responded slowly to pleasurable stimuli. He soon was not lifting his head and was unable to eat. He had two more episodes of pneumonia and several bronchial infections. A gastrostomy was done when Justin was 13 months old and a tube for feeding was placed. Testing was done while Justin was hospitalized, and the resulting diagnosis of MLD ensued. Justin began having generalized tonic-clonic seizures at age 2.

At age 4, Justin is totally nonambulatory and dependent on caregivers meeting his physical, psychological, and educational needs. He has no oral intake and is tube-fed. He has grown 1.5 inches and gained 5 pounds in the last year. Currently, he will not require tube feeding at school because he is enrolled in the half-day early childhood program. He has been free of respiratory infection for the last 4 months. He requires oral suctioning as needed. He usually requires suctioning at least three or four times while at school. Justin's seizures are fairly well controlled with Depakote, 250 mg tid. Justin is incontinent of bowels and urine and is diapered. Justin's mother does not have any relatives to help her because the family was transferred here 2 years ago. She does have many friends who help and support her to the best of their ability. Justin's father does not want to discuss Justin's condition and avoids interaction with school personnel and caregivers if possible. Alex seems well adjusted, but Mom would like to spend more time with him because she feels he is being given a minimum of attention on account of of the energy required to care for Justin.

### IEP Recommendations for an MLD Student Based on the Above Case Study

Justin must be watched closely because of his seizure disorder, compromised respiratory status, and need for suctioning. One classroom staff member should be assigned primary responsibility to monitor Justin while he is at school.

At least two classroom staff members working with Justin should be trained in CPR.

Justin must have a trained aide on his bus or be transported in a "Care Cab" (a vehicle staffed with emergency-trained personnel).

### Weekly School Nursing Time Required

| | | |
|---|---|---|
| Weekly/biweekly conferences/phone calls with parents, physician—indirect services | = | 30 minutes |
| Weekly observations and discussion of condition with teachers paraprofessionals, transportation personnel (as appropriate)—indirect services | = | 1 hour 30 minutes |
| Classroom observation—indirect services | = | 30 minutes |
| Total weekly nursing needs—indirect services | = | 2 hours 30 minutes |

# Metachromatic Leukodystrophy

| Assessment Data | Nursing Diagnosis | Goals | Nursing Interventions | Expected Outcomes |
|---|---|---|---|---|
| Skin care needed for gastrostomy stoma.<br><br>Skin care for needed for genital area.<br><br>History of tonic-clonic seizures. | Risk for impaired skin integrity at gastrostomy stoma site.<br><br>Total incontinence related to neurologic dysfunction.<br><br>Risk for aspiration during seizure. | Justin will maintain skin integrity with assistance.<br><br>Justin will not aspirate during seizure. | Provide in-service for staff in how to care for gastrostomy stoma.<br><br>Provide in-service for staff in diapering, skin care, signs and symptoms of potential skin breakdown.<br><br>Position Justin on side during seizure. See ECP. | Justin will maintain skin integrity around gastrostomy stoma site with assistance.<br><br>Justin will remain free from skin breakdown due to incontinence and pressure, with assistance from staff.<br><br>Justin will not aspirate during seizure. |
| Compromised respiratory status. | Ineffective breathing pattern related to neurologic/muscular impairment.<br><br>Risk for ineffective airway clearance related to inability to clear oral secretions.<br><br>Risk for impaired gas exchange related to increased mucus production and/or inability to clear oral secretions. | Justin will maintain optimal breathing pattern and pulmonary function. | Provide in-service and supervise educational and support staff (including bus drivers) regarding:<br>• signs of respiratory distress<br>• proper oral suctioning procedure<br>• proper positioning for ease of breathing<br>• when emergency intervention may be necessary<br><br>Staff will be qualified to perform CPR if necessary. CPR training for at least 2 classroom staff and 1 transportation employee.<br><br>Develop ECP to address what to do if breathing problems develop. | Justin will breathe comfortably during the school day, with staff intervention as needed. |

| Assessment Data | Nursing Diagnosis | Goals | Nursing Interventions | Expected Outcomes |
|---|---|---|---|---|
| Susceptibility to respiratory infections, pneumonia. Has been free from respiratory infections the past 4 months. | Risk for infection related to inability to clear secretions or aspiration and ineffective breathing pattern. | Justin will have minimal respiratory infections during the school year. | Provide in-service for staff on infection-control practices, especially hand washing. Monitor frequently to ensure proper infection-control practices are being followed. Monitor respiratory secretions (color, consistency, and amount). | Justin will remain free of respiratory infection. Justin will maintain good school attendance pattern. |
| History of tonic-clonic seizures fairly well controlled. Medication: Depakote, 250 mg tid. | Risk for injury during seizure. | Prevent injury during seizure. | Develop ECP for a seizure. Provide in-service for staff: • generalized tonic-clonic seizure • how to protect student during seizure: move sharp objects, loosen clothing if possible, etc. • positioning of student during seizure • when to call 911 • document all seizure activity Side effects of student's seizure medication—notify parents and school nurse if side effects occur. | Justin will remain safe during seizure. Justin will not aspirate secretions during a seizure. |

# Emergency Care Plan
## Metachromatic Leukodystrophy

Date: _____     School: _____

Student: _Justin_____     Grade: _____

Date of birth: _____

Parent(s)/Guardian(s): _____     Home telephone: _____

_____     Father's work: _____

_____     Mother's work: _____

Primary Care Provider: _____     Telephone: _____

Specialist: _____     Telephone: _____

Contact: _____

Medical condition(s): _Metachromatic leukodystrophy_____

## Conditions that may require emergency care:

Seizure lasting longer than 5 minutes or seizure where student is not breathing and turns blue:
- Turn student on side.
- Call school nurse and 911.

Student is unable to breathe or breathing with difficulty:
- Call school nurse.
- Suction as trained.
- Call 911 if no resolution.

Student is not breathing and has no pulse:
- Call school nurse.
- Call 911.
- Administer CPR (or honor DNR as appropriate).

Evacuation.
- Student will be taken from school/classroom in wheelchair by designated person.

# References

Balslev, T., Cortez, M. A., Blaser, S. I., & Haslam, R. H. (1997). Recurrent seizures in metachromatic leukodystrophy. *Pediatric Neurology, 17*(2), 150–154

Gieselmann, V., Kreysing, J., & von Figura, K. (1994). Genetics of metachromatic leukodystrophy. *Gene Therapy, 1*(Suppl. 1), S87.

Kaye, E. M. (2001). Update on genetic disorders affecting white matter. *Pediatric Neurology, 24*(1), 11–24.

Landrien, P., Blanche, S., Vanier, M. T., Metral, S., Husson, B., Sandhoff, K., et al. (1998). Bone marrow transplantation in metachromatic leukodystrophy caused by saposin-B deficiency: A case report with a 3-year follow-up period. *Journal of Pediatri*cs, *133*(1), 129–132.

Malde, A. D., Naik, L. D., Pantvaidya, S. H., & Oak, S. N. (1997). An unusual presentation in a patient with metachromatic leukodystrophy. *Anaesthesia, 52*(7): 690–694.

Malm, G., Kingden, O., Wintarski, J., et al. (1996). Clinical outcome in four children with metachromatic leukodystrophy treated by bone marrow transplantation. *Bone Marrow Transplant, 17*(6), 1003–1008.

McDonald, C. (1999). Electrodiagnosis in pediatrics. In G. E. Molnar & M. A. Alexander (Eds.), *Pediatric rehabilitation* (3rd ed., p. 91). Philadelphia: Hanley & Belfus.

MedlinePlus. (2003). *Medical encyclopedia: Metachromatic leukodystrophy.* Retrieved August 21, 2003, from http://www.nlm.nih.gov/medlineplus.htm

MLD Foundation. (2003). MLD 101—*An overview of metachromatic leukodystrophy for the layperson.* Retrieved August 20, 2003, from http://www.mldfoundation.org/MLD101html

NANDA International. (2003). *Nursing diagnoses: Definitions & classification 2003-2004.* Philadelphia: Author.

National Institutes of Health, National Institute of Neurological Disorders and Stroke. Metachromatic leukodystrophy. Retrieved September 1997 from ninds.nih.gov/healinfo/DISORDER/metachrom.leuk/meta.leuko.htm

National Institute of Neurological Disorders and Stroke (NINDS). (2003). *Metachromatic leukodystrophy information.* Retrieved August 20, 2004, from http://www.ninds.nih.gov/health_and_medical/disorders/meta_leu_doc.htm

Nevo, Y., Pestronk, A., Lopate, G., & Carroll, S. L. (1996). Neuropathy of metachromatic leukodystrophy: Improvement with immunomodulation. *Pediatric Neurology, 15*(3), 237–239.

National Organization for Rare Diseases (NORD). (2003). *Leukodystrophy, metachromatic.* Retrieved August 20, 2003, from http://www.rarediseases.org

Ohashi, T., Watabe, K., Sato, Y., Saito, I., Barranger, J. A., & Matalon, R. (1996). Gene therapy for metachromatic leukodystrophy. *Acta Paediatrica Japonica 38*(2), 193–201.

Ouvrier, R. A., McLeod, J. G., & Pollard, J. D. (1999). *Peripheral neuropathy in childhood* (2nd ed.). London: MacKeith Press.

Peters, C., & Steward, C. G. (2003). Hematopoietic cell transplantation for inherited metabolic diseases: An overview of outcomes and practice guidelines. *Bone Marrow Transplant 31*(4): 229–239.

Shapiro, E.G., Lockman, L. S., Balthazor, M., & Krivit, W. (1995). Neuropsychological outcomes of several storage diseases with and without bone marrow transplantation. *Journal of Inherited Metabolic Disease, 18*(4), 413–429.

Tylki-Szymanska A. T., Czartoryska B., & Lugowska A. (1998). Practical suggestions in diagnosing metachromatic leukodystrophy in probands and in testing family members. *European Neurology, 40*(2), 67–70.

United Leukodystrophy Foundation. (2003). *Introduction to leukodystrophy.* Retrieved August 21, 2003, from http://www.ulf.org/ulf/intro/index.htm

Zlotogora, J., Back, G., Bosenberg, C., Barak, Y., von Figura, K., & Gieselmann, V. (1995). Molecular basis of late infantile metachromatic leukodystrophy in the Habbanite Jews. *Human Mutations, 5*(2), 137–143.

# Bibliography

Hootman J., & Carpenito L. J. (1996). *Nursing diagnosis: Application in the school setting.* Scarborough, ME. National Association of School Nurses.

Johnson, M., Bulechek, G., Dochterman, J. M., Maas, M., & Moorhead, S. (Eds.). (2001). Nursing diagnoses, outcomes, and interventions. NANDA, NOC and NIC linkages. St. Louis, MO: Mosby.

Kim T. S., Kim I. O., & Kim, W. S., et al. (1997). MR of childhood metachromatic leukodystrophy. *American Journal of Neuroradiology, 18*(4), 733–738.

Molnar, G. E., & Alexander, M. A. (Eds.). (1999). *Pediatric rehabilitation* (3rd ed.). Philadelphia: Hanley & Belfus.

*Publication Manual of the American Psychological Association* (5th ed). (2001). Washington, DC: American Psychological Association.

## Resources

ARC of the United States
500 East Border Street
Suite 300
Arlington, TX 76010
817-261-6003

Association for Neuro-Metabolic Disorders
5223 Brookfield Lane
Sylvania, OH 43560-1809
419-885-1497
VOLK4OLKS@aol.com

Hunter's Hope Foundation, Inc.
3859 North Buffalo Street
Orchard Park, NY 14127
716-667-1200
1-877-984-4673
hunters@huntershope.org
http://www.huntershope.org

National Institute of Neurological Disorders and
    Stroke
PO Box 5801
Bethesda, MD 20824
301-496-5751
1-800-352-9424
http://www.ninds.nih.gov/

National Lipid Diseases Foundation
1201 Corbin Street
Elizabeth, NJ 07201
908-527-8000
1-800-527-8005

National Organization for Rare Disorders
PO Box 1968
55 Kenosia Avenue
Danbury, CT 06813-1968
203-744-0100
203-798-2291 (fax)
orphan@rarediseases.org
http://www.rarediseases.org

National Tay-Sachs & Allied Diseases Association
2001 Beacon Street
Suite 204
Boston, MA 02135
617-277-4463
1-800-906-8723
info@ntsad.org
http://www.NTSAD.org

United Leukodystrophy Foundation
2304 Highland Drive
Sycamore, IL 60178
815-895-3211
1-800-728-5483
815-895-2432 (fax)
ulf@tbcnet.com
http://www.ulf.org/
4/27/05

Metachromatic Leukodystrophy

*Chapter Fifty-four*

# Migraine Headache

MaryAnn Tapper Strawhacker

## Introduction

Migraine headache prevalence is 17.2% for females and 6.0% for males in the general population (Lipton et al., 2002). Onset is often during childhood, with 20% starting before age 10 and 45% before age 20. The prevalence of migraine in children is between 8% and 9% (Silverboard, 2001). The ratio of males to females is equal prior to puberty. After puberty, female migraineurs outnumber males 3:1. When both parents have migraines, a child's risk is 70%. The risk drops to 45% when only one parent has migraines (Evans, 2000).

## Pathophysiology

Migraines are a neurologic condition of unknown origin (Beers & Berkow, 1999). Pain associated with migraines is thought to result from vasodilation of meningeal blood vessels. This vasodilation activates the trigeminovascular system, causing the release of neuropeptides that promote neurogenic inflammation and intensify headache pain. Recent research suggests that brainstem activation may also play a role in migraines. Treatments for acute migraine now focus on interrupting trigeminal pain mechanisms by effecting 5-HT receptors. These receptors act to constrict large cranial vessels and inhibit peripheral trigeminal nerve branches (National Institute of Neurological Disorders and Stroke [NINDS], American Academy of Neurology [AAN], American Headache Society [AHS], & National Headache Foundation [NHF], 2001).

In 1988, the International Headache Society (IHS) developed a classification system that is still in use today. Headaches are classified into two groups based on structural origin: primary, which are those unassociated with lesions, and secondary, which are those associated with trauma or lesions.

Migraines are a type of primary headache with at least four distinct phases: prodrome, aura, headache, and resolution. Up to 25% of migraineurs experience prodrome symptoms up to 24 hours before an attack. Changes in mood, neurologic symptoms, and physical symptoms may occur. Approximately 15% of migraine attacks will then follow with an aura. An aura is a preceding neurologic event usually resolving within 60 minutes. Symptoms of an aura are usually visual but may include auditory, sensory, language, or motor disturbances as well. The headache phase lasts up to 72 hours and is usually characterized by a throbbing unilateral pain of moderate to severe intensity (NINDS, AAN, AHS, & NHF, 2001). To meet IHS migraine criteria, a headache without aura must be accompanied by at least one of the following symptoms: nausea, vomiting, light sensitivity, or sound sensitivity. Resolution, the final phase, is often characterized by deep sleep. Fatigue may continue up to 24 hours after the headache has resolved (NINDS, AAN, AHS, & NHF, 2001).

In children, the duration of headache may be as short as 1 hour and is often bilateral temporal. To address differences in children, revised IHS pediatric criteria have been proposed (Evans, 2000). These criteria lessen the required minimum number of attacks per year and length of headache and allow variation in location of the headache, associated symptoms, and description of pain experienced. Early trials with these revised criteria improved diagnostic sensitivity significantly across pediatric age levels (Winner, Rothner, Putman, & Asgharnejad, 2003).

Results from the Glaxo Wellcome clinical trial's database shed new light on adolescents with migraines. Average age of participants in the database is 14.1 years, with a range of 11 to 18 years. The majority suffer from migraines without aura (67%). Pain is most often described as unilateral (58%) and pulsating (74%). Physical activity aggravated migraines in 88% of participants. The majority of attacks (76%) start between 6 a.m. and 6 p.m., with a higher proportion occurring Monday through Wednesday. Those with aura treated their migraines somewhat more quickly. Whereas pretreatment nausea occurred in 53% of attacks, vomiting was reported by only 5%. Sensitivity to light, sound, or both was reported by 80%. Migraine-related school absences are usually less than 3 days per year; however, reduced productivity associated with various phases of migraine may occur despite attendance (Winner et al., 2003).

The role of trigger mechanisms in development of migraines is not well understood. It is thought that for some individuals, triggers may influence pathophysiology at one or more phases of a migraine. Studies vary widely as to the percentage of migraineurs experiencing triggers. Reported food triggers include cheese, chocolate, citrus fruits, processed and cured meats, alcoholic drinks, dairy products, caffeinated beverages, food dyes, additives, and aspartame. Elimination diets may prove to be a useful alterative for some sensitive individuals but are difficult to maintain. A well-balanced diet is generally encouraged as well as an avoidance of potential triggers. Other types of triggers include stress, fasting, fatigue, exercise, sleep deprivation, bright lights, head trauma, infection, menstruation, and contraceptives (Millichap & Yee, 2003).

Five pediatric migraine equivalents are currently recognized: benign paroxysmal torticollis, benign paroxysmal vertigo, abdominal migraines/cyclical vomiting, acephalgic migraines, and acute confusional migraines. Equivalents may represent up to 10% of identified pediatric migraines. Episodes are periodic, involve a sudden onset, are without headache, but are thought to have a migrainous etiology. Benign paroxysmal torticollis begins during infancy and usually resolves by early to middle childhood. Characterized by torticollis with or without other symptoms, it lasts somewhere between 4 hours and 4 days. Onset of benign paroxysmal vertigo is between 1 and 3 years, with brief episodes lasting between 1 and 5 minutes. Characteristics include unsteadiness, pallor, and sometimes fear. Episodes usually resolve within 2 years of onset.

Abdominal migraines and cyclical vomiting usually occur between the ages of 4 and 10 years. Crampy, periumbilical pain or extreme nausea and vomiting with high-frequency emesis of small volume is typical of these episodes. Duration is usually longer than 1 hour. Resolution most often occurs within 2 years of onset. Between the ages of 5 and 12 years, acephalgic migraines occur. Episodes usually last less than 10 minutes and are similar to migrainous auras but fail to progress to headaches. Acute confusional migraines have an onset typically during late childhood to adolescence. Children appear confused and agitated with memory disturbances; often this is the initial presentation in a child that is predisposed to other types of migraines. Minor head trauma may precede this type of episode. Rarely, a headache may accompany symptoms. Duration of the episode is up to 8 hours (Al-Twaijri & Shevell, 2002).

## Management

Treatment depends on frequency, duration, and intensity of the migraines. Primary medication management is divided into two categories: acute and preventive. The goal of acute therapy is to treat the attack and restore function with minimal side effects. Agents include antiemetics, painkillers, nonsteroidal anti-inflammatory drugs, and migraine-specific medications, among others. Prompt intervention with rest and/or simple analgesics often alleviates symptoms. Side effects of nonprescription analgesics may include cramps, diarrhea, dizziness, drowsiness, heartburn, nausea, vomiting, or headaches. Those unable to take oral drugs on account of nausea and/or vomiting may be prescribed injections, nasal sprays, or suppositories (NINDS, AAN, AHS, & NHF, 2001). Newer studies suggest that early intervention while headache is still mild may interrupt the progression of symptoms (Winner et al., 2003).

Preventive therapy is indicated under the following circumstances: when attacks cause significant life impact despite use of acute treatments, with increased frequency of attacks causing risk for overuse of acute treatments, or when acute therapies are contraindicated or have failed. Medications used for prevention include beta-blockers, anticonvulsants, and antidepressants, among others. These medications have a variety of drug interactions, side effects, and precautions. Most are prescribed in different dosage than the recommendations for original indications. Many have not been tested on children. Use of acute medications should not exceed 3 days per week because of the risk of dependency or rebound headaches (NINDS, AAN, AHS, & NHF, 2001; Silverboard, 2001). For these reasons, it is important to consult with the student's physician or pharmacist to obtain current drug information and parameters for medication monitoring.

Rescue medications are used to lessen the severity and/or shorten the duration of migraine symptoms once other therapies have failed. They must be used early in the attack to be effective. Common types of abortive agents include ergotamine tartrate and dihydroergotamine (Migranal, DHE45). These medications should not be taken more that 2 days per week, and doses should be taken at least 5 days apart. Possible side effects of ergot alkaloids include nausea, vomiting, diarrhea, dizziness, leg cramps, rebound headaches, and chest discomfort. Triptans, which are selective serotonin agonists, have possible side effects of dizziness, drowsiness, muscle aches, nausea, vomiting, chest or throat tightness, warmth, and tingling. Specific medications in this category include sumatriptan (Imitrex), naratriptan (Amerge), rizatriptan (Maxalt), and zolmitriptan (Zomig). Isometheptene mucate (Midrin) is a combination drug that acts to constrict inflamed blood vessels in the head, relieves pain, and helps the student relax. One of the few side effects is drowsiness (NINDS, AAN, AHS, & NHF, 2001; Silverboard, 2001; Evans, 2000). Consult with the student's physician or pharmacist for medication monitoring parameters. Depending on the severity and duration of pain, emergency medical treatment may become necessary.

In addition to, or in place of, pharmaceuticals, other therapies are growing in popularity. Relaxation therapy is a training process to reduce sympathetic outflow and muscle activity. This approach may be used with biofeedback or alone. The goal of these behavioral therapies is to help migraineurs identify and manage factors associated with headaches. Effective treatment teaches the student techniques and then provides guidance and support for application (NINDS, AAN, AHS, & NHF, 2001). Families may also try a combination of natural and alternative therapies, the effects of which may be unknown. It is important to monitor changes in health status and be alert to signs of worsening symptoms. Suboptimal management is associated with having three or more headaches per month, absence from work or school, daily medication for headaches, and visiting the emergency room within the previous 6 months (Chatterton et al., 2002).

# Individualized Healthcare Plan

## Assessment

### History
- Date of last complete physical examination
- Age diagnosis made
- Presence of other health concerns
- Family history of migraines

### Current Status and Management
- Frequency, severity, and duration of attacks
- History of auras and presenting symptoms
- Typical signs of a migraine
- Associated symptoms with migraines
- Identified potential triggers, such as food, environmental, or hormonal
- Dietary or environmental restrictions
- Healthcare providers involved in the student's care (physicians, specialists, practitioners)
- Medical treatment plan (medications, biofeedback, relaxation therapy)
- Use of alternative therapies
- Effectiveness of treatment to manage attacks and associated symptoms
- Tools used to rate/describe a migraine attack
- Home use of logs, headache diaries, pain scale ratings to document migraines
- Tolerance of treatment, including medication side effects
- Use of over-the-counter medications or herbal remedies
- Supplies/medications/equipment needed during the school day
- Preferred mode of notification when medication refills are needed at school
- Changes noticed in the student's general activity level/tolerance before, during, or after an attack
- Experience with disruption of sleep patterns
- Student's dietary habits, include whether eats regularly, skips meals, and variety of food intake

### Self-care
- Medications/treatments/procedures administered independently at home and with supervision
- Self-management skills currently taught at home
- Student's ability to anticipate signs and symptoms of an impending migraine
- Need for adult guidance to identify early signs and symptoms of a migraine
- Student's ability to participate in selection of appropriate treatments based on symptom severity

### Psychosocial Status
- Family and student perception of overall health status
- Family and student's ability to cope with migraine diagnosis
- History or suspicion of substance abuse
- Experience with activity disruption
- Disclosure of student's diagnosis with peer group and peer response
- Concerns expressed regarding peer reactions
- Participation in extracurricular activities with peers
- Experience with teasing at school or in the community as a result of diagnosis
- Existence of social support from extended family or community
- Community resource(s) currently in use and remaining unmet needs

### Academic Issues
- Past school attendance record, including patterns of absences and reason for absences
- Student's academic history; note any decline in scores/grades since diagnosis
- Modifications, accommodation, adaptations made for the student during the school day
- Additional modifications, accommodation, adaptations needed during the school day
- Existence of 504 plan or an individualized education program to address health and educational needs at school
- Training school staff requires to meet student needs
- Provisions made for migraine management at school

## Nursing Diagnoses (N.D.) (NANDA, 2003)

**N.D.1** Pain (NANDA 00133) related to migraine symptoms

**N.D.2** Activity intolerance (NANDA 00092) related to:
- migraine symptoms (headache; nausea; vomiting; sensitivity to light, sound, or movement)
- medication side effects
- frequency, severity, or duration of attacks

**N.D.3** Knowledge deficit (NANDA 00126) related to:
- recent diagnosis of migraines
- complicated management of migraines

**N.D.4** Ineffective family therapeutic regimen management (NANDA 00080) related to:
- multiple caregiver demands
- inability to select appropriate treatments based on symptoms
- inconsistent primary caregiver
- knowledge deficit

**N.D.5** Ineffective therapeutic regimen management (NANDA 00078) related to:
- denial of early warning signs of impending attack
- inadequate follow-up of relaxation and biofeedback training
- multiple changes in medications/treatments
- knowledge deficit

**N.D.6** (Risk for) noncompliance with prescribed treatment (NANDA 00079) related to:
- denial of need for medication/ treatment
- perceived ineffectiveness of medication/ treatment
- undesirable side effects of medication
- knowledge deficit

**N.D. 7** Ineffective coping (NANDA 00069) related to:
- fear of future attacks
- stress imposed by migraines and their management
- altered role performance
- pain

**N.D.8** Ineffective role performance (NANDA 00055) related to:
- absence from school/ class due to migraines
- symptoms of migraines
- management of migraines

**N.D.9** Situational low self-esteem (NANDA 00120) related to:
- frequency, severity, or duration of attacks
- ineffective coping
- altered role performance

## Goals

The student will demonstrate improved physical activity tolerance. (N.D.1, 2)

The student will experience an increased level of comfort, allowing active participation in school activities. (N.D. 1, 2, 4, 5)

The student will attend school/class and participate with modifications made as needed. (N.D. 1, 2, 4, 5, 8, 9)

The student, in association with the parent and physician, will develop a mutually agreeable medical treatment plan. (N.D. 1–9)

The student will seek treatment for migraines at first sign of an attack. (N.D. 1, 3, 5, 6, 8)

The student will perform relaxation and biofeedback strategies with assistance as needed. (N.D. 1, 4–9)

The student will demonstrate increased knowledge of migraine management. (N.D. 3, 4)

The student will demonstrate increased knowledge of migraine pathophysiology. (N.D. 3, 5)

The student will participate in planning and implementing the migraine treatment plan at school. (N.D. 4–9)

The student will progress toward adapting to living with a chronic condition. (N.D. 4–9)

The student will comply with prescribed migraine treatment plan. (N.D. 6)

The student will demonstrate effective use of coping strategies (N.D. 7)

The student will demonstrate improved self-esteem. (N.D. 7–9)

## Nursing Interventions

Obtain a signed release of information to obtain pertinent medical orders and records and to share information with the medical provider. (N.D. 1–9)

Obtain parental and student permission to share relevant medical information with school personnel. (N.D. 1–9)

Provide emotional support to the student and family. (N.D. 1–9)

- Provide support and encouragement to student.
- Develop trusting, open communication with the student, encouraging verbalization of feelings of anger, frustration, depression, concerns, and fears.
- Establish a preferred mode of scheduled communication with parents/guardians to facilitate coordination of medical treatment and to monitor the student's social and emotional adjustment.
- Refer family to counseling resources as needed to facilitate student's adaptation to living with a chronic condition.

Provide pain management. (N.D. 1–9)

- Observe the student for signs of discomfort.
- Assist student with decision making during acute episodes.
- Standardize, in association with the student and family, an individual pain-rating scale for school use.
- In association with the family, assemble a list of comfort measures and help the student to select appropriate choices based on level of discomfort.
- Instruct the student to use prescribed treatment before symptoms are severe.
- Reinforce learned biofeedback and relaxation therapy techniques.
- Support the family while exploring alternative treatment options.
- Locate a quiet, dark place for the student to rest during acute attacks.
- Determine the impact of discomfort on the student's school performance.
- In association with the student, family, and medical team, evaluate the effectiveness of present comfort measures.
- Modify environmental factors that may contribute to the student's discomfort.
- Assist the family/student to identify possible triggers where appropriate.
- Make referrals to support groups and outside resources as appropriate.
- In collaboration with the medical provider, family, and student, develop a school migraine treatment plan based on symptoms.

Reinforce or provide additional migraine education to the student/family. (N.D. 1–5)

- Assess the student/primary caregiver's knowledge of migraines.
- Determine the readiness and ability of caregivers/student to learn the necessary skills.
- Review the known pathophysiologic processes with the student at a developmentally appropriate level.
- Provide current migraine resources as needed.
- Reinforce teaching with the student/primary caregiver on an ongoing basis.

Provide medication management. (N.D. 1–6)

- Determine medication required and administer per physician's orders.
- Monitor student's ability to self-medicate.
- Facilitate self-medication administration when appropriate and in accordance with district policy.
- Review medication actions and side effects.
- Instruct student to report any unusual side effects to the school nurse.
- Monitor effectiveness of medications.
- Monitor for adverse drug effects.
- Review with the student/family appropriate use of over-the-counter as well as prescription medications.
- Review medication administration technique for nasal and parenteral routes.
- Discuss use of herbals and alternative therapies that may interact with over-the-counter or prescription medication.
- Monitor student's medication/treatment compliance and assist in removing existing barriers.
- Provide consultation with other healthcare providers regarding results of treatment and necessary modifications.
- Instruct student to consult with physician regarding medication management.

Provide migraine educational materials to designated school personnel and allow time for questions. (N.D. 1–9)

Assist teacher(s) in monitoring the student's activity tolerance and making adjustments in scheduling as needed. (N.D. 1, 2, 7–9)

Provide opportunities for student/family/nurse to educate classmates about migraines. (N.D. 1–3, 6–9)

Refer to building student assistance team or 504 coordinator if not already involved. (N.D. 1–9)

Outline for school staff possible student medical accommodations, such as: (N.D. 1–7)
- Quiet place to rest during an acute attack
- Modified work load if attacks are severe and frequent
- Shortened school day if attacks are severe and difficult to control
- Mentor assigned to assist coordination of missed schoolwork
- Teach activity organization and time-management techniques to assist student with work completion during times of exacerbation.

Promote family management of therapeutic plan. (N.D. 4–6)
- Determine student's level of dependency on family members.
- Identify family's expectations for management.
- Assess need for reinforcement teaching and notify primary care provider as needed.
- Assist primary caregiver to identify strengths and challenges with current management strategies.
- Collaborate with primary caregiver to set goals for school management.
- Support primary caregiver through active listening.
- Assist to resolve conflicts between the student and family that serve as barriers to treatment.

Assist the family to minimize disruption of their daily life due to migraine management. (N.D. 4–6)
- Determine impact of the family's cultural practices and beliefs on the student's migraine management.
- Determine, in association with the primary caregiver, the scope of family disruption.
- Assist family to adapt prescribed treatment into their lifestyle.
- Assist family to focus on the student's strengths and not on migraine symptoms.
- Encourage the student's participation in age-appropriate activities.
- Encourage parents to set age-appropriate limits and expectations for the student.
- Discuss strategies for managing acute attacks in a variety of settings.
- Identify and promote family's use of adaptive coping mechanisms.
- Assist primary caregiver to advocate for student in a variety of settings.
- Encourage family to seek and maintain a social support network.
- Assist primary caregiver to locate and utilize existing community resources as needed.
- Make referrals to outside agencies as appropriate.

Facilitate student participation in the therapeutic plan. (N.D. 5–9)
- Determine student's current level of participation.
- Set goals in collaboration with student and primary caregiver.
- Explore strategies with the student to progress toward goal attainment.
- Break down treatment plan into discrete teachable components.
- Maintain consistency in student supervision through written protocol and support staff training.
- Encourage student to participate in monitoring progress toward goal attainment.
- Provide ongoing feedback to primary caregiver regarding student's progress toward goal attainment.
- Provide positive reinforcement to the student.
- Provide student with choices in migraine management, whenever possible.
- Review goals with student and modify plan of care as needed.

Promote self-esteem enhancement. (N.D. 7–9)
- Facilitate an environment that encourages self-esteem.
- Assist student to identify the impact of migraines on self-concept.
- Assist student to examine negative self-perceptions and reasons for self-criticism.
- Monitor self-critical statements.
- Assist student to identify self-destructive behaviors.
- Assist student to problem-solve situations made difficult because of migraines.
- Encourage increased level of self-care and responsibility.
- Encourage student to discuss the impact of peer group on feelings of self-worth.
- Facilitate self-expression with peers.
- Monitor student for signs of social isolation.
- Assist student to identify strengths and reinforce examples of those strengths when observed.
- Convey confidence in the student's abilities.

Assist student to adapt to the stress of migraines and their management. (N.D. 7–9)
- Provide an attitude of unconditional acceptance.
- Assist student to develop an objective appraisal of his/her migraine status.
- Assist student to identify his/her own strengths and challenges.
- Discuss alternative responses to stress.
- Encourage constructive outlets for expression of frustration and anger.

- Facilitate acceptance of others' limitations.
- Evaluate student's decision-making ability related to treatment.
- Teach new coping and problem-solving skills.
- Introduce student to an adult mentor, with family approval, who successfully manages his or her chronic condition.
- Encourage use of spiritual resources as appropriate.

## Expected Student Outcomes

The student will:
- Report an improved level of comfort after interventions. (N.D. 1)
- Participate in development of the migraine treatment plan. (N.D. 1–9)
- Improve school attendance with accommodations as needed. (N.D. 1–8)
- Recognize the early warning signs of an oncoming migraine. (N.D. 1–5, 7–9)
- Progress toward self-monitoring of comfort interventions. (N.D. 1, 3–6)
- Receive consistent management of migraines. (N.D. 1, 3–6)
- Utilize biofeedback and/or relaxation therapy techniques in pain management. (N.D. 1, 5, 6)
- Demonstrate an understanding of the migraine process and utilize that knowledge to make health management decisions. (N.D. 3–6)
- Actively participate in making migraine treatment choices. (N.D. 3–6)
- Self-administer medications in compliance with prescribed orders and district policy/procedures. (N.D. 3–9)
- Comply with the medically prescribed treatment. (N.D. 6)
- Obtain counseling as needed. (N.D. 6-9)
- Attend his/her school health planning meetings. (N.D. 6–9)
- Identify and utilize existing community resources as needed. (N.D. 6–9)
- Demonstrate a reduction in self-destructive behavior. (N.D. 6–9)
- Demonstrate the use of adaptive coping skills. (N.D. 7–9)
- Demonstrate a reduction in self-critical comments. (N.D. 7–9)

# Case Study

Lindsey Newell is a 16-year-old girl diagnosed 5 years ago with migraines without aura. Usual symptoms are nausea; vomiting; sensitivity to light, noise, movement; and headache. No food or environmental triggers have ever been identified. Up until the last 2 years, Lindsey was able to control her migraine pain with the use of over-the-counter medication and the occasional use of Migranol. In the past year, however, Lindsey has gone from one to two migraines per month to migraines occurring almost weekly. She has missed 36 school days this year and has been hospitalized twice for pain management. School health office visits average four to five times per week, and counselor visits average one to two times per week. Lindsey's grade-point average has dropped this semester, and she has quit band and pep squad. Current treatment prescribed by the neurologist includes biofeedback and relaxation therapy. Medication options include Excedrin Migraine, Naproxen, and Imitrex. Her parents disagree on medical treatment approach. Lindsay is an only child whose parents recently divorced. Custody is shared on an every-other-week basis. Both parents travel out of town routinely for business. Lindsey's maternal grandparents live in a nearby suburb and are actively involved in her care. Lindsey denies having any other chronic health conditions or taking any additional medications. Last month Lindsey was given an in-school suspension for possession of alcohol on school grounds.

## Migraine

| Assessment Data | Nursing Diagnosis | Goals | Nursing Interventions | Expected Outcomes |
|---|---|---|---|---|
| • Neurologist appointment management plan outlined, orders received.<br><br>• Medications prescribed include Imitrex, Naproxen, Excedrin, and Migranal. Stadol NS was added.<br><br>• Herbal supplements will be discontinued.<br><br>• Relaxation therapy and biofeedback training will continue.<br><br>• Family is scheduled for a pain-management seminar at the community college next weekend. | Knowledge deficit related to complicated management of migraines. | Lindsey will demonstrate an increased knowledge of migraine management. | 1. Obtain a signed release of information to obtain pertinent medical orders and records and to share information with the medical provider.<br>2. Assess the student and primary caregiver's knowledge of migraines.<br>3. Determine the readiness and ability of caregivers/student to learn the necessary skills.<br>4. Review the known pathophysiologic processes with Lindsey at a developmentally appropriate level.<br>5. Provide current migraine resources as needed.<br>6. Reinforce teaching with Lindsey on an ongoing basis.<br>7. Monitor student's ability to self-medicate.<br>8. Facilitate self-medication administration when appropriate and in accordance with district policy.<br>9. Review medication actions and side effects.<br>10. Instruct Lindsey to report any unusual side effects to the school nurse. | Lindsey will demonstrate an understanding of the migraine process and utilize that knowledge to make health management decisions. |

*Chapter Fifty-four: Migraine Headache*

| Assessment Data | Nursing Diagnosis | Goals | Nursing Interventions | Expected Outcomes |
|---|---|---|---|---|
| • Lindsey has expressed confusion over which medication to select.<br><br>• Lindsey has not utilized the relaxation therapy or biofeedback training she received several years ago, according to her mother.<br><br>• Lindsey does not currently utilize a pain rating scale, although she was given a copy of one at her last neurologist visit.<br><br>• Once a migraine begins, Lindsey prefers to call her family to take her home.<br><br>• Lindsey reports frequently having difficulty falling asleep at night and "often waking up with a headache."<br><br>• Lindsey reports that occasionally she does skip breakfast, but she eats lunch and dinner regularly. | Pain related to migraine symptoms. | Lindsey will experience an increased level of comfort, allowing active participation in school activities. | 1. In association with the student, family, and medical team, evaluate the effectiveness of present comfort measures through interview and review of records.<br><br>2. In collaboration with the medical provider, family, and student, develop a school migraine-treatment plan based on symptoms.<br><br>3. Observe the student for signs of discomfort.<br><br>4. Standardize, in association with the student and family, an individual pain rating scale for school use.<br><br>5. In association with the family, assemble a list of comfort measures and help Lindsey to select appropriate choices based on level of discomfort.<br><br>6. Instruct the student to use prescribed treatment before symptoms are severe.<br><br>7. Reinforce learned biofeedback and relaxation therapy techniques.<br><br>8. Support the family while exploring alternative treatment options.<br><br>9. Locate a quiet, dark place for Lindsey to rest during acute attacks. | Lindsey will participate in development of the migraine treatment plan.<br><br>Lindsey will recognize the early warning signs of an oncoming migraine. |

| Assessment Data | Nursing Diagnosis | Goals | Nursing Interventions | Expected Outcomes |
|---|---|---|---|---|
| | | | 10. Determine the impact of discomfort on the student's school performance.<br>11. Modify environmental factors that may contribute to Lindsey's discomfort.<br>12. Assist the family/student to identify possible triggers where appropriate.<br>13. Make referrals to support groups and outside resources as appropriate. | |
| • Lindsey has stated, "I just want it all to go away…. I don't want to live my life like this…. Why can't things be the way they were?"<br><br>• In-school suspension last month for possession of alcohol on school grounds<br><br>• Parents express concern over Lindsey's "rebellious attitude."<br><br>• Grade point has dropped from an A-B average to C-D.<br><br>• Currently failing in algebra.<br><br>• Dropped out of band and pep squad this semester. | Ineffective coping related to stress imposed by migraines and their management. | Lindsey will demonstrate effective use of coping strategies. | 1. Obtain a signed medical release to obtain pertinent mental health records and to provide progress updates.<br>2. Evaluate student's decision-making ability related to treatment.<br>3. Assist student to adapt to the stress of migraines and their management.<br>4. Provide an attitude of unconditional acceptance.<br>5. Assist student to develop an objective appraisal of her migraine status<br>6. Assist Lindsey to identify strengths and reinforce examples of those strengths when observed.<br>7. Discuss alternative responses to stress.<br>8. Encourage constructive outlets for expression of frustration and anger. | Lindsey will demonstrate a reduction in self-destructive behavior.<br><br>Lindsey will demonstrate a reduction in self-critical comments. |

| Assessment Data | Nursing Diagnosis | Goals | Nursing Interventions | Expected Outcomes |
|---|---|---|---|---|
| • Parents have taken Lindsey to see a private therapist on a weekly basis for the last 2 years. | | | 9. Facilitate acceptance of others' limitations.<br><br>10. Teach new coping and problem-solving skills.<br><br>11. Introduce student to an adult mentor, with family approval, who successfully manages his or her own chronic condition.<br><br>12. Encourage use of spiritual resources as appropriate for family's values.<br><br>13. Encourage Lindsey to seek and maintain a social support network.<br><br>14. Provide opportunities for student/family/nurse to educate classmates about migraines.<br><br>15. Refer to building student-assistance team for potential evaluation. | |

## References

Al-Twaijri, W. A., & Shevell, M. I. (2002). Pediatric migraine equivalents: Occurrence and clinical features in practice. *Pediatric Neurology, 26*, 365–368.

Beers, M. H., & Berkow, R. (Eds.). (1999). *The Merck manual* (17th ed., pp. 1376–1377). Whitehouse Station, NJ: Merck Research Laboratories.

Chatterton, M. L., Lofland, J. H., Shechter, A., Curtice, W. S., Hu, H., Lenow, J., et al. (2002). Reliability and validity of the migraine therapy assessment questionnaire. *Headache, 42*, 1006–1015.

Evans, R. W. (2000). Headaches during childhood and adolescence. In R. W. Evans & N. T. Matthew (Eds.), *Handbook of headache* (pp. 139–149). Philadelphia: Lippincott-Williams & Wilkins.

Lipton, R. B., Scher, A. I., Kolodner, K., Liberman, J., Steiner, T. J., & Stewart, W. F. (2002). Migraine in the United States: Epidemiology and patterns of health care use. *Neurology, 58*, 885–894.

Millichap, J. G., & Yee, M. M. (2003). The diet factor in pediatric and adolescent migraine. *Pediatric Neurology 28*(2), 9–15.

National Institute of Neurological Disorders and Stroke, American Academy of Neurology, American Headache Society, & National Headache Foundation. (2001). 21st century prevention and management of migraine headaches. *Clinician, 19*(11), 1–35.

NANDA International. (2003). *Nursing diagnosis: Definitions & classification 2003–2004*. Philadelphia: Author.

Silverboard, G. (2001). Childhood migraine: A practical review. *Medscape Neurology*. Retrieved February 26, 2001, from http://pediatrics.Medscape.com/Medscape/Neurology/journal/2001/v03.n01/mn0202.silv/pnt-mn0202.silv.html

Winner, P., Rothner, A. D., Putman, D. G., & Asgharnejad, M. (2003). Demographic and migraine characteristics of adolescents with migraine: Glaxo Wellcome clinical trial's database. *Headache 43*, 451–457.

## Bibliography

Bauman, R. J. (2002). Behavioral treatment of migraine in children and adolescents. *Pediatric Drugs, 4*(9), 555–561.

Edmeads, J., & Mackell, J. A. (2002). The economic impact of migraine: An analysis of direct and indirect costs. *Headache, 42*, 501–509.

Gibbs, T. S., Fleischer, A. B., Feldman, S. R., Sam, M. C., & O'Donovan, C. A. (2003). Health care utilization in patients with migraine: Demographics and patterns of care in the ambulatory setting. *Headache, 43*(4), 330–335.

Kolar, K. R., Fisher, W., & Gordon, V. (2001). Nurse, my head hurts: A review of childhood headaches. *Journal of School Nursing, 17*(3), 120–125.

Linder, S. L., & Winner, P. (2001). Pediatric headache. *Medical Clinics of North America, 85*(4), 1037–1053.

Matthew, N. T. (2001). Pathophysiology, epidemiology, and impact of migraine. *Clinical Cornerstone, 4*(3), 1–17.

Mathew, N. T. (2002). Use of rescue medication in trials of almotriptan versus placebo in the treatment of acute migraine. *Clinical Therapeutics, 24*(4), 520–529.

McCloskey, J. C., & Bulechek, G. M. (Eds.). (2000). *Nursing interventions classification (NIC)* (3rd ed.). St. Louis, MO: Mosby Yearbook.

Smith, M. S., Martin-Herz, S. P., Womack W. M., & Marsigan, J. L. (2003). Comparative study of anxiety, depression, somatization, functional disability, and illness attribution in adolescents with chronic fatigue or migraine. *Pediatrics 111*(4 Pt 1), 376–381.

# Resources

American Council for Headache Education
19 Mantua Road
Mt. Royal, NJ 08061
856-423-0258
856-423-0082 (fax)
http://www.achenet.org

American Headache Society
19 Mantua Road
Mount Royal, NJ 08061
856-423-0043
856-423-0082 (fax)
ahshq@talley.com
http://www.ahsnet.org

International Headache Society
Oakwood
9 Willowmead Drive
Prestbury
Cheshire SK10 4BU, UK
+44 (0)1625 828663
+44 (0)1625 828494 (fax)
http://www.i-h-s.org

MAGNUM (Migraine Awareness Group: a National
    Understanding for Migraineurs)
113 South Saint ASAPH
Suite 300
Alexandria, VA 22314
1-703-739-9384
1-703-793-2432 (fax)
http:// ww.migraines.org

National Headache Foundation
820 North Orleans
Suite 217
Chicago, IL 60610
1-888-NHF-5552
773-525-7357 (fax)
info@headaches.org
http://www.headaches.org

National Institute of Neurological Disorders and
    Stroke
National Institutes of Health (NIH)
Office of Communications and Public Liaison
Bethesda, MD 20892-2540
301-496-5751
1-800-352-9424
301-402-2186 (fax)
http://www.ninds.nih.org

# Chapter Fifty-five

# Mitochondrial Disorders

Katherine J. Cuddy

## Introduction

Mitochondrial disorders have been described and spoken of only within the last 10 years. These disorders are inherited mainly from the mother, but both parents may pass them on to their children. Mitochondrial disorders are primarily energy disorders. The reduced production of energy at the mitochondrial level results in a multifaceted impact on health, performance, and behavior. The disorders can affect the central nervous system, the musculoskeletal system, the heart, the kidneys, and the liver. The degree of involvement varies.

Depending on the degree of involvement, some children might appear to be well, whereas others may be wheelchair-bound and tremulous. The mitochondrial diseases are now considered as common as childhood cancers that affect the cell's ability to produce life-sustaining energy (United Mitochondrial Disease Foundation, 2003). The mitochondrial group of diseases generally results in death in childhood or young adulthood (Bailey, 1995; Klehm, 1995; Portales, 1995). Some of the various mitochondrial diseases are Leigh disease, Barth syndrome, Pearson's syndrome, and Alpers' disease. These disorders are progressive, but the speed of progression varies from individual to individual (Bailey; Klehm; Portales).

## Pathophysiology

Every cell in the body, except red blood cells, contains mitochondria. Mitochondria are small and complex structures within the cell. Mitochondria carry their own DNA that is separate from the cell's DNA. Each cell contains one to hundreds of mitochondria. Mitochondria are called the "power house" of the cell, because they are required to produce the majority of energy (90%) used for growth and vital functioning of the body. Mitochondria produce this energy by changing the by-products of food we eat into adenosine triphosphate, which is energy for the body. The higher the energy need of the organ, the more dependent the organ is on properly functioning mitochondria. The organs requiring the highest energy levels are the brain, heart, skeletal muscle, kidney, liver, and bone marrow (Downie, 1998).

A metabolic disease develops when a significant number of mitochondria malfunction within the cells. The cells with the abnormal mitochondria vary in number from organ to organ and cell to cell. The malfunctioning of the mitochondria causes an interruption in the Krebs cycle. The disease also leads to an increase in the organic acids of the body, which can result in acidosis. Lactic acid is one of the organic acids that is commonly found to be increased in mitochondrial diseases, especially in the blood and spinal fluid. Mitochondrial diseases affect the functions of the brain, heart muscles, liver, and/or bone marrow. There is a wide range of body systems involved and symptoms.

In many cases, there are no affected family members. There are many questions regarding inheritance in these cases. Some "models" of inheritance are autosomal recessive, maternal, X-linked recessive, and autosomal dominant. Commonly, mitochondrial diseases are inherited from the maternal side of the family. The reason for this is that the mitochondria are given to the fetus from the mother's egg (Washington University School of Medicine, 1998).

Because of the varying symptoms and ages at onset, diagnosis of a mitochondrial disease is sometimes difficult. Even within the same family, siblings may present with different symptoms and at an older or younger age. The diagnosis of mitochondrial disease should be considered if three or more organ systems are involved, setbacks or flare-ups with a chronic disease occur with infections, and/or a common illness has atypical features that separate it from the group.

In addition to a complete history and physical examination, samples of blood and urine are taken for specific tests, and brain magnetic resonance imaging and muscle biopsy are done to make a final diagnosis. Spinal taps may also be used as a diagnostic tool. Once the diagnosis is made, the child should be referred to a healthcare center that specializes in mitochondrial disorders.

## Management

There is no cure for mitochondrial diseases. The goals of treatment are to alleviate the symptoms and to slow the progression of the disease. Individuals with a mitochondrial disease receive treatment for the signs and symptoms, such as cardiac arrhythmias, seizure disorder, or hypoglycemia. An experimental drug, dichloroacetate, is used to lower lactic acid levels. Most physicians prescribe a regimen of cofactors and vitamins, thinking these will help the metabolic process. Some of these medicines include coenzyme Q, carnitine, niacin, thiamine, and riboflavin. Some patients are placed on special diets, ranging from high fat to high carbohydrate to low fructose, and these are thought to help. Fasting should be avoided. Small, frequent meals and snacks are thought to be very beneficial. Stress should be avoided.

The effectiveness of treatment varies from patient to patient, largely depending on the severity of the illness. Treatment cannot reverse any damage done. Genetic counseling for the child's parents is also necessary. Education about the disease process, treatments, and prognosis is essential for the child and family. Research to find a more effective treatment and a cure is currently being conducted.

## Individualized Healthcare Plan

### Assessment
*History*
- Onset of signs and symptoms
- Diagnosis and medical testing
- Primary care physician and specialists seen
- Seizure activity and neurologic involvement
- Respiratory involvement and signs and symptoms
- Growth and development history
- Nutritional supplements or interventions used during mealtime
- Food likes and dislikes
- Toileting, any assistance needed, or diapered
- Mobility, limitations, tone and strength of extremities
- Other system involvement—cardiac, liver, gastrointestinal, or urinary
- Allergies to insects, food, or medicine
- Visual or auditory concerns or problems
- Sleep pattern: Does the student sleep through the night; if not, why and how long is he or she awake; bed time, rising time
- Migraines, head or abdominal, and if so, any aura
- Frequent colds or viruses
- Immunization history
- Communicable disease history
- Activity likes and dislikes
- Parent or guardian's knowledge of the disease process and treatment
- Student's knowledge of the disease process and treatment (if applicable)

*Current Status and Management*
- Baseline neurologic assessment
- Baseline respiratory assessment
- Baseline cardiac assessment
- Baseline height and weight
- Baseline skin integrity assessment
- Mobility needs, wheelchair or walker
- Physical ability: strength, range of motion, tremors, and use of orthotics
- Mealtime: amount of time needed, any special utensils or dishes, any assistance needed in feeding
- Toileting: frequency, any assistance needed, and incontinence
- Stools: type, any constipation or diarrhea, and if so, treatment
- Speech and language ability: Is it understandable, does the child speak in phrases or sentences, what language is used at home, what language does the child understand
- Current medications: name, dose, schedule, and route of administration
- Dietary supplements or snacks, type, amount, and times
- Treatments needed
- Therapy schedules and routines, if applicable
- Example of current routine day
- Signs and symptoms of impending illness: temperature, crying, lethargy, headache or stomachache
- Activity tolerance: amount of activity or class time the child is able to tolerate before needing rest periods
- Fine motor: any assistance needed from a modified pencil to computer equipment
- Special seating, glasses, or hearing aids needed
- Child's best and worst time of the day

- Signs and symptoms of fatigue: may need more rest periods or naps on certain days due to constantly changing energy level, may need modified activities, may need to eliminate activity
- Access to healthcare providers and services, facilities, insurance or financial needs
- Individual supplies needed
- Caretakers at home, at daycare, before or after school

### Self-care
- Ability to dress self
- Ability to feed self
- Ability to toilet self or signal when toileting is necessary
- Ability to carry out personal hygiene
- Knowledge of activity limits and when rest periods are needed
- Child knowledge of the signs and symptoms to watch for that signal the onset of illness
- Ability to self-administer medications, experience at home
- Decision-making skills

### Psychosocial Status
- Child's perception of his/her health status
- Interaction with child's peers: specific activities in school, church, and community
- Child's age and developmental level
- Child's reaction to doctor's visits and/or hospitalizations
- Participation in counseling, past or present
- Classes and subjects that the child enjoys
- Motivators that encourage the child
- Behavioral issues: school and home
- Parent's/guardian's perception of child's current health status
- Support at home for the student with homework
- Family participation in community resources for psychosocial issues regarding the child and his/her health status

### Academic Status
- Individualized education program (IEP) or 504 plan
- Therapy needed in school programs: speech, occupational, or physical therapy
- School attendance and reason for absences: past and present
- Preferential seating needed: due to vision or hearing disabilities
- Need for modified schedule: allow for rest periods and more important classes in the morning
- Need for a modified school day: early release, late start
- Mobility needs around school (stairs, long distances)
- Nursing care needed during school
- Assistance needed for toileting, eating, mobility, or writing
- Transportation needs: to and from school
- Therapies needed during school
- Out-of-school educational program: homebound, hospital-based
- Modifications needed: schedule, curriculum, assignments, testing
- Academic performance: past and present

## Nursing Diagnoses (N.D.) (NANDA, 2003)

N.D. 1 Imbalanced nutrition: less than body requirements (NANDA 00002 ) related to:
- high energy requirements
- inability to ingest or digest food or absorb nutrients due to biological factors

N.D. 2 Impaired urinary elimination (NANDA 00021) related to:
- sensory motor impairment

N.D. 3 Risk for decrease in cardiac output (NANDA 00029) related to:
- altered stroke volume and altered contractility

N.D. 4 Risk for ineffective breathing pattern (NANDA 00032) related to:
- neuromuscular dysfunction
- respiratory muscle fatigue

**N.D. 5** Risk for ineffective tissue perfusion: cerebral (NANDA 00024) related to:
- seizure activity
- stroke-like symptoms

**N.D. 6** Risk for chronic pain (NANDA 00133) related to:
- frequent migraines, head and/or abdominal

**N.D. 7** Risk for injury (NANDA 00035) related to:
- trauma
- seizure activity
- stroke-like symptoms
- fatigue
- low muscle tone and strength

**N.D. 8** Delayed growth and development (NANDA 00111) related to:
- high energy need, effects of physical disability
- poor nutritional intake

**N.D. 9** Risk for impaired skin integrity (NANDA 00046) related to:
- physical immobilization
- excretion and/or secretions
- orthotics
- G-tube placement, moisture
- altered fluid and nutritional intake

**N.D. 10** Risk for disturbed sensory perception (NANDA 00122) related to:
- visual function/vision deficit
- sensory-neural hearing loss/hearing deficit

**N.D. 11** Risk for impaired verbal communication (NANDA 00051) related to:
- speech delay, weakening of musculoskeletal system
- student's understanding of class/material
- student's decreased self-confidence

**N.D. 12** Deficient knowledge (NANDA 00126) related to:
- absences from school/school attendance pattern
- decreased academic achievement
- amount of incomplete work
- activity tolerance
- lack of help/support from home
- school schedule in relation to activity tolerance/fatigue

**N.D. 13** Risk for impaired physical mobility (NANDA 00085) related to:
- low muscle tone and strength, musculoskeletal, neuromuscular impairment
- low energy level
- decreased activity tolerance, decreased strength and endurance

**N.D. 14** Risk for activity intolerance (NANDA 00092, 00093) related to:
- fatigue and low energy

**N.D. 15** Risk for ineffective individual coping: student and family (NANDA 00069) related to:
- resources of the family, inadequate
- student's age
- student and/or parent knowledge deficit

**N.D. 16** Impaired social interactions (NANDA 00052, 00053) related to:
- decreased self-esteem
- school absences/attendance pattern
- fatigue and limited physical mobility

**N.D. 17** Self-care deficit: bathing/hygiene, dressing/grooming, and feeding (NANDA 00108, 00109, 00102) related to:
- neuromuscular impairment
- weakness and tiredness
- knowledge deficit regarding the disease
- knowledge deficit regarding self-care activities
- healthcare procedures, treatments
- medication administration

## Goals

The student will eat a balanced diet. ( N.D. 1, 8, 9)

The student will maintain a stable weight and will not lose weight. (N.D. 1, 8)

The student will maintain proper fluid intake. (N.D. 1, 2, 9)

The student will increase knowledge of the signs and symptoms of the disease to report and the causes for the signs and symptoms. (N.D. 2, 3, 4, 5, 6)

The student will avoid triggers of pain, cough, or illness. (N.D. 2, 4, 6)

The student will ask for assistance, when needed. (N.D. 2, 3, 4, 5, 6, 7)

The student will increase knowledge of what activities to avoid and why. (N.D. 6, 7)

The student will maintain good urinary and bowel elimination pattern. (N.D. 2, 9)

The student will perform regular position changes. (N.D. 9)

The student will maintain proper/prescribed use of orthotics. (N.D. 9)

The student will report any hearing or visual change. (N.D. 10)

The student will wear prescribed glasses, or hearing aids, or use preferential seating as needed. (N.D. 10)

The student will communicate needs to teachers, peers, and caregivers. (N.D. 11, 16)

The student will maintain a good school attendance pattern. (N.D. 12, 16)

The student will know and communicate the need for a rest period or possible changes in schedule. (N.D. 12, 17)

The student will ask for extra help, when needed. (N.D. 12, 15)

The student will follow his/her prescribed exercise program from physical therapy. (N.D. 13, 15, 17)

The student will demonstrate good decision-making skills in choosing activities—in school, after school, and/or in the community—that do not exceed his/her physical limitations. (N.D. 13, 14)

The student will increase his/her knowledge about his/her disease. (N.D. 15, 16, 17)

The student will participate in the development of his/her schedule and care plan. (N.D. 15, 16, 17)

The student will comply with his/her medical management plan. (N.D. 15, 17)

## Interventions

### Teaching: Individual/learning facilitation

Monitor academic performance. (N.D. 12)

- Watch academic progress: grades, ability to participate, increase in skills and knowledge.
- Make a referral for 504 assessment, if needed.
- Make a referral for special education assessment, if needed.

Assist the special education team to assess the student and develop an IEP for student. (N.D. 1–17)

- Include student, parent or guardians, healthcare providers, teachers, and other staff in assessment and IEP development process.
- Coordinate home care with school care, incorporating necessary treatments into the school day.
- Participate in IEP assessment plan, incorporating required health-related services into the assessment summary report and the IEP.
- Review IEP with team members yearly and as needed.
- Reconvene special education team for additional services, if needed.

Assist teachers to modify curriculum, as needed. (NANDA 10, 11, 12, 13)

- Avoid any excess writing for assignments, both in school and for homework.
- Use multiple choice, opposed to essay, questions for testing.
- Use computer in school or photocopy student's work or have someone assist student to write out assignments.
- Provide a longer time for specific assignments.

### Staff development

Educate teachers and other school staff. (N.D. 1–17)

- Describe what mitochondrial disorder is.
- Explain possible symptoms involved.
- Describe common symptoms.
- Relate importance of rest periods or shortened classes.
- Explain treatment and medication schedule during the school day.
- Describe ways to minimize energy use.
- Restrict, modify or alternate activities for the student.
- State importance of listening to student and reporting any symptoms.
- Describe signs and symptoms to watch for and report to the school nurse.

- Specify actions to take if a seizure occurs.
- Illustrate alternate learning techniques in class that may be needed.
- Detail need for good communication with the home.
- Make plan for make-up work, for frequent or prolonged absences.
- Arrange for special measures for transportation, recess, and field trips.

Assist physical education teachers or adaptive physical education teachers to understand the need to provide activities that use little energy. (N.D. 13, 14)
- Assist them to observe the student's muscle strength and tone.
- Discuss possible modifications of activities or alternate activities that use less energy but promote flexibility and muscle tone.
- Avoid any climbing or swimming due to possible seizure.
- Include student in the choosing of activities.
- Encourage inclusion of a few friends to do alternate activities with student.

Provide a list of staff members trained in the care of the student to teacher, nurse, and administrator. ( N.D. 1–17 )

Assist teachers in understanding the social benefits of a student being in a regular education class with peers either full-time or for appropriate subject matter. (N.D. 16)
- Describe class modifications that may be required.
- Provide assistance of an adult.

### Emergency care

Develop an emergency care plan for seizures that occur at school or on field trips, as needed.

Provide staff with emergency phone numbers and emergency contacts. ( N.D. 7)

### Documentation

Assist in obtaining medical releases signed to allow information to be shared between school and healthcare provider throughout the year. ( N.D. 1–17 )

Obtain orders and authorization for any treatments, medication, and special diet, if necessary, from both parent and physician. (N.D. 1–10, 13)
- Daily and "as needed" medications
- Special dietary intake and supplements
- Nursing treatments needed throughout the school day
- Special instructions for administering medication to the student
- Specific side effects to monitor for
- Any change in medication or treatments must be obtained in writing from the doctor and parent.

### Energy management

Monitor activity tolerance, level of fatigue, and any contributory factors. (N.D. 1, 3, 4, 5, 6, 7, 8, 12, 13, 14)
- Develop a daily schedule with student, parent, and teacher.
- Avoid long walks to and from class or to the bathroom.
- Use the elevator instead of stairs.
- Assign a hall buddy and/or staff person to stop and rest with student and to carry his/her books.
- Allow student to have a second set of books at home to avoid carrying them back and forth to school.
- Provide alternate activities for student during gym period and recess, if necessary.
- Provide a rest or nap time, if necessary.
- Modify school schedule, as needed.
- Provide a quiet, designated area for resting.
- Encourage student to voice how he/she is feeling.
- Document the occurrence of any signs of fatigue and notice if there is a pattern.
- Notify parent and healthcare provider of a change in condition.
- If student uses a wheelchair, provide a travel friend between classes, to and from the bus, and to and from lunch and recess.
- Assign a staff person for responsibility and supervision of transporting the student.
- Develop an emergency plan (fire or other emergency), whether the student is ambulatory or in a wheelchair.

### Nutrition management

Provide a well-balanced, nutritious diet. (N.D. 1, 8)
- Incorporate the student's likes and dislikes pertaining to food.
- Know how student is able to drink.

- Provide texture of food student is able to tolerate (grind, cut).
- Provide adaptive equipment, as needed.
- Allow student sufficient time for eating.
- Assist the student by preparing meals for eating (open cartons, cut meat, etc.).
- Give supplements as ordered.
- Provide a snack, if needed.
- If fed through G-tube, administer the prescribed formula at the set rate.
- Note any signs of abdominal distention and notify parent and physician.
- Monitor intake of fluids and solids.
- Thicken liquids, if necessary.
- Provide access for good hydration during the school day.
- Document any change in intake and notify parent and physician.
- Monitor student's need for a short rest period during meals.
- Note any signs of dysphasia and report to parent and physician.
- If student must be fed, instruct the person doing the feeding in proper feeding technique; allow ample time between bites for chewing and swallowing, train person in Heimlich maneuver (require a demonstration of skill).
- Weigh student monthly and record.
- Notify parent and physician of any weight loss and change weight checks to every 2 weeks.
- Avoid periods of fasting.

*Urinary elimination management/bowel management*
Monitor student's output. (N.D. 2)
- Discuss with parent and/or student: urine and bowel frequency at home.
- Toilet student at regular intervals and when needed.
- Provide staff to assist with toileting, if needed.
- If needed, ask parent to send a change of clothing to school.
- If diapered, change at regular times and when needed.
- Assist parents to provide needed supplies (diapers, clothes, etc.).
- Note color, odor, and amount of urine and stool.
- Document baseline urine and stool outputs.
- Notify parent and healthcare provider of any changes or concerns regarding output; document.
- Note any edema; document and notify parent and doctor.
- Note any change in stools, diarrhea or constipation, and notify parent and physician.

*Cardiac care*
Monitor student's cardiac status. (N.D. 3)
- Obtain baseline apical pulse, rate and rhythm, and blood pressure and document assessment.
- Check pulse and blood pressure weekly, notify parent and physician of any change.
- If student complains of chest pain, assess type and location of pain and monitor vital signs and notify parent.

*Respiratory monitoring*
Monitor respiratory status. (N.D. 4)
- Obtain baseline assessment of respiratory rate, rhythm, and breath sounds and document.
- Check respiratory rate and breath sounds weekly and as needed, document assessment.
- Note any change in respiratory rate, rhythm, or breath sounds; notify parent and physician.
- Administer treatments and medications as ordered.
- Reassess student after treatment.
- Document response to treatment.
- Position child for optimal air exchange.
- Refer child to physician for new-onset cough or congestion.
- Keep child away from others with respiratory infections.
- Note activities that cause child to become short of breath, and avoid these or shorten the time to allow for rest.
- If suctioning is ordered, suction for increased congestion to maintain a patent airway.
- Avoid any allergens that might lead to respiratory congestion.

*Self-care assistance: Dressing*
Assist student to dress appropriately for the weather, especially cold and rainy climates. (N.D. 4)

*Pain management*
Monitor complaints of pain. (N.D. 6, 7)
- Assess type of pain and location.
- Assess for trauma that may be causing pain.
- Provide comfort measures, especially those that have worked in the past.
- Determine if this is new-onset or chronic pain.
- Try to determine factors precipitating pain and plan to avoid factors in the future.
- Provide medication for pain, as ordered.
- Document pain, type, onset, known causes, and relief.
- Document specific regimens that help alleviate the student's pain.
- Notify parent and physician of any new or increase in pain.

*Seizure precaution/seizure management*
Monitor seizure activity and neurologic status. (N.D. 5, 6)
- Do a baseline neurologic assessment and document.
- Communicate with parent to keep school informed of any seizure activity changes in medication, and any alteration in neurologic status.
- Maintain a seizure record.
- Reassess neurologic signs monthly and as needed.
- Notify parent and/or physician of any change in neurologic status.
- Have student wear helmet, if needed, for ambulation.
- Make any accommodations, if student has weakness or immobility of one side.
- Take seizure precautions—stairs, swimming, and climbing.
- Note any specific time of day or activity that coincides with seizures. Inform parent and physician, and plan to avoid activities that precipitate seizures in the future.

*Communication enhancement: Visual deficit*
Monitor vision status. (N.D. 10)
- Provide vision screening yearly.
- Refer any visual complaints to healthcare provider.
- Preferential classroom seating (as needed).
- If student has glasses, assist the student to wear them in school.
- Inform the staff of the possible involvement of the mitochondrial disease on the eye.
- Discuss special education visual-impaired services with special education team, if needed.
- Offer extra help in short intervals of time. Encourage incorporating alternate methods of learning, use keyboard, tape recorder, and large-print books in the classroom, as needed.
- Assist the student and teacher to obtain a reading buddy to read to student, as needed.
- Speak before approaching student.

*Communication enhancement: Hearing deficit*
Monitor hearing status. (N.D. 10)
- Provide audiological screening yearly.
- Refer student to healthcare provider, if indicated.
- Obtain records from audiologist, if assessed or under care.
- Preferential seating in class, (if needed): away from window, door, projectors, ventilation system, and other noise-making areas in the classroom.
- If student is to wear hearing aids or an FM transmitter, assist the student to wear the hearing device in school and monitor function of the device daily.
- Speak slowly and clearly.
- Look at student when talking.

*Emotional support/counseling*
Encourage student to verbalize needs. (N.D. 11, 15-17)
- Refer student to speech clinician for evaluation, as needed.
- Assist the student to feel comfortable with surroundings and staff and peers.

- Provide a place with privacy.
- Listen carefully to child.
- Observe for facial expressions and grimaces.
- Coordinate services to provide the student with consistent care providers so the child can develop a relationship.
- Provide counseling as needed.
- Maintain student confidentiality; explain to the student that some information must be shared with parents, physicians, and/or teachers and the reason for it.
- Help educate the student on the disease process and symptoms to be aware of. (N.D. 1–17)
- Assist the student to report the symptoms to his or her parents and healthcare providers.

*Family mobilization*
Assist parents in understanding the social benefits of a student being in a regular education class with peers either full-time or for appropriate subject matter. (N.D. 16)
- Describe class modifications that may be required.
- Provide assistance of an adult.
- Assist the parent to observe the class.
Encourage the parent to communicate with school nurse and classroom teacher regularly or with any change in student's condition or treatment. (N.D. 15)
- Discuss need for change in schedule.
- Discuss need for increased health condition management needs at school.
- Develop a communication notebook.
- Provide one contact for healthcare providers, for necessary information to and from them.
- Encourage parents to inform school of upcoming appointments with healthcare providers.
Educate parent on school attendance policy and appropriate absences. (N.D. 15)
- Call school when child is absent.
- Send note upon student's return.
- Notify school nurse of any illness.
- Discuss signs and symptoms or complaints to listen to and keep child home.
- Contact the teacher or school for make-up work and/or tutoring.
Monitor attendance pattern and reasons for absences. (N.D. 12)
Arrange to have parent send in required equipment and/or supplies on a regular schedule. ( N.D. 1, 2, 9, 17)

*Self-care assistance*
Assist the child in self-care activities, treatments, and medications that he/she can participate in. (N.D. 15, 17)
- Monitor student's ability to perform self-care skills.
- Provide privacy for administration of medications or treatments.
- Discuss with the student the purpose and benefit of the treatment and/or medication.
- Reinforce proper technique in self-care activities.
- Assist student to store and access supplies.
- Help student identify positive and negative aspects of self-care.
- Minimize or alleviate negative aspects of self-care.
- Highlight positive aspects of self-care.

*Health education*
Provide health education to student's peers, if they choose. (N.D. 15, 16)
- Obtain parental permission and student permission.
- Discuss information that the parent and student want shared and information they do not want shared.
- Discuss any fears with the student and/or peers.
- Help the student feel more comfortable with peers.

*Decision-making support*
Assist student, counselors, and parents to plan electives and schedule, when applicable. (N.D. 15, 16, 17)
- Identify and discuss with student alternate choices, when available.
- Educate the student on alternate activities that require low energy.

*Exercise therapy: Muscle control, joint mobility*
Monitor changes in physical mobility. (N.D. 13)
- Compare to student's baseline strength and limitations of mobility.
- Physical therapy involvement: progress toward and attainment of goals.
- Occupational therapy involvement: progress toward and attainment of goals.
- Assist with the scheduling and/or provision of range-of-motion exercises: Develop a weekly schedule and give to teacher, parent, and student.
- Teach student and caregivers proper exercises and frequency.
- Educate the student and parent on the purpose of the exercises.
- Help the student choose strengthening and endurance activities.
- If the student is able, encourage participation in team, including academic team activities, and contact sports.

*Body image enhancement*
Assist the student to maintain a positive body image. (N.D. 15- 17)
- Provide privacy and assistance with toileting, if needed.
- Provide oral care during feeding.
- Provide oral care for drooling (avoid use of bibs).
- Elaborate on student's strengths and abilities.
Offer counseling for student. (N.D. 15, 16)

## Expected Student Outcomes

The student will:
*Student health status*
- Participate in regular education classes, when able. (N.D. 12, 15, 16)
- Participate in regular physical education classes with modifications made, as needed. (N.D. 3-7, 13, 14)
- Maintain a good school attendance record. (N.D. 12- 15)

*Adaptation to physical disability*
- Identify and choose alternate activities, if unable to participate in regular gym class or recess. (N.D. 7, 13, 14)
- Demonstrate alternate ways to carry out activities. (N.D. 7, 13)

*Knowledge of disease process*
- Describe the disease process and list reasons for medications and treatments. (N.D. 2, 3, 15, 17)
- List signs and symptoms of a respiratory or viral illness. (N.D. 2, 4)
- Describe physical limitations due to disease. (N.D. 13- 15)

*Nutritional status*
- Eat a balanced diet. (N.D. 1, 8, 14)
- Demonstrate normal fluid intake during the school day. (N.D. 1, 8, 14)

*Participation in healthcare decisions*
- Participate in prioritizing school-day activities. (N.D. 12, 15)

*Compliance behavior*
- Report signs and symptoms of having a respiratory infection to parents and school nurse. (N.D. 4)
- Do exercises as prescribed and instructed. (N.D. 13, 14)
- Assist in monitoring his or her weight. (N.D. 1, 8)
- Follow prescribed rest and exercise plan. (N.D. 1, 3, 4, 6, 7, 13, 14, 17)
- Wear orthotics, if needed.

*Health promotion behavior*
- Dress appropriately for the weather. (N.D. 4)

*Knowledge of body mechanics*
- Describe the need for regular physical therapy. (N.D. 13, 14)

*Vision compensation behavior*
- Report any changes in vision. (N.D. 10)
- Wear glasses as prescribed. (N.D. 10)

*Hearing compensation behavior*
- Report any changes in hearing. (N.D. 10)
- Wear hearing devices, if prescribed. (N.D. 10)

*Energy conservation*
- Rest for regular intervals, as needed. (N.D. 7, 13- 15)
- Demonstrate ability to modify rest and exercise plan based on activity tolerance. (N.D. 1, 3, 4, 6, 7, 13, 14, 17)

*Risk control*
- Demonstrate avoidance of exposure to respiratory and other infections. (N.D. 4)

*Pain control*
- Report migraine or pain when it occurs. (N.D. 6)
- Follow prescribed pain management plan, if migraine or pain occurs. (N.D. 6)

*Personal safety behavior*
- Wear helmet, if needed. (N.D. 7, 13)

*Body positioning: self-initiated*
- Make regular position changes. (N.D. 9, 13, 17)

*Communication: expressive*
- Communicate needs to teacher, aide, nurse, and parents. (N.D. 11, 15-17)
- Demonstrate speaking slowly and clearly. (N.D. 11)
- Participate in speech therapy if needed. (N.D. 11)

*Student health status*
- Finish all assigned class work with modifications made, as needed. (N.D. 12)
- Ask for extra class help, when needed. (N.D. 12)

*Sleep*
- Demonstrate compliance with a consistent bedtime. (N.D. 14)

*Coping*
- Participate in counseling, if needed. (N.D. 15)
- Express, feelings, questions, or concerns regarding disease and/or treatments to parents, school nurse, and/or physician. (N.D. 15)

*Social involvement*
- Interact with peers in school. (N.D. 16)
- Assist in choosing appropriate work or travel buddies. (N.D. 16)

*Self-care status*
- Demonstrate ability to self-care. (N.D. 17)

*Self-care: hygiene*
- Assist in caring for his or her skin. (N.D. 9)
- Demonstrate proper hand washing. (N.D. 2, 4, 9, 17)

*Self-care: toileting*
- Participate in creating a toileting and/or changing schedule. (N.D. 2)
- Notify the staff when it is necessary to be toileted and/or changed. (N.D. 2 )

## Case Study

Sarah is a 10-year-old girl who was diagnosed with Leigh disease at age 4 years. She has one older sibling who was also diagnosed with this disease. Sarah lives at home with her mother and sees a specialist at Boston Children's Hospital

Sarah's sitting, crawling, and walking developed slowly. She crawled at 9 months and walked at 16 months. She was toilet trained at 3 1/2 years of age. She became unsteady and began to fall regularly at age 3 1/2. After multiple tests and a muscle biopsy, she was diagnosed with Leigh disease. Since that time she has been gradually weakening. She was placed on carnitine, coenzyme Q and vitamin C, and carbamazepine (Tegretol).

Sarah appears to be happy and answers questions appropriately. Her speech is difficult to understand. She drools continuously. She is small for her age and has very thin arms and legs. She has constant fine tremors in her arms. She is able to follow commands. Breath sounds are clear. Apical pulse is 94 and regular. Blood pressure is 102/58 mm Hg. Abdomen is soft and nontender with good bowel sounds. She is diapered. Her urine is clear amber. Bowel movements are once every 2 to 3 days. She is wheelchair-bound and nonambulatory but can stand to pivot, with assistance. She wears ankle-foot orthoses on both lower extremities. Her last tonic-clonic seizure was 1 year ago. She enjoys school. She attends some special education and some regular education classes.

## Mitochondrial Disorders

| Assessment Data | Nursing Diagnosis | Goals | Nursing Interventions | Expected Outcomes |
|---|---|---|---|---|
| Small for age<br>Weight: 55 lbs<br>Extremities: very thin arms and legs. | Alteration in nutritional status related to difficulty chewing and fatigue. | Sarah will maintain good hydration and nutrition. | Monitor Sarah with meals at school.<br><br>Provide nutritional supplements and snacks at school per physician order.<br><br>Monitor for difficulty with swallowing. Notify parent and physician if it occurs.<br><br>Provide proper food consistency and size to enhance Sarah's ability to chew and swallow foods.<br><br>Monitor weight monthly. Notify parent and physician of any weight loss.<br><br>Monitor hydration needs closely, especially on hot days. | Sarah will eat a balanced diet, including snacks, food supplements.<br>Sarah has good hydration throughout the school day.<br>Sarah demonstrates a slow, steady weight gain. |
| Breath sounds are clear<br>Short of breath after some activities.<br><br>Occasional dry cough.<br>No cyanosis. | Ineffective breathing pattern related to lung involvement and low energy level. | Sarah will increase knowledge of activities that cause shortness of breath.<br><br>Sarah will avoid activities that cause breathing difficulty or choose alternative activities. | Assist Sarah to position herself for optimal respiratory effort.<br><br>Assess breath sounds, rate and rhythm, or respiration weekly and as needed.<br><br>Notify parent and physician of any change in respiratory status.<br><br>Allow Sarah to rest as needed.<br><br>With Sarah's teachers and parents, modify activities that are known to cause shortness of breath, and identify activities that may be alternative activities. | Sarah will identify activities that cause shortness of breath.<br><br>Sarah does not participate in activities that cause shortness of breath.<br><br>Sarah will participate in alternative activities that do not cause shortness of breath. |

| Assessment Data | Nursing Diagnosis | Goals | Nursing Interventions | Expected Outcomes |
|---|---|---|---|---|
| Tonic-clonic seizures—last one was a year ago Medication: Tegretol, daily, at home. | Risk for injury related to seizure activity. | Sarah will remain safe if a seizure occurs at school or on a field trip. | With Sarah's parents, develop an emergency care plan (ECP) for seizure activity that occurs at school or on field trips.<br><br>Obtain any medication and authorization from the parent and physician for administration of the medication.<br><br>Provide in-service training for teachers and other staff working with Sarah about her seizures, the ECP, and what to do if a seizure occurs at school or on a field trip. | Sarah will not incur any injuries if a seizure occurs.<br><br>Sarah will participate with staff in practicing what to do if a seizure occurs. |
| Sarah has fine, constant tremors in her arms Able to follow commands Speech slightly garbled. | Ineffective tissue perfusion: cerebral resulting in neurologic symptoms. | Sarah will participate in classroom activities, with assistance as needed.<br><br>Sarah effectively communicates needs to others.<br><br>Sarah will utilize resources for assistance, if needed. | Document baseline neurologic status (information from observations, parents, and physician).<br><br>Reassess neurologic status monthly, including need for increased assistance in the classroom as reported by teachers and aides.<br><br>Notify parent and physician of any changes in neurologic status or increased tremors. See IEP. | Sarah participates in regular education class activities, with assistance as needed.<br><br>Sarah participates in physical education classes, with modifications made as necessary.<br><br>Sarah demonstrates effective communication with teachers and aides.<br><br>Sarah completes assigned class work with modifications and assistance as needed. |

| Assessment Data | Nursing Diagnosis | Goals | Nursing Interventions | Expected Outcomes |
|---|---|---|---|---|
| Sarah is diapered for stool and urine.<br><br>Frequent drooling.<br>Wheelchair for mobility.<br>Wears ankle-foot orthoses. (AFOs) on lower extremities. | Risk for impaired skin integrity related to incontinence, immobility, and wearing orthotics. | Sarah will maintain good skin integrity. | Change diapers every 3 hours and as needed.<br><br>Provide proper cleaning and skin care with each diaper change.<br><br>Check for skin breakdown with each diaper change. If it occurs, document and notify parent.<br><br>Remove AFOs for 1 hour each day and check skin for irritation or breakdown.<br><br>If any redness occurs from AFOs, rub the area with alcohol and recheck in 15 minutes.<br><br>If redness persists, notify parent.<br><br>Practice weight shifts with Sarah.<br><br>Encourage her to do at least one weight shift per class period. | Sarah will shift her weight once per class period, as observed by teacher or aide. |

# Emergency Care Plan
# Mitochondrial Disorders

Date: January 18, 1999

Student: Sarah Jones

Date of birth: _____

School: _____

Grade: _____

Parent(s)/Guardian(s): _____

_____

_____

Home telephone: _____

Father's work: _____

Mother's work: _____

Emergency contact: _____

Healthcare provider: _____

Hospital preferred: _____

Telephone: _____

Telephone: _____

Telephone: _____

## Child-Specific Emergencies

| If you see this | Action to take |
|---|---|
| Seizure activity:  New onset<br><br>Prolonged<br><br>Cyanosis present | 1. Remove from danger.<br><br>2. Maintain airway.<br><br>3. Activate 911 system.<br><br>4. Provide nursing care as needed.<br><br>5. Notify parent.<br><br>6. Transport to hospital with nurse.<br><br>7. Send a copy of the student's medical history, medications, and emergency contacts to the hospital. |

Signatures:

Emergency Care Plan written by: _____ Date _____

School Nurse _____ Date _____

Parent/guardian (if required) _____ Date _____

Student Signature (if appropriate) _____ Date _____

Mitochondrial Disorders

# Emergency Evacuation Plan
## Mitochondrial Disorders

Name: <u>Sarah Jones</u>                    Staff Person: _____

Room No.: _____        Back-up staff person: _____


Any equipment necessary: _____

Mode of transportation: _____

Two staff are assigned and trained in how to safely evacuate the student, in case of an emergency or a drill. They are given a copy of the student's schedule.

If assistance will be needed, the fire department is to be notified.

There is an emergency bag ready to take (located _____), for continued care of the student, containing such things as diapers, equipment, meds, etc.

# References

Bailey, I. *Living with mitochondrial disorders.* (1995 May). Paper presented at the Conference of Mitochondrial Disorders, Boston Children's Hospital, Boston, MA.

Downie, J. *Mitochondrial diseases,* Retrieved August 4, 1998, from www.hmtnet.com/users/cobrown

Klehm, M. *Medications for patients with mitochondrial disease.* (1995 May). Paper presented at the Conference of Mitochondrial Disorders, Boston Children's Hospital, Boston, MA.

NANDA International. (2003). *NANDA nursing diagnoses: Definitions & classification 2003-2004.* Philadelphia: Author.

Portales A. *Neurodevelopmental and educational issues of mitochondrial disease.* (1995 May). Paper presented at the Conference of Mitochondrial Disorders, Boston Children's Hospital, Boston, MA.

United Mitochondrial Disease Foundation. (2003). *Redefining hope.* Retrieved September 17, 2003, from http://www.umdf.org/index-mainframe.html

Washington University School of Medicine. (1998). *Mitochondial disorders.* Retrieved August 4, 1998, from http://www.neuro.wusl.edu/neuromuscular/mitosyn.html

# Bibliography

Boles, R., & Mason, T. (2003). *The genetics of mitochondrial disease.* Retrieved September 17, 2003, from http://www.umdf.org/mitodisease/genetics.html

Cohen, B. (2003). *Mitochondrial disease diagnostic testing.* Retrieved September 17, 2003, from http://www.umdf.org/mitodisease/testing.html

Cohen, B. (2003). *Mitochondrial disease: Treatment.* Retrieved September 17, 2003, from http://www.umdf.org/mitodisease/treatment.html

Harbor UCLA Medical Center. (1998). *Mitochondial diseases.* Retrieved August 4, 1998. from http://www.humc.edu

McLance, K. L., Huether, S. E. ( 2002 ). *Pathophysiology: The biologic basis for disease in adults and children* (4th ed.). Philadelphia: Mosby.

MDA News. (2002). *New directions in mitochondrial diseases.* Retrieved September 20, 2003, from www.mdausa.org/news/98042/mito.html

Naviaux, R. K. (2003). *Mitochondrial disease: Diagnosis.* Retrieved September 17, 2003, from http://www.umdf.org/mitodisease/diagnosis.html

Preston P. (1998) *Mitochondrial diseases: Information for patients and parents.* Retrieved August 4, 1998, from www.netcentral.co.uk/last

# Resources

Kennedy Krieger Institute
707 North Broadway
Baltimore, MD 21205
1-800-873-3377
433-923-9405 (fax)
http://www.kennedykrieger.org

Muscular Dystrophy Association
1140 Avenue of the Americas
Suite 1801
New York, NY 10036
212-689-9040
212-689-0269 (fax)
http://www.mdausa.org

National Information Center for Children and Youth With Disabilities
PO Box 1492
Washington, DC 20013
1-800-695-0285
http://www.nichcy.org

United Mitochondrial Disease Foundation
8085 Saltsburg Road
Suite 201
Pittsburgh, PA 15239
412-793-8077
412-793-6477 (fax)
http://www.umdf.org

## Chapter Fifty-six

# Neurofibromatosis

Sally Zentner Schoessler

## Introduction

Neurofibromatosis is a genetically determined developmental disorder that is present at birth. Neurofibromatosis takes many forms in that many patients have very mild cases with few symptoms, whereas other patients display dramatic and disfiguring effects. The disorder seems to be a result of a defect that alters peripheral nerve differentiation and growth (Wong, Hockenberry-Eaton, Wilson, Winkelstein, & Kline, 2003). It affects equal numbers of males and females with no common racial, ethnic, or geographic denominators (Neurofibromatosis, 2002).

The severity and complications of each form of neurofibromatosis create unique challenges for the school nurse caring for an affected child. Each case must be evaluated on an individual basis with an individualized plan of care.

## Pathophysiology and Management

Neurofibromatosis has several distinct characteristics. Although these distinguishing findings are indicative of the disorder, it is important to stress that the symptoms will vary in severity in each child. The condition derives its name from *neurofibroma,* the most common type of tumor seen in the condition.

Neurofibromatosis is categorized into two distinct disorders. They are both autosomal dominant genetic disorders, and although approximately half of the cases of neurofibromatosis are passed to the child from a parent, about half of all cases of NF1 represent new mutations (Freidman, 2003).

Neurofibromatosis type 1 (NF1), also called peripheral neurofibromatosis, is the most prevalent form of neurofibromatosis and has been associated with von Recklinghausen's disease. The following are characteristics of NF1:

- Incidence of 1 in 4,000 births
- Multiple café-au-lait spots
- Neurofibromas under the skin
- Enlargement of bones and bone deformity
- Scoliosis
- Tumors of the brain and spinal cord

- Learning disabilities (National Neurofibromatosis Foundation, 2004)

Neurofibromatosis type 2 (NF2), or bilateral acoustic neurofibromatosis, occurs in 1 in 40,000 births. Characteristics are as follows:

- Multiple tumors of the cranial and spinal nerves
- Other lesions of the brain and spinal cord
- Tumors of both auditory nerves (National Neurofibromatosis Foundation, 2004)

Café-au-lait spots become prominent in over 90% of patients with neurofibromatosis. These flat, pigmented spots are usually present at birth or appear by the child's second birthday and increase in number and darken in color throughout childhood. Axillary freckling is also present in most cases (Behrmann & Klingman, 2004).

In addition, Lisch nodules develop on the iris surface; these appear as clear to yellow or brown elevations and increase in number as the child grows older (Wong et al., 2003). Lisch nodules have no effect on vision and appear at puberty. Whereas they are an indicator of neurofibromatosis, they have no medical significance.

Many complications can be present with neurofibromatosis. These include:

- Disfigurement from tumors
- Visual abnormalities due to optic nerve tumors
- Auditory difficulties due to auditory nerve tumors
- Scoliosis
- Learning disabilities
- Bone defects, including an absence of the orbital wall and congenital bowing of the tibia and fibula (pseudarthrosis is often seen if bones are fractured)
- Hypertension caused by renal artery stenosis

Treatment tends to be symptom-specific, but the student must be treated in a holistic manner to provide care for all aspects of neurofibromatosis. Many children with neurofibromatosis can function well within the school setting with slight modifications in their activity. The school nurse needs to be attentive to the physical limitations of each child and be aware of the psychosocial issues involved when the child's condition is obviously disfiguring.

# Individualized Healthcare Plan

## Assessment

*History*
- Symptoms that led to the diagnosis of neurofibromatosis
- Age at which the child was diagnosed
- Genetic link to neurofibromatosis
- Course the condition has taken to this time
- Treatments that have been used
- Child's surgical history
- Current medical management
- Use of any orthotic devices: Type: _____
- Child's prognosis at this time

*Current Status and Management*
- Presence of neurofibromas
- Presence of café-au-lait spots and/or axillary freckling
- Presence of iris nevi and other complications
- Student's visual acuity
- Student's hearing acuity
- Student's scoliosis screening results
- Student's current height and weight
- Student's understanding of neurofibromatosis
- Student's and family's knowledge of disease process
- Management program and student's understanding of the management plan
- Current treatments being used
- Schedule that the child sees his/her specialist(s) and/or healthcare provider

*Self-care*
- Knowledge about health condition
- Ability to demonstrate correct and appropriate use of any orthotic devices

*Psychosocial Status*
- Student's perception of his/her health
- Presence of any outwardly disfiguring symptoms
- Student's ability to verbalize feelings about symptoms
- Fears the student has about how others will react toward him/her
- Child's verbalization of feelings about course of condition
- Self-esteem status (based on positive versus negative comments about self)
- Student relationship to peers, siblings, parents
- Activities the child is involved in with peers outside of school, in sports, religious organization, community
- Student and family feelings about the condition
- Student feelings about wearing orthotic device at school
- Peer group relationships, friends at school, in classes, at lunch

*Academic Status*
- Student's academic achievement
- Student's attendance pattern, reasons for absences
- Use of orthotic device at school
- Participation in after-school activities
- Modifications needed in physical education program
- Plan for modifications or accommodations, special instruction

**Nursing Diagnoses (N.D.)** (NANDA, 2003)

**N.D. 1** Risk for injury (NANDA 00035) related to:
- bone abnormalities
- pseudarthrosis

**N.D. 2** Disturbed sensory perception, visual, (NANDA 00122) related to (potential) tumors of the optic nerve

**N.D. 3** Disturbed sensory perception, auditory, (NANDA 00122) related to (potential) tumors of the auditory nerve

**N.D. 4** Risk for disproportionate growth (NANDA 00113) related to (potentially) progressive skeletal abnormalities and complications

**N.D. 5** Disturbed body image (NANDA 00118) related to:
- numerous neurofibroma tumors
- numerous café au-lait spots
- numerous skeletal abnormalities

**N.D. 6** Chronic self-esteem disturbance (NANDA 00119) related to altered body appearance, physical limitations, and/or learning difficulties

**N.D. 7** Deficient knowledge (NANDA 00126) regarding effective treatment of symptoms and possible progression of disease

## Goals

The student will not experience injury or reinjury at school. (N.D. 1)

The student will develop and use/demonstrate adaptations that are needed to attain and maintain academic and social success in the school setting. (N.D. 1)

The student will maintain maximum potential for vision and hearing. (N.D. 2, 3)

The student will assist in identifying any visual or auditory problems in early stages to promote early intervention. (N.D. 2, 3)

The student will assist in identifying symptoms of skeletal involvement of tumors and/or scoliosis to promote early intervention in care. (N.D. 4)

The student will demonstrate (increased) acceptance of and psychological comfort with body image. (N.D. 5)

The student will demonstrate (increased) self-acceptance and positive self-esteem. (N.D. 6)

The student will increase knowledge of disease process and possible progression of disease (as is age-appropriate). (N.D. 7)

The student will increase involvement in school activities/community groups. (N.D. 7)

## Nursing Interventions

Assist teacher to modify physical education program as needed. (N.D. 1)

Encourage participation in activities that do not increase risk for injury. (N.D. 1)

Monitor use of brace or orthotic device in physical education and all physical activities (as prescribed). (N.D. 1)

Review care of brace or orthotic device with student (as needed). (N.D. 1)

Observe for signs of pressure on skin underneath brace. (N.D. 1)

Instruct the student on injury-prevention methods that will help prevent injuries or reinjuries. (N.D. 1)

Review injury-prevention measures with physical education teacher(s) to decrease risk of injury. (N.D. 1)

Review injury-prevention measures with faculty and staff to decrease risk of injury. (N.D. 1)

Screen student's vision twice a year and as needed. (N.D. 2)

Screen student's hearing twice a year and as needed. (N.D. 2)

Encourage student to report any problems with his or her ability to see to their teacher, parent, or school nurse. (N.D. 2)

Encourage student to report any problems hearing in the classroom to their teacher, parent, or school nurse. (N.D. 3)

Notify parents and assist them in accessing their healthcare provider if any alterations in vision, hearing or scoliosis results are noted. (N.D. 2, 3, 4)

Request teachers to inform you if they suspect the student has visual or hearing difficulties in the classroom. (N.D. 2)

Assist teachers to make modifications in the classroom if vision or hearing deficits occur (preferential seating, etc.) (N.D. 3, 4)

Screen student for scoliosis as agreed upon with parent and healthcare provider. (N.D. 4)

Monitor student's height and weight. (N.D. 4)

Allow student to verbalize feelings about condition and body alterations. (N.D. 5, 6)

Arrange for private dressing area when changing clothes for physical education. (N.D. 5)

Provide positive feedback to student as needed. (N.D. 6)

Assist family in accessing healthcare, counseling, and other community resources as needed. (N.D. 6)

Encourage student to become active in school activities and community groups (appropriate to activity limitations). (N.D. 6)

Provide student with age-appropriate information about neurofibromatosis. (N.D. 7)

Discuss prognosis with family and student, help student to understand the potential body changes of adolescence as indicated. (N.D. 7)

Discuss treatment options that are available with family and student, as indicated. (N.D. 7)

## Expected Student Outcomes

The student will:
- Not experience injury. (N.D. 1)
- Participate in school activities with modifications as needed. (N.D. 2, 6)
- Identify measures necessary to prevent injuries. (N.D. 1)
- Wear brace or orthotic device during physical education classes and other activities that have potential for injury. (N.D. 1)
- Demonstrate use of injury-preventative measures when participating in school activities. (N.D. 1)
- Assist in maintaining good visual acuity as his/her condition allows (N.D. 2)
- Assist in maintaining good auditory acuity as his/her condition allows. (N.D. 3)
- Assist in bringing vision, hearing, and scoliosis information to parents and healthcare provider. (N.D. 2, 3, 4)
- Participate in scoliosis screening. (N.D. 4)
- Demonstrate adequate growth and development. (N.D. 4)
- Demonstrate positive feelings about body and body image. (N.D. 5)
- Verbalize feelings about body and self-image. (N.D. 6, 7)
- Participate in school activities and/or community groups. (N.D. 7)
- Describe his/her condition and prognosis in age-appropriate terms. (N.D. 7)

## Case Study

Elizabeth Clarke is a 12-year-old student who was diagnosed with neurofibromatosis as an infant. She has numerous neurofibromas and café-au-lait spots, but they are not pronounced on the visible parts of her body.

The primary cause for concern for Elizabeth's medical and nursing management is a pseudarthrosis of the left tibia. She has had numerous fractures of the bone and has been surgically treated several times, including bone grafting. The last procedure was performed when Elizabeth was 5 years old and involved an Ilizarov brace, which corrected the nonunion of the bone and allowed for proper growth of the left leg. She wears a brace at all times to protect her left leg. Her physical education activities need to be limited to noncontact, nonstress sports. She is allowed to run and enjoys modified physical activities.

Elizabeth has a yearly examination by a pediatric neurologist, which includes magnetic resonance imaging every other year. Her parents have provided the school health office with the phone numbers of her doctors and emergency instructions should her leg become injured or should she report symptoms such as dizziness.

## Neurofibromatosis

| Assessment Data | Nursing Diagnosis | Goals | Nursing Interventions | Expected Outcomes |
|---|---|---|---|---|
| Elizabeth's left leg is suscepti-ble to fractures. Elizabeth has had several surgeries, includ-ing use of the Ilizarov tech-nique, to left leg. | Risk for injury related to bone abnormalities and pseudarthrosis. | Elizabeth will not experience injury or reinjury at school.<br><br>Elizabeth will develop and use/demonstrate adaptations that are needed to attain and maintain academic and social success in the school setting. | Assist teacher to modify phys-ical education program as needed.<br><br>Monitor use of leg brace in physical education and all physical activities.<br><br>Encourage participation in activities that do not increase risk for injury.<br><br>Review injury-prevention measures with physical edu-cation teacher to decrease risk of injury.<br><br>Review brace or orthotic care with Elizabeth (as needed).<br><br>Observe for signs of pressure on skin underneath brace. Screen Elizabeth's vision twice a year and as needed. | Elizabeth will not experience injury.<br><br>Elizabeth will participate in school activities with modifi-cations as needed.<br><br>Elizabeth will wear brace or orthotic device during physi-cal education classes and other activities that have potential for injury.<br><br>Elizabeth will demonstrate use of injury preventative measures when participat-ing in school activities. |
| Elizabeth is at risk for decreases in visual and audi-tory function. | Disturbed sensory percep-tion–visual– related to (poten-tial) tumors of the optic nerve.<br><br>Disturbed sensory percep-tion–auditory–related to (potential) tumors of the audi-tory nerve. | Elizabeth will maintain maxi-mum potential for vision and hearing.<br><br>Elizabeth will assist in identify-ing any visual or auditory problems in early stages to promote early intervention. | Encourage Elizabeth to report any problems with her ability to see to her teacher, parent, or school nurse.<br><br>Screen Elizabeth's hearing twice a year and as needed.<br><br>Encourage Elizabeth to report any problems hearing in the classroom to her teacher, par-ent, or school nurse. | Elizabeth will assist in main-taining good visual acuity as her condition allows.<br><br>Elizabeth will assist in main-taining good auditory acuity as her condition allows. |

**Neurofibromatosis**

| Assessment Data | Nursing Diagnosis | Goals | Nursing Interventions | Expected Outcomes |
|---|---|---|---|---|
| | | | Notify parents and assist them in accessing their healthcare provider if any alterations in vision or hearing results are noted. | |
| Elizabeth is at an increased risk to develop scoliosis. | Risk for disproportionate growth related to (potentially) progressive skeletal abnormalities and complications. | Elizabeth will assist in identifying symptoms of skeletal involvement of tumors and/or scoliosis to promote early intervention in care. | Screen Elizabeth for scoliosis twice a year and as needed.<br><br>Notify parents and assist them in accessing their healthcare provider if any alterations in scoliosis results are noted. | Elizabeth will participate in scoliosis screening.<br><br>Elizabeth will assist in bringing scoliosis information to parents and healthcare provider. |

# References

Behrmann, R. E., & Klingman, R. M. (2004) *Nelson essentials of pediatrics* (17th ed.). Philadelphia: Saunders.

NANDA International. (2003). *Nursing diagnoses: Definitions & classification 2003-2004.* Philadelphia: Author.

National Neurofibromatosis Foundation. *Common signs of NF type 1.* (2004). Retrieved June 5, 2004, from http://www.nf.org/manimage/manimage.htm

Neurofibromatosis Inc. *What is NF?* (2002). Retrieved June 5, 2004, from http://www.nfinc.org/whatisnf.html

Freidman, J. (2003). *All about neurofibromatosis type 1.* Retrieved August 29, 2004, from http://www.nf.org/nf_professionals/nf/nf1.htm

Wong, D. L., Hockenberry-Eaton, M., Wilson, D., Winkelstein, M. L., & Kline, N. E. (2003). *Whaley and Wong's nursing care of infants and children* (6th ed.). St. Louis, MO: Mosby.

# Bibliography

Barton, B., & North, K. (2004). Social skills of children with neurofibromatosis type 1. *Developmental Medicine and Child Neurology, 46*(8), 553–563.

Beers, M. (2003). *Merck manual of medical information* (2nd home ed.) Whitehouse Station, NY: Merck.

Kuzier, B., Erb, G., Berman, A., & Snyder, S. (2004). *Fundamentals of nursing* (7th ed.). Upper Saddle River, NJ: Pearson, Prentice Hall

*Professional guide to signs and symptoms* (4th ed.). (2003). Philadelphia: Lippincott, Williams & Wilkins.

*Serving students with special care needs.* (1992). Hartford, CT: State of Connecticut Department of Education.

Towers, R. (2004). The physical and psychological implications of neurofibromatosis. *Nursing Times, 100*(27), 34–36.

# Resources

National Institute of Neurological Disorders and Stroke
NIH Neurological Institute
PO Box 5801
Bethesda, MD 20824
1-800-352-9424
http://www.ninds.nih.gov/health_and_medical/disorders/neurofibro.htm

National Neurofibromatosis Foundation, Inc.
95 Pine Street
16th Floor
    New York, NY 10005
212-344-6633
1-800-323-7938
NNFF@nf.org
http://www.nf.org/

Neurofibromatosis, Inc.
9320 Annapolis Road
Suite 300
Lanham, MD 20706-3123
320-918-4600
http://www.nfinc.org/

## Chapter Fifty-seven

# Organ Transplant

Mary Jo Martin

## Introduction

Solid organ transplant has become an increasingly acceptable treatment for children with end-stage organ failure. The three most prevalent solid organ transplants for children are liver, kidney, and heart replacement. With the introduction of the immunosuppressive drug cyclosporine in 1983 and better surgical techniques, the number of organ transplant procedures has increased dramatically. However, this number has reached a plateau in the last 5 years (Caplan, 1999). This plateau is related to the shortage of organ donors and is an unfortunate situation for those candidates awaiting lifesaving transplantation.

Successful kidney transplantation was first performed in the 1960s. Kidney transplantation is now more successful than ever using both living donor and cadaver organs. Estimates indicate that the 1-year and 2-year survival rates of living donor transplants are 90% and 86%, respectively. For cadaver donors, 1-year and 2-year survival rates are 78% and 72% (Stanford University School of Medicine, 2002).

Renal transplantation clearly provides the optimum therapy for children with end-stage renal failure. Causes of kidney failure include congenital diseases such as renal hypoplasia or dysphasia; acquired diseases such as glomerulonephritis; and hereditary diseases such as Alport's syndrome and juvenile nephrophthisis. Clinical manifestations include electrolyte abnormalities, hyperglycemia, anemia, congestive heart failure, and peripheral neuropathy.

In 1963, the first pediatric liver transplantation was performed on a child with biliary atresia. The 1-year survival rate in the 1960s was 34%. Pediatric liver transplantation and survival rates have increased in recent years with the development of reduced-size liver (cadaver donors) and living-related donor transplants. It is now estimated that the 1-year survival rate for children receiving partial livers from living-related donors is 92%. The survival rate for those who receive livers from cadavers is approximately 75% (Humar, Hertz, & Blakemore, 2002).

Liver transplantation may result from the complications of acute or chronic liver failure. Common clinical manifestations include jaundice, ascites, hepatomegaly, hypoglycemia, hormone imbalance, and encephalopathy. Rapid progression of symptoms over days to a few months is characteristic of acute-onset liver disease. Fulminant liver failure or acute hepatitis may be the cause.

Chronic liver disease may progress more slowly, with symptoms appearing gradually over a few months. Causes of chronic liver failure include biliary atresia, cystic fibrosis, Wilson's disease, and Alagille syndrome.

Heart transplantation also began in the 1960s. In recent years, it has become a treatment option for infants and children with worsening heart failure and a limited life expectancy despite maximum medical and surgical management. The International Society for Heart Transplantation registry data on survival of cardiac transplant recipients since 1982 indicate a 1-year survival rate of approximately 73% and a 3-year survival rate of 66%. Indications for heart transplantation in children include cardiomyopathy and end-stage congenital heart defects. Clinical manifestations include respiratory distress, congestive heart failure, cardiomegaly, arrhythmias, and growth retardation (Jackson & Vessey, 2000).

### Pathophysiology

Transplantation for children with end-stage organ failure is a hope for survival and a better quality of life. Evaluation for the procedure involves multiple diagnostic tests, blood work, and radiologic examination. Each child is evaluated individually, and the child's compatibility for the particular organ is weighed against the presence of other ongoing health conditions (Jackson & Vessey, 2000). Once approved to be a candidate, the child is matched for donor tissue. Kidney and partial liver organ donations come from either a living donor or a cadaver donor soon after death. The closer the genetic relationship between the donor and recipient, the better the chances for long-term survival (Wong, 2001). Donor matching for heart transplants is primarily by ABO blood type and body size (Jackson & Vessey, 2000).

Once a child is typed and matched, his or her medical criteria for transplantation are entered into a computerized database. The United Network for Organ Sharing (UNOS) maintains a centralized computer network linking all organ procurement organizations and transplant centers. When an organ becomes available, the information about the donor's organ is entered and a list of possible recipients is generated (UNOS, 2003). The pediatric transplant team reviews the list, considers several factors, and decides what would be best for their individual patient.

## Management

Posttransplant care involves not only the physical recovery from the surgery but the possibility of problems associated with immunosuppression and organ rejection. Immunosuppression is the artificial suppression of the immune response, usually through drugs, so that the body will not reject a transplanted organ or tissue. Immunosuppression is vital for long-term survival of the donated organ. Prednisone and cyclosporine are used, along with other drugs specific to the type of transplant. However, the administration of these drugs is not without risk. Children are at risk for infection because the therapy not only suppresses the immune response to the grafted tissue but also suppresses the body's ability to fight off other infectious agents. Studies have shown that over 80% of these patients do not get serious infections and have the same risk as the general population. Ten percent become infected with viruses such as cytomegalovirus, Epstein-Barr virus, or the hepatitis B or C virus (Fishman & Rubin, 1998).

Initially, immunosuppresion drugs are administered intravenously for 14 days after the transplant. However, for long-term survival, the transplanted child must take the drugs for the rest of his or her life. Careful monitoring of the possible side effects of cyclosporine and prednisone is required. Some of the more common side effects of cyclosporine are hypertension, renal dysfunction, gum hyperplasia, hirsutism, diarrhea, seizures, and tremors. Prednisone can interfere with calcium absorption and retard linear growth. Other corticosteroid-induced side effects include the characteristic cushingoid face, cataracts, fluid and sodium retention, gastric ulcer, and obesity (Wong, 2001).

Despite successful transplantation, rejection of the new organ is a leading cause of graft failure (Jackson & Vessey, 2000). It occurs when the body makes antibodies that work to eliminate the transplanted organ. Rejection can be one of three types—hyperacute, acute, or chronic. Hyperacute happens immediately or within a few hours of the surgery and is irreversible. This type of rejection is usually seen in second transplant cases where the individual's body has already built up a supply of antibodies against the new tissue.

Acute rejection usually occurs between the first few days to 6 months after transplantation but can occur as long as 1 or 2 years later. These symptoms of rejection are very similar to the symptoms of organ failure. Early detection is essential to successful reversal of acute rejection. The child must be closely monitored in all settings, and the transplantation team should be notified of any concerns.

Chronic rejection is characterized by a gradual deterioration of organ function and typically begins 6 months or more after transplantation. Typically, this type of rejection is not reversible and is also a response to the child's immune system. Some organs lose complete function over time; some lose only partial function and are able to provide adequate function. The best way to prevent chronic rejection is by taking antirejection medications exactly as prescribed (Virtual Hospital, 2003).

Symptoms of rejection are particular to the type of organs involved. Rejection of a transplanted kidney is characterized by fever, decreased urine output, weight gain over 2 pounds per day, hypertension, and pain over the site. Rejection can be determined by decreased blood flow on a renal flow scan. Signs and symptoms of liver rejection include fever, fatigue, jaundice, darkening of urine, clay-colored stools, and pain. A liver biopsy is used to confirm the rejection process. Cardiac rejection is complicated by the fact that rejection has progressed to moderate or severe levels before signs and symptoms appear. Manifestations include congestive heart failure, cardiomegaly, fever, arrhythmias, ventricular dysfunction, and pericardial effusion. Myocardial biopsy and laboratory and radiologic tests help confirm rejection (Jackson & Vessey, 2000; Virtual Hospital, 2003).

The school nurse is the recipient's advocate and health manager in the school setting. Posttransplantation care is demanding and complex. The physical and emotional needs of the child and family need to be continually monitored. A multidisciplinary approach to care is needed so that all needs can be assessed and met. Good communication skills are the key to establishing trust with the child, family, and transplantation team. Compliance with posttransplant medications and treatments will give the child the second chance at life, which he or she deserves.

# Individualized Healthcare Plan

## Assessment

*History*

- Symptoms experienced during end-stage organ failure
- Review of medical records and testing
- Immunization history
- Growth and development history
- Review of previous illness
- Hospital experiences
- Age of child at the time of diagnosis
- Date of transplant
- Posttransplant health status
- Medical management routine
- Individual response of child to treatment
- History from family
  - family's knowledge base of posttransplantation care
  - family's concerns and needs
  - family's coping abilities

*Current Status and Management*

- Current symptoms
  - related to transplant
  - related to other health conditions
- Management plan
  - medications
- Diet plan
- Healthcare procedures that need to be done in the school setting
  - medications
- Physical limitations in school environment
- Vision and hearing assessment
- Healthcare providers
  - transplant team contact
  - pediatrician/primary care physician

*Self-care*

- Self-care abilities (independent, assisted, supervised, done by parent)
- Posttransplantation care compliance
- Motivators to self-care and compliance
- Barriers to self-care

*Psychosocial Status*

- Life stressors: terminal illness, hospitalization, medication requirements, physical activity limitations
- Coping abilities: successful coping strategies
- Level of knowledge
- Body image: changes related to
  - scars
  - drug side effects (obesity, cushingoid face)
- Interaction with peers
- Peer acceptance
- Level of self-esteem
- Family coping
  - Support persons and systems being utilized by the student and family

- Developmental and academic level and progress
- Consult with teacher, counselor, physical therapist, occupational therapist, or any other member of multidisciplinary team
  - assess current, or need for, 504 plan and/or individual education program (IEP)
  - Physical activity limitations needed in the school environment.
- Physical activity tolerance during the school day, including transportation to and from school
- Attendance pattern, past and current
- School health services needed: medication management, nutrition/hydration plan, healthcare procedures, monitoring for signs and symptoms of infection or rejection, emergency healthcare plan

## Nursing Diagnoses (N.D.) (NANDA, 2003)

**N.D. 1** Risk for disproportionate growth (NANDA 00113) related to:
- poor or loss of appetite
- pain (abdominal)
- infection
- depressed body defenses
- effects of chronic condition
- long-term effects of corticosteroids after transplantation

**N.D. 2** Risk for infection (NANDA 00004) related to:
- alteration in immune response
- immunosuppression
- medication (side effects)
- exposure to pathogens
- organ rejection
- infections in the school environment

**N.D. 3** Risk for injury (NANDA 00035) related to:
- lack of safety precautions
- lack of safety education
- photosensitive skin

**N.D. 4** Risk for activity intolerance (NANDA 00094) related to:
- fatigue
- chronic health condition

**N.D. 5** Risk for impaired adjustment (NANDA 00070) related to:
- actual change in body part
- side effects of medication
- verbalization of:
  - fear of reaction by others
  - negative feelings about body
  - feelings of helplessness and hopelessness
  - lack of privacy
  - depression

**N.D. 6** Risk for situational low self-esteem (NANDA 00153) related to:
- child's chronic health condition
- fear of organ rejection
- psychosocial stressors:
  - feelings of isolation
  - family disruption
  - financial burdens

Organ Transplant

## Goals

The student will maintain adequate nutritional intake. (N.D. 1)
The student will remain free of infections. (N.D. 2)
The student will demonstrate good personal hygiene skills. (N.D. 2)
The student will remain free of injury. (N.D. 3)
The student will decrease energy expenditure as needed based on activity tolerance level. (N.D. 4)
The student will maintain adequate growth pattern. (N.D. 4)
The student will demonstrate positive behaviors that indicate a good body image. (N.D. 5)
The student will participate in school/classroom activities, with modifications as needed. (N.D. 1-6)
The student will maintain academic progress. (N.D. 1–5)
The student will develop and/or maintain effective individual and family coping behaviors. (N.D. 6)
The student will seek, obtain, and maintain community support for self and his/her family. (N.D. 6)

## Nursing Interventions

*Nutritional management*
Discuss diet guidelines with student and family. (N.D. 1, 4)
Implement prescribed diet at school. (N.D. 1)
Monitor eating habits. (N.D. 1, 5)
Assist student to maintain diet guidelines at school, (e.g., refrigerator available, not missing lunch). (N.D. 1)

*Environmental management*
Monitor for and teach staff to recognize signs and symptoms of bacterial, fungal, viral, and protozoan infections. Signs and symptoms include fever, fatigue, pain. (N.D. 2)
Monitor school environment for infectious diseases, especially chickenpox, influenza, pneumonia, pertussis. (N.D. 2)
Teach students, classmates, and staff good hand-washing and illness prevention techniques. (N.D. 2)

*Risk control*
Encourage student to bring own water bottle, and instruct him/her not to drink from drinking fountains. (N.D. 2)
Coordinate communication between medical care provider, organ transplant team, parents, and school staff. (N.D. 3)
Inform teachers that certain activities are not recommended for students having had solid organ transplant; these include contact sports, downhill sledding, and hanging from the waist on a bar. (N.D. 4)
Encourage sun safety measures, such as use of a sunscreen with sun protection factor of at least 15, avoiding exposure to direct sunshine, and wearing a hat. (N.D. 3)
Notify parent of any signs or symptoms of infection that occur. Decide with parent whether student goes home or stays in school. (N.D. 3)
Notify parents if student is exposed to measles, mumps, varicella, shingles, herpes, or influenza. (N.D. 2)

*Emergency care*
Develop emergency care plan (ECP) regarding what to do if signs of possible rejection or infection occur. (N.D. 3)
Maintain current emergency information with current emergency contacts (e.g., phone or pager number of parents, medical care providers). (N.D. 3)

*Energy management*
Assist staff in modifying activities appropriate to activity tolerance. (N.D. 3)
Encourage exercise within child's limitations. (N.D. 4)
Inform staff about student's limitations. (N.D. 4)
Inform staff of signs and symptoms to report, such as respiratory difficulties, cyanosis, and fatigue. (N.D. 4)
Discuss with student signs and symptoms that need to be reported to the teacher or health office as soon as they occur. (N.D. 4)
Assist student to set own physical limitations based on tolerance. (N.D. 4)
Assist student to rest as needed. (N.D. 4)

*Health screening*
Monitor height and weight as requested by parent and/or healthcare provider. (N.D. 1, 4)
Assess vision and hearing annually. (N.D. 4)

*Oral health promotion*
Encourage routine dental visits with prophylactic antibiotics administered before dental work to prevent infection. (N.D. 2, 4)
Monitor gums for signs and symptoms of gum hyperplasia in children taking cyclosporine. (N.D. 5)

*Coping enhancement*
Assess change in:
  • social involvement with family, peers, and school staff
  • verbalization of negative body image
  • signs of depression and noncompliance with health plan (N.D. 5)
Assess student for successful coping mechanisms, reinforce as needed. (N.D. 5)
Establish caring atmosphere to keep communication open. (N.D. 5)
Demonstrate sense of acceptance regardless of health condition. (N.D. 5)
Encourage interactions with peers and other students with same diagnosis (i.e., support group). (N.D. 5)
Encourage verbalization of feelings. (N.D. 5)
Assist the student to share his/her feelings about self and body image with family and staff. (N.D. 5)
Encourage student to verbalize feelings of self and body image to family. (N.D. 5)

*Family support*
Facilitate positive family dynamics, communication, and coping patterns. (N.D. 6)
Monitor need for student and family to seek counseling to help deal with stressors. (N.D. 6)

*Family mobilization*
Refer to community resources and local organ transplant support group as needed. (N.D. 6)
Supply information and emotional support to cope with fears, future milestones, and other aspects of organ transplant to student and family. (N.D. 6)

## Expected Student Outcomes

The student will:
*Nutritional status*
  • Maintain a well-balanced diet as prescribed. (N.D. 1, 4)

*Risk control*
Self-monitor for signs and symptoms of infection. (N.D. 2)
Remain free of infection in the school setting. (N.D. 2)
Not experience physical injury in the school setting. (N.D. 3)
Comply with activity limitations as prescribed. (N.D. 4)
Assist in notifying parents if signs and symptoms of infection/organ rejection develop. (N.D. 2, 5)

*Personal well-being*
  • Demonstrate good (independent, assisted) personal hygiene skills. (N.D. 2)
  • Demonstrate compliance with activity limitations as prescribed. (N.D. 2, 4, 5)

*Energy conservation*
  • Assist in modifying activities based on activity tolerance. (N.D. 4)
  • Rest as needed. (N.D. 4)

- Participate in school/classroom activities with modifications made as needed. (N.D. 4)
- Maintain academic progress. (N.D. 1–4)

*Body image*
- Be able to verbalize feelings of body image. (N.D. 5)
- Develop and demonstrate positive coping strategies. (N.D. 5)

*Social support*
- Utilize community resources and support persons and groups, as needed. (N.D. 5)
- Identify persons who provide caring and support. (N.D. 6)

# Case Study

Emily, born on May 15, 1999, is now 5 years, 4 months old. Her history was obtained from Emily's parents at an informational meeting on September 2, 2003, and from a review of health records.

Emily was delivered at 40 weeks via cesarean section after a prolonged labor. Apgar scores were 7 at 1 minute and 9 at 5 minutes. Records show a slightly elevated serum bilirubin level. The physician told Emily's parents to put her in the sunlight for a couple of hours a day. Mother and baby were discharged 48 hours after birth.

Mom describes Emily as a "fussy" baby. Feeding was difficult, and she slept for only short periods of time. Her stomach seemed bloated, and her parents thought she had colic. The yellow color of her skin was a concern to her doctor, and tests were conducted at age 4 weeks. Blood and urine studies, ultrasound, and a liver biopsy confirmed that Emily had biliary atresia (inflammation and obstruction of the ducts that carry the bile from the liver to the intestine). On June 20, 1999, a Kasai procedure was performed.

Emily seemed to "feel better" after the surgery. Her parents describe this time as stressful, and they were concerned about her growth. She was initially put on a low-fat diet with vitamin supplements but progressed to a regular diet in 6 months. She took a variety of medications, including oral antibiotics, diuretics, and phenobarbital. Developmental milestones included sitting up at 9 months, crawling at 11 months, and walking at 18 months. Dad states that Emily began cooing at 3 months and said her first word at 10 months.

Her parents' concerns grew greater when, at the age of 3 1/2, Emily's weight had dropped to 28 pounds. She had increasing episodes of stomachaches, loss of appetite, and fatigue. Medical tests found Emily's liver to be damaged further. Records show that complications from cirrhosis would require a liver transplant

Emily received one fourth of her mother's liver on November 28, 2002. Recovery was described as slow, but Emily has now regained her strength and has gained 10 pounds in the past 18 months.

Currently, Emily has no known allergies. Her immunizations are up to date. Early childhood screening records indicate that Emily passed her vision and hearing screening 6 months ago. Emily currently attends a morning kindergarten program and has never been in a day-care setting.

Emily eats a low-fat diet. She is described as a "picky" eater and often has to be encouraged to eat. She takes medication daily, including cyclosporine and prednisone. Her parents describe her as an active child who sometimes becomes tired after a lot of physical activity. After a short rest period, Emily is then able to resume activity. Emily is described as a good "sleeper." She falls asleep easily and sleeps 8 to 10 hours per night.

## Organ Transplant

| Assessment Data | Nursing Diagnosis | Goals | Nursing Interventions | Expected Outcomes |
|---|---|---|---|---|
| Emily has had a liver transplant 2 years ago (Nov. 2002) | Risk for infection related to:<br>1. immunosupression;<br>2. medication (side effect);<br>3. exposure to pathogens in the school environment;<br>4. organ rejection | Emily will remain free of infection. | Monitor for and teach staff to recongnize signs and symptoms of bacterial, fungal, viral, and protozoan infections, including fever, fatigue, pain.<br><br>Monitor school environment for infectious diseases, especially chickenpox, influenza, pneumonia, pertussis.<br><br>Notify parents if student is exposed to measles, mumps, varicella, shingles, herpes, or influenza.<br><br>Teach student, classmates, and staff good hand-washing and illness prevention techniques.<br><br>Encourage student to bring own water bottle and instruct him/her not to drink from drinking fountains. | Emily will remain free of infection in the school setting.<br><br>Emily will demonstrate good (independent, assisted) personal hygiene skills. |
| Emily attends school. She takes immunosuppression medication daily and continually needs to be monitored for signs and symptoms of infection and/or organ rejection. | Risk for injury related to:<br>1. lack of safety precautions;<br>2. lack of safety education;<br>3. photosensitive skin | Emily will remain free of injury. | Maintain current emergency information with current emergency contacts.<br><br>Coordinate communication between medical care provider, organ transplant team, parents, and staff.<br><br>Develop an emergency care plan regarding what to do if signs/symptoms of possible rejection or infection occur. | |

| Assessment Data | Nursing Diagnosis | Goals | Nursing Interventions | Expected Outcomes |
|---|---|---|---|---|
| | | | Notify parents of any signs/symptoms of infection that occur. Decide with parent whether student should remain in school or not.

Assist staff in modifying activities appropriate to activity tolerance.

Encourage sun safety measures, such as: use sunscreen with sun protection factor of at least 15, avoid exposure to direct sunshine, wear a hat. | Emily will not experience physical injury in the school setting.

Emily will use sunscreen and wears a hat for all outdoor activities. |

# References

Caplan, A. L. (1999). Fairness in organ transplantation. *Pediatric Ethicscope, 10,* 1–8.

Fishman, J. A., & Rubin, R. H. (1998). Infection in organ transplant recipients. *New England Journal of Medicine, 17,* 1244–1245.

Humar, A., Hertz, M., & Blakemore, L. (2002). Pediatric liver transplantation. In *Manual of liver transplant medical care* (chap. 6). Retrieved September 22, 2003, from http://www.medscape.com

Jackson, P. L., & Vessey, J. A. (2000). *Primary care of the child with a chronic condition* (3rd ed.). St. Louis, MO: Mosby-Yearbook.

NANDA International. (2003). *Nursing diagnoses: Definitions & classification, 2003-2004.* Philadelphia: Author.

Stanford University School of Medicine. (2002, October 10). *Survival boost for tiniest transplant patients* [News Release]. Retrieved September 22, 2003, from http://med.news.standford.edu

United Network for Organ Sharing (2003). *How the transplantation system works: Matching donors and recipients.* Retrieved September 22, 2003, from www.unos.org

Virtual Hospital. (2003). *Rejection.* Retrieved on September 23, 2003, from http://www.vh.org/adult/patient/surgery/rejection

Wong, D. L. (2001) *Wong's essentials of pediatric nursing.* St. Louis, MO: Mosby.

# Bibliography

Blue, L., & Hasse, J. (2002). *Comprehensive guide to transplant nutrition.* Chicago, IL: American Dietetic Association.

Gaedeke, N., & House, M. (1991). *Organ and tissue transplantation: Nursing care from procurement through rehabilitation.* New York: Davis.

Harmon, W., Fine, R., & Tejani, A. (2000). *Solid organ transplantation.* Boston, MA: Blackwell Science.

Johnson, M., Bulechek,G., Dochterman, J., Maas, M., & Moorhead, S. (2003). *Nursing Diagnosis, Outcomes, & Interventions: NANDA, NOC, & NIC Linkages, Nursing Interventions Classification 4e, Nursing Outcomes Classification 3e, 2nd Edition.* St. Louis: Mosby.

Parr, E., & Mize, J. (2001). Coping *with an organ transplant: A practical guide to understanding, preparing for, and living with an organ transplant.* New York: Avery Penguin Putnam.

Schroeder, R.,Johnson, L.,& Kuo, P. (2001). *Clinical management of the transplant patient.* Cary, NC: Oxford University Press.

# Resources

American Heart Association
National Center
7272 Greenville Avenue
Dallas, TX 75231
1-800-AHA-USA1
http://www.americanheart.org

American Kidney Fund, Inc.
6110 Executive Boulevard
Suite 1010
Rockville, MD 20852
1-800-638-8299
http://www.akfinc.org

American Liver Foundation
75 Maiden Lane
New York, NY 10038
1-800-GO-LIVER
http://www.liverfoundation.org

American Lung Association
61 Broadway
Sixth Floor
New York, NY 10006
212-315-8700
http://www.lungusa.org

Children's Heart Information Network
1561 Clark Drive
Yardley, PA 19067
215-493-3068
http://www.tchin.org

Children's Organ Transplantation Association
2501 Cota Drive
Bloomington, IN 47403
1-800-366-2682
http://www.kintera.org

National Kidney Foundation
30 East 33rd Street
New York, NY 10016
1-800-622-9010
http://www.kidney.org

Trans Web
1327 Jones Drive
Suite 201
Ann Arbor, MI 48105
734-998-7314
http://www.transweb.org

United Network for Organ Sharing
700 North 4th Street
Richmond, VA 23219
804-782-4800
1-888-894-6391

## Chapter Fifty-eight

# Osteogenesis Imperfecta

Valeria S. Baldocchi

## Introduction

Osteogenesis imperfecta (OI), also known as "brittle bone disease," is a hereditary genetic disorder characterized by bones that easily break. It affects the production of type 1 collagen, which is the major protein in the body's connective tissue. Collagen gives bones and other connective tissue their strength and structure. It acts as a scaffolding and is why bones regenerate and heal after an injury. The faulty gene that causes OI instructs the body to make either too little type 1 collagen or collagen that is of poor quality. The result is bones that break easily, often for little or no apparent reason. There is a wide range of severity and symptoms of the disorder, and school-aged children will have variable needs and limitations, depending on the degree to which they are affected by OI. Children with OI typically are of normal to above average intelligence and integrate easily into a regular education classroom. Some children with milder forms of OI may have no visible signs of the disorder and have infrequent fractures, whereas others may be more severely affected and need mobility supports to effectively ambulate in the school setting. It is estimated that between 20,000 and 50,000 people in the United Stated have osteogenesis imperfecta (National Institutes of Health, Fast Facts, August, 2004).

### Pathophysiology

There are four recognized types of osteogenesis imperfecta. They were categorized by Dr. D. O. Silence and colleagues in 1979 and are now known as the Silence classification (**Table 1**). A wide variation in symptoms and severity is found even among people with the same type. The definitions are based on subjective observations of clinical features, and determining the type is not always straightforward. Biochemical (collagen) or molecular (DNA) testing can help confirm the diagnosis, but neither test is 100% accurate and may give false-negative results.

Two novel types of OI, type V and type VI, have been identified but are clinically within the Silence type IV group (National Institutes of Health, Novel Forms of Osteogenesis, October, 2002).

**Table 1. Four Types of Osteogenesis Imperfecta Based on Sillence Classification**

| Classification | Clinical Features |
|---|---|
| Type I | • Mildest and most common type<br>• Near-normal life span<br>• Bones fracture easily; most fractures occur before puberty<br>• Easily bruisable<br>• Stature normal or near normal<br>• Hyperextensibility of large joints<br>• Blue, purple, or gray tint to the sclera<br>• Tendency toward mild scoliosis<br>• Little or no deformity of the bones<br>• Dental problems (brittle teeth) possible<br>• Hearing loss frequently occurs, usually beginning early 20s or 30s<br>• Structure of collagen is normal but amount is less than normal |

| Classification | Clinical Features |
|---|---|
| Type II | • Most severe form<br>• Infants often succumb at or shortly after birth, usually due to cardiac and respiratory problems<br>• Severe bone deformity, numerous fractures, underdeveloped lungs, small stature<br>• Improperly formed collagen |
| Type III | • Progressively deforming<br>• Many fractures throughout lifetime, sometimes several hundred<br>• Fractures often present at birth<br>• Very short in stature; adult height may reach only 3 feet<br>• Blue, purple, or gray tint to the sclera, becoming white in late childhood<br>• Decreased muscle development in arms and leg; loose joints<br>• Barrel-shaped rib cage<br>• Triangular shape to the face<br>• Dental problems<br>• Possible hearing loss<br>• Spinal curvature<br>• Bone deformity, often severe<br>• Possible respiratory problems<br>• Improperly formed collagen |
| Type IV | • Tends to fall between type I and type III in severity<br>• Numerous fractures; most occur before puberty<br>• Shorter-than-average stature<br>• Sclera normal in color<br>• Spinal curvatures<br>• Barrel-shaped rib cage<br>• Triangular shape to the face<br>• Dental problems: more than with type I<br>• Possible hearing loss<br>• Loose joints<br>• Improperly formed collagen |

## Genetics

Osteogenesis imperfecta usually occurs from a dominant mutation of one of the two genes that carry the instructions for making type 1 collagen. When a gene with a dominant mutation pairs with a normal gene, the mutated gene dominates the normal gene and a genetic defect occurs. In OI types II, III, and IV, the quality of the collagen is affected. In OI type I, the quantity of the collagen is affected. There are three ways for the mutation typically to occur. One is by direct inheritance, which occurs when a parent passes on a faulty gene to the child. Another is by a new, dominant mutation, which occurs by a spontaneous mutation of the sperm or egg cell prior to conception. The third way is by mosaicism, which is a mutation of the cells that give rise to the multiple sperm or eggs of the parent (National Institutes of Health: Genetics, April, 2004).

## Management

Osteogenesis imperfecta is primarily managed by promoting mobility and independence and caring for fractures when they occur. Some people affected with OI require very little modification of their activities of daily living (ADLs), whereas others may require the use of braces, crutches, walker, or wheelchair. Physical therapy (PT) may be necessary to assist with muscle weakness and motor skill delay. Occupational therapy (OT) may help develop fine motor skills and provide for necessary adaptive equipment. Some children benefit from a surgical procedure called rodding to give bones extra support. Most medication therapy has not proved to be effective, but the bisphosphonate drugs (intravenous Aredia, oral Fosamax) have been studied and may prove to be helpful. Promoting a healthy lifestyle of proper nutrition, weight management, and exercise will go far in assisting the person with

OI to become independent in all major life functions. Modification of the school curriculum may be necessary so the child can participate in regular school activities, including physical education (PE) and recess, to the fullest extent possible.

When a fracture is suspected or does occur, there should be minimal handling of the affected limb, and school personnel should be trained in the care of the injury until the child's parent or guardian arrives. Fractures can occur in children with OI spontaneously and with no explanation that an incident occurred. There may be some confusion between OI and child abuse, because the same types of fractures are typically observed in both situations. Parents are advised to carry a letter from their child's doctor documenting the diagnosis. The diagnostic information should be placed in the child's school health records, and key school personnel should be notified of the diagnosis if the parents desire (OI Foundation: A Guide for Nurses, 2003).

## Individualized Healthcare Plan

### Assessment

*History*
- When was the diagnosis made?
- What type of OI is the child affected with?
- Is there a family history of the disorder? Who is affected?
- What signs and symptoms of the disorder does the student have currently and chronically?
- How many previous fractures have occurred? Which bones were affected?
- Have any surgical procedures been done? Are any planned?
- Are there any acute or chronic mobility concerns?
- Have any medication therapies been tried?
- Any other health concerns?
- How are the family dynamics affected by having a child with OI?

*Current Status and Management*
- Are growth and development affected by OI?
- What is the prognosis?
- To what degree of severity is the student affected by the OI?
- Is there a plan of care? How effective is it?
- Are there any respiratory, auditory, or dental concerns?
- Are any modifications to the daily activity schedule required?
- Is a personal assistant required in the school setting? If yes, what percentage of the school day and what qualifications does this person need to have?
- How is the student's mobility affected by OI?
- Are any assistive devices required for ambulation or ADLs?
- Are any modifications of the curriculum or assistive devices needed in the school setting?
- Who are the student's significant others, and how involved are they in his/her care?
- Who are the student's healthcare providers? How often does the student need care?
- What type of medical insurance coverage does the child have?

*Self-care*
- What do the student, family, and school personnel know about OI?
- What do the student, family, and school personnel know about fracture identification, fracture care, respiratory hygiene, hearing loss, and first aid?
- What do the student, family and school personnel know about fracture prevention? What activities are considered an acceptable risk for the student?
- To what extent are the student, family, and school personnel involved in designing/implementing the care plan?
- How knowledgeable are the student, family, and school personnel about the need and use of assistive devices?
- How well can the student manage ADLs?
- Are there any barriers that prevent self-care?
- How motivated is the student to provide self-care?
- How much self-care does the student provide at home?

## Psychosocial Status

- What is the current developmental stage of the student?
- What is the current developmental stage of the family?
- What level of acceptance of the disability have the student and family reached?
- How does the student feel about having OI?
- How do the student's significant others feel about having a family member with OI?
- How does the student perceive his/her health, abilities, and disabilities?
- How does the family perceive the student's health, abilities, and disabilities?
- What coping mechanisms do the student and family use?
- What is the status of the student's emotional health?
- How well can the student interact with family, peers, and school personnel?
- How strong is the student's and family's support system?
- What level of acceptance do school personnel have about the student's disability?
- What level of acceptance do school personnel have about disabled children in general being in the regular education classroom?
- What are the school personnel's fears, anxieties, and concerns about the student?
- What support systems are in place for school personnel who have special-needs students in their classrooms?

## Academic Issues

- What level of cognitive functioning does the student have? Does the child have any learning problems or other special education needs, such as speech/language, PT, or OT?
- What are the student's academic strengths and weaknesses?
- How have the student's attendance patterns been? How much absence is due to OI issues?
- What is the student's level of academic performance? Have there been any significant changes in the performance?
- Does the student have an individualized education program (IEP) or 504 plan? If yes, when and where was it written?
- Does the student have any behavioral or emotional health concerns?
- Does the student like school?
- What are the school personnel's perceptions of the student's academic abilities?
- What extracurricular activities is the student involved in?
- Are any assistive devices or personnel necessary?
- Are there any architectural barriers that may need to be considered in the school building or grounds?
- Are any modifications to the PE curriculum necessary? Are there any concerns regarding recess and playground equipment?
- Does the child require special transportation?
- What plans need to be implemented in the event of a building emergency and/or evacuation?

## Nursing Diagnosis (N.D.) (NANDA, 2003)

**N.D. 1** Impaired physical mobility (NANDA 00085) related to:
- musculoskeletal, neuromuscular impairment
- intolerance to activity/decreased strength and endurance
- decreased muscle strength, control, and/or mass
- loss of integrity of bone structure

**N.D. 2** Activity intolerance (NANDA 00092) related to:
- generalized weakness
- potential for injury

**N.D. 3** Disturbed body image (NANDA 00118) related to:
- musculoskeletal, neuromuscular impairment
- functional impairment
- effects of physical disability
- fear of rejection or reaction of others
- complexity of therapeutic regimen

**N.D. 4** Risk for injury (NANDA 00035) related to:
- musculoskeletal, neuromuscular impairment
- design, structure, and/or arrangement of building facilities

**N.D. 5** Risk for disuse syndrome (NANDA 0040) related to:
- mechanical immobilization

**N.D. 6** Delayed growth and development (NANDA 00111) related to:
- effects of physical disability

**N.D. 7** Chronic pain (NANDA 00133) related to:
- chronic physical/psychosocial disability

**N.D. 8** Risk for impaired skin integrity (NANDA 00047) related to:
- physical immobility
- developmental factors
- use of assistive devices

**N.D. 9** Ineffective breathing pattern (NANDA 00032) related to:
- musculoskeletal impairment
- body position

**N.D. 10** Impaired dentition (NANDA 00048) related to:
- genetic predisposition

**N.D. 11** Disturbed sensory perception (auditory) (NANDA 000122) related to:
- reported or measured change in sensory acuity

**N.D. 12** Risk for imbalanced body temperature (NANDA 00005) related to:
- altered metabolic rate
- illness or trauma affecting temperature regulation

**N.D. 13** Risk for situational low self-esteem (NANDA 00153) related to:
- disturbed body image
- functional impairment
- decreased power/control over environment

**N.D. 14** Impaired adjustment (NANDA 00070) related to:
- negative attitudes toward health behavior
- intense emotional state
- disability or health status change requiring change in lifestyle
- lack of motivation to change behaviors
- absence of intent to change behavior

**N.D. 15** Caregiver role strain (NANDA 00061) related to:
- illness severity
- illness chronicity
- increasing care needs/dependency
- unpredictability of illness course
- 24-hour care responsibilities
- years of care giving
- inability to fulfill one's own or other's expectations

**N.D. 16** Compromised family coping (NANDA 00074) related to:
- prolonged disease or progression of disability that exhausts supportive capacity of significant people

## Goals

The student will acquire the necessary adaptations in the school setting to accommodate impaired physical immobility and activity intolerance. (N.D.1, 2)

The student will develop and maintain skills necessary for maximum independence related to the ADLs. (N.D. 1–3, 5, 6, 13, 14)

The student will have a safe school environment. (N.D. 4)

The student will become comfortable with and accept physical limitations while still being given the opportunity to acquire greater intellectual, social, and mobility skills. (N.D. 3, 5-7, 13, 14)

The student will develop and maintain positive relationships with peers and school personnel (N.D. 13, 14)

The student will have normal or near-normal respiratory status. (N.D. 9)

The student will maintain maximum hearing potential (N.D. 11)

The student will maintain normal body temperature. (N.D. 12)

The student will develop effective coping skills and express optimism and hope toward student's condition. (N.D. 14-16)

The student will monitor skin for areas of redness or breakdown. (N. D. 8)

The student will maintain intact skin, free from breakdown. (N. D. 8)

The student will participate in good oral health care at school. (N. D. 10)

## Nursing Interventions

Assess student's self-management skills and collaborate with key school personnel (PT, OT, administration, special education teacher, PE teacher, classroom teacher) regarding any necessary accommodations. (N.D. 1, 2)

Tour the school building and grounds to determine if there are any architectural barriers that will restrict the student's ability to participate in school activities. (N.D. 1, 2, 4)

If architectural barriers exist, confer with necessary school personnel to address accommodations or changes that need to be arranged. This could include portable ramps, wheelchair lifts, lowering shelves or lockers, special desks or tables, rearrangement of space, providing for a personal assistant. (N.D. 1, 2, 4)

Collaborate with school and OT/PT staff to arrange assistive devices that may be necessary. This may include special desks, laptop computer, typing systems, a standing frame, etc. Monitor their use and effectiveness. (N.D.1, 2)

Educate appropriate staff about OI. Explain that fractures may occur and that they should follow guidelines for activity and assistance of the student. (N.D. 13, 14)

Refer student to committee on special education or 504 committee to determine if a complete evaluation is needed. Address any academic modifications to the curriculum. (N.D. 6, 13, 14)

Consult with regular education PE teacher and adaptive PE teacher to provide any necessary modifications or accommodations in the PE curriculum. (N.D. 1, 2, 5)

Determine if special transportation is needed, and speak with necessary personnel to arrange this. (N.D. 1, 2)

Monitor student's ability to perform self-management skills. (N.D. 1, 2)

Instruct student on ways to improve and increase potential for learning. (N.D. 1, 2)

Determine if crowded hallways pose a problem or safety concern for the student. Suggest interventions such as preferred seating arrangements, early/late arrival to class, personal escort. It may be useful to enlist peers to assist student in maneuvering the building when necessary. (N.D. 1, 2, 4)

Arrange for a separate set of books to be given to the student for home use to avoid the need to carry heavy books. (N.D. 1, 2, 4)

Screen hearing, if appropriate. Refer student for a full hearing evaluation, if necessary. Confer with necessary personnel (speech/language pathologist, hearing impairment specialist, teachers, administrators) to provide any necessary accommodations. (N.D. 11)

Educate appropriate staff about OI. Explain that fractures may occur and that no one, including staff and students, are at fault when this occurs. (N.D. 13, 14)

Encourage family to have student wear clothing that will help maintain normal body temperature. A change of clothes may be necessary for excessive sweating. Take a baseline temperature to determine student's normal body temperature to gauge when a febrile state has occurred. (N.D. 12)

Maintain regular communication with student and his/her family. (N.D. 1, 2, 14-16)

Act as a liaison between school and other healthcare and service providers to assist in continuity of care between school, home, and healthcare providers. (N.D. 14-16)

Educate appropriate staff members about identification and immediate care of fractures. Consult with parent about how transportation should be provided in the event of a suspected fracture. Some parents may want an ambulance called only as a last resort. (N.D. 4)

With permission from student and family, arrange to speak to the other students regarding OI. (N.D. 3, 13, 14)

Assess for any respiratory concerns. Monitor and teach respiratory hygiene skills. Attempt to limit student's exposure to infectious disease. Notify parent of any unusual occurrence of infectious diseases in the school. (N.D. 1, 2, 9)

Monitor for signs of skin breakdown. Instruct student/staff on early signs of skin breakdown. Enlist preventive measures to prevent skin breakdowns. (N.D. 1, 2, 5, 8)

Help arrange for home tutoring for prolonged absences due to fractures or surgery. (N.D. 1, 2, 7, 14, 15)

Promote age-appropriate peer relationships. Encourage parents to support inclusion of student in extracurricular clubs and events. Emphasize to extracurricular event leaders importance and value of allowing student to participate. (N.D. 3, 13, 14)

Assist student to develop a high level of self-esteem. Encourage student to identify his/her strengths/weaknesses. Reinforce positive attitudes and behaviors. Encourage student to share feelings about OI and disability. Facilitate strategies to handle teasing, questions about disability, and discrimination. (N.D. 3, 13, 14)

Promote wellness by emphasizing proper nutrition, hydration, sleep, hygiene, and exercise. (N.D. 1, 4-7, 14)

Support family members by listening and encouraging them to express concerns, fears, and anxieties of caring for a disabled child. Refer student/family to support groups, counseling, family therapies, clergy. Assist in identifying any social service resources the school district provides. Reinforce student's strengths to family members and highlight progress achieved. ( N.D. 13-16)

Students less affected by OI need subtle yet careful monitoring of activities to prevent fractures while still maintaining normal school and extracurricular activities. Assist student and family to weigh risks versus benefits of an activity when making choices. (N.D. 1, 2, 4, 14)

Develop an emergency plan related to fracture identification and management. (N.D. 1, 2, 4)

Develop an emergency plan for a building emergency and/or evacuation. (N.D. 1, 2, 4)

Explain to parent and student about Medic Alert bracelets and the appropriateness of wearing one. (N.D. 4)

Develop an individualized healthcare plan that addresses the student's academic, social, and physical needs. (N.D. 1–16)

Participate as a member of the interdisciplinary team to develop an IEP or 504 plan, if necessary. (N.D. 1–16)

Have knowledge about regulations of the Health Insurance Portability and Accountability Act (HIPAA) and the Family Educational Rights and Privacy Act (FERPA). Take precautions to give health information only to those who need to know about the student's condition. Encourage and teach others about confidentiality issues and the legal implications. (N.D. 14, 15)

## Expected Student Outcomes

The student will:

- Have full access to all necessary areas in the school building and grounds. (N.D. 1, 2, 4)
- Maintain mobility in the school and on the school grounds. (N.D. 1, 2, 4-7)
- Attend all classes and school-related activities with modifications made as needed. (N.D. 1, 2, 4, 5 )
- Have few or no occurrences of bone fractures. (N.D. 1, 2, 4)
- Receive assistance for activities that require intervention/assistance. (N.D. 2, 4, 8)
- Utilize special transportation if needed. (N.D. 1, 2, 4)
- Be given and trained in, and utilize, assistive devices that may be necessary. (N.D. 1, 2, 4, 5)
- Receive necessary school-based therapies with minimal disruption of the school schedule. (N.D. 1–8, 11, 13, 14 )
- Receive and correctly use hearing devices or interventions so hearing loss will not negatively impact academic success. (N.D. 11)
- Achieve growth and developmental milestones within normal limits of his/her type of OI. (N.D. 6)
- Demonstrate good oral hygiene skills. (N.D.10)
- Have few or no respiratory problems. (N.D. 9 )
- Report signs/symptoms of skin irritation or breakdown and perform or be assisted with repositioning techniques. (N.D. 2, 5, 8)
- Notify school staff of signs/symptoms that a fracture may have occurred. (N.D. 1, 2, 4-7)
- Actively participate in PE class and recess activities as appropriate. (N.D. 1–6, 13, 14)
- Make correct choices regarding his/her ability to participate in an activity and accept staff members' recommendations and accommodations if the activity seems too hazardous. (N.D. 1, 2, 4, 6, 7, 13, 14)
- Be able to share feelings about having OI with staff, family, and peers. (N.D. 3, 13, 14)
- Be able to develop and maintain appropriate relationships with family, peers, and school personnel. (N.D. 3, 6, 13, 14)
- Have positive feelings about himself/herself and capabilities. (N.D. 3, 6, 13, 14)
- Be included in appropriate extracurricular activities. (N.D. 1–4, 6, 13, 14)
- Have staff members who are knowledgeable about OI and can give assistance if necessary. (N.D. 1, 4, 5, 7-9, 11, 13, 14)
- Have good support from family/significant others. The family will feel supported by the school system. (N.D. 13-16)
- Be safe during building emergencies and/or evacuations and during drills for the same. (N.D. 1, 2, 4, 6)
- Be encouraged to wear a medical alert bracelet. (N.D. 4, 15)
- Have any curricular modifications updated regularly to reflect changes in status of the OI. (N.D. 1–16)
- Have skin that is intact and healthy. (N.D. 8)
- Have healthy teeth and gums. (N.D. 10)

# Case Study

Katie S. is a 6-year-old girl with a diagnosis of osteogenesis imperfecta type III. She was diagnosed at 18 months of age after having sustained several unexplained fractures. Prior to the diagnosis, Katie's parents had been questioned by authorities for possible child abuse charges. This has made them distrustful of healthcare providers and wary to seek assistance. They have, however, established a good relationship with a local children's hospital and orthopedic staff, so Katie has received proper care for the OI. Katie is an only child, and her parents have chosen to not send her to preschool or kindergarten. She will be attending first grade at the local public school. Katie's mother is a former teacher and has been home-schooling her daughter. Katie has acquired many of the academic skills of a typical first grader and is an enthusiastic student.

In spite of good medical and home care, Katie has many health concerns due to the OI. She has sustained fractures about five times each year, and x-ray evidence reveals other healed, undiagnosed fractures. The fractures have mostly been of the radius/ulna or the tibia/fibula, but she has also fractured her right femur and had a skull fracture at the age of 3 years. Both the femur fracture and skull fracture required surgical intervention. Katie is 28 inches tall and weighs 24 pounds, which is below the third percentile on the CDC growth charts. Her arms and legs are short, and she is barrel-chested. A curvature of the spine is noted, and she will someday need surgery to correct this, including the insertion of a rod. Her muscle tone is low and weak. Katie's baseline temperature is 99.4°F; she sweats excessively and is sensitive to temperature extremes. Katie's teeth are also affected by the OI and are discolored. She will potentially need dental crowns. Katie is very susceptible to respiratory infections and has several a year, especially during the winter months. On three occasions, the respiratory infections required that she be hospitalized. To treat the OI, Katie is taking Aredia as prescribed by her orthopedic doctor.

Katie's mother requested a meeting with the school nurse, classroom teacher, and an administrator prior to the beginning of the school year. Katie was present for part of the meeting. She has a motorized wheelchair for ambulation and proficiently uses it. She cannot bear weight on her legs or use her arms for transferring from her wheelchair. Though she has full bowel and bladder control, someone must pick her up and put her on the toilet and assist her with hand washing. Katie is worried about this because her parents have been her only caretakers. She is also worried about how the other children will respond to her, because she has never been in a school setting. Mrs. S. is quite anxious about her daughter starting school and wants to be sure that staff are properly informed and trained in caring for Katie. She is requesting a teaching assistant who can help with Katie's physical needs as well as her academic needs due to the OI.

## Osteogenesis Imperfecta

| Assessment Data | Nursing Diagnosis | Goals | Nursing Interventions | Expected Outcomes |
|---|---|---|---|---|
| Katie S. has type III OI. She has weak muscle tone and has sustained many fractures. Katie cannot bear weight on her legs, and her arms tire easily. She uses a motorized wheelchair.

Katie will need accommodations for her physical and activity intolerance needs for both curricular and extracurricular activities. | Impaired physical mobility related to musculoskeletal impairment, intolerance to activity/decreased strength and endurance.

Loss of integrity of bone structure.

Activity intolerance related to generalized weakness.

Risk for disuse syndrome related to mechanical immobilization.

Risk for impaired skin integrity related to physical immobilization, developmental factors. | Student will maintain mobility throughout the school with the use of a wheelchair and assistive personnel.

Student will acquire necessary adaptations to accommodate impaired physical immobility and activity intolerance.

Student will develop and maintain skills necessary for independence related to ADLs.

Student will have a safe school environment with few or no occurrences of fractures.

Student will be free of skin breakdowns. | Collaborate with OT and PT for use of assistive devices and monitor their use. Assist in arrangements for transportation to and from school.

Consult with teachers, including regular and adaptive PE staff and administrators, to provide any necessary modification or accommodation to curriculum, recess, and extracurricular activities.

Refer student to the 504 committee to determine if an evaluation is needed.

Speak with parents on specific transfer technique; teach key personnel this technique.

Instruct student/staff on early signs of skin breakdown and enlist preventive measures. | Assistive devices will be acquired from home and school and used appropriately.

Wheelchair-adapted bus will be used for transportation.

Student will perform as many activities independently as possible.

Student will be able to attend all classes and/or activities.

Key staff members will be trained in care of student, including transfer and toileting technique.

Student will routinely reposition self in wheelchair with aid of assistant to prevent skin breakdowns. |
| Katie has a history of frequent respiratory infections. Her anatomic and physiologic impairments contribute to this. | Ineffective breathing pattern related to musculoskeletal impairment and body position. | Student will have few or no respiratory infections. | Monitor health of student and peers.

Encourage frequent hand washing of all students and staff. Teach student/staff/parents respiratory hygiene exercises and expect student compliance every 2 to 3 hours. Have student maintain hydration. | Student will have few or no respiratory infections.
Student will demonstrate effective airway clearing.

Student will drink 4 to 6 glasses of fluid per day.

Students and staff will wash their hands several times a day. |

| Assessment Data | Nursing Diagnosis | Goals | Nursing Interventions | Expected Outcomes |
|---|---|---|---|---|
| Katie is at risk for fractures. School staff require knowledge of fracture assessment and management. | Risk for injury related to musculoskeletal, neuromuscular impairment and the design, structure, and/or arrangement of the facility. | Student will have a safe school environment with few or no occurrences of fractures. | Speak with parents and medical team on specific transfer technique.<br><br>Write care plan for potential fracture care. | Key staff members will be trained in care of student, including transfer and toileting technique.<br><br>Staff members will recognize and respond correctly to potential fractures. |
| Katie has a higher than normal body temperature, excessive sweating, and sensitivity to temperature extremes. | Risk for imbalanced body temperature related to altered metabolic rate, illness, or trauma affecting temperature regulation | Student will maintain proper body temperature. | Encourage family to have student wear lightweight cotton clothing to help maintain proper body temperature.<br><br>Try to have student stay in cooler parts of the building and school grounds. Obtain a baseline oral temperature reading. | Student's body temperature will stay within her normal limits.<br><br>Student will feel comfortable in clothing worn to school. A change of clothing will be available as needed if clothing becomes wet from sweating.<br><br>Student's normal body temperature will be known as a baseline to determine febrile state. |
| Katie and her family have fears and concerns regarding the physical and psychosocial aspects of starting school. | Disturbed body image related to biophysical, developmental changes, psychosocial illness, illness treatment.<br><br>Risk for situational low self-esteem related to disturbed body image, functional impairment, decreased power/control.<br><br>Caregiver role strain related to illness severity, illness chronicity, increasing care needs/dependency/unpredictability of illness course. | Student and family will be able to express fears and concerns effectively with staff members.<br><br>Student and family will develop and maintain relationships with peers, staff, and other school families.<br><br>Student and family will enjoy being in the school setting and feel confident about educational, physical, and emotional support given. | Listen to student and family's concerns and fears. Write care plan with parent and healthcare provider input.<br><br>Facilitate student in interacting with others and making friends.<br><br>Refer family to support groups both in and out of the school setting. | Student and family will verbalize concerns about school, past experiences, peers, emergency care.<br><br>Student and family will participate in activities and functions and feel included in the school community.<br><br>Student and family will receive counseling, if needed. |

| Assessment Data | Nursing Diagnosis | Goals | Nursing Interventions | Expected Outcomes |
|---|---|---|---|---|
| | 24-hour care responsibilities, years of care giving.<br><br>Compromised family coping related to prolonged disease or progression of disability that exhausts supportive capacity of significant people. | | | |

# Emergency Safety Plan
## Osteogenesis Imperfecta
### Katie S.

Katie S. has osteogenesis imperfecta type III, a collagen production disorder causing bones that easily break. She is unable to walk or stand and uses a wheelchair for ambulation. In the event of a building emergency, the following care plan will be in place:

**Evacuation from the first floor:** Katie will leave the building in her wheelchair through the closest exit door accompanied by a designated adult. An adult will stay with her at all times.

**Evacuation from the second floor:** An adult trained in transferring technique will pick Katie up and carry her down the stairs. Another adult will bring her wheelchair downstairs. Katie will then be placed in her wheelchair and exit the building from the closest door. An adult will stay with her at all times.

**Tornado emergency:** Katie will be brought to the designated area in her wheelchair. An adult will assist in providing protective head cover per school routine.

**Confinement emergency:** If there is a confinement emergency (such as an intruder, act of war, neighborhood emergency), Katie will be brought to the designated area of the building in her wheelchair per school emergency plan to await further instructions. An adult will be with her at all times.

Copies of this plan were distributed to the following school personnel: (name school personnel who received a copy, including parent)

Local emergency services personnel have been notified of Katie's disability and special evacuation needs.

**Signatures:**

School Nurse _____ Date _____

Parent _____ Date _____

Administrator _____ Date _____

Osteogenesis Imperfecta

# Emergency Care Plan
## Suspected Bone Fracture
### Katie S. — First Grade

Katie S. has osteogenesis imperfecta type III, a collagen production disorder causing bones that easily break. She is unable to walk or stand and uses a wheelchair for ambulation. Katie's bones break very easily, and she has sustained many fractures throughout her life, including a skull fracture. The following care plan is in place if an injury is suspected:

1. Katie and her parents feel that the benefits of participation in school activities outweigh the risks and would like her to be included in as many activities as possible. They understand that fractures will inevitably happen to her.

2. Listen to Katie's assessment of an injury. She will advise you on where her pain is and what her immediate needs are.

3. Do not move Katie out of the area unless it is absolutely necessary to protect her from harm.

4. Have the other children leave the area; leave only necessary staff to stay with Katie.

5. Call a parent. It is their request that they be called first instead of emergency personnel because of the cost. An ambulance should be called only as a last resort or if the injury is potentially life-threatening. School nurse and parents will establish criteria for calling an ambulance.

6. Notify the school nurse.

7. Keep Katie warm and comfortable. Do not give her food or fluids.

8. If Katie must be moved before a parent has arrived, protect the injury from movement. This can be done by manual splinting (someone gently holding the affected injured area while Katie is being moved) or using makeshift splints made from pillows or towels. Several staff members should be taught the immobilization techniques and only those trained should attempt to move her.

9. If a serious head and/or neck injury is suspected, emergency medical transportation will be necessary. Call an ambulance and Katie's parent. Do not move her or allow her to move herself. Keep Katie warm, still, and as quiet as possible. Be prepared to start CPR, if necessary.

10. Comfort/support Katie and the other children who may be upset by the event.

Copies of this plan were distributed to the following school personnel: (name school personnel who received a copy, including parent)

Local emergency services personnel have been notified of Katie's disability and special evacuation needs.

**Signatures:**

School Nurse _____  Date _____

Parent _____  Date _____

Administrator _____  Date _____

# References

NANDA International. (2003). *Nursing diagnosis: Definitions and classification 2003-2004.* Philadelphia: Author.

National Institutes of Health Osteoporosis and Related Bone Diseases, National Resource Center. (2004, August). *Fast facts on osteogenesis imperfecta.* Retrieved September 15, 2004, from http://www.osteo.org/oi.html

National Institutes of Health Osteoporosis and Related Bone Diseases, National Resource Center. (2002, October). *Novel forms of osteogenesis imperfecta: Types V & VI.* Retrieved July 16, 2003, from http://www.osteo.org/oi.html

National Institutes of Health Osteoporosis and Related Bone Diseases, National Resource Center. (2002, April). *OI issues: Genetics.* Retrieved July 16, 2003, from http://www.osteo.org/oi.html

Osteogenesis Imperfecta Foundation. (2003, September). *Osteogenesis imperfecta: A guide for nurses.* Retrieved October 16, 2003, from http://www.oif.org

# Bibliography

Arnold, M. J., & Silkwood, C. K. (1999). *The school nurse's source book of individualized healthcare plans* (Vol. 2). North Branch, MN: Sunrise River Press.

Clark, C. (2001). Osteogenesis imperfecta: An overview. *Nursing Standard, 16*(5), 47–53.

D'Ambra, P., & Jack, J. G. (1997–2000). *Nursing assessment of school age youth.* Musculoskeletal (Home Study Module Number 5). Scarborough, ME: National Association of School Nurses.

Dawson, P. A., & Marini, J. C. (2000). Osteogenesis imperfecta. In M. J. Econs (Ed.), *The genetics of osteoporosis and metabolic bone disease* (pp. 75–93). Totowa, NJ: Humana Press.

Falk, M. J., Heeger, S., Lynch, K. A., DeCaro, K. R., et al. (2003). Intravenous bisphosphonate therapy in children with osteogenesis imperfecta. *Pediatrics, 111*(3), 573–578.

Marini, J. C. (1998). Osteogenesis imperfecta—Managing brittle bones [Editorial]. *New England Journal of Medicine, 339*(14), 986–987.

Marini, J. C., & Chernoff, E. J. (2001). Osteogenesis imperfecta. In S. B. Cassidy & J. E. Allanson (Eds.), *Management of genetic syndromes* (pp. 281–300). New York: Wiley-Liss.

National Center for Health Statistics. (2004, May). *2000 CDC growth charts: United States.* Retrieved June 28, 2004, from http://www.cdc.gov/growthcharts

National Institutes of Health Osteoporosis and Related Bone Diseases, National Resource Center. (2002, April). *OI issues: Child abuse.* Retrieved July 16, 2003, from http://www.osteo.org/oi.html

National Institutes of Health Osteoporosis and Related Bone Diseases, National Resource Center. (2002, April). *OI issues: Education.* Retrieved June 28, 2004, from http://www.osteo.org/oi.html

National Institutes of Health Osteoporosis and Related Bone Diseases, National Resource Center. (2002, April). *OI issues: Genetics.* Retrieved July 16, 2003, from http://www.osteo.org/oi.html

National Institutes of Health Osteoporosis and Related Bone Diseases, National Resource Center. (2003, May). *Osteogenesis imperfecta: A guide for medical professionals, individuals, and families affected by OI.* Retrieved July 16, 2003, from http://www.osteo.org/oi.html

National Institutes of Health Osteoporosis and Related Bone Diseases, National Resource Center. (2004, August). *Fast facts on osteogenesis imperfecta.* Retrieved September 15, 2004, from http://www.osteo.org/oi.html

Osteogenesis Imperfecta Foundation. (1998). *Plan for success: An educator's guide to students with osteogenesis imperfecta.* Retrieved July 16, 2003, from http://www.oif.org

Osteogenesis Imperfecta Foundation. (2002, October). *Questions and answers about bisphosphonates.* Retrieved July 16, 2003, from http://www.oif.org

Osteogenesis Imperfecta Foundation. (2003, September). *Osteogenesis imperfecta: A guide for nurses.* Retrieved October 16, 2003, from http://www.oif.org

Rauch, F., & Glorieux, F. (2004). Osteogenesis imperfecta. *Lancet, 363,* 1377–1385.

Sillence, D. O., Senn, A., & Danks, D. M. (1979). Genetic heterogeneity in osteogenesis imperfecta. *Journal of Medical Genetics, 16,* 101–116.

Silverwood, B. (2001). Osteogensis imperfecta: Care and management. *Paediatric Nursing, 13*(3), 38–42.

## Resources

National Institutes of Health
Osteoporosis and Related Bone Diseases
National Resource Center
2 AMS Circle
Bethesda, MD 20892-3676
202-223-0344
1-800-624-2663
202-293-2356 (fax)
202-466-4315 (TTY)
Osteoinfo@osteo.org
http://www.osteo.org

Osteogenesis Imperfecta Foundation
804 West Diamond Avenue
Suite 210
Gaithersburg, MD 20878
301-947-008
1-800-981-2663
301-947-0456 (fax)
bonelink@oif.org
http://www.oif.org

Shriners Hospital for Children
1529 Cedar Avenue
Montreal, Quebec, Canada H3G 1A6
514-842-5964

*Chapter Fifty-nine*

# Posttraumatic Stress Disorder

Margarita Fernan Granthom

## Introduction

Formal recognition of the diagnosis of posttraumatic stress disorder (PTSD) occurred in 1980, but at that time little was known about PTSD in children and adolescents. PTSD is a debilitating condition that often follows a terrifying physical or emotional event, causing the person who survived the event to have persistent, frightening thoughts and memories, or flashbacks, of the ordeal. Not every individual who is traumatized develops PTSD (American Psychiatric Association [APA], 2000). All children and adolescents experience stressful events, which can emotionally and physically affect them. A child or adolescent who experiences a catastrophic event may develop PTSD. Such an event involves a situation in which someone's life has been threatened or severe injury has occurred (i.e., being a victim or a witness of physical abuse, sexual abuse, violence in the home or in the community, automobile accidents, natural disasters such as flood, fire, or earthquakes; being diagnosed with a life-threatening illness) (APA).

Traumatic experiences are not common in the lives of most children and adolescents, but approximately 3 million children each year are diagnosed with PTSD. The incidence of PTSD in children and adolescents is estimated to be as high as 40% in violence-ridden neighborhoods. Children and adolescents are more at risk of exposure to violence at home or on the streets than in school. One million children are confirmed victims of child abuse each year. Eighty-seven percent of inner-city elementary school-aged boys have seen someone arrested, 84% have heard guns being fired, and 25% have seen someone get killed (Cincinnati Children's Hospital Medical Center, 2003).

### Pathophysiology

Events that can trigger PTSD include:
- something that occurred in the person's life
- something that occurred in the life of someone close to him or her
- something the person witnessed (APA, 2000)

The risk for developing PTSD is often affected by the child's or teen's proximity and relationship to the trauma, the severity of the trauma, the duration of the traumatic event, the recurrence of the traumatic event, the resiliency of the child, the coping skills of the child, and the support resources available to the child from the family and community following the events (American Academy of Child and Adolescent Psychiatry [AACAP], 1999).

Examples of catastrophic, life-threatening events that may cause PTSD in a child or adolescent include the following:
- serious accidents (car, train, or bus crashes, falling from a height)
- natural disasters (floods, earthquakes, tornados, fire, hurricanes)
- man-made tragedies (bombings, a plane crash)
- violent personal attacks (beating, mugging, rape, torture, being held captive, kidnapping)
- physical abuse
- sexual assault
- sexual molestation
- emotional abuse
- neglect (AACAP, 1999)

Following trauma, children may initially show agitated or confused behavior, intense fear, helplessness, anger, sadness, horror, or denial. Children experiencing repeated trauma may develop a kind of emotional numbing to deaden or block the pain and trauma. They may also become less responsive emotionally, depressed, withdrawn, and more detached from their feelings. Symptoms may last from several months to many years (APA, 2000).

The most common symptoms of PTSD in children and adolescents are the following (APA, 2000):
- Sleep disturbances (insomnia, night terrors, nightmares, bed-wetting)
- Depression
- Feeling jittery or "on guard"
- Being easily startled
- Loss of interest in things formerly enjoyed; detachment; general lack of responsiveness; feeling numb
- Difficulty feeling affectionate
- Irritability, acting more aggressive than before, or even violent
- Avoiding certain places or situations that bring back memories
- Flashbacks or intrusive images (flashbacks can come in the form of images, sounds, smells, or feelings; a person usually believes that the traumatic event is happening all over again)

- Losing touch with reality
- Reenactment of an event for a period of seconds or hours or, very rarely, days
- Problems in school; difficulty concentrating
- Worry about dying at an early age
- Regressive behaviors; acting younger than one's age (i.e., thumb sucking, bed-wetting)
- Physical symptoms (i.e., headaches, stomachaches)

Criteria for PTSD now include age-specific features for some symptoms (Hamblen, 1998). Very young children may present with few PTSD symptoms, because eight of the PTSD symptoms require a verbal description of one's feelings and experiences. Young children may report more generalized fears, such as stranger or separation anxiety, avoidance of situations that may or may not be related to the trauma, sleep disturbances, and a preoccupation with words or symbols that may or may not be related to the trauma. These children may also display posttraumatic play in which they repeat themes of the trauma. Children may also lose an acquired developmental skill (i.e., toilet training) as a result of experiencing a traumatic event (Hamblen, 1998).

Elementary school-aged children may not experience visual flashbacks or amnesia for aspects of the trauma. They do experience "time skew" and "omen formation," which are not typically seen in adults. Time skew is when a child mis-sequences trauma-related events when recalling the memory. Omen formation is a belief that if they are alert enough, they will recognize warning signs and avoid future traumas. School-aged children also exhibit posttraumatic play or reenactment of the trauma in play, drawings, or verbalizations. Posttraumatic play is literal representation of the trauma; it involves compulsively repeating some aspect of the trauma and does not tend to relieve anxiety. Posttraumatic reenactment is more flexible and involves behaviorally recreating aspects of the trauma (Hamblen, 1998).

PTSD in adolescents may begin to more closely resemble PTSD in adults. They engage in traumatic reenactment, in which they incorporate aspects of the trauma into their daily lives. Adolescents are more likely to exhibit impulsive and aggressive behaviors (Hamblen, 1998).

## Diagnostic Evaluation

PTSD is diagnosed only if symptoms persist for more than 1 month and are adversely affecting the child's life and level of functioning (APA, 2000). Symptoms may begin within 3 months following the trauma but can also start months or years later. A qualified mental health professional usually diagnoses PTSD in children or adolescents following a comprehensive psychiatric evaluation. Seeking early evaluation is extremely important.

## Management

Early detection and intervention can reduce the severity of symptoms, enhance the child's normal growth and development, and improve the quality of life. Treatment should always be based on a comprehensive evaluation of the child and family. Support from parents, school, and peers is important (Hamblen, 1998). Emphasis needs to be placed on establishing a feeling of safety. Treatment recommendations may include the following:

- *Cognitive behavioral therapy.* This is the most effective approach. It focuses on helping the child or adolescent learn skills to manage his or her anxiety and to help him or her master the situations that contributed to PTSD. It involves the child directly discussing the traumatic event (exposure), anxiety management techniques such as relaxation and assertiveness training, and correction of inaccurate or distorted trauma-related thoughts. There is some controversy in exposing children to the events that scare them; exposure-based treatments seem to be most relevant when memories or reminders of the trauma distress the child. Children can be exposed gradually and taught to learn to relax while recalling their experiences. A majority of studies have found that cognitive behavioral therapy is safe and effective for children with PTSD (Hamblen, 1998).
- *Psycho-education and parental involvement.* This therapy primarily involves parents and uses education about PTSD symptoms and their effects as its approach. Parents and caregivers must understand the effects of PTSD. When parents cope with the trauma, they support their children, and their children will function better. It is extremely important for parents to seek treatment for themselves to develop the necessary coping skills to help their children (Hamblen, 1998).
- *Play therapy.* This is used to treat young children with PTSD who are not able to deal with the trauma more directly. Games, drawings and other techniques are used to help the children process their traumatic memories (APA, 2000).
- *Psychological first aid.* This is prescribed for children exposed to community violence and can be used in schools and traditional settings. It involves clarifying trauma-related facts, normalizing the children's PTSD reactions, encouraging the expression of feelings, teaching problem-solving skills, and referring the most symptomatic children for additional treatment (Hamblen, 1998).
- *Twelve-step approaches.* These approaches are prescribed for adolescents with substance abuse problems and PTSD.
- *Eye movement desensitization and reprocessing.* This is a combination of cognitive therapy with directed eye movements. Shown to be effective in treating both children and adults with PTSD, studies indicate that it is the cognitive intervention, rather than the eye movements, that accounts for change (Hamblen, 1998).
- *Medications.* Some children and adolescents may

also benefit from treatment with antidepressant or antianxiety medication. Because of lack of research in this area, it is too early to evaluate the effectiveness (APA, 2000).

- *Specialized interventions.* These may be needed for children exhibiting particularly problematic behaviors or PTSD symptoms.

## Preventive Measures
- Teach children that it is okay to say "No" to someone who tries to touch their body or approach them in any way that makes them feel uncomfortable.
- Teach children that it is okay to tell an adult they trust right away if someone makes them feel uncomfortable.
- Encourage violence prevention programs within your community or local school system.
- Assist in fostering school programs to assist children and adolescents with severe emotional distresses (Hamblen, 1998).

## Individualized Healthcare Plan

### Assessment

*History*
- PTSD diagnosed (date)
- Traumatic event that caused PTSD
- Risk factors: severity of the traumatic event, the parental reaction to the traumatic event, and the physical proximity to the traumatic event
- Differences in levels of exposure and the number of traumatic events experienced in the past
- Family support and parental coping
- Symptoms affecting the child's life and level of functioning
- Repeated reliving of the trauma (i.e., nightmares and disturbing recollections during the day)
- PTSD symptoms

*Current Status and Management*
- Child's age
- General health
- Current healthcare providers including mental health
- Appropriate examination for the presenting physical complaint; extent of symptoms
- Vital signs; weight and height measurement and compare to previous measurements
- Sleep pattern: including sleep disturbances, problems falling or staying asleep; concentrating
- Nutritional pattern: appetite, problems
- Current medication: medication results, side effects
- Current therapy: counseling, play therapy, cognitive behavioral therapy, etc.
- Current symptoms:
  - agitated or confused behavior
  - intense fear, helplessness, anger, sadness, horror, or denial
  - emotional numbing to deaden or block the pain and trauma that may develop (dissociation)
  - avoidance of situations or places that remind them of the trauma
  - less responsive emotionally, depressed or withdrawn and more detached from their feelings
  - reexperiencing the traumatic event by having frequent memories of the event, having upsetting and frightening dreams, acting or feeling like the experience is happening again, developing repeated physical or emotional symptoms when reminded of the event
  - worry about dying at an early age
  - loss of interest in activities
  - sudden and extreme emotional reactions; angry outbursts or irritability
  - acting younger than their age (i.e., clingy, shy behavior, thumb sucking)
  - increased alertness to the environment
  - repeating behavior that reminds them of the trauma
- Expectations for the course of the disorder

*Self-care*
- Ability to recognize symptoms and seek assistance from trusted adults when they occur
- Locus of control
- Decision-making abilities

*Psychosocial Status*
- Student's perception and understanding of having PTSD
- Parent's perception and understanding of having PTSD
- Student's general temperament and coping ability
- Family interaction
- Participation in family activities
- Participation with peers: sports, church, community
- Family support systems: relatives, healthcare providers, community resources

*Academic Issues*
- Current and past academic performance
- Current and past attendance patterns, including reasons for absences
- Special education services needed
- Section 504 accommodations needed
- Involvement in school and classroom activities with peers

## Nursing Diagnoses (N.D.) (NANDA, 2003)

**N.D. 1** Disturbed sleep pattern (NANDA 00095) related to:
- problems falling or staying asleep (insomnia)
- nightmares/night terrors

**N.D. 2** Acute confusion (NANDA 00128) related to:
- agitated or confused behavior
- fluctuation in sleep pattern

**N.D. 3.** Posttrauma syndrome (NANDA 00141) related to:
- response due to physical or psychological trauma

**N.D. 4** Anxiety (NANDA 00146 ) related to:
- past physical or psychological trauma
- death of someone close to them

**N.D. 5** Ineffective coping (NANDA 00069) related to:
- inadequate choice or practiced effective responses
- inability to use available resources
- sleep disturbances

**N.D. 6** Fear (NANDA 00148) related to:
- real or perceived threat
- separation from support system
- unfamiliar environment

**N.D. 7** Chronic sorrow (NANDA 00137) related to:
- perceived loss or trauma
- recurrent feelings of sadness

**N.D. 8** Acute pain (NANDA 00132) related to:
- headaches and stomachaches
- expressive behavior: irritability, agitated behavior
- protective behavior

**N.D. 9** Social isolation (NANDA 00053) related to:
- need to relocate (new town/school, etc)
- absence of supportive significant others

**N.D. 10** Disturbed thought processes (ND 00130) related to:
- difficulty concentrating
- decreased academic progress
- decreased decision-making ability
- sleep disturbances

## Goals

The student will identify sources of fear and anxiety and utilize effective coping strategies that reduce or eliminate them. (N.D. 1, 4-6)

The student will increase knowledge of the PTSD symptoms and treatment plan. (N.D. 1, 3, 4, 6, 7, 9, 10)

The student will effectively communicate feelings to parents/guardians and school personnel. (N.D. 3-9)

The student will decrease severity/frequency of physical symptoms related to anxiety and fear. (N.D. 1, 4, 6, 8)

The student will learn and utilize decision-making skills. (N.D. 2, 5, 10)

The student will effectively interact and participate in activities with peers. (N.D. 5, 9, 10)

The student will maintain sufficient sleep for age. (N.D. 1, 5, 6, 10)

The student will achieve and maintain good academic performance. (N.D. 5, 10)

The student will seek assistance from significant others as needed to reduce symptoms. (N.D. 1-10)

## Interventions

Establish a relationship with the student that shows sincere interest, acceptance, caring, positive attitude, and support. (N.D. 1-10)

Allow student to express feelings: especially feelings of fear, anxiety, sadness, confusion, helplessness, etc. (N.D. 2-9)

Assist the student to feel safe in the school environment. (N.D. 2-5, 8)
- Orient the student to the school building and staff.
- Identify places the student can go if fear, anxiety, or other symptoms occur (health office, counseling office, etc.)
- Allow student to connect with parent/guardian, psychologist if they need assistance with reassurance or reinforcement during the school day.
- Assist in providing a secure building, especially if an order for protection is in place.

Collaborate with school staff to review educational and behavioral assessments, observations, and recommendations with the student and parent. (N.D. 1, 2, 4-10)

Provide opportunities for the student to learn and utilize decision-making skills. Assist student through the process, as needed. (N.D. 5, 10)

Assist student to identify adults or adult resource persons at school they feel comfortable talking to, especially when feeling fear and anxiety. (N.D. 4-6, 10)

Educate student regarding PTSD, including risk factors, symptoms, management, and prevention (N.D. 3)

Monitor the student's self-care ability: hygiene, dress, homework completion, sleeping pattern. (N.D. 1-3, 7, 8)

Assist the student to attain and maintain sufficient sleep for age: allow them to rest/sleep in health office, as needed. (N.D. 1, 2, 5, 10)

Administer medication in school, if needed: antidepressant or anti-anxiety medications (N.D. 2, 4, 7, 8, 10)
- Obtain medication orders and authorization for medications needed at school from parent and physician.
- Assist in monitoring and ensuring compliance with medication regimen.
- Monitor for potential medication side-effects.

Provide in-service for school staff about PTSD, including: (N.D. 3, 10)
- causes
- symptoms
- management
- support needed at school

Collaborate with other school personnel (school counselor, school social worker, classroom teacher, etc.) in providing the school-related portion of the child's treatment plan, for example, attendance, symptom monitoring, preferential seating, modification of student's educational program due to known triggers (e.g., alternative activities instead of discussions or stories of abuse or torture). (N.D. 1-10)

Assist in fostering school programs and support networks to deal with severe emotional distress. (N.D. 2-4, 6, 7, 9)

Provide extra support for planned and unplanned school events. (N.D. 4-6)
- Fire drills, tornado drills, school lock-down drills, loss of electricity: Keep the student close to the teacher and provide information and supportive interactions.
- For younger students especially: If the teacher has a planned absence, encourage the teacher to inform the parents and student that he/she will be gone and a substitute teacher will be there in his/her place.

Provide educational opportunities for parents/guardians to learn about PTSD: printed resources, community resources, internet access. (N.D. 3)

Assist parent/guardian and student to keep mental health/counseling appointment: release from school for appointments, assist in getting missed homework. (N.D. 1, 2, 4-10)

Assist parent/guardian to arrange for referral and follow-up care for the student, as needed. (N.D. 1, 2, 4-10)

Assist parent/guardian in their supportive role in the treatment process and emphasize that recovery is influenced by the support available within the family environment and community resources (mental health, healthcare providers, religious support, cultural support). (N.D. 3)

## Expected Student Outcomes

The student will:
- Identify (number) stressors that cause feelings of fear and anxiety. (N.D. 1, 4-6, 8, 10)
- Identify effective coping strategies that reduce anxiety or fear. (N.D. 1, 4-6, 8, 10)
- Use effective coping strategy to reduce anxiety or fear. (N.D. 1, 3-6, 8)
- Student reports and demonstrates a decrease in physical symptoms related to PTSD. (N.D. 1, 2, 4-6, 8)
- Name his/her friends. (N.D. 9, 10)
- Participate in school/class activities with peers. (N.D. 9, 10)
- Complete classroom and homework assignments within required timelines. (N.D. 5, 10)
- Ask for assistance with assignments from teachers, as needed. (N.D. 5, 10)
- Rest in health office, if needed. (N.D. 1, 8)
- Identify two adults at school they feel comfortable talking with. (N.D. 2-10)
- Identify two supportive adults (family, community, healthcare providers, etc.) he/she can utilize for support and assistance. (N.D. 1-10)
- Ask for assistance from others, as needed, to decrease symptoms. (N.D. 1- 10)
- Utilize supportive adults to assist in decreasing feelings of fear and anxiety. (N.D. 1, 4, 6, 8)
- Demonstrate positive, effective interactions with (staff, peers, family members). (N.D. 5, 9, 10)
- Demonstrate appropriate decision-making skills. (N.D. 2-5, 10)
- Appropriately manage a school event (that is/may be related to a trigger event experience), with assistance from others as needed. (N.D. 3, 4, 6)

## Case Study

About a month ago, Mica, who is 11 years old, and Michael, who is 6 years old, were involved in a motor-vehicle accident. Their father died instantly at the accident site. Initially, both Mica and Michael were very agitated: Mica jumped out of the car to check on her father's injuries, and Michael was confused and kept on asking why his father had to die. They had watched the firemen and highway patrolmen do CPR on their father while they were waiting for the other ambulance to arrive. The children, with their mother, were treated for minor physical injuries in the emergency room of the local hospital. Mica reports that during this time there were intense feelings of fear, helplessness, and horror.

In the weeks that followed, Mica stated that she felt like the experience was happening again. She has had upsetting and frightening dreams at night that wake her up, and she has a hard time getting back to sleep. Mica reports that she also has had a lot of headaches and stomachaches. Mica has missed parts of several classes in the past 3 to 4 weeks for these symptoms. Mica says she feels anxious right before the symptoms start. Mica's teachers report that she has become less responsive in the classroom setting and appears depressed, withdrawn, and tired. They also report that she seems fearful and even angry at times. Mica verbalized that she worries about dying at an early age.

## Posttraumatic Stress Disorder (PTSD)

| Assessment Data | Nursing Diagnosis | Goals | Nursing Interventions | Expected Outcomes |
|---|---|---|---|---|
| Mica states she has upsetting and frightening dreams that cause her to wake up at night and she has a hard time getting back to sleep. | Disturbed sleep pattern related to upsetting and frightening dreams. | Mica increases and maintains sufficient sleep for age. | Monitor for symptoms of tiredness at school.<br><br>Discuss this issue with Mica's mother and suggest she share these symptoms with Mica's healthcare provider.<br><br>Assist Mica in coping, reducing, or eliminating fears that are interfering with her ability to fall or stay asleep.<br><br>Explore with Mica things that help her relax and fall asleep and encourage her to try them.<br><br>Allow Mica to rest in the health office, as needed. | Mica (and her mother) will report that Mica is demonstrating:<br>• less waking at night due to bad dreams<br>• increased uninterrupted sleep<br><br>Mica will appear well rested in school. |
| Mica has a lot of headaches and stomachaches during the day. | Acute pain related to anxiety. | Mica will reduce the occurrences of physical symptoms during the school day.<br>Mica will increase her knowledge of PTSD symptoms and her treatment plan. | Assist Mica to identify things that decrease her symptoms of headaches and stomachaches—rest, relaxation exercises, talking with her mother or school staff member.<br>Assist Mica to eat well during the school day—breakfast and lunch. | Mica will report a decrease in physical symptoms.<br><br>Mica will decrease absences from class due to physical symptoms.<br><br>Mica will state (2) symptoms that occur when she feels anxious.<br><br>Mica demonstrates (1) effective strategy that decreases anxiety. |

| Assessment Data | Nursing Diagnosis | Goals | Nursing Interventions | Expected Outcomes |
|---|---|---|---|---|
| Mica worries about dying at an early age.<br><br>Mica appears fearful, angry, depressed, and sad. | Anxiety related to recent psychological trauma. | Mica will effectively communicate her feelings to her mother and school staff. | Assist Mica to discuss her feelings with her mother.<br><br>Assist Mica's mother to set up an appointment to consult with Mica's healthcare provider (and community resources, if needed), for assistance in dealing with Mica's anxiety symptoms.<br><br>Assist Mica's mother to meet with and work with Mica's teachers and other supportive school personnel (school counselor, school psychologist, etc.) to assist Mica in coping with and decreasing symptoms during the school day. | Mica will identify 2 school staff members that she feels comfortable talking with.<br><br>Mica will utilize school staff to assist her in decreasing her anxiety (when she feels she needs to).<br><br>Mica will effectively communicate her feelings to her mother, as reported by Mica and her mother. |
| Mica has become less responsive and withdrawn in school and classes. | Ineffective coping related to inadequate, practiced, effective coping responses. | Mica develops an effective coping skill to manage her feelings effectively in the school setting.<br><br>Mica increases her active participation in classroom activities with peers. | In collaboration with Mica's school psychologist and counselor:<br>• Assist Mica to identify feelings that make it hard to participate in class.<br>• Assist Mica to learn a coping skill that allows her to effectively manage her feelings and also participate in classroom activities.<br><br>Encourage Mica to let her teacher know when she feels she needs assistance from others in helping her cope. | Mica will demonstrate an effective coping skill in the classroom setting when she feels she needs to use it.<br><br>Mica will demonstrate active participation in classroom activities.<br><br>Mica tells her teacher when she needs assistance from someone to help her with her feelings. |

| Assessment Data | Nursing Diagnosis | Goals | Nursing Interventions | Expected Outcomes |
|---|---|---|---|---|
| | | | If she needs to leave the classroom to manage symptoms: with assistance from the teacher, assist Mica to reenter the classroom setting and begin participating in activities. | |
| | | | Encourage Mica's teacher to share behavior observations with Mica's mother. | |
| | | | Encourage Mica's mother to share the teacher's behavior observations with Mica's healthcare provider. | |

# References

American Psychiatric Association (APA). (2000). *Diagnostic and statistical manual of mental disorders* (5th ed). Washington, DC: Author

American Academy of Child and Adolescent Psychiatry. (1999). *Facts for families: No. 70. Posttraumatic stress disorder.* Retrieved October 4, 2004, from http://aacap.org/publications/factsfam/ptsd.70.htm

Cincinnati Children's Hospital Medical Center. (2003). *Child and adolescent mental health: Posttraumatic stress disorder.* Cincinnati, OH: Cincinnati Children's Hospital Medical Center.

Hamblen, J. (1998). Practice parameters for the assessment and treatment of children and adolescents with posttraumatic stress disorder. *Journal of the American Academy of Child and Adolescent Psychiatry*, 37(10).

NANDA International. (2003). *Nursing diagnoses: Definitions & classification (2003-2004).* Philadelphia: Author.

# Bibliography

Adelman, H., & Taylor, L. (1997–2000). *Nursing assessment of school age youth. Psychosocial screening* (Home Study Module Number 3). Scarborough, ME: National Association of School Nurses.

Bergren, M. D. (2002). Child and adolescent mental health Web resources. *Journal of School Nursing*, 18(4), 226–228.

Delaney, K. R., Belmonte-Mann, F. (2001). Identifying the mental health needs of preschool children. *Journal of School Nursing*, 17(4), 222–226.

Denehy, J. (2002) The mental health needs of children and adolescents. *Journal of School Nursing*, 18(4), 189–190.

DeSocio, J., Hootman, J. (2004). Children's mental health and school success. *Journal of School Nursing*, 20(4), 189–196.

Hootman J. (1996). *Quality nursing interventions in the school setting: Procedures, models, and guidelines.* Scarborough, ME: National Association of School Nurses.

Hootman, J., Houck, G. M., King, M. C. (2002). A program to educate school nurses about mental health interventions. *Journal of School Nursing*, 18(4), 191–195.

Knafl, K., & Santacroce, S. (2004). Chronic conditions and the family. In P. J. Allen & J. A. Vessey (Eds.), *Child with a chronic health condition* (chap. 3). St. Louis, MO: Mosby.

Marx, E., Wooley, S., & Northrop, D., (Eds.). (1998). *Health is academic: A guide to coordinated school health programs.* New York: Teachers College Press.

National Association of School Nurses. (n.d.). *Addressing the mental health needs of children and adolescence* [Education program]. Retrieved November 7, 2004, from http://nasn.org/education/education.htm

National Association of School Nurses. (2000). *Issue Brief: Mental health and illness.* Scarborough, ME: Author.

National Association of School Nurses. (Revised 2000). *Position Statement: Mental health of students.* Scarborough, ME: Author.

Wong, D., Hockenberry, J. J., Wilson, D., Winkelstein, L., & Kline, N. E. (Eds.). (2003). *Nursing care of infants and children.* St. Louis, MO: Mosby.

# Resources

American Academy of Child and Adolescent Psychiatry
3615 Wisconsin Avenue, NW
Washington, DC 20016-3007
202-966-7300
202 966-2891 (fax)
http://www.aacap.org

American Academy of Family Physicians
PO Box 11210
Shawnee Mission, KS 66207-1210
913-906-6000
http://www.aafp.org

Child Trauma Academy
5161 San Felipe
Suite 320
Houston, TX 77056

281-932-1375
713-481-9821 (fax)
http://www.childtrauma.org

Cincinnati Children's Hospital Medical Center
3333 Burnet Avenue
Cincinnati, OH 45229-3039
513-636-4200
http://www.cincinnatichildrens.org

National Center for PTSD
VA Medical Center (116D)
215 North Main St
White River Junction, VT 05009
802-296-6300
http://www.ncptsd.org

# Chapter Sixty

# Prader-Willi Syndrome

Linda L. Solum

## Introduction

Prader-Willi syndrome (PWS) is a neurobehavioral genetic disorder affecting one in 10,000 to 15,000 live births (Goldberg, Garrett, Van Riper, & Warzak, 2002). The most dominant characteristics of PWS include insatiable appetite (resulting in obesity), developmental delays, mental retardation, and behavioral problems.

In 1956, Prader, Labhart, and Willi described a new syndrome characterized by obesity (due to hyperphagia), short stature, lack of muscle tone in infancy, undescended testicles, and mental retardation. Since then, other researchers have noted additional characteristics of a tendency toward diabetes, strabismus, orthopedic problems (scoliosis and hip dislocation among others), gross motor developmental delay, and severe personality problems (Prader-Willi syndrome [online], 1994).

It is interesting to note that in 1680, a 6-year-old girl who weighed 120 pounds was the subject of a painting by Juan Carreno de Miranda, a painter to the Spanish Court. The painting, entitled *Eugenia Martinez Vallejo, La Monstrua,* was ordered by King Charles II and depicts some of the common features of PWS: obesity, small triangular mouth, and small hands and feet. The painting is located in the Prado Museum in Madrid, Spain (Prader-Willi syndrome [online], 1994).

## Pathophysiology

Individuals with PWS have a genetic defect, which occurs during embryonic development, involving chromosome 15. Genes that should have been inherited from the father on chromosome 15 are missing, and the person with PWS inherits two copies of the mother's chromosome 15. When the father's genes are missing, PWS develops. Parents of individuals with PWS almost always have normal chromosomes (Barrett, 1999).

Prader-Willi syndrome has two distinct clinical stages.
- Stage 1: Failure to thrive. Infants with PWS have a low birth weight and may be referred to as "floppy babies." Along with weak muscles (hypotonia), these babies often are unable to suck and demonstrate delayed developmental progress in lifting their head, sitting up, crawling, walking, and speaking.
- Stage 2: Thriving too well. An insatiable appetite and excessive weight gain usually become apparent during toddler years. Children with PWS do not feel full and can eat great amounts of food without becoming nauseated. They also gain weight on relatively few calories. Between the ages of 3 and 5 years, behavior problems may develop, including stubbornness, temper tantrums, acts of violence, and perseveration, or the uncontrollable repetition of a particular word, phrase, or gesture. These behaviors may be spontaneous or initiated by withholding food.

People with PWS also share some common physical features. They may have almond-shaped eyes, narrow forehead, down-turned mouth, thin upper lip, small chin, and small hands and feet. Other common features that may be present include a tendency to pick at their skin, thick saliva, scoliosis, daytime sleepiness, sleep abnormalities due to obesity, small penis in boys, and small clitoris in girls.

## Management

The one thing that all people with PWS need is 24-hours-a-day supervision of their access to food and consumption of food. They have been known to gorge, hoard, and forage for food. Families have reported that whole batches of cookies have disappeared and raw hamburger that was defrosting was eaten. Cupboards, refrigerators, freezers, and garbage cans need to be locked up. People with PWS may also steal money to have access to more food. Even though people with PWS may have a lower IQ, they can demonstrate cleverness in seeking food.

Everyone in the child's food environment needs to be aware of monitoring food intake. Children with PWS may ask others for food or trade food at lunchtime. They cannot use school snack bars, and they need to be monitored during school lunch. Special occasions like parties at school should be planned in advance so children with PWS can eliminate 50 to 100 calories a day for a week ahead of the social.

Other considerations in the school setting may include adaptations to physical education because of orthopedic concerns, weight loss or maintenance, and special education involvement because of the tendency to have a lower IQ and negative behavior issues.

# Individualized Healthcare Plan

## Assessment

### History

- Healthcare provider involvement
- Age of child at time of PWS diagnosis
- Involvement of support systems/groups for child and family
- Past experiences concerning obsession with food
- Past experiences concerning behavior problems/issues
- Past growth pattern
- Management methods concerning food intake that are successful
- Medications: types, reason, efficacy
- Behavioral issues management, behavior modification, social skills training

### Current Status and Management

- Current symptoms
- Last assessment with healthcare providers
- Knowledge of student's general health
- Level of intellectual functioning
- Sleep pattern and current management of sleep disturbances
- Current behavioral issues and current management plan
- Current height and weight
- Current daily caloric intake
- Activity tolerance, physical limitations
- Activity interests and abilities
- PWS management plan, including problems and successes in:
- Medication
- Behavior management
- Counseling/therapy
- Child/family education
- Current scoliosis screen
- Presence of orthopedic problems
- Skin integrity

### Self-care

- Student's decision-making skills
- Student's perception about PWS
- Student's level of cooperation and participation in food management plan
- Student's level of personal self-care—oral hygiene, bathroom cues, skin picking
- Child's motivation to be involved in self-care, self-management

### Psychosocial Status

- Student's locus of control—health, school, activities of daily living
- Student's concerns about health condition, behaviors, sleep problems
- Student's concerns about peer's reaction to, weight and eating behaviors
- Parent's and teacher's concerns about peers reaction to weight and eating behaviors

### Academic Issues

- Barriers to food management control in school
- Individualized education program or section 504 plan
- Monitoring food intake in school classroom/education/hallway-locker, etc.
- Staff awareness and knowledge of PWS
- Behavior-management issues/plan (inclusion of teachers, psychologist, social worker, paraprofessionals, etc.)

**Nursing Diagnoses (N.D.)** (NANDA, 2003)

**N.D. 1** Risk for imbalanced nutrition: more than body requirements (NANDA 00003) related to excessive appetite (PWS)

**N.D. 2** Noncompliance (NANDA 00079) with food management plan related to:
- behavior patterns
- lack of ability to feel satiety

**N.D. 3** Disturbed thought processes (NANDA 00130) related to:
- appropriate eating behaviors
- mental retardation (mild to severe)

**N.D. 4** Deficient knowledge (NANDA 00126) related to:
- mental retardation (mild to severe).

**N.D. 5** Risk for other-directed violence (NANDA 00140) or risk for self-directed violence (NANDA 00138) related to aberrant behaviors associated with PWS

**N.D. 6** Risk for disproportionate growth (NANDA 00113) related to lack of adolescent growth spurt in PWS

**N.D. 7** Fatigue (NANDA 00093) related to:
- sleep disturbances
- decreased metabolic rate

**N.D. 8** Impaired physical mobility (NANDA 00085) related to:
- skeletal impairments associated with PWS

**N.D. 9** Risk for activity intolerance (NANDA 00094) related to:
- obesity
- decreased physical stamina/endurance
- gross motor delay
- hypotonicity

**N.D. 10** Risk for impaired skin integrity (NANDA 00047) related to skin-picking behaviors

**N.D. 11** Risk for situational low self-esteem (NANDA 00153) related to:
- looking different from peers

**N.D.12** Social isolation (NANDA 0053) related to:
- obesity
- aberrant behaviors

## Goals

The student will participate and cooperate in food-management plan in the school setting. (N.D. 1, 2)
The student will increase compliance with food-management plan. (N.D. 1, 2)
The student will increase appropriate eating behaviors. (N.D. 1, 2)
- Choice of food
- Amount of food

The student will make appropriate decisions regarding food choices. (N.D. 1, 2)
The student will maintain stable and appropriate weight. (N.D. 1, 6)
The student will participate in physical education activities, with modifications made as needed. (N.D. 1, 8)
The student will participate in classroom activities, with modifications made as needed. (N.D. 3, 4, 5, 8)
The student will increase knowledge of PWS and increase knowledge in alteration in growth and development. (N.D. 3, 4, 6)
The student will decrease violent/injurious behavior to others. (N.D. 5)
The student will decrease self-injurious behavior (skin-picking). (N.D. 5, 10)
The student will prevent fatigue during the school day. (N.D. 7)
The student will decrease sleeping in the classroom. (N.D. 7)
The student will increase activity tolerance. (N.D. 9)
The student will maintain skin integrity and prevent infection. (N.D. 10)
The student will participate in social club activities with peers. (N.D. 11, 12)

## Nursing Interventions

Encourage parents to send appropriate school lunches from home to control portions. (Standard school lunches are usually too high in calories). (N.D. 1)

Monitor weight on a basis agreed upon with parents and healthcare provider and alert family of weight gain. (N.D. 1)

Inform staff that educational plan should include 30 minutes of daily physical activity to prevent fatigue, raise metabolism, and help maintain or promote weight loss, and discuss possible ways of scheduling physical activity into the student's schedule. (N.D. 1-3)

Inform staff and administration that one-to-one supervision during the school day may be necessary to monitor food intake, especially in the cafeteria, and discuss possible ways of providing supervision. (N.D. 1-3)

Assist the student to learn which behaviors are associated with PWS. (N.D. 1-5)
• gorging, hoarding, and foraging for food
• stubbornness
• temper tantrums
• acts of violence
• perseveration
• skin-picking

Assist student to learn and understand the limits or boundaries that are needed to: (N.D. 1-4, 7, 9)
• control food intake
• control behavior
• promote adequate sleep
• exercise

Educate everyone working with the student about PWS and the PWS management plan, including food restriction, food-related activities, behavior-modification, and physical activity. (N.D. 1-3, 5, 9)

Update healthcare plan annually to provide current student concerns. (N.D. 1–12)

Assist the student in realistic goal setting and positive, effective problem solving regarding the condition. (N.D. 2-4)

Communicate with family regarding behavior modification techniques that are successful, and inform staff of these interventions in the school setting. (N.D. 2-5)

Initiate collaboration between families and educators regarding educational plan, which should be based on intellectual functioning and behavioral needs. (N.D. 2-5)

Develop and implement measures for behavior modification plan that are consistent and oriented toward intervention and prevention. (N.D. 3-5)

Refer to special education team for assessment if behaviors significantly impact ability to learn or if the student is having difficulty academically. (N.D. 4, 5)

Assist the student to learn what PWS is:
• a genetic disorder resulting in a desire to eat food without control (N.D. 4, 11)

Assist the student to learn alterations in growth and development associated with PWS: (N.D. 6)
• delayed growth spurt

Screen for scoliosis annually or as necessary. (N.D. 8)

Review student's daily schedule. (N.D. 9)
• academic classes
• movement around the school environment
• pattern of activities: sitting, moving around, physical education

Assist student to identify and participate in activities with peers outside of class time, for example: school newspaper, student bulletin board, after-school sports (adaptive sports). (N.D. 9, 11)

Observe, clean, and bandage skin lesions as necessary. (N.D. 10)

**Expected Student Outcomes**

The student will:
- Maintain a stable weight or appropriate weight as defined by his or her healthcare provider. (N.D. 1)
- List three or more behaviors associated with PWS. (N.D. 1-5)
- Cooperate with the food- and behavior-management plan in the school setting. (N.D. 2, 3)
  - Does not take food from other students
  - Does not get food from the snack bar
  - Does not trade his or her food for other people's food
- Describe alterations in his/her growth and development related to PWS (at the level of the student's understanding). (N.D. 4, 6)
- Describe what PWS is. (N.D. 4, 11)
- Not demonstrate self-injurious or inappropriate behaviors in the school setting. (N.D. 5)
- Not sleep in school. (N.D. 7)
- Follow the physical activity plan to prevent fatigue. (N.D. 7)
- Describe his/her physical limitations. (N.D. 8)
- Participate in physical education activities (with modifications as needed). (N.D. 8, 9)
- Be involved in activities with other students outside of the school day. (N.D. 8, 9, 11, 12)
- Self-manage activities and mobility in the school setting. (N.D. 9)
- Decrease skin-picking episodes. (N.D. 10)

## Case Study

Peter is 12 years old and in the fifth grade. Currently his height is 59 inches and his weight is 150 pounds. When Peter was born, he was a "floppy baby" with poor muscle tone. When he was around 2 years old, he gained 20 pounds in 4 months. He was then diagnosed with Prader-Willi syndrome. Since then, he has needed to be on a strictly monitored diet.

Because of the neurologic disabilities associated with Prader-Willi syndrome, Peter demonstrates poor judgment and difficulty understanding abstract concepts. He has been known to crawl out of his bedroom window in the middle of the night to walk to a grocery store to get extra food. He also struggles with obsessive-compulsive behaviors, skin-picking, temper tantrums, and a tendency to be argumentative. His mental abilities are at the level of a 7-year-old. At times he is frustrated because of the inability to live a normal lifestyle.

# Prader-Willi Syndrome

| Assessment Data | Nursing Diagnosis | Goals | Nursing Interventions | Expected Outcomes |
|---|---|---|---|---|
| Excessive continual overeating leading to obesity. | Risk for imbalanced nutrition: more than body requirements related to excessive appetite. | Risk for imbalanced nutrition: more than body requirements related to excessive appetite.<br><br>Peter will make appropriate decisions regarding food choices. | Inform staff and discuss with administration that one-to-one supervision during the school day may be necessary to monitor food intake. (Meals monitored by a school staff member.)<br><br>Record weights weekly and alert family of weight gain.<br><br>Food intake must be monitored in the school setting, especially during school lunch.<br><br>The student cannot use the school snack bar. | Peter will cooperate with the food- and behavior-management plan in the school setting.<br><br>Peter will maintain a stable weight or appropriate weight as defined by his healthcare provider.<br><br>Peter does not use the snack bar during lunch. |
| The student has been known to ask the other students for food, trade food, and badger other students for food. | Disturbed thought processes related to: inappropriate eating behaviors and mental retardation (mild). | Peter will increase compliance with the food management plan. | Educate everyone working with the student about PWS, the management plan including food restrictions, food-related activities, behavior modification, and physical activity. | Peter will cooperate with the food and behavior management plan in the school setting: will not take food from other students; will not trade food with other students. |
| It is difficult for the student to understand PWS and the boundaries that need to be followed during the school day. | Knowledge deficient related to mental retardation (mild). | Peter will increase knowledge of PWS. | Assist the student to learn and understand what PWS is and the limits or boundaries that are needed to control food intake boundaries. | Peter will describe what PWS is at appropriate development level. |

# References

Barrett, J. (1999). Prader-Willi syndrome. *Gale encyclopedia of medicine* (pp. 2333–2337). Retrieved August 18, 2003, from the Infotrac database (item No. A54823541).

Goldberg, C. L., Garrett, C. L. , Van Riper, C., & Warzak, W. J. (2002). Coping with Prader-Willi syndrome. *Journal of the American Dietetic Association, 102*(4), 537–543. Retrieved August 18, 2003, from the Infotrac database (item No. A85005762).

NANDA International. (2003). *Nursing diagnoses: Definitions & classification.2003-2004.* Philadelphia: Author.

Prader-Willi syndrome online, (1994). Prader-Willi syndrome. Retrieved October 29, 2003, from the PEDBASE database: http://www.icondata.com/health/pedbase/files/PRADER-W.HTM

# Bibliography

Psychiatric and behavioral problems found in youth with Prader-Willi syndrome. (2002). *The Brown University Child and Adolescent Behavior Letter, 18*(7). Retrieved August 18, 2003, from the Infotrac database (item No. A89807689): http://web2.infotrac.galegroup

Hanchett, J., & Greenswag, L. Health care guidelines for individuals with Prader-Willi syndrome. Retrieved October 25, 3003, from http://pwsusa.org/postion/HCGuide/HCG_doc.htm [MOLLY: I'm not sure what this is, but I couldn't retrieve it]

Whaley, L. F., & Wong D. L. (1999). *Nursing care of infants and children.* St. Louis, Mo: Mosby.

Weber, R. (1993). Physical education for children with Prader-Willi syndrome. *Palaestra, 9*(3), 41–47. Retrieved October 25, 2003, from the Infotrac database

# Resources

Prader-Willi Syndrome Association
5700 Midnight Pass Road
Sarasota, FL 34242
941-312-0400
1-800-926-4797
941-312-0142 (fax)
national@pwsausa.org
www.pwsausa.org

*Chapter Sixty-one*

# Pregnancy, Adolescent

### Anne L. Hedges

## Introduction

Adolescent pregnancy and births in the United States are declining but continue to be among the highest in Western industrialized nations. About 1 million girls become pregnant every year, and almost half of these adolescents become parents. Teenagers who do not become pregnant until they have completed adolescent development and completed high school are socially and economically better prepared to become parents (Hockenberry, Wilson, Winkelstein, & Kline, 2003; National Network of Child Care, n.d.). Pregnancy places grave responsibilities in the hands of schoolchildren at a time when their formal education is midcycle or incomplete. According to the Council of Chief State School Officers (2003), adolescents who engage in sexual activity that results in pregnancy are more likely to perform poorly in the school setting. Only about 3 in 10 adolescent mothers ever complete high school (National Network of Child Care). Single parenthood leads to an increase in poverty, reliance on the welfare system, and limited academic achievement. The negative aspects of adolescent childbearing place the heaviest burden, socially and financially, on the mother. The mother and child are likely to live in poverty for most of the child's formative years (Sawhill, 2000). Menschke and Bartholomae (1998) found that the children of unmarried adolescent mothers tend to have lower cognitive ability and academic achievement, as well as social behavior problems.

Adolescent pregnancy continues to be a cause for concern for families, policy makers, and social service providers. Adolescents who give birth tend to be more successful if they have extended families that offer a positive level of caring and support (Meschke & Bartholomae, 1998). With the early coordination of social services, access to welfare benefits such as Aid to Families with Dependent Children; Medicaid; Special Supplemental Nutrition Program for Women, Infants and Children (WIC Program); and other support programs, adolescents are better able to manage the burdens of adolescent pregnancy (USDA Food and Nutrition Services, 2004). Educators, guidance counselors, and healthcare providers have an opportunity to influence adolescents to remain in school while pregnant, and then return to school after delivery. School nurses have a pivotal role in supporting the pregnant student during the pregnancy and by encour-aging the student upon return to school. Maternal physiology and adolescent development knowledge is basic to effective nurse interventions.

## Pathophysiology

Many normal changes occur during pregnancy. Some signs or symptoms seen in pregnancy can also be indicators of disease in the nonpregnant female. Therefore, having a suspected pregnancy confirmed early is important in order to provide proper care. Pregnancy has a systemic effect on the female anatomy. Changes occur in the adolescent at a time when the body is still growing and developing, which sometimes leads to adverse effects on the mother and infant.

Pregnancy carries significant physical and psychosocial risks for teens; the younger the teen, the more likely she is to have physical complications during pregnancy. These include fetopelvic incompatibility, premature and prolonged labor, toxemia associated with hypertension, hemorrhage, spontaneous abortion, and even death (Hockenberry et al., 2003; Meschke & Bartholomae, 1998). Infant mortality rates for adolescent pregnancies are markedly higher than those among women in their 20s.

### Physiologic Changes and Effects

While acknowledging that the mother and baby need to be assessed and treated as a whole, it is helpful to consider physiologic changes that occur in the mother's body.

### Gastrointestinal

- Nausea and vomiting, especially during the first trimester, is not unusual, and may or may not require medical intervention; nausea and vomiting beyond the middle of the second trimester requires medical evaluation.
- Gastric volume and the digestive process may be adversely affected as the uterus enlarges to accommodate the baby.

### Respiratory

- Anatomic and functional changes occur during pregnancy; for example, the enlargement of the uterus changes the subcostal angle, with an increase in the circumference and diameter of the chest.
- Mild dyspnea or some hyperventilation and a rela-

tive decrease in exercise tolerance may occur as a result of altered pulmonary functions.

- Activities may cause shortness of breath as pregnancy progresses.

### Cardiovascular
- Pregnancy results in a 40% increase in cardiac output.
- Oxygenation increases to provide improved flow of nutrition to the fetus (Beckmann et al., 2002).

### Hypertensive
- Pregnancy-induced hypertension develops in 5% to 10% of pregnancies beyond the first trimester. Substantial risks may occur in the mother and fetus despite prenatal care.
- The cause of hypertension unique to pregnancy is unknown; hypertension is associated with preeclampsia and eclampsia.
- Persistent headaches or visual disturbances warrant referral for care.

### Hematologic
- Plasma volume increases around the sixth week of pregnancy.
- Physiologic anemia develops in pregnancy as a result of a 15% dilution in blood volume due to an increase in red cell mass volume versus a higher increase in plasma volume (Beckmann et al., 2002).

### Urinary Tract
- Urinary tract changes occur as a result of a decrease in bladder tone, increasing the likelihood of infection or urinary frequency.
- Glucose excretion is common; therefore, urine glucose measurements in diabetic patients are a poor reflection of glucose levels.
- Hypertension or a preeclamptic condition promotes development of proteinurea.

### Skin
- Skin changes are due to an increase in levels of estrogen during pregnancy. This can result in vascular spiders or palmar erythema. Striae gravidarium are either purple or pink lines that initially appear on the breasts, lower abdomen, and thighs. These are the result of stretching skin and fade to become white or silvery in color.
- Hyperpigmentation is due to elevated estrogen and melanocyte-stimulating hormone levels.
- Hair growth may be affected, with hair loss occurring 2 to 4 months after pregnancy (Beckmann et al., 2002).

### Breasts
- Breast size increases as the breasts grow to support lactation.
- Breast-feeding provides health, nutritional, and economical benefits to the mother and baby.

### Musculoskeletal
- These changes are due to the secretion of relaxin and progesterone, resulting in some laxity of the ligaments.
- Gait may become unsteady because of changes in the center of gravity.
- Backache may occur because of compensatory lordosis of the spine.
- Elevated parathyroid hormone levels keep the skeleton maintained, reducing the risk of bone density loss (Beckmann et al., 2002).

### Ophthalmic
- Blurred vision may occur as a result of the lens becoming edematous; this usually returns to normal after delivery.
- Abnormal changes in vision, such as sensitivity to light or repeated headaches, could be related to eclampsia or preeclampsia (Beckmann et al., 2002).

### Reproductive Tract and Abdominal Wall
- Vascularity increases, resulting in vulvae varicosities. Vaginal secretions also increase, resulting in a thick vaginal discharge with the cervix forming a mucous plug as a barrier against infection.
- Uterine weight and volume increase, causing pressure on the bladder and abdominal wall (Beckmann et al., 2002).

### Endocrinologic
- Insulin resistance may occur on account of hormonal changes throughout the pregnancy.

### Drug Use
Drugs, legal and illegal, affect the mother and fetus. The pregnant teen should not take any illegal drugs or alcohol during the pregnancy. She should take only medications prescribed or recommended by a healthcare provider who is aware of her pregnancy.

Caffeine consumption should be limited during pregnancy because of the stimulant effects.

Nicotine should be totally avoided during pregnancy. It interferes with the supply of oxygen to the fetus. It is implicated in retarded fetal growth (weight, length, chest and head circumference), lower Apgar scores at birth, and preterm labor. Nicotine is passed through breast milk. There are detrimental effects of secondhand smoke (Hockenberry et al., 2003).

Safe levels of alcohol intake have not been established at any stage during pregnancy. Students who are pregnant should not drink alcoholic beverages at all. Alcohol is harmful to the baby by increasing the risk of mental retardation, learning disabilities, and major birth defects, such as fetal alcohol syndrome (Beckman, 2002).

Marijuana use interferes with the supply of oxygen to the fetus. Cocaine use reduces the appetite, which can lead to impaired fetal growth and cardiac function and suppression of fetal immune system. Cocaine also increases the risk of spontaneous abortion or premature rupture of the membranes (Beckmann et al., 2002; Hockenberry et al., 2003). Narcotic use is associated with low birth weight, hyperactivity, and irritability in infants (Hockenberry et al.).

### Nutritional Needs

As in the case of any pregnancy, there is need for nutritional intake to meet the growth needs of the mother and the unborn baby. Teen girls who are pregnant have food preferences, eating habits, and lifestyle behaviors similar to those of teen girls who are not pregnant. Many may choose foods that are high in fat and low in essential nutrients, which results in lower intake of calcium, iron, zinc, folic acid, and vitamins A, B₆, and C, all of which are vital to fetal development.

### Infectious Agents and Environmental Factors

Screening and monitoring should be done during prenatal care for toxoplasmois, hepatitis, rubella, cytomegalovirus, herpes simplex virus, bacterial infections, and HIV/AIDS (Hockenberry et al., 2003).

## Management

"In most cases, with early care, teenage pregnancy is no longer considered to be biologically disadvantageous to the child. However, teenage parenting is still regarded as socially, educationally, psychologically, and economically disadvantageous to both the mother and the child" (Hockenberry et al., 2003, p. 805).

The school adolescent pregnancy management program may include elements of prevention education to assist teens in avoiding unplanned pregnancy, early referral and continuing care for the student who is pregnant while supporting her as a student, and the care of the mother and child when the mother returns to school. This chapter focuses on the adolescent who is pregnant through postpartum planning.

Community norms and school district policy may determine to some extent the questions the nurse may ask, as well as counseling information the nurse can provide. It is imperative that the school nurse understands laws and policies related to sexual abuse, sex education, and confidentiality issues regarding healthcare and counseling of a minor.

The well-being of the pregnant and parenting students influences the physical cognitive behavioral and emotional status of their children. Students who are pregnant are at risk for dropping out of school. School nurses should assist students in providing solutions to meet their health and social needs through referral to adolescent-friendly healthcare and teen parenting programs. Many school districts offer school-based programs that support parenting teens. Participation in these programs helps facilitate learning, keeping the student in school while providing childcare for the student. Through collaboration with the student, family, school staff, and medical provider, the school nurse can have a significant role in the health and well-being of the student (Hechinger, 1992). In addition to nursing care, the role of the school nurse includes connecting students with school and community resources to assist with the developmental, physical, social, emotional, and economic needs of the student (National Association of School Nurses [NASN], 2004).

Once pregnancy has been established, the school nurse's role is to focus on:

- identifying students in the school setting who are pregnant and make early referrals for prenatal care
- developing a supportive, trusting, and nonjudgmental relationship with the student to maximize health outcomes
- using each assessment opportunity or intervention as a vehicle to provide health education and information
- providing support and interventions as the pregnancy progresses with modifications for the well-being of the student
- encouraging the student to maintain good physical and mental health during pregnancy
- collaborating with the healthcare provider to monitor the student's healthcare needs for the pregnancy and any other health issues the student may have (Hockenberry et al., 2003; NASN, 2004).

More specific management strategies, which address the physical and emotional issues that occur as a result of the pregnancy, as described in the pathophysiology section of this chapter, might include the following:

- Gastrointestinal issues managed with nutritional counseling; for example:
  - Promote good dietary habits, such as frequent small meals, with avoidance of foods that exacerbate the nausea.
  - Assist the student in choosing a healthy and balanced diet (USDA, 2004).
  - Encourage the student to take vitamins and minerals as prescribed by the healthcare provider.
  - Stress the importance of avoiding the use of illegal and illicit drugs and alcohol, and excessive amounts of caffeine and drugs that have not been approved by the healthcare provider (Beckmann et al., 2002).
- Respiratory issues managed by monitoring existing conditions, such as asthma. The pregnant student with asthma should be evaluated by her asthma specialist and monitored throughout the pregnancy. The student with severe asthma should maintain her prepregnancy medical regimen as directed by her physician (Beckmann et al., 2002). The school nurse should provide ongoing assessment for additional respiratory concerns that may develop during pregnancy. Severe or unresolving respiratory symptoms and infections should be referred immediately for proper care. Smoking cessation should be encouraged to reduce the risks to the infant (Beckmann et al.).
- Cardiovascular issues managed by careful monitoring of any preexisting cardiac diseases and ongoing assessment of changes that are occurring during the pregnancy. Collaborating with the student's health-

care provider allows the student to stay in school. For example, the school nurse can monitor blood pressure and report results to the clinic. The student may not miss any or only a few minutes of class, whereas if she went to the doctor's office, she may miss considerable school time.

- Musculoskeletal issues managed by observation and counseling. As the pregnancy continues, the student may benefit from discussion of body mechanics and practice of approved exercises.

The nurse should monitor the student's general mental well being by

- observing the student for signs of physical, emotional, or medical abuse
- assessing the student for concerns related to cultural folklore, rituals, or behaviors associated with pregnancy
- assessing the student for feelings of isolation or alienation from family or peers.

If the student is going to keep and parent the baby, the nurse should refer the student and other significant person(s) (her birthing coach, parents, father of the baby) to birthing and parenting classes. Stress the benefits of breast-feeding. Research has shown that there is no better food than breast milk for a baby's first year of life. Breast-feeding provides many health, nutritional, economic, and emotional benefits to mother and baby (USDA Food and Nutrition Services, 2004). Within the school, the nurse should provide a therapeutic environment for talking, listening, and addressing concerns of the student and for reinforcing the teachings provided by her healthcare provider, such as preparation for labor, delivery, and breast-feeding.

The school nurse should be alert to those signs and symptoms that warrant an immediate referral, such as persistent headaches, blurred vision, and changes in elevated blood pressure, protein urea (if checking), and any severe pain or bleeding.

## Individualized Healthcare Plan

### Assessment
*History*
- Reason for visit to the health room today
- Experiencing any pain; if so, describe
- Date of last menstrual period; describe normal menstrual cycle
- Sexual activity, method of contraception, condom use
- Sexually transmitted diseases
- Date of last sexual encounter, possibility of pregnancy
- Signs to indicate pregnancy, such as nausea or vomiting, breast tenderness, tiredness, dietary changes
- Pregnancy tests results
- Feelings related to being pregnant
- Student's living arrangements
- Relationship with sexual partner/father of the baby, father supportive
- Feelings of happiness in school and at home
- Emotional, physical, or sexual-abuse history
- Forced to have sex
- Parents/family/guardian knowledge of pregnancy
- Use of chemical before or at the time of becoming pregnant

*Current Status and Management*
- Confirmation of pregnancy
- Health insurance—to determine proper referral
- Healthcare provider referral needed
- Medications—prescription and nonprescription
- Nutritional assessment
- Date of prenatal appointment with doctor
- Developmental, social, emotional, and economic concerns
- Health status, including medical complexities
- Establish extent of student's support system with family and peers
- Use of chemicals such as tobacco, alcohol, marijuana, other
- Need for nurse to facilitate meeting of student with her parent/guardian
- Student/parent consent for nurse to collaborate with healthcare provider

*Self-care*
- Knowledge of pregnancy, including related medical complexities
- Ability to verbalize importance of self-care and prenatal care
- Ability to address social, emotional, physical care of self
- Motivation to seek health and social services
- Ability to monitor and measure dietary intake maintaining well-balanced diet
- Motivation to exercise, participate in prenatal programs to prepare for delivery of infant
- Motivate to refrain from smoking, alcohol, or drug use

*Psychosocial Status*
- Developmental maturity, decision-making skills
- Coping strategies related to pregnancy
- Current psychosocial status, challenges/risks
- Perception of family support
- Reaction to family support
- Adequacy of social support, relationship with peers
- Family stability relative to student's pregnancy
- Ability to care for the infant
- Barriers to balancing time and energy between self, infant, and partner/family

*Academic Issues*
- Attendance patterns
- Academic standing
- Interested in a parenting program that includes academics at another school location
- Accommodations needed to maintain good attendance and complete academic requirements—physical education class, lunchtime, food selection, rest time, etc.
- Need for 504 plan

## Nursing Diagnoses (N.D.) (NANDA, 2003)

**N.D. 1** Imbalanced nutrition: less than body requirements (NANDA 00002) related to:
- nausea and/or vomiting resulting in deficit fluid volume
- increased nutritional needs during pregnancy
- knowledge deficiency related to nutritional and fluid volume needs

**N.D. 2** Ineffective health maintenance (NANDA 00099) related to:
- lack of adaptive behaviors to internal environmental change: pregnancy
- lack of health-seeking behaviors
- lack of material/financial resources
- lack of communication skills
- lack of ability to make deliberate and thoughtful judgment associated with immaturity/adolescence
- psychosocial barriers
- avoidance of prenatal visits to healthcare provider
- lack of consistent compliance with therapeutic care regimen prescribed by healthcare provider

**N.D. 3** Activity intolerance (NANDA 00092) related to:
- enlargement of the uterus and increased abdominal pressure
- imbalance between oxygen supply/demand caused by cardiovascular changes associated with pregnancy, needing accommodation in school scheduling
- exertion discomfort or dyspnea
- verbal report of fatigue or weakness
- altered self-confidence associated with physical changes of pregnancy

**N.D. 4** Deficient knowledge (NANDA 00126) related to:
- lack of maturity to accept pregnancy and to understand the process
- physiologic and psychologic changes in female body during pregnancy
- fetal growth and development
- labor and delivery process

- stress, anxiety, and fear
- inability to verbalize concerns/problems
- exaggerated behaviors (agitated, hysterical) related to pregnancy

**N.D. 5** Impaired adjustment (NANDA 00070) related to:
- low state of optimism
- intense emotional state
- negative attitudes toward health behavior/status
- multiple stressors associated with _____
- absence of family and/or social support
- health status change requiring change in lifestyle
- lack of motivation to change behaviors

**N.D. 6** Ineffective coping (NANDA 00069) related to:
- impaired adjustment to pregnancy
- inadequate social support created by characteristics of relationships
- inadequate resources available
- high decrease of threat (real or perceived)
- situational or maturational crisis
- disturbance in appraisal of threat
- fear of current circumstances

**N.D. 7** Impaired verbal communication (NANDA 00151) related to:
- developmental age associated with readiness for enhanced communication
- psychosocial barriers
- lack of information/knowledge
- stress
- alteration in self-esteem or self-concept
- diagnosed communication disorder (speech/language deficit)

**N.D. 8** Risk for impaired parenting (NANDA 00057) related to:
- normal maturation process of mother/father
- developmental age of baby's parent(s)
- anxiety associated with the parent role
- inability to meet personal needs
- physical barriers
- lack of knowledge
- sleep deprivation
- perception of parenting role
- impact academics have on parenting role
- child-care issues
- attachment and conflicts associated with perceived peer expectations in academic setting, family dynamics, or relationship with baby's father
- lack of resources

**N.D. 9** Compromised family coping (NANDA 00074)
- significant person (foster mother) displays protective behavior disproportionate to student's ability for autonomy
- significant person attempts assistive or supportive behaviors with unsatisfactory results due to a lack of knowledge base
- temporary family disorganization and role changes due to student's inability to recognize and appreciate significant people's support of daily activities

**N.D. 10** Impaired social interaction (NANDA 00052) related to:
- pregnancy during adolescence
- dysfunctional daily routine
- self-concept disturbance
- limited physical mobility
- sociocultural dissonance associated with _____.
- communication barriers
- lack of anger control associated with anger, frustration, denial

**N.D. 11** Anxiety (NANDA 00146) related to:
- situational/maturational crises: adjustment to pregnancy
- unmet needs

- potential loss of baby: planned termination, spontaneous abortion, stillbirth
- potential for infant adoption
- distress related to family relationship

N.D. 12 Sexual dysfunction (NANDA 00059) related to:
- normal adolescent development
- lack of knowledge related to sexuality issues and sexual function
- seeking confirmation of desirability related to vulnerability and ineffectual or absent role models
- sociocultural dissonance associated with sexual activity
- values conflict
- psychosocial abuse (harmful relationships)
- physical abuse

N.D. 13 Readiness for enhanced family processes (NANDA 00159) related to:
- risk for impaired parenting
- socially expected behavior patterns related to family interrelationships
- expressed desire for self and family to adapt to change in positive ways

N.D.14 Readiness for enhanced parenting (NANDA 00164) related to:
- enrolled in parenting classes offered in school or community
- student expresses a willingness to enhance parenting
- providing an environment for child that is sufficient to nurture growth and development

## Goals

The student will acquire and apply knowledge in making decisions related to pregnancy for self and baby. (N.D. 2, 4–9, 11, 13, 14)

The student will engage in a healthy lifestyle regarding food/drink, exercise, rest, and personal safety. (N.D. 1–4, 8, 12, 14)

The student will describe normal physical and psychological changes in female body during pregnancy. (N.D. 1, 3, 4, 7)

The student will describe fetal growth and development. (N.D. 4, 7, 8, 14)

The student will describe labor and delivery process. (N.D. 4, 5, 11)

The student will prepare physically and psychologically for childbirth. (N.D. 1, 2, 4, 6, 7, 9, 11)

The student will openly communicate feelings, fears, anxieties, and need for knowledge associated with pregnancy. (N.D. 4–12)

The student will utilize positive support of family, peers, and school community. (N.D. 3, 5–10, 12, 13, 14)

The student will foster positive relationship development with family, peers, and other caring adults. (N.D. 5–11, 14)

The student will seek counsel and guidance in making and honoring decisions to: (N.D. 4–8, 10–12)
- terminate the pregnancy
- offer the baby for adoption
- keep the baby
- continue education

The student will seek counsel and guidance to deal with feelings of loss and separation, value conflict, in the event of psychosocial or physical abuse. (N.D. 5, 6, 8, 9, 11, 12,)

The student will regularly attend school during and after pregnancy. (N.D. 3–9, 13, 14)

## Nursing Interventions

Facilitate decision-making process regarding pregnancy outcomes. (N.D. 4–7, 9, 11–13)
- Encourage the student to involve support system during decision making.
- Discuss the student's reaction to her pregnancy (and that of the father of the baby).
- Discuss families' reaction to pregnancy.
- Offer to meet with the student when she tells her parents.
- Role-play with the student how disclosure of pregnancy could occur.
- Provide referral information to allow the student and significant other to explore options about the outcome of the pregnancy, including termination, adoption, or keeping the infant.
- Provide open communication to foster discussion of all alternatives.

If the student elects to terminate the pregnancy or has a spontaneous abortion:
- Manage the physical and psychological needs of the student undergoing a spontaneous or elective termination. (N.D. 4–7, 9, 11, 12)

- Clarify information about contraceptive use. (N.D. 4, 12)
- Determine if more in-depth crisis intervention is needed. (N.D. 5, 6, 7, 9, 10, 11)

If the student elects to deliver the baby and then offer it for adoption: (N.D. 4–7, 10)
- Provide support for grieving, loss, and separation.
- Observe the student for signs of loss and grief, such as anxiety, depression, or crying.
- Refer for counseling and guidance for assistance with the grieving process.
- Assist her in locating an adoption agency and in establishing a relationship with the agency's nurse or social worker.

If the student chooses termination or adoption, focus attention on long-term outcomes to project the student into the future. (N.D. 4, 5, 12, 13)

Determine the student's decision regarding the pregnancy.
- Monitor for possibility that she may change her mind, have serious misgivings about her decision to keep the infant, give the baby for adoption, or terminate the pregnancy. (N.D. 5, 6, 7, 11)
- Encourage her to talk with trusted adult (parents/family, school nurse, school counselor, teacher), the father of the infant, and/or a religious advisor about these misgivings. (N.D. 5, 6, 7, 11)

If student plans to deliver baby:
- Meet with family to discuss school plan during pregnancy. (N.D. 2–11)
  – Demonstrate interest in student's academic and physical well-being.
  – Advocate for student in a mother-baby learning environment.
  – Stress the importance of academics on student's future.
  – Assist the student in developing a plan of action that is realistic and that is attainable for the student.
- Assist the student to minimize barriers to healthcare, such as financial hardship or accessibility, which prevent the student from obtaining primary healthcare. (N.D. 2)

Collaborate with healthcare provider (N.D. 1–4 )
- Provide nursing assessment as requested by healthcare provider and requested by student.
- Refer to primary healthcare provider for assessment: vomiting, elevated blood pressure, edema, bleeding.

Encourage self-management of prescribed therapeutic regimen related to prenatal care. (N.D. 1, 2, 4- 6, 11)
- Keeping prenatal appointments
- Compliance with prescribed and recommended over-the-counter medication regimen, avoiding all other drugs and alcohol
- Follow recommended schedule for rest, exercise, and nutritional plan

Provide support through referral to school district resources, such as guidance/behavioral health counselor to maintain/improve academic standing and social growth. (N.D. 3, 5- 7, 10, 11)

Monitor student's academic progress and attendance patterns related to pregnancy. (N.D. 2- 4, 8, 9, 11)

Facilitate accommodations for student during school day, such as bathroom breaks, visits to school nurse or guidance counselor, rest periods, health room visits, shortened day, physical education/team sports, availability of food and water. (N.D. 2, 3, 6, 11)

Provide/reinforce education in areas of _____.
- Negative effects of smoking, alcohol, and drugs on the unborn fetus. (N.D. 2, 4)
- Assist the student in understanding the physiologic and psychologic changes that will occur throughout the pregnancy. (N.D. 3, 4)
- Prenatal healthcare. (N.D. 2, 4)
- Labor and delivery. (N.D. 2, 4)
- Fetal development. (N.D.4, 8, 14)
- Importance of nutrition to the fetus during pregnancy. (N.D. 1, 2, 14)
- Assist the student to develop a meal plan and food budget, and encourage her to practice proper nutrition. (N.D. 1, 2, 4)
- Teach the family and father (if present) about the physical and psychological changes that occur during pregnancy. (N.D. 3, 4, 13, 14)
- Teach the student concepts of personal hygiene, exercise, rest, nutrition, and breast care. (N.D. 1-4, 14)

Provide developmentally appropriate cooperative learning situations where the student can assess the opportunities and problems and make decisions based on factual information. (N.D. 14)

Refer to health, social service, and educational resource agencies and support system referrals to assist the student to attain her goal, such as WIC Program, daycare center, women's center, counseling service, and religious group. (N.D. 2, 8, 13, 14)

Facilitation of the development of the parent-infant relationship. (N.D. 4, 8, 9, 11, 14)

Refer to agencies that provide peer-group sessions for social support, mutual problem solving, and affirmation of program goals. (N.D. 5, 6, 10)

Direct the student to classes, demonstrations, and literature that increase the student's knowledge and choices for care. (N.D. 8, 14)

Discuss parenting program that includes academics, parenting classes, and childcare. (N.D. 4, 8, 10, 14)

Encourage student to return to school postpartum. (N.D. 8, 10, 14)

Discuss alternative educational plans/placement as the need arises in order to assist the student to become self-sufficient and continue in school. (N.D. 3, 5, 9, 10)

Instruct/reinforce teaching the student in the nutrients and the calories needed in the daily diet to maintain a healthy mother and fetus: determine the food likes and intake of the student. (N.D. 1, 4)

Assess the student for mood changes and level of self-esteem. (N.D, 6, 7, 10)

Encourage the student to express her concerns and needs. (N.D. 4, 5, 7-11)

Assist the student in choosing and obtaining childcare prior to delivery. (N.D. 4, 13, 14)

Encourage student to stay in school and graduate from high school. (N.D. 5, 6, 14)

Determine student's understanding of her behavior relative to male students. (N.D. 4, 10, 12)

Encourage student to seek counseling to assist in resolution of behavior. (N.D. 10, 12)

Encourage student to participate in appropriate school and community activities. (N.D. 3, 5, 6, 10)

Reinforce counseling strategies on how to curb her outbursts of anger, coach student to use forms of coping that impede adaptive behavior. (N.D. 6, 7, 10)

Encourage student to attend birthing classes with whoever plans to be with her during labor and delivery. (N.D. 4, 8, 11)

Stress the importance of using birth control to avoid unplanned pregnancy while breast-feeding. (N.D. 12)

## Expected Student Outcomes

The student will:
- Demonstrate application of knowledge in decision making related to pregnancy for self and baby. (N.D. 2, 4–9, 11, 13, 14)
- Increase her knowledge regarding pregnancy evidenced by ability to (N.D. 4)
  - Describe physiologic and psychological changes that are occurring in her body during each of the three trimesters.
  - Describe fetal development from conception to birth.
  - Describe stages and process of labor and delivery.
- Ask for clarification or reinforcement to explanation of teaching if she doesn't understand or forgets. (N.D. 4).
- Attend birthing classes (with whomever will be with her during labor). (N.D. 4)
- Participate in school or community social activity group(s). (N.D. 5, 9, 10)
- Utilize community resources as an integral part of her support network. (N.D.1, 2, 4, 6, 8, 9, 14)
- Name at least two peer-age friends with whom she interacts who are supportive of her plan to keep the baby and continue in school. (N.D. 5, 9, 10)
- Engage in healthy lifestyle practices to benefit self and baby—nutritional plan, exercise, rest, and personal safety behaviors—and keep prenatal appointments. (N.D.1–4, 8, 12, 14)
- Tolerate changes in activity patterns as pregnancy progresses toward term, allowing her to attend classes throughout the school day with accommodations as needed. (N.D. 3, 4, 10, 11)
- Understand the roles and expectations of a new mother regarding self-care and the care of her newborn baby. (N.D. 4-6, 8, 9, 14)
- Provide a safe and nurturing environment for the child. (N.D. 4, 14)
  - Describe the physical and psychological needs of a newborn. (N.D. 4, 14)
  - Recognize and identify age-appropriate infant behaviors. (N.D. 4, 14)
  - Be aware of strengths and weakness, utilizing community resources to assist with caring for newborn. (N.D. 4, 8, 14)

If keeping the baby:
- Form a bonding relationship with infant. (N.D. 5)

If adoption or termination of pregnancy occurs:
- Is able to verbalize her loss. (N.D. 5, 6, 9, 11)
- Believes that the decision she made was the best decision for her at this time; gradually resumes her role as student and teenager. (N.D. 6)
- Seeks and continues counseling as needed during pregnancy and in postpartum period for guidance in decision-making process. (N.D. 2, 4-6, 9, 11)
- Fosters positive relationships with family, peers, and other caring adults. (N.D 4-6, 9, 11)
- Prevents future unintended pregnancies. (N.D 4, 12)

# Case Study

Reola is an 18-year-old student in good physical health with normal physical growth and development. However, emotionally she is quite fragile, demonstrating deviations from the norms of her age group. Reola has a history of hyperactivity treated with psychostimulants when she was younger. Reola is constantly in motion, exhibiting frequent outbursts of temper and disruptive behavior. Her temper tantrums enhance a pronounced speech deficit (stuttering).

Reola lives with her biological aunt as a foster child. The Department of Children and Families placed her with her aunt when she was 5 years old following neglect and abandonment by her mother. Her father has never been part of her life. The home is shared with her aunt, her aunt's boyfriend, and three other foster children.

Reola is a high school senior. She is pregnant and physically healthy with no significant physical complaints. Her psychological and social functioning has a negative effect on her lifestyle in the school setting. She has been diagnosed with speech, language, and emotional disabilities; she shares a classroom with 11 other students who have emotional handicaps or other medical exceptionalities. Reola constantly flirts with male students on campus, antagonizing her female counterparts. She has received counseling in the past with little effect.

Reola has good rapport with the school nurse, who has known Reola since elementary school. She seems quite receptive to advice and counseling on health matters and is very happy about her pregnancy. The father of her baby is a senior at another local high school. He is described by Reola as kind and is supportive of her and the pregnancy. His mother has committed to taking care of the baby when Reola returns to school. Her aunt is supportive but is frequently impatient with Reola. The news of the pregnancy resulted in Reola being evicted from the home and moving to the boyfriend's home for a while. Her aunt forgave her, so she is now back at home.

She appears receptive to advice but is slow to follow up with referrals to healthcare providers. Referrals to the WIC Program have been problematic. Despite interventions from the school nurse and Reola's caseworker, she still has not kept her appointments. Transportation is not a problem. Reola visits the school nurse before and following prenatal appointments.

Reola's teachers report that she has been late to class several times during the past 2 weeks. Reola says it is hard for her to get through the crowded hall because she is getting bigger. She says she bumps into people and moves slower because she gets "winded" if she tries to keep up with crowd. No edema of the feet is noted. She seems to be comfortable around other students that she knows, but says she doesn't like being in the hallways with so many students she doesn't know looking at her "big belly."

She has many questions regarding the birthing process. Reola qualifies for Medicaid and has chosen to receive services at the health department. She reports that she takes vitamins and iron and does not take any harmful substances. The school nurse monitors Reola on a regular basis in conjunction with the midwife appointments at the health department.

One of Reola's concerns was the child birthing process. She shows little understanding of anatomy and physiology or what to expect from the labor and delivery process. The school nurse also used textbook illustrations to explain in simple terms about the process of birthing a baby. The nurse refers her to the clinic for reinforcement of the birthing information and for additional information regarding use of pain medication during labor and delivery. The nurse encouraged Reola to place her trust in the labor and delivery staff and physician because they were experts in pregnancy and childbirth. The school nurse also discussed a program named Operation Baby Safe, which is a program for mothers who find it hard to care for their baby or don't want their baby. In that event, the mother can leave the baby at a hospital, fire house, or police department.

It is difficult to predict how Reola will cope with the care of her infant. She has assisted in the care of infants within the family, so she feels very comfortable with children. Academically, Reola requires one more semester of high school in the fall. The hope is that she will return to school for the final semester. Failing that, she would need to take the general educational development (GED) examination to receive her high school diploma. Obtaining the diploma will increase her chances of employment in the future. The baby is due in June, and Reola is confident that she will return to school for two classes a day in the fall.

The nurse recognizes there are many issues that will require assistance and guidance. Based on the information available, the nurse prioritizes the following issues to be addressed in a healthcare plan for the remainder of this school year:

Activity intolerance related to the pregnancy in the school setting
Impaired social interaction with adults and peers
Deficient knowledge regarding pregnancy, labor, delivery, and child care
Risk for impaired parenting when the baby arrives

# Adolescent Pregnancy

| Assessment Data | Nursing Diagnosis | Goals | Nursing Interventions | Expected Outcomes |
|---|---|---|---|---|
| Reola has been late getting from one class to another. She says it is hard for her to get through the crowded hall because she is getting bigger. She says she moves slower because she gets "winded" if she tried to keep up with the crowd. No edema of the feet is noted. Reola seems to have a more difficult time moving about as the pregnancy progresses to term.<br><br>Reola seems to be comfortable around other students that she knows, but says she doesn't like being in the hallways with so many students she doesn't know looking at her 'big belly.' | Activity intolerance related to enlargement of uterus, exertion discomfort or dyspnea, and altered self-confidence associated with physical changes of pregnancy. | Reola will engage in a healthy lifestyle regarding exercise and rest to address activity-intolerance issues. | Monitor student's academic progress and attendance patterns and facilitate accommodations for Reola during the school day:<br>• Provide a pass allowing student to leave class 2 minutes early in order to arrive at the next class safely and on time without feelings of insecurity.<br>• Encourage slow walking as tolerated at other times of the day with a friend or family member.<br>• Continually monitor for additional signs of activity intolerance and address with appropriate interventions, such as resting with feet elevated when sitting.<br><br>Discuss needed accommodations with teachers. | Reola will tolerate changes in activity patterns as pregnancy progresses toward term, allowing her to attend classes throughout the school day. |
| Reola doesn't have good relationship with some peers, and doesn't like being around crowds of students she doesn't know. She sometimes has hyperactive tendencies interspersed with uncontrollable emotional outbursts related to educational difficulties, speech impairment and social adversities. | Impaired social interaction related to self-concept disturbance, limited physical mobility, communication barriers, and lack of anger control. | Reola will foster positive relationship development with peers and caring adults in the school and community. | Provide support through referral to school district's resources/guidance counselor to improve social growth.<br><br>Encourage Reola to participate in appropriate school and community activities<br>• Continue the ones she participated in prior to pregnancy if physically appropriate. | Reola will participate in at least one school or community social activity group.<br><br>Reola will name at least two peer-age friends with whom she interacts who are supportive of her plan to keep the baby and continue in school. |

| Assessment Data | Nursing Diagnosis | Goals | Nursing Interventions | Expected Outcomes |
|---|---|---|---|---|
| | | | • Choose new ones as physical condition allows.<br><br>Refer to agencies that provide peer-group session for social support and mutual problem solving.<br>• Encourage Reola to strengthen current friendships and develop new ones that can support her during and after her pregnancy.<br><br>Discuss alternative educational plans/placements that include academics, parenting classes, and childcare to assist Reola to be more self-sufficient. | |
| Reola lacks knowledge about physiologic and psychological changes that occur to the mother during pregnancy, fetal development, and the process of labor and delivery. | Deficient knowledge related to lack of maturity to understand pregnancy process, anxiety, and fear of the unknown, and inability to verbalize concerns. | The student will describe<br>• normal physical and psychological changes in the female body during pregnancy<br>• fetal growth and development<br>• labor and delivery process<br>The student will prepare physically and psychologically for childbirth.<br><br>Reola will openly communicate feelings, fears, anxieties, and need for knowledge associated with pregnancy. | Asses the student for mood changes and level of self-esteem.<br><br>Provide/reinforce education in areas of physiologic and psychological changes that will occur throughout the pregnancy, prenatal healthcare, fetal development, and labor and delivery.<br><br>Encourage Reola to attend birthing classes with whoever plans to be with her during labor and delivery. | Reola will describe physiologic and psychological changes that are occurring in her body during each of the 3 trimesters.<br><br>Reola will describe fetal development from conception to birth.<br><br>Reola will describe stages and process of labor and delivery.<br><br>Reola will ask for clarification or reinforcement or explanation of teaching if she doesn't understand or forgets. |

| Assessment Data | Nursing Diagnosis | Goals | Nursing Interventions | Expected Outcomes |
|---|---|---|---|---|
| | | | Encourage Reola to express her needs and concerns about pregnancy, fetal development, and the birthing process.<br><br>Facilitate the development of the parent-infant relationship | Reola will attend birthing classes (with aunt and father of the baby). |
| Reola's aunt asked her to leave the house upon learning of pregnancy. Reola is back with her aunt now. Currently, the father of the baby and Reola are in a relationship. The paternal grandmother plans to care for the baby when Reola returns to school. | Risk for impaired parenting related to developmental age of Reola, lack of knowledge, impact academics have on parenting role, attachment, and potential conflicts related to relationship with baby's father and his family. | The student will utilize positive support of family, peers, and school community. | Refer to health, social service, and educational resource agencies and support-system referrals to assist the student to attain her goal, such as WIC Program<br><br>Direct student to classes, demonstrations, and literature that increase knowledge of family dynamics<br><br>Encourage student to return to school postpartum; assist her in developing a plan addressing her needs and care for the child.<br><br>Encourage student to express her needs and concerns related to care for the child | Reola will understand the roles and expectations of a new mother regarding self-care and the care of her newborn baby.<br><br>Reola will be aware of strengths and weakness, utilizing community resources to assist with caring for newborn.<br><br>Reola will provide a safe and nurturing environment for the child. |

# References

Beckmann, C. R. B., Ling, F. W., Laube, D. W., Smith, R. P., Barzansky, B. M., & Herbert, W. N. P. (2002). *Obstetrics and gynecology* (4th ed., chapters 4 & 5). Baltimore: Lippincott, Williams & Wilkins.

Council of Chief State School Officers. (2003). Why support school-based teen pregnancy prevention? *A primer for action.* (A 4-part kit.) Washington, DC: Author. Retrieved from www.ccsso.org

Hechinger, F. M. (1992). *Babies born to children: Fateful choices: Healthy youth for the 21st century.* Carnegie Council on Adolescent Development, Carnegie Corporation of New York. New York: Hill & Wang.

Hockenberry, M. J., Wilson, D., Winkelstein, M. L., Kline, N. E. (Eds.). (2003). *Wong's nursing care of infants and children* (7th ed.). St. Louis, MO: Mosby.

Meschke, L., & Bartholomae, S. (1998). Examining adolescent pregnancy. *Human Development and Family Life Bulletin, 3*(4). Retrieved April 1, 2004, from http://www.hec.ohio-state.edu/famlife/bulletin/volume.3/bull34f.htm

NANDA International. (2003). *Nursing diagnoses: Definitions & classification 2003-2004.* Philadelphia: Author.

National Association of School Nurses. (2004). *Position Statement: The role of the school nurse in supporting adolescent parents.* Scarborough, ME: Author. Retrieved February 7, 2005, from www.nasn.org

National Network of Child Care. (n.d.). *Kids having kids. Youth & family violence prevention information update.* Washington, DC: Cooperative Extension System's NNCC. Retrieved February 14, 2005, from http://www.nncc.org/Release/kidswkids.html

Sawhill, I. V. (2000) *Welfare reform and reducing teen pregnancy.* Washington, DC: Brookings Institute. Retrieved April 1, 2004, from http://www.brook.edu/dybdocroot/views/articles/sawhill/winter2000.htm

USDA Food and Nutrition Services. (2004). *Nutrition assistance programs: Special supplemental nutrition program for women, infants and children (WIC).* Alexandria, VA: Author. Retrieved February 28, 2005, from http://www.fns.usda.gov/fns/menu/PROGRAMS.htm

# Bibliography

Hoyt, H. H., & Broom, B. L. (2002). School-based teen pregnancy prevention programs: A review of the literature. *Journal of School Nursing, 18*(1), 11–17.

Logsdon, M. C., Cross, R., Williams, B., & Simpson, T. (2004). Prediction of postpartum social support and symptoms of depression in pregnant adolescents: A pilot study. *Journal of School Nursing, 20*(1), 36–42.

National Association of School Nurses. (Adopted 2002). *Position Statement: Reproductive health education.* Scarborough, ME: Author.

National Association of School Nurses. (2004*). Issues Brief: The role of the school nurse in supporting adolescent parents.* Scarborough, ME: Author.

Perrin, K. M., & Dorman, K. A. (2003). Teen parents and academic success. *Journal of School Nursing, 19*(5), 288–293.

Spear, H. J. (2002). Reading, writing, and having babies: A nurturing alternative school program. *Journal of School Nursing, 18*(5), 293–300.

# Chapter Sixty-two

# Prenatal Alcohol and Drug Exposure

## Mariann Smith

## Introduction

Historically, society has always used herbs, plants, and other substances to relieve pain and/or alter mental perceptions. Prior to the passage of the Harrison Narcotics Act in 1914 (which made narcotics illegal), opium was a common ingredient in patent medications easily obtained without prescriptions and given to women to prevent miscarriages (Lewis, 1995). This increased the incidence of addiction in women because of the standard of practice at the time.

Today, women are still abusing drugs—before, during, and after pregnancy. According to the National Survey of Drug Use and Health (Substance Abuse and Mental Health Services Administration, 2002), 3.3% of women of childbearing age (15 to 44 years) reported using illicit drugs, 9.1% reported using alcohol with 3.1% binge drinking, and 17.3% reported smoking in the month prior to participating in this survey. Alcohol (which many in society do not consider a drug) continues to be a concern. The National Organization of Fetal Alcohol Syndrome (2003) and the American Academy of Pediatrics (AAP) (2000) identify prenatal exposure to alcohol as the leading preventable cause of birth defects, mental retardation, and neurodevelopmental disorders. Prenatal exposures to alcohol can result in fetal alcohol syndrome, alcohol-related neurodevelopmental disorder, and alcohol-related birth defects. The latter two terms are now used to replace the term *fetal alcohol effects*, which lacked specificity and absence of definitive diagnostic criteria (AAP, 2000).

Substance abuse covers all socioeconomic groups and has become a very costly burden on our social, health, and educational services. Treatment of these women continues to be a problem because many of the treatment facilities do not accept pregnant women or their children. These children are often shifted from foster family to foster family while the mother is in treatment. Grandparents and other relatives also may be asked to take over the care of these children.

One study concluded that 25% of drug-affected children have developmental delays and 40% have neurologic abnormalities that might affect their ability to socialize and function appropriately in a school setting (US General Accounting Office, 1991). It is estimated that 42% to 53% of these children will need special education services (Kansas Department of Social and Rehabilitation Services, 1990). Using the Vineland Adaptive Behavior Scales, a study of adolescents and adults who were born drug-affected found that overall adaptive functioning was only at the level of a 7-year-old (Streissguth, 1994).

## Pathophysiology

Alcohol interferes with normal fetal development, including growth retardation and brain damage. A defect in craniofacial development (abnormal features of the eyes, face, and head) may also occur. It is not the degree of alcohol intake of the mother that is related to the presence of abnormalities in the fetus. Rather, it is the amount consumed in excess of the fetal liver's ability to detoxify it (Wong et al., 2003). When the fetal liver receives more alcohol than it is able to handle, the excess is continually recirculated until it can be converted to carbon dioxide and water. Circulating alcohol has a special affinity for brain tissue.

Exposure to cocaine can result in decreased uterine blood flow, especially in the placenta (Wagner, Katikaneni, Cox, & Ryan, 1998). This can lead to uterine irritability, abruptio placenta, and premature birth. Cerebral infarcts in the infant can occur after birth (Scherer, Anyaegbunam, & Onyeije, 1998), as well as hypertonia and tremors (Scher, Richardson, & Day, 2000; Morrow et al., 2001). Often, pregnant women who are using drugs have a general lack of interest in self-care, and because of the fear of being discovered using illegal drugs, they often avoid the medical system and receive little or no prenatal care.

Maternal smoking is related to significant deficits in birth weight. Twenty-one percent to 39% of the incidence of low-birth-weight infants is attributable to maternal smoking (Slotkin, 1998; Wong, et al., 2003). Smoking also results in more miscarriages, premature births, increased perinatal mortality, and respiratory concerns. Exposure to marijuana is similar to the effects of tobacco smoking. There is also some increase in precipitate labor and meconium staining.

Heroin exposure often results in first trimester spontaneous abortions, premature delivery, intrauterine growth retardation, and meconium aspiration. Maternal and/or neonatal infections are also prevalent (sexually transmitted diseases, hepatitis, human immunodeficiency virus, cytomegalovirus, herpes, chlamydia, etc.).

Prenatal exposure to alcohol, tobacco, and illegal drugs is harmful to babies. These babies may be born prematurely and may have a low birth weight, a small head circumference, cardiac concerns, and neurologic concerns. They may have mental retardation. They are often hyperactive, irritable, and highly sensitive to sensory stimuli. They may have to remain in the hospital longer following their birth. Bonding and feeding problems are common. These problems, along with the mother's continued substance abuse, place these babies at an increased risk for physical abuse and/or neglect.

During the preschool years, drug-affected children are affectionate but also distractible. Many display poor fine-motor skills. As these children enter elementary school, they often have inadequate communication skills, are impulsive, and have difficulty with social interactions. When these same students enter adolescence, they may exhibit poor judgment, trouble with abstract reasoning, and limited problem-solving skills (**Table 1**).

## Management

Managing students exposed to prenatal substance abuse is challenging. Substance abuse does not occur in a vacuum. The child may have been exposed to a combination of drugs, often in a chaotic and violent environment. Ensuring a safe, loving environment that meets the physical and psychological needs of these children is critical. The optimal intervention would be to assist the mother to accept and successfully complete the necessary treatment to become and remain sober and drug-free. Assisting with social, financial, and medical supports to the family would be another important, and tandem, intervention. If this is not possible, out-of-home placement in foster care or in the care of a relative may be needed. In both of these cases, training in caring for the children with special needs is essential (Weiner & Morse, 1994; Wunch, Conlon, & Scheidt, 2002; Kuehne & Reilly, 2004).

A consistent, highly structured routine, as well as consistent limits on behavior, is very important at home and school. Classroom stimuli and noise need to be kept to a minimum. Pictures and other clues need to be posted throughout the classroom to provide information on how to use materials, etc. (Kuehne & Reilly, 2004).

Many of these students have cardiac, neurologic, visual, hearing, speech, and perceptual concerns. Medical management involves monitoring and treating the various symptoms in order to maximize the child's potential. Medical management for any of these problems may be lifelong.

Because of numerous health and/or developmental concerns, these students usually require special education services, including health-related services such as medication administration. The student's teachers will need to know each student's health status, activity restrictions, medication effects, and possible side effects.

The school nurse is the critical liaison between the educational and the medical community and the child's parents/guardians. Close communication with the parents/guardians, teachers, and healthcare providers is necessary so that the most appropriate health and educational programs can be developed and implemented. The school nurse is also an important member of the special education team if special education services are needed or as part of a 504 team if a 504 plan is needed.

**Table 1. Characteristics Often Observed in Students**

| Exposed to Prenatal Substance Abuse | Executive functioning (planning, sequencing) deficits |
|---|---|
| Mental retardation or learning disabilities | Expressive and receptive language difficulties |
| Growth retardation | Visual/motor difficulties |
| Microcephaly | Low tolerance for frustration |
| Hearing problems | Poor peer interactions |
| Congenital abnormalities | Hyperactivity/impulsiveness |
| Craniofacial abnormalities | Heightened response to sensory/motor stimuli |
| Developmental delays | Distractibility |
| Fine and gross motor delays | Behavioral difficulties |
| Memory difficulties | |

Adapted from "Substance Abuse: A Preventable Threat to Development," in *Children With Disabilities*, by M. J. Wunsch, C. J. Conlon, and P. C. Scheidt, 2002, Baltimore: Paul H. Brooks.

# Individualized Healthcare Plan

## Assessment
### History
- Prenatal care
- Type of prenatal substance abuse of mother
- Birth weight
- Birth trauma
- Length of baby's hospital stay
- Physical abnormalities
- Neurologic abnormalities
- Cardiac abnormalities
- Attainment of developmental milestones
- Social and Rehabilitation Services involvement (e.g., foster care)
- Concurrent diagnoses (e.g., attention deficit hyperactivity disorder [ADHD], oppositional defiant disorder [ODD], obsessive compulsive disorder)
- Any early medical/educational interventions

### Current Status and Management
- Developmental levels and abilities: physical, cognitive, social, and communication/language
- Healthcare provider(s)
- Current medications: effectiveness and/or side effects
- Current health status
- Vision and hearing status
- Sleep pattern
- Nutrition pattern
- Student's developmental level

### Self-care
- Student's ability level in independent activities of daily living
- Student's level of responsibility in complying with medication plan
- Student's willingness and interest in participating in self-care activities
- Student's decision-making skills

### Psychosocial Status
- Peer relations
- Self-esteem level
- Family support systems: extended family, support groups, respite care
- Family coping strategies and effectiveness
- Family's expectations regarding health conditions
- Family's expectations about educational conditions
- Student's perception of strengths and abilities
- Student's perception of disabilities

### Academic Issues
- Early educational interventions
- School attendance patterns
- Academic performance patterns
- Current classroom participation and performance
- Modification needed: classroom, curriculum, activity limitations and supervision, academic assistance, etc.
- School staff perceptions of student's abilities and disabilities

### Nursing Diagnoses (N.D.) (NANDA, 2003)

N.D. 1 Disturbed body image (NANDA 0018) related to:
- physical and/or neurologic anomalies
- developmental delays

N.D. 2 Risk for impaired child/parent attachment (NANDA 00058) related to:
- lack of attachment
- behavior disorders
- difficult temperament
- poor cognitive development
- unrealistic expectations regarding health and education concerns

N.D. 3 Impaired verbal communication (NANDA 00051) related to:
- developmental delays
- neurologic anomalies
- hearing concerns

N.D. 4 Risk for delayed development (NANDA 00112) related to:
- prenatal substance abuse of mother with questionable prenatal care
- physical and/or neurologic anomalies
- vision and/or hearing concerns
- mental retardation/learning disabilities

N.D. 5 Risk for injury (NANDA 00035) related to:
- developmental delay
- hyperactivity/impulsiveness/distractibility

N.D. 6 Chronic low self-esteem (NANDA 00119) related to:
- lack of success in activities at home, school, and in the community

N.D. 7 Disturbed sensory perceptions in all areas (NANDA 00122) related to:
- neurologic abnormalities from prenatal drug exposure
- hyperreaction of sensory stimuli
- irritability

N.D. 8 Impaired social interaction (NANDA 00052) related to:
- low tolerance for frustration
- dysfunctional social interaction with peers

N.D. 9 Disturbed thought processes (NANDA 00130) related to:
- developmental delays
- hyperactivity/impulsiveness/distractibility

N.D.10 Deficient knowledge (NANDA 00126) related to:
- long-term effects of prenatal drug exposure

N.D. 11 Ineffective therapeutic regimen management (NANDA 00078) related to:
- concurrent diagnoses with frequent changes in medical management
- student's decision-making skills
- student's developmental level and ability to comply with health plan
- family's coping skills and ability to comply with health plan

### Goals

The student will increase knowledge about physical and/or neurologic disabilities. (N.D. 1, 4, 7, 9, 10)

The student will be safe at school. (N.D. 5)

The student will maintain good school attendance pattern. (N.D. 2, 3, 6, 8)

The student will participate in medication plan at school. (N.D. 2, 11)

The student will participate in development and implementation of healthcare plans at school. (N.D. 1–11)

The student will increase self-awareness and acceptance of self. (N.D. 1, 3, 4, 6, 7, 9)

The student will increase appropriate interactions with others. (N.D. 6, 8)

The student will utilize school support systems to increase effective coping skills. (N.D. 6, 8)

The student will participate in school activities to enhance and refine verbal and language skills (N.D. 3)

The student will develop trusting, nurturing, and stable relationship with caregivers. (N.D. 2)

## Nursing Interventions

Establish trusting, open communication with student to discuss health concerns, increase acceptance of self, identify strengths and abilities, determine effective ways to cope with disabilities, and comply with medication plan (N.D.1–11)

In-service school staff about effects of exposure to prenatal substance abuse. (N.D. 1–11)
- Outline characteristics of students who are prenatally exposed to drugs
- Discuss methods of restructuring classroom environment to minimize distractions.
- Stress need for routine and calmness.
- Identify specific health needs, including medications and specific healthcare needs for the student.
- Identify specific educational needs for the student if applicable.
- Discuss student's psychosocial needs.

Collaborate with school staff in developing appropriate school curriculum and activities in order to maximize student's potential. (N.D. 3-9)

Provide student with opportunities to identify his/her strengths and abilities at home and school. (N.D. 1, 3, 4, 6, 7, 9)

Collaborate with school staff in providing appropriate opportunities for student to have successful interactions with peers. (N.D. 6, 8)

Collaborate with multidisciplinary team to document possible academic/behavior/developmental/sensory concerns and need for further assessment (special education). (N.D. 3, 4, 7-9)

Obtain written authorization from healthcare provider(s) for medication and specialized healthcare procedures, if indicated. (N.D. 4, 7-9)

Include student, parents/guardians, appropriate school personnel, and healthcare provider(s) in development and implementation of an individualized healthcare plan. (N.D. 1–11)

Assist parents to maintain supply of medication at school. (N.D. 4, 7-9)

Assist student to comply with his/her healthcare plan. (N.D. 4, 7-9)

Provide health counseling session to identify safety rules at school. (N.D. 5, 7-9)

Establish trusting, open communication with parents/caregivers. (N.D. 1–11)
- Provide opportunities to discuss student's physical and psychosocial needs.
- Provide opportunities to discuss realistic goals and expectations.
- Educate regarding respite care and utilization of community support systems.
- Encourage compliance with medical management of health concern.
- Encourage daily school attendance unless student is ill.

## Expected Student Outcomes

The student will:
- Comply with medication plan at school (e.g., taking medication on time each day). (N.D. 11)
- Demonstrate self-acceptance by working toward maximizing his/her potential (educational and psychosocial). (N.D. 1, 3, 4, 6-9)
- Maintain regular school attendance, missing less than 10 days per school year. (N.D. 2, 3, 6-9)
- Maintain academic progress, with modification made as needed. (N.D. 3, 4, 6-9)
- Identify and demonstrate the use of safety rules at school. (N.D. 5)
- Identify his/her strengths and abilities. (N.D. 1, 3, 6-9)
- Demonstrate his/her abilities and strengths to other peers and adults. (N.D. 4, 6, 8)
- Identify and demonstrate effective ways to cope with disabilities. (N.D. 1, 3, 4, 7, 9-11)
- Interact appropriately with others (peers, staff, family members). (N.D. 3-8)
- Participate in all school activities with modifications as necessary. (N.D. 1, 3-5, 7-9)

# Case Study

Janson is a 6-year-old kindergarten student at Place Elementary School. Jason was exposed prenatally to his biological mother's frequent binge drinking. Janson is short for his age. He had frequent episodes of otitis media when younger resulting in intermittent hearing loss with delays in language development. Diagnoses of ADHD, ODD, language delays, and gross/fine motor skills delays were made after being evaluated by a developmental pediatrician. Various medications have been tried in the past. Currently, Ritalin and Tegretol are prescribed. Side effects from these medications cause Janson to have difficulty going to sleep at night. He also has a poor appetite.

Janson currently lives with his third set of foster parents. His biological mother is incarcerated because of cocaine dealing. The whereabouts of the biological father is unknown.

Janson is having difficulty in school because of his impulsive behavior, very short attention span, and delays in language development. In addition, he often hits and/or kicks other children but denies that he did it. He also frequently uses inappropriate language and does not respond well when corrected. He hates school and everyone at school.

The pediatrician has recommended that Janson and his family participate in private family counseling to work on anger management issues, but foster parents have not yet followed through with this recommendation. They have also not been able to attend several school-sponsored parent workshops where math and reading games, etc., can be made to be used at home. They have tried to be consistent in maintaining the medication plan; however, they do admit that it is a challenge trying to get Janson to take his medications. He often hides them in his mouth and then spits them out when they are not looking.

Lately, Janson has complained of frequent headaches and/or stomachaches in the morning and tries to convince his foster mother that he needs to stay home from school. When at school, Janson frequently visits the health room with minor complaints. Janson and his school nurse are beginning to trust each other and have decided to decrease health room visits through a reward system and contract. In addition, school staff have decided to meet to plan the most appropriate education placement, including possible special education services or 504 services.

## Prenatal Alcohol And Drug Exposure

| Assessment Data | Nursing Diagnosis | Goals | Nursing Interventions | Expected Outcomes |
|---|---|---|---|---|
| Janson was prenatally exposed to alcohol. | Disturbed body image. | Janson will increase his knowledge about and accept his physical and neurological disabilities. | Provide in-service training of staff regarding long-term effects of prenatal drug exposure and student's specific health and educational needs. | Janson will identify and demonstrate his strengths and abilities. |
| Janson has short stature. | Risk for delayed development. | | | Janson will identify and demonstrate effective methods to cope with disabilities. |
| Janson has developmental delays. | Disturbed sensory perception related to prenatal alcohol exposure, resulting in hyperreaction to sensory stimuli. | Janson will increase self-awareness and acceptance of self. | Establish trusting, open communication with student to discuss concerns, to increase acceptance of self, and to identify strengths and abilities and effective ways to cope with disabilities. | |
| Janson has hyper reactions to sensory stimuli. | Deficient knowledge related to long-term effects of prenatal drug exposure. | | Provide Janson with opportunities to identify his strengths and abilities at home and school. | |
| Janson has physical and neurological anomalies. | | | | |
| Student lives with new foster family. | Risk for impaired child/parent attachment related to lack of attachment, behavior disorders, difficult temperament, poor cognitive development, and unrealistic expectations regarding health and education concerns. | Janson will develop a trusting, nurturing, and stable relationship with his new foster parents. | Establish trusting, open communication with foster parents to provide opportunities to discuss realistic health and education goals and expectations. | Janson will interact with foster parents appropriately. |
| Side effects of medication cause difficulty sleeping and poor appetite. | | | Encourage parents to utilize community and school support systems. | Janson will comply with family rules. |
| Janson denies behavior problems and does not respond appropriately when corrected. | | | | |
| Janson's foster parents have not been able to attend any school-offered parent workshops. | | | | |

| Assessment Data | Nursing Diagnosis | Goals | Nursing Interventions | Expected Outcomes |
|---|---|---|---|---|
| Janson had frequent episodes of otitis media with intermittent hearing loss and delays in language development. | Impaired verbal communication related to developmental delays and hearing loss. | Janson will participate in school activities that will enhance and refine his verbal and language skills. | Monitor hearing status quarterly and refer when appropriate.<br><br>Collaborate with school staff in developing appropriate school curriculum and activities to maximize student's potential (e.g., need for preferential seating close to instruction, decreased distractions in classroom, and transition time between activities).<br><br>Collaborate with multidisciplinary team to document possible academic/behavior/hearing/developmental concerns and for further assessment. | Janson will maintain academic progress with modifications made as needed. |
| Janson has short attention span and is very impulsive. Student has gross and fine motor delays. | Risk for injury related to impulsiveness and developmental delays. | Janson will be safe at school. | Health counseling with Janson to identify safety rules at school and to reinforce safety rules, etc., learned in physical education class. | Janson will identify and demonstrate use of 10 general safety rules at school. |
| Janson "hates" school and often hit or kicks classmates.<br><br>Janson is frequently seen in the health room with vague complaints.<br><br>Janson frequently complains of headaches and stomachaches and wants to stay home from school. | Impaired social interaction related to low tolerance for frustration and dysfunctional social interaction with peers.<br><br>Chronic low self-esteem related to lack of success in school. | Janson will increase appropriate interactions with peers.<br><br>Janson will increase acceptance of self.<br><br>Janson will utilize school support systems to increase coping skills.<br><br>Janson will maintain a good school attendance pattern. | Collaborate with school staff in providing appropriate opportunities for student to have successful interactions with peers.<br><br>Implement contract or reward system to encourage fewer health room visits, resulting in more learning time in the classroom. | Janson will demonstrate self-acceptance by working toward maximizing his potential (educational and psychosocial).<br><br>Janson will interact appropriately with peers at school with no hitting or kicking episodes. |

| Assessment Data | Nursing Diagnosis | Goals | Nursing Interventions | Expected Outcomes |
|---|---|---|---|---|
| Private family counseling has been recommended to deal with anger management issues but has not yet been implemented. | | | Refer student to school counselor and/other support personnel. | Janson will participate in all school activities with modifications as necessary. |
| | | | Work with community resources and foster parents to obtain family counseling with a community resource. | Janson will receive private family counseling to enhance efforts of school counseling. |
| | | | Encourage school counselor and other appropriate school personnel to meet with student, in addition to participating in family counseling. | Janson will maintain regular school attendance, missing less than 10 days per school year. |
| | | | Encourage parent to send student to school every day unless ill. | |
| Janson is diagnosed with ADHD, ODD, and developmental delays.<br><br>Janson will need to take Ritalin and Tegretol at school.<br><br>Janson frequently spits out medications when foster parent is not looking. | Ineffective therapeutic regimen management related to concurrent diagnoses, frequent medication changes, student's developmental ability to comply with health plan, and family's coping skills and ability to comply with health plan. | Janson will participate in the development and implementation of healthcare plans at school.<br><br>Janson will participate in medication plan at school. | Provide in-service training for school staff regarding medication need and side effects.<br><br>Health counseling with student regarding need for medication and how medication can help improve behavior and school work.<br><br>Implement contract or reward system to encourage and help student comply with need for medication.<br><br>Encourage foster parent to send supply of medication to school when needed. | Janson will comply with his medication plan at school.<br><br>Janson will swallow his medication immediately upon taking it at school. |

# References

American Academy of Pediatrics (AAP). (2000). Policy *statement: Fetal alcohol syndrome and alcohol-related neurodevelopmental disorders (RE9948).* Retrieved August 12, 2003, from http://www.aap.org/policy/re9948.html

Kansas Department of Social and Rehabilitation Services. (1990). *Alcohol and other drug exposed babies: A preventable tragedy.* Topeka, KS: Kansas Dept of Social & Rehabilitation Services.

Kuehne, E. A., & Reilly, M. W. (2004). Prenatal cocaine exposure. In P. J. Allen & J. A. Vessey (Eds.), *Primary care of the child with a chronic condition* (4th ed). St. Louis, MO: Mosby.

Lewis, K. D. (1995). *Infants and children with prenatal alcohol and drug exposure: A guide to identification and intervention.* North Branch, MN: Sunrise River Press.

Morrow, C. E., Bandstra, E. S., Anthony, J. C., Ofir, A. Y., Xue, L., & Reyes, M. L. (2001). Influence of prenatal cocaine exposure on full-term infant neurobehavioral functioning. *Neurotoxicology and Teratology, 23*, 533–544.

NANDA International. (2003). *Nursing diagnoses: Definitions & classification 2003-2004.* Philadelphia: Author.

National Organization on Fetal Alcohol Syndrome (NOFAS). (2003). *What is fetal alcohol syndrome?* Retrieved September 12, 2003, from http://www.nofas.org/main/what_is_FAS.htm

Scher, M. S., Richardson, G. A., & Day, N. L. (2000). Effects of prenatal cocaine/crack and other drug exposure on electroencephalographic sleep studies at birth and one year. *Pediatrics, 105*, 39–48.

Scherer, D. M., Anyaegbunam, A., & Onyeije, C. (1998). Antepartum fetal intracranial hemorrhage, predisposing factors and prenatal sonogram: a review. *American Journal of Perinatology, 15*, 431–441.

Slotkin, T. A. (1998). Fetal nicotine or cocaine exposure: Which one is worse? *Journal of Pharmocology and Experimental Therapeutics, 285*, 931–945.

Streissguth, A. P. (1994). A long-term perspective of FAS. *Alcohol Health and Research World, 18*(1), 74–81.

Substance Abuse and Mental Health Services Administration (SAMHSA). (2002). 2002 *national survey on drug use and health (NSDUH).* Retrieved September 9, 2003 from http://www.samhsa.gov/oas/nhsda/2K2nsduh/Results/2K2Results.htm

US General Accounting Office. (HRD 90-138). (1991). *Drug exposed infants.* Washington, DC: Author.

Wagner, C. L., Katikaneni, L. D., Cox, T. H., & Ryan, R. M. (1998). The impact of prenatal drug exposure on the neonate. *Obstetrics and Gynecology Clinics of North America*, 169–194.

Weiner, L., & Morse B. A. (1994). Intervention and the child with FAS. *Alcohol Health and Research World, 18*(1), 67–72.

Wong, D. L., Hockenberry, M. J., Wilson, D., Winkelstein, M. L., & Kline, N. E. (2003). *Wong's nursing care of infants and children.* (7th ed.). St. Louis, MO: Mosby.

Wunsch, M. J., Conlon, C. J., & Scheidt, P. C. (2002). Sustance abuse: A preventable threat to development. In M. L. Batshaw (Ed.), *Children with disabilities.* Baltimore: Paul H. Brooks.

## Bibliography

James, S. R., Ashwell, J. W., & Droske, S. C. (2002) *Nursing care of children principles and practice* (2nd ed., pp. 1004–1005). Philadelphia: Saunders.

Lewis, K. D., & Bear, B. J. (2002). *Manual of school health* (2nd ed., pp. 219–223). Philadelphia: Saunders.

Lewis, K.D. (1995). *Infants and children with prenatal alcohol and drug exposure: A guide to identification and intervention.* North Branch, MN: Sunrise River Press.

Odom, S. E., Herrick, C., Holman, C., Crowe, E., Clements, C. (1994). Case management for children with attention deficit hyperactivity disorder. *Journal of School Nursing, 10*(3), 17–21.

# Resources

American Academy of Pediatrics
141 Northwest Point Boulevard
Elk Grove Village, IL 60007-1098
847-434-4000
1-800-842-7777
www.aap.org

Children and Adults With Attention Deficit Disorder
8181 Professional Place
Suite 150
Landover, MD 20785
1-800-233-4050
www.chadd.org

National Institute on Drug Abuse
National Institutes of Health
6001 Executive Boulevard
Room 5213
Bethesda, MD 20892-9561
300-443-1124
www.nida.nih.gov

National Organization on Fetal Alcohol Syndrome
900 17th Street, NW
Suite 910
Washington, DC 20006
1-800-666-6327
www.nofas.org

US Department of Health and Human Services
Substance Abuse and Mental Health Services
   Administration
Room 12-105 Parklawn Building
5600 Fishers Lane
Rockville, MD 20857
301-443-4795 (Office of Administrator)
www.samhsa.gov

*Chapter Sixty-two: Prenatal Alcohol and Drug Exposure*

## Chapter Sixty-three

# Rett Syndrome

### Charlotte R. Gorun

## Introduction

Rett syndrome is a neurodevelopmental disorder that usually affects females regardless of race or ethnic background. It was first described by a German physician, Dr. Andreas Rett, in a presentation of a paper in 1966 (Braddock, Braddock, & Graham, 1993). Since Dr. Rett's presentation, more research has been done and more attention has been focused on this disorder.

The child's physician, following the established criteria, makes the diagnosis of Rett syndrome. Parents are very aware of their child's development and may begin to notice changes in the child's skills and growth. After the diagnosis has been established, a multidisciplinary approach must be developed and implemented to maintain optimal health. As the stages progress, the child's medical and educational needs will need to be reassessed and changes will need to be made in the child's healthcare management and educational programming.

## Pathophysiology

There are several theories as to the cause of Rett syndrome. Dr. Rett suspected elevated ammonia levels. Another theory suggested an abnormal neurotransmitter function (Iyama, 1993). In 1999, the gene *MECP2* was identified as the gene that causes Rett syndrome (National Institute of Child Health & Human Development,I 1999). The *MECP2* gene is carried on the X chromosome. The mutated *MECP2* gene occurs spontaneously and does not occur through heredity. The *MECP2* gene interferes with the maturation of the brain, thereby making Rett syndrome a developmental disease (International Rett Syndrome Association [IRSA], 2003). The frontal, motor, and temporal cortexes, brainstem, basal forebrain, and basal ganglia, as well as the portions of the brain that control motion and emotion, are affected by Rett syndrome. The discovery of the gene *MECP2* has provided an opportunity for the development of definitive testing for identification of Rett syndrome. The discovery may also assist researchers in the discovery of a cure for this disease in the future.

In spite of this discovery, at present Rett syndrome must still be considered a clinical diagnosis, because children may still have Rett syndrome even if they do not have the mutated gene. Therefore, at a conference in 2001, the diagnostic criteria were reestablished to clearly outline the characteristics a physician should follow in diagnosing a child (Hagberg, Hanefeld, Percy, & Skjeldal, 2002). **Table 1** lists the revised criteria as it appeared at the conference in Germany on September 11, 2001.

Diagnosis is made through a comprehensive history, documentation of developmental milestones, and elimination of other developmental and metabolic disorders. A definitive diagnosis is usually not made until 2 to 5 years of age to avoid a misdiagnosis.

Diagnosis of Rett syndrome is dependent upon meeting the diagnostic criteria established by Hagburg and associates (Hagberg et al., 2002). The infant develops normally for approximately 6 to 18 months. The infant has a normal head circumference at birth, but the head's growth rate slows between 3 months to 4 years of age. The child loses the ability for expressive, communicative, and receptive language. There is a decline in acquired skills between 6 and 30 months. The classic appearance of hand wringing, squeezing, clapping together, mouthing, and rubbing take the place of purposeful hand movements. The child's gait becomes stiff-legged and unsteady, and the habit of toe-walking develops.

Other symptoms also support the initial diagnosis. Breathing dysfunction such as periodic apnea while awake, intermittent hyperventilation, and forced expulsion of air or saliva occur. Abnormalities in electroencephalographic testing, with the possible development of seizures, contractures of limbs related to muscle rigidity and spasticity, scoliosis, growth retardation, and decreased body fat and muscle mass also occur. A child may also experience abnormal sleep patterns and irritability and agitation. Eating becomes difficult on account of difficulty with chewing and swallowing. Because of poor circulation, the extremities may feel cold and develop a bluish discoloration. Constipation becomes an issue, as does decreased mobility (IRSA, 2003).

The progression of Rett syndrome is identified through clinical stages that were established by Hagberg. Stage I, known as early onset, occurs from ages 6 to 18 months. Symptoms of Rett syndrome may begin but are often difficult to detect. Parents may describe a child as

**Table 1. Revised Criteria for Diagnosis of Rett Syndrome**

| Inclusion criteria | 1. Meet at least 3 of the 6 main criteria<br>2. Meet at least 5 of 11 supportive criteria |
|---|---|
| Main criteria | 1. Absence or reduction of hand skills<br>2. Reduction or loss of babble speech<br>3. Monotonous pattern to hand stereotypes<br>4. Reduction or loss of communication skills<br>5. Deceleration of head growth from first years of life<br>6. Rett syndrome disease profile: a regression stage followed by recovery of interaction, contrasting with slow neuromotor regression |
| Supportive criteria | 1. Breathing irregularities<br>2. Bloating/air swallowing<br>3. Bruxism, harsh-sounding type<br>4. Abnormal locomotion<br>5. Scoliosis, kyphosis<br>6. Lower limb amyotrophy<br>7. Cold, purplish feet, usually growth impaired<br>8. Sleep disturbance, including night screaming outbursts<br>9. Laughing/screaming spells<br>10. Diminished response to pain<br>11. Intense eye contact/eye pointing |

Adapted from "An Update on Clinically Applicable Diagnostic Criteria in Rett Syndrome," by B. Hagberg, H. Folker, A. Percy, and O. Skjeldal, 2002, *European Journal of Paediatric Neurology*, 6(5), p.293-297)

easygoing. The baby may lose interest in toys and exhibit decreased eye contact. Developmental milestones may be delayed. The characteristic hand wringing may begin, and head growth slows.

Stage II, or rapid destructive stage, may occur from ages 1 to 4 years and last for weeks to months. Symptoms during this stage may progress rapidly or gradually. Purposeful hand skills are lost with the increase of hand wringing or mouthing of hands. These movements do not occur in sleep. Acquired verbal communication skills are lost. Breathing characteristics of apnea, irritability, and hyperventilation occur. Ambulating skills decline and become unsteady. The child with Rett syndrome becomes irritable at times, has frequent crying spells, and has difficulty sleeping (IRSA, 2004).

Stage III, or plateau stage, occurs from 2 to 10 years of age and may last for years. This stage is characterized by increased difficulty performing automatic movements; motor coordination is poor and seizures may occur. There appears to be less autistic-type behavior, and irritability and crying decrease. There may be more awareness of the environment and a willingness to interact with others (IRSA, 2004).

Stage IV, or late motor deterioration, is divided in two subcategories: (1) where the child is presently walking, and (2) where the child has never walked (IRSA, 2004).

Stage IV begins when stage III ends, which could be up to 25 years. Some children may never exit stage III, and stage IV may last for decades. The child will stop walking. There is leveling off of cognitive, communication, and hand skills. The characteristic hand movements may decrease. Scoliosis may develop. Overall rigidity and spasticity are common, which will affect ambulating skills.

## Management
Management of Rett syndrome consists of the following:
- Modification of environment—eliminating barriers to prevent injury, maintain body temperature
- Medication: anticonvulsant for seizure control; laxative for bowel elimination management, drooling
- Behavior such as crying, self-injurious, and withdrawal are managed by behavior modification, facilitated communication, and staff's awareness of student's needs

Physical therapy: negotiating school environment safely
- Occupational therapy: for motor planning, fine-motor control, self-care skills, and adaptive equipment
- Speech therapy: establish communication system to express wants and needs
- Nutritional modification: to accommodate risk of aspiration; increase fiber and fluid

- Assistance with activities of daily living—hygiene, grooming, dressing
- Parent/guardian education for maintenance of health
- Counseling: assist student and family in coping with Rett syndrome
- Staff and peer education for understanding Rett syndrome

## Individualized Healthcare Plan

### Assessment

*History*
- Date diagnosis was made? Which stage is child in?
- Respiratory status: apnea, reaction to upper respiratory tract infection, hyperventilation
- Level of ambulating mobility, orthotic use, need for wheelchair
- Level of fine-motor coordination
- Nutritional status; difficulty swallowing or chewing; reflux; need for gastrostomy tube feedings
- Type of seizure activity; duration of seizure; behavior observed prior to the seizure
- History of bowel and bladder training
- Sleep patterns
- Physical development, growth pattern

*Current Status and Management*
- Current status of seizure activity: duration, frequency, behavior observed
- Current seizure management plan, including medication
- Current medication's therapeutic effects and adverse side effects
- Nutritional status: assess type of food toleration for texture, consistency, ability to chew, ability to swallow, oral feedings, hydration
- Bowel and urinary elimination pattern: toileting schedule; frequency of diaper changes
- Current height and weight
- Current respiratory status: periods of apnea; hyperventilation; coloration of skin
- Dental status
- Scoliosis
- Level of activity tolerance
- Mobility status: walking or wheelchair mobility
- Verbal communication skills—need for facilitated communication
- Emergency information with current contact names, phone numbers, medical needs
- Emergency care plan (ECP): seizures, apnea, hyperventilation

*Self-care*
- Toileting: assistance needed
- Dental hygiene: assistance needed
- Meals and snacks: assistance needed
- Ambulation or wheelchair mobility: assistance needed
- Ability to communicate needs
- Ability of child to participate in decisions about himself/herself

*Psychosocial Status*
- Orientation to time and place, especially after seizure
- Ability to participate in classroom activities, especially activities with other children, groups
- Interactions with peers: in and outside of school
- Assistance needed in activities with other students to prevent accidental injury
- Targeted socialization activities with staff and peers

*Academic Issues*
- Mobility around the school and classroom: assistance needed
- Transportation needs to and from school
- Classroom environment: safety for ambulation and seizure activity
- Communication needs: assistance needed, speech/language therapy, facilitated language—implement facilitated communication

- Ability to process information and respond
- Nutritional needs during the school day: snacks, lunch
- Bathroom facilities: privacy, assistance, storage of supplies, equipment needed
- Academic schedule: courses in morning; better able to attend
- Functional skills development
- Academic classes
- Physical education: modification needed, assistance needed
- Special education services: school health services needed
- Implement facilitated communication
- Adaptations needed for field trips

## Nursing Diagnoses (N.D.) (NANDA, 2003)

**N.D. 1** Imbalanced nutrition: less than body requirements (NANDA 00002) related to biological factors

**N.D. 2** Risk for constipation (NANDA 00015) related to functional factors

**N.D. 3** Ineffective breathing pattern (NANDA 00032) related to hyperventilation and apnea

**N.D. 4** Risk for injury (NANDA 00035) related to external and internal factors due to seizure disorder

**N.D. 5** Risk for aspiration (NANDA 00039) related to impaired swallowing and seizure disorder

**N.D. 6** Impaired verbal communication (NANDA 00051) related to loss of expressive language

**N.D. 7** Impaired social interaction (NANDA 00052) related to:
- communication barriers
- limited physical mobility

**N.D. 8** Social isolation (NANDA 00053) related to:
- decreased mobility
- delay in accomplishing developmental tasks
- altered state of wellness

**N.D. 9** Impaired physical mobility (NANDA 00085) related to neuromusculosketal impairment and need for wheelchair

**N.D. 10** Fatigue (NANDA 00093) related to interruption of sleep cycle at night

**N.D. 11** Feeding, self-care deficit (NANDA 00102) related to neuromuscular impairment

**N.D. 12** Impaired swallowing (NANDA 00103) related to neuromuscular impairment

**N.D. 13** Dressing/grooming, self-care deficit (NANDA 00109) related to neuromuscular impairment with loss of purposeful hand movement

**N.D. 14** Toileting, self-care deficit (NANDA 110) related to neuromuscular impairment with loss of purposeful hand movement

**N.D. 15** Delayed growth and development (NANDA 00111) related to effects of physical disability

**N.D. 16** Impaired wheelchair mobility (NANDA 00089) related to inability to operate wheelchair independently

## Goals

The student will participation in school/classroom activities with modifications made as needed. (N.D. 7, 8, 9)

The student will maintain communication through facilitated language. (N.D. 6, 7)

The student will remain safe during seizure activity, with assistance. (N.D. 4)

The student will prevent injury during interactions with peers, with assistance when needed. (N.D. 9, 10)

The student will prevent injury from aspiration, with assistance. (N.D. 1, 3, 5, 12)

The student will prevent choking while eating. (N.D. 1, 5, 12)

The student will maintain good personal care, with assistance as needed. (N.D. 2, 11, 13, 14)

The student will maintain adequate nutrition and hydration. (N.D. 1, 11, 15)

The student will utilize periods of relaxation between activities as needed. (N.D. 3, 9, 10)

The student will maintain ambulation/mobility in the school/classroom setting with assistance. (N.D. 9, 16)

The student will maintain adequate bowel elimination pattern. (N.D. 1, 2, 14)

The student will maintain adequate urinary elimination pattern. (N.D. 14)

The student will maintain effective breathing pattern. (N.D. 3, 5)

## Nursing Interventions

- Assist student with all areas of personal care (toileting, dental care, grooming, applying outerwear). (N.D. 13, 14)
- Monitor eating behaviors, food tolerance. (N.D. 1, 5, 11, 12)
- Instruct paraprofessionals working with student on assistance required with meals and snacks. (N.D. 5, 11, 12)
- Monitor height and weight. (N.D. 1)
- Collaborate with therapists to instruct staff on proper feeding technique. (N.D. 3, 5, 9, 11, 12)
- Develop ECP for seizures: Instruct school staff working with the student on what to do if a seizure occurs. (N.D. 4, 5)
- Develop ECP: apnea, hyperventilation. (N.D. 3, 5)
- Assess nutritional intake and hydration. (N.D. 1, 2, 15)
- Assist teachers to establish relaxation periods between work sessions. (N.D. 3, 9, 10)
- Monitor activity tolerance. (N.D. 3, 4, 9, 10)
- Monitor respiratory status during activities, which require increased energy expenditure. (N.D. 3)
- Assess and modify classrooms for safe environment, barrier-free. (N.D. 4, 9, 16)
- Develop emergency evacuation plan to ensure safe and expedient exit from the school building if needed. (N.D. 4, 9, 16)
- Participate in the school multidisciplinary team regarding special educational services required and development of individualized education program. (N.D. 4, 6, 8, 9, 15)
- Assist in determining and providing appropriate bathroom facilities: storage of supplies, privacy room, assistance with toileting needs. (N.D. 2, 9, 14)
- Assist in establishing appropriate activity guidelines in cooperation with parent/guardian and physician to prevent injury. (N.D. 3, 4, 9, 10, 15)
- Allow student adequate time to process and respond to information. (N.D. 6, 7)
- Utilize facilitated communication when interacting with student. (N.D. 6, 7, 8)
- Encourage parent/guardian to maintain semiannual dental evaluation with dentist. (N.D. 5)
- Screen for scoliosis annually, if not done by physician. (N.D. 9)
- Instruct staff working with student on how to perform Heimlich maneuver in case of choking. (N.D. 3, 4, 5, 6)
- Obtain medication orders from physician. (N.D. 4, 5)
- Administer prescribed medication. (N.D. 4, 5)
- Monitor therapeutic and adverse effects of medication. (N.D. 4, 5)
- Assist educational team to maintain communication with parent/guardians regarding child's adjustment to school activities, and modify school programs as needed. (N.D. 6, 7, 8, 9, 15, 16)
- Maintain communication with parents regarding the student's healthcare needs at school (N.D. 1–5, 9–15)
- Provide only two choices in assisting the student to make decisions. (N.D. 6, 7, 8)

## Expected Student Outcomes

The student will:
- Not aspirate during meal and snack periods. (N.D. 3, 5, 12)
- Use facilitated communication to interact with staff and peers. (N.D. 6, 7, 8)
- Participate in school/classroom activities with peers. (N.D. 6, 7, 8, 9)
- Maintain good hygiene with assistance as needed. (N.D. 11, 13, 14)
- Participate in classroom activities without injury to self and with assistance from staff as needed. (N.D. 3, 4, 9, 10)
- Participate in health screenings. (N.D. 1, 15)
- Maintain good nutrition and hydration orally or by gastrostomy feedings. (N.D. 1, 5, 12, 15)
- Be mobile in the school/classroom environment. (N.D. 9, 16)
- Exit the school building safely and quickly in an emergency (fire, etc.). (N.D. 9, 16)
- Maintain effective breathing pattern during the school day. (N.D. 3)
- Maintain good bowel-elimination pattern. (N.D. 2, 14)
- Participate in classroom activity, with assistance as needed. (N.D. 7, 8, 9, 10, 15)
- Participate in resting/relaxation measures between activities at school. (N.D. 3, 10)
- Participate in dressing and grooming activities, with assistance as needed. (N.D. 13)

## Case Study

The individualized healthcare plan was initiated for Anne, who is 10 years old. She was diagnosed as having Rett syndrome at 18 months. Prior to this age, she was achieving the normal developmental milestones. According to Anne's mother, she was speaking in two- to three-word phrases and feeding herself. One morning the child was participating in a routine interaction with her mother, asking for a pretzel, but she only stared at the cabinet and was unable to verbalize the request. Self-injurious behavior began, which consisted of banging her head on the cabinet. She lost the ability to create phrases. Eye contact diminished. She became incontinent after having been toilet-trained prior to this episode.

The child was examined by several physicians. A complete physical examination was performed, including an electroencephalogram and was diagnosed with Rett syndrome. Starting at age 25 months, she was enrolled in an early intervention program. During the early stage, Anne had periods of irritability, crying, and screaming. She also lost purposeful hand skills. At age 3, she was enrolled in a private school for special needs students, which she still attends. At the age of 9 years and 6 months, she was diagnosed with partial complex seizures, and she is currently taking medication for the seizures, which appears to be effective. Eye contact has improved, and periods of irritability have also diminished. The student is able to ambulate while in school, with assistance. She uses a wheelchair during family outings that require longer periods of ambulation. Complete care is required for all activities of daily living. The school district has arranged for a one-to-one classroom aide. Her educational program is multidisciplinary, involving a physical therapist, occupational therapist, speech therapist, and music therapist, as well as a classroom teacher experienced with special needs students. Anne's placement is in an out-of-district school specific to students with special needs.

# Rett Syndrome

| Assessment Data | Nursing Diagnosis | Goals | Nursing Interventions | Expected Outcomes |
|---|---|---|---|---|
| Partial-complex seizures.<br><br>Frequency 6-8 times per hour.<br><br>Occurs daily. Behavior displayed: staring spell, stops activity, blinks eyes (similar to daydreaming).<br><br>Unable to determine if child experiences aura.<br><br>No loss of consciousness. | Risk of injury related to seizure activity. | Anne will remain safe during seizure activity with assistance.<br><br>Anne will maintain an effective breathing pattern. | Develop ECP for seizures.<br><br>Provide in-service for staff working with Anne: seizure disorder ECP.<br><br>Establish appropriate activities with necessary adaptations.<br><br>Maintain seizure log in school.<br><br>Communicate seizure activity to parents.<br><br>Monitor activity tolerance after seizure. | Anne will not experience injury during seizure activity.<br><br>Anne will maintain effective breathing pattern during the school day. |
| Frequent drooling.<br><br>Needs to eat small amounts of food at a time.<br><br>Gag reflex present at this time. | Risk of aspiration related to impaired swallowing and seizure disorder. | Anne will prevent injury from aspiration with assistance. | Monitor eating behaviors, food tolerances.<br><br>Assist with eating activities—small portions.<br><br>Consult with parents as to which foods are appropriate.<br><br>The parents will supply appropriate meals.<br><br>Instruct paraprofessionals working with student on assistance needed for meals. | Anne will not aspirate during meals and snacks. |
| Anne utilizes picture exchange communication board created by speech department. | Impaired social interaction related to communication barriers and limited physical mobility. | Anne will maintain communication through use of facilitated language. | Anne's communication board will be situated appropriately for student.<br><br>Assess classrooms for safe environment, barrier-free. | Anne will utilize facilitated communication to interact with staff and peers. |

| Assessment Data | Nursing Diagnosis | Goals | Nursing Interventions | Expected Outcomes |
|---|---|---|---|---|
| Anne is unable to use verbal communication. Anne has consistent paraprofessional help on daily basis. Anne is able to visually cue response. | | | Allow student adequate time to process and respond to information. Provide only two choices in assisting the student to make decisions. Utilize facilitated communication when interacting with student. | Anne will participate in classroom activities with peers. |
| Anne must be assisted with ambulation. Anne requires wheelchair for extensive periods of walking, such as a field trip. Anne becomes tired during long periods of ambulation. During periods of hyperventilation Anne becomes tired. Lips become bluish in color. | Impaired physical mobility related to neuromusculoskeletal impairment. | Anne will be able to participate in school/classroom activities with modifications, as needed. Anne will utilize periods of relaxation between activities, as needed. | Assess classroom/school for barriers for ambulation. Instruct staff in correct handling of wheelchair. Monitor activity tolerance. Collaborate with occupational therapy/physical therapy (OT/PT) with correct method of ambulation. Assist is establishing appropriate activity guidelines with parent/guardian and OT/PT. Conduct annual scoliosis examination. Assist in determining appropriate toileting facilities with necessary accommodations and assistance, as needed. | Anne will participate with classroom/ school activities. Anne will participate in school health screenings. |

# References

Braddock, S. R., Braddock, B. A., & Graham, J. M., Jr, (1993). Rett syndrome: An update and review for the primary pediatrician. Clinical Pediatrics, 32, 613–626.

Hagberg, B., Hanefeld, F., [AU: Second author's name has been changed per PubMed] Percy, A., & Skjeldal, O. (2002). An update on clinically applicable diagnostic criteria in Rett syndrome. European Journal of Paediatric Neurology, 6, 293–297. Retrieved September 13, 2003, from http://www.idealibrary.com

International Rett Syndrome Association. (2003). Rett syndrome: Rosetta stone of neurologic diseases. Retrieved September 13, 2003, from http://www.rettsyndrome.org/main/update-on-rett-syndrome.htm

International Rett Syndrome Association. (2004). Stages of Rett syndrome. Retrieved on August 21, 2004, from http://www.rettsyndrome.org/main/stages.htm

Iyama, C. M. (1993). Rett syndrome. Advances in Pediatrics, 40, 217–245.

NANDA International (2003). Nursing diagnoses: Definitions & classification 2003-2004. Philadelphia: Author.

National Institute of Child Health & Human Development. (1999). NICHD funded researchers discover gene for Rett syndrome (NIH News Alert September 30, 1999). Retrieved September 13, 2003, from http://www.nichd.nih.gov/new/release/retgene.cfm

# Bibliography

Batshaw, M. L. (2002) Children with disabilities. Baltimore: Paul H. Brooks.

Hootman, J. (1996). Quality nursing interventions in the school setting: Procedures, models, and guidelines. Scarborough, ME: National Association of School Nurses.

Kline, F. M., Silver, L. B., & Russell, S. C. (2001). The educator's guide to medical issues in the classroom. Baltimore: Paul H. Brooks.

Tams-Little, S., & Holdgrafer, G. (1996). Early communication development in children with Rett syndrome. Brain and Development, 18, 376–378.

# Resources

International Rett Syndrome Association
9121 Piscataway Road
Suite 2-B
Clinton, MD 20735
301-856-3334
1-800-818-RETT
301-856-3336 (fax)
http://www.rettsyndrome.org

## Chapter Sixty-four

# School Refusal Behavior

Elaine D. Level and Tona L. Leiker

## Introduction

Children of all ages experience normal fear at each developmental stage of life. Poor school attendance creates dilemmas and difficult choices for students, parents, and school personnel. It is estimated that approximately 2 in 5 children become reluctant to attend school at some point in their K–12 school experience (Schor, 1999; National Association of School Psychologists [NASP], 2003).

The NASP prefers the term "school refusal" because it reflects the multiplicity of explanations for the condition. The reasons that children refuse to go to school "range from mental illness and learning problems to general defiance and a desire for attention" (NASP, 2003). Unfortunately, parents, whether there is personal awareness or not, often contribute to the reluctance of the child to attend school (Brand & O'Connor, 2004; Jellineck, Patel, & Froehle, 2002). Therefore, an interdisciplinary team approach is essential in creating a consistent treatment approach. School refusal is often complicated by other health-related factors, such as fatigue, illness, or injury. Thus a cycle of avoidance, increased anxiety, feelings of being overwhelmed, and, potentially, depression creates a complex problem requiring a multifaceted treatment approach.

### Pathophysiology

Elementary school refusal behaviors may begin following an illness or vacation. Separation anxiety disorder, depression, or a mixed diagnosis of anxiety and depression may be the underlying cause. Adolescents with school refusal behaviors often present with other precipitating events, prior to the onset of the current behavior or health-related concerns. The school nurse is in a key role to differentiate between illness, avoidance, fear of rejection, or a combination of these factors.

The *Diagnostic and Statistical Manual of Mental Disorders* (DSM-IV-TR) of the American Psychiatric Association (APA) does not recognize school phobia as a psychiatric disorder. However, components of school phobia, school refusal, or school avoidance are noted in the criteria of generalized anxiety disorders and social phobias, as follows: excessive anxiety and concern (apprehensive expectation), occurring more days than not for at least 6 months, about a number of events or activities such as school or work performance (APA, 2000).

In the school environment, young students, prekindergarten through elementary school, may experience a separation anxiety disorder, which needs to be treated as such to prevent future educational compromise or grade level retention or dropout status. On the other end of the spectrum are older students, especially high school students, who may be avoiding school because of a traumatic event, including harassment and/or bullying, lengthy or chronic illness, prolonged recovery from an accident, or perceived rejection or conflict with peers, parents, and/or teachers (Brand & O'Connor, 2004). Fear of failure, not being selected for an activity or team, and unrealistic parental expectations are common precipitating events to school-avoidance behaviors. Both ends of the age spectrum may indeed experience any of these anxiety-related issues.

Avoidance behaviors may seem to be a temporary solution to the problem, but the real issues are not being addressed and the long-term sequelae become even more devastating for the student and his or her family. Anxiety disorders arise out of a physiologic response to stressors, resulting in an autonomic nervous system response, including elevated pulse and blood pressure, narrowed ability to problem-solve, and increased agitation, that is, the typical fight-or-flight reaction to stress. Research during the past 50 years has led to increased understanding of the physiologic and neurochemical basis for anxiety, sleep, and mood disorders. Serotonin balance is believed to be a key component to effective adaptation. Norepinephrine, dopamine, and histamine neurotransmitter systems in the brain influence a student's ability to adapt to anxious and/or fearful life events. When an imbalance occurs, a student may be seen in the school health office describing or exhibiting various somatization illnesses, such as headaches, stomachaches, vomiting, diarrhea, rapid heartbeat, and sweating (Antai-Otong, 2003; Jellineck et al., 2002).

### Management

The school nurse is in a key position to assess the situation, monitor attendance, and initiate the development of a collaborative team to openly address the problems created by school avoidance behaviors. Additional team members should include the student, parents, teachers, counselor (school and/or private), administrators, and any other school personnel working with the student.

Thorough assessment should be completed, including a parental assessment of the issues at hand, a teacher assessment of academic ability and performance, and an administrative assessment of other school-related behaviors, concerns, or attendance. Parental acceptance that this issue will not improve with continued school avoidance/absenteeism is central to problem resolution. The student's perceptions are critical to creating a plan of care that is workable and one that the student will adopt in an effort to strive for compliance.

Students with other comorbid disorders require a coordinated effort to maximize student potential, yet not support school avoidance or school withdrawal. Early intervention and school attendance are critical to the student's academic success and preservation of self-esteem. If the student's school avoidance lasts more than 1 week, the student may need professional assistance to deal with it. Refer the student and family to the pediatrician or other primary healthcare provider. At times, parental referral to a child psychiatrist or psychologist for professional guidance and counseling may be suggested to address avoidance fears and dysfunctional family dynamics (Schor, 1999).

School refusal behavior impacts not only the student and the parents but the school-based support team as well. The cycle of anxiety, school refusal behavior, and resulting frustration must be broken. For positive change to occur, the student and the parents must admit that there is a school refusal problem. To assist the student in developing effective coping skills and ensuring appropriate school attendance and overall academic success, the student, parents, school nurse, teachers, counselors, administrators, and other identified members of the school-based support team must be active participants in planning and implementing appropriate interventions.

Home-based school services should not be recommended or implemented (Brand & O'Connor, 2004). Rather, appropriate school interventions developed and implemented by the student, parents, and school-based support team should include:

- No provision for home-based services
- Mandatory daily school attendance
- Positive reinforcement for attendance
- Modification of the educational environment to decrease stressors
- Limiting student visits to the health office, counselor's office, library, etc., to decrease out-of-classroom time

Appropriate parental interventions should include:

- Parental support and enforcement of mandatory daily school attendance, to include the parents physically bringing the student to school
- Counseling services to enhance family function
- Undesirable consequences for the student (i.e., loss of personal privileges) who displays school refusal behavior. Consequences are clearly delineated and are consistently applied by parents.

---

## Individualized Healthcare Plan

### Assessment

*History*

- Student's complete health history, including any major illness or injury
- Date of last physical examination or visit to primary healthcare provider
- Date of last mental health examination
- History of any major illness, injury, or chronic health issue with immediate family member
- Student's past response to stress, including avoidance, anxiety, somatic complaints
- School attendance, including previous year(s) and current school year
- Previous issues with separation from parents, to include setting, duration, and outcome
- Any major changes in the student's home life or school activities, such as relocation, divorce, having been dropped from athletic team, conflict with teacher
- Academic standing prior to onset of school refusal behavior
- Onset and duration of school refusal behavior, including somatic complaints
- Activities and behavior outside the school setting

*Current Status and Management*

- Current academic standing
- Current treatment plan for any diagnosed chronic illness or mental health issues
- Medications at home or during school hours
- Parental response, including enforced consequences, for school refusal behavior
- Student and parent description of current family processes and impact of school refusal behavior on family dynamics
- Parental reaction to separation difficulties
- Parental attitude toward school, including support for attendance policies, academic requirements, and consequences

*Self-care*
- Student's acknowledgment of school refusal behavior as an ineffective coping mechanism
- Student's ability to verbalize and identify the source of anxiety or fear
- Student's ability to utilize relaxation methods to decrease physiologic responses to anxiety

*Psychosocial Status*
- Student's opinion of academic achievement
- Student's perception of parental expectations
- Student's perception of personal losses, i.e., peer conflict, dropped from athletic team, failed relationship with significant other
- Student's home environment and impact on school attendance

*Academic Issues*
- Effect of poor attendance on academic achievement
- Classroom modifications required to decrease stress and anxiety
- Vigilance on the part of the school-based team to encourage/support student to attend classes and participate in classroom activities

## Nursing Diagnoses (N.D.) (NANDA, 2003)

**N.D. 1** Anxiety (NANDA 00146) related to the school setting resulting in school refusal behaviors

**N.D. 2** Fear (NANDA 00148) of attending school related to:
- fear of failure
- separation anxiety

**N.D. 3** Health-seeking behaviors (NANDA 00084) related to somatic complaints

**N.D. 4** Interrupted family processes (NANDA 00060) related to:
- unrealistic parental expectations
- difficulty in child/parent separation
- stress of poor school attendance and possible poor academic performance on the parent/child relationship
- conflict between parent and child

**N.D. 5** Acute pain (NANDA 00132) related to physiologic response to anxiety

**N.D. 6** Ineffective role performance (NANDA 00055) related to ineffective coping skills, which result in school refusal behavior

**N.D. 7** Impaired social interaction (NANDA 00052) related to poor school attendance resulting in limited opportunities for age-appropriate social interaction

**N.D. 8** Ineffective coping (NANDA 00069) related to inability to form a valid appraisal of current stressors, inadequate choices of responses, and/or inability to use available resources

## Goals

The student will recognize the source of anxiety and fear. (N.D. 1, 2)
The student will verbalize the source of fear. (N.D. 2)
The student will employ relaxation methods to decrease anxiety. (N.D. 1, 2, 8)
The student will decrease use of the health room as an avoidance behavior. (N.D. 3)
The student will accurately describe physical symptoms of anxiety. (N.D. 3, 5)
The student will experience fewer physical symptoms associated with anxiety. (N.D. 3, 5)
The student will improve school attendance and participation in classroom activities. (N.D. 6, 7)
The student will identify stressors in family processes that result in school refusal behaviors. (N.D. 4, 8)
The student will participate in school activities, which increases her interaction with peers. (N.D. 7).
The student will request assistance with and make use of school and community resources for increasing effective coping skills. (N.D. 4, 6, 7, 8)

## Nursing Interventions

Develop relationships with other school- and/or community-based professionals to provide a team-based approach for working with the student and parents. (N.D. 1–7)

Help the student voice and identify fears and anxieties, as well as the source of the anxiety, i.e., parental expectations, peer conflicts, separation anxiety, personal safety issues, conflict with teachers. (N.D. 1, 2, 8)

Facilitate changes to decrease or eliminate the source of the fear or anxiety. (N.D. 1, 2)

Negotiate with the student to limit health room visits that interfere with classroom attendance. (N.D. 1, 3, 5, 6)

Allow student to verbalize feelings associated with physical symptoms of anxiety in a safe and supportive environment. (N.D.1, 5)

Teach student anxiety-reduction methods, such as desensitizing the student to school/campus, and relaxation techniques, such as deep breathing, visualization, and positive affirmations and other methods (N.D. 1, 2, 3, 5, 8)

Assist the student and parents in mutual goal setting, leading to the student attending all classes. A phased-in approach with multiple steps may be advised. (N.D. 1, 4, 6)

Assist student in identifying her/his positive attributes and talents (N.D. 2, 4, 6, 8).

Recognize and praise student's efforts to adapt and maintain appropriate coping mechanisms. (N.D. 3, 6, 7)

Discuss with parents the need for a thorough physical examination to rule out acute or chronic illness as cause of pain; assist parents in finding medical resources, if necessary. (N.D. 5)

Follow up on the results of the physical examination and make appropriate school plan. (N.D. 5)
- If acute or chronic illness is the root cause of poor attendance, complete an individualized healthcare plan (IHP) that addresses the health needs of the student and supports school attendance. (N.D. 5)
- If mental health is the cause of the school refusal, complete an IHP that supports the treatment plan, to include medication administration, if ordered. (N.D. 5)
- If no physical or mental health issues are the cause of school refusal, complete an IHP that specifies interventions to decrease anxiety, decrease somatic complaints, and increase school attendance. (N.D. 5)

Meet with the student's teachers, counselors, and administrators to implement the team's plan for improving the student's attendance pattern, including: (N.D. 3–7)
- Interventions to decrease stress in the classroom
- Services to be provided by counselor, psychologist or social worker
- Health office visits: assess and treat physical symptoms, returning student to class in a timely manner
- Required attendance
- Ongoing communication of success or failure of interventions with team, student, and parents
- facilitation of a reward system for the student that includes classroom attendance, participation, and completion of assignments

Set up ongoing communication with the student's parents and private therapist (if applicable) to discuss the school refusal problem and effectiveness of school-based interventions and home-based interventions. (N.D. 4, 6)

Collaborate with faculty members to identify the student's interests and talents, as well as appropriate school activities, programs, or clubs that will increase peer-to-peer interaction and assist in developing friendships. (N.D. 7)

Provide support for the parents regarding how the student's school refusal has affected family dynamics. (N.D. 4)

Facilitate communication with the parents to include staff conferences, status of student's health, and any changes that would impact school attendance. (N.D. 4, 6)

Refer the student and family to community-based support services as appropriate. (N.D. 4, 8)

## Expected Student Outcomes

The student will:
- Verbalize and identify the source(s) of anxiety and fear. (N.D. 1, 2, 3)
- Differentiate between effective and ineffective methods of coping with anxiety. (N.D. 1, 8)
- Describe physiologic responses to anxiety and fear. (N.D. 3, 5)
- Decrease frequency of visits to the health office, and experience a decrease in physical symptoms associated with anxiety. (N.D. 3, 5)
- Experience a decrease in painful physical symptoms associated with anxiety. (N.D. 1, 5)
- Utilize school and community resources to assist in reducing school refusal behaviors. (N.D. 4, 6, 7, 8)
- Identify stressors in family processes that result in school refusal behaviors. (N.D. 4, 8)
- Return to previous level of academic success. (N.D. 6)
- Attend classes on a daily basis. (N.D. 1, 2, 6, 7)
- Increase interactions with peers and develop age-appropriate relationships. (N.D. 7)

In order to support the student's academic success, the parent(s) will:
- Accept that a school refusal problem does exist. (N.D. 4, 6)
- Maintain communication with the school-based support team. (N.D. 4, 6)
- Identify the impact of school refusal behavior on the family. (N.D. 4)
- Verbalize their feelings regarding their child's school refusal behavior. (N.D. 4)
- Consistently employ consequences for school refusal behavior. (N.D. 4)
- Encourage the child to attend school activities and develop friendships. (N.D. 7)
- Attend follow-up meetings and conferences regarding their child. (N.D. 4)
- Access appropriate healthcare resources to support, treat, and care for their child and themselves. (N.D. 4)
- Request assistance with and make use of school and community resources for increasing effective coping skills. (N.D. 4, 6, 7)

## Case Study

Courtney is a 17-year-old junior in a suburban high school. She maintains a 3.5 grade point average and has been active in choir, theater, debate, and community theatre since sixth grade, often cast in leading roles. She auditioned for the lead role in the school's fall musical production, but was chosen as the understudy. Courtney was upset about the casting decision and engaged in several verbal disagreements with the theater teacher. Recently, Courtney competed at the state vocal music festival and received a "2" rating. Courtney dropped her theater class for spring semester and told the school counselor that her older brother was arrested last month for drug possession. Courtney's friends report that she has dropped out of their group.

Courtney's attendance over the last 9 weeks has been sporadic at best. Her grades have fallen on account of missing or incomplete work. Attempts by teachers and the school counselor to contact her parents have been unsuccessful. When Courtney does attend school, she often spends an hour or more resting in the health office. She tells the nurse that she becomes very anxious, is afraid to go to theater or choir class, and complains of headaches and nausea. Courtney has also left the school grounds without permission on numerous occasions.

The school principal recently sent an attendance concern letter via registered mail to Courtney's parents. They agreed to bring Courtney to the district administration center and attend a meeting with the principal, school counselor, several teachers, and the school nurse. During the meeting, her parents stated, "Courtney has always been our 'good girl,' the perfect child. We don't understand why she would disappoint us with this type of behavior."

The following items were addressed during the meeting:
1. Courtney verbalized she feels "overwhelming anxiety" when she enters the school building. Attending choir and theater classes contributes to the anxiety.
2. Her parents were concerned about Courtney's headaches and nausea and agreed she should be examined by her family physician. The results of the examination will be communicated to the school nurse.
3. Courtney is expected to attend classes on a daily basis unless her mother or father calls and speaks directly with the principal or school nurse regarding absences.
4. Her parents will bring Courtney to school and wait until she enters the building before leaving campus.
5. Courtney may not bring her cell phone to school and must call her parents from the health office or counselor's office.
6. If Courtney is absent from her scheduled class, the office will be notified immediately.
7. Parents stated that if Courtney is absent without permission, she will lose her car driving privileges.
8. The school psychologist will work with Courtney to utilize relaxation techniques to decrease her anxiety.
9. If Courtney feels overwhelmingly anxious or wants to leave campus, she may visit the health office or counselor's office for 10 minutes to discuss her anxiety.
10. The family was referred to a local counseling center that provides family therapy services for a nominal fee.

## School Refusal

| Assessment Data | Nursing Diagnosis | Goals | Nursing Interventions | Expected Outcomes |
|---|---|---|---|---|
| Courtney states that she feels "overwhelming anxiety" when she attends school. | Anxiety related to the school setting resulting in school refusal behavior. | Courtney identifies the source of anxiety. | Help the student voice and identify anxieties, as well as the source, i.e. parental expectations, peer conflicts, or separation anxiety.<br><br>Allow student to verbalize feelings associated with physical symptoms of anxiety in a safe and supportive environment<br><br>Teach student anxiety-reduction methods such as desensitizing the student to school/campus, and relaxation techniques, such as deep breathing, visualization, and positive affirmations, and other methods.<br><br>Facilitate changes in the school environment to decrease or eliminate the source of anxiety. | Courtney verbalizes and identifies the source(s) of anxiety and fear.<br><br>Courtney will differentiate between effective and ineffective methods of coping with anxiety.<br><br>School attendance and participation in school activities improve. |
| Courtney verbalizes that her fear and anxiety increase when she attends a theater or choir class. | Fear of attending school related to fear of failure. | Courtney will verbalize the source of fear. | Help the student voice and identify fears and anxieties, as well as the source of the anxiety, such as conflict with a teacher or fear of failing at a vocal music competition.<br><br>Assist Courtney in identifying her positive attributes and talents. | Courtney will attend classes on a daily basis. |

| Assessment Data | Nursing Diagnosis | Goals | Nursing Interventions | Expected Outcomes |
|---|---|---|---|---|
| Frequent health office visits, interfering with class attendance. | Health-seeking behavior related to somatic complaints. | The student will decrease use of the health room as an avoidance behavior.<br><br>The student will experience fewer physical symptoms associated with anxiety. | Negotiate with the student to limit health room visits that interfere with classroom attendance—limiting visits to before school, during break or lunch time, or after school as appropriate, unless emergency situation.<br><br>Recognize and praise the student's efforts to adopt and maintain appropriate coping mechanisms. | Courtney will decrease frequency of visits to the health office and experience a decrease in physical symptoms associated with anxiety. |
| Frequent complaints of headache, diaphoresis, and nausea when Courtney attends school. | Acute pain related to physiologic response to anxiety and fear. | Courtney accurately describes physical symptoms of anxiety. | Discuss with parents the need for a thorough physical examination to rule out acute or chronic illness as cause of pain; assist parents in finding medical resources, if necessary.<br><br>Follow up on the results of the physical examination and make appropriate school IHP plan, to addresses the health needs of the student and support school attendance.<br><br>Meet with the student's teachers, counselors, and administrators to implement the team's plan for improving the student's attendance pattern, including that in the case of health office visits, physical symptoms will be assessed and treated, returning student to class in a timely manner | Courtney will describe physiologic responses to anxiety and fear.<br><br>Courtney experiences a decrease in painful physical symptoms associated with anxiety. |

| Assessment Data | Nursing Diagnosis | Goals | Nursing Interventions | Expected Outcomes |
|---|---|---|---|---|
| Parents state that Courtney has always been a "perfect child." They are frustrated that Courtney engages in school refusal behavior. | Interrupted family processes related to unrealistic parental expectations, conflict between parent and child, and stress of poor attendance on family roles. | Courtney will identify stressors in family processes that result in school refusal behaviors. | Set up ongoing communication with the student's parents and private therapist (if applicable) to discuss the school refusal problem and effectiveness of school-based interventions and home-based interventions. Develop relationships with other school- and/or community-based professionals to provide a team-based approach for working with the student and parents. Refer the student and family to community-based support services as appropriate. | Parents accept that a school refusal problem exists. Parents consistently apply consequences when Courtney engages in school refusal behavior. Courtney engages in school refusal behavior. Courtney's parents access appropriate healthcare resources to support, treat, and care for their child and themselves. |
| Courtney's grades are currently below her previous academic performance. | Ineffective role performance related to ineffective coping skills. | Courtney will improve school attendance and participate in classroom activities. | Meet with the student's teachers, counselors, and administrators to implement the team's plan for improving the student's attendance pattern, including facilitation of a reward system for the student that includes classroom attendance, participation, and completion of assignments. | Courtney returns to her previous level of academic success. |
| Courtney's friends report that she has "dropped out" of their peer group. | Impaired social interaction related to poor school attendance resulting in limited opportunities for age-appropriate social interaction. | Courtney participates in school activities, which increases her interaction with peers. | Collaborate with faculty members to identify the student's interests and talents, as well as appropriate school activities, programs, or clubs that will increase peer-to-peer interaction and assist in developing friendships. | Courtney will utilize school and community resources to assist in reducing school refusal behaviors. Courtney increases her interactions with peers and develops age-appropriate relationships. |

# References

American Psychiatric Association. (2000). *Diagnosis and statistical manual of mental disorders text revision* (4th ed., text revision). [CD ROM]. Washington, DC: Author.

Antai-Otong, D. (2003). *Psychiatric nursing: Biological & behavioral concepts.* Clifton Park, NY: Delmar Learning.

Brand, C., & O'Connor, L. (2004). School refusal: It takes a team. [Electronic version]. *Children and Schools, 26,* 54–64. Retrieved February 14, 2004, from ProQuest Nursing Journals database. http://proquest.umi.com/pqd-web?index=4&sid=2&srchmode=3&vinst=PROD&fmt=6&startpage=-1&clientid=66947&vname=PQD&RQT=309&did=523461271&scaling=FULL&ts=1115408687&vtype=PQD&aid=1&rqt=309&TS=1115408696&clientId=66947

Jellinek, M., Patel, B. P., & Froehle, M. C. (Eds.), (2002). *Bright futures in practice: Mental health.* Georgetown University Arlington, VA: National Center for Education in Maternal and Child Health.

NANDA International. (2003). *Nursing diagnoses: Definitions & classification 2003–2004.* Philadelphia: Author.

Schor, E. L. (1999). *Caring for your school-age child: Ages 5–12.* New York: Bantam. Available from American Academy of Pediatrics at http://www.aap.org/pubed/ZZZXEV1OQ7C.htm?&sub_cat=1

Wimmer M. B. (2003). *School refusal: Assessment & intervention within school setting.* Bethesda, MD: National Association of School Psychologists. Available from http://www.nasponline.org/bestsellers/schoolrefusal.html

# Bibliography

Adelman, H., & Taylor, L. (1997–2000). *Nursing assessment of school age youth. Psychosocial screening* (Home Study Module Number 3). Scarsborogh, ME: National Association of School Nurses.

Bergren, M. D. (2002). Child and adolescent mental health Web resources. *Journal of School Nursing, 18*(4), 226–228.

Denehy, J. (2002). The mental health needs of children and adolescents. *Journal of School Nursing, 18*(4), 189–190.

DeSocio, J., Hootman, J. (2004). Children's mental health and school success. *Journal of School Nursing, 20*(4), 189–196.

Hootman, J., Houck, G. M., & King, M. C. (2002). A program to educate school nurses about mental health interventions. *Journal of School Nursing, 18*(4), 191–195.

National Association of School Nurses. (n.d.). *Addressing the mental health needs of children and adolescence* [Education Program]. Retrieved November 7, 2004, from http://nasn.org/education/education.htm

National Association of School Nurses. (2000). *Issue Brief: Mental health and illness.* Scarborough, ME: Author.

National Association of School Nurses. (Revised 2000). *Position Statement: Mental health of students.* Scarborough, ME: Author.

*Psychosocial screening* (Home Study Module Number 3). Scarborough, ME: National Association of School Nurses.

# Resources

American Academy of Pediatrics
141 Northwest Point Boulevard
   Elk Grove Village, IL 60007-1098
   847-434-4000
   847-434-8000 (fax)
www.aap.org

Bright Futures Project
   Georgetown University
Box 571272
   Washington, DC 20057-1272
202-784-9556
   202-784-9777 (fax)
www.brightfutures.org

National Association of School Psychologists
4340 East West Highway
Suite 402
Bethesda, MD 20814
301-657-0270
http://www.nasponline.org/

National Center for Education in Maternal and Child
   Health
Georgetown University
Box 571272
Washington, DC 20057-1272
202-784-9770
www.ncemch.org

## Chapter Sixty-five

# Scoliosis

Sally Zentner Schoessler

## Introduction

Scoliosis is a condition that results from alterations in a child's spinal alignment. It is the most common spinal deformity (Wong, Hockenberry-Eaton, Wilson, Winkelstein, & Kline, 2003). The child is typically an otherwise healthy child, and the spinal curvature is usually an isolated health concern. The cause of scoliosis is unknown, although it can be congenital, secondary to an underlying neuromuscular disorder, or a compensatory disorder resulting from a discrepancy in the lengths of the child's legs (Behrmann & Klingman, 2004).

## Pathophysiology

Scoliosis is defined as a curvature of the spine (Children's Hospital, 2005). Although the exact cause of the condition is unknown, the primary age at onset of scoliosis is between 10 and 15 years, and 2% to 3% of the population of the United States are affected. There is an increased incidence in young females, who are also more prone to having the problem progress to the point that treatment will be required. Some cause for concern also exists if there is a family history of spinal abnormalities. Heredity plays a part in the diagnostic process, because approximately 20% of children with scoliosis have a family member who has scoliosis (Children's Hospital, 2005). There are few complications with scoliosis; however, respiratory function may be impacted if the curvature is severe.

Scoliosis can be classified into two types—structural and functional—each with unique characteristics. It is very important that the child is carefully examined to determine the origin and severity of the spinal curvature as well as how the condition impacts the child's general health and mobility. Diagnosis is made by direct observation of the child's exposed back and by radiographic evaluation.

## Structural Scoliosis

### 1. *Idiopathic*

This is the most common form of scoliosis and is a painless disorder that is most commonly characterized by a right thoracic curve (Behrmann & Klingman, 2004). It occurs more often in children over the age of 10 (Wong, Hockenberry, Wilson, Winkelstein, Ahmann & Divito-Thomas, 1999) and is the form of scoliosis most often diagnosed following a positive finding from school screenings. Many idiopathic spinal deformities are nonprogressive and never advance to the stage where medical intervention is required.

### 2. *Congenital*

In congenital scoliosis, spinal abnormalities have their origin in the first trimester of fetal formation. The symptoms of spinal problems are evident early in the child's life. There can be a partial or complete curvature of the spine, and the scoliosis may be a single deformity or in combination with other bone or soft tissue anomalies. The risk for progression is dependent on many factors specific to the child's overall condition.

### 3. *Neuromuscular*

Neuromuscular scoliosis is caused by a muscle imbalance and is often only one factor involved with the child's disabilities. This category usually presents along with Duchenne's muscular dystrophy, cerebral palsy, or another significant health problem that is part of the child's overall condition (Behrmann & Klingman, 2004).

Students who are ambulatory tend to have a milder spinal deformity than those who are wheelchair-dependent. Students who are nonambulatory can suffer changes in their pulmonary function as a result of the drastic changes that their spinal curvature can cause. The treatment plan for this category of student should involve maintaining the student's current condition and preventing increased spinal abnormality.

### 4. *Neurofibromatosis*

Neurofibromatosis has many clinical facets, but the orthopedic complications, which usually appear early, include spinal deformities such as scoliosis. Additional orthopedic complications that are seen include congenital bowing and pseudoarthrosis of the tibia and the forearm, overgrowth phenomenon of the extremity, and soft tissue tumors (Crawford, 2002).

### 5. *Traumatic*

Trauma to the spine, including fracture, irradiation for treatment of a tumor, or surgical displacement, can also cause the condition (Wong et al., 2003).

### 6. Mesenchymal Disease

Congenital disorders, such as mesenchymal disease, dwarfism, and connective tissue and bone diseases can be responsible for spinal curvatures. Rheumatoid arthritis is an example of an acquired disorder responsible for a diagnosis of scoliosis (Wong et al., 2003).

### 7. Miscellaneous

Finally, a child may present with idiopathic spinal symptoms, for several other reasons: tumor, inflammation, nutritional deficit (rickets), metabolic (renal osteodystrophy), and intraspinal conditions (Wong et al., 2003).

## Functional Scoliosis

Functional scoliosis is caused by a nonspinal condition, such as unequal leg length. The curve is flexible, and correction is seen on bending or in compensating for the unequal leg length.

Some states require scoliosis screening for students annually (between 8 and 16 years of age), whereas other states do not make this the responsibility of the school's health services. There is some controversy as to whether or not the school nurse (or physical education department) should be using his or her time to screen for scoliosis. On the other hand, the school nurse is a valuable indi- vidual to be assessing questionable spinal curvatures because he or she has a high level of contact with the student and is able to identify and confirm students at risk for developing problems related to scoliosis.

## Therapeutic Management
### Nonoperative

Treatment for cases of scoliosis that are progressive may include the use of braces, or orthotics, which can be an effectual nonsurgical method of correcting a worsening spinal curve or serve to stabilize the spine. Orthotics, including use of the "Milwaukee brace" (which is to be worn 23 hours a day), can be effective, but the adolescent student often exhibits a low compliance level with this form of therapy. In cases where the scoliosis is caused by a specific condition, treatment of that underlying condition is necessary to correct the scoliosis.

### Operative

Several surgical methods can be employed to straighten and secure the spine. These often include the implantation of metal rods or a form of spinal fusion to correct the misalignment. Recovery time for these procedures varies and can impact the student's mobility and physical education and/or sports program for up to a full school year.

---

## Individualized Healthcare Plan

### Assessment
*History*
- Family history of scoliosis (Member of the family has been diagnosed with scoliosis)
- Age at which the alteration in the student's spine was first noticed
- Age at which the student was diagnosed with scoliosis
- Curve attributes: thoracic, lumbar, or sacral
- Presence of kyphosis (an accentuated backward rounding of the upper spine)
- Presence of lordosis (an accentuated forward curvature of the lower spine)
- Use of orthotics
- Surgical history
- Student's general health, especially symptoms related to scoliosis

*Current Status and Management*
- Current scoliosis findings: location of curve, kyphosis, lordosis, severity
- Skin integrity related to orthotics use, pressure points, preventative measures used
- Activity status: limitations, recommended exercise program

*Self-care*
- Student knowledge of scoliosis and scoliosis management plan
- Appropriate use orthosis
- Measures used to prevent skin breakdown if wearing a brace
- Ability to get into and out of orthotic independently, need for assistance
- Student's ability to self-monitor skin integrity

*Psychosocial Status*
- Student's perceptions of body and body image
- Student's feelings about the diagnosis of scoliosis

*Academic Issues*
- Physical education modifications
- Postsurgical homework assistance needed, modified school day
- Need for private physical education changing area, safe storage of orthosis
- Chair and desk modifications needed (orthosis comfort, proper alignment in postsurgical period)
- Need for homebound instruction (postsurgically)

## Nursing Diagnoses (N.D.) (NANDA, 2003)

**N.D. 1** Impaired physical mobility (NANDA 00085) related to:
- spinal alignment abnormalities and /or
- use of orthotic brace,
- spinal surgery,
- instrumentation

**N.D. 2** Disturbed body image (NANDA 00118) related to:
- defect in body structure
- pronounced spinal curves
- scarring from surgical procedures

**N.D. 3** Self-esteem disturbance (NANDA 00120) related to:
- visible spinal abnormalities
- potential long-term treatment of condition

**N.D. 4** Deficient knowledge (NANDA 00126) related to:
- pathophysiology
- scoliosis
- treatment plan

**N.D. 5** Risk for impaired skin integrity (NANDA 00046) related to orthotic brace.

## Goals

The student will retain or attain maximum level of physical mobility with classroom/school modifications in activities as needed. (N.D. 1)

The student will participate in physical education classes and sports with modifications as needed. (N.D. 1)

The student will demonstrate use of orthotic and describe its therapeutic value. (N.D. 1)

The student will express feelings about his/her body. (N.D. 2, 3)

The student will express feelings about how his/her scoliosis affects his/her feelings about self. (N.D. 3)

The student will demonstrate understanding of scoliosis and treatment modalities. (N.D. 4)

The student will demonstrate understanding of his/her scoliosis treatment plan. (N.D. 4)

The student will demonstrate understanding of use of orthotics and/or appropriate surgical procedures. (N.D. 4)

The student will demonstrate methods to prevent skin irritation and breakdown with use of orthotic brace. (N.D. 5)

## Nursing Interventions

Screen student, as agreed upon with parent and physician, to assess condition of spine and/or curvature. (N.D. 1)

Assist parent and student to access their healthcare provider as needed for assessment of positive screening findings. (N.D. 1)

Communicate with healthcare provider, with parental permission, to document treatment plan and prognosis for student's condition. (N.D. 1)

Encourage student to identify and discuss activities that are difficult and/or strenuous for him/her due to spinal abnormalities. (N.D. 1)

Encourage student to identify and discuss activities that are difficult and/or strenuous for him/her due to limitations from use of orthotics. (N.D. 1)

Encourage student to identify and discuss activities that are difficult and/or strenuous for him/her due to limitations due to spinal surgery instrumentation. (N.D. 1)

Encourage student to identify and discuss activities that are pleasurable and manageable for him/her. (N.D. 1)

Encourage student to identify and discuss activities that are pleasurable and manageable for him/her even with the use of orthotics. (N.D. 1)

Collaborate with physical education teachers to modify physical education activities as needed per activity limitations by physician. (N.D. 1)

Arrange for extra books as needed so the student does not have to carry books to class or home. (N.D. 1)

Arrange for early release between classes and at the end of the day (for 2 to 4 weeks) following surgery to avoid getting bumped or pushed in the hallway. (N.D. 1)

Arrange for use of elevator, as needed. (N.D. 1)

Assist in arranging for homebound services, as needed, following surgery. (N.D. 1)

Encourage student to verbalize feelings about body image and self as related to scoliosis. (N.D. 2, 3)

Encourage student to verbalize feelings about body image and self as related to use of orthotic brace. (N.D. 2, 3)

Encourage student to write a journal to record his/her feelings about his/her condition and treatment and how it relates to his/her life. (N.D. 2, 3)

Encourage student to share his/her understanding of his/her condition and treatment with his/her parents and the school nurse. (N.D. 4)

Assist student and parents to understand the scoliosis management plan appropriate to age and level of understanding. (N.D. 4)
- Screening procedure
- Screening results
- Pathophysiology of scoliosis
- Treatment options
- Personal treatment plan
- Use of orthotics prescribed and self-care as related to their use (if appropriate)
- Surgical procedures and recovery process (if appropriate)

Discuss school scoliosis management plan with parents, as needed. (N.D. 4)

Review and revise school scoliosis management plan as needed with parents and student to provide a unified approach to management. (N.D. 4)

Discuss with student and parent the need to monitor skin integrity and proper care of areas of skin irritation. (N.D. 5)

Assist student to notify parents of any alteration in skin integrity related to orthotic use. (N.D. 5)

## Expected Student Outcomes

The student will:
- Attend classes regularly without absences related to scoliosis symptoms. (N.D. 1)
- Participate in classroom and school activities with modifications made as needed. (N.D. 1)
- Participate in regular physical education classes with modifications in activities as needed. (N.D. 1)
- Use orthotic with 100% reliability as prescribed. (N.D. 1)
- Demonstrate proper use of his/her orthotic. (N.D. 1, 4)
- Verbalize feelings about body image. (N.D. 2)
- Write feelings about body image. (N.D. 2)
- Verbalize positive feelings about himself/herself and what he/she is capable of doing well. (N.D. 3)
- Write positive feelings about himself/herself and what he/she is capable of doing well. (N.D. 3)
- Accurately describe what scoliosis is. (N.D. 4)
- Demonstrate appropriate self-limitation of activities based on scoliosis management plan in physical education classes/sports activities. (N.D. 4)
- Accurately describe his/her treatment plan. (N.D. 4)
- Describe, to the school nurse, any changes made in the treatment plan. (N.D. 4)
- Describe methods utilized to prevent skin breakdown (when using the orthotic). (N.D. 4)
- Explain any surgical procedure(s) that he/she has undergone or will undergo. (N.D. 4)
- Describe the postoperative course he/she can expect to experience. (N.D. 4)
- Express his/her concerns about upcoming scoliosis treatments. (N.D. 4)
- Experience minimal skin breakdown due to proper use of orthotic brace. (N.D. 5)
- Experience minimal skin breakdown due to early identification and intervention. (N.D. 5)
- Report skin irritation problems to his/her parents or school nurse, upon occurrence. (N.D. 5)
- Assist in preventing skin breakdown. (N.D. 5)

# Case Study

Stephanie Blake is a 16-year-old girl who underwent several surgeries at ages 5 months and 18 months to repair a cleft lip and palate, as well as surgery at 14 months to remove and repair her toes. She continues to have minimal facial scarring from these surgeries but is a student who is bright and quick to smile despite her ongoing health concerns.

Stephanie was screened annually for scoliosis from age 8 until the current time. Her screening results were negative until age 12, at which time the school nurse found her to have an 8- to 9-degree thoracic spinal curvature using a scoliometer. A referral was sent home and returned with the report that an orthopedic scoliosis specialist had already seen her after the curvature was noticed by her healthcare provider at her seventh-grade physical. She has had a series of x-rays as well as a computed tomographic scan. At the time of examination, the specialist stated that no restrictions on her activity were indicated but that she would be followed up and evaluated for possible surgical intervention. Her parents indicated that they would be seeking a second and third opinion in the coming months.

In the summer preceding this school year, Stephanie underwent surgery to have a full metal rod inserted along her spine. She has been recuperating in a brace and can expect to wear the brace for 2 to 4 months. Her surgeon has requested no physical education classes or sports for the full school year. Stephanie should also avoid lifting heavy objects. It has been arranged to issue her three sets of books so that she will not need to carry any textbooks. She may use the stairs, but an elevator pass has been issued for use as she feels the need.

## Scoliosis

| Assessment Data | Nursing Diagnosis | Goals | Nursing Interventions | Expected Outcomes |
|---|---|---|---|---|
| Stephanie has difficulty ambulating and maneuvering with brace in place at school. | Impaired physical mobility related to spinal alignment abnormalities and/or use of orthotic brace. | Stephanie will retain or attain maximum level of physical mobility with classroom/school modifications in activities as needed.<br><br>Stephanie will demonstrate use of orthotic and describe its therapeutic value. | Communicate with healthcare provider, with parental permission, to document treatment plan and prognosis for Stephanie's condition.<br><br>Encourage Stephanie to identify and discuss activities that are difficult and/or strenuous for her due to limitations from use of orthotics.<br><br>Encourage Stephanie to identify and discuss activities that are pleasurable and manageable for her.<br><br>Collaborate with physical education teachers to modify physical education activities as needed per activity limitations by physician.<br><br>Arrange for extra books as needed so that Stephanie does not have to carry books to class or home.<br><br>Arrange for use of elevator, as needed. | Stephanie will attend classes regularly without absences related to scoliosis symptoms.<br><br>Stephanie will participate in classroom and school activities with modifications made as needed.<br><br>Stephanie will participate in regular physical education classes with modifications in activities as needed.<br><br>Stephanie accurately describes why her orthotic is needed and how it is helping therapeutically.<br><br>Stephanie will use orthotic with 100% reliability as prescribed. |
| Stephanie has had numerous surgeries with resulting scarring. | Disturbed body image related to scarring from surgical procedures. | Stephanie will express feelings about her body. | Encourage Stephanie to verbalize feelings about body image and self as related to scoliosis. | Stephanie will verbalize feelings about body image.<br><br>Stephanie will write down her feelings about body image. |

| Assessment Data | Nursing Diagnosis | Goals | Nursing Interventions | Expected Outcomes |
|---|---|---|---|---|
| | | | Encourage Stephanie to write a journal to record her feelings about her condition and treatment and how it relates to her life. | |
| | | | Encourage Stephanie to verbalize feelings about body image and self as related to use of orthotic brace. | |
| Stephanie occasionally asks questions about treatment plan. | Deficient knowledge related to pathophysiology, scoliosis, and treatment plan. | Stephanie will demonstrate understanding of her scoliosis treatment plan.<br><br>Stephanie will demonstrate understanding of use of orthotics and/or recent surgical procedures. | Encourage Stephanie to share her understanding of her condition and treatment with her parents and the school nurse<br><br>Assist Stephanie and parents to understand the scoliosis management plan appropriate to age and level of understanding.<br><br>Review and revise school scoliosis management plan as needed with parents and Stephanie to provide a unified approach to management. | Stephanie will accurately describe her treatment plan.<br><br>Stephanie will describe, to the school nurse, any changes made in the treatment plan.<br><br>Stephanie will demonstrate proper use of her orthotic.<br><br>Stephanie will describe methods utilized to prevent skin breakdown when using the orthotic.<br><br>Stephanie will explain the surgical procedure that she has undergone.<br><br>Stephanie will describe the postoperative course she can expect to experience. |

# References

Behrmann, R. E., & Klingman, R. M. (2004). *Nelson essentials of pediatrics.* (17th ed.). Philadelphia: Saunders.

Children's Hospital, Oakland, CA. (2005). *Scoliosis treatment.* Retrieved May 18,2005, from http://www.scoliosisrx.com

Crawford, A. (2002). *Neurofibromatosis.* Retrieved August 29, 2004, from http://www.emedicine.com/orthoped/topic525.htm

NANDA International. *(2003). Nursing diagnoses: Definitions & classification 2003–2004.* Philadelphia: Author.

Wong, D., Hockenberry, M., Wilson, D., Winkelstein, M., Ahmann, E., & DiVito-Thomas, P. (1999). *Whaley & Wong's nursing care of infants and children* (6th ed.). St. Louis, MO: Elsevier

Wong, D. L., Hockenberry-Eaton, M., Wilson, D., Winkelstein, M. L., & Kline, N. E. (2003). *Whaley and Wong's nursing care of infants and children.* (6th ed.). St. Louis, MO: Mosby.

## Bibliography

Beers, M. (2003). *Merck manual of medical information* (2nd home ed.). Whitehouse Station, NY: Merck.

Bell, S., Calandra, J., & Snowden, L. (2000). *Mosby's pediatric nursing reference* (5th ed.). St. Louis, MO: Mosby.

Bowen, J. R., Keeler, K. A., & Pelegie, S. (2001). Adolescent idiopathic scoliosis managed by a nighttime bending brace. *Orthopedics, 24*(10), 967–970.

Donnelly, M. J., Dolan, L. A., Grande, L., & Weinstein, S. L. (2004). Patient and parent perspectives on treatment for adolescent idiopathic scoliosis. *Iowa Orthopaedic Journal, 24,* 76–83.

Dutton, M. (2004). *Orthopaedic examination, evaluation and intervention.* New York: McGraw Hill.

Litin, S. (2003). *Mayo Clinic family health book* (3rd ed.). New York: Harper.

MedHelp International. *What is scoliosis? And how is it treated?* Retrieved September 20, 2003, from http://www.medhelp.org/lib/scolio.htm

Nettina, S. (2001). *Lippincott manual of nursing practice* (7th ed.). Philadelphia: Lippincott, Williams & Wilkins.

Reichel, D., & Schanz, J. (2003). Developmental psychological aspects of scoliosis treatment. *Pediatric Rehabilitation 6*(3-4), 221–225.

Vandal S., Rivard C. H., & Bradet R. (1999). Measuring the compliance behavior of adolescents wearing orthopedic braces. *Issues in Comprehensive Pediatric Nursing, 22*(2–3), 59–73.

## Resources

National Scoliosis Foundation
5 Cabot Place
Stoughton, MA 02072
1-800-673-6922
NSF@scoliosis.org
www.scoliosis.org
Biannual newsletter: *The Spinal Connection*

Scoliosis Research Society
611 East Wells Street
Milwaukee, WI 53202-3892
1-414-289-9107
tjackson@execinc.com
www.srs.org

*Chapter Sixty-six*

# Seizures

Sarah Kiel and Elisabeth Barclay

## Introduction

Seizures are neurologic events that may be idiopathic or may be acquired at any time during a person's life span. The incidence of epilepsy in childhood is 100 to 200 in 100,000 (Hauser, 2001), and approximately 315,000 schoolchildren through the age of 14 have epilepsy (Epilepsy Foundation of America, 2004a). It is estimated that 5% of the U.S. population will have one seizure by the age of 20 (Hauser, 2001). There is a 1% overall risk of developing epilepsy in childhood and adolescence (Annegers, 2001). Children with neurodevelopmental disorders such as autism, cerebral palsy, and mental retardation have an increased risk of developing epilepsy (O'Dell, 2004a). The specific etiologies of hypoxic brain injury that may result in cerebral palsy and mental retardation may also contribute significantly to the risk of seizure disorders; these include stroke (e.g., intrauterine, sickle cell, vascular lesion), head trauma, infection (meningitis, encephalitis, congenital cytomegalovirus, etc.), and brain tumors (National Institutes of Health, 2000).

Approximately 50% of all people who have a seizure will have it during their school years, and an estimated 120,000 children will have their first convulsion before the age of 18 (Epilepsy Foundation of America, 2004a). Therefore the potential exists for students with no known seizure disorder to have a first seizure while in the school setting.

The following terms are associated with seizures:

*Aura:* a feeling or sensation that occurs just prior to the onset of a known seizure. Level of awareness (consciousness) is not altered in the aura.

*Automatism:* an automatic, nonpurposeful behavior that occurs in the course of a seizure. Examples: lip smacking, chewing, eye blinking, picking at clothes or random objects, wandering (Arunkumar, Kotagal, & Rothner, 2001).

*Impairment in consciousness:* an alteration in a child's awareness, any change from the student's usual baseline behavior. There does not need to be a state of unconsciousness before an impairment in consciousness is recognized (Arunkumar et al., 2001).

*Todd's paralysis:* the sustained weakness of the involved side after the seizure resolution. Duration may be minutes to days (Arunkumar et al., 2001).

## Pathophysiology

Seizures are the result of abnormal or excessive electrical activity within the neurons of the cerebral cortex. O'Dell (2004a, p. 11) has defined seizures as "sudden and stereotyped alterations in motor activity, sensation, behavior, or consciousness" and epilepsy as "the chronic neurological condition characterized by recurrent epileptic seizures unprovoked by systemic neurological insults." The underlying cause of seizures can be quite variable and include hypoxic injury (perinatal or vascular insult, near drowning), tumor, infection, traumatic brain injury, metabolic disorders, and genetic malformations of cortical development (Annegers, 2001). Idiopathic seizures are those with no known cause (Arunkumar et al., 2001). Comorbid neurodevelopmental disorders, such as cerebral palsy and mental retardation, are thought to put children at a higher risk for developing epilepsy (Annegers).

Most seizures are self-limiting and spontaneously resolve within 2 to 3 minutes (Shinnar, Berg, Moshe, & Shinnar, 2001). Clinical manifestations of seizures reflect the location within the cortex in which they originate (Arunkumar et al., 2001).

Seizures may be nonrecurrent (acute) or recurrent (chronic) and can be provoked by various factors. Common seizure triggers include illness, sleep deprivation, fatigue, menses, bright and/or flashing lights (photic stimulation), stress, and noncompliance with medication (O'Dell, 2004a). Anticonvulsants are usually prescribed on the basis of a child's weight; therefore, a rapidly growing student may easily outgrow a therapeutic dose. If there is an otherwise unexplained increase in seizure activity, this should be taken into consideration.

Reflex epilepsies are less common but include seizures that can be provoked by thinking (particularly arithmetic), reading, speaking, writing, listening to music, isolated body movements, eating, and being startled (Zifkin & Andermann, 2001).

## Seizure Classification

The current classification of seizures was last revised in 1989 by the International League Against Epilepsy (ILEA,1989). Seizures are classified into two types, partial and generalized (**Table 1**). The terminology is defined and the epilepsy syndromes common in children and adolescents are described in **Tables 2** and **3**.

**Table 1. Classification of Seizures**

| Partial | Generalized (Primary generalized) | |
|---|---|---|
| Simple partial<br>Complex partial<br>Secondary generalized | Absence<br>Atonic<br>Clonic | Myoclonic<br>Tonic<br>Tonic-clonic |

**Table 2. Seizure Classification Definitions**

| | |
|---|---|
| **I. Partial** | A seizure with its onset within one cerebral hemisphere (Arunkumar et al.,2001) |
| 1. Simple partial | Most commonly presents as sensory or motor involvement without impairment in consciousness. Clinical symptoms are usually confined to one side of the body. Example: tingling or burning sensation limited to right arm or progressive to entire right side of body. An aura, often called a warning, is the particular sensation that occurs just prior to a seizure that involves an alteration in consciousness. Auras are simple partial seizures. Example: déjà vu, nausea, or other gustatory sensation is frequently associated with temporal lobe seizures. (Arunkumar et al., 2001) |
| 2. Complex partial | Sensory and/or motor seizure with alteration in awareness. May include behavioral arrest, blank staring, or automatisms. May progress into a secondary generalized tonic-clonic seizure (Arunkumar et al., 2001). Formerly referred to as "psychomotor" or "temporal lobe" seizures. |
| 3. Secondary generalized tonic-clonic | A partial seizure that evolves into tonic-clonic activity on both sides of the body (Arunkumar et al., 2001; Dreifuss & Nordli, 2001) |
| **II. Generalized** | Seizures involving both cerebral hemispheres simultaneously at onset. First clinical sign may be alteration in awareness. Primary generalized seizures include: absence, atonic, myoclonic, tonic, clonic, and tonic-clonic. (Dreifuss & Nordli, 2001) |
| 1. Absence | Episodes of behavioral arrest and prolonged staring. May be associated with automatisms. May be provoked by hyperventilation. Children with absence seizures may be accused of daydreaming. Occasionally still referred to as petit mal seizures. (Dreifuss & Nordli, 2001) |
| 2. Atonic | Loss of tone. Also called "drop attacks." Falls resulting from these seizures are a frequent cause of facial injury. Can be quite recalcitrant to medical therapies. (Farrell, 2001) |
| 3. Clonic | Rapid jerking of single or multiple extremities. (Dreifuss & Nordli, 2001) |
| 4. Myoclonic | Quick, sudden, brief jerks. (Dreifuss & Nordli, 2001) |
| 5. Tonic | Stiffening of single or multiple extremities. (Dreifuss & Nordli, 2001) |
| 6. Tonic-clonic | A seizure episode with loss of consciousness and intervals of symmetrical stiffness and jerking (tonic-clonic activity) of all extremities. May include bladder and/or bowel incontinence (Fisch & Olejniczak, 2001). Occasionally still referred to as grand mal seizure or convulsion. |

**Table 3. Epilepsy Syndromes and Seizure Types Common in School-Aged Children and Adolescents**

| | |
|---|---|
| **Benign rolandic epilepsy** | Age at onset is between 3 and 13 years, with peak age at onset being 9 to 10. Seizures in this syndrome are resolved by age 15. Seizures occur most frequently during sleep, typically start as a partial seizure with sensory symptoms, but may evolve into generalized tonic-clonic seizure. Has diagnostic EEG pattern. (Dreifuss & Nordli, 2001) |
| **Childhood absence epilepsy** | A primary generalized seizure type. Onset is typically in school-aged children. More frequent in females than males. Staring episodes usually occur daily. Seizures may remit in adolescence. (Dreifuss & Nordli, 2001; O'Dell, 2004a) |
| **Gelastic seizures** | A subclass of partial seizures that presents as unprovoked laughing episodes. Usually not accompanied by feelings of mirth. Often mistaken for inappropriate behavior. (Arzimanoglou, Guerrini, & Aicardi, 2004) |
| **Febrile seizures** | Convulsive episodes associated with acute febrile illness, typically occurring in children from 6 months to 5 years of age (Shinnar & O'Dell, 2004). The most common cause of status epilepticus in children (Shinnar et al., 2001). |
| **Juvenile absence epilepsy** | Similar to childhood absence epilepsy but with an onset closer to puberty. Absence episodes are more sporadic than in childhood absence. May be associated with generalized tonic-clonic seizure. Occurs equally in males and females. (Dreifuss & Nordli, 2001) |
| **Juvenile myoclonic epilepsy** | A primary generalized epilepsy that begins in childhood or early adulthood and is characterized by early morning myoclonic seizures. Also includes generalized tonic-clonic and absence seizures. Children are typically of normal development and intelligence. This syndrome usually responds well to treatment with valproic acid/valproate. (Dreifuss & Nordli, 2001) |
| **Landau-Kleffner syndrome** | Seizures associated with a progressive inability to process receptive or expressive speech. May also be associated with behavioral disturbances. Some children may have noticeable partial seizures (e.g., motor involvement) in addition to the difficulties in language processing that characterize this syndrome. (Dreifuss & Nordli, 2001) |
| **Lennox-Gastaut syndrome** | Onset is usually in early childhood and is defined by a characteristic pattern on EEG. Children have multiple seizure types, including atonic, myoclonic, generalized tonic-clonic seizures, absence and partial seizures. The atonic seizures typically occur numerous times daily, and the resulting falls have the potential to be particularly dangerous to these cognitively impaired children. (Dreifuss & Nordli, 2001) |

EEG, electroencephalogram.

## Comorbidities in Childhood Epilepsy

The occurrence of comorbid disorders is higher in children with epilepsy than in the general pediatric population. These disorders include attention deficit hyperactivity disorder, behavioral disorders, learning disorders, depression, mental retardation/cognitive impairment, and cerebral palsy (O'Dell, 2004a; Pellock, 2004c; Austin et al., 2002). As previously discussed, children with cognitive impairment or cerebral palsy have an increased risk of developing seizures (Annegers, 2001).

## Status Epilepticus

In 1981, the ILEA defined status epilepticus as "a seizure that persists for a sufficient length of time or is repeated frequently enough that recovery between attacks does not occur" (ILEA, 1989). Status epilepticus is a medical emergency that requires prompt intervention. Children are at a higher risk of developing status epilepticus than adults; most children who present to the emergency department in convulsive status epilepticus do not have a history of epilepsy (DeLorenzo et al., 1996).

Most convulsive seizures are self-limiting and resolve within 2 to 3 minutes, with nearly all stopping by 5 minutes. A *prolonged seizure* is one that lasts longer than 5 to 10 minutes (Shinnar et al., 2001). *Acute repetitive seizures*, also called cluster seizures, occur in such a frequency that there is insufficient time for recovery in between (Mitchell et al., 1999; Kriel et al., 1999).

## Management

An overview of available treatment options for seizure disorders is provided, including antiepileptic drugs (AEDs), the ketogenic diet, the vagus nerve stimulator (VNS), and epilepsy surgery. It should be noted that prior to the arrival of automated external defibrillators, *AED* has long been the preferred abbreviation for *antiepileptic drugs* in neuroscience and the field of epilepsy (even commonly used by the National Institutes of Health and National Institutes of Neurological Disorders and Stroke). There are no plans at the current time to alter this practice. In this chapter, *AED* is the abbreviation for *antiepileptic drugs*.

### Medications

Many AEDs have U.S. Food and Drug Administration (FDA) indication for adjunctive therapy in the use of partial seizures in people 12 years of age and older and are used off-label in younger children. This reflects the practice of pharmaceutical clinical trials rather than specific difficulties or contraindications with any of these drugs in younger populations. All of the anticonvulsants presented in this chapter are standard in the armamentarium used in the medical treatment of children with seizure disorders. A table with more detailed discussion of the most commonly used anticonvulsant medications is included as the Appendix.

Of note, several AEDs have the potential for idiosyncratic rash that may evolve into life-threatening Stevens-Johnson syndrome. This rash usually presents within the first 2 to 8 weeks of starting a new drug, although it can occur with prolonged treatment as well. Any rash in children taking anticonvulsants warrants prompt evaluation by the child's primary care provider or prescribing neurologist. AEDs most likely to cause a rash include carbamazepine, lamotrigine, oxcarbazepine, and phenytoin. Of course, this does not exclude the possibility of rash occurring as a result of other anticonvulsants or for other reasons common in childhood (Sharp & Wilder, 2001).

Diastat (diazepam rectal gel) has the FDA indication for the treatment of acute recurrent or prolonged seizures outside of the hospital setting, making it the only rescue medication approved for use by nonlicensed caregivers (Pellock, 2004b) (Table 4). Other treatment options (e.g., intravenous diazepam or lorazepam) require administration by licensed personnel, typically in an acute care setting (e.g., hospital or emergency medical services [EMS]). Local school districts, as well as individual state boards of nursing and education, may regulate the administration of Diastat in the school setting (Kiel, 2004).

**Table 4. Dosing Chart for Diastat (diazepam rectal gel)**

| 2 to 5 years 0.5 mg/kg | | | 6 to 11 years 0.3 mg/kg | | | ≥12 years 0.2 mg/kg | | |
|---|---|---|---|---|---|---|---|---|
| Weight (kg) | Weight (lb) | Dose (mg) | Weight (kg) | Weight (lb) | Dose (mg) | Weight (kg) | Weight (lb) | Dose (mg) |
| 6-11 | 13-24 | 5 | 10-18 | 22-40 | 5 | 14-27 | 31-60 | 5 |
| 12-22 | 25-50 | 10 | 19-37 | 41-82 | 10 | 28-50 | 61-110 | 10 |
| 23-33 | 51-73 | 15 | 38-55 | 83-121 | 15 | 51-75 | 111-166 | 15 |
| 34-44 | 74-97 | 20 | 56-74 | 122-163 | 20 | 76-111 | 167-245 | 20 |

Adapted from *Seizure Emergencies: Are You Prepared?* [Patient education material], 2003. Xcel Pharmaceuticals.

## Ketogenic Diet

The ketogenic diet is a nonpharmacologic option for the treatment of intractable epilepsy. It is prescribed by a physician and overseen by a registered dietitian experienced in its management. The diet is high in fat and low in carbohydrates and protein, forcing the body to convert its primary source of metabolism from carbohydrates to fats. One of the by-products of fat metabolism is ketones, and the presence of excessive ketones produces ketosis (the metabolic state of using fat for energy). Ketosis that results from the ketogenic diet has an anticonvulsant effect. Potential side effects of the ketogenic diet include hypoglycemia, dehydration, renal stones, osteoporosis, and thinning of hair (Nordli & De Vivo, 2001). Best, Franz, Gilbert, Nelson, and Epstein (2000) have reported some cardiac complications in children on the diet, including prolonged Q-T interval and cardiac enlargement. The diet should be treated as an antiepileptic drug in regard to compliance. It should be stopped gradually because abrupt discontinuation, or sudden administration of glucose, may provoke seizures and even induce status epilepticus (Nordli & De Vivo, 2001).

## Vagus Nerve Stimulator

The VNS is a device used in the treatment of seizures that have been refractory to medications. Approved by the FDA in 1997 for use in partial seizures in patients 12 years of age and older, in practice VNS is also commonly used to treat all seizure types in children as young as 6 months of age. VNS is a two-piece system that is implanted by a surgeon (i.e. neurosurgeon, an otolaryngologist, or cardiothoracic surgeon).

Similar in size to a cardiac pacemaker, the device's generator is implanted in the left upper quadrant of the chest just below the clavicle, anterior to the axilla. The surgeon works within the carotid sheath to place the electrode coils around the vagus nerve via an incision on the left lateral neck. An insulated lead wire is tunneled under the skin and plugged into the generator, connecting the two parts.

The generator is set to deliver preprogrammed cycles of electrical stimulation to the vagus nerve at intervals ranging from less than 1 second to every 30 minutes. These delivery parameters are set by the treating neurologist using a programming wand and hand-held or laptop computer. The settings cannot be changed without deliberate intent.

The mechanism of action for the VNS is not clearly understood. It is theorized that the electrical stimulation delivered via the left vagus nerve (cranial nerve X) serves to desynchronize epileptiform activity and, over time, provides an overall inhibitory effect on seizures. Only the left vagus nerve is used, because its afferent nerve fibers transmit visceral sensory information to the central nervous system. The remaining 20% of afferent fibers primarily innervate the gastrointestinal system. The fibers of the right vagus nerve innervate the heart and are responsible for the vasovagal response and associated bradycardia (Valencia, Holder, Helmers, Madsen, & Riviello, 2001).

Side effects of the VNS are often transient and most commonly related to the dose of stimulation the patient receives. These include hoarse voice, coughing, shortness of breath, and a tingling sensation in the neck generally synchronized with the delivery of stimulation (Valencia et al., 2001).

The third component of treatment with VNS is the small, hand-held magnet. In addition to the continuous stimulation provided by the implanted generator, the VNS magnet gives the student or caregiver an external mode of control in the event of an acute seizure or seizure cluster. As such, it should be readily available for rapid use. Approximately the size of a large pencil eraser (3.5 cm X 6 cm X 1 cm), the magnet comes with a pager-type belt clip or a Velcro wristband. To abort an acute seizure episode, the magnet should be swiped slowly over the generator implanted in the left chest for 2 seconds to initiate an additional stimulation within the first few seconds after the onset of the seizure.

The goal of magnet use is to abort a seizure completely or to lessen its intensity, duration, and postictal recovery time. There are no side effects of using the VNS magnet; it can be used as often as necessary. It is recommended that the magnet not be stored near electronic data that may be erased (e.g., discs, credit cards). The VNS can be turned off in an emergency by holding the magnet in place over the device for 65 seconds. The magnet can be taped securely over the device, and the device will remain off until the magnet is removed (Valencia et al., 2001). Events that may warrant turning off the VNS device include direct trauma to the neck with subsequent pain consistent with the timing of stimulation cycles and severe, cyclical coughing, choking, or dyspnea consistent with stimulation cycles.

## Epilepsy Surgery

Many school-aged children and adolescents are being evaluated for and undergoing resective surgery for the treatment of their medically intractable seizures. These children have chronic seizures despite treatment with multiple medications. The comprehensive presurgical evaluation for epilepsy surgery candidates may require multiple, and possibly extended, school absences for these students. Once surgery is complete, these students will be absent for their recovery period (generally about 2 weeks) and then ease back in to school and their regular activities.

There are several neurosurgical options for the treatment of epilepsy, and the surgical approach is specifically tailored for each individual child and his or her needs (Harkness, 2001). The following section is a broad overview of techniques used in epilepsy surgery. In addition to the referenced sources, more detailed resources are available for further knowledge (Devinsky, 2002; Epilepsy Foundation of America, 2004c).

Focal resections concentrate on the removal of the smallest amount of cerebral cortex responsible for generating recurrent seizures. In multiple subpial transections, the epileptogenic horizontal nerve fibers are surgically disrupted without the removal of any cortical tissue (Wyler,

2001). Multiple subpial transections are often completed in combination with focal resections in areas of eloquent cortex (e.g., language, sensory, motor cortex) that would otherwise leave the child with a significant neurologic deficit if removed.

Hemispherectomy is an aggressive surgical approach reserved for a child with catastrophic partial epilepsy originating within the confines of one abnormal cerebral hemisphere. These children frequently present with neurologic impairment as a result of the seizing hemisphere (e.g., hemiparesis on the contralateral side or a visual field cut), so the disconnection of the seizing hemisphere is not likely to impart additional significant deficit. A functional hemispherectomy does not remove any tissue but disconnects the hemisphere, leaving it nonfunctional. This approach reduces the risk of hydrocephalus that is associated with a traditional hemispherectomy (Holthausen & Pieper, 2001).

Corpus callosotomy is the surgical separation of the corpus callosum, the large midline white matter fiber tract that connects the two cerebral hemispheres (Devinsky, 2002). The corpus callosum serves as the conduit for electrical impulses and transfer of information between the two hemispheres. In the case of generalized seizures, it also serves to rapidly distribute the epileptogenic impulses throughout the brain. In a callosotomy, the corpus callosum is surgically split, thereby preventing the spread of these seizure-generating impulses from hemisphere to hemisphere (Roberts & Siegel, 2001). An "anterior callosotomy" is typically performed in higher-functioning children to preserve cognitive function, whereas a "complete callosotomy" can be performed in children with more severe developmental and neurocognitive disabilities (Roberts & Siegel). Many children who undergo this procedure have multiple seizure types. However, atonic seizures or "drop attacks," which can occur up to 100 times daily in some children and be quite recalcitrant to medical treatment, typically respond rather well to intervention with corpus callosotomy, often improving the child's overall quality of life (Roberts & Siegel). Whereas the advent of VNS has reduced the number of procedures done, the corpus callosotomy remains a viable surgical treatment option for the appropriate patient.

### Treatment Plan

Not every seizure is a medical emergency that warrants initiation of EMS. Prolonged or repetitive seizures are medical emergencies that require prompt medical intervention. Acute management reduces the morbidity and mortality associated with status epilepticus (Wheeless, 2004). All children with known seizure disorders should have a treatment plan on file and readily available in order to minimize the time between seizure onset and delivery of first aid or medical care (O'Dell, 2004b). This plan should be a coordinated effort between the treatment team (physician and/or nurse practitioner), parents/legal guardians, school representatives, and, where appropriate,

the students themselves (Kiel, 2004). The school nurse should initiate and coordinate this process. Several forms for this purpose are already available (Epilepsy Foundation of America, 2004b; Xcel Pharmaceuticals, 2004).

The comprehensive written treatment plan should clearly define the student's normal baseline behavior against which activity that might indicate seizures can be compared. It should describe the student's typical seizure activity, including frequency, duration, provoking factors, postictal behavior, and recovery time (Kiel, 2004; O'Hara, 2004). The child's medication regimen should be noted even if routine medications are not administered at school. It should describe measures for intervention, including basic seizure first aid, administration of maintenance or emergency medications, use of the vagus nerve stimulator magnet, parameters for parental notification, and initiation of EMS (O'Dell, 2004b).

Primary goals of acute medical intervention in the event of prolonged or repetitive seizures should include minimizing the risk of injury to the student and rapid termination of seizure activity. In addition, care should be given to provide medical intervention in a manner that is respectful of the child's privacy and, if possible, enables the child to return to normal classroom activities and minimizes the disruptive effects on other students (O'Hara, 2004).

### First Aid for Seizures

When a student is having a convulsive (generalized tonic-clonic) seizure, the following should be done (Epilepsy Foundation of America, 2005):

1. Remove objects that may cause injury if hit during seizure. Cushion head, remove glasses, loosen tight clothing.
2. Turn the student on his/her side (recovery position) and keep the airway clear.
3. Do not put anything in the student's mouth. (The student is unable to swallow his/her tongue. The recovery position will use gravity to keep the tongue from occluding the airway and prevent aspiration of saliva.)
4. Do not restrain the student during a seizure. This may cause more injury to extremities and is not necessary.
5. If the student has a VNS implant, use the VNS magnet as outlined in the emergency treatment plan.
6. Observe the duration and characteristics of the seizure.
7. If the seizure does not stop within 5 minutes, administer rescue medication (Diastat), if ordered, as outlined in the emergency treatment plan.
8. Initiate EMS according to the emergency treatment plan.
9. If this is the student's first seizure, notify EMS.
10. Notify the student's parents as outlined in the emergency treatment plan.

## Postictal Care

After the seizure, in the postictal period, students should be observed for level of awareness, respiratory effort, excessive secretions, and the possibility of injury or recurrence of seizures.

When a student is having a nonconvulsive seizure (partial, absence, atonic, myoclonic) (Epilepsy Foundation of America, 2005):

1. Keep the student in a safe environment. Do not restrict the student's movement unless he or she is in danger.

2. Observe the duration and characteristics of the seizure.
3. Observe for secondary generalization.
4. If the student has a VNS, use the VNS magnet as outlined in the emergency treatment plan.

School nurses can expect to encounter children with seizures and seizure disorders consistently throughout the educational spectrum. School nurses are equipped to implement both routine and emergency care for the student with epilepsy, thereby facilitating the educational experience and contributing to the student's dynamic neurodevelopmental process.

# Individualized Healthcare Plan

## Assessment

### History

- Significant perinatal history (prenatal, delivery, newborn period)
- Developmental history, including growth parameters and timeline of milestone achievements
- Seizure history
  - seizure type(s)
  - age of the student at his/her first seizure
  - description of student's seizures; changes in course of seizure
  - longest seizure-free period
  - seizures longer than 5 minutes
  - medications used to treat seizures; effect of medication

### Current Status and Management

- Describe current seizures; length of usual seizure; time of day
- Typical resolution of seizures; whether intervention is required to stop seizure activity
- Time needed for the student to return to their normal baseline
  - Describe postictal period
- Aura or behaviors that indicate seizure activity is about to occur
  - Student awareness of aura or behaviors
  - Child's typical response when this occurs (e.g., seeks out help or lies down)
- Antiseizure medications regimen: medication, time given, reaction, plan for missed or late dose
- For students with the VNS:
  - Student ability to use the magnet himself/herself
  - Storage location of magnet(s)
- Seizure pattern warranting parent notification: who and how to notify (current emergency contact information)
- Student's longest seizure-free period in the past year
- Student's use of medical-alert identification

### Self-care

- Student's awareness of the need for medication and compliance with medication regimen. Student's use of prompts to remember to take medication as prescribed
- Student's ability to recognize aura or to identify behaviors and activities that trigger seizures
- Student's ability to avoid these seizure triggers, either independently or when prompted to avoid such activities
- Student's ability to recognize certain activities (e.g., swimming without supervision, climbing in high places) as being unsafe in the event of a seizure and adherence to safety guidelines for seizure precautions

### Psychosocial Status

- Student's sensitivity to the chronic diagnosis of epilepsy and feeling different from peers as evidenced by denial of diagnosis, noncompliance with medical interventions (e.g. medications), refusal to adhere to safety guidelines, and lack of peer relationships, etc.
- School problems the student attributes to the seizure disorder or to seizure medication
- Student's desire and ability to tell any classmates or teachers (adults) about the seizure disorder. Student's feelings about others' reaction.

- Ask student to identify how he would like to be treated by classmates, teachers and other school personnel during seizure events or in routine interactions
- Evidence of depression related to seizure disorder, self-esteem issues, or peer interactions. Evidence of hyper-activity or disruptive behaviors, sadness, apathy, and sleep and appetite changes

*Academic Issues*
- Change in the student's academic performance that overlaps with a change in seizure activity or adjustments in medications
- Classroom modifications required to assist the student in achieving academic goals

## Nursing Diagnoses (N.D.) (NANDA, 2003)

**N.D. 1** (Risk for) ineffective therapeutic regimen management (NANDA 00078) related to inadequate information regarding seizure disorder treatment options

**N.D. 2** (Risk for) ineffective health maintenance (NANDA 00099) related to inadequate information regarding need for compliance and follow-up for seizure disorder

**N.D. 3** (Risk for) total urinary (NANDA 00014) and/or bowel incontinence (NANDA 00021) related to seizure activity

**N.D. 4** (Risk for) ineffective breathing pattern (NANDA 00032) related to seizure activity

**N.D. 5** (Risk for) disturbed thought process (NANDA 00130) related to seizure activity

**N.D. 6** (Risk for) fear (NANDA 00148) related to unknown seizure activity pattern

**N.D. 7** Risk for injury NANDA 00035) from falling during seizure activity

**N.D. 8** (Risk for) fatigue (NANDA 00093) related to:
- type of seizure activity
- frequency of seizure activity
- severity of seizure activity

**N.D. 9** (Risk for) noncompliance (NANDA 00079) related to beliefs regarding seizure disorder

**N.D. 10** Risk for delayed development (NANDA 00112) related to:
- type of seizure activity and associated disorders
- frequency of seizure activity and associated disorders
- severity of seizure activity and associated disorders

**N.D. 11** Risk for situational low self-esteem (NANDA 00153) related to seizure disorder.

**N.D. 12** (Risk for) social isolation (NANDA 00053) related to unknown seizure activity pattern

**N. D.13** (Risk for) aspiration (NANDA 00039) related to seizure activity

**N.D. 14** Ineffective coping (NANDA 00069) related to seizure condition

**N.D. 15** Deficient knowledge (NANDA 00126) related to:
- information misinterpretation
- cognitive limitations
- lack of information resources

**N.D. 16** Disturbed sensory perception (NANDA 00122) related to seizure condition (Santilli 2001)

## Goals

The student will (if developmentally able) demonstrate safety measures, when aura presents prior to seizure, in order to prevent injury. (N.D. 4-7, 13, 15)

The student will appropriately and successfully interact in social settings in the school, home, and community. (N.D. 11, 12, 14)

The student will (as developmentally appropriate) assist in the decision-making process regarding health management issues at school. (N.D. 1- 5, 7-9, 11, 13, 14)

The student will describe abilities and disabilities realistically. (N.D. 5, 7, 11, 12, 14-16)

The student will maintain scheduled therapeutic regimen, meal, sleep, and rest patterns during the week and on weekends. (N.D. 1, 2, 8, 9, 11, 14, 15)

The student will provide an extra set of clothing at school. (N.D. 3)

The student will (as developmentally appropriate) understand methods being used to control seizures. (N.D. 1, 2, 4, 7, 9, 13, 15)

The student will use VNS appropriately. (N.D. 1, 2, 7, 9, 11, 12, 14, 15)

The student will (as developmentally appropriate) increase knowledge and understanding of the seizure disorder type and treatment options. (N.D. 1, 2, 9, 11, 14, 15)

The student will identify and participate in developmentally appropriate and safe extracurricular activities. (N.D. 7, 11, 12, 14, 15)

The student will (as developmentally appropriate) assist in the decision-making process regarding health management choices. (N.D. 1, 2, 7, 8, 9)

The student will (as developmentally appropriate) correctly identify situations and circumstances where the student is in control. (N.D. 6, 10, 11, 12, 14)

The student will (as developmentally able) communicate effectively with others. (N.D. 5, 8, 10-12, 14, 16)

The student will identify school and community resources that can provide support. (N.D. 11, 12, 14)

The student will wear medical alert jewelry. (N.D. 1, 2, 4, 5, 7-9, 12, 13, 16)

## Nursing Interventions (Santilli, 2001)

Reduce or remove factors that may cause or contribute to injury during a seizure. (N.D. 4, 6, 7, 13, 15, 16)

Provide student-specific information to selected school personnel for student: (N.D. 1-5, 7, 8, 11, 14, 16)
- Type of seizure, treatment regimen, including medication side effects
- Precautions, safety issues
- First aid care for immediate and recovery care
- Vegas nerve stimulator magnet application
- Seizure log documentation
- Emergency plan of care and follow-up
- Evacuation plan

In cooperation with student, parents, and other school personnel, participate in development of individualized education plan (IEP) as indicated, or 504 plan as needed to address accommodations needed in the school setting. (N.D. 1, 2, 4, 5, 7-10, 13, 14, 16)

Provide educational opportunities for peers regarding seizure activity and management options for the student. (N.D. 1-5, 7, 9, 14-16)

Provide space for supplies, including extra clothing, to be stored at school. (N.D. 1-3, 9, 15)

Encourage student to tell an adult when an aura presents. (N.D. 5-7, 11, 12, 14, 16)

Encourage student to position self in safe position if aura presents or ask for assistance in going to the nurse's office. (N.D. 4-7, 13, 15)

Encourage student to communicate needs related to seizure activity: (N.D. 2, 3, 5-8, 11, 14-16)
Recovery time
Repeat instructions
Extra time to complete assignment
Peer relationships
Physical needs
"Buddy" system in hallways, restrooms, bus, etc.

Assist student to safe position when seizure activity or alteration in awareness is observed, especially in the event that student cannot notify the nurse, teacher, or other staff member by himself/herself. (N.D. 5-7, 11, 12)

Develop and implement use of a seizure activity log sheet in the school setting. (N.D. 1, 2)

Encourage the student to actively participate in recreational, social, and/or self-help groups within the school or community. (N.D. 10-12)

Support the student in expressing emotional needs to adults. (N.D. 10-12, 14)

Provide opportunities where the student can make decisions regarding seizure disorder management in the school setting. (N.D. 1, 2, 9, 11)

Stress importance of the student's strengths and abilities. (N.D. 11, 12)

Provide student and parents with medical alert jewelry resources. (N.D. 1, 2, 5, 7, 11)

Encourage student to wear medical alert jewelry at all times. (N.D. 2, 4, 5, 7, 8, 13, 15, 16)

Assist student to identify need for assistance and/or referral to: (N.D. 11, 12, 14, 15)
Guidance counselor
Social worker
Vocational rehabilitation services
Mental health care
Community resource

Discuss changes, limitations, and alterations in daily living caused by student's seizure disorder. (N.D. 2, 3, 5, 7, 8, 14, 15)

Discuss with student ways of handling other's reaction to seizure activity. (N.D. 6, 11, 12, 14)

## Expected Student Outcomes

The student will:
- Ask the teacher for clarification of instructions or directions that were missed on account of seizure activity (if student is aware that a seizure has occurred). (N.D. 5, 8,10-12)
- Not sustain injury during seizure while at school. (N.D. 2, 4, 5, 7, 13)
- Reduce the risk of potential injury (as developmentally appropriate) by demonstrating the appropriate way and understanding of when to position self in a safe position or ask to be assisted to the nurse's office prior to a seizure. (N.D. 4, 7, 11, 15)
- (If developmentally able) describe symptoms that accompany an aura. (N.D. 1, 2, 7, 16)
- Use the VNS appropriately. (N.D. 1, 2, 9, 11, 12, 14, 15)
- Follow schedule that allows for regular meals, sleep, and rest times. (N.D. 8)
- Keep extra clothing at school in case of incontinence episode. (N.D. 3)
- Describe and discuss situations that are associated with the feeling of fear related to seizure pattern. (N.D. 6)
- (If developmentally able) describe and follow medication regimen and other methods being used to control seizure activity as prescribed by healthcare provider. (N.D. 1, 2, 9, 11, 14)
- Wear a medical alert bracelet. (N.D. 1, 4, 5, 7-9, 12, 13, 16)
- (As developmentally able) share information about specific seizure disorder with peers and others in the school and community setting. (N.D. 6, 11, 12, 14, 15)
- Verbalize age-appropriate acceptance of seizure disorder. (N.D. 2, 11, 12, 14, 16)
- Develop positive coping mechanisms. (N.D. 1, 2, 5, 8, 9, 11, 12, 14, 15)
- Verbalize frustrations, anger, fears related to seizure disorder limitations. (N.D. 6, 9, 11, 12, 14, 15)
- Participate in at least one recreational, social, or self-help group within the school or community. (N.D. 11, 12, 14)

## Case Study

Clark is a 9-year-old boy who will begin fourth grade at TJ Elementary School in the fall. Clark is a pleasant boy who has complex partial seizures. Clark and his mother shared the following information during a conference: He has a history of staring episodes and a change in his level of consciousness. A typical seizure for him includes a feeling of extreme drowsiness where he may fall asleep at his desk. Clark is sometimes aware of an impending seizure and tries to get himself into a safe position. Occasionally, when this drowsiness occurs, Clark recognizes that as a sign his seizure is about to occur. In such a case he may ask to go to the nurse's office so he can lie down and rest. He may also appear to be "day-dreaming" or "staring into space"; these symptoms are typical of one of his seizures. He may be mildly disoriented when he wakes up. He is usually lethargic for at least an hour after a seizure. He currently takes Depakote at home to control his seizure activity.

In addition to his seizure disorder, Clark has a diagnosed learning disability. He will be placed in a special education instructional class for math and be mainstreamed in co-taught classes for his other academic classes. His academic needs will be addressed in his IEP. Health goals may also be included in the IEP to address health concerns.

During the conference, Clark said he thinks his teachers should know about his seizure patterns. He doesn't feel comfortable telling his peers. He is afraid they will tease him.

The following is a list of health concerns related to Clark's seizure disorder to be addressed in the plan for this school year:
1. Experiences episodes of extreme drowsiness.
2. May have episodes of "day dreaming" or "staring into space."
3. May miss instructions and directions given in class, may need instructions repeated and/or extra time to complete assignment.
4. Need for monitoring/supervision in and outside of the classroom (halls, restroom, bus).
5. Need for improved coping skills related to peer relationships.

## Seizures

| Assessment Data | Nursing Diagnosis | Goals | Nursing Interventions | Expected Outcomes |
|---|---|---|---|---|
| Clark's mother reports that his complex partial seizure pattern includes drowsiness causing him to fall asleep, or to have the appearance of "day dreaming," and "staring into space" episodes. Clark does sometimes recognize the feeling of extreme drowsiness as the start of seizure activity. | Risk for injury related to seizure activity.<br><br>Fatigue related to seizure activity. | The student will (if developmentally able) demonstrate safety measures when aura presents prior to seizure in order to prevent injury.<br><br>The student will wear medical alert jewelry.<br><br>The student will (as developmentally appropriate) assist in the decision-making process regarding health management issues at school: identify need for rest/sleep, ask to go to health room to rest. | Provide student-specific information to selected school personnel for student:<br>• Type of seizure<br>• Precautions, safety issues<br>• First aid care<br>• Seizure log<br>• Emergency plan of care and follow-up<br>• Evacuation plan<br><br>Encourage student to position self in safe position if aura presents or ask for assistance in going to the nurse's office.<br><br>Encourage Clark to communicate his needs to school personnel. | Clark will reduce the risk of potential injury (as developmentally appropriate) by demonstrating the appropriate way and understanding of when to position self in a safe position or ask to be assisted to the nurse's office prior to a seizure.<br><br>The student will wear a medical alert bracelet. |
| Upon coming out of the seizure, Clark is lethargic for about an hour and sometimes mildly disoriented. He won't recall what the conversation/instructions were just previous to the seizure. | Disturbed thought process related to seizure activity. | Clark will assist in the decision-making process regarding health management choices in the school setting: asking for assistance, time to rest in health room, clarification of instruction, extra time to do assignment when his mind is not clear. | In cooperation with student, parents, and other school personnel, participate in development of individualized education plan (IEP) to address health and educational needs in the school setting: rest time, additional time to do assignments, repeat of instructions, etc. | Clark will ask the teacher for clarification of instructions or directions that were missed due to seizure activity when the student is aware that a seizure has occurred. |

| Assessment Data | Nursing Diagnosis | Goals | Nursing Interventions | Expected Outcomes |
|---|---|---|---|---|
| Clark is okay with letting adults know about his seizure condition but is shy about letting classmates know. He doesn't like to be treated differently. Sometimes he will try activities that are not safe for him to do without a "buddy." | Ineffective coping related to limitations to social interactions related to seizure condition. | Clark will identify and participate in developmentally appropriate and safe extracurricular activities.<br><br>Clark will assist in the decision-making process regarding health management choices in the school setting.<br><br>The student will (as developmentally able) communicate effectively with peers about his seizure condition and how to help. | Discuss with student ways of handing other's reaction to seizure activity.<br><br>Support the student in expressing emotional needs to adults.<br><br>Provide educational opportunities regarding seizure activity and management options for the student and peers. | Clark will develop positive coping mechanisms regarding health management in the school setting.<br><br>Clark will share information about specific seizure disorder with peers and others in the school and community setting. |

# Emergency Care Plan
## 2004–2005 School Year

Date: _____

Student: Clark _____

Date of birth: 9-6-94 _____

Parent(s)/Guardian(s): Harry and Carey _____

_____

_____

School: _____

Grade: 4 _____

Home telephone: 555-1234 _____

Work: 555 1167 _____

Cell: 555-2318 _____

Home Address: 100 Addison Place _____

Medical Diagnosis: Seizure disorder: complex partial _____

| Symptom | Action |
|---------|--------|
| Complaints of extreme drowsiness | 1. Clark will be assisted to the nurse's office by an adult (if time allows). If time does not allow, then:<br>2. Assist Clark to floor and place in a safe position for duration of seizure. |
| Found sleeping with head on desk | 1. Check Clark's breathing pattern and respiration rate. If not normal, activate emergency procedures. If normal, then:<br>2. Let Clark continue to sleep at his desk as this is typical of one of his seizures and he should awaken within 20 to 30 minutes. Upon awakening, ask Clark if he needs to rest in the nurse's office. He may be disoriented at first and need time to re-collect himself. Prior instructions or directions may need to be repeated.<br>3. Teacher, teacher aid, nurse, or other school personnel must remain with Clark throughout the duration of his seizure and recovery time.<br>4. Teacher will document seizure activity on the log sheet that is sent home in the assignment notebook each night.<br>5. If unable to reorient Clark, he should be escorted to the nurse's office for further evaluation. |
| Sleeping in the nurse's office | 1. Allow Clark to sleep until he awakens on his own. Reorient to surroundings when he wakes.<br>2. Nurse will track seizure activity on log sheet.<br>3. Parent(s) must be notified if unable to reorient Clark after a seizure. It may be necessary for him to go home from school early.<br>4. Seizure log should be sent home on daily basis for parent(s) to sign. |

| Symptom | Action |
|---|---|
| Day-dreaming or staring into space | 1. This may signal that Clark is going to have a seizure.<br>2. It may be possible to use verbal prompts and cues and attempt to get Clark back on task.<br>3. If getting Clark back on task is not possible, then assist him to a safe position in case he has a seizure and falls asleep.<br>4. Seizure log should be sent home on daily basis for parent(s) to sign. |
| Illness | 1. Notify Clark's parent(s) if he complains of being ill while at school. Leaving school early and additional medical attention may be needed. |
| Injury | 1. Notify Clark's parent(s) if he injures himself during a seizure. Additional medical attention may be needed. |
| Incontinence | 1. If Clark experiences incontinence during a seizure, it will be necessary to provide a private place for him to change his clothes. Extra clothing is stored in the nurse's office and provided by his parents.<br>2. Soiled clothes should be sent home in a plastic bag, and Clark's parents will send a clean set to school on the next school day. |

At this time, the above symptoms are the most common symptoms Clark experiences related to his seizure disorder. Incontinence has never been an issue at school but is noted for reference. Please review this periodically and keep with your substitute teacher lesson plans in case you are absent. Stop by my office if you have questions, comments, or concerns.

**Signatures:**

School Nurse_____ Date_____

Parent/guardian (if required)_____ Date_____

# Emergency Evacuation Plan
## Seizures

**Student:** Clark  
**Disability Area:** Physically Impaired  
**Deficit Area:** Seizure Disorder  

**School:** TJ Elementary School  
**Grade:** 4

**Concerned Personnel:** Teachers, Administrators, Support Personnel (i.e., Nurse, Counselor, Case Manager, Social Worker, Bus Driver, Custodian)

**Concern:** Clark has a seizure disorder and a learning disability and may need special assistance in leaving the building during an emergency situation in the school setting.

**Plan:** Activate this plan if Clark is experiencing a seizure during an emergency evacuation situation in the school setting.

1. Manually transport Clark out of the building via the school's evacuation wheelchair with restraint straps secured around his body. (Location of wheelchair: _____ )
2. Once at the designated safe location, Clark can be moved to the ground and placed in the traditional left-sided recovery position until his seizure subsides.
3. The school nurse, classroom teacher (s), school administrator, or support personnel should remain with him until the seizure subsides.

# References

Annegers, J. F. (2001). The epidemiology of epilepsy. In E. Wyllie (Ed.), *The treatment of epilepsy: Principles & practice* (3rd ed.). Philadelphia: Lippincott, Williams & Wilkins.

Arunkumar, G., Kotagal P., & Rothner, A. D. (2001). Localization-related epilepsies: Simple partial seizures, complex partial seizures, benign focal epilepsy of childhood, and epilepsia partialis continua. In J. M. Pellock, W. E. Dodson, & B. F. D. Bourgeois (Eds.), *Pediatric epilepsy: Diagnosis & therapy* (2nd ed.). New York: Demos.

Arzimanoglou, A., Guerrini, R., & Aicardi, J. (2004). *Aicardi's epilepsy in children* (3rd ed.). Philadelphia: Lippincott, Williams & Wilkins.

Austin, J. K., Dunn, D. W., Caffrey, H. M., Perkins, S. M., Harezlak, J., & Rose D. F. (2002). Recurrent seizures and behavior problems in children with first recognized seizure: A prospective study. *Epilepsia, 43,* 1564–1573.

Best, T. H., Franz, D. N., Gilbert, D. L., Nelson, D. P., & Epstein, M. R. (2000). Cardiac complications in pediatric patients on the ketogenic diet. *Neurology, 54,* 2328–2330.

DeLorenzo, R. J., Hauser, W. A., Towne, A. R., Boggs, J. G., Pellock, J. M., Penberthy, L., et al. (1996). A prospective, population-based epidemiologic study of status epilepticus in Richmond, Virginia. *Neurology, 46*(4), 1029–1035.

Devinsky, O. (2002). *Epilepsy: Patient & family guide* (2nd ed.). Philadelphia: Davis.

Dreifuss, F. E., & Nordli, D. R. (2001). Classification of epilepsies in childhood. In J. M. Pellock, W. E. Dodson, & B. F. D. Bourgeois (Eds.). *Pediatric epilepsy: Diagnosis & therapy* (2nd ed.). New York: Demos.

Epilepsy Foundation of America. (2004a). Epilepsy and Seizure Statistics Retrieved August 14, 2004, from www.efa.org/answerplace/statistics.cfm

Epilepsy Foundation of America (2004b). Forms for School Nurses and Parents Retrieved December 28, 2004, from www.epilepsyfoundation.org/answerplace/Social/education/schoolforms.cfm_

Epilepsy Foundation of America (2004c). Surgery Types: Benefits and Risks Retrieved December 30, 2004, from www.epilepsyfoundation.org/answerplace/Medical/treatment/surgery/benefitsrisks.cfm

Epilepsy Foundation of America. (2005). *First aid.* Retrieved May 1, 2005, from http://www.epilepsyfoundation.org/answerplace/Medical/firstaid/index.cfm

Farrell, K. (2001). Tonic and atonic seizures. In Wyllie, E. (Ed.). *The treatment of epilepsy: Principles & practice* (3rd ed.). Philadelphia: Lippincott, Williams & Wilkins.

Fisch, B. J., & Olejniczak, P. W. (2001). Generalized tonic clonic seizures. In E. Wyllie (Ed.). (2001). *The treatment of epilepsy: Principles & practice* (3rd Ed.). Philadelphia: Lippincott, Williams & Wilkins.

Harkness, W. F. J. (2001). How to select the best surgical procedure for children with epilepsy. In H. O. Luders & Y. G. Comair (Eds.). *Epilepsy surgery* (2nd ed.). Philadelphia: Lippincott, Williams & Wilkins.

Hauser, W. A. (2001). Epidemiology of epilepsy in children. In J. M. Pellock, W. E. Dodson, & B. F. D. Bourgeois (Eds.). *Pediatric epilepsy: Diagnosis & therapy* (2nd ed.). New York: Demos.

Holthausen, H., & Pieper, T. (2001). Complications of hemispherectomy. In H. O. Luders & Y. G. Comair (Eds.), *Epilepsy surgery* (2nd ed.). Philadelphia: Lippincott, Williams & Wilkins.

International League Against Epilepsy (1989). *Commission on classification and terminology of the International League Against Epilepsy: Proposal for revised clinical and electroencephalographic classification of epileptic seizures.* In E. Wyllie (Ed.). (2001). *The treatment of epilepsy: Principles & practice* (3rd ed.). Philadelphia: Lippincott, Williams & Wilkins.

Kiel, S. (2004 July). *Safety of providing medication in schools: Legal issues and treatment plans.* Poster session presented at the annual meeting of the National Association of School Nurses, Seattle, WA.

Kriel, R. L., Cloyd, J. C., Pellock, J. M., Mitchell, W. G., Cereghino, J. J., & Rosman, N. P. (1999). Rectal diazepam gel for treatment of acute repetitive seizures. The North American Study Group. *Pediatric Neurology, 20,* 282–288.

Mitchell, W. G., Conry, J. A., Crumrine, P. K., Kriel, R. L., Cereghino, J. J., Groves, L., et al. (1999). An open-label study of repeated use of diazepam rectal gel (Diastat) for episodes of acute breakthrough seizures and clusters: Safety, efficacy, and tolerance. North American Study Group. *Epilepsia, 40,* 1610–1617.

NANDA International. (2003). *Nursing diagnoses: Definitions & classifications 2003–2004.* Philadelphia: Author.

National Institutes of Health. (2000). NIH publication No. 00-156. In O'Dell, C. (2004 July). *The Epidemiology and classification of seizures in children.* In *Acute seizure management: Treatment options in the school setting.* Symposium conducted at the annual meeting of the National Association of School Nurses, Seattle, WA.

Nordli, D. R., & De Vivo, D. C. (2001). The ketogenic diet. In J. M. Pellock, W. E. Dodson, & B. F. D. Bourgeois, B.F.D (Eds.) *Pediatric epilepsy: Diagnosis & therapy* (2nd ed.). New York: Demos.

O'Dell, C. (2004a July). *The epidemiology and classification of seizures in children. Acute seizure management: Treatment options in the school setting.* Symposium conducted at the annual meeting of the National Association of School Nurses, Seattle, WA.

O'Dell, C. (2004b, July). *The epidemiology of seizures in children: Risk factors, prognosis and care.* Poster session presented at the annual meeting of the National Association of School Nurses, Seattle, WA.

O'Hara, K. (2004, July). *The importance of a seizure emergency treatment plan.* Poster session presented at the annual meeting of the National Association of School Nurses, Seattle, WA.

Pellock, J. M. (2004a). New pharmacotherapies for pediatric seizures. *Pediatric Annals, 34*(6) 385–391.

Pellock, J. M. (2004b). Safety of Diastat, a rectal gel formulation of diazepam for acute seizure treatment. *Drug Safety, 27*(6) 383–392.

Pellock, J. M. (2004c). Understanding comorbidities affecting children with epilepsy. *Neurology, 62*(5) S17–23.

Roberts, D. W. & Siegel, A. M. (2001). Corpus callosotomy. In H. O. Luders & Y. G. Comair (Eds.). *Epilepsy surgery* (2nd ed.). Philadelphia: Lippincott, Williams & Wilkins.

Santilli, N. (2001). *Students with seizures: A manual for school nurses* (2nd ed.). Landover, MD: Epilepsy Foundation of America.

Sharp, G. B., & Wilder, B. J. (2001). *Quick reference guide: Epilepsy and the use of antiepileptic drugs.* Florence, KY: Shire Richwood.

Shinnar, S., Berg, A. T., Moshe, S. L., & Shinnar R. (2001). How long do new-onset seizures in children last? *Annals of Neurology, 49*(5) 659–664. In Wheeless, J.W. (2004) Treatment of status epilepticus in children. *Pediatric Annals, 33*(6) 377–383.

Shinnar, S., O'Dell, C. (2004). Febrile seizures. *Pediatric Annals, 33*(6) 394–401.

Taketomo, C. K., Hoddin, J. H., & Kraus, D. M. (2003). *Pediatric dosage handbook* (10th ed.). Hudson, OH: Lexi-Comp.

Valencia, T., Holder, D. L., Helmers, S. L., Madsen, J. R., & Riviello, J. J. (2001). Vagus nerve stimulation in pediatric epilepsy: A review. *Pediatric Neurology, 25*(5), 368–376.

Wyler, A. R. (2001). Multiple subpial transections. In H. O. Luders & Y. G. Comair (Eds.). *Epilepsy surgery* (2nd ed.). Philadelphia: Lippincott, Williams & Wilkins.

Wheeless, J. W. (2004). Treatment of status epilepticus in children. *Pediatric Annals, 33*(6), 377–383.

Willmore, L. J., Wheeless, J. W., & Pellock, J. M. (2001). Adverse effects of antiepileptic drugs. In J. M. Pellock, W. E. Dodson, & B. F. D. Bourgeois, (Eds.), *Pediatric epilepsy: Diagnosis and therapy* (2nd ed.). New York: Demos.

Xcel Pharmaceuticals, Inc. (2003). *Seizure emergencies: Are you prepared?* (Patient education material). Author.

Xcel Pharmaceuticals, Inc. (2004). *Treatment order and emergency seizure plan: Back to school kit.* (Patient education material). Author.

Zifkin, B., & Andermann, F. (2001). *Epilepsy with reflex seizures.* In E. Wyllie (Ed.) *The treatment of epilepsy: Principles and practice* (3rd ed.). Philadelphia: Lippincott, Williams & Wilkins.

## Bibliography

Allen, P. J., & Vessey, J. A. (2004). *Child with a chronic condition* (4th ed.). St. Louis, MO: Mosby

*Captain Bio encounters a brainstorm.* (1994). Gladstone, NJ: Tim Peters.

Child Neurology Foundation & Child Neurology Society (2004). *Exceptional parent resource guide* [Brochure]. Author.

*Dotty the dalmatian has epilepsy.* (1995). Gladstone, NJ: Tim Peters.

Filipps, T. (2001). *Chris plays basketball.* [Brochure]. USA: Novartis Pharmaceuticals.

Freeman, J., Vining, E. P. G., & Pillas, D. J. (2002). *Seizures and epilepsy in childhood: A Guide for parents* (3rd ed.). Baltimore: Johns Hopkins University Press.

Gosselin, K. (1996). *Taking seizure disorders to school.* Valley Park, MO: JayJo Books.

Santilli, N. (1996). *Managing seizure disorders: A handbook for health care professionals.* Philadelphia: Lippincott-Raven.

Wong, D. L., Hockenberry, M. J., Wilson, D., Winkelstein, M. L., & Kline, N. E. (2003). *Nursing care of infants and children* (7th ed.). St. Louis, MO: Mosby.

# Resources

American Association of Neuroscience Nurses
4700 West Lake Avenue
Glenview, IL 60025
847-375-4733
1-888-557-2266
877-734-8677 (fax)
www.aann.org
Publishes *Journal of Neuroscience Nursing*

American Epilepsy Society
342 North Main Street
West Hartford, CT 06117-2507
860-586-7505
www.aes.net

Association of Child Neurology Nurses
www.aacn.org

Child Neurology Society
1000 West County Road E.
Suite 290
Saint Paul, MN 55126
651-486-9447
651-486-9436 (fax)
www.childneurologysociety.org

Child Neurology Foundation
1821 University Avenue West
Suite N-188
Saint Paul, MN 55102
651-645-4319
651-645-4349 (fax)
www.childneurologyfoundation.org

Citizens United for Research in Epilepsy
730 North Franklin
Suite 404
Chicago, IL 60610
312-255-1801
www.CUREepilepsy.org

Cyberonics, Inc.
100 Cyberonics Boulevard
Houston, TX 77058
1-800-332-1375
281-218-9332 (fax)
www.cyberonics.com
Produces Vagus Nerve Stimulator device for epilepsy

Epilepsy Foundation of America
4351 Garden City Drive
Landover, MD 20785-7223
1-800-332-1000
www.epilepsyfoundation.org or www.efa.org

Epilepsy Institute
257 Park Avenue South
New York, NY 10010
212-677-8550
www.epilepsyinstitute.org

Exceptional Parent Magazine
65 East Route 4
River Edge, NJ 07661
877-372-7368
www.eparent.com

National Institute of Neurological Disorders and
   Stroke
NIH Neurological Institute
P.O. Box 5801
Bethesda, MD 20824
1-800-352-9424
301-468-5981 (TTY)
www.ninds.nih.gov

National Organization for Rare Disorders
P.O. Box 1968
55 Kenosia Avenue
Danbury, CT 06813-1968
203-744-0100
1-800-999-6673
203-798-2291 (fax)
www.rarediseases.org

# Appendix – Anticonvulsant Medications

| Trade Name | Generic Name | Seizure Type/Syndrome | Dose | Therapeutic Level | Common Side Effects |
|---|---|---|---|---|---|
| Ativan | lorazepam | Rescue for breakthrough seizures | Not standard for oral use. | N/A | Somnolence. Note: not commonly used as maintenance antiepileptic drug |
| Carbatrol | carbamazepine | Partial seizures | 10-30 mg/kg/day | 4-12 | Gastrointestinal complaints, somnolence, dizziness, decreased white blood cells, hyponatremia, rash. Can exacerbate primary generalized seizures. Can decrease levels of ethosuximide, felbamate, lamotrigine, phenobarbital, primidone, tiagabine, topiramate, zonisamide, and valproic acid. Can increase phenytoin levels. |
| Depakote, Depakene | valproic acid, valproate sodium | Partial and generalized seizures, including absence | 15-60 mg/kg/day | 50-100 | GI complaints, weight gain, hair loss, tremor, pancreatitis, liver failure. Can increase lamotrigine and phenobarbital levels. May decrease phenytoin levels. |
| Diastat | diazepam | Acute repetitive seizures, prolonged seizures (status epilepticus) | 0.2-0.5 mg/kg/dose | N/A | Somnolence, confusion (usual postictal symptoms). Note: different safety profile than intravenous diazepam. No respiratory suppression. |
| Dilantin | phenytoin | Partial and generalized seizures | 4-8 mg/kg/day | 10-20 | Somnolence, rash, nystagmus, ataxia, hursuitism, gingival hyperplasia. Can exacerbate absence seizures in juvenile myoclonic epilepsy. Can decrease levels of carbamazepine, ethosuximide, felbamate, lamotrigine, phenobarbital, primidone, tiagabine, topiramate, zonisamide, and valproic acid. |
| Felbatol | felbamate | Partial and generalized seizures, especially Lennox-Gastaut syndrome | 15-45 mg/kg/day | 20-135 | Anorexia, aplastic anemia. Can decrease carbamazepine levels but increase carbamazepine by-product responsible for central nervous system side effects. Can increase phenytoin, valproic acid, phenobarbital, and lamotrigine levels. Not commonly used. |
| Gabitril | tiagabine | Partial seizures | 0.5-1 mg/kg/day | 20-70 | Somnolence, dizziness, knee buckling. Can decrease valproic acid levels. Not too commonly used in pediatrics. |
| Keppra | levetiracetam | Partial, absence, and myoclonic seizures | 10-50 mg/kg/day | N/A | Somnolence, dizziness, agitation, behavioral changes |

| Trade Name | Generic Name | Seizure Type/ Syndrome | Dose | Therapeutic Level | Common Side Effects |
|---|---|---|---|---|---|
| Klonopin | clonazepam | Generalized seizures, especially Lennox-Gastaut | 0.01-0.2 mg/kg/day | N/A | Somnolence, ataxia, behavioral changes, agitation, excessive salivation |
| Lamictal | lamotrigine | Partial and generalized seizures | 1-15 mg/kd/day | 2-20 | Dizziness, diplopia, headache, ataxia, nausea, somnolence, vomiting, rash (may be serious, life-threatening rash, especially with concomitant valproic acid); can worsen myoclonic seizure with encephalopathic epilepsy. May affect oral contraceptives. Can decrease valproic acid levels. |
| Mysoline | primidone | Partial and generalized seizures | 10-25 mg/kg/day | 2-12 (20-40 PB level) | Somnolence, dizziness, ataxia, hyperactivity. Metabolizes into phenobarbital |
| Neurontin | gabapentin | Partial seizures | 20-100 mg/kg/day | N/A | Somnolence, dizziness, fatigue, ataxia, weight gain, behavioral changes |
| Phenobarbital | phenobarbital | Partial and generalized seizures | 2-5 mg/kg/day | 20-40 | Somnolence, dizziness, ataxia, hyperactivity, behavioral changes |
| Tegretol, Tegretol XR | carbamazepine | Partial seizures | 10-30 mg/kg/day | 4-12 | GI complaints, somnolence, dizziness, decreased white blood cells, hyponatremia, rash. Can exacerbate primary generalized seizures. Can decrease levels of ethosuximide, felbamate, lamotrigine, phenobarbital, primidone, tiagabine, topiramate, valproic acid and zonisamide. Can increase phenytoin levels. |
| Topamax | topiramate | Partial and generalized seizures | 6-8 mg/kg/day | N/A | Psychomotor slowing, cognitive dulling, anorexia, weight loss, renal stones, decreased sweating, hyperthermia, may affect oral contraceptives. Can increase phenytoin levels and decrease valproic acid levels. |
| Trileptal | oxcarbazepine | Partial and secondarily generalized seizures | 10-60 mg/kg/day | N/A | Somnolence, headache, dizziness, ataxia, mild hyponatremia. May increase phenytoin levels. |
| Zarontin | ethosuximide | Absence seizures | 20 mg/kg/day | 40-80 | Gastrointestinal complaints. |
| Zonegran | zonisamide | Partial and generalized seizures | 2-12 mg/kg/day | N/A | Somnolence, ataxia, anorexia, cognitive dulling, irritability. |

Adapted from "New Pharmacotherapies for Pediatric Seizures," by J. M. Pellock, 2004a, Pediatric Annals, 34, pp. 385–391; Pediatric Dosage Handbook (10th ed.), by C. K. Taketomo, J. H. Hoddin, and D. M. Kraus, 2003, Hudson, OH: Lexi-Comp; and Pediatric Epilepsy: Diagnosis and Therapy (2nd ed.), by L. J. Willmore, J. W. Wheeless, and J. M. Pellock, 2001, New York: Demos.

# Seizure Activity Log Sheet
## (Name Of School)

Student Name _____ Grade _____ D.O.B. _____

Date of seizure _____ Time of onset _____ Total time involved _____

| Observation Before Seizure | Cries out | Complaints of headache | Complaints of aura feeling (describe) | Other |
|---|---|---|---|---|
| **Observation During Seizure** *Extremity involvement* | **Arms affected** | Right<br>Left<br>Straight<br>Bent<br>Stiff<br>Limp | **Head** | Turned right<br>Turned left<br>Turned down<br>Hyperextended back<br>Nodding |
| | **Legs affected** | Right<br>Left<br>Straight<br>Bent<br>Stiff<br>Limp | **Body-trunk** | Rigid<br>Limp<br>Sitting<br>Laying<br>Trembling<br>Jerking<br>Standing |
| | **Verbal sounds** | Before<br>During | **Skin color** | Pale<br>Grey<br>Blue<br>Red (flushed) |
| | **Face twitching** | | | |
| | **Mouth** | Open<br>Closed<br>Grimacing<br>Drooling<br>Vomiting | **Breathing** | Difficulty during<br>Difficulty after<br>Length of difficulty |
| | **Eye movement** | Staring<br>Open<br>Closed<br>Fluttering<br>Rolled back | **Incontinent** | Bladder<br>Bowels |
| **Observation After Seizure** | Drowsy<br>Confused<br>Sleep (length of time) | | Other<br>Injury (explain)<br>School nurse called<br>Parent called<br>911 called | |

Reporter's Signatures: _____ Reporter's Initals: _____

| Seizure Description | Date | Time | Date | Time | Date | Time | Date | Time | Date | Time |
|---|---|---|---|---|---|---|---|---|---|---|
| Length | | | | | | | | | | |
| Loss of Awareness | | | | | | | | | | |
| Confusion | | | | | | | | | | |
| Falling Down | | | | | | | | | | |
| Jerky Motions | | | | | | | | | | |
| Numbness | | | | | | | | | | |
| Stiffness | | | | | | | | | | |
| Unusual Smell or Taste | | | | | | | | | | |
| **Medication** | | | | | | | | | | |
| Last Dose of Medication | | | | | | | | | | |
| **Other** | | | | | | | | | | |
| Lack of Sleep | | | | | | | | | | |
| Use of any OTC Medication | | | | | | | | | | |
| Female LMP | | | | | | | | | | |
| Changes in Diet | | | | | | | | | | |
| Extreme Stress | | | | | | | | | | |
| Illness | | | | | | | | | | |

**Additional Comments:** _____

_____

_____

Seizures

**Signature:** _____ Date_____

## Chapter Sixty-seven

# Sickle Cell Disease

Carolyn F. Holman

## Introduction

Sickle cell disease is an inherited chronic illness that affects approximately 72,000 Americans of African decent. In the African American population, 1 in 500 live births have sickle cell anemia (HbSS), 1 in 835 live births have hemoglobin SC disease (HbSC), and 1 in 1,667 live births have sickle beta-thalassemia disorders. The Hispanic American population averages 1 case of sickle cell anemia in every 1,000 to 1,400 births. Other ethnic groups that are affected include people from South America, Cuba, Central America, Saudi Arabia, India, Turkey, Greece, and Italy (US Department of Health and Human Services [USDHHS], Public Health Service [PHS], & National Heart, Lung, and Blood Institute [NHLBI], 1996; NHLBI, 2002)

Children with sickle cell anemia require careful monitoring and coordination of their care. The signs and symptoms of sickle cell disease can range from mild to life-threatening. Knowledge and appropriate management of this disease can have a significant impact on the life of the child with sickle cell disease.

Recent advances include a decrease in infant morbidity and mortality caused by overwhelming pneumococcal infections. The administration of prophylactic penicillin from the ages of 2 months to 5 years is responsible for this decrease (USDHHS, PHS, & NHLBI, 1996). Bone marrow transplants have been reported to cure some patients of their disease (USDHHS, PHS, & NHLBI). Improved testing of blood products has decreased the number of complications resulting from blood transfusions (USDHHS, PHS, & NHLBI; NHLBI, 2002). Administration of hydroxyuria has been shown to decrease the incidence of painful events and acute chest syndrome as well as reduce the number of transfusions needed by the patient with sickle cell disease (USDHHS, PHS, & NHLBI).

Hydroxyuria is an anticancer drug that appears to stimulate the production of fetal hemoglobin, which seems to reduce the sickling of red blood cells (USDHHS, PHS, & NHLBI, 1996). Red blood cells containing fetal hemoglobin also appear to live longer in the bloodstream (USDHHS, PHS, & NHLBI). Erythropoietin is a genetically engineered hormone that stimulates red blood cell production. If used in conjunction with hydroxyuria, a smaller dose of the hydroxyuria may be effective.

Butyrate, a simple fatty acid, is also being investigated for use to stimulate fetal hemoglobin production. Clotrimazole is under investigation to determine its effectiveness in preventing water loss from the red blood cells. Clotrimazole is an over-the-counter medication used to treated fungal infections (USDHHS, PHS, & NHLBI).

The use of regular blood transfusions (every 3 weeks) for children at high risk of stroke has been proven to reduce the incidence of stroke in children with sickle cell disease. (USDHHS, PHS, & NHLBI, 1996; NHLBI, 2002; Information Center for Sickle Cell and Thalassemic Disorders, 2000). The goal is to keep the hematocrit under 30%, which reduces the viscosity of the blood. Transcranial Doppler (TCD) screening tests are used to identify children at risk for stroke. Such screening is recommended by the NHLBI for all children with sickle cell disease between 2 and 16 years of age. It is recommended that the screening be done at a comprehensive sickle cell program site, so that comparisons can be made to the information from the Stroke Prevention Trial in Sickle Cell Anemia (STOP). The STOP Trial was to determine if medical intervention could prevent a stroke in a child with sickle cell disease. One hundred and thirty subjects with sickle cell disease, ages 2-16 years, were selected for the study due to their high risk for stroke, based on elevated cerebral blood flow per TCD screening tests. Approximately one half of the subjects received simple or exchange transfusions every 3 to 4 weeks in an effort to maintain the Hb S level below 30%. The remainder of the subjects received standard supportive care. At the end of one year, the data revealed 10 of the subjects in the standard care group had suffered a cerebral infarction compared to 1 child in the transfusion group. Based on this evidence, the study was stopped on September 2, 1997. All fourteen of the participating study centers were notified so the children in the standard care group could be offered the effective treatment to prevent first-time stroke (Adams, et al., 1998) Intervals for TCD screening have not yet been determined; however, every 6 months is considered reasonable (NHLBI; Information Center for Sickle Cell and Thalassemic Disorders).

Pulmonary hypertension is also a serious complication of sickle cell disease. Pulmonary hypertension is not related to the blood pressure measured with a cuff on an extremity. It is caused by excess pressure in the blood vessels that supply the lungs. Narrowing and thickening of these vascular walls cause the increased pressure. The heart works harder to meet the oxygen demands of the body. When it cannot keep up with demands, the person becomes tired, dizzy, and short of breath. If a cause for pulmonary hypertension cannot be identified, it is called primary hypertension. If a preexisting disease such as sickle cell disease triggers this phenomenon, it is called secondary hypertension. Secondary hypertension can be found in most hereditary and chronic anemias that are caused by hemolysis or destruction of red blood cells. Recent research has identified secondary hypertension in approximately one third of adults with sickle cell disease. This may explain sudden deaths in adults with sickle cell disease in the absence of cardiovascular disease. Doppler echocardiography can be used as a screening tool to identify this problem in adults. Interventions such as oxygen and nitric oxide, blood exchanges through transfusion, and use of vasodilator drugs may open these blood vessels or arteries (National Institutes of Health, 2004).

## Pathophysiology

*Sickle cell disease* is the term used to describe a group of genetic disorders characterized by the presence of abnormal sickle hemoglobin S (HbS), hemolytic anemia, and acute and chronic tissue injury, secondary to blockage of blood flow by abnormally shaped erythrocytes. Sickle cell anemia is the most prevalent type of sickle cell disease (USDHHS, PHS, & NHLBI, 1996; NHLBI, 2002; Information Center for Sickle Cell and Thalassemic Disorders, 2000).

Normal hemoglobin (HbA) is composed of two alpha globin chains. In HbS, the alpha chain is the same as in HbA. The beta chain is different on account of the substitution of valine for glutamic acid on the sixth position (USDHHS, PHS, & NHLBI, 1996; NHLBI, 2002; Information Center for Sickle Cell and Thalassemic Disorders 2000).

Chronic hemolytic anemia is caused by the amino acid substitution on the beta globin of HbS. This results in the polymerization of the HbS molecules within the erythrocyte upon deoxygenation. A change is then produced in the erythrocyte's shape, from a biconcave disc to a crescent or sickle shape. When the erythrocyte is reoxygenated, it initially resumes a normal shape, but with repeated cycles of "sickling and unsickling," the erythrocyte is damaged permanently and hemolyzes. The anemia is the result of this hemolysis, which reduces the normal life span of the erythrocyte from 120 days to 10 to 20 days (USDHHS, PHS, & NHLBI, 1996; NHLBI, 2002; Information Center for Sickle Cell and Thalassemic Disorders, 2000).

The lowered hematocrit actually helps reduce the blood viscosity and deoxygenation, which decreases the incidence of polymerization of HbS to its abnormal form. Hypoxemia, acidosis, erythrocyte dehydration, hyperosmolality of the renal medulla (which dehydrates the erythrocyte), and viral infections can result in increased sickling. Other risk factors that affect the above are hemoglobin (Hgb) level higher than 8.5 g/dl, elevated reticulocyte count, cold weather, fever, menstruation, sleep apnea, obstructive snoring, infection, pregnancy, and deoxygenation (i.e., high altitude) (NHLBI, 2002).

The acute and chronic tissue injury is a result of hypoxia, secondary to vaso-occlusion caused by the abnormally shaped erythrocytes. All tissues within the body are susceptible to damage. At greatest risk are the spleen, bone marrow, eye, head of the femur, and humerus. The lung may be at special risk for vaso-occlusion and infarction since receives any deoxygenated erythrocytes that leave the spleen or bone marrow. Acute hypoxic injury may present as painful events or acute chest syndrome. Aseptic necrosis of the hip and sickle cell retinopathy are examples of insidious hypoxic injury. Acute and/or chronic tissue injury usually results in organ damage, especially as the person ages (USDHHS, PHS, & NHLBI, 1996; NHLBI, 2002; Information Center for Sickle Cell and Thalasemic Disorders, 2000).

## Management

A definitive diagnosis should be made on the basis of clinical history, blood counts, peripheral blood smear, and hemoglobin electrophoresis, including measurement of the minor hemoglobins $A_2$ and $F_1$. Family studies that include electrophoresis and measurement of Hb $A_2$ and Hb $F_1$ are helpful if available. (USDHHS, PHS, & NHLBI, 1996; NHLBI, 2002; Information Center for Sickle Cell and Thalasemic Disorders, 2000).

The suggested schedule for routine laboratory work is shown in **Table 1**.

**Table 1. Suggested Routine Laboratory Tests for Patients With Sickle Cell Disease**

| Test | Age | Frequency |
|---|---|---|
| CBC with WBC differential, reticulocyte count | 3–24 months<br>>24 months | Every 3 months<br>Every 6 months |
| Percent Hb F | 6–24 months<br>>24 months | Every 6 months<br>Annually* |
| Renal function (creatinine, BUN, urinalysis) | ≥12 months | Annually |
| Hepatobiliary function (ALT, fractionated bilirubin) | ≥12 months | Annually |
| Pulmonary function (transcutaneous O2 saturation) | ≥12 months | Every 6 months* |

ALT = Alanine Transaminase; BUN = blood urea nitrogen; CBC = complete blood count; WBC = white blood cell.
*Frequency may vary according to patient's clinical course.

Adapted from *The Management of Sickle Cell Disease* (4th ed.), 2002, Bethesda, MD: National Institutes of Health; NIH publication 02-2117.

Immunizations should follow current guidelines for hepatitis B, polio, diphtheria, pertussis, tetanus, *Haemophilus influenzae* type b, measles, mumps and rubella. Children with sickle cell disease require additional immunizations with Prevnar, the 7-valent pneumococcal conjugated vaccine (PCV7), and (PPV23), the 23 valent pneumococcal polysaccharide vaccine (**Table 2**).

**Table 2. Guidelines for Immunization of Children with Sickle Cell Disease**

| Age | Vaccine |
|---|---|
| Birth (or first visit) | Hepatitis B vaccine #1 or hepatitis B immunoglobulin if the mother is HBsAg |
| 1 month (or 4 weeks after first visit) | Hepatitis B vaccine #2 |
| 2 months | DTaP #1, HbcV #1 or Tetrammune, IPV #1, Prevnar #1 |
| 4 months | DTaP #2, HbcV #2 or Tetrammune, IPV #2, Prevnar #2 |
| 6 months | DTaP #3, HbcV #3 or Tetrammune, IPV #3, hepatitis B vaccine #3 (or 6 months after hepatitis #2 vaccine), Prevnar #3 |
| 12 to 15 months old | MMR (measles, mumps, rubella) #1, Prevnar #4 |
| 15 months old | HbcV booster |
| 15 to 18 months old | DTaP #4, IPV #3 (if not previously given) |
| 24 months old | Pneumococcal (PPV23) vaccine |
| 4 to 6 years old | DTaP #5, pneumococcal (PPV 23) vaccine booster, IPV #4, MMR booster |
| 14 to 16 years old | Td booster, annual influenza vaccine * |

Adapted from *Facts About Sickle Cell Anemia*, 1996, Bethesda, MD: US Department of Health and Human Services, Public Health Service, National Heart, Lung, and Blood Institute; NIH publication 96-4067; *The Management of Sickle Cell Disease* (4th ed.), 2002, Bethesda, MD: National Institutes of Health; NIH publication 02-2117; and *Management of Patients With Sickle Cell Disease*, 2000, Information Center for Sickle Cell and Thalassemic Disorders, available at: http://sickle.bwh.harvard.edu/scdmanage/html.

It is recommended that the varicella vaccine be given anytime at or after the age of 12 months, to any child who has not had a documented case of chickenpox. Children 13 years of age or older who have not had chickenpox should receive two doses of the varicella vaccine given at least 4 weeks apart. Although the varicella vaccine is not addressed specifically in the sickle cell literature, all references indicate children with sickle cell disease should have the recommended childhood immunizations, which includes varicella, in addition to the PPV23 listed in Table 2 (Centers for Disease Control and Prevention [CDC], 2002).

Oral prophylactic penicillin is recommended starting at 2 months of age. Pen VK, 125 mg twice a day, is given until 3 years of age. Pen VK, 250 mg, is given twice a day from 3 years until 5 years of age. Tablets are used whenever possible because of the increased shelf life over liquid penicillin. Injectable Bicillin can be used intramuscularly if indicated. Erythromycin ethylsuccinate (20 mg/kg) is used for children allergic to penicillin (USDHHS, PHS, & NHLBI, 1996; NHLBI, 2002; Information Center for Sickle Cell and Thalassemic Disorders, 2004).

Maintaining adequate hydration is very important to reduce sickle cell episodes (painful events) and vaso-occlusive complications. Because of the inability to concentrate urine, the child will need access to fluids throughout the day and restroom privileges as well. Fluid requirements are calculated on the basis of 150 ml/kg per day. Water and juices containing electrolytes are recommended. An illness with vomiting and/or diarrhea could have serious consequences if appropriate care is not provided (NHLBI, 2002). It is essential that the child and teacher understand their responsibilities related to this and work together.

Many times the child will know that a health problem is beginning. The child should feel comfortable discussing this with parent, teacher, or school nurse so appropriate interventions can be taken. Utilizing a self-rating scale for pain management is helpful. It is important for the child with sickle cell disease to access medical care if his/her temperature exceeds 101°F (38.5°C). Early treatment of infections is imperative, because septicemia in patients with sickle cell disease can be fatal within a few hours (USDHHS, PHS, & NHLBI, 1996; NHLBI, 2002; Information Center for Sickle Cell and Thalassemic Disorders, 2000). Care providers should be aware that nonsteroidal anti-inflammatory drugs (NSAIDs) are not indicated for fever, without medical evaluation. They could mask a significant fever (temperature, >101°F), which could delay medical evaluation and intervention (Information Center for Sickle Cell and Thalassemic Disorders, 2000). Acetaminophen, NSAIDs (ibuprofen), and mild opioids (codeine) are used for pain management in young children. Older children require stronger NSAIDs and opioids for severe pain (NHLBI, 2002).

A decline in academic performance could indicate the presence of cardiovascular disease and the need for further medical evaluation. If the child is hospitalized, absent frequently, or taking narcotic pain medications, changes in performance may be noted. An individualized education program (IEP) may recommend tutoring, homebound, or hospital-based instruction.

The sickle cell crises action plan shown in **Table 3** is a resource for the school setting. Priapism is a painful, prolonged penile erection that was not included in this action plan. The initial intervention for this problem is to empty the bladder and increase fluid intake. Taking a warm bath and/or using exercise to divert blood flow may also be helpful. If the painful erection persists for several hours, it is considered a medical emergency. The condition can adversely affect the reproductive function in males (NHLBI, 2002; Information Center for Sickle Cell and Thalassemic Disorders, 2000).

Dietary counseling should recommend a well-balanced diet. No supplemental iron is recommended. Folic acid (1 mg, by mouth, daily) is recommended to prevent risk of bone marrow aplasia, if the child has chronic hemolysis. Extensive nutritional counseling may be necessary if the child comes from a high-risk environment, such as limited education or low income (NHLBI, 2002).

Regular dental care, including topical fluoride, is needed. Prophylactic antibiotics are indicated prior to procedures to reduce the risk of rheumatic fever, septicemia, or sepsis. Blood transfusions may be necessary if general anesthesia or extensive surgery is needed.

Blood pressure screening is recommended every 6 months after the age of 2 years (Information Center for Sickle Cell and Thalassemic Disorders, 2004).

Routine hearing and vision screening are indicated for young children. Older children and adolescents should have yearly eye examinations by an ophthalmologist because of the increased risk of retinopathy. Periodic tuberculosis skin tests are also recommended (NHLBI, 2002; Information Center for Sickle Cell and Thalassemic Disorders, 2004).

Counseling should include the dangers of illicit drugs, tobacco, and alcohol use. Abstinence, safe sex, and contraception should also be discussed (NHLBI, 2002). Contraception for the female with sickle cell disease may include low-dose-estrogen birth control pills, because of a theoretical risk of thrombosis. Progesterone-only pills can also be helpful since progesterone stabilizes the red blood cell membrane. Depo-Provera is preferred and is given every 12 weeks intramuscularly, may have inhibitory effects on sickling with improved hematologic function during treatment. The decrease in menstrual flow may decrease the anemia. Other benefits include reduced risk of pelvic inflammatory disease, endometriosis, uterine fibroids, ectopic pregnancies, and ovarian cysts. The diaphragm and gel are less effective for contraception than the oral or intramuscular medications. Intrauterine devices are not recommended for women with sickle cell disease because of the risk of bleeding and infections. Condoms are unreliable for contraception but do offer barrier protection against sexually transmitted diseases. Abstinence should be strongly advocated with preteens and adolescents (NHLBI, 2002). Genetic counseling is recommended at the appropriate developmental level.

Sickle Cell Disease

Academic and vocational counseling is needed to assist the individual in making life choices. The goal is for the child to reach his or her potential as an independent and productive member of society (USDHHS, PHS, NHLBI, 1996; NHLBI, 2002; Information Center for Sickle Cell and Thalassemic Disorders, 2000). Counseling resources are available through the comprehensive sickle cell centers as well as in many school settings.

Patients with sickle cell disease also need information on recreational activities, which can help them develop positive self-esteem and self-image and promote self-reliance. They need guidance on travel arrangements that are appropriate for their situation. Parents, family, and the school community should be counseled on the advantages of treating children with sickle cell disease as normally as possible (USDHHS, PHS, NHLBI, 1996; NHLBI, 2002; Information Center for Sickle Cell and Thalassemic Disorders 2000).

**Table 4** provides a concise overview of the primary care needs of a child with sickle cell disease.

**Table 3. SICKLE CELL CRISES ACTION PLAN**

| Symptoms | Plan of Action |
|---|---|
| **Vasco Occlusive Episode or Painful Crisis**<br>*Altered Peripheral/Vascular Tissue Perfusion* | |
| Pain in hands or feet: may have edema (younger children)<br><br>Bone pain in arms, legs, back or chest (older children)<br><br>Abdominal pain | • Acetaminophen as prescribed for pain (no aspirin)<br>• Encourage fluids; daily fluid requirements for weight are:<br>   0 25 pounds   = 1 1/2 to 1 3/4 quarts<br>   26 50 pounds  = 2 to 2 1/2 quarts<br>   51 75 pounds  = 2 1/4 to 3 quarts<br>   76 100 pounds = 2 1/2 to 3 1/2 quarts<br>• Heating pad or warm compress may be used at site if helpful<br>• Rest until medication takes effect<br>• Acetaminophen with codeine if needed; a small amount may be kept on hand and used as prescribed<br>• Use coping strategies for pain management<br>  - divert attention from pain<br>  - use calming self statements<br>  - reinterpret pain sensations (do not discount pain)<br>• Return to class if pain is controlled<br>• Notify parents of episode, treatment, and results |
| **Fever and/or Infection**<br>*Potential for Infection* | |
| Fever over 101°F | • Notify parent to seek medical attention<br>• Assist parent to access medical care if needed |
| **Pulmonary Manifestations/Acute Chest Syndrome**<br>*Altered Cardiopulmonary Tissue Perfusion* | |
| Cough, pain in chest, fever, bone pain, hypoxia | • Notify parent to seek medical care<br>• Anticipate child being absent approximately 2 weeks; arrange for schoolwork appropriately<br>• Expect 1 week of limited activity when child returns to school; make necessary arrangements for schedule or activity modifications |
| **Inability to Concentrate Urine**<br>*Altered Urinary Elimination* | |
| Urinary frequency, enuresis | • Adequate fluid intake is essential; refer to daily requirements provided above<br>• Access to restroom as needed<br>• Communication among teacher, nurse, parent and child may be necessary to avoid abuse of these privileges |
| **Stroke**<br>*Altered Cerebral Tissue Perfusion* | |
| Loses balance, falls more than usual, weakness in a limb or limbs on one side, altered gait, c/o headache, visual disturbances, change in behavior, unexplained change in academic performance, first seizure | • Contact parent to seek medical evaluation<br>• In the event of neurological or physical impairment, provide appropriate individualized school services as needed |

Sickle Cell Disease

| Symptoms | Plan of Action |
|---|---|
| **Aplastic Episode, Severe Anemia**<br>*Altered Peripheral Tissue Perfusion* | |
| Pallor (nail beds, conjunctiva), lethargy (often accompanies viral illness) | • Notify parent to seek medical evaluation |
| **Splenic Sequestration Altered**<br>*Altered Cardiovascular Tissue Perfusion* | |
| Pallor, weakness, lethargy; swollen, painful abdomen; perspiration<br>May go into shock and die | • MEDICAL EMERGENCY. Activate EMS plan for this child |

Reprinted, with permission from Holman.7 For educational materials that may be used in the school setting, contact your local Sickle Cell Disease Association or: National Association for Sickle Cell Disease, 3345 Wilshire Boulevard, Suite 1106, Los Angeles, CA 90010 1880, (800) 421 8453.

**Table 4. Summary of Primary Care Needs for the Child With Sickle Cell Disease**

## Health Care Maintenance

### Growth and development
These children tend to weigh less and be shorter than their peers; weight is affected more than height, and males are affected more than females.
Puberty is delayed for both sexes.
Developmental impairment varies.

### Diet
Diet should be well balanced with a generous amount of fluid; fluid intake should be increased during illness. Supplemental folate requirements may be met with folate tablets, 1 mg daily. Children who are receiving chronic transfusions should limit their oral intake of vitamin C rich foods to limit iron overload.

### Safety
Ingestion of narcotics could lead to respiratory depression.
Alcohol may dehydrate and potentiate narcotics.
Narcotics may impair driving or safe use of machinery.
Recreational activities that involve prolonged exposure to cold, prolonged exertion, or exposure to high altitudes should be avoided. Ice should not be used to treat injuries.
A medical alert bracelet may be helpful.

### Immunizations
Routine standard immunizations are recommended.
*Haemophilus influenzae* type b vaccine is given at 2, 4, and 6 months; immunogenic response is not reliable.
Pneumococcal vaccine is given at 24 months, with boosters given every 3 to 5 years thereafter.

Hepatitis vaccine is strongly recommended.
Influenza vaccine given annually is strongly recommended.

### Screening
*Vision.* Routine screening is recommended until 10 years of age, then an annual retinal examination is recommended to rule out sickle retinopathy.
*Hearing.* Yearly audiologic examination is recommended.
*Dental.* Routine screening is recommended.
*Blood pressure.* Blood pressure should be measured every 6 months after 2 years of age.
*Hematocrit.* Hematocrit is deferred because of condition-specific screening.
*Urinalysis.* Urinalysis is deferred because of condition-specific screening.
*Tuberculosis.* Routine screening is recommended.

### Condition-specific screening
*Hematologic screening.* A CBC with differential, reticulocyte count, and RBC smear should be checked every 6 months.
*Renal function screening.* The BUN and creatinine levels should be checked and a urinalysis done on a yearly basis.
*Lead poisoning.* Lead screening using the EP level is unreliable; the serum lead level must be determined.
*Scoliosis.* Screening should be extended to the late teens because of delayed puberty.
*Cardiac function.* Both ECG and ECHO should be used every 1 to 2 years after age 5.
*Liver function.* Serum liver function tests should be done yearly, The gallbladder should be assessed using ultrasound every 2 years after age 10.

## Common Illness Management

### Differential diagnosis
*Fever*

*Age 5 years or less*

TEMPERATURE LESS THAN 38.5°C

Outpatient management may be considered if the source of the fever can be identified, appropriate antibiotics are given, and follow-up is ensured.

TEMPERATURE MORE THAN 38.5°C

The child should be admitted to the hospital for fever workup, parenteral antibiotics, and observation.

*Age 5 years or more*

The child's condition, compliance with therapy, and ability to obtain followup determine whether or not he or she should receive inpatient or outpatient care.

*Urinary Tract Infections (UTI's).* UTI's, pyelonephritis, and asymptomatic bacteria are more common in SCD. Blood cultures are needed to rule out bacteremia with a diagnosis of UTI. Treatment of the cultured organisms with appropriate follow up is necessary.

### Acute gastroenteritis
Significant dehydration may occur quickly and lead to acidosis and sickling. If oral intake is inadequate, IV hydration is needed.

### Abdominal pain
Abdominal pain crisis may be differentiated from surgical problems by evaluating fever, hematologic changes, peristalsis, and response to symptomatic, supportive therapy.

### Anemia
Hemoglobin and hematocrit levels significantly lower than baseline levels may reflect aplastic crisis, hyperhemolytic crisis, or splenic sequestration. Splenic sequestration may be life-threatening.

### Respiratory distress
It is important to evaluate the patient for acute chest syndrome, which may be fulminant and require exchange transfusion.

### Neurologic changes
Neurologic changes may indicate stroke. Rapid, through evaluation is critical. Exchange transfusion should be performed as quickly as possible if stroke occurs.

### Drug interactions
Antihistamines and barbiturates may potentiate narcotics. Diuretics and bronchodilators, which may have diuretic effects, may cause dehydration and sickling.

## Developmental Issues
### Child care
The caregiver needs to be mindful of fluid requirements and the importance of maintaining normal body temperature and must be able to administer medicines.

### Discipline
Expectations should be consistent, fair, and similar to those of peers and siblings.

### Toileting
Enuresis is frequently a longterm issue because of a large volume of dilute urine.

Nocturia may persist.

### Sleep patterns
Routine care is recommended.

### School issues
The child may have frequent, unpredictable absences. While at school, the child needs access to fluids and liberal bathroom privileges. He or she may participate in mainstream physical education.

### Sexuality
Puberty may be delayed. Men may have fertility problems. Women usually have normal fertility but have some special contraceptive concerns.

### Special family concerns
Because sickle cell disease is genetically transmitted, there is a need for genetic counseling, as well as support for feelings of guilt and responsibility.

---

BUN = blood urea nitrogen; CBC = complete blood count; ECG = electrocardiography; ECHO = echocardiography; EP = erythrocyte protoporphyrin; RBC = red blood cell.

Adapted, with permission, from *Primary Care of the Child with a Chronic Health Condition* (4th ed,. p. 763–764), by P. J. Allen and J. A. Vessey, 2004, Philadelphia: Mosby

# Individualized Healthcare Plan

## Assessment

### History

- Date of diagnosis of sickle cell disease
- Specific type of sickle cell disease child has
- Primary healthcare provider
- Specialist or special clinics
- Immunizations child has received
- Growth and development pattern
- Daily fluid requirements
- Problems with temperature regulation due to environmental temperatures, increased activity, poor hydration, past management
- Problems, hospitalizations, or emergency department visits child has experienced
- Modifications to his/her school program
- Child's special achievements

### Current Status and Management

- Current general health
- Current problems
- Current management routine at home, including medications and fluid requirements
- Child's pain rating scale
- Diversional activities used in his/her pain management plan
- Pain management interventions needed while your child is at school
- Current emergency care plan: need for changes
- Include medical phone numbers in case of an emergency
- Immunization status: required immunizations this school year
- Sensory status: vision and hearing
- Blood pressure
- Growth pattern
- Current sleep/rest pattern
- Nutrition and hydration status
- Current activity tolerance, activity limitations
- Therapeutic regimen: meets an appropriate level of care
- Community's available resources to provide and/or improve care
- Family resources to access and implement appropriate healthcare

### Self-care

- Care the child manages alone
- Student's knowledge about sickle cell disease: age-appropriate
- Student's perception about sickle cell disease
- His/her locus of control.
- Student's knowledge about risk factors
- Student's knowledge of preventive measures to decrease risk factors for complications (diet, fluid requirements, rest, exercise, hygiene, reporting symptoms promptly)
- Student's self-care skills
- Student's barriers to self-care, self-medication and self-treatment
- Student's motivators to self-care and compliance with treatment plan
- Student's readiness to enhance his/her personal knowledge of sickle cell disease
- Student's readiness to enhance his/her self-concept
- Student's readiness for enhanced fluid management
- Parts of care plan parent/guardian does or manages

### Psychosocial Status

- Student's strengths
- Student's adjustment to the problems he/she experiences with sickle cell (medical visits, medications, other related problems)
- Family support system for this child

- Child's friends
- Social activities he/she enjoys

*Academic Issues*
- Student's academic progress (identify strengths and problem subjects)
- Student's attendance record (total and for sickle cell issues)
- Student's fluid requirements during the school day and need for increased/unlimited restroom privileges
- Student's participation in extracurricular activities.
- Student's need for health assessment, medication, and management of symptoms, in the school setting and on field trips
- Need for academic support
- Student's need for homebound and/or hospital instruction
- Student's need for modified physical education program
- Need for modified classroom instruction
- Need for modifications in the school environment
- Need for emergency care plan (ECP).
- Regular or advanced academic school program
- Special education program for homebound or other alternative instruction
- Attendance problems
- Strongest subjects
- Weakest subjects
- Child's special interests or favorite activities in and outside of the school setting
- Previous individualized healthcare plan (IHP)
- Previous IEP

## Nursing Diagnoses (N.D.) (NANDA, 2003)

**N.D. 1** Ineffective tissue profusion—renal, cerebral, cardiopulmonary, gastrointestinal, or peripheral vascular (NANDA 00024)

**N.D. 2** (Risk for) peripheral neurovascular dysfunction (NANDA 00086)

**N.D. 3** Deficient fluid volume (NANDA 00027)

**N.D. 4** Impaired urinary elimination (NANDA 00016)

**N.D. 5** Risk for infection (NANDA 00004)

**N.D. 6** (Risk for) ineffective thermoregulation (NANDA 00005)

**N.D. 7** Ineffective role performance (NANDA 00055) (student) related to absence from school/class due to sickle cell disease symptoms

**N. D. 8** (Risk for) Impaired adjustment (NANDA 00070)

**N. D. 9** Deficient diversional activity (NANDA 00097)

**N. D. 10** Impaired social interaction (NANDA 00052)

**N. D. 11** Social isolation (NANDA 00053)

**N. D. 12** Acute pain (NANDA 00132), chronic pain (NANDA 00133)

**N. D. 13** Deficient knowledge (NANDA 00126) related to cause, treatment, and diagnosis of sickle cell disease

**N. D. 14** Delayed growth and development (NANDA 00111)

**N. D. 15** Impaired dentition (NANDA 00048)

**N. D. 16** Ineffective health maintenance (NANDA 00099)

**N. D. 17** Risk for activity intolerance (NANDA 00092)

**N. D. 18** Disturbed thought processes (NANDA 00130) related to:
- pain management
- risk of cerebral vascular accidents

**N.D. 19** Risk for impaired skin integrity (NANDA 00047) related to peripheral vascular complications

**N.D. 20** Risk for injury (NANDA 00035) if complications of stroke or seizures occur

**N.D. 21** Impaired physical mobility (NANDA 00085) if complication of aseptic necrosis of joints occurs

**N.D. 22** Disturbed sensory perception (NANDA 00122) related to increased risk of visual disturbances

**N.D. 23** Impaired gas exchange (NANDA 00030) related to increased risk of pulmonary infections and pulmonary emboli

**N.D. 24** Ineffective health maintenance (NANDA 00099) related to:
- knowledge deficit
- perceived ineffectiveness of interventions

- denial of need for interventions
- poor self-care skills
- difficult access to care
- poor decision-making and/or problem-solving skills

**N.D. 25** Death anxiety (NANDA 00147)
**N.D. 26** Readiness for enhanced knowledge (NANDA 00161)
**N.D. 27** Readiness for enhanced self-concept (NANDA 00167)
**N.D. 28** Readiness for enhanced fluid balance (NANDA 00160)
**N.D. 29** Effective therapeutic regimen management (NANDA 00082)
**N.D. 30** Ineffective therapeutic regimen management (NANDA 00078)
**N.D. 31** Readiness for enhanced therapeutic regimen management (NANDA 00162)

## Goals

The student will attain and maintain adequate hydration. (N.D.1–4, 28)
The student will assist in preventing/decreasing the number of painful sickle cell events. (N.D. 1–4, 6, 12, 13, 17, 25)
The student will participate in developing and utilizing the pain management plan. (N.D. 12)
The student will assist in preventing/decreasing occurrences of infections. (N.D. 5, 15, 24, 26, 31)
The student will attain and maintain current immunizations as recommended for student with sickle cell disease. (N.D. 5, 16, 24-26, 31)
The student will demonstrate age-appropriate knowledge of diagnosis, symptoms, prescribed interventions, and medication. (N.D. 13, 24, 26-28, 31)
The student will demonstrate increased knowledge and increase self-care skills. (N.D. 16, 24, 26-31)
The student will demonstrate improved decision-making/problem-solving skills. (N.D.13, 16, 24, 26, 27, 29-31)
The student will demonstrate good school attendance pattern. (N.D. 7, 9, 10)
The student will demonstrate good class attendance and participation. (N.D. 7, 9, 10)
The student will assist in developing and implementing an action plan for each potential complication of sickle cell disease, including an emergency care plan for life-threatening symptoms. (N.D. 1–7, 9, 10, 12–14, 16–23, 30)
The student will participate in regular school/class activities, including physical education, with modifications made as necessary. (N.D. 1–12, 14, 17, 30)
The student will demonstrate compliance with sickle cell health management program. (N.D. 8, 13, 24, 26–29, 31)
The student will maintain preventative oral hygiene pattern. (N.D. 15)
The student will good respiratory status during the school day. (N.D. 23)
The student will learn and utilize coping skills that eliminate or reduce anxiety related to their sickle cell disease. (N.D. 25)

## Nursing Interventions

Develop an individualized sickle cell action plan. (N.D. 1–8, 12, 13, 16–18, 20–29, 31)
- Include student, parent/guardian, teacher, and healthcare providers in the development process.
- Coordinate with and incorporate the sickle cell home management plan with parent/guardian and healthcare providers.
- List and describe management measures to follow for each type of potential sickle cell-related problem.
- Include considerations for field trips and other extracurricular school activities.
- Establish guidelines for seeking assistance, including what to do with early warning signs, if medications or interventions have been used within the last hour, if symptoms subside and reappear, when to notify parent/guardian and/or healthcare provider, including telephone numbers.
- Establish criteria for handling medical emergencies related to sickle cell disease.
- Modify plan as needed.

Obtain medical orders for medications and/or interventions needed at school, including modifications needed in the school program. Work with parent/guardian and healthcare provider. (N.D. 1–7, 12–23, 29, 31)
- For preventive management of sickle cell
- For management of sickle cell events
- Anticipate needs for homebound and/or hospital instruction.

Keep accurate records of sickle cell events. (N.D. 1–7,12–23, 29, 31)
- Time of onset of symptoms
- Time symptoms were reported to teacher, health office, or other school personnel and who reported the information

- Describe presenting symptoms—pain and location, not feeling well, difficulty breathing, change in behavior or level of consciousness
- Action taken—temperature, fluids, medication, rest, relaxation techniques, notification of parent and/or healthcare provider, emergency response
- Effectiveness of intervention used
- Name of person notified of the event, time of notification, who made the contact and what was the response or further instructions

In-service teachers and other appropriate school personnel. (N.D. 1–7, 12–23, 29, 31)
- What is sickle cell disease
- What increases risk of problems with sickle cell disease
- What are the preventive measures needed at school
- Note importance of acknowledging and recognizing early warning symptoms
- What to do in the event of symptoms
- Describe importance of prompt management
- Detail problems related to pain management

Work with physical education teachers to modify physical education requirements as indicated. (N.D. 1–14, 16–23, 29)
- Consider contract with older children to self-limit activities only when needed.

Assist parents/guardians, teachers, and healthcare providers in understanding the need for student to participate in regular classroom activities. (N.D. 1–14, 16–23, 26–29, 31)
- Consider classroom and restroom privilege modifications that may be needed.
- Consider modifications to promote self-care and maintain self-esteem.

Encourage and assist parents/guardians to talk with the student's teachers about the child and his/her sickle cell disease. (N.D. 1–31)
- What previous problems the child has experienced
- What preventive measures are used at home
- What treatment/interventions the child requires
- How to handle symptoms that occur at school
- Any modifications in the classroom/school/field trips the child may require (seat near door to facilitate needed restroom facilities, access to sports bottle for fluid requirements during day, avoidance of extreme temperatures, ability to self-limit physical activities as needed)
- Discuss criteria for when child will not be able to attend school and how teacher(s) will be notified.
- Need for assignments if child is absent, possible need for intermittent homebound or hospital-based instruction

Assist the student to administer prescribed medications and/or interventions appropriate for his/her knowledge and skills according to school district policy and legal mandates. (N.D. 1–8, 12–24, 26–29, 31)
- Fluids and restroom facilities will be easily accessible.
- Medications will be easily accessible and administered according to prescribed orders and school district policy and procedures (controlled substances will be handled according to legal mandates as well).
- Physical activities will be self-limited according to symptoms.
- Diet modifications will be made in the child nutrition program if needed for dentition abnormalities.
- These activities will be done with the least amount of disruption to promote optimum participation in the school program.
- These activities will be monitored and/or supervised by the school nurse.

Discuss with the student: (N.D. 1–8, 10–13, 16–24, 26–29, 31)
- Importance of participating in class activities and physical education as much as possible
- Importance of advising adult of overexertion from activity intolerance
- Importance of advising adult of heat or cold intolerance due to thermoregulation problems
- Responsibilities for fluid intake and appropriate use of restroom privileges
- Symptoms that he/she should report to appropriate adult for further evaluation/intervention
- Responsibilities of notifying appropriate adult(s) when symptoms first appear
- What to do if a sickle cell event begins

Provide health education opportunities for individual or group instruction related to: (N.D. 1–31)
- What is sickle cell disease
- How is sickle cell transmitted
- What are signs and symptoms of sickle cell disease
- What can be done to reduce the risk of some of these problems
- What to do when symptoms occur
- Relaxation and guided imagery techniques for mild pain management
- What may be needed to handle moderate and severe pain

- Psychosocial issues related to pain management
- Options for recreational activities/travel
- Growth and development issues
- Counseling on career choices
- How to get help, if needed

Assist the student to identify motivators and barriers to self-care. (N.D. 7, 9, 10, 11, 13, 16, 24, 26–31)

Assist the student to select motivators and implement them to promote self-care. (N.D. 7, 9, 10, 11, 13, 16, 24, 26–31)

Remove as many barriers to self-care as possible. (N.D.13, 24, 26–29)

Assist the student to develop self-care skills. (N.D. 13, 24, 26–29)

- Discuss fluid requirements.
- Discuss responsibility with restroom privileges.
- Discuss hygiene, including rest and nutrition.
- Discuss activity levels and physical education participation.
- Discuss pain management including self-rating pain scale, relaxation techniques, nonsteroidal pain relievers, and controlled substances.
- Discuss adolescent changes when age-appropriate.
- Discuss factors to consider in decision-making process.
- Monitor self-care skills, encourage appropriate actions, reinforce areas needing improvement.

Assist the student to develop appropriate decision-making skills. (N.D. 13, 23, 26–29)

Assist the student to participate in his/her sickle cell management measures. (N.D. 13, 23, 26–29)

- Allow the student to have control over designated areas.

Discuss with the student: (N.D. 13, 23, 26–29)

- The need to take medications as prescribed (on time, at designated intervals, proper dose, method and documentation)
- The need to implement interventions as recommended to decrease risk factors for potential problems
- The importance of his/her participation in the management of medications and interventions
- Benefits of compliance
- Consequences of noncompliance
- Motivators and barriers to compliance

Assist the student to choose and implement motivators for compliance. (N.D. 13, 23, 26–29)

Remove as many barriers to compliance as possible. (N.D. 13, 23, 26–29)

Monitor student's compliance with medications and interventions as prescribed. (N.D. 13, 23, 26–29)

Monitor classroom and physical education activity tolerance. (N.D. 17)

Assist the teacher to adjust activity participation based on activity tolerance and current problems. (N.D. 7)

Monitor attendance patterns and reasons for absences. (N.D. 7)

Monitor need for and use of hospital or homebound services. (N.D. 7)

Monitor utilization of alternative instruction arrangements, if needed. (N.D. 7)

Monitor academic performance. (N.D. 7)

- Refer for evaluation as appropriate.
- Participate in IEP development as indicated.

## Expected Student Outcomes

The student will:

- Participate in regular classroom activities, with modifications made as necessary (hospital or homebound instruction when needed). (N.D. 7, 10, 11, 14, 17, 21, 22)
- Demonstrate good hygiene practices, including hand washing. (N.D. 5, 16, 19)
- Participate in regular physical education activities, with modifications as needed. (N.D. 7, 9, 10, 12, 14, 17, 20-21, 23-24, 29, 31)
- Define what sickle cell disease is (at a developmentally appropriate level). (N.D. 13, 24-26, 31)
- List his/her risk factors. (N.D. 13, 24, 26)
- List his/her preventive measures. (N.D. 13, 15-16, 24, 26, 28, 29, 31)
- List his/her warning signs of a sickle cell event. (N.D. 13, 24-25)
- Maintain adequate hydration as defined in the prescribed health maintenance plan. (N.D. 3-4, 6, 16, 24, 26, 28, 29, 31)
- Recognize his/her warning signs of a sickle cell event and stop activity. (N.D. 1-3, 5, 6, 12, 17-18, 26, 29)
- Describe what to do if a sickle cell event occurs. (N.D. 18, 20, 23, 26, 29, 31)

- Inform his/her teacher (and/or other personnel) when he/she is having sickle cell symptoms. (N.D. 18, 27, 29, 31)
- Initiate and perform his/her action plan (dependent on demonstrated knowledge, skill, school district policy, and legal mandates). (N.D. 27, 29, 31)
- Name the medications, fluid requirements, and interventions he/she uses for management of his/her sickle cell disease. (N.D. 24, 26-29, 31)
- Explain why he/she needs each of the above medications, fluids, or interventions. (N.D. 4, 24, 26-29,31)
- Demonstrate use of self-rating pain scale. (N.D. 12, 26, 29, 31)
- Demonstrate proper procedure for administering medication (as prescribed according to school district policy and legal mandates: check label, dose, interval, time, documentation). (N.D. 26, 27, 29, 31)
- Demonstrate alternative pain management techniques (rest, relaxation, guided imagery). (N.D. 12, 24, 26, 27, 29, 31)
- Describe how he/she participates in his/her sickle cell disease management. (N.D. 27)
- Participate in his/her sickle cell disease management (dependent on demonstrated knowledge, skill, school district policy, and legal mandates). (N.D. 8, 26, 27, 29, 31)
- Describe the benefits of each management plan intervention. (N.D. 8, 26, 27, 29, 31)
- Describe the consequences of not using these management plan interventions. (N.D. 8, 24, 30)
- List motivators and barriers to compliance with prescribed medications and interventions. (N.D. 8, 24, 26, 27, 29, 31)
- Demonstrate compliance with his/her sickle cell management plan (maintenance and emergency). (N.D. 8, 19, 25, 29, 31)
- Demonstrate a good attendance pattern (number of days absent depends on severity of child's disease, a decrease in number from preceding school year). (N.D. 7, 29, 31)
- Have minimal disruptions in his/her educational program due to sickle cell disease. (N.D. 7-8, 29, 31)

## Case Study

James Arnold is a 9-year-old African American boy with sickle cell disease. He was born September 5, 1989. He is 57 inches tall and weighs 48 pounds (both measurements are slightly below the fifth percentile for age). His blood pressure is 106/66 mm Hg, which is within normal limits for his age. Immunizations are up-to-date, including hepatitis B series, MMR booster, and pneumococcal booster. His primary care provider is Dr. Sam Jones, and his pediatric hematologist is Dr. Tom White. His mother talks with Nancy Brown, the nurse practitioner at Dr. White's office (sickle cell center) if she has questions or if problems arise during office hours.

Mrs. Arnold states that James has never been hospitalized for sickle cell events. He was treated in the emergency department for diarrhea and vomiting last year. He had several ear infections as a preschool child, but they resolved with antibiotic therapy. He is no longer taking prophylactic antibiotics unless he goes to the dentist. He eats a well-balanced diet with the rest of the family (parents and two older brothers). He is not taking folate or other medications at this time.

His fluid requirements are approximately 3.5 quarts a day. He prefers cranberry juice, orange sports drink, and water. He has marked containers in the refrigerator at home, and he is responsible for his fluid intake through the day (summertime). He tries not to drink anything after 6 p.m. so he will not have problems with nocturnal enuresis. He likes to feel "in control" of this because he "wants to be like his older brothers and take care of himself."

The only symptoms he has experienced so far are painful events (vaso-occlusive episodes) in his arms and legs. Several episodes were precipitated by hot weather, poor fluid intake, and increased outdoor activity (playing basketball with his older brothers). His pain management plan includes resting, taking three acetaminophen chewable tablets, and increasing fluid intake. He had to use Tylenol 2 with codeine on one occasion last summer.

James has not missed many days of school. He is doing well with his studies. He has never had an IHP before. He enjoys his friends and joined the Cub Scouts at church last year. His maternal grandparents live nearby and help with after-school activities because both parents work outside the home. They try to treat him like all the other grandchildren and don't make a fuss over his health condition.

## Sickle Cell Disease

| Assessment Data | Nursing Diagnosis | Goals | Nursing Interventions | Expected Outcomes |
|---|---|---|---|---|
| Mother reports history of sickle cell events, usually occurring in summer or extremely hot weather with increased activity. | Ineffective tissue perfussion related to sickle cell disease resulting in need to decrease participation in activities to prevent or manage a sickle cell event. | Prevent/decrease sickle cell events. Maintain adequate hydration. | Obtain medical orders for interventions needed at school, including modifications needed in student's school program. Develop a sickle cell action plan to manage events that occur at school.

Keep accurate records of sickle cell events. Provide in-service training for teachers and other identified school personnel regarding sickle cell events that occur at school.

Collaborate with the physical education teachers to modify physical education requirements, as indicated.

Assist parents, teachers, and healthcare providers in understanding the need for James to participate in regular classroom activities. | James will attend school unless symptoms are present that indicate he should not attend (according to criteria established by physician, parents, and school.) Teacher/other school personnel will initiate action plan if an episode occurs at school. James will participate in regular physical education activities, with modifications made as needed. James will have minimal disruptions in his educational program on account of his health condition. |
| History of painful sickle cell events in arms and legs. | Risk for alteration in comfort/pain, related to vaso-occlusive events associated with sickle cell disease. | Improve and maintain good pain management during occurrences of sickle cell events at school. | Monitor classroom and physical education activity tolerance.

Assist teachers in modifying activities based on tolerance.

Obtain medical orders for medication to manage pain associated with sickle cell events. | James will participate in regular classroom activities, with modifications made as needed.

Medication is available in the health office for use during sickle cell episodes. |

| Assessment Data | Nursing Diagnosis | Goals | Nursing Interventions | Expected Outcomes |
|---|---|---|---|---|
| | | | Discuss with James: signs and symptoms of sickle cell disease; what to do if the symptoms occur; relaxation and guided imagery techniques for mild pain management; medications that may be needed for moderate to severe pain management; responsibility for notifying an appropriate adult when symptoms first occur. | James recognizes the signs and symptoms of sickle cell disease. James tells his teacher or the school nurse if signs and symptoms occur at school. |
| | | | Encourage and assist parents to talk with James about his sickle cell disease. | James identifies two methods to decrease pain/discomfort during a sickle cell event. James utilized methods of decreasing pain/discomfort during a sickle cell event. |
| | | | Discuss with James: his responsibilities for fluid intake and use of the restroom; importance of participating in classroom and physical education activities; symptoms he should report to teachers, the school nurse, or other school personnel if they occur; responsibility for notifying appropriate adult when symptoms first appear; what he should do when a sickle cell event begins. | James will participate in regular classroom activities, with modifications made as needed.

James will participate in homebound or hospital-based instruction, if needed.

James will drink 8 oz of fluids per hour while at school.

James will recognize his warning signs for a sickle cell event, stop activity, and notify his teacher if they occur. |
| | | | Provide health education opportunities for James, individual and group. Monitor classroom and physical education activity tolerance. | James will initiate sickle cell action plan if an episode occurs at school. James participates in sickle cell education opportunities. |

| Assessment Data | Nursing Diagnosis | Goals | Nursing Interventions | Expected Outcomes |
|---|---|---|---|---|
| | | | James demonstrates the use of guided imagery to manage mild pain.<br><br>James demonstrates proper administration of medication to manage moderate to severe pain. | Assist James to participate in guided imagery techniques in school to use for management of mild pain during sickle cell events.<br><br>Assist parents to provide medication for management of pain during school hours. Medication is stored and administered according to school policy and procedures.<br><br>All doses of medication given are properly documented. |

# Letter to Schools about Physical Education
## from Healthcare Provider

Date: _____

Re: Patient's name_____

     Medical record number _____

     Date of birth _____

To Whom It May Concern: _____ is currently under my care for sickle cell disease.

    Please allow him/her to participate in the regular physical education program. It will be necessary for him/her to self-limit participation at times due to the effects of sickle cell disease. When this becomes necessary, please allow for alternate activities to promote participation.

    Dehydration, extreme temperatures, and heavy exercise may precipitate a sickle cell event. An individualized healthcare plan is on file in the school for this child, which should be helpful to you.

    Please contact me if you have further questions or concerns regarding this student.

Sincerely,

_____

_____

Printed Name

Phone number_____

Fax number_____

# References

Adams, R.J, Makie, V.C., Brambilla, D., Carl, E., et al. (1998). Stroke prevention in sickle cell anemia. *Control Clinical Trials* 19: 110-129.

Centers for Disease Control and Prevention (CDC). (2002). Recommended childhood immunization schedule—United States 2002. *Morbidity and Mortality Weekly Report, 51*(02). Retrieved May 25, 2004, from http://www.cdc.gov/mmwr/preview/mmwrhtml/mm5102a4.htm

Information Center for Sickle Cell and Thalassemic Disorders. *Management of patients with sickle cell disease.* (2000). Retrieved March 29, 2004, from http://sickle.bwh.harvard.edu/scdmanage.html

National Institutes of Health. (2004, February 25). High blood pressure in the lungs a major risk for death in adults with sickle cell disease. *NIH News.* Retrieved March 21, 2004 from http://www.nih.gov/news/pr/feb2004/cc-25.htm

NANDA International. (2003). *Nursing diagnoses: Definitions & classification 2003-2004.* Philadelphia: Author.

National Heart, Lung, and Blood Institute. (2002). *The management of sickle cell disease* (4th ed.). Bethesda, MD: National Institutes of Health. NIH publication 02-2117. Retrieved March 21, 2004, from http://www.nhlbi.nih.gov/health/prof/blood/sickle/sc_mngt.pdf

U.S. Department of Health and Human Services, Public Health Service, National Heart, Lung, and Blood Institute. (1996 November). *Facts about sickle cell anemia* (pp.1–6). NIH publication 96-4067. Retrieved March 21, 2004, from http://www.nhlbi,nih.gov/health/public/blood/sickle/sca_fact.pdf

# Resources

American Sickle Cell Anemia Association
www.ascaa.org/

Comprehensive Sickle Cell Centers
Public information Web site
www.rhofed.com/sickle/

National Heart, Blood, and Lung Institute
Information Center
P.O. Box 30105
Bethesda, MD 20824-0105
www.nhlbi.nih.gov
301-592-8573

International Association of Sickle Cell Nurses and
    Physician Assistants
http://www.iascnapa.org/

Joint Center for Sickle Cell and Thalassemic
    Disorders
http://sickle.bwh.harvard.edu

Sickle Cell Disease Association of America
16 South Calvert Street
Suite 600
Baltimore, Maryland
410-528-1555
1-800-421-8453
410-528-1495 (fax)
scdaa@sicklecelldisease.org
http://sicklecelldisease.org/

*Sickle Cell Disease: Information for Health
    Professionals*
http://www.sicklecellsociety.org/education/healthpr.htm

Special Child Health and Early Intervention Services
New Jersey Department of Health and Senior
    Services
P.O. Box 364
Trenton, NJ 08625-0364
609-292-1582
609-943-5752 (fax)
http://www.state.nj.us/health/fhs/sicklecell/index.html
Publishes guide: *Sickle Cell Disease: Information for
    School Personnel*

Sickle Cell Information Center
P.O. Box 109
Grady Memorial Hospital
80 Jessie Hill Jr. Drive Southeast
Atlanta, GA 30303
404-616-3572
404-616-5998 (fax)
aplatt@emory.edu
http://www.SCInfo.org

The Sickle Cell Disease Program
Division of Blood Diseases and Resources
National Heart, Lung, and Blood Institute
11 Rockledge Centre
6701 Rockledge Drive
MSC 7950
Bethesda, MD 20802-7950
301-435-0055

# Chapter Sixty-eight

# Skin Disorders

Sue Boos

## Introduction

The skin is the largest organ of the body and is the primary protective barrier to the outside environment (Ball & Bindler, 2003). Its main purpose is to protect inner layers of the body from infectious organisms and from injury caused by temperature extremes and chemical burns; from mechanical damage causing scrapes, bruises, or cuts; and from perforations by foreign objects. Other purposes include sealing the body from outside chemicals and sealing the inner environment of the body from excessive fluid and electrolyte loss. The vascularity of the skin allows it to be the main temperature regulator of the body, as well as an organ of expression, as seen from blushing due to embarrassment or sweating due to fear. Also, the skin is a sensory organ where the perceptions of temperature, texture, and pain are felt. On different parts of the body, the skin differs in texture and color, with each variation being an adaptation to its particular location. Some areas, such as the bottom of the feet and the palms of the hands, are thicker and tougher, whereas delicate areas, such as around the eyes, are thinner and therefore more fragile and pliable.

## Pathophysiology

Skin structures include the outer layer, or epidermis, which itself is composed of five layers. Skin cells are continually produced from its lowest level and progressively migrate to the surface, where they thicken, eventually die, and are constantly sloughed off to be replaced by new cells approximately every 4 weeks (James, Ashwill, & Droske, 2002). The tough epidermis is nourished by blood vessels within the next lower level of skin, the dermis, which is the thickest skin layer. This layer is more firm than the epidermis and gives skin its flexibility. It has an elaborate network of blood vessels and nerves within its connective tissue mass. Below the dermis is the thick, subcutaneous fat tissue layer, which is the cushion for major vessels, nerves, and lymphatics. This is the layer that gives contour to the body and protects and insulates against cold and absorbs trauma (Hockenberry, Wilson, & Kline, 2003). Hair follicles, as well as sweat and sebaceous glands, originate within this layer.

Different structures, such as sweat glands and hair follicles, are more concentrated in certain parts of the body and are very sparse in others. The concentration of various skin structures in different locations is often the determining factor regarding the type of skin disorder found on various parts of the body (Hockenberry et al., 2003).

Skin lesions have various causes. They may be the result of (1) trauma from injury, infectious organisms, temperature extremes, or toxic chemicals; (2) an allergic reaction due to an insect bite or from contact with an individual allergen or irritant; (3) a hereditary condition; or (4) a systemic disease with a skin manifestation (Hockenberry et al., 2003). Distinctive reactions may differ from child to child and from age to age with a specific child.

More than half of all dermatologic disorders constitute a variety of dermatitis (Hockenberry et al., 2003). Common and acute reactions cause erythema with or without vesicles, edema, and inflammation. The location and type of reaction are often distinctive to the particular disorder. Without subsequent infection from itching and scratching, they are often easily treated and the skin recovers with no lasting marks (Hockenberry et al., 2003). This may not be true of chronic conditions.

Wounds are the disruption of the integrity of the skin. They are classified as (1) partial-thickness, meaning that the epidermis and some portions of the dermis are compromised; (2) full-thickness, which is more serious, meaning that damage extends through the epidermis, the entire dermis, and into the subcutaneous tissue; and (3) complex, those which extend into muscle or bone (Hockenberry et al., 2003). Acute wounds are those that will heal uneventfully in an expected manner and time frame barring infection or other complications. Chronic wounds are those that fail to heal as anticipated on account of other complications. Children with mobility problems, paralysis, or paresthesia are prone to skin breakdown when pressure from braces or wheelchairs presses on soft skin over bony protuberances.

Many factors influence the healing of wounds of all kinds. Good, overall health and the quality of nutrition, with sufficient protein, calories, and vitamin C, in particular, are necessary for the healing of serious assaults to the skin. An adequate intake of water and other fluids is needed to maintain skin hydration (Hockenberry et al., 2003). Certain chemicals commonly used as antiseptics, such as hydrogen peroxide and povidone-iodine solutions, have been found to have only minimal disinfectant properties and may be damaging to healthy cells, and may possibly be absorbed through the skin (Hockenberry et al.).

Because of the very large and visible nature of skin disorders, they can be a source of great emotional discomfort, as well as painfully and physically distressing. Other children may reject a child who "looks funny or strange" or fear that they may "catch" the disorder regardless of its cause. For acute, short-lived and, usually, easily treated conditions, this does not present a long-term problem. But for children who suffer from chronic or severely disfiguring conditions, the psychological effects may be more devastating than the physical.

## Management

Treatment for skin disorders may be topical or systemic. Bland ointments are used topically to avoid further irritation and reduce absorption through broken or inflamed skin lesions. To reduce stimuli causing itching in many disorders, avoid hot or cold applications. Instead, tepid or cool applications of soaks or lotions soothe the skin surface and protect from external stimuli. The anti-inflammatory effects of glucocorticoids ease minor allergic skin reactions. These topical over-the-counter ointments are often used incorrectly by families for *all* skin manifestations. Other topical treatments include antibiotics for localized and minor infections and antifungals for localized fungal infections.

Systemic treatment, usually corticosteroids and antibiotics, is often used as an adjunct to topical treatment for skin disorders (Ball & Bindler, 2003). To avoid excessive absorption, topical treatments are used cautiously for skin lesions that are serious and/or long-term or for those covering a large amount of body surface (Fox, 2002).

If the offending causative factor is thought to be allergic in nature, it must be eliminated from the child's environment. Many common household remedies can further irritate dermatitis and must be identified and eliminated. If the skin disorder is chronic, nursing care must be sensitive to the ongoing regularity of treatment and the psychosocial disturbances caused by visible flare-ups.

Commonly used dressings serve many functions, including (1) protection from infection and further injury; (2) compression to stop bleeding and reduce swelling; (3) maintenance of a moist, healing environment; (4) reduction of pain; (5) absorption of drainage; and (6) application of medication (Hockenberry et al., 2003). Not only does the traditional sterile gauze pad used on an open wound offer little protection from infection, it also may cause further damage by allowing a wound to become dry and crusted, or by sticking to the wound itself, disrupting healing when the dressing is removed.

In the school setting, nursing management is directed toward preventing further damage, preventing infection or other complications, and providing pain relief and protection during healing.

## Individualized Healthcare Plan

## Assessment

*History*
*Wounds:*
- Date injury occurred
- Cause of injury
- Injury treatment plan to date: effectiveness, compliance with treatment plan both at home and at school, ability of parent or guardian to manage treatment plan—healthcare access, financial ability to comply, hygiene facilities at home and school, barriers to compliance both at home and at school.
- Medical or home management of the wound to date
- Previous skin problem history
- Other injuries associated with the wound

*Skin Conditions*
- Date first noticed
- Date medical diagnosis made
- Healthcare provider
- Appearance since onset
- Subsequent spread to other areas
- Cause: infection, environmental or chemical irritant, mechanical trauma, allergen, inherited trait
- Objective symptoms: inflammation, lesions, rash, dryness, scaling, scarring, hair loss, discoloration, affected locations on the body
- Subjective symptoms: itching, burning, stinging, soreness, aching, tingling, more or less than when first noticed
- Use of any skin products: lotions, creams, soaps, shampoos
- Daily appearance: same or evolving, changes since first identified, spread
- Symptoms interfering with activities of daily living: eating, sleeping, playing, sports, socializing with peers
- Family or friends with similar symptoms
- Past skin conditions

- Connection to any other medical treatment: medications (prescription or over-the-counter), treatments, conditions
- Medical treatment plan to date: effectiveness, compliance, ease of adapting medical regimen to daily life of child and family/school, easing or worsening of condition

## Current Status and Management
- Current subjective symptoms
- Current objective findings and appearance
- Current discomfort or pain associated with the skin condition/injury
- Known allergies
- Current behavioral manifestations: scratching, rubbing, splinting to avoid movement, crying, irritability, distractibility, sleeplessness, decrease in appetite, decrease in physical activity
- Current medical treatment plan, including medications, dressings, dietary requirements or restrictions, hydration needs, infection prevention measure needed, other interventions
- Effectiveness of medical treatment plan
- Current home remedy treatments: ointments, lotions, medications
- Effectiveness of home remedies
- Other associated current symptoms: erythema, odor, fatigue, lack of appetite, depression, fever, joint pain, malaise, headache
- Skin indications of physical or sexual abuse, such as bruises in several stages of healing; patterns of marks, cuts, or bruises; frequent health room visits; designation as an "accident-prone student," etc.
- Depth of the injury into lower tissue levels
- Cleanliness and/or signs of infection
- Evidence of healing.

## Self-care
- Student's knowledge of the cause, treatment, and prevention of the skin condition
- Parents'/guardians' knowledge of the cause, treatment, and prevention of the skin condition
- Student's self-care skills: hygiene and hand washing, diet and hydration needs, medication administration, treatment plan, dressing changes, prevention, knowledge of signs and symptoms of infection
- Student's motivation to do self-care
- Student's ability to follow medical treatment plan
- Student's willingness to comply with treatment plan at home and school and during other activities away from home
- Barriers at home and school to performing self-care daily
- Student participation in treatment plan and associated self-care: independent, semi-independent, dependent

## Psychosocial Status
(Primarily for chronic or seriously disfiguring skin disorders)
- Age and developmental level of the student
- Family developmental level
- Student's perception of general health
- Student's perception of his/her skin disorder
- Student's feelings and concerns about the skin condition
- Student's perceptions of what his peers think about his skin condition
- Student's level of interaction and comfort level with peers
- Changes in social relationships with peers as a result of the skin condition: isolation, avoidance
- Student's efforts to hide his/her skin condition: clothing, make-up, hats, long hair
- Student's social behaviors at school: classroom interaction, avoidance of physical education, cafeteria, playground, sports, changes in bus behavior, recipient of bullying behavior or taunting
- Student's support network: family, friends, church, school, support groups

## Academic Issues
- School attendance patterns, in relation to skin condition/injury
- Academic performance
- Teacher's perception of the student's classroom performance and behaviors in relation to academic ability
- Participation in physical education and extracurricular activities: activity limitations if needed

- Classroom or other environmental modifications or adaptations needed
- Health services needed during the school day

## Nursing Diagnoses (N.D.) (NANDA, 2003)

**N.D. 1** (Risk for) impaired skin integrity (NANDA, 00046, 00047) related to:
- environmental agents
  - chemicals
  - unclean water
- mechanical trauma
  - repeated friction over skin surface (such as from braces or wheelchairs)
  - scratching or picking at affected skin
- compromised immunologic factors
  - other systemic chronic illness or disease
  - recent viral illness
- infective agents
  - childhood communicable disease (such as chickenpox, fifth disease, *Strep* infection)
- allergens
  - known food allergen for this student (such as peanuts, chocolate, milk, strawberries)
  - known or suspected seasonal allergies (such as grass, molds, pollens)
  - other symptoms thought to be allergic in nature (such as a runny nose, husky voice, scratchy throat, and/or hearing difficulties)
- inherited traits
  - family history of allergies (to food, pets, dust mites, pollens, molds, etc.)
  - family history of severe acne (at and during puberty)

**N.D. 2** Risk for infection (NANDA, 00004) related to:
- presence of bacterial, viral, or fungal infective agents within school population (such as chickenpox, *Strep* infection, plantar warts, athlete's foot, ringworm)
- pruritus (itching) and scratching
- inadequate hand washing and general hygiene
- ineffective or inadequate treatment plan
- noncompliance with treatment plan
- improper care of medications (such as not washing hands before opening ointments or salves, leaving medication containers open after use)

**N.D. 3** Pain, acute or chronic (NANDA, 00132, 00133) related to:
- skin lesions
- pruritus/itching
- underlying disease process
- secondary infection
- noncompliance with treatment plan

**N.D. 4** Risk for disturbed body image (NANDA, 00118) related to:
- inaccurate perception of appearance
- avoidance of peer relationships (due to fear of reaction of others/peers and personal feelings about appearance)
- unpredictable nature of chronic skin outbreaks
- scarring from repeated lesions

**N.D. 5** Risk for deficient knowledge (NANDA, 00126) related to:
- lack of knowledge of current management plans and information about healing
- continuous nature of treatment for chronic skin conditions
- importance of hand washing and general hygiene
- relationship of nutrition and hydration to healing
- ways to avoid or reduce contact with allergens
- pain-reduction techniques (both pharmacologic and nonpharmacologic)

**N.D. 6** Risk for ineffective therapeutic regimen management, individual or family (NANDA, 00078) related to:
- knowledge deficit
- improper use of medications
- perceived ineffectiveness of medication
- chronic nature of some skin disorders leading to necessity of long-term adherence to treatment plan

- complexity and regularity of treatments
- inability of student and/or family to demonstrate proper care skills and behavior
- noncompliance with management/therapeutic/medical plan
- perceived financial or transportation barriers

## Goals

The student will attain and maintain (normal) skin appearance and integrity. (N.D. 1)

The student will increase/maintain compliance with treatment plan. (N.D. 6)

The student will increase independent self-care skills, including proper hand washing, glove use, and proper technique with medications and treatments. (N.D. 2, 3, 5, 6)

The student will increase knowledge about his/her known allergens. (N.D. 5, 6)

The student will maintain an improved self-image. (N.D. 4)

The student will increase and/or maintain academic achievement. (N.D. 4)

The student will increase ability to manage itching, soreness, and/or pain. (N.D. 3)

The student will participate in age-appropriate activities with peers and family. (N.D. 4)

The student will make wise food choices to enhance healing. (N.D. 1, 2, 5, 6)

The student will continue treatment and medical care, as needed. (N.D. 1, 5, 6)

The student will maintain good nutrition and hydration (N.D. 5)

## Nursing Interventions

Develop an IHP (N.D. 1–6)
- Include student, parents/guardians, teachers, and healthcare provider.
- Coordinate home and school management.
- Determine if known allergens or triggers are present at school.
- Determine time and place for daily treatments needed at school.
- Identify a place to keep medications and treatment supplies secure and clean.
- Identify place and proper method of disposal for used gloves, treatment, and/or dressing supplies.
- Modify plan as needed.

Keep accurate treatment records. (N.D. 1–6)
- Changes in skin appearance
- Treatments and medications, time, dose, route of administration
- History of effective and ineffective medications and treatments
- Supplies used and/or needed
- Psychosocial adjustment of student
- Pain management techniques

Provide in-service training for teachers and other school personnel working with the student. (N.D. 1, 2, 4, 5, 6)
- General skin disorder information and skin disorder information specific to student
- Medication and treatments necessary on a daily basis
- Signs and symptoms of a secondary skin infection
- Importance of regular and continuing treatment, including medications and treatments that must be administered during the school day (allowing for input from teachers on how to avoid an impact on learning or social relationships for the time missed from the classroom and peer contact)
- Allergic components (if pertinent), including known triggers for this student
- If food allergies are suspected or identified, ensure that classroom teacher and lunchroom personnel are notified
- Detail importance of avoidance of known triggers
- Importance of good hand washing and good hygiene in general
- Importance of well-balanced nutrition to enhance healing. If severe acne is the diagnosis, stress that food is rarely implicated as a cause.

Observe and monitor medication and treatment administration. Teach and reinforce proper technique when needed. (N.D. 2, 5, 6)
- Periodically inspect affected skin.
- Have student practice and demonstrate proper technique.
- Discuss treatments, including proper storage, use, and disposal of medications and treatment supplies. Observe periodically.
- Modify treatment plan as needed.

Refer for medical evaluation, diagnosis, and treatment, if indicated. (N.D. 1, 2, 3)
- Assist parent and student to access healthcare.
- Assist parent to access skin specialist (dermatologist).
- Encourage periodic follow-up with healthcare provider.
- Assist family to decrease barriers (financial, transportation) to continued healthcare.

Obtain medication and treatment orders from student's healthcare provider and parental authorization. (N.D. 1, 2, 6)
- Administer medications and treatments in accordance with prescribed orders.
- Encourage positive skin care procedures and general hygiene measures to promote skin healing.
- Encourage compliance with prescribed treatments.
- Teach developmentally appropriate self-care with treatments, medications, and supplies.
- Assist student to prevent secondary infection.
- Obtain accurate information of known allergens.
- Assist student to maintain proper technique with treatments and medication.

Develop health education plan for student and family to encourage compliance with proper and continuing treatment at home and at school. (N.D. 1–6)
- Develop plan to increase student's and family's level of knowledge on causes of skin disorder and treatments needed.
- Assess student's knowledge about medications.
- Stress importance of and encourage regular school attendance and participation.
- Stress importance of social relationships and support.
- Stress importance of regular peer interaction.
- Monitor classroom performance and academic achievement. Refer as needed.

Assist student to properly treat skin condition at school and at home. (N.D. 2, 4, 5, 6)
- Assess level of skill with supplies and medications.
- Teach, encourage, and periodically monitor and reinforce proper hand-washing technique.
- Stress importance of keeping hands away from affected skin.
- Keep healthy skin that is near affected skin dry and clean to prevent its breakdown from moisture.
- Teach and periodically reinforce proper glove technique.
- Reinforce safe disposal of all dressings and supplies used, including gloves, to prevent possible spread of germs and infection to self or others.
- Ensure privacy for treatments, with secure storage of medications.
- Determine how to decrease disruption of the regular school day as much as possible.

Discuss with student/family and periodically reinforce (N.D. 1, 2, 5, 6), as needed:
- Importance of regular school attendance.
- Regular and normal peer interactions and relationships.
- Full participation in school-day activities, including physical education.
- Understanding the need to avoid known allergens.
- Importance of proper nutrition, hydration, and diet to enhance and promote healing.
- Importance of adequate intake of water to enhance hydration.
- Modification of treatment plan, in collaboration with healthcare provider, student, family, and teachers.

Assist student/family to identify barriers to continued treatment. (N.D. 5, 6)
- Assist with removing barriers

Assist student to identify motivators to continued self-care. (N.D. 4, 6)
- Implement motivators

Discuss and periodically reinforce with student: (N.D. 1-6)
- Understanding of causes of disorder
- Knowledge of and responsibilities for self-care
- Identification of known allergens and ways to avoid or reduce contact with irritants
- Self-care skill level, acknowledging good care
- Knowledge and recognition of signs and symptoms of infection
- Importance of adherence to regular treatment protocols (when, where, how, proper medications and disposal of used supplies)
- Consequences of noncompliance
- Motivators and barriers to compliance
- Importance of participation in normal school and peer activities
- Perceptions of self-image

Assist student to participate in management of skin disorder treatment plan, as appropriate. (N.D. 4, 5, 6)
- Allow student input into daily schedule (dependent upon age, developmental level, and knowledge of and skill level for treatments).
- Increase student independence in medication and treatment administration, as appropriate.
- Monitor student, family, teacher perceptions of student's self-care ability and responsibility level to adhere to treatment protocol.
  - Implement nondrug or medication pain reduction techniques (such as using lukewarm rather than hot water, loose clothing made from natural fibers [avoidance of wool], and washing irritants from skin quickly with cool water).
- Modify plan accordingly.

Assist student to recognize and verbalize positive social and peer interactions. (N.D. 4)
- Encourage increased participation in extracurricular activities
- Recognize student achievement in classroom and social activities.

Promote confidence through emphasis on past successful coping. (N.D. 4)
- Identify and encourage use of past successful coping skills.
- Identify and eliminate unsuccessful coping skills.
- Assist student to learn and utilize coping strategies that are more successful.

Encourage persistence with treatments through frequent and regular interactions with the student and family. (N.D. 6)

## Expected Student Outcomes

The student will:
- Accurately describe steps in wound healing. (N.D. 5)
- Correctly identify known allergens. (N.D. 5)
- Independently avoid allergic irritants. (N.D 1 and 5)
- Identify and describe signs and symptoms of secondary skin infection, such as redness, increased temperature (systemically or at site of lesion), oozing, increased size or distribution of lesions, etc. (N.D. 2)
- Verbalize absence, reduction, or control of pain or itching. (N.D. 3)
- Exhibit no evidence of discomfort or continued scratching. (N.D. 3)
- Demonstrate regular school attendance. (N.D. 4)
- Participate fully with peers and family, in age-appropriate activities, including physical education. (N.D. 4)
- Verbalize and manifest positive self-image by active participation in management of, and compliance with, treatment modalities. (N.D. 4, 5)
- Demonstrate active social participation with peers in school, extracurricular, community (church, groups, clubs, etc.) and home/neighborhood activities during free time. (N.D. 4)
- Consistently demonstrate proper self-care, hand-washing and glove technique. (N.D. 2, 5, 6)
- Demonstrate proper disposal of medications/ointments/soaks, gloves, and any applicators and/or dressings. (N.D. 2, 5, 6)
- Demonstrate good hygiene practices. (N.D. 2, 5, 6)
- Demonstrate wise nutrition choices in cafeteria at lunch and snacks to enhance healing. (N.D. 1, 2, 5, 6)
- Continue treatment and medical care as needed. (N.D. 1, 5, 6)

The student's affected skin will:
- Show signs of healing, lessening of allergic reaction, or maintenance of control of chronic or inherited condition. (N.D. 1, 2)
- Show no signs of impaired skin integrity or evidence of secondary infection. (N.D. 1, 2)
- Demonstrate good nutrition and hydration intake at school. (N.D. 1, 2)

## Case Study

Josh is a rough-and-tumble 11-year-old boy with a history of asthma and chronic atopic dermatitis (eczema) seen on the flexor surfaces of elbows and knees and on the backs of both hands. His type of manifestation and body distribution is the most common for his age. He lives in the sunny western part of the United States where the weather is frequently windy and dry with long hot summers. The dermatitis is exacerbated from mid spring to late fall, when the boys and girls play soccer and football, with the attendant number of scrapes and cuts that occur from falls on the turf and rolling along the ground. Because of his age, careful hand washing usually is minimal, so secondary infection from scratching with dirty fingernails is common.

More than half of children with atopic dermatitis have a family disposition toward allergic conditions, including asthma. The skin of affected children usually has a strong inflammatory response to allergens or other irritants, causing swelling and erythema that aggravate pruritus. Because of excessive scratching from intense itching, skin infections often accompany atopic dermatitis.

The typical appearance of the child is one of a tired and cranky child with dry and itchy skin that shows a pattern of exacerbation and healing. When infected, the skin may be oozing or crusted. A diagnosis is made by a positive family history, the type and body distribution of the lesions, intense itching and scratching, and the elimination of scabies as a cause. The goals of treatment are control of the itching, hydration, prevention or control of secondary infection, and avoidance of allergens or irritants.

# Skin Disorders

| Assessment Data | Nursing Diagnosis | Goals | Nursing Interventions | Expected Outcomes |
|---|---|---|---|---|
| Josh has chronic, but periodic, itchy, weepy skin sores on his elbows and hands related to seasonal allergies. | Impaired skin integrity related to: allergies and inherited traits; sensitive and easily irritated skin; frequent trauma to the skin related to rambunctious nature of Josh. | Josh will learn age- and developmentally appropriate self-care. | Refer to physician for complete medical evaluation, if information is not current and available. | Josh's skin has normal appearance and integrity. |
| Family history of allergic symptoms and conditions. | | Josh will appropriately avoid known allergic triggers. | Secure physician orders and parent authorization for medication and treatment. | Josh demonstrates age- and developmentally appropriate self-care. |
| Josh's skin is dry and easily becomes itchy, red, and weepy in response to many irritants, environmental contacts, and some food allergies. | | Josh will drink water regularly to enhance hydration. | Determine if known allergens are present in the school environment. | Josh avoids known allergic triggers and skin irritants routinely (daily). |
| Josh is a very active boy who frequently has cuts and scrapes on his skin. | | Josh will learn ways to avoid injuries on the playground. | Coordinate care plan at home and school to promote healing. | Josh demonstrates a decrease in playground injuries and other cuts and scrapes. |
| | | Josh will assist in prevention of skin irritation. | Keep accurate records of skin appearance and treatments including effective and ineffective. | Josh's fluid and water intake consistently maintains hydration. |
| | | | Schedule and oversee prescribed treatments at school as needed. | |
| | | | Periodically inspect all affected skin and document appearance. | |
| | | | Encourage Josh and parent to comply with continued treatment. | |

| Assessment Data | Nursing Diagnosis | Goals | Nursing Interventions | Expected Outcomes |
|---|---|---|---|---|
| Josh has frequent secondary infection from playing soccer and football during times of skin breakout. | Risk for infection related to: itching and scratching, causing open sores that are easily contaminated with germs; inadequate hygiene and hand washing; nonuse of gloves for treatment; improper care and disposal of medication and treatment supplies; frequent skin trauma due to Josh's rambunctious nature. | Josh will learn signs and symptoms of skin infection. | Teach signs and symptoms of infection. | Josh's skin shows no evidence of secondary infection. |
| Josh's hands and fingernails don't appear clean. | | Josh will learn and practice good hygiene in general, with hand washing being a high priority. | Teach and encourage: good hygiene, hand washing, and use of gloves for treatments. | Josh consistently demonstrates good hygiene and proper hand washing. |
| His hand-washing skills are poor. | | Josh will stop scratching behaviors to relieve itching. | Proper storage, use, and disposal of treatment supplies. | Josh identifies and treats any secondary infection quickly and promptly. |
| Josh frequently scratches his skin until it is open and bleeding. | | Josh will practice age- and developmentally appropriate self-care. | Age- and developmentally appropriate self-care. | Josh's skin is intact and shows no evidence of scratching. |
| Medication tubes and bottles are left open and not kept in clean containers. | | Josh will keep medications and supplies clean and in closed containers. | Explore behavior modification plan to acknowledge and reward NOT scratching. | Josh demonstrates proper use, storage and disposal of medication and supplies without prompting. |
| Josh doesn't understand that scratching with dirty fingernails will lead to secondary infection. | | | | Josh's self-care practices are consistent with age and developmental level. |
| Josh doesn't know how to properly take care of and dispose of medications and treatment supplies, to minimize risk of secondary infection. | | | | |
| J. says skin is itchy and sore. | Pain related to: a) weepy and itchy skin sores; b) underlying disease process; c) secondary infection; d) incomplete treatment. | J. will: increase compliance with prescribed treatments. | Teach non-pharmacologic techniques to avoid further irritating skin. | J. demonstrates several non-pharmacologic pain reduction techniques when needed. |
| | | J. will: increase his ability to manage itching and soreness. | Teach age- and developmentally appropriate pain management techniques. | J. demonstrates compliance with prescribed treatments consistently. |
| | | J. will: identify and avoid known allergies and irritants. | Administer medication and treatment as prescribed | |

| Assessment Data | Nursing Diagnosis | Goals | Nursing Interventions | Expected Outcomes |
|---|---|---|---|---|
| | | J's skin will be intact consistently. | Encourage continued self-care to promote healing and lessen itchy lesions. | J's skin is intact with no evidence of scratching.<br><br>J. can correctly identify and avoids known skin irritants. |
| Josh expresses embarrassment over skin appearance.<br><br>Josh is aggressive due to anger and rejects his friends when skin disorder is present.<br><br>Josh's school attendance is poor when disorder is apparent.<br><br>Josh avoids his friends and social activities at school and with family. | Risk for body image disturbance related to: inaccurate perception of appearance; inaccurate perception of friends' thinking and feeling about Josh; avoidance of social activities; poor school attendance. | Josh will maintain a high self-image.<br><br>Josh will attend school regularly and participate fully in class activities, including physical education class.<br><br>Josh will maintain normal peer relationships.<br><br>Josh will maintain age-appropriate social relationships with peer and adults. | Provide privacy and increasing independence with self-care.<br><br>Allow age- and developmentally appropriate control over scheduling of treatments.<br><br>Schedule health/treatment related activities to minimize classroom disruption and learning interruption.<br><br>Regularly monitor psychosocial adjustment, participation in, and behavior during classroom and playground activities.<br><br>Monitor school attendance and academic performance.<br><br>Encourage and promote positive coping skills. | Josh freely verbalizes feelings and concerns appropriately.<br><br>Josh attends school regularly and participates fully in activities.<br><br>Josh demonstrates active participation with peers in school and extracurricular/social activities. |
| Josh doesn't understand why treatment must be continued for long periods of time.<br><br>Josh doesn't practice good food choices.<br><br>Josh forgets to wash his hands. | Risk for knowledge deficit related to: underlying disease process; chronic nature of treatment; relationship of good nutrition, adequate hydration, and hygiene to healing; identification and avoidance of allergens; non-pharmacologic pain reduction. | Josh will independently follow treatment regimen.<br><br>Josh will maintain effective treatment management.<br><br>Josh will learn good hygiene and hand-washing technique. | Develop educational plan for Josh by first assessing knowledge level and deficits.<br><br>Teach signs and symptoms of infection and disease process. | Josh consistently demonstrates proper treatment technique and management.<br><br>Josh recognizes signs and symptoms of infection.<br><br>Josh accurately describes the disease process of his skin condition. |

## Skin Disorders

| Assessment Data | Nursing Diagnosis | Goals | Nursing Interventions | Expected Outcomes |
|---|---|---|---|---|
| Josh's fingernails are often long and dirty.<br><br>Josh forgets to use gloves, and when he does, he forgets to dispose of them properly.<br><br>Josh's skin is dry and scaly-looking, with poor turgor. | | Josh will learn and make proper food choices.<br><br>Josh will learn and maintain proper gloving technique and disposal.<br><br>Josh will learn and maintain proper disposal of used supplies.<br><br>Josh will learn avoidance of known allergens.<br><br>Josh will drink enough water and fluids for adequate hydration. | Teach and periodically monitor proper technique for treatment, medication storage, and disposal of supplies.<br><br>Teach importance of hand washing and good hygiene, proper nutrition, and adequate hydration.<br><br>Teach recognition and avoidance of allergens. | Josh demonstrates proper hand washing and gloving.<br><br>Josh demonstrates proper medication storage and disposal of supplies.<br><br>Josh accurately demonstrates wise food choices and maintains adequate hydration.<br><br>Josh identifies his known allergens and ways to avoid them. |
| Because of periodic, but chronic, nature of skin condition, treatment isn't continuous and is frequently abandoned before symptoms are resolved.<br><br>Josh doesn't understand that treatment may be complex and long-term.<br><br>Josh gets tired of constant treatment regimens.<br><br>Josh doesn't use good treatment technique and doesn't properly dispose of supplies. | Risk for ineffective management of therapeutic regimen related to: chronic nature of allergic skin disorders; improper use, storage, and disposal of medication and supplies; complexity, regularity, and continuity of treatment protocols; poor self-care skill; noncompliance. | Josh will maintain compliant and age-appropriate self-care management.<br><br>Josh will consistently avoid known allergic triggers and allergens.<br><br>Josh will independently use proper self-care skills.<br><br>Josh will consistently use good treatment technique and disposal of supplies. | Secure privacy for self-care treatment.<br><br>Aid student to recognize barriers to continued treatment protocols.<br><br>Teach and monitor proper treatment technique.<br><br>Monitor long-term compliance with complex regimens.<br><br>Motivate student to continue compliance.<br><br>Allow student input into daily scheduling of treatments during the school day.<br><br>Give increasing independence in treatment regime as compliance increases. | Josh explains his skin condition and states the reasons for prolonged and persistent treatment.<br><br>Josh is compliant with treatment regimen through age-appropriate self-care.<br><br>Josh demonstrates and maintains proper treatment technique.<br><br>Josh demonstrates proper disposal of gloves and supplies.<br><br>Josh avoids contact with known allergic triggers and allergens. |

*Chapter Sixty-eight: Skin Disorders*

# References

Ball, J., & Bindler, R. (2003). *Pediatric nursing: Caring for children* (3rd ed.). Upper Saddle River, NJ: Prentice Hall.

Fox, J. A. (2002). *Primary health care of infants, children, and adolescents* (2nd ed.). St. Louis, MO: Mosby.

Hockenberry, M. J., Wilson, D., & Kline, N. E. (2003). *Wong's nursing care of infants and children* (7th ed.). St. Louis, MO: Mosby.

James, S. R., Ashwill, J. W., & Droske, S. C. (2002). *Nursing care of children: Principles & practice* (2nd ed.). Philadelphia: Saunders.

NANDA International. (2003). *Nursing diagnoses: Definitions & classification 2003 – 2004*. Philadelphia: Author

# Bibliography

Adinoff, A , & Clark, R. (1996). Atopic dermatitis. In C. W. Bierman, D. Pearlman, G. Shapiro, & W. Busse (Eds.), *Allergy, asthma, and immunology from infancy to adulthood* (pp. 613–632). Philadelphia: Saunders.

Bryant, R., & Doughty, D. (1998). *Acute and chronic wounds: Nursing management* (2nd ed.). St. Louis: Mosby.

Carpenito, L. J. (2002). *Nursing diagnosis: Application to clinical practice* (9th ed.). Philadelphia: Lippincott.

Cohen, B. A. (2000). *Pediatric dermatology* (2nd ed.). Philadelphia: Saunders.

Hanifin, J. M. (2003). An overview of atopic dermatitis. *Dermatology Nursing, 15*(4), S6–9.

Kristal, L., & Klein, P. (2000). Atopic dermatitis in infants and children. *Pediatric Clinics of North America, 47*(4), 877–896.

LeBoit P. E. (Ed.). (1997). *Primary care dermatology* (pp. 48–51). Philadelphia: Saunders.

McLeod, R. P. (2004). Lumps, bumps, and things that go itch in your office! *Journal of School Nursing, 20*(1), 57–59.

Nichol, N. H. (2002). Managing atopic dermatitis in children and adults. *Nurse Practitioner, 25*(4), 58–79.

Nichol, N. H. (2003). Evolution in the treatment of atopic dermatitis: New approaches to managing a chronic skin disease. *Dermatology Nursing, 15*(4), S4–5.

Potts, N. L., & Mandleco, B. L. (2002). *Pediatric nursing: Caring for children and their families*. Clifton Park, NY: Delmar.

Singleton, J. K. (1997). Pediatric dermatoses: Three common skin disruptions in infancy. *Nursing Practice, 22*(6), 32–50.

Weston, W., & Bruckner, A. (2000). Allergic contact dermatitis. *Pediatric Clinics of North America, 47*(4), 897–908.

# Resources

About Allergies Web site
www.allergies.about.com

About Pediatrics Web site
www.Pediatrics.about.com

American Academy of Dermatology
P.O. Box 4014
Schaumburg, IL 80188-4014
847-330-0230
847-330-0050 (fax)
http://www.aad.org

*Dermatology Online Journal*
http://dermatology.cdlib.org

Health Information Service of the National Library of Medicine and National Institutes of Health
http://www.medlineplus.gov

Medscape Dermatology Web site
www.dermatology.medscape.com/Home/Topics/Dermatology/Dermatology.html

Society for Pediatric Dermatology
5422 North Bernard
Chicago, IL 60625
773-583-9780
http://www.pedsderm.net

## Chapter Sixty-nine

# Spina Bifida

Maureen C. Maguire

## Introduction

Spina bifida (SB), a condition in which the neural tube fails to close and fuse completely during fetal life, is the most common birth defect affecting the central nervous system (Hockenberry, 2003). The rates are higher in females and in whites than in African Americans. The incidence in the United States recorded through 1990 was approximately 1,500 newborns annually (Centers for Disease Control and Prevention [CDC], 1992). The cause in over 50% of the cases is now known to be a deficiency of folic acid while the child is in utero; in the other cases, the cause is multifactorial (Hockenberry). Starting in 1992, the U.S. Public Health Service (USPHS), the CDC, and other organizations launched extensive campaigns to advise women of childbearing years to consume 0.4 mg of folic acid daily to reduce the incidence of this serious birth defect (CDC, 2003a). In January 1998, mandatory enrichment of cereal grains with folic acid was begun, resulting in a 31% reduction of reported cases of spina bifida by December 1999. Experts think that the prevalence could be decreased by 70% if all women took folic acid during pregnancy (CDC, 2004)

### Pathophysiology

The neural tube forms between the 17th and 30th days of embryonic life. It develops into the baby's central nervous system. In spina bifida the distal end of the tube does not close, resulting in failure of the spinal cord and column to form correctly (CDC, 1992). There are degrees of seriousness of the condition.

*Spina bifida occulta* is the mildest form of spina bifida. There is an opening in one or more of the vertebrae but without damage to the spinal cord (National Dissemination Center for Children With Disabilities [NDCCD], 2003) and is not visible externally. It is most common in the lumbosacral area. It may go undetected, but there may be some cutaneous signs such as a dimple, hair tufts, or port-wine angiomatous nevi. There is usually no neurologic involvement (Hockenberry, 2003).

*Meningocele* occurs when the meninges, contained in a sac, push through the opening in the vertebrae but without involving the spinal cord. About 4% of infants with manifested spina bifida have this type of defect. It can be readily repaired surgically and should result in little or no damage to nerve pathways (NDCCD, 2003).

*Myelomeningocele (or meningomyelocele)* is the most severe form of spina bifia; the terms are often used interchangeably. With this problem, a portion of the spinal cord, along with the meninges, protrudes through the spine (NDCCD, 2003). Most of these defects occur in the lumbar or lumbosacral region of the spine. The size of the defect and the level of spinal cord involvement determine the severity of the neurologic manifestations. There is a loss of motor and sensory function below the defect, which includes loss of bowel and bladder control if nerves in the sacral area are involved, and often orthopedic deformities of the spine and hips (Hockenberry, 2003). Between 70% and 90% of children with myelomeningocele will have a secondary hydrocephalus, which requires surgical shunting to relieve cerebrospinal fluid pressure on the brain (NDCCD). Hydrocephalus can cause seizures. Some children with spina bifida and hydrocephalus have an Arnold-Chiari II malformation, in which the cerebellum of the brain protrudes into the spinal canal (National Institute of Neurological Disorders and Stroke, 2004)

Many children with severe spina bifida develop tethered cord syndrome from scar tissue following the surgery to close the defect. With this condition, the spinal cord becomes attached to the bones of the spine, preventing the cord from sliding normally. If this creates symptoms, the cord needs to be surgically released (University of Missouri Health Care, 2004). Other complications of spina bifida include obesity, urinary tract disorders/infections, psychological issues, and learning problems (Australian Spina Bifida & Hydrocephalus Association, 2004).

Fetal surgery to close the defect is being done experimentally at some medical centers. It is hoped that such procedures will improve the neurologic functioning of the affected children (Hockenberry, 2003).

It is estimated that up to 73% of children and adolescents with myelomeningocele have sensitivity to latex (American Association of Nurse Anesthetists, 2005). Symptoms range from mild, such as watery eyes, to anaphylactic shock (Spina Bifida Association of America, 2003). No specific cause has been identified, but it is thought that repeated exposure, early in life, to rubber products during surgeries, diagnostic tests, and elimination programs may result in this immune response (Poley & Slater, 2000). In one study the investigators found that 47% of children with myelomeningocele in their study had antibodies to latex, as compared to 2.7% of well controls (Pittman et al., 1995). There are many potential sources for latex exposure in and around schools, ranging from rubber bands in classrooms to reconstructed tire flooring in play areas. If there is a child with spina bifida in a school, latex gloves should not used by the school nurse when caring for any children, because the powder from latex gloves can become airborne and represent a risk for the child with spina bifida (Meeropol, 2003).

Some studies have found an increased incidence of learning problems in children with spina bifida with and without hydrocephalus (Lollar, 1995). Vachha and Adams (2004) compared children with myelomeningocele and shunted hydrocephalus with a group of normal controls. They found that the affected children did significantly worse on verbal, nonverbal, and information prioritizing tasks. Another study showed a greater number of nonverbal learning disabilities in children with myelomeningocele and hydrocephalus (Yeates, Loss, Colvin, & Enrile, 2003). However, providers at the Mayo Clinic (2003) who work with children with spina bifida stress that many children with the condition have normal intelligence and can do well in school with adequate educational support.

## Management

Children with spina bifida require multidisciplinary care. A variety of medical specialties (such as pediatrics, neurosurgery, and orthopedics), specialized nursing care, physical therapy, and social work are needed. Initial care consists of surgically closing the defect, treating hydrocephalus if present, and preventing complications such as infection. At the same time, attention needs to be given to the family through support and education.

The lifelong care of these children is complicated because multiple systems are affected. Many hospitals have developed multidisciplinary outpatient centers to coordinate the physical, rehabilitation, and emotional needs of the children and to help their families cope with their many new responsibilities.

One major area that needs to be addressed is locomotion. The level of neurologic deficit determines what functional status can be achieved. Children with cord damage at L2 or above will usually be confined to a wheelchair. Those with lower injuries are often able to ambulate with braces and crutches. All children will need extensive physical therapy for mobility and occupational therapy for bracing.

Up to 90% of children with myelomeningocele have problems with urinary functioning, including urine retention and stress incontinence. Those with neuropathic bladder can develop urinary system distress with urinary tract infections that can progress to ureterohydonephrosis, vesicoureteral reflux, and renal insufficiency. Severe urinary distress, especially early in infancy, often requires surgical interventions such as vesicostomy or augmentation enterocystoplasty. Many children, however, can be managed through a program of clean intermittent catheterization and medications such as antispasmodics and possibly anticholinergics.

Some degree of bowel continence can be achieved in most children with myelomeningocele. The children require dietary modification, often with fiber supplementation, and a program of regular evacuation using suppositories, laxatives, and enemas (Hockenberry, 2003).

## Individualized Healthcare Plan

### Assessment
*History*
- What is the vertebral level of the student's deficit?
- What surgical procedures has the student had and at what age?
  - Closure of the myelomeningocele?
  - Shunt for hydrocephalus?
  - Ventriculoperitoneal or ventriculoatrial?
  - Bladder or bowel diversion or reconstruction?
  - Orthopedic reconstruction of spine, hips, or lower extremities?
- What therapies has the student received and where?
  - Physical, occupational, ostomy, psychiatric?
- What complications has the student experienced and when?
  - Infection or blockage of hydrocephalic shunt?
  - Infection at the site of any surgical diversions?
  - Seizures?
  - Urinary incontinence?
  - Urinary tract infections?
  - Constipation or fecal impaction?
  - Skin breakdown?
  - Psychological problems?

- If there were complications, how were they managed?
- Does the student have latex allergy?
  - What symptoms?
  - Ever had an anaphylactic reaction? When?
  - How are symptoms managed?
- What has been the student's response to his/her limitations?
  - Adaptive ability?
  - Psychological coping?
- How has the family dealt with the stresses of having a disabled child?
  - Interpersonal/marital?
  - Daily care?
  - Home structure?
  - Financial?
  - Support systems?
- What was the student's previous educational experience (if any) and adaptation?
  - Public, private, or home school?
  - Any learning disabilities?
  - Ability to navigate in building structure?
  - Assistance provided by school personnel?
  - Attitude of teachers and other students to the child?
  - Student's emotional response to attending school?

*Current Status and Management*
- Physical assessment
  - Level of diminished sensation
  - Level of impaired mobility
  - Skin: scars from surgical procedures, skin breakdown
  - Presence of any ostomy sites and condition of stoma(s)
  - Orthopedic deformities of spine, hips, legs, or feet
  - Contractures of any joints
  - Visible presence of hydrocephalic shunt bulb or tubing
  - Odor of urine or feces
  - Signs of abuse
- What assistive devices does the student use to ambulate?
  - Orthotics (braces, splints, stabilizers)
  - Mobility equipment (wheelchair, walker, crutches, wheel board)
- What human assistance does student need to ambulate?
  - Opening doors
  - Carrying books and study materials
  - Carrying cafeteria tray or lunch bag
- Bladder and bowel regimen
  - Frequency of emptying/evacuating
- Need unlimited permission to go to bathroom?
  - Any ostomy? Bags?
  - Clean intermittent catheterization?
  - What equipment/medication must be kept at school to aid child?
  - How independent is student with managing regimen?
- What specific assistance does student require with toileting at school?
- Activities of daily living in school—abilities and needs
  - Mobility, toileting, classroom and learning activities, recreational activities
- Emergency plan in place and communicated to members of school community
- Student's knowledge about condition and specials needs
- Family's status in caring for child with disability
  - Caregivers knowledgeable and skillful in dealing with child's needs?
  - Physical environment adapted for child's special needs
  - Interpersonal relationships among family members
  - Financial concerns
  - Sources of support

– Opportunities for socialization and recreation for all family members
– Any specific stressors present at this time

### Self-care
- Degree to which student can manage with little or no assistance
  – Mobility throughout the school
  – Participation in classroom activities
  – Carrying school books and supplies
  – Toileting
  – Medication management
  – Eating lunch and/or snacks
  – Socialization with other students
  – Ability to identify situations requiring adult intervention
- Transportation needs to and from school
  – Transported by parent?
  – Handicapped accessible van?
  – Public transportation via mobility van or lift-equipped bus?
  – Need assistance to get to and from the transportation vehicle
- School building accessibility for handicapped students
  – Doorways wide enough
  – Ramps or elevator
  – Toilet stalls large enough
  – Adequate classroom space/aisles
  – Desk and cafeteria table high enough to accommodate wheelchair
  – Access to nurse's office

### Psychosocial Status
- Student's age and developmental level
- Student's feelings about condition and limitations
- Student's recognition of abilities
- Student's self-esteem
- Attitude of teachers and other students
- Student's perception of how others perceive him/her
- School activities available in which student can participate
- Friends in school?
- Availability of support services: nurse, teachers, school administrators, counselor/social worker, other students
- Availability of support systems outside of school: family, church, healthcare institutions, community organizations, churches, public/governmental resources
- Signs or symptoms of emotional distress

### Academic Issues
- Intellectual ability
- Documented or suspected learning disabilities
- Availability of special education coordinator for the district
- Individualized education program (IEP)
- Appropriate grade placement
- Availability of resource teachers/services
- Pattern of absence from school
- Communication between school and family
- Physical education activities within student's capabilities

## Nursing Diagnosis (N.D.) (NANDA, 2003)

**N.D. 1** Impaired physical mobility (NANDA 00085) related to:
- damage to spinal cord and spinal nerves
- need for orthotic/mobility equipment

**N.D. 2** Altered sensory perception, tactile, (NANDA 00122) related to damage to spinal cord and spinal nerves

**N.D. 3** Risk for constipation (NANDA 00015) related to:
- altered peristalsis secondary to lack of enervation to sphincters
- hard feces secondary to inappropriate diet and lack of sufficient fluid intake due to fear of incontinence

**N.D. 4** Risk for delayed growth and development (00112) related to:
- inability to walk
- increased dependence

**N.D. 5** Risk for injury (NANDA 00035) related to:
- possibility for falling
- latex allergy
- increased intracranial pressure

**N.D. 6** Risk for infection (NANDA 00004) related to:
- altered urinary and bowel elimination
- skin breakdown

**N.D. 7** Disturbed personal identity (NANDA 00121) related to inability to participate in age-appropriate physical activities

**N.D. 8** Risk for body image disturbance (NANDA 00118) related to:
- muscle atrophy below spinal defect
- need for assistive devices

**N.D. 9** Risk for chronic low self-esteem (NANDA 00119) related to:
- inability to achieve full independence
- altered toileting regimen
- possibility of odor of urine/feces

**N.D. 10** Risk for impaired skin integrity (NANDA 00046) related to:
- lack of sensation below defect
- orthotic devices
- possible incontinence

**N.D. 11** Risk for social isolation (NANDA 00053) related to:
- inability to participate in peer activities
- use of orthotic/mobility devices
- altered lower body appearance
- possible lack of peer experiences in earlier life
- possible overprotectiveness of family

**N.D. 12** Risk for toileting self-care deficit (NANDA 00110) related to alteration in methods for achieving urine and fecal elimination

**N.D. 13** Risk for ineffective role performance (NANDA 00055) related to:
- physical restrictions
- low self-esteem
- prolonged dependence on family
- possible learning disabilities

**N.D. 14** Risk for bowel incontinence (NANDA 00014) related to nonformed feces secondary to inappropriate diet

**N.D. 15** Risk for ineffective management of therapeutic regimen (NANDA 00078) related to:
- multiple and complex needs
- immaturity

**N.D. 16** Risk for ineffective individual coping (NANDA 00069) related to increased physical, emotional, intellectual demands imposed by condition

**N.D. 17** Risk for activity intolerance (NANDA 00092) related to needing to move about school building(s)

## Goals

The student will demonstrate ability to use adaptive devices to increase mobility. (N.D. 1)

The student will use safety measures to minimize injury. (N.D. 1, 5)

The student will take part in activities to increase the strength of upper body. (N.D. 1)

The student will take measures to prevent skin breakdown (e.g., wheelchair push-ups, modify orthotics to prevent pressure points, keep skin clean and moisturized, monitor skin condition. (N.D. 2, 5, 10)

The student will master procedure to evacuate bowel. (N.D. 3)

The student will describe causative factors for constipation or incontinence. (N.D. 14, 15)

The student will eat a diet appropriate to prevent constipation or incontinence. (N.D. 14, 15)

The student will demonstrate age-appropriate behaviors in physical, social, and cognitive activities within the scope of physical limitations. (N.D. 4, 11, 13)

The student will identify factors/situations that increase risk for injury. (N.D. 5)

The student will use safety measures to prevent injury (e.g., use wheelchair brakes, not move onto unstable surfaces). (N.D. 5)

The student will demonstrate thorough and appropriate hand washing. (N.D. 6)

The student will demonstrate knowledge of risks for infection imposed by condition. (N.D. 6)

The student will practice appropriate precautions to prevent infection, especially during toileting activities. (N.D. 6)

The student will verbalize feelings of self-worth. (N.D. 7)

The student will demonstrate healthy adaptation and coping. (N.D. 7, 16)

The student will verbalize/demonstrate acceptance of appearance. (N.D. 8)

The student will modify unrealistic self-expectations. (N.D. 7, 9)

The student will verbalize acceptance of limitations. (N.D. 7, 9, 11, 13)

The student will identify positive personal attributes. (N.D. 7-9, 11, 13, 16)

The student will identify factors that contribute to skin breakdown. (N.D. 10)

The student will identify problematic behaviors that interfere with socialization. (N.D. 11, 13, 17)

The student will seek opportunities for peer interaction. (N.D. 11)

The student will make use of supports in school to foster social interactions (e.g., clubs, games). (N.D. 11)

The student will use proper techniques in managing elimination. (N.D. 12, 6)

The student will demonstrate acceptable school performance. (N.D. 13)

The student will describe and incorporate the measures needed to manage the restrictions imposed by condition. (N.D. 16)

The student will comply with measures to maintain his/her health and safety. (N.D. 16)

The student will verbalize feelings of anxiety, fear, and depression. (N.D. 16

The student will identify coping strategies. (N.D. 16)

The student will accept support from nurse, teachers, and counselor. (N.D. 15, 16)

The student will identify activities that increase fatigue and work with school personnel to modify them. (N.D. 17)

## Nursing Interventions

*Positioning wheelchair*
Position student in wheelchair to maintain the angle of hips at 100 degrees, knees at 150 degrees, and ankles at 90 degrees, with heels resting flat on footrests (N.D. 2, 5, 10)

Facilitate small shifts of weight frequently (N.D. 2, 10)

Instruct student how to transfer to and from wheelchair as appropriate (N.D. 2, 5)

Instruct student on exercises to increase upper body strength (N.D. 2, 17)

*Exercise therapy: Ambulation*
Monitor student's use of assistive devices (N.D. 1)

*Self-care assistance*
Monitor student's ability for self-care. (N.D. 12, 13, 16)

Assist student in accepting dependency needs. (N.D. 4, 12, 13, 16)

Encourage student to perform normal activities of daily living to level of ability. (N.D. 12, 13, 16)

Encourage independence but intervene when necessary. (N.D. 12, 13, 15, 16)

Determine need for safety-related changes in school facility. (N.D. 5, 12, 13, 16)

Assist student in establishing a daily school routine. (N.D. 12, 13, 16)

Determine student's ability to use assistive devices. (N.D. 12, 13, 15, 16)

*Self-care: Toileting*
Determine student's ability to follow elimination procedures. (N.D. 12)

Determine what assistive devices student needs for elimination. (N.D. 12)

Assist student to remove/put on clothing as needed. (N.D. 1, 12)

Provide privacy during elimination. (N.D. 12)

*Lower extremity monitoring*
Determine what devices are needed to assist mobility. (N.D. 1, 2, 5, 10)

Inspect skin for redness or breakdown. (N.D. 2, 10)

Monitor condition of orthotics/assistive devices. (N.D. 2, 10)
Perform ongoing surveillance to determine need for referral. (N.D. 2, 5, 10)

## Bowel training
Determine if student will evacuate bowel at school on a routine basis. (N.D. 3, 14)
Determine student's knowledge of bowel program. (N.D. 3, 14, 15)
Assess student's abdomen for palpable stool in colon. (N.D. 3, 14)
Determine student's dietary pattern with particular attention to fiber and fluid. (N.D. 3, 14, 15)
Assist student with bowel evacuation as necessary (e.g., administer suppository, perform digital dilation). (N.D. 3, 14)
Facilitate hygiene after elimination. (N.D. 3, 6, 14)

## Developmental enhancement: child
Build trusting relationship with student. (N.D. 9)
Assist student to understand his/her importance as an individual. (N.D. 7, 8, 9)
Identify how special needs can be met in school environment. (N.D. 4, 11, 13)
Facilitate student's integration with peers. (N.D. 4, 11)
Collaborate with school team to encourage student's interaction with other children. (N.D. 11, 13)
Encourage student to express feelings. (N.D. 7, 8, 9)

## Environmental management: Safety
### Fall prevention: Surveillance
Identify safety needs of student based on abilities and limitations. (N.D. 1, 5)
Alert members of school community that there is a student at risk for falling. (N.D. 5)
Identify safety hazards in the environment. (N.D. 5)
Determine student's awareness of risks. (N.D. 1, 5)
Confer with others in school community in order to reduce risks. (N.D. 5)
Modify environment to minimize hazards as much as possible. (N.D. 5)
Monitor condition of assistive devices. (N.D. 1, 5, 17)
Instruct other members of school community how to assist student in emergency. (N.D. 5)
Monitor student's neurologic status. (N.D. 1, 2)

## Latex precautions
Question student/family to determine if student has had any reaction when exposed to natural rubber (latex) products and what signs and symptoms occurred. (N.D. 5)
Record allergy on school records. (N.D. 5)
Have student wear medical alert tag. (N.D. 5)
Inform other members of the school community about allergy. (N.D. 5)
Survey environment for latex products. (N.D. 5)
Remove any latex products from health room and other areas student will be in regularly. (N.D. 5)
Have emergency treatment medications and equipment on hand. (N.D. 5)
Instruct other members of school community about signs/symptoms of allergic reaction and necessity of prompt action. (N.D. 5)

## Infection protection
### Infection control
Monitor for generalized and localized signs/symptoms of infection. (N.D. 6)
Teach student and members of school community about signs/symptoms of infection. (N.D. 6)
Teach student how to avoid infection. (N.D. 6)
Notify family of suspected infection. (N.D. 6)
Institute standard precautions. (N.D. 6)

## Self-esteem enhancement
Monitor student's statements of self-worth. (N.D. 7, 8, 9)
Encourage student to identify strengths. (N.D. 9, 13, 16)
Reinforce accurate perception of strengths. (N.D. 7, 8, 9)
Encourage eye contact when communicating with others. (N.D. 7, 9, 13)

Cooperate with school community in providing experiences that increase student's autonomy to the degree possible. (N.D. 7, 13, 17)
Assist student to identify positive responses from others. (N.D. 7, 11, 16)
Refrain from negative criticism. (N.D. 9)
Convey confidence in student's ability to handle new situations. (N.D. 7, 9, 16)
Assist student in setting realistic goals that will increase self-esteem. (N.D. 9)
Assist student in accepting dependence on others when appropriate. (N.D. 16, 15)
Encourage increased responsibility for self as appropriate. (N.D. 13, 16)
Assist student to identify the impact of peer group on feelings of self-worth. (N.D. 11, 13, 16)
Explore previous achievements. (N.D. 7, 13)
Explore reasons for self-criticism. (N.D. 13)
Praise student for progress in accomplishing goals. (N.D. 7, 13)
Monitor frequency of self-negating statements. (N.D. 7, 13)
Monitor goal achievement. (N.D. 13, 16)
Make positive statements about student. (N.D. 16)

*Skin surveillance*
Monitor for sources of pressure and friction. (N.D. 2, 10)
Monitor for presence of skin redness or breakdown. (N.D. 2, 5, 10)

*Role enhancement*
Facilitate discussion about student's role in school. (N.D. 4, 13)
Facilitate role rehearsal by having student anticipate reactions from others in school. (N.D. 13)
Facilitate opportunities for student to role-play new behaviors. (N.D. 13)
Facilitate discussion of expectations of student in school. (N.D. 13)

*Coping enhancement*
Appraise student's adjustment to condition, body image, and limitations. (N.D. 16)
Appraise student's understanding of neurologic condition. (N.D. 16)
Use calm, reassuring approach. (N.D. 16)
Provide an atmosphere of acceptance. (N.D. 16)
Seek to understand student's perception of school. (N.D. 16)
Encourage relationships with others who have common interests. (N.D. 16)
Encourage social activities. (N.D. 16)
Confront student's feelings of depression or anger. (N.D. 16)
Foster constructive outlets for emotions. (N.D. 16)
Assist student in identifying realistic goals. (N.D. 16)
Appraise student's need for support. (N.D. 16)
Assist student to identify support resources in school. (N.D. 16)
Assist the student to identify positive strategies to deal with limitations. (N.D. 16)
Instruct the student in relaxation techniques as appropriate (N.D. 16)

*Energy management*
Arrange physical activities to conserve energy. (N.D. 17)
Encourage alternating activity with rest. (N.D. 17)
Encourage physical activity. (N.D. 17)
Instruct student to recognize signs/symptoms of fatigue that require rest. (N.D. 17)

## Expected Student Outcomes

The student will:
*Ambulation: Wheelchair*
   • Transfer to and from wheelchair. (N.D. 1)
   • Propel wheelchair safely. (N.D. 1)
Maneuver wheelchair up ramps and curbs and through doorways. (N.D. 1)

*Body positioning: Self-initiated*
- Do exercises to increase upper body strength. (N.D. 1)
- Using upper body, move body in wheelchair to avoid pressure areas. (N.D. 1, 2)

*Bowel elimination*
*Self-care toileting*
- Effectively evacuate stool and pass urine. (N.D. 3, 12, 14)
- Have stools that are neither hard nor liquid. (N.D. 3, 14, 15)
- Eat a diet that prevents constipation and incontinence. (N.D. 3, 14, 15)
- Describe appropriate procedures for elimination. (N.D. 3, 12)
- Use proper techniques in managing elimination. (N.D. 3, 12, 14)

*Child development: Middle childhood*
*Coping*
- Perform in school to level of ability. (N.D. 4, 16)
- Develop friendships. (N.D. 4, 11, 16)
- Express feelings constructively. (N.D. 4, 16)
- Identify with same gender peer group. (N.D. 4, 11)
- Assume responsibilities for schoolwork. (N.D. 4, 16)
- Participate in extracurricular activities. (N.D. 4, 11)
- Follow safety rules. (N.D. 4, 5)
- Understand right from wrong. (N.D. 4)
- Comprehend increasingly complex ideas. (N.D. 4)

*Fall prevention behavior*
*Knowledge: Personal safety*
Risk control
- Use assistive devices correctly. (N.D. 5, 15)
- Use safe transfer procedure. (N.D. 5, 15)
- Acknowledge risk factors. (N.D. 5, 15)
- Identify personal behaviors that increase risk of injury. (N.D. 5, 15)
- Identify situations that increase risk of injury. (N.D. 5, 15)
- Avoid situations that increase risk of falling. (N.D. 5, 15)
- Follow risk-control strategies. (N.D. 5, 15)

*Knowledge: Infection control*
- Describe how infection is spread. (N.D. 6)
- Identify factors contributing to acquiring an infection. (N.D. 6)
- Practice behaviors to prevent acquiring an infection. (N.D. 6)
- Describe signs/symptoms of infection. (N.D. 6)
- Comply with treatment of infection. (N.D. 6)

*Self-esteem*
*Adaptation to physical disability*
- Verbalize self-acceptance. (N.D. 7-9, 13)
- Accept limitations. (N.D. 7-9, 13)
- Fulfill appropriate roles in school. (N.D. 7-9, 13, 16)
- Describe successes in school and social groups. (N.D. 7-9, 13, 16)
- Confront others appropriately. (N.D. 7-9, 13, 16)
- Express feelings of self-worth. (N.D. 7-9, 13, 16)
- Verbalize reconciliation to disability. (N.D. 7-9, 16)
- Adapt to physical limitations. (N.D. 7-9, 13, 16)
- Use strategies to reduce stress related to disability. (N.D. 7-9, 13, 16)
- Identify plan to accomplish activities of daily living. (N.D. 7, 9, 13, 16)
- Identify risk of complications associated with disability. (N.D. 5)
- Accept need for physical assistance. (N.D. 4, 7, 9, 13, 17)

- Use available support. (N.D. 9, 13, 16, 17)
- Identify ways to increase independence appropriately. (N.D. 7, 9, 11-13, 16)
- Identify ways to cope with limitations. (N.D. 7-9, 13, 16)
- Report increased psychological comfort. (N.D. 7, 9, 16)

*Immobility consequences: Physiological*
- Prevent pressure sores. (N.D. 10)

*Social interaction skills*
*Social involvement*
- Exhibit receptiveness to others. (N.D. 11)
- Cooperate with others. (N.D. 11)
- Be assertive as appropriate. (N.D. 11)
- Exhibit consideration for others. (N.D. 11)
- Engage others. (N.D. 11)
- Interact with peers and adults. (N.D. 11)
- Participate in school/extracurricular activities. (N.D. 11)

*Activity tolerance*
- Avoid situations leading to excessive fatigue. (N.D. 17)
- Exhibit no signs/symptoms indicating oxygen deprivation or excessive muscle fatigue. (N.D. 17)
- Not become excessively breathless during school activities. (N.D. 17)

## Case Study

Jane is a 7-year-old girl with a myelomeningocele at L4 that was closed at birth. She had hydrocephalus requiring the placement of a ventriculoperitoneal (VP) shunt. She has had no problems with shunt malfunction or infection. She is wheelchair-dependent for mobility and has splints on legs to maintain positioning. She has good upper body strength and can reposition herself in the chair and propel the wheelchair. Jane has had training in bowel/bladder management.

Jane and her family have just moved into this school district. She attended regular first grade in her previous school, where she did well academically. She had several friends in school and liked to participate in craft activities. The school nurse reports that Jane has basic self-care skills but requires some assistance with toileting. She does not evacuate her bowel during the school day, but does do self-catheterization for urine. She needs reminding about leaning over in her chair and going too fast. She has a history of rash when exposed to latex in the hospital.

Jane is outgoing and seems to have adapted well to her limitations. Her parents say they try not to be overprotective and to allow Jane to be as independent as possible, but they worry how she is going to deal with being in a new school.

Spina Bifida

# Spina Bifida

| Assessment Data | Nursing Diagnosis | Goals | Nursing Interventions | Expected Outcomes |
|---|---|---|---|---|
| Jane is paralyzed from L4 down and is dependent on wheelchair for ambulation. She sometimes leans over too far and goes too fast. She has a VP shunt that works well. She has had a rash from contact with latex. | Impaired physical mobility related to damage to spinal cord and spinal nerves. | Jane will: <br> • Demonstrate ability to use wheelchair safely to move about in the school | Determine that Jane is properly positioned in chair to maintain angle of 100 degrees for hips, 90 degrees for knees, 150 degrees for ankles with feet flat on foot rests. | Jane will: <br> • Propel wheelchair safely <br><br> • Maneuver wheelchair up ramps and curbs and through doorways |
|  | Risk for injury related to leaning over and going too fast in chair, potential increased intracranial pressure, and latex allergy. | • Do activities to strengthen upper body | Instruct Jane on exercises to strengthen upper body. | • Achieve mobility without injury <br><br> • Self-initiate exercises to increase upper body strength |
|  |  | • Identify situations that increase risk for injury | Monitor Jane's use of wheelchair. | • Identify personal behaviors that increase risk of injury |
|  |  | • Use safety measures to minimize injury | Identify safety needs. | • Identify situations that increase risk of injury |
|  |  | • Identify signs/symptoms of increased intracranial pressure | Identify safety hazards throughout school. | • Avoid situations that increase risk of injury |
|  |  | • Avoid exposure to latex | Alert school community of presence of child with increased risk for injury. | • Follow risk-control strategies |
|  |  |  | Confer with school community in order to reduce risks/hazards. | • Recognize risks related to exposure to latex and avoid |
|  |  |  | Monitor Jane's neurologic status. |  |
|  |  |  | Monitor signs/symptoms of increased intracranial pressure. |  |
|  |  |  | Record latex allergy on school records. |  |
|  |  |  | Have Jane wear a medical alert tag. |  |

# Spina Bifida

| Assessment Data | Nursing Diagnosis | Goals | Nursing Interventions | Expected Outcomes |
|---|---|---|---|---|
| | | | Inform school community about latex allergy. | |
| | | | Instruct members of school community about signs and symptoms that require prompt action. | |
| | | | Survey environment for presence of latex. | |
| | | | Remove latex products from areas child frequents. | |
| | | | Have emergency medication and equipment on hand. | |
| Jane has no sensation below level of defect. This puts her at risk for pressure sores. She is confined to a wheelchair and has splints on her legs. | Altered sensatory perception, tactile related to damage to spinal cord and nerves.<br><br>Risk for impaired skin integrity related to sitting in wheelchair and having splints. | Jane's skin will remain warm, pink, and without lesions/breakdown.<br><br>Jane will:<br>• Identify behaviors that lead to skin breakdown<br><br>• Take measures to prevent skin breakdown | Facilitate small changes in position frequently.<br><br>Monitor skin at sacrum and under splints to observe for redness or signs of breakdown.<br><br>Monitor chair and splints for need of repair. | Do wheelchair pushups and initiate frequent position changes.<br><br>Position splints to prevent pressure over bony prominences.<br><br>Keep skin clean and moisturized.<br><br>Have no skin damage. |
| Jane requires help when doing self-catheterization. She is not expected to do bowel evacuation in school. | Risk for toileting self-care deficit<br><br>Risk for infection related to improper catheterization procedure | Jane will:<br>• Demonstrate thorough and appropriate hand washing<br><br>• Demonstrate knowledge of risks for infection imposed by condition | Practice standard precautions.<br><br>Determine Jane's ability to follow elimination procedure.<br><br>Determine what equipment Jane needs to have in bathroom. | Jane will:<br>• Describe correct procedure for catheterization<br><br>• Use proper techniques for catheterization<br><br>• Avoid urinary tract infection |

| Assessment Data | Nursing Diagnosis | Goals | Nursing Interventions | Expected Outcomes |
|---|---|---|---|---|
| | | • Practice appropriate precautions to prevent infection | Monitor Jane to observe for breaks in technique that could lead to urinary tract infection.<br><br>Assist Jane during toileting as needed.<br><br>Provide for privacy.<br><br>Monitor for signs/symptoms of urinary tract infection.<br><br>Notify family of any suspicion of infection. | |
| Jane is outgoing by nature. She established friendships at her previous school but is now in a new school situation and in a higher grade, where expectations will be higher. | Risk for delayed growth and development related to entering new school and increased educational challenges.<br><br>Risk social isolation related to having no friends/social groups in new school. | Jane will:<br>• Demonstrate age-appropriate behaviors in physical, social, and cognitive activities within the scope of her limitations<br><br>• Seek opportunities for peer interaction<br><br>• Make use of school activities/clubs<br><br>• Identify own behaviors that might interfere with socialization | Build a trusting relationship with Jane.<br><br>Encourage Jane to express feelings.<br><br>Identify how her special needs can be met in school.<br><br>Facilitate Jane's integration into peer group.<br><br>Collaborate with other school personnel to encourage her interaction with other children. | Jane will:<br>• Express feelings constructively<br><br>• Assume responsibility for schoolwork<br><br>• Comprehend increasingly complex ideas<br><br>• Develop friendships<br><br>• Identify with same-gender peer group<br><br>• Take part in extracurricular activities |

# Emergency Care Plan

Ascertain names and phone numbers of student's medical providers.

Keep current list of phone numbers for family.

Have emergency supplies for first aid.

Have emergency medications to manage allergic reaction.

Identify type of transport needed if student must go to emergency department.

Identify person in school who will accompany the student if student must be transported.

# Evacuation Plan

Have up-to-date schedule of student's regular classes/activities.

Inform all school personnel that there is a special-needs student to be evacuated.

Designate a teacher/administrator to check that student has been evacuated (in addition to nurse).

Identify school personnel with physical strength to carry student down stairs and out of building if necessary.

# References

American Association of Nurse Anesthetists. (2005). AANA latex protocol. Parkrigdge, IL : Author.

Australian Spina Bifida & Hydrocephalus Association. (2004). Spina bifida explained. Retrieved March 11, 2005 from http://www.asbha.org.au

Centers for Disease Control and Prevention. (1992). Spina bifida incidence at birth—United States, 1983–1990. *Morbidity and Mortality Weekly Report 41*(27), 497–500.

Centers for Disease Control and Prevention. (2003a). *Folic acid now fact sheet.* Government NCBDDD publication 8000d615. Atlanta, GA: Author.

Centers for Disease Control and Prevention. (2003b). Information for health professionals—folic acid recommendations. Government NCBDDD publication 800523d6. Atlanta, GA: Author.

Centers for Disease Control and Prevention. (2004). Spina bifida and anencephaly before and after folic acid mandate—United States, 1995–1996 and 1999–2000. *Morbidity and Mortality Weekly Report 53*(17), 362–365.

Hockenberry, M. J. (2003). *Wong's nursing care of infants and children* (7th ed., pp. 425–441). Philadelphia: Mosby.

Lollar, D. J. (1995). *Learning among children with spina bifida.* Washington, DC: Spina Bifida Association of America.

Mayo Foundation for Medical Education and Research. (2003). *Spina bifida.* Retrieved February 15, 2005, from http://www.mayoclinic.com/printinvoker.cfm?objectid+CB5F085A-6152-42FC-8CFC55380EF705A2

Meeropol, E. (2003, July/August). Keeping your child latex-safe in school. (Back-to-School Pullout.) *Insights Into Spina Bifida.* NANDA International. (2003). *Nursing diagnoses: Definitions & classification 2003–2004.* Philadelphia: Author.

NANDA International. (2003). *NANDA nursing diagnosis: Definitions & classification 2003-2004.* Philadelphia: Author.

National Dissemination Center for Children with Disabilities. (2003). *Spina bifida fact sheet 12.* Retrieved January 28, 2004, from http://www.nichcy/org/pubs/factshe/fs12txt.htm

National Institute of Neurological Disorders and Stroke. (2004). *NINDS Chiari malformation information page.* Retrieved January 4, 2005, from http://www.ninds.nih.gov/disorders/chiari/chiari.htm

Pittman, T., Kiburz, J., Gabriel, K., Steinhardt, G., Williams, D., & Slater, J. (1995). Latex allergy in children with spina bifida. *Pediatric Neurosurgery, 22*(2), 96–100.

Poley, G. E., & Slater, J. E. (2000). Latex allergy. *Journal of Allergy and Clinical Immunology, 105*, 1054–1062.

Spina Bifida Association of America (SBAA). (2003). *An overview of latex (natural rubber) allergy in spina bifida.* Retrieved March 12, 2004, from http://www.sbaa.org/site/PageServer?pagename=asb_latex

University of Missouri Health Care Neuromedicine. (2004). *Tethered cord syndrome.* Retrieved January 4, 2005, from http://www.muhealth.org/~neuromedicine/tetheredcord.shtm

Vachha, B., & Adams, R. (2004). Learning efficiency in children with myelomeningocele and shunted hydrocephalus. *Cerebrospinal Fluid Research, 1*(Suppl. 1), S62.

Yeates, K. O., Loss, N., Colvin, A. N., & Enrile, B. J. (2003). Do children with myelomeningocele and hydrocephalus display nonverbal learning disabilities? An empirical approach to classification. *Journal of the International Neuropsychology Society, 4*, 653–662.

# Bibliography

Benner, B. (2002, Summer). Spina bifida: managing bowel dysfunction in the school-aged child. *See/Hear*

Carpenito-Moyet, L. J. (2003) *Nursing diagnosis: Application to clinical practice* (10th ed.). Philadelphia: Lippincott.

*Coordinating spina bifida care.* (n.d.) Retrieved February 8, 2004, from http://www,schoolnurse.com/med_info/coordination_spina.htm

*Creating a safe school for latex-sensitive children.* (2002). Press release of the American Association of Nurse Anesthetists. http://www.aana.org

Dochterman, J. M., & Bulechek, G. M. (Eds.). (2004). *Nursing interventions classification (NIC)* (4th ed.). Philadelphia: Mosby.

*Learning problems in children with spina bifida and hydrocephalus.* (n.d.) Retrieved January 27, 2004, from http://www.waisman.wisc.edu/~rowley/lollor.html

Moorhead, S., Johnson, M., & Maas, M. (Eds.). (2004). *Nursing outcomes classification (NOC)* (3rd ed.). Philadelphia: Mosby.

National Association of School Nurses. (Adopted 2000). *Position Statement: Natural rubber latex allergy.* Scarborough, ME: Author.

*Spina bifida general checklist: Working with schools.* (2004). Baltimore, MD: Kennedy Krieger Institute.

# Resources

March of Dimes Birth Defects Foundation
1275 Mamaroneck Avenue
White Plains, NY 10605
914-428-7100
www.marchofdimes.com

National Rehabilitation Information
8455 Colesville Road
Suite 935
Silver Spring, MD 20910
1-800-227-0216
www.naric.com

Spina Bifida Association of America
4590 MacArthur Boulevard, NW
Suite 250
Washington, DC 20007
1-800-621-3141
www.sbaa.org

# Chapter Seventy

# Spinal Cord Injury

Cynthia K. Silkworth

## Introduction

Spinal cord injuries are not common in children. Such injuries in children from birth to 15 years of age account for only 4.5% of all spinal cord injuries (Massagli, 2000). The majority of spinal cord injuries, about 55%, occur between the ages of 16 and 30 (National Spinal Cord Injury Statistical Center, 2001).

Causes of spinal cord injury vary with age. Motor vehicle accidents, including automobile-bicycle accidents and all-terrain vehicle and snowmobile accidents, are the leading cause of spinal cord injury in children and adolescents. Other known causes of spinal cord injuries in children and adolescents include falls from heights; recreational activities, such as horseback riding; and sports injuries, such as in gymnastics, diving, and downhill skiing. Birth injuries can occur during delivery from traction and angulation or torsion of the spine. Spinal cord injuries may also be caused by acts of violence, such as gunshot or stabbing wounds and shaking of infants. Diseases, such as polio, spina bifida, and tumors, can also cause spinal cord injury (Massagli, 2000; Wong, Hockenberry, Wilson, Winkelstein, & Kline, 2003).

## Pathophysiology

The spinal cord transmits motor and sensory signals between the brain and the body. An injury to the spinal cord affects the sending and receiving of signals across the site of the injury and results in a loss of motor and sensory function below the site (**Table 1**). Depending on the level of the injury, a person who sustains a spinal cord injury may also experience impairments in regulating respiration, temperature, and blood pressure and in bowel, bladder, and sexual function. Unless a head injury was also sustained, a person with a spinal cord injury will not have intellectual or cognitive impairment as a result of the injury. Spinal cord injuries can occur at any level on the spinal cord or at multiple levels. Spinal cord injuries are described by the level of injury and amount of damage:

*Level of the spinal cord injury*: The level of injury is described as the lowest point on the spinal cord below which there is a decrease or absence of feeling and/or movement. In general, the higher the level of injury, the greater the degree of loss of sensation and movement.

*Amount of damage to the cord*: Complete injuries usually lead to total loss of functional motor and sensory loss below the level of injury. Incomplete injuries may result in varying degrees of motor and sensory loss below the site of the injury (National Spinal Cord Injury Association, 2003).

Definitions associated with spinal cord injury include the following:

*Tetraplegia (quadriplegia):* injury to the spinal cord at the level C1-T1; causes loss of feeling and/or movement in the neck, shoulders, arms, upper chest, abdomen, legs, and diaphragm; bowel and bladder and sexual function will be affected.

*Paraplegia:* injury to the spinal cord at the thoracic and sacral levels, (T2–S5); can include loss of feeling and/or movement of the lower parts of the body (middle of the chest, stomach, hips, legs, feet, toes); bowel, bladder and sexual function may be affected.

*Hemiplegia:* loss of sensation and/or movement on one side of the body.

*Flaccid paralysis:* paralysis with decreased or absent reflexes and muscle tone.

*Spastic paralysis:* paralysis with involuntary contraction of muscles associated with increased reflexes and muscle tone.

**Table 1. Functional Ability Associated with Spinal Cord Injury**

| Highest Intact Cord Level | Functional Ability |
|---|---|
| **C1-C3**<br>Muscle innervation: head and neck muscles | Limited head and neck movement<br>No voluntary control below chin<br>Respiratory paralysis complete, ventilator-dependent<br>May cause bradycardia or tachycardia<br>Requires electric wheelchair using mouth stick, head/chin control<br>Talking is difficult, limited or impossible<br>Totally dependent for activities of daily living (ADLs) |
| **C4**<br>Muscle innervation: intact sternocleidomastoid, trapezius, upper cervical paraspinous muscles | Usually has head and neck control<br>No voluntary function of upper extremities, trunk, or lower extremities<br>Respirator-dependent<br>Requires electric wheelchair<br>Talking is normal<br>Totally dependent for ADLs |
| **C5**<br>Muscle innervation: partial deltoid, biceps, major muscles of rotator cuffs at shoulders, diaphragm | Has head and neck control<br>Can shrug shoulder and has shoulder control<br>Can bend elbows and turn palms face up<br>Abdominal respiration<br>Requires electric wheelchair, with hand control<br>With assistance in setting up and adaptive equipment, can perform eating, drinking, face washing, brushing teeth, and hair care independently. |
| **C6**<br>Muscle innervation: pectoralis major, serratus anterior, latissimus dorsi muscles, complete deltoid and brachioradialis muscles, partial triceps muscle | Has movement in head neck, shoulders, arms, and wrists<br>Can bend elbows, turn palms up and down, and extend wrists<br>Can use manual wheelchair for daily activities, may use power chair for greater distances<br>Can independently do transfers, may require sliding board<br>With some adaptive equipment, has greater independence with ADLs<br>Can independently do pressure relief |
| **C7**<br>Muscle innervation: triceps and finger flexor muscles, shoulder depressor muscles | Added ability to straighten elbows<br>Able to lift body weight and can transfer with greater ease<br>Daily use of manual wheelchair<br>Needs fewer adaptive aids for ADLs<br>Able to do wheelchair pushups for pressure relief |
| **C8-T1**<br>Muscle innervation: hand intrinsic muscles | Full use of upper extremities<br>Added strength and precision of finger movements that result in limited to normal hand function<br>Uses manual wheelchair, transfers independently<br>Can live independently<br>Independent with ADLs without assistive devices |
| **T2-T6**<br>Muscle innervation: upper extremity muscles, upper back and chest muscles | Normal motor function in arms, hands, and fingers<br>Increased use of rib and chest muscles<br>Increased trunk control<br>Independent with all activities |

| Highest Intact Cord Level | Functional Ability |
|---|---|
| **T7-T12**<br>Muscle innervation: full abdominal and upper back muscle control | Good trunk balance<br>Added motor function with increased abdominal control |
| **L1 – L5**<br>Muscle innervation: hip flexors, pelvic girdle muscles, quadriceps muscle, partial gluteus and hamstring muscles, ankle dorsiflexors, intrinsic foot muscles | Additional return of motor movement in hips and thighs<br>Walking can be done with specialized leg and ankle braces |
| **S1 – S5**<br>Muscle innervation: leg flexor muscles, ankle plantar flexors, posterior thigh muscles, anal sphincter, groin muscles | Increased ability to walk with fewer or no supportive devices<br>May be various degrees of return of voluntary bladder, bowel, and sexual function |

Adapted from "The Child with Neuromuscular and Muscular Dysfunction," in *Nursing Care of Infants and Children* (7th edition, p. 1854), by D. L. Wong, M. J. Hockenberry, D. Wilson, M. L. Winkelstein, and N. E. Kline, 2003, St. Louis, MO: Mosby; and *Understanding Spinal Cord Injury and Functional Goals,* by K, Lindsey, P. Klebine, & M. J. Wells, 2000, Birmingham, AL: University of Alabama at Birmingham, available at: http://www.spinalcord.uab/edu.

## Autonomic Dysreflexia

In autonomic dysreflexia, a stimulus, either internal or external, causes a generalized spread of sympathetic and parasympathetic activity that leads to increased blood pressure in a person with a spinal cord injury at or above T6. The body is unable to recognize or take the necessary action to decrease the stimulus and blood pressure because of the spinal cord injury (McCluer, 1995; Senelick & Dougherty, 1998; Rehabilitation Institute of Chicago—Spinal Cord Injury Team, 2002).

**Autonomic dysreflexia is a medical emergency that requires immediate intervention.**

Stimuli that may cause an episode of autonomic dysreflexia include:

- distended or spastic bladder
- bladder infection
- distended bowel or impaction
- pressure areas on skin, such as irritating clothing
- skin temperature changes
- uterine contractions associated with menstrual cramps

Symptoms include the following:

- pounding headache that begins all of a sudden
- flushing of the face and/or red splotches on skin (above the site of the spinal cord injury)
- sweating (above the site of the spinal cord injury)
- sudden high blood pressure
- tachycardia or bradycardia (abnormally fast or slow heartbeat)
- nasal stuffiness
- blurred vision
- nausea
- anxiety

Management of an episode requires identifying and removing the cause as quickly as possible:

- Check the bladder for distention or spasms; empty the bladder.
- Check the bowels for distention or impaction; remove the stool or impaction.
- Change the position to relieve skin pressure.
- Loosen tight or constricting clothing.
- Check the skin for irritation or infection.

## Management

A complex, interdisciplinary team of people is needed to provide a comprehensive approach to rehabilitation and management. The child and the family need to work collaboratively with the medical and school teams to identity the child's needs and to plan and implement realistic goals, interventions, and outcomes. Members of the medical team include physicians (primary and specialists), rehabilitation nurse, physical therapist and occupational therapist, respiratory therapist, dietitian, recreational therapist, social worker, psychologist, and vocational counselor.

Members of the team at school include the school nurse, teacher(s) (regular education), special education teacher with physically impaired certification, physical education teacher with developmental and adaptive physical education certification, physical therapist, occupational therapist, administrator, and paraprofessionals who will be working directly with the student.

Management and rehabilitation of the child with a spinal cord injury involve setting and changing goals based on the child's age, development, and expectations. It is critical that the medical and school teams work collaboratively to assist the child to achieve optimal development, academic, self-care, and independence outcomes.

Management measures may include the following (Dudgeon, Massagli, & Ross, 1997; Massagli, 2000; Wong, Hockenberry, Wilson, Winkelstein, & Kline, 2003):

- Respiratory care—maintaining good airway clearance and ventilation; child with a high-level injury, C1-C4, will require ventilatory assistance, most often a tracheostomy and ventilator; care may include positioning for optimal chest expansion, chest physiotherapy, breathing exercises, medications
- Temperature regulation—maintaining normal body temperature by use of clothing and environmental measures added or removed, depending on body temperature, and monitoring for fever and signs of infection
- Skin care—maintaining clean and dry skin and monitoring for signs of pressure areas
- Autonomic dysreflexia—prevention of episodes and quick assessment and intervention to remove the causes and resolve the episodes
- Mobility—maintaining mobility in the home and community, including proper fit and use of wheelchair, walker or crutches, braces, orthoses; environmental accessibility issues
- Bladder management—preventing overextension of the bladder and urinary retention; control of urinary tract infections
- Bowel management—including training to control defecation until in an appropriate, usually planned, time and place
- Physiotherapy—maintaining proper body alignment, range-of-motion exercises, preventing pressure sores, repositioning and transferring techniques
- Psychosocial rehabilitation—assisting the child or adolescent to develop a realistic definition of interdependent living, express feelings, build a positive self-image, and participate in educational and vocational opportunities and programming

# Individualized Healthcare Plan

## Assessment

*History*
- Development and health prior to the spinal cord injury
- When the spinal cord injury occurred
- Age of the student when the injury occurred
- How the injury occurred
- Level of the spinal cord injury and amount of damage to the spinal cord
- Initial care after the injury
- Rehabilitation program
- Complications or infections related to the spinal cord injury
- Prognosis
- Most recent reevaluation

*Current Status and Management*
- Level of function—motor and sensory
- Mobility—wheelchair use, orthoses, braces
- Respiratory care—need for ventilatory assistance (type), tracheostomy, and trach care needed, use of oxygen and humidification, chest physiotherapy or breathing exercises, cough reflex and strength
- Autonomic dysreflexia—prevention, common causes, interventions used
- Skin care—skin breakdown prevention measures, monitoring of pressure areas
- Bladder elimination—pattern, during school hours, catheterization (indwelling, sterile, self-catheterization), use of diapers or pads, other monitoring for urinary tract infections
- Bowel elimination program—pattern, needs during school hours
- Temperature regulation—environmental needs
- Medications—at home, during school hours
- Nutrition—meal pattern, snacks, assistance needed with eating, fluid intake needs
- Growth—height and weight
- Daily activity schedule—energy use, need for rest
- Current therapy—physical, occupational, recreational, speech

*Self-care*
- Knowledge about current health status, abilities, and disabilities
- Student's perception of his/her abilities and disabilities and health status
- Parent's perception of student's abilities and disabilities and health status
- Student's decision-making skills
- Student's ability to participate in self-care activities—activities of daily living (ADLs)
- Participation in ADLs—at home, in school
- Ability to transfer—in and out of wheelchair, in and out of stander, etc.
- Independent skills—physical, psychosocial, cognitive
- Independent mobility skills—manual wheelchair, power wheelchair
- Motivation to participate in self-care
- Barriers to participating in self-care

*Psychosocial Status*
- Student's contact and interaction with family, peers, and adults
- Student's locus of control
- Participation in family, peer, school, and community activities
- Involvement with support persons, groups, and services

*Academic Issues*
- Past and current academic achievement
- Schools the student has attended, including hospital-based and homebound educational programs
- School health services needed: specialized healthcare procedures and or medications required during the school day

- School environment issues: building temperature, space for wheelchair mobility in classroom, table/desk to fit with wheelchair, access in and out of the building, access to media center, cafeteria, auditorium, etc.
- School and classroom modifications needed: computer utilization; assistance with locker, books, lunch, and getting between classes; management aide assistance in the classroom; schedule; assistance from peers; access to media center books and resource materials
- Curriculum modifications: amount of work, types of activities required, expectations of performance, testing (oral versus written tests)
- Special educational services: past services, current needs
- Emergency evacuation from the building
- Transportation issues: special busing, need for health services on the bus

## Nursing Diagnoses (N.D.) (NANDA, 2003)

N.D. 1 Impaired physical mobility (NANDA 00085) related to:
- paraplegia
- quadriplegia

N.D. 2 Risk for disuse syndrome (NANDA 00040) related to spinal cord injury/neuromuscular impairment/paralysis

N.D. 3 Risk for injury (NANDA 00035) related to:
- paralysis/immobility
- sensory deficit (tactile)

N.D. 4 Risk for impaired skin integrity (NANDA 00046) related to immobility

N.D. 5 Ineffective airway clearance (NANDA 00031) related to impaired ability to cough

N.D. 6 Impaired spontaneous ventilation (NANDA 00033) related to spinal cord injury

N.D. 7 Risk for autonomic dysreflexia (NANDA 00010) related to autonomic nerve function

N.D. 8 Risk for body temperature: imbalanced (NANDA 00005) related to autonomic nerve dysfunction

N.D. 9 Impaired urinary elimination pattern (NANDA 00016) related to neuromuscular impairment

N.D. 10 Bowel incontinence (NANDA 00014) related to lack of voluntary sphincter control due to neuromuscular impairment

N.D. 11 Risk for constipation (NANDA 00015) related to neuromuscular impairment

N.D. 12 Self-care deficit related to physical disability:
- feeding (NANDA 00102)
- bathing/hygiene (NANDA 00108)
- dressing/grooming (NANDA 00109)
- toileting (NANDA 00110)

N.D. 13 Risk for chronic low self-esteem (NANDA 00119) related to perception of physical disability

N.D. 14 Risk for powerlessness (NANDA 00152) related to:
- physical impairment
- dependence on others for ADLs at home and school

## Goals

The student will maintain independence with mobility in the school setting. (N.D. 1, 2)

The student will increase independence with mobility in the school setting. (N.D. 1, 2, 13)

The student will assist in development and implementation of an emergency evacuation plan (EEP). (N.D. 1, 2)

The student will assist in prevention of physical injuries. (N.D. 3)

The student will utilize prevention methods to prevent skin breakdown and pressure areas. (N.D. 4)

The student will assist in prevention of respiratory infections. (N.D. 5, 6)

The student will maintain open airway, effective breathing pattern, and air exchange. (N.D. 5, 6)

The student will assist in development of emergency care plan (ECP) for management of an autonomic dysreflexia episode at school. (N.D. 7)

The student will assist in management of episodes of autonomic dysreflexia effectively. (N.D. 7)

The student will maintain body temperature within normal range. (N.D. 8)

The student will dress appropriately for body temperature and environmental conditions, with assistance as needed. (N.D. 8)

The student will assist in prevention of bladder distention and incontinence during the school day. (N.D. 9)

The student will assist in prevention of urinary tract infections. (N.D. 9)

The student will maintain adequate dietary and fluid intake. (N.D. 9, 10, 11)

The student will assist in prevention of bowel incontinence during the school day. (N.D. 10)

The student will participate verbally/physically in: (specify ADLs). (N.D. 12)

The student will increase self-care skill(s) (specify what skill). (N.D. 12)

The student will maintain optimal hygiene, with assistance as needed. (N.D. 12, 13)

The student will utilize healthy adaptation and coping skills. (N.D. 13)

The student will describe abilities, disabilities, and appearance realistically. (N.D. 13)

The student will make decisions regarding health management, assistive care, school, and peer activities. (N.D. 12, 14)

The student will communicate effectively with parent(s) and teachers. (N.D. 14)

The student will demonstrate responsibility and control of (identify factor(s) in his/her life). (N.D. 14)

## Nursing Interventions

*Environmental management*

Orient student to the school building, make note of rooms or areas that are inaccessible, such as the media center, band room, auditorium, etc., and modifications that need to be made to make them accessible. (N.D. 1, 2)

With the student, check all classrooms to make sure there are desks or tables that will accommodate the student's needs, such as the wheelchair being able to fit under the desks or tables. (N.D. 1, 2)

Educate teachers and management assistants on assistive measures that will be needed in the classroom, such as accessing books and materials that are needed, assistance with writing for assignments and tests, assistance with completing special assignments or experiments, etc., based on student need and preference. (N.D. 1, 2)

Inform teachers and others working with the student of tactile deficit and need to protect skin from pressure and harmful environments, such as chemicals, hot and cold. (N.D. 4)

Develop an EEP that clearly indicates how the student will be evacuated from the building in case of an emergency situation. All persons who will be involved with the student during the school day, as well as the student, should be involved in developing and practicing the plan. (N.D. 1, 2)

Monitor environment for possible contact with environmental hazards, such as chemicals, heat/cold, slippery floor or sidewalk surfaces, etc. Utilize measures to prevent exposure. (N.D. 3).

*Energy management*

With the student, check the time it takes to get from class to class, class to lunch, and last class to bus home, and make modification in release times if needed. (N.D. 1, 2)

*Positioning: wheelchair*

Assist the student to maintain proper body positioning in his/her wheelchair. (N.D. 1, 2, 3, 4)

Discuss with the student factors that increase risk of injury. (N.D. 3)

Instruct student to use safety equipment, properly, at all times, such as having the wheelchair belt securely fastened. Monitor use. (N.D. 3)

Utilize correct techniques for moving, transferring, and transporting the student. (N.D. 3)

Handle extremities carefully when turning and positioning. (N.D. 3)

Monitor for signs of contracture deformity. Inform parents if signs are noticed. (N.D. 3)

*Pressure ulcer prevention*

Discuss with student: (N.D. 4)
- what skin breakdowns are
- ways to prevent skin breakdown and pressure areas, such as shifting weight at least once every class period
- signs and symptoms of skin breakdown
- what to do if signs and symptoms are present

Assist student to notify parent(s) if signs or symptoms of a skin breakdown or pressure area occur. (N.D. 4)

Assist the student to keep skin and clothing clean and dry. (N.D. 4)

Inspect skin for signs and symptoms of skin breakdown, especially when putting on or removing braces or orthotic devices, doing catheterization procedures, when cleaning anal area after a bowel movement, or changing the student's clothing. (N.D. 4)

*Respiratory monitoring*

Discuss with student: (N.D. 5)
- how regular breathing exercises can assist in maintaining good respiratory function
- signs and symptoms of a respiratory infection

- ways to minimize risk of contracting a respiratory infection
- what to do if signs and symptoms are present

Encourage the student and family to consult their healthcare provider about yearly influenza immunization. (N.D. 5, 6)

Assist the student to demonstrate and utilize effective coughing. (N.D. 5)

### Artificial airway management

Provide tracheostomy care as prescribed and as needed. (N.D. 6)

Maintain an adequate supply of tracheostomy care equipment and supplies. (N.D. 6)

If the student is ventilator-dependent, develop knowledge and understanding of the function of the particular ventilator the student is on and what to do if a malfunction occurs. A manual ventilation bag must always be immediately available. (N.D. 6)

If the student has a diaphragmatic pacemaker, develop a knowledge and understanding of the function of the pacemaker and what to do if the pacemaker malfunctions. An extra supply of batteries for the student's pacemaker and a manual ventilation bag must always be available. (N.D. 6)

Develop an ECP to manage occurrences of ventilator or diaphragmatic pacemaker malfunction. (N.D. 6)

### Dysreflexia management

Develop an ECP to manage dysreflexia episodes at school with the student, parent(s), and healthcare provider. (N.D. 7)

Follow ECP if an episode occurs. (N.D. 7)

Provide in-service training to the student's teachers and other staff who work with him/her regarding dysreflexia and what to do if an episode occurs. Include a copy of the ECP. (N.D. 7)

Discuss with the student: (N.D. 7)
- what causes dysreflexia episodes
- signs and symptoms of a dysreflexia episode and how he/she feels when an episode occurs
- what to do if an episode occurs at school, during after-school activities, and on field trips

### Temperature regulation

Encourage the student to dress appropriately for the weather and school environment. (N.D. 8)

If the student is exposed to significant temperature changes during the school day, assist the student to adjust clothing accordingly. Provide extra coverage with blankets, if appropriate. (N.D. 8)

### Urinary elimination management

Encourage the student to maintain adequate fluid intake. (N.D. 9, 11)

### Urinary catheterization

If the student has an indwelling catheter, assist the student to drain the bag at a mutually agreed upon time during the school day. (Note color, amount, and clarity of urine, patency of catheter.) (N.D. 9)

### Urinary catheterization: intermittent

If the student requires sterile catheterization, provide a private area for the procedure to be done. Arrange for an adequate supply of equipment to be kept at school. (Note color, amount and clarity of urine.) (N.D. 9)

If the student is able to self-catheterize, provide a private bathroom that is handicap-accessible and easily accessible for the student. Provide a place for the student to store catheters and other supplies. (N.D. 9)

Inform the student's teachers of the student's need for catheterization and, if needed, extra time out of class for the procedure to be done. (N.D. 9)

Assist student to have and store extra clothing and supplies in school in case urinary incontinence/bowel incontinence occurs. (N.D. 9, 10)

Provide a private space/bathroom for the student to use for cleaning and clothing change, if urinary incontinence or a bowel movement occurs at school. (N.D. 9, 10)

### Infection status

Monitor for signs and symptoms of a urinary tract infection. (N.D. 9)

Discuss with the student: (N.D. 9)

- signs and symptoms of a urinary tract infection
- what to do if the signs and symptoms occur

Assist the student to notify his/her parent(s) if any signs or symptoms of a urinary tract infection occur. (N.D. 9)

### Bowel management

Discuss the current bowel elimination program with the student and parent(s). (N.D. 10, 11)

Discuss with student and parent(s) what to do if a bowel movement occurs at school. (N.D. 10)

### Self-care assistance: bathing/hygiene, dressing/grooming, feeding, toileting, transfer

Promote participation in feeding, hygiene, toileting, and dressing activities. (N.D. 11, 14)

With the student and parents, determine areas for potential increase in participation in self-care activities. (N.D. 12, 14)

Provide opportunities for the student to increase his/her self-care skills, such as choosing which clothes to wear, getting his/her own drink of water, opening his/her own locker after it has been unlocked by a peer or adult, etc. (N.D. 12, 14)

During care activities, provide choices and request preferences from the student. (N.D. 12, 14)

### Body image enhancement

Encourage the student to express how he/she feels and thinks or views him/herself, and to ask questions at home and school. (N.D. 13)

Clarify any misconceptions the student has about himself/herself and his/her care and education. (N.D. 13)

Assist the student to ask for and accept assistance from others when it is appropriate. (N.D. 12, 14)

Encourage good hygiene, grooming, and dress. (N.D. 12, 13)

Encourage involvement with peers in school and community activities. (N.D. 13)

If the student's perception of body image is strongly distorted or negative, discuss it with the student's parents and refer them to their healthcare provider or community mental health resources for further assessment. (N.D. 13)

### Self-esteem enhancement

Provide the student with opportunities to make decisions regarding health management, assistive care, and school and peer activities. (N.D. 14)

Respect and follow the student's decision if you have given him/her options. (N.D. 14)

Provide opportunities for the student to take on responsibility and control of identified factors in his/her life, such as relaying information to teachers or parents, getting homework done and turned in on time, getting missed assignments if he/she is absent, and being in class on time. (N.D. 14)

Emphasize the student's strengths and abilities. (N.D. 12, 13, 14)

Assist the student to maintain good communication with his/her parents and teachers. (N.D. 13,14)

## Expected Student Outcomes

The student will:

### Ambulation: wheelchair
- Demonstrate independent mobility in the school setting. (N.D. 1, 2)
- Demonstrate increase in independent mobility in the school setting. (N.D. 1, 2)
- Utilize adaptive devices to increase mobility in the school setting. (N.D. 1, 2 )

### Body positioning
- Maintain proper body positioning in wheelchair (percent of time). (N.D. 3, 4)

### Risk control
- Identify factors that increase the risk of injury. (N.D. 3)

### Personal safety behavior
- Utilize safety measures to prevent injury (specific measure). (N.D. 3)
- Propels wheelchair safely in the school environment and on field trips. (N.D 3)

### Respiratory status: airway patency, ventilation
- Demonstrate maintenance of an open airway and effective breathing pattern and air exchange. (N.D. 5, 6)
- Demonstrate effective coughing. (N.D. 5)

*Participation in healthcare decisions*
- Assist in development of ECP for dysreflexia episodes. (N.D. 7)
- Assist to develop ECP for occurrence of ventilator or diaphragmatic pacemaker malfunction, date: _____. (N.D. 6)
- Assist to develop and implement an EEP. (N.D. 1, 2)

*Knowledge: disease process*
- Identify causes of skin breakdown and pressure areas. (N.D. 4)
- Identify prevention methods that can be used to prevent skin breakdown. (N.D. 4)
- Describe what causes dysreflexia episodes. (N.D. 7)
- Identify early signs and symptoms of a dysreflexia episode. (N.D. 7)
- Describe how regular breathing exercises can assist in maintaining good respiratory function. (N.D. 5)
- Identify the signs and symptoms of a urinary tract infection. (N.D. 9)

*Knowledge: treatment procedure*
- Describe what to do if a dysreflexia episode occurs. (N.D. 7)
- Demonstrate effective management of dysreflexia episodes, when they occur. (N.D. 7)
- Demonstrate proper technique and utilization of breathing exercises. (N.D. 5)
- Describe what to do if signs and symptoms of a urinary tract infection occur. (N.D. 9)

*Health promotion behavior*
- Dress appropriately for the weather and school environment, with assistance as needed. (N.D. 8)

*Urinary continence*
- Self-catheterize every 4 to 6 hours. (N.D. 9)
- Participate in catheterization plan. (N.D. 9)
- Experience no urinary incontinence during the school day. (N.D. 9)

*Compliance behavior*
- Accurately report signs and symptoms of a urinary tract infection to his/her parent(s). (N.D. 9)
- Demonstrate adequate fluid intake, as observed by parent(s) and reported by student. (N.D. 9, 10, 11)

*Bowel continence*
- Follow bowel elimination program, as reported by student and parent(s). (N.D. 10,11)
- Experience no bowel incontinence during the school day. (N.D. 10)

*Self-care: feeding, hygiene, toileting, dressing, grooming, ADLs*
- Demonstrate active participation in feeding, hygiene, toileting, and dressing and grooming activities. (N.D. 12, 14)
- Make choices and request preferences with caregivers, as observed by school personnel and parent(s). (N.D. 12, 14)
- Demonstrate increase in self-care skill (specific increase, specific skill). (N.D. 12)
- Demonstrate good hygiene and appearance in school, with assistance as requested or needed. (N.D. 12, 13)

*Body image*
- Identify and describe his/her abilities, disabilities, and appearance (age-appropriate, as observed by: school staff, parent(s). (N.D. 13)

*Self-esteem*
- Ask for and accept assistance, when needed. (N.D. 12, 13, 14)
- Identify factors in his/her life over which he/she has control. (N.D. 14)
- Demonstrate responsibility for (identify the factor). (N.D. 14)

- Participate in one activity with peers in school, in the community (specify number and organization). (N.D. 13)
- Demonstrate good communication with parent(s), as reported by student and parent(s). (N.D. 14)
- Demonstrate good communication with teachers, as reported by student and teachers. (N.D. 14)

*Decision making*
- Make decisions regarding school and peer activities in school, as observed by teachers and other school staff. (N.D. 14)

# Case study

Karen is an 11-year-old girl who will begin at Central Middle School this fall. Karen is a bright, articulate sixth grader who has tetraplegia caused by a birth injury. She uses a power wheelchair for mobility. She has recurrent urinary infections and bronchial stenosis, which places her at higher risk for respiratory infections. Karen also has severe osteoporosis, especially in her legs and hips, due to tetraplegia and no weight-bearing activities.

Karen will be placed on a mainstream sixth grade team. Other than assistance with setting up the materials she needs for her classes and adapted physical education, Karen does not require any direct academic assistance. She will need assistance getting her lunch and opening her milk carton and with her coat and locker at the beginning and end of the day.

Karen and her parents came to visit the school yesterday. In meeting with them, several health-related issues and concerns were discussed:

1. Karen will need to be catheterized after lunch every day. The parents want the school nurse to use sterile technique and they will provide all the supplies that are needed in school. Because she has a history of recurrent urinary tract infections, her parents would like the school nurse to report any signs of an infection to them as soon as possible so appropriate antibiotic therapy can be initiated.
2. Because Karen has tetraplegia, she has a potential for developing autonomic dysreflexia (sudden increase in blood pressure). It is a medical emergency and requires immediate action.
3. Central Middle School is a multifloor building. Karen will use the elevator to get between floors of the building as needed. However, if she is on the second floor and an emergency evacuation of the building is needed, she will not be able to use the elevator. Plans for safe and expedient evacuation from the building are a big concern to both Karen and her parents.
4. Because of her severe osteoporosis, Karen should remain in her wheelchair throughout the school day, except during catheterization and as needed to evacuate the building. When she is rolled to remove her thoracic lumbar sacral orthosis (TLSO) for catheterization, she needs to be log-rolled to prevent twisting of joints, which may lead to fractures. She must also remain properly positioned in her wheelchair.
5. On account of her bronchial stenosis, Karen's respiratory status can change quickly if she has a respiratory infection. Karen will receive an influenza vaccine again this year; however, her parents would like to be notified if there are numerous cases at school or if school personnel notice Karen coughing or having other respiratory symptoms. Karen has missed numerous school days in the past several years on account of severe respiratory infections.

# Spinal Cord Injury

| Assessment Data | Nursing Diagnosis | Goals | Nursing Interventions | Expected Outcomes |
|---|---|---|---|---|
| C7 tetraplegia related to birth injury<br><br>Dysreflexia episodes—usually caused by bladder distention and need for bowel movement | Risk for autonomic dysreflexia related to tetraplegia, usually resulting from a distended bladder or need for bowel movement. | Karen will assist in the development of an Emergency Care Plan (ECP) for management of an autonomic dysreflexia episode at school and on field trips and other school-related activities.<br><br>Karen will assist in the prevention of bladder distention during the school day. | Develop an ECP with Karen and her parents (see attached). Provide in-service training for Karen's teachers on autonomic dysreflexia and the ECP.<br><br>Discuss with Karen:<br>• potential and known causes of dysreflexia episodes for her, signs and symptoms of a dysreflexia episode. | Karen participates in the ECP planning meeting. ECP date:<br><br>Karen identifies 3 causes of dysreflexia episodes, including her 2 most common causes.<br><br>Karen describes how she feels (signs and symptoms) when a dysreflexia episode occurs.<br><br>Karen demonstrates what to do when a dysreflexia episode occurs.<br><br>Karen follows the ECP when a dysreflexia episode occurs. |
| C7 tetraplegia<br><br>Power wheelchair for mobility around the school and community<br><br>Does have very limited manual mobility of wheelchair | Impaired physical mobility related to tetraplegia resulting in need for power wheelchair for mobility and need for assistance in evacuating the building safely in an emergency. | Karen will assist in developing and implementing an Emergency Evaluation Plan (EEP) plan.<br><br>Karen will evacuate the building quickly and safely in an emergency. | Develop an EEP with Karen, her parents, and school staff (see attached).<br><br>Hold a trial evacuation and make any changes to the plan that are needed.<br><br>Provide in-service for staff on what to do if an emergency evacuation is needed. | Karen participates in the EEP planning meeting.<br><br>Karen actively participates in the trial evacuation.<br><br>Karen successfully evacuates the building in a safe and timely manner.<br><br>Date of fire drill: _____ |
| Severe osteoporosis, especially in hips and legs<br><br>Tetraplegia | Risk for injury related to severe osteoporosis (especially lower extremities). | Karen will assist in maintaining proper positioning in her wheelchair. | Inform Karen's teachers of her increased risk for fractures. | Karen will maintain proper positioning in her wheelchair, with assistance from staff. |

| Assessment Data | Nursing Diagnosis | Goals | Nursing Interventions | Expected Outcomes |
|---|---|---|---|---|
| No weight bearing on legs.<br><br>Twisting of joints may cause fractures.<br><br>Wears thoracolumbosacral orthosis (TLSO) at all times when she is sitting to provide proper trunk support. | | Karen will have no fractures of her lower extremities.<br><br>Karen assists in describing to care givers how she needs to be log-rolled to prevent lower extremity fractures. | With the assistance from the physical therapist, inform teachers and paras what to do if Karen does not have proper body alignment in her wheelchair.<br><br>Parents will position Karen properly in her wheelchair before she leaves for school.<br><br>Karen will remain in her wheelchair during the school day, except when she is transferred to the hi-low cot for catheterization.<br><br>Karen's wheelchair belt needs to be monitored for secure fastening several times per day because she likes to loosen it up at times.<br><br>Maintain proper alignment when transferring Karen to the cot.<br><br>Maintain proper alignment when Karen is lying on the cot for catheterization; needs to be log-rolled when removing and putting on clothing. | Karen will demonstrate her ability to accurately describe how she needs to be transferred and log-rolled.<br><br>Karen will wear her wheelchair belt securely fastened at all times. |
| | | | Discuss with Karen the importance of shifting her weight often (1 or 2 times per class period) to prevent pressure sites. | Karen will identify 3 causes of pressure points and skin breakdown. |

| Assessment Data | Nursing Diagnosis | Goals | Nursing Interventions | Expected Outcomes |
|---|---|---|---|---|
| Stays in wheelchair throughout the school day, except during catheterization.<br><br>Wears orthoses on trunk and lower legs, ankles and feet to help maintain proper alignment. | Risk for impaired skin integrity related to tactile deficit due to tetraplegia and need to wear orthoses | Karen will assist in preventing pressure areas and skin breakdown by utilizing preventive measures.<br><br>Karen increases her knowledge of skin breakdown and what to do if she or someone notices it occurs. | Assist Karen to practice and demonstrate how to shift her weight and still maintain proper alignment.<br><br>Discuss with Karen:<br>• What is skin breakdown<br>• Signs and symptoms<br>• What needs to be done if it occurs<br><br>Monitor skin under TLSO daily when it is removed for catheterization.<br><br>Make sure to smooth clothing and make sure there is cloth padding between the orthoses and her skin.<br><br>Assist Karen to notify her parents of any changes in her skin condition.<br><br>Inform teachers of Karen's tactile deficit and the need to protect her skin from pressure and harmful environments (hot and cold). | Karen will identify 3 causes of pressure points and skin breakdown.<br><br>Karen will shift her weight in her wheelchair at least once per class period, as observed by teacher or para.<br><br>Karen will accurately describe what skin breakdown is.<br><br>Karen identifies 3 or 4 signs and symptoms of skin breakdown.<br><br>Karen describes what needs to be done if skin breakdown occurs.<br><br>Karen will accurately inform her parents when signs or symptoms of skin breakdown occur. |
| Doesn't always wear appropriate clothing for the outside weather to school, especially in the winter<br><br>She leaves home with proper clothing, but takes off her hat, mittens, and/or scarf on the bus on the way to school. | Ineffective thermoregulation related to autonomic nerve dysfunction. | Karen will wear appropriate clothing to maintain her body temperature and for environmental conditions.<br><br>Karen will maintain optimal body temperature. | Before Karen leaves school every day, para or teacher will check to determine if she is dressed appropriately for the outside weather and make adjustments as needed.<br><br>Assist Karen to adjust clothing indoors during the school day, based on the indoor school environment. | Karen will dress appropriately for the outside weather and indoor school environment, with assistance as needed. |

| Assessment Data | Nursing Diagnosis | Goals | Nursing Interventions | Expected Outcomes |
|---|---|---|---|---|
| C7 Tetraplegia Recurrent urinary tract infections (UTIs)–does not have indwelling catheter due to recurrent UTIs.<br><br>Sterile urinary catheterizations after lunch, at school, every day. | Impaired urinary elimination pattern related to tetraplegia, requiring the need for urinary catheterization and resulting in frequent UTIs. | Karen will maintain good urinary elimination pattern.<br><br>Karen will assist in prevention of bladder distention and incontinence during the school day.<br><br>Karen will assist in the prevention of UTIs. | Sterile urinary catheterization, every day, after lunch at school and as needed for bladder distention.<br><br>Provide:<br>• Private space<br>• Storage area for supplies (provided by parents)<br><br>Monitor urine for color, amount, clarity, smell.<br><br>Assist Karen to notify parents if signs or symptoms of a UTI occur.<br><br>Inform Karen's teachers of need for urinary catheterization, which will cause her to miss 10 minutes of her 6th mod class.<br><br>Assist Karen to obtain drinks of water as requested.<br><br>Karen may also carry a water bottle with her if she wishes to | Karen will independently come to the health office every day after lunch for catheterization.<br><br>Karen will experience no episodes of bladder distention or incontinence during the school day.<br><br>Karen will demonstrate good fluid intake during the school day. |
| Decreased pulmonary function due to bronchial stenosis and C7 tetraplegia.<br><br>Upper respiratory infections usually lead to complications such as pneumonia. | Risk for infection related to decreased pulmonary function due to bronchial stenosis and tetraplegia. | Karen will assist in the prevention of respiratory infections this school year. | Observe daily for signs and symptoms of a respiratory infection.<br><br>Assist Karen to notify parents if she is coughing or has signs of a respiratory infection. | Karen will demonstrate decrease in the number of missed school days due to respiratory infections this school year.<br><br>Karen will demonstrate good dietary and fluid intake patterns. |

| Assessment Data | Nursing Diagnosis | Goals | Nursing Interventions | Expected Outcomes |
|---|---|---|---|---|
| Has missed numerous school days the past several years due to respiratory infections. | | | Monitor school environment for increased number of cases of respiratory illnesses. | Karen receives influenza vaccine this school year. |
| | | | Notify Karen's parents if it occurs to discuss possible ways to prevent absences from school. | Karen demonstrates effective quad-cough technique. |
| | | | Encourage parent to get yearly influenza immunization. | |
| | | | Encourage Karen to cough, with quad-cough technique when she does have a cough or respiratory infection. | |

# Emergency Care Plan
# Spinal Cord Injury

Date: _____       School: _____

Student: <u>Karen</u>                     Grade: _____

Date of birth: _____

Parent(s)/Guardian(s): _____       Home telephone: _____

                      _____       Father's work: _____

                      _____       Mother's work: _____

Primary Care Provider: _____       Telephone: _____

Specialist: _____       Telephone: _____

Contact: _____

Health Condition: <u>Spinal Cord Injury (Tetraplegia): Risk for Autonomic Dysreflexia</u>

| Indication of Need | Actions to Take |
|---|---|
| *Autonomic Dysreflexia*<br><br>Usually experiences **sweating** as the first Sign.<br><br>In addition, she may experience:<br>  Flushing of her face (redness)<br>  Pounding headache<br>  Slow or fast heart rate<br>  Distended neck veins<br>  Shivering or chills<br><br>Autonomic dysreflexia is a medical emergency that occurs in persons with quadriplegia.<br><br>There is a potential risk for her blood pressure to suddenly increase. This may lead to a stroke or death. Immediate action is necessary to determine and remove the cause of the dysreflexia episode. | Karen will shift her weight in her wheelchair to attempt to relieve any episodes caused by pressure on a part of her body.<br><br>If sweating or other symptoms continue:<br>• Karen will notify her teacher<br>• Karen will come to the health office immediately accompanied by a staff member or student<br>• School Nurse or Health Aide will assist Karen to transfer herself from her wheelchair to a lying down position on a cot.<br>• School Nurse will assist Karen to find the source of the stimulus and remove it.<br>  – Skin irritation<br>  – Need for catheterization<br>  – Need for bowel movement<br><br>If the episode is relieved, Karen may return to classes.<br><br>If the episode continues to be unrelieved, notify her parents.<br><br>If needed, notify her physician and call 911 for assistance. |

Signatures:

School Nurse_____ Date_____

Parent/guardian (if required)_____ Date_____

# Emergency Evacuation Plan
## For Students With Disabilities

**Student:** Karen                    **School:** Pine Valley Elementary
**Disability Area:** Physically Impaired     **Grade:** 6
**Medical Diagnosis:**                **Teacher:**

**Concerned Personnel:** Teachers, Administrators, Student, Counselor, Parents, Social Worker, Paraprofessionals working with Karen

**Concern:** Karen is physically impaired (tetraplegia) and may have difficulty evacuating the building in an emergency situation. She uses an electric wheelchair for mobility around school and uses the elevator to get between first and second floor. (The elevator cannot be used in an emergency evacuation.)

**Plan:** For emergency evacuation from first floor (mods 2–10):
   Karen, accompanied by school nurse (or designated person), will exit the building by her wheelchair, out the front door or annex door.
For emergency evacuation from second floor (mod 1):
   Karen will go to the main stairway at the north end of the building.
   The School Nurse and 3 designated teachers will carefully remove Karen from her wheelchair, place her in the carrying sling, transport her down the stairs and out the door. (The wheelchair will be left in the building.)
On cool days, a space blanket will be placed over Karen for warmth. (Space blanket will be kept in the pack on the back of her chair at all times.)
(The school psychologist will cover for the school nurse when she is out of the building.)

**Case Manager**_____
cc: Case Manager, Parent(s), Paraprofessional, Health Services, Classroom Teachers, Principal

**Spinal Cord Injury**

# References

Dudgeon, B. J., Massagli, T. L., & Ross, B. R. (1997) Educational participation of children with spinal cord injury. *American Journal of Occupational Therapy, 51,* 553–561.

Lindsey, L., Klebine, P., & Wells, M. J. (2000). *Understanding spinal cord injury and functional goals. Spinal cord injury infosheets 4 and 5.* Retrieved October 21, 2003, from http://www.spinalcord.uab.edu/show.asp?durki=22408

Massagi, T. L. (2000). Medical and rehabilitation issues in the care of children with spinal cord injuries. *Physical Medicine and Rehabilitation Clinics of North America, 21*(1), 169–182.

McCluer, S. (1995). Autonomic dysreflexia. Factsheet 25. Retrieved September 16, 2003, from http://www.spinal-cord.uab.edu/show.asp?durki=21542

NANDA International. (2003). *Nursing diagnoses: Definitions & classification 2003–2004.* Philadelphia: Author.

National Spinal Cord Injury Association. (2003). *More about spinal cord injury.* Retrieved October 22, 2003, from http://www.spinalcord.org/html/factsheets/spinalstat.php

National Spinal Cord Injury Statistical Center. (2001) *Spinal cord injury: Facts and figures at a glance.* Retrieved September 16, 2003, from http://www.spinalcord.uab.edu/show.asp?durki=21446

Rehabilitation Institute of Chicago—Spinal Cord Injury Team. (2002). Spinal cord injury complications: Autonomic dysreflexia. Chicago, IL: Rehabilitation Institute of Chicago.

Senelick, R. C., & Dougherty, K. (1998). *The spinal cord injury handbook: For patients and their families.* Birmingham, AL: HealthSouth Press.

Wong, D. L., Hockenberry, M. J., Wilson, D., Winkelstein, M. L., & Kline, N. E. (2003). The child with neuromuscular and muscular dysfunction. In *Nursing care of infants and children* (7th ed., pp. 1852–1862). St. Louis, MO: Mosby.

# Bibliography

Denehy, J. (2004). *Using nursing languages in school nursing practice.* Castle Rock, CO: National Association of School Nurses.

Dochterman, J. M., & Bulechek, G. M. (Eds.). (2004). *Nursing interventions classification (NIC)* (4th ed.). St. Louis, MO: Mosby.

Keating, R. F., Spence, C. A., & Lynch, D. (2002). The brain and nervous system: Normal and abnormal development. In M. L. Batshaw (Ed.), *Children with disabilities* (5th ed., pp. 256–257). Washington, DC: Paul H. Brooks.

Medical College of Wisconsin Model SCI System. (1999). *Take it from us: Strategies and ideas about going back to school.* Milwaukee, WI: Medical College of Wisconsin Model SCI System.

Morehead, S., Johnson, M., & Maas, M. (2004). *Nursing outcomes classification (NOC).* St. Louis, MO: Mosby.

Palmer, S., Kriegsman, K. H., & Palmer, J. B. (2000). *Spinal cord injury: A guide for living.* Baltimore: Johns Hopkins University Press.

University of Alabama & Medical RRTC in secondary complications in SCI. (2001). *Autonomic dysreflexia—A possible life threatening situation.* Retrieved October 22, 2003, from http://www.spinalcord.uab.edu/show.asp?durki=21426&site=1021&return=21541

Young, W. (2003). *Spinal cord injury levels and classification.* Retrieved October 22, 2003, from http://carecure.rutgers.edu/Spinewire/Articles/SpinalLevels/SpinalLevels.html

# Resources

American Spinal Injury Association
345 East Superior Avenue
Room 1436
Chicago, IL 60611
312-238-1242
http://www.asia-spinalinjury.org

National Information Center for Children and Youth with Disabilities
P.O. Box 1492
Washington, DC 20013
1-800-695-0285
nichcy@aed.org
http://www.nichcy.org

National Spinal Cord Injury Association
6701 Democracy Boulevard
Suite 300-9
Bethesda, MD 20817
301-588-6959
1-800-962-9629
resource@spinalcord.org
http://www.spinalcord.org

National Spinal Cord Injury Statistical Center
619 19th Street South
SRC 544
Birmingham, AL 35249-7330
205-934-3320
NSCISC@uab.edu
http://www.spinalcord.uab.edu

## Chapter Seventy-one

# Substance Abuse

Brenda Kay Lenz

## Introduction

Adolescence is a critical period when lifelong health behaviors and lifestyle choices are established. It is also a time when health risks and problems result from these lifestyle choices. According to the Centers for Disease Control and Prevention (CDC), only a few behaviors account for the majority of the mortality, morbidity, and social problems in adolescents. These behaviors are drug and alcohol use; tobacco use; sexual behavior; behaviors that result in unintentional or intentional injuries; diet; and physical inactivity (Kann et al., 1996; Grunbaum et al., 2002). Specifically, the use and abuse of alcohol, tobacco, and other drugs contributes to one of the major public health problems for adolescents today and for their future.

## Pathophysiology

The substance abused by the adolescent will depend on the availability of the substance, the cost, peer or social influences, and parental acceptance of the drug used (James, Ashwill, & Droske, 2002). Alcohol and tobacco are the drugs most commonly abused by adolescents. The CDC (Grunbaum et al., 2002) reported that the percentage of students who used any tobacco during the preceding 30 days ranged from 43.3% in 1997 to 33.9% in 2001, and the percentage who smoked cigarettes on 20 or more of the preceding 30 days ranged from 12.7% in 1991 to 13.8% in 2001. For alcohol, the percentage of students having at least one drink in the previous 30 days ranged from 50.8% in 1991 to 47.1% in 2001 (Grunbaum et al., 2002), and those having five or more drinks in a row in 2001 (within a couple of hours) was approximately 31%. This is referred to as binge drinking (Grunbaum et al., 2002; Lundy & Janes, 2001).

In the past 10 years, the rate of marijuana use has been increasing, but it is still used less often than alcohol and tobacco. Marijuana use in the preceding 30 days ranged from 14.7% in 1991 to 23.9% in 2001 (Grunbaum et al., 2002) **(Table 1)**. Illicit drugs such as cocaine, heroin, club drugs (e.g., ecstasy), and methamphetamines are used less frequently and by fewer adolescents than alcohol, tobacco, and marijuana. Students who reported any use of cocaine in their lifetime ranged from 5.9% in 1991 to 9.4% in 2001, and of methamphetamines, 1.7% in 1991 to 4.2% in

2001. In addition, a smaller percentage of adolescents used inhalants and over-the-counter medications such as cold preparations (ephedrine) for mood-altering intentions. The amount of any of the substances used varies depending on gender, ethnicity, age, and geographic area.

**Table 1. Percentage of Students Reporting Substance Use, 1991 and 2001**

| Substance and time period | 1991 | 2001 |
|---|---|---|
| Any tobacco use past 30 days | 43.3% | 33.9% |
| At least one drink past 30 days | 50.8% | 47.1% |
| Any marijuana use past 30 days | 14.7% | 23.9% |
| Any cocaine use in lifetime | 5.9% | 9.4% |
| Any methamphetamine use in lifetime | 1.7% | 4.2% |

Adapted from material taken from "Youth Risk Behavior Surveillance—United States, 2001," by J. A. Grunbaum, L. Kann, S. Kinchen, B. Williams, J. G. Ross, R. and Lowry, et al., 2002, Morbidity and Mortality Weekly Report, 51(SS-4), p. 1-64

Age is a prime indicator of the likelihood of substance abuse. Experimentation may begin as early as the preteen years, but as teens progress through adolescence, the more likely they are to abuse substances. Twelfth graders consistently have the highest rates of tobacco, alcohol, and marijuana use among all adolescent age groups. For example, from the Minnesota Student Survey, the prevalence of any cigarette use in the previous 30 days was 3.5% among sixth graders, 18.7% among ninth graders, and 34.7% among seniors (Minnesota Department of Children, Families, and Learning, 2001). Similar findings, regarding the increase in tobacco use with increasing age, were described in the Youth Risk Behavior Surveillance (Grunbaum et al., 2002).

Adolescent substance use can range from experimentation to recreational use to compulsive use or progression (Winkelstein, 2003; Chatlos, 2001). Peer acceptance is typically the goal for adolescents who are experimenting or using the substance intermittently. The goal may be intox-

**Table 2. Classes of Common Drugs and Their Side Effects**

| Drug Classes and Common Examples | Physical Signs | Behaviors |
|---|---|---|
| **Stimulants**<br>Nicotine<br>Amphetamine<br>Caffeine<br>Cocaine<br>Methamphetamine<br>Ecstasy | Increased alertness, increased activity, tachycardia, hypertension, weight loss over time, sleep problems | Restlessness, agitation, sweating, dilated pupils, dry mouth, diarrhea |
| **Depressants**<br>Barbiturates<br>  Phenobarbital<br>  Secobarbital<br><br>Nonbarbiturates<br>  Quaalude<br>  Placidyl<br><br>Ethanol/alcohol<br>  Beer<br>  Wine | Slurred speech<br>  Slowed reflexes<br>  Constricted pupils (barbiturates)<br><br>Dilated pupils (nonbarbiturates)<br>  Poor coordination<br>  Ataxia, confusion, slurred speech<br><br>Lethargy<br>  Poor coordination | Short attention span<br>  Impaired judgment<br>  Combativeness, violence<br><br>Hyperexcitability<br>  Euphoria<br><br><br>Impaired judgment<br>  Loss of inhibitions<br>  Aggressiveness, lethargy |
| **Narcotics/opiates**<br>Morphine<br>Heroin<br>Methadone<br>Hallucinogens<br>LSD, PCP, and<br>THC<br><br>Cannibis/marijuana | Physical signs similar to barbiturates<br><br>Dilated pupils, reddened eyes, occasionally hypertension<br><br>Delayed response time, poor coordination | Drowsiness, poor muscle control, nausea, confusion<br><br>Hallucinations<br>  Perceptual changes<br>  Euphoria, confusion<br>  Simple euphoria, mild intoxication, drowsiness |
| **Organic solvents**<br>Glue<br>Cleaning fluid<br>Aerosol sprays<br>Gasoline<br>Lighter fluid | Nonspecific<br><br>May observe sore throat, runny nose, cough | Euphoria, confusion, impaired perception and coordination, restlessness, loss of consciousness |
| **Minor tranquilizers**<br>Valium<br>Librium | Nonspecific | Decreased anxiety, occasional loss of inhibition |

Adapted from Nursing Care of Infants and Children (7th ed., p. 886), by D. L. Wong, M. J. Hockenberry, D. Wilson, M. L. Winkelstein, and N. E. Kline, 2003, St. Louis, MO: Mosby.

Substance Abuse

ication for compulsive users who engage in periodic heavy use or binges. Adolescents whose patterns of use involve high doses of the substance, with the threat of dependence, withdrawal symptoms, and altered lifestyle, are the greatest concern. Dependence or addiction is defined by Haspeslagh & Barton (2001) as, "When there are physiological symptoms that occur with withdrawal of the substance" (p. 466). Substances or drugs can be classified according to the risk of dependence, and the risk of dependence is greatest for nicotine (tobacco), amphetamines, and alcohol.

A second classification method is by chemical or drug action. **Table 2** lists the classes of drugs and common examples along with the more common physical signs and behaviors associated with their use.

The consequences of substance abuse include both physical and social problems for the person abusing the substance. According to Haspeslagh and Barton (2001), substance abusers are at increased risk for death as a result of automobile accidents and violence. They state that substance use is strongly associated with other high-risk behaviors and put the substance abuser at greater risk for unprotected sexual encounters, pregnancy, and sexually transmitted diseases. As the substance abuser ages, he or she is more likely to develop chronic health problems associated with long-term use, such as emphysema, hypertension, or pancreatitis. These social and physical problems strain parent and family relationships. Finally, society suffers from substance abuse. Drugs and alcohol cost taxpayers millions in unnecessary healthcare costs, automobile crashes, crime, lost productivity (school and employment), and extra law enforcement (Haspeslagh & Barton).

School problems associated with substance abuse may begin with subtle attitude changes. Lane, Gerstein, Huang, & Wright (2001) reported that adolescents who were approached to purchase marijuana were more likely to have used marijuana in the past year, and those with friends who tried or used marijuana and had more favorable attitudes toward the drug were more likely to have used it. As curiosity evolves into experimentation followed by regular use, the adolescent may experience excessive dependence on peer influence, changing peer groups, changing style of dress, loss of interest in former hobbies and sports, poor school performance, irregular school attendance, deterioration of relationships with family members, and aggressive or rebellious behavior (Stanhope & Knollmueller, 2001; James et al., 2002). As substance abuse frequency and amount increase to the dependence stage, students may experience school failure, law enforcement involvement, changes in eating and sleeping behaviors, and violence.

In addition, adolescents who use drugs may have comorbid conditions. In some cases, the drug use may be a marker for mental health problems and other conditions (Light, Grube, Madden, & Gover, 2003). Mental health problems associated with substance abuse may include depression, anxiety, attention deficit hyperactivity disorder, conduct disorders, suicidal ideology, and other problems.

The etiology of substance abuse is multifaceted. Substance abuse and substance dependence tend to cluster in families (James et al., 2002). There is some evidence that substance abuse may be an adolescent's attempt to cope with anxiety generated by low self-esteem, poor social skills, poor interpersonal relationships, or lack of adaptive behaviors. Both risk and protective factors associated with substance abuse have been researched. Schiffman (2004) has grouped these factors into five domains, including community (availability of drugs); family (discipline, conflict, attitudes, communication); peer (individual's delinquency, perception of risk, friends' attitudes and use toward drugs); school (attendance and grades); and general (participation in activities, religious beliefs). The pattern of risk and protective factors is similar for all substance abuse, although the strength of the associations may vary by substances.

Since the use of all substances is illegal for adolescents under the age of 18 years, teens most frequently gain access to drugs through peers or by social access (Lenz, 2003). Studies of access indicate adolescents initiate use at parties and social gatherings, where peers may allow another to have a cigarette or drink or to smoke marijuana. Other means to access substances include having a young adult just over the legal age purchase the legal substance for the underage teen and stealing from a family member's supply (Muscari, 1999). Research of the initiation of substance use for adolescents consistently demonstrates peer or social use. "Young people smoke because they are around people who smoke," according to McFeely (2001, p.6). Peer or social pressure was once thought of as a contributing factor for only the young adolescents (12 to 15 years of age) to begin using drugs. Yet, studies have demonstrated that social factors also contribute to substance abuse in late adolescence and young adulthood (Lenz).

In the past, substance abuse interventions were based on the type of substance used. For example, when inhalant use was first discovered, schools rushed to provide education to adolescents and parents strictly about inhalants. Through research, professionals have learned that it is not about the substance per se, but about the behavior and the underlying needs associated with those behaviors. Throughout time there has always been, and there always will be, a new drug, but the behaviors, lifestyle choices, and causes of those choices associated with the abuse and use of substances remain constant. Intervention efforts must focus on evidence-based prevention methods rather than the substance.

School nurses can play an integral role in the prevention of substance abuse. Nursing assessment should include the prevalence and trends of substance abuse nationally, regionally, and locally (Schiffman, 2004). In planning prevention and intervention programs, the nurse needs to support an evidence-based approach because it improves student outcomes and is fiscally responsible. Evidence-based approaches require nurses to stay abreast of current research, clinical practice guidelines, and standards of practice. Informatics and technology are ever-evolving, making it easier and more convenient to find evidence by simply searching the Internet at one's workplace or local library. The bibliography at the end of this chapter contains suggests for evidence-based databases and other resources.

## Management

School nurses with formal education in public health nursing have a unique knowledge base that allows them to respond to substance abuse at two distinct levels. The familiar role is case finding: to identify individual students at risk and provide nursing interventions that include communication with parents, referral for diagnosis and treatment, and collaboration with providers to coordinate care when the teen returns to school. In this role, the school nurse must consider the boundaries of the professional nursing license. The role of the nurse in caring for an individual suspected of being under the influence of a chemical is assessment and referral, whereas the physician's role is diagnosis and treatment. When communicating with parents about findings, the nurse should choose words wisely, to avoid crossing professional boundaries. The role of case finding and referral is addressed in the individualized healthcare plan.

A second role, sometimes forgotten in the business of daily work, is the crucial role of providing community-focused or public health nursing care for all students. Substance abuse is a common community health problem that can be addressed successfully through community-focused assessment, surveillance, and interventions aimed at the entire school. Evidence-based prevention is the most effective way to reduce the overall incidence of substance abuse, and school nurses are in an excellent position to make positive impact on the school community as a whole.

In either role, nurses need to be familiar with federal and state privacy laws dealing with drug and alcohol evaluation and treatment. Federal law provides confidentiality protection to persons, including minors, who seek evaluation and treatment from a federally assisted drug or alcohol program (Schwab, Gelfman, & Cohn, 2001). Drug- or alcohol-related information about a student might be confidential and protected, even from parents. The nurse should consult with the school's legal representative or other legal sources to insure she fully understands the current legal confidentiality requirements. See the bibliography section for suggested legal resource.

### School as "Community" Assessment

Many school districts participate in the Safe and Drug-Free Schools Prevention Activities. The U.S. Department of Education Office of Safe and Drug-Free Schools provides financial assistance to state and local education agencies for drug and violence prevention activities that promote the health and well-being of students in elementary and secondary schools. This program is fre-

quently administered through state departments of education. Funded school districts designate a Safe and Drug-Free School coordinator. State departments of education have requirements that districts must meet in order to quality for the prevention grants. Nurses are encouraged to check with their school district and state department of education to learn more about the Safe and Drug-Free Schools program in their district. School nurses, if educated in public health nursing, have the expertise to serve as the Safe and Drug-Free Schools Program Coordinator.

To qualify for the funding, school districts may have to comply with periodic school-based assessments of student behaviors related to substance abuse, violence, sexual activity, and other lifestyle behaviors. These assessments are an excellent source of information to use in planning schoolwide interventions. For example, in Minnesota, the Minnesota Student Survey is completed every 3 years by school districts receiving money for Safe and Drug-Free Schools Programs. Findings from the assessment are released to each individual school district, the county health department, and local libraries and are posted on the Minnesota Department of Education's Web site.

If this information is not available from the state or local level, national assessment data, such as the Youth Risk Behavior Surveillance conducted by the CDC, can be used as a basis for program planning. National substance abuse assessment data are available through several Web sites, and addresses are given in the resources at the end of this chapter.

If only national assessment data are available for use, the nurse should collect local data about students' substance abuse through other methods. Data collection methods include informant interviews, observation, constructed surveys, focus groups, group meetings, and secondary analysis of records, documents, and other previously collected data. The nurse should attempt to collect data using several different methods to eliminate bias (Lundy & Janes, 2001). The nurse is encouraged to consult a community health nursing textbook or the CDC regarding further details of conducting a community assessment.

### School as Community-Based Nursing Diagnoses

Community-based nursing diagnoses are based on assessment findings and include (1) risk (a specific problem or health risk in the school community), (2) among (the specific group affected by the risk/problem), and (3) related to (strength or weaknesses in the community that influence the specific risk) (Lundy & Janes, 2001). Diagnoses should be based on assessment findings and may differ from district to district. The diagnoses of the North American Nursing Diagnosis Association (NANDA) (Doenges, Moorhouse, & Geissler-Murr, 2004) are usually not used for community-level problems because they were developed in acute care nursing and focus more on individual and family problems. Sample community-based diagnoses are given below.

- Risk of substance abuse by ninth-grade boys related to lack of after-school activities for nonathletes
- Risk of tobacco use by eighth graders related to unattended over-the-counter tobacco displays (easy to shoplift) at local gas stations where middle school students walk to attend school
- Risk of alcohol abuse by 12th grade students related to unsupervised in-home parties following prom

## School as Community-Based Interventions

Community interventions must be based on assessment data. Below are some possibilities.

### Primary Prevention Efforts

The goal is to prevent substance abuse before drug abuse occurs.

Reaching parents:

- Informal teaching can take place during any parent contact. Include developmentally appropriate anticipatory guidance throughout adolescence, provide information about home access to substances of abuse, and discuss the importance of the physical presence of parents after school and in the home (Muscari, 1999).
- Take advantage of parent-teacher conferences to provide parent education and support sessions on substance abuse to parents. Parents can form a "parent communication network" to keep each other informed about their adolescents' activities.
- Support families whose students are using drugs by finding opportunities to follow up and guide the student and family to get the needed services and make changes in their lifestyle choices and behaviors. Behavior change is never easy, and if the nurse can support these families, success is more likely.

Create a safe and supportive school environment for students:

- Implement school policies that make children and adolescents feel safe and comfortable with peers, teachers, and administration. For example, tobacco-free policies promote a nonsmoking norm (Von Bothmer, 2001). Students found in possession or use of tobacco on school grounds are ticketed and as a consequence attend a class after school. Drug-free policies for after-school activities and drug-free dances should be included.
- Strengthen social bonding by providing support groups for at-risk students. For example, weekly support groups can provide skill building, education, and emotional support for these adolescents. In a study by Houck, Darnell, and Lussman (2002), students who participated in a weekly support group experienced a decrease in stress, family distress, and suicidal ideation and became engaged in formal treatment for the first time.

- Use opportunities when working with students to discuss substance abuse. For example, when putting on a bandage to a minor cut, talk about tobacco and alcohol use. In each interaction with a student, the nurse has an opportunity to make a difference in the life of this young person.
- Support nontraditional after-school activities. Not all students are comfortable participating in traditional after-school activities. Disparities exist between participants and nonparticipants regarding risk-taking behaviors. Crime rates and risk-taking activities occur more frequently after school. Changes in after-school programming and activities can be made to be more inclusive than traditional activities requiring athletic and academic talents. Nurses can educate parents about the after-school time period.
- Change the perception of the school. Frequently, students believe that "everyone uses" substances. Contrary to that myth, the majority of students do not use. A social norms campaign to decrease this perception will build a more healthy school perception.

Curriculum:

- Search for curriculums that are "evidence-based" or have demonstrated effective student outcomes. One source for this information is the U.S. Department of Education Office of Safe and Drug-Free Schools. For example, Project Alert has been found to be exemplary by the Department of Education as it strengthens life skills and drug refusal skills. (See the resources at the end of this chapter.)
- Intervene early, at appropriate developmental stages, and during transitions.
- Reinforce interventions over time and throughout the adolescence years. As seen from the prevalence studies, more adolescents begin to use as they progress through high school. Initiatives should not stop with the middle grades but include high school students through periodic "boosters" of prevention interventions and education.

Community interventions and initiatives:

- Search for evidence-based interventions to provide for the most effective student outcomes. Examples of ineffective interventions include speakers, displays of car wrecks, and other one-time attractions. These activities develop student awareness, but do not have a lasting impact on behavior or change behavior.
- Facilitate community-wide initiatives for substance abuse reduction. Start at the grassroots level. Grant dollars may be available for community initiatives. The resource section offers a list of possible sources for grant dollars. For example, the school nurse, along with students, attends the local city council

meeting to change city ordinances regarding selling of tobacco products or works with local media to change tobacco billboard advertisements.

• Monitor and evaluate initiatives for outcomes.

### Secondary Prevention Efforts

The goal is to detect and stop substance abuse before the person becomes physically addicted and the problem becomes chronic (Lundy & Janes, 2001). Individual-based assessment and intervention should be implemented.

• Efforts should be made to detect the problem as soon as possible.
• Get the abuser into treatment to prevent addiction.

Treatment facilities include:

– Drug-free programs. These programs are administered by a variety of organizations. They can include residential facilities or highly intensive nightly group meetings or camps.
– Therapeutic communities. These are community-based residential treatment programs. Adolescents in these programs have usually had previous treatment experiences and are frequently referred by the criminal justice system.
– Residential adolescent treatment programs. These are operated by profit-making corporations and include trained staff. Adolescents frequently spend time preparing them for long-term recovery.

• Day-care programs. These programs provide less structured drug-free outpatient programs and may also provide alternative schooling.

### Tertiary Prevention Efforts

The goal of tertiary prevention is to prevent reactivation of substance-abusing behaviors. Individual-based assessment and intervention should be implemented as described previously.

• Ongoing support must be available.
  – Aftercare. These programs are designed and carried out to reinforce and continue support once formal treatment has been completed.
• Community-based support groups. See the resources section at the end of this chapter.

### School as Community-Based Outcomes

To evaluate the effectiveness of implementations, the nurse evaluates the response of the community to the intervention. Questions the nurse needs to ask are: Was the plan carried out? Was it acceptable to the community? Was the health problem changed? Was the program effective? What are the recommendations for future community health promotion? (Lundy & Janes, 2001).

## Individualized Healthcare Plan

### Assessment

#### History

• A history of current and past drug use should be obtained, if possible. Provide a nonthreatening environment and ensure confidentiality within appropriate limits, because this will enable students to discuss their substance abuse more openly. Questions about tobacco are usually less threatening and serve as a good lead-in, followed by questions regarding alcohol use, and finally questions about other drugs.
• The history should include:
  – Friends' use of tobacco, alcohol, and drugs; history of use
  – Age when initiated use for the first time
  – All substances ever experimented with and current substances used
  – Use with peers or use alone
  – Frequency and time of use; use before or after school; weekday use and weekend use
  – Amount of substance used during a party or event
  – Amount of substance used at the beginning of a party or event and feelings associated with initial use at party or event
  – Withdrawal symptoms experienced when not using
  – Reasons for use by student; may include socialization, relaxation, or to forget about problems
  – Lying about use and the amount used; legal trouble; school and job performance; parent and friendship relationships
  – Memory problems associated with use; using substances when not planning to; blacking out indicates high blood level of substance and is safety hazard
  – Feelings about self and self-identity; suicide attempts; feeling about self during chemical use
• A family and social history, medical history, and legal history should be obtained, if possible.
  – Parent or family use of alcohol, marijuana, tobacco, or other chemicals, including frequency, amount, and substance
  – Consequences of parent or family use, such as missing work; problems substance use has created for student, parent, or family
  – Treatment history of parent or family; response to treatment; illness or death of family member associated with alcohol or drug use, for example, liver cirrhosis or pancreatitis

- Home environment; student relationship with parents and family; problem-solving methods
  - Parent or family legal problems associated with substance abuse; for example: driving while intoxicated, possession, selling of drugs, manufacturing of drugs

*Current Status and Management*
- For students who are suspected of being under the influence of a substance, a physical assessment is indicated. Physical assessment should include the adolescent's respiration rate, heart rate, blood pressure, activity level, mood, affect, judgment, speech, sensory responses, and memory (James et al., 2002).
- When other components of the history or physical assessment suggest substance abuse, assess for symptoms indicative of snorting substances, such as inflammation of the nose, runny nose, and reddened eyes, because these symptoms may indicate snorting or abusing chemicals (Sloand & Thate, 2004). However, be cautious and do not prematurely assume that all adolescents with allergy symptoms are abusing substances.
- Pupil size is not an accurate indicator of substance abuse, because lighting, prescription medications, and eye conditions can affect pupil size.
- Observe the student's behavior as objectively as possible, and keep a written description. Keep out personal bias and values. This is often valuable if the student is transferred to a medical facility.
- A physical assessment is not necessary for students not suspected of being under the influence and may cause distrust and limit self-disclosure during the history.

*Psychosocial Status*
- Indicators of risk are valuable predictors of potential problems. Not every adolescent who uses drugs is addicted. The occasional use of alcohol or marijuana at a party is not automatically abuse (McWhirter, McWhirter, McWhirter, & McWhirter, 1993); rather, there is a continuum of substance abuse. The Five-Stage Model of Substance Use (**Table 3**) is one model to assist health professionals in determining the possible extent of the adolescent's substance abuse (Stanhope & Knollmueller, 2001).

**Table 3. Five-Stage Model of Substance Use**

| Stage 1: Curiosity | The individual at this stage is curious but does not use any drugs. Behaviors include risk taking and a desire for acceptance. |
|---|---|
| Stage 2: Experimentation | This stage includes the use of tobacco, alcohol, and marijuana. The frequency is weekend use for recreational purposes. Behaviors observed include lying, but little other behavior change. |
| Stage 3: Regular use | Additional drugs may be added, including amphetamines, hashish. The frequency of use increases to midweek use with the purpose to get high. The person displays behaviors of mood swings, faltering school performance, truancy, changing peer groups, changing style of dress. |
| Stage 4: Psychological or chemical dependence | Stimulants and hallucinogens are added to the other drugs. The frequency of use is daily. Behaviors observed include pathologic lying, school failure, family fights, law enforcement involvement, truancy, shoplifting, driving under the influence, and violence. |
| Stage 5: Uses drugs to feel normal | Any drugs that are available will be used. Frequency of use is all day, or any way possible. Behaviors include drifting, repeated failures, blackouts, amnesia, fatigue, malnutrition, and symptoms of paranoia, aggression, and frequent overdosing. |

Adapted from Handbook of Public and Community Health Nursing Practice (2nd ed.), by M. Stanhope and R. N. Knollmueller, 2001, St. Louis, MO: Mosby.

*Self-care*
- Student's perception of his or her own chemical use, peer use, family use, or exposure to chemicals
- Decision-making and refusal skills
- Student's perception of social or peer pressure to use chemicals
- Student's level of knowledge of chemicals and consequences of use
- Family's understanding of chemicals, consequences, and needs

*Academic Issues*
- Review the student's actual academic record for signs of decline. Keep in mind that student's self-report may differ dramatically from what is factual. Falling grades and changes in friendships are indicators of risk.
- Review the student's attendance record for increase in absenteeism and tardiness, or leaving before the end of the day.
- Information from classmates and peers should be used cautiously. Student perception can be biased, inflated, and negatively motivated. Substantiating information from teachers and support staff is always advisable.
- Review any other student records or files, such as police reports. Some states have laws that allow police departments to disclose police reports to the school district involving minor alcohol consumption violations, marijuana use and possession, and other law violations.
- Review the student's discipline records, including emotional and behavioral difficulties, attention-getting behaviors, explosive temper, disregard for rules, inappropriate social skills, poor concentration, and delayed maturation.

## Nursing Diagnoses (N.D.) (NANDA, 2003)

**N.D. 1** Ineffective coping (NANDA 00069) related to:
- own chemical use
- exposure to peer and/or family use of chemicals

**N.D. 2** Impaired social interaction (NANDA 00052) related to…
- own chemical use
- exposure to others' use and limited social skills

**N.D. 3** Situational low self-esteem (NANDA 00120) related to:
- limited social skills
- ineffective coping skills
- a poor sense of self-management
- own chemical use or exposure to others' chemical use

**N.D. 4** Compromised family coping (NANDA 00074) related to chemical use.

**N.D. 5** Risk for injury (NANDA 00035) related to:
- own chemical use or overdose
- exposure to chemical use in environment

**N.D. 6** Deficit in knowledge (NANDA 00126) regarding consequences of chemical use related to maturity/experience.

## Goals

The student will cope effectively in social interactions without use of substances in the school setting. (N.D. 1–4)

The student will have positive self-esteem or self-regard in the school setting. (N.D. 3)

The student will remain injury-free from chemical use or exposure to chemicals in school setting. (N.D. 5)

The student will demonstrate knowledge of consequences of chemical use in school setting. (N.D. 6)

The student (and family) will demonstrate knowledge of community resources to assist in diagnosis, treatment, and support for chemical abuse. (N.D. 4)

## Nursing Interventions

If student is currently under the influence, stay alert to life-threatening consequences of drug toxicity. Transfer to a medical facility immediately if indicated. (N.D. 5)

Determine possible extent of substance abuse using the Five State Model of Substance Abuse.
- Students at stage 1 or 2:
  - Provide accurate education about the social and personal costs of drug use. (N.D. 1–3, 6)
  - Provide assertiveness training, teach refusal skills, and allow time to role-play refusal skills. (N.D. 1–3, 6)
  - Teach and role-play decision-making strategies by defining the nature of the choice, giving a number of

alternatives, and discuss benefits and consequences of each alternative. (N.D. 1–3, 6)
  – Provide peer-cluster involvement through trained peer facilitators who can engage students in skills necessary to stop using drugs. (N.D. 1–3, 6)
- Students moving into stage 3 or higher:
  – If the nurse is the first to encounter the abuse, notify family and/or student's support system as directed by school policy and federal and state privacy laws. (N.D. 5)
  – Educate families about stages of substance abuse and correlate to nursing assessment and history findings. (N.D. 6)
  – Refer student for diagnosis and treatment. (N.D. 4, 5)
  – Provide emotional and psychological support for student (and family) as they process first through awareness and later through acknowledgment of student's risk-taking behaviors. (N.D. 4)
  – Provide student and family with current list of local treatment options. Include services offered, cost of program, payment source (county program, private pay, or bill insurance), credentials of staff, age of clients, and program's reputation and success or recidivism (return to treatment) rate. (N.D. 4, 6)
- Students returning to school following treatment:
  – Meet with student and family to plan for possible school accommodations.
  – Educate teachers and support staff regarding accommodations, keeping in mind student and family confidentiality needs.
  – Encourage families and student to maintain active, long-term involvement in support groups. (N.D. 1–4)
  – Refer to appropriate resources that support long-term changes in student's social and emotional patterns of relating. See resource list at end of this chapter. (N.D. 1–4)
  – Provide school-based "after-care" support groups for students returning from treatment. (N.D. 1–3)
  – Collaborate with School Support Services (social worker, psychologist, counselor) to support students. (N.D. 1–3)
- For students whose parent is involved in drug possession, manufacturing, and trafficking:
  – Refer to child protection services. (N.D. 4, 5)
  – Refer for evaluation regarding possible toxic chemical exposure from home drug manufacturing process. (N.D. 5)
  – Refer for psychological evaluation, diagnosis, and treatment as needed. (N.D. 5)
  – Collaborate with School Support Services (social worker, psychologist, counselor) to support students. (N.D. 1–3)
  – Assist family members (not involved in chemicals) to make appropriate and safe choices through education, informative referral, and support. (N.D. 4, 5)
  – Provide peer-cluster involvement through trained peer facilitators who can engage students in skills necessary to resist drugs and to gain peer acceptance. (N.D. 1–3, 6)

## Expected Student Outcomes

The student will:
- Identify ineffective coping behaviors and consequences as evidenced by ability to identify stressors leading to substance abuse. (N.D. 1)
- Meet psychological needs as evidenced by participation in alternative activities, identification of options involving alternative peers and social situations that do not involve substance abuse. (N.D. 1)
- Verbalize awareness of factors and identify feelings that cause or promote poor social interactions as evidenced by self-report. (N.D. 2)
- Develop effective social support system and use of resources that do not involve substance abuse. (N.D. 2)
- Verbalize understanding of individual factors that precipitated substance abuse or exposure to peer use of chemicals. (N.D. 3)
- Experience positive self-appraisal, as evidenced by self-report of having a positive attitude toward himself or herself in regard to not using substances. (N.D. 3)
- Verbalize understanding of individual factors that contribute to possibility of injury related to substance abuse. (N.D. 5)
- Demonstrate behaviors, lifestyle changes to protect self from injury related to substance abuse. (N.D. 5)
- Be free of injury related to substance abuse. (N.D. 5)
- Verbalize understanding of substance abuse and its consequences by direct report and by behavior change as evidenced by improvements in school performance (N.D. 6)
- Experience an increase in school attendance, school performance, and participation in school activities related to reduced substance abuse or no substance abuse. (N.D. 1–3)

- Verbalize knowledge and understanding of substance abuse. (N.D. 4)
- Identify need for outside support for substance abuse. (N.D. 4)
- Identify or verbalize resources to deal with substance abuse. (N.D. 4)

## Case Study

Justin is a 15-year-old boy in the ninth grade at Centennial High School. Three times during the past week and a half, he has complained to the health assistant that he is not feeling well and she has had him rest in the health office. On the third visit, the licensed school nurse is present and takes note of his frequent health office visits. The school nurse reviews his academic record in the computer and learns that he is failing a number of his classes, although in previous semesters he was a B and C student.

The school nurse asks Justin how he is feeling. She learns that he is tired because of what happened in his home earlier this morning. He relates that the police were in his home and then realizes that he has given out too much information. However, the nurse continues to question Justin in a non-threatening manner and finds out that his father was arrested for manufacturing methamphetamine. The police did not remove Justin from the home, even though he was left home alone. He is unsure why he was not removed from the home and speculates that perhaps the police did not notice his young age.

The nurse brings Justin into her office and continues to interview him about his own chemical use in a confidential manner. He denies use. He relates that his mother and grandparents live in another part of the community but he does not get along with them.

1. Following the interview, the school nurse discusses the situation with the police liaison officer. She is concerned about child protection issues because Justin is a minor and has been exposed to the manufacturing of illegal chemicals by the custodial parent. Also, Justin has been left on his own while his father is under arrest.

2. The police officer and the school nurse contact Justin's mother and discuss his needs. Justin is referred for a chemical evaluation to a licensed health provider. The mother consents to take him for the evaluation. She also has Justin move into her home.

3. The chemical evaluation results are negative. It was found that Justin does not abuse any substances, and he returns to school.

4. The school nurse, counselor, social worker, and police liaison officer meet to develop a plan to support Justin during the school day. This includes peer cluster involvement and mentoring. In addition, the school nurse visits with Justin regularly on a one-to-one basis to convey support.

## Substance Abuse

| Assessment Data | Nursing Diagnosis | Goals | Nursing Interventions | Expected Outcomes |
|---|---|---|---|---|
| Frequent visits to health office Complaints of being tired, and grades falling below passing. | Ineffective coping related to chemical use. | Student will cope effectively. | Determine possible extent of substance abuse using the Five State Model of Substance Abuse.<br><br>Collaborate with School Support Services (social worker, psychologist, counselor) to support student. | Justin will experience an increase in school attendance, school performance, and participation in school activities. |
| Student reports his father was removed from home by police for illegal drug manufacturing. | Risk for injury related to exposure to chemical use in the environment. | Student will remain injury-free from exposure to chemicals. | Refer to child protection services.<br><br>Assist family members (not involved in chemicals) in making appropriate and safe choices through education, informative referral, and support.<br><br>Refer for evaluation regarding possible toxic chemical exposure from home drug manufacturing process. | Justin will be free of injury related to substance abuse. |
| Student reports that father has sole custody of student Father currently in jail for illegal activity.<br><br>Student coping with family chemical use by spending time away from classes and sleeping in health office. | Situational low-self esteem related to exposure to chemical use by others. | The student will have positive self-esteem or self-regard in the school setting. | Collaborate with School Support Services (social worker, psychologist, counselor) to support student.<br><br>Provide peer-cluster involvement through trained peer facilitators who can engage students in skills necessary to resist drugs and to gain peer acceptance. | Justin will experience positive self-appraisal, as evidenced by self-report of having a positive attitude toward himself. |

| Assessment Data | Nursing Diagnosis | Goals | Nursing Interventions | Expected Outcomes |
|---|---|---|---|---|
| Student living in home alone Noncustodial parent unaware of custodial parent's arrest.<br><br>Student is minor (15 years of age).<br><br>Student has mother who resides in community. | Compromised family coping related to chemical use. | The family will demonstrate knowledge of chemical use and exposure to chemicals and the effects of use on the student's health and safety and knowledge of community resources. | Refer to child protection services.<br><br>Assist family members (not involved in chemicals) in making appropriate and safe choices through education, informative referral, and support. | Family will verbalize knowledge and understanding of substance abuse.<br><br>Family will identify or verbalize resources to deal with substance abuse. |

# References

Chatlos, J. C. (2001). Substance use and abuse: The impact on academic performance. In F. M. Kline, L. B. Silver, & S. C. Russell, (Eds.), The educator's guide to medical issues in the classroom (pp. 65-79). Baltimore: Paul H Brookes.

Doenges, M. E., Moorhouse, M. F., & Geissler-Murr, A. C. (2004). Nurse's pocket guide: Diagnoses, interventions, and rationales (9th ed.). Philadelphia: F.A. Davis.

Grunbaum, J. A., Kann L., Kinchen, S., Williams, B., Ross, J. G., Lowry, R., et al. (2002). Youth risk behavior surveillance—United States, 2001 .Morbidity and Mortality Weekly Report, 51(SS-4), 1–64. Retrieved March 23, 2004, from http://www.cdc.gov/nccdphp/dash/yrbs Haspeslagh, J., & Barton, J. A. (2001). Substance abuse as a community health problem. In K. S. Lundy, & S. Janes, (Eds.), Community health nursing: Caring for the public's health (pp. 464–491). Boston: Jones and Bartlett.

Houck, G. M., Darnell, S., & Lussman, S. (2002). A support group intervention for at-risk female high school students. Journal of School Nursing, 18(4), 212–218.

James, S. R., Ashwill, J. W., & Droske, S. C. (2002). Nursing care of children principles and practice (2nd ed.). Philadelphia: Saunders.

Kann, L., Warren, C. W., Harris, W. A., Collins, J. L., Williams, B. I., Ross, J. G., et al. (1996). Youth risk behavior surveillance—United States, 1995. Morbidity and Mortality Weekly Report, 45(SS-04), 1–83. Retrieved month day, year from http://www.cdc.gov/nccdphp/dash/yrbs

Lane, J., Gerstein, D., Huang, L., & Wright, D. (2001). Risk and protective factors for adolescent drug use: findings from the 1997 National Household Survey on Drug Abuse. Rockville, MD: National Clearinghouse for Alcohol and Drug Information.

Lenz, B. K. (2003). Correlates of young adult tobacco use: Application of a transitionframework. Journal of School Nursing, 19(4), 135–139.

Light, J. M., Grube, J. W., Madden, P. A., & Gover, J. (2003). Adolescent alcohol use and suicidal ideation: A nonrecursive model. Addictive Behaviors, 28, 705–724.

Lundy, K. S., & Janes, S. (2001). Community health nursing: Caring for the public's health. Boston: Jones and Bartlett.

McFeely, S. (2001). Young people's pathway to smoking cessation. Nursing Standard, 16(2), 39–42.

McWhirter, J. J., McWhirter, B. T., McWhirter, A. M., & McWhirter, E. H. (1993). At risk youth: A comprehensive response. Belmont, CA: Brooks/Cole.

Minnesota Department of Children, Families, and Learning, & Minnesota Department of Human Services. (2001). Minnesota student survey key trends 2001 (MS-1882, 9-01). Roseville, MN: Minnesota Department of Children, Families, and Learning.

Muscari, M. E. (1999). Prevention: Are we really reaching today's teens? American Journal of Maternal/Child Nursing, 24(2), 87–91.

NANDA International. (2003). Nursing diagnoses: Definitions & classification 2003-2004. Philadelphia: Author.

Schiffman, R. F. (2004). Drug and substance use in adolescents. American Journal of Maternal/Child Nursing, 29(1), 21–27.

Schwab, N., Gelfman, M., & Cohn, S. (2001). Fundamentals of U.S. law. In N. Schwab, & M. Gelfman, (Eds.), Legal issues in school health services. (pp. 249–250). North Branch, MN: Sunrise River Press.

Sloand, E., & Thate, J. (2004) Allergies. In P. J. Allen & J. A. Vessey, (Eds.), Primary care of the child with a chronic condition (4th ed., pp. 155–173). St. Louis, MO: Mosby.

Stanhope, M., & Knollmueller, R. N. (2001). Handbook of public and community health nursing practice (2nd ed.). St. Louis, MO: Mosby.

Von Bothmer, M. (2001). Promoting a tobacco-free generation: Who is responsible for what? Journal of Clinical Nursing, 10(6), 784–792.

Winkelstein, M. L. (2003). Behavioral health problems of adolescents. In D. L. Wong, M. J. Hockenberry, D. Wilson, M. L. Winkelstein, & N. E. Kline, (Eds.), Nursing care of infants and children (7th ed., pp. 884–895). St. Louis, MO: Mosby.

# Bibliography

Bergren, M. D. (2002). Child and adolescent mental health Web resources. Journal of School Nursing, 18(4), 226–228.

Maharaj, K., Ternullo, S. (2001). Using nicotine replacement therapy in treating nicotine addiction in adolescents. Journal of School Nursing, 17(5), 278–282.

National Association of School Nurses. (2000). Issue Brief: Substance use and abuse. Scarborough, ME: Author.

National Association of School Nurses. (Adopted 2001). Position Statement: Controlled substances in the school setting. Scarborough, ME: Author.

National Association of School Nurses. (Adopted 2003). Position Statement: The role of the school nurse regarding drug testing in schools. Scarborough, ME: Author.

NIDA Notes. Reports on advances in the drug abuse field; identifies resources; promotes the exchange of information; and improves communication among clinicians, researchers, administrators, and policymakers. (Available from the National Institute on Drug Abuse, National Institutes of Health, 6001 Executive Boulevard, Room 5213, Bethesda, MD, 20892.)

The Prevention Researcher. Each single-theme issue focuses on an at-risk youth topic from prevention standpoint. (Available from Integrated Research Services, Inc., 66 Club Road, Suite 370, Eugene, OR 97401.)

Schwab, N., & Gelfman, M. (Eds.). (2001). Legal issues in school health services. North Branch, MN: Sunrise River Press.

# Resources

## Support Organizations

Many substance abuse support organizations have national and/or state Web sites. The Web page for these organizations will have the most current information, including workshops, support groups, available print material, and more. A partial list of examples is included here.

Al-Anon Family Group Headquarters Inc.
1600 Corporate Landing Parkway
Virginia Beach, VA 23454
1-888-4-AL-ANON

Alcoholics Anonymous
Grand Central Station
PO Box 459
New York, NY 10163

Narcotics Anonymous
P.O. Box 9999
Van Nuys, CA 91409
818-773-9999

Tough Love
P.O. Box 1069
Doylestown, PA 18901
215-348-7090

### Government Organizations
Centers for Disease Control and Prevention
1600 Clifton Road
Atlanta, GA 30333
1-800-311-3435
http://www.cdc.gov/tobacco
Web site offers information about tobacco intervention and prevention; guidelines for school programs based on evidence-based information for tobacco prevention and other adolescent health issues; and links to other sources.

http://www.cdc.gov/healthyouth/yrbs/index.html
Web site for Youth Risk Behavior Surveillance System.

Drug Policy Information Clearinghouse
P.O. Box 6000
Rockville, MD 20849–6000
1-800–666–3332
http://www.whitehousedrugpolicy.gov/prevent/practice.html
The Office of National Drug Control Policy is required to develop and implement a set of research-based principles upon which prevention programming can be based.

National Institute on Drug Abuse
National Institutes of Health
6001 Executive Boulevard
Room 5213
Bethesda, MD, 20892
301-443-1124
http://www.drugabuse.gov
http://www.nida.nih.gov/about/organization/ICAW/ICA.html
Prevention principles, funding, and grant opportunities.

U.S. Department of Education
Office of Safe and Drug-Free Schools
400 Maryland Avenue, SW
Washington, DC 20202
1-800-872-5327
http://www.ed.gov/about/offices/list/osdfs/index.html

**Other Organizations**
American Academy of Pediatrics (AAP)
141 Northwest Point Boulevard
Elk Grove Village, IL 60007
847-434-4000
http://www.aap.org/visit/cmte35.htm
The Committee on Substance Abuse of the AAP provides professional and public education in the area of
   substance abuse. It produces materials for use by
   physicians and works with governmental, public, and
   private organizations to address problems and
   advance goals.

American Lung Association
61 Broadway
Sixth Floor
New York, NY 10006
1-800-548-825
http://www.lungusa.org/tobacco/
Provides educational resources.

National Association of School Nurses
Eastern Office:
P.O. Box 1300 (163. U.S. Route 1)
Scarborough, ME 04070
877-627-6476
nasn@nasn.org

Statements and briefs from the National Association of
School Nurses are official positions taken by the
organization on issues related to health or to school
nursing.

Monitoring the Future
University of Michigan
Ann Arbor, MI 48109
734-764-1817
http://www.monitoringthefuture.org/
An ongoing study of behaviors, attitudes, and values
   includes an annual survey of secondary school students.

Project Alert
725 South Figueroa Street
Suite 1825
Los Angeles, CA 90017
1-800-ALERT-10
http://www.projectalert.best.org/
Substance abuse prevention curriculum for the middle
   grades, sponsored by the Best Foundation.

## Chapter Seventy-two

# Systemic Lupus Erythematosus

### Jean Mientus

## Introduction

Systemic lupus erythematosus (SLE) is a chronic, inflammatory, multisystem disorder of the immune system (National Institutes of Health [NIH], National Institute of Arthritis and Musculoskeletal and Skin Diseases [NIAMS], 2001). The immune system normally protects the body against invading foreign material, such as viruses and bacteria. In lupus, the body's immune system develops antibodies that react against the body's normal tissue. This response can range from mild to severe and, depending on the extent of the inflammation and organ system(s) involved, can be very damaging.

The term *lupus* is derived from Latin, meaning "wolf." With the cutaneous (skin) manifestations of the disease, the facial rash that frequently accompanies lupus has been known to resemble the bite of a wolf. Other organs that may be involved include joints, kidneys, heart, lung, brain, and blood system (NIH, NIAMS, 2001).

More than 16,000 Americans develop lupus each year (NIH, NIAMS, 2001). Adult women are affected 10 to 15 times more frequently than adult men, and people of African American, Indian, and Asian descent are more likely to develop lupus than Caucasian women (Lupus Foundation of America [LFA], 2001a).

For most people, lupus is a manageable disease, affecting only a few organ systems, but for some, it can be life-threatening (LFA, 2001a). The disease is characterized by flares and remissions and may be unpredictable and individualized.

## Pathophysiology

Lupus is considered an autoimmune disorder. The body makes antibodies against its own tissue, which are known as *autoantibodies* (NIH, NIAMS, 2001). The autoantibodies that are typically found in lupus patients often bind to the cell's nucleus and are known as antinuclear antibodies, because their target is usually the complexes that are found inside the cell's nucleus. Other antibodies in lupus bind to cell surface membranes and can damage the cell directly (LFA, 2001b). Most people with lupus will test positive for a variety of autoantibodies.

When these autoantibodies attack the antigen—in this instance, the body's own healthy tissue—they form immune complexes. These immune complexes are then deposited in various tissues in the body, resulting in inflammation and possible tissue damage.

The cause of this autoimmune dysfunction remains unknown. Research to date suggests that genes may play a role in the etiology of this disease (NIH, NIAMS, 2001). This is supported by the high incidence of lupus among first- and second-degree relatives as well as identical twins (Sullivan, 1999). Environmental agents have also been shown to be a contributing factor in individuals with a genetic predisposition (NIH). Sunlight (UVA, UVB rays), stress, certain viruses, and chemical substances have been shown to influence the development or course of the disease. Hormones also influence lupus disease activity. The disease is more prevalent in women during their reproductive years and can exacerbate during pregnancy and/or the postpartum period.

## Disease Classification

SLE can be classified into three disease groups:
- Discoid lupus: involving the skin only, rarely leading to SLE
- SLE: involving more than one system
- Drug-induced lupus: developing after use of certain drugs and gradually subsiding after the offending drug is discontinued (NIH, NIAMS, 2001)

Lupus symptoms vary according to the body system affected (NIH, NIAMS, 2001). It is therefore difficult to make an accurate, timely diagnosis of the disease. Symptoms may be generalized or involve specific organs. There is no single laboratory test that can accurately diagnose lupus. The diagnosis includes an accurate family history, evaluation of presenting symptoms, and the presence of laboratory abnormalities. The American College of Rheumatology has developed a set of 11 diagnostic criteria to aid in the diagnosis of lupus (**Table 1**). If at least 4 of the 11 criteria develop, a probable diagnosis of lupus may be made. However, the presence of fewer than four symptoms does not exclude the diagnosis, and these patients should be observed for development over time of other symptoms.

**Table 1. The Eleven Criteria Used for the Diagnosis of Lupus**

| Criterion | Definition |
|---|---|
| Malar rash | Rash over the cheeks, flat or raised, tending to spare the nasolabial folds |
| Discoid rash | Red raised patches |
| Photosensitivity | Reaction to sunlight, resulting in the development or increase in skin rash |
| Oral ulcers | Ulcers in the nose or mouth, usually painless |
| Arthritis | Nonerosive arthritis involving two or more peripheral joints (arthritis in which the bones around the joints do not become destroyed) characterized by tenderness or swelling |
| Serositis | Pleuritis or pericarditis (inflammation of the lining of the heart or lung) |
| Renal disorder | Excessive protein in the urine (greater than 0.5 gm/day or 3+ on test sticks) and/or cellular casts (abnormal elements in the urine, derived from red and/or white cells and/or kidney tubule cells) |
| Neurologic disorder | Seizures (convulsions) and/or psychosis in the absence of drugs or metabolic disturbances which are known to cause such effects |
| Hematologic disorder | Hemolytic anemia or leukopenia (white blood cell count below 4,000 per cubic millimeter) or lymphopenia (less than 1,500 lymphocytes per cubic millimeter) or thrombocytopenia (less than 100,000 platelets per cubic millimeter). The leukopenia and lymphopenia must be detected on two or more occasions. The thrombocytopenia must be detected in the absence of drugs known to induce it. |
| Immunologic disorder | Positive anti-double stranded DNA test, positive anti-Sm test, positive antiphospholipid antibody such as anticardiolipin or false-positive syphilis test (VDRL) |
| Antinuclear antibody | An abnormal titer for antinuclear antibodies in the absence of drugs known to induce it |

Adapted from "The 1982 Revised Criteria for the Classification of Systemic Lupus Erythematosus (SLE)," by E. M. Tan, A. S. Cohen, & J. F. Fries, et al., 1982, in *Arthritis and Rheumatism, 25,* pp. 1271–1277

## Symptoms

Early symptoms of lupus are generalized and vague and may be confused with a variety of other conditions that may not merit an immediate trip to the physician. Symptoms usually present themselves based on the body system or organ presented (**Table 2**) (NIH, NIAMS, 2001). The intensity and duration may vary and individual symptoms may often appear independent of one another.

## Management

Management of lupus is individualized and based on the specific needs and systems involved. Because the disease is highly variable, treatment differs significantly among individuals. For the majority of people, prompt, effective treatment can minimize symptoms and reduce inflammation (LFA, 2001c). The goal of an effective treatment plan is to reduce the inflammation and, in more complicated cases, suppress the immune system abnormalities that produce the inflammation. Treatment plans are often complex and need to be completely explained to encourage compliance and reduce the chance of dangerous side effects. Medications used in the treatment of lupus may include the following:

- *Nonsteroidal anti-inflammatory drugs (NSAIDs):* Used to treat the pain and inflammation associated with the musculoskeletal involvement of lupus.

**Table 2. Symptoms of Lupus**

| General manifestations | Fatigue, fever, weight loss, lymphadenopathy, psychological and emotional changes |
|---|---|
| Dermatologic | Facial butterfly rash, photosensitivity, discoid lupus lesions, hypopigmentation/hyperpigmentation, alopecia, pruritus, bruising, mouth ulcers |
| Musculoskeletal | Arthralgias, arthritis, soft-tissue inflammation |
| Hematologic | Anemia, decreased white blood cell count, thrombocytopenia, circulating lupus anticoagulants, false-positive VDRL, elevated sedimentation rate, low serum complement levels |
| Cardiopulmonary | Pleuritis, pericarditis, myocarditis, vasculitis, valvular heart disease, pulmonary fibrosis |
| Renal | Cellular casts, proteinuria, high blood pressure, fluid and electrolyte imbalance, urinary tract infections, focal, diffuse, and membranous renal involvement |
| Central nervous system | Changes in mentation, headaches, seizures, cerebritis, cranial neuropathies, stroke |
| Gastrointestinal | Anorexia, intestinal or mesenteric vasculitis, ascites, pancreatitis |
| Ophthalmologic | Conjunctivitis, dry eyes, cytoid bodies, glaucoma, cataracts |

Adapted from *Lupus: A Patient Care Guide for Nurses and Other Health Professionals* (pp. 28–32), by J. Freeman, A. B. Rodgers (Eds.), 2001, Bethesda, MD: National Institutes of Health.

Usually the drug of choice in mild cases without serious organ involvement.

- *Corticosteroids:* Highly effective in reducing inflammation not controlled by NSAIDs and for suppressing the immune system. In higher doses, they are effective in controlling major organ involvement, especially with central nervous system and renal involvement. People with lupus must be monitored carefully during administration because side effects of the medication and abrupt discontinuation of treatment can lead to complications.
- *Antimalarials:* Used to treat the joint pain, skin rashes, and fatigue associated with lupus. They are especially effective in the treatment of discoid lupus erythematosus.

- *Immunosuppressives:* Agents normally used to reduce rejection of transplanted organs and in the treatment of certain cancers have been used in lupus to suppress inflammation that is not effectively managed by other medications. They may reduce the need for high doses of corticosteroids.

In addition to use of medications, a multidisciplinary treatment approach that includes rest, joint protection, energy conservation, avoidance of known disease aggravators, good nutrition, and good communication with healthcare professionals is important in maintaining health and preventing disease flares.

# Individualized Healthcare Plan

## Assessment

*History*
- When was the diagnosis made
- What were the presenting criteria
- What is the family history of autoimmune disorders
- What systems are involved
- What are the laboratory markers
- At what age were steroids introduced

*Current Status and Management*
- Disease process: remission or exacerbation
- Specialists involved in the care of the student
- Present steroid dose and taper schedule
- Degree of immunosuppression: relating to steroids or thrombocytopenia
- Current chemotherapy course: hospital versus outpatient
- Nutritional support: dietary restrictions and requirements
- Level of fatigue
- Active arthritis in any joints
- Most recent sedimentation rates, compliment levels
- Fluid restriction based on the renal involvement
- Risk of bleeding related to thrombocytopenia

*Self-care*
- Awareness of activity tolerance related to fatigue
- Ability to follow dietary regimen within the school setting
- Ability to identify signs, symptoms of an impending flare
- Ability to participate in gym activities relating to arthritis, thrombocytopenia, fatigue

*Psychosocial Status*
- Signs of isolation related to altered body image
- Participation in peer activities versus isolation due to altered body image
- Participation in disease-related support groups
- Involvement with school guidance personnel
- Identification of altered mental status possibly relating to disease, medication, or depression

*Academic Issues*
- School and classroom accommodations needed: altered school schedule, alternative gym activities, access to elevator, peer support within classroom
- Current academic achievement
- Implementation of 504 service agreement
- Emergency evacuation plan

## Nursing Diagnoses (N.D.) (NANDA, 2003)

**N.D. 1** Fatigue (NANDA 00093) related to:
- depressed body defenses (disease or chemotherapy driven)
- depression
- poor nutritional intake
- proximal muscle weakness due to prolonged steroid use
- disease process (fever, inflammation, depressed blood counts)

**N.D. 2** Chronic pain (NANDA 00133) related to:
- arthralgias/arthritis
- oral mucosal ulcers
- steroid-induced muscle weakness
- systemic inflammation

**N.D.3** Impaired skin integrity (NANDA 00046) related to:
- photosensitivity
- alopecia
- skin rash
- oral ulcers
- increased bruising
- medications
- altered nutritional state

**N.D. 4** Ineffective protection (NANDA 00043) related to:
- abnormal blood profiles
- inadequate nutrition
- drug therapies, corticosteroid, chemotherapeutic
- disease process

**N.D. 5** Ineffective tissue perfusion, renal, (NANDA 00024) related to:
- elevated blood urea nitrogen/creatinine, positive serologic markers such as anti-DNA, low serum complement levels
- proteinuria

**N.D.6** Risk for infection (NANDA 00004) related to:
- immunosuppression: disease process, immunosuppressants
- chronic disease state
- skin rash, oral ulcers

**N.D.7** Imbalanced nutrition, less than body requirements, (NANDA 00002) related to:
- side effects of chemotherapy (nausea, vomiting, fever, dehydration, anorexia)
- oral ulcers, bleeding gums, dry mouth

**N.D.8** Disturbed body image (NANDA 00118) related to:
- side effects of steroid use (cushingoid syndrome, increased facial hair, muscle atrophy,
- skin rash, photosensitivity
- decreased physical activity
- fatigue
- side effects of chemotherapy (alopecia)

**N.D. 9** Impaired social interaction (NANDA 00052) related to:
- medication side effects (self-concept disturbance)
- prolonged absence
- photosensitivity
- isolation from peers because of immunosuppression

**N.D. 10** Deficient knowledge of disease, medications, (NANDA 00126) due to:
- fear of disease process
- unfamiliarity of resources

## Goals

The student will be able to perform activities without excessive fatigue or pain. (N.D.1, 2)

The student will participate in an energy-conservation plan for completing school activities. (N.D. 1, 2, 8, 10)

The student will participate in an exercise program developed in conjunction with school personnel to protect joints, maintain range of motion, and reduce pain and stiffness. (N.D. 1, 2, 10)

The student will follow an emergency evacuation plan as developed by school personnel. (N.D. 1, 2)

The student will be protected against impaired skin integrity. (N.D. 2, 3, 6, 7)

The student and family will be notified of increased incidence of communicable diseases such as flu and strep infection by (according to school district procedure). (N.D. 3, 4, 6, 7)

The student will maintain adequate and proper dietary intake. (N.D. 2-4, 6, 7)

The student will understand and participate in food management plan as developed by school. (N.D. 3, 6, 7, 10)

The student will be protected against injury while on school property. (N.D. 1, 2, 4, 6)

The student will have a decrease in pain related to joint inflammation. (N.D. 2)

The student will have an increased understanding of lupus and treatment regimens. (N.D. 9, 10)

The student will successfully follow the prescribed treatment plan. (N.D. 8-10)

The student will develop a support network within the school setting. (N.D. 9, 10)

The student will maintain adequate renal status while in the school setting. (N.D. 5, 7, 9)

## Nursing Interventions

Collaborate with the student, parents, and other school staff to develop a 504 plan. (N.D. 1-3, 6)

Meet with guidance counselor, teacher to arrange class schedule that will provide adequate rest periods in the day. (N.D. 1, 2)

Provide a hall pass to enable the student to leave classes 5 minutes early, allowing adequate time to change classes and to prevent injury due to crowded hallways. (N.D. 1, 2)

Provide student with an elevator pass allowing access to school elevator if available. (N.D. 1, 2)

Request that teachers assign student a "travel buddy," who will carry books, ride the elevator, and accompany student in hallways. (N.D. 1, 2, 4)

Meet with physical education instructor(s) and principal to suggest adaptations in gym curriculum, providing alternative activities when contact or high-endurance units are being taught. (N.D. 1, 2)

Collaborate with school physical and occupational therapists for in-school therapy to maintain muscle tone, improve activities of daily living, and instruct staff and student on energy-conservation and joint-protection techniques. (N.D. 1, 2, 10)

Allow student to rest in the health room (during study hall, nonacademic classes, etc). (N.D. 1, 2)

Facilitate application of sunscreen SPF 15 or higher to sun-exposed areas when in direct sunlight or near fluorescent or halogen lighting. (N.D. 3)

Inform principal and scheduling counselors that classrooms with fluorescent and halogen lighting should be avoided when possible. (N.D. 3)

Encourage student to wear long-sleeved shirts and wide-brimmed hats when out in the sun (N.D. 3, 8)

Assist student in menu selection, avoiding spicy or acidic foods and allowing choices that are low-odor, soft, and nutritionally adequate. (N.D. 3, 7, 8)

Provide student with warm saline oral rinses as needed for mouth ulcers. (N.D. 3)

Collaborate with cafeteria staff and teacher to allow student to eat frequent, nutritious snacks during day. (N.D. 3, 7, 8)

Assist and instruct student in keeping a food diary with fluid, food intake. (N.D. 5, 7)

Arrange for student to keep a water bottle at desk during day. (N.D. 3, 5, 7)

Meet with gym teachers to stress the importance of avoiding contact activities in gym class. (N.D. 2-4)

Give student and family an application for medical alert bracelet and have her wear at all times. (N.D. 4, 6, 10)

Instruct staff to identify and observe for signs of internal/external bleeding: (N.D. 2-4, 6)
- Pain, swelling at pain site
- Abdominal rigidity
- Signs of shock
- Gum, nasal bleeding
- Petechiae of skin
- Increased bruising

Provide student with soft bristled toothbrush to be used at school and instruct on the avoidance of razors. (N.D. 4, 6)

Notify the student and family when there is an increased incidence of strep and/or flu by _____(school district procedure). (N.D. 4, 6)

Notify the family of any fevers or injuries. (N.D. 3, 4, 6)

Reinforce/teach student to recognize the signs and symptoms of infection. (N.D. 6, 10)

Teach hand-washing technique. (N.D. 6, 10)

Monitor school environment for communicable/infectious diseases. (N.D. 6)

Provide ongoing nursing assessment as indicated by signs and symptoms:
- Monitor for any facial or extremity edema. (N.D. 5)
- Monitor blood pressure and record. (N.D. 5)
- Weigh patient daily and log weight gain if requested to do so by healthcare provider. (N.D. 5, 7)
- Assess breath sounds if student complains of breathing problems. (N.D. 5)

Meet with dietary department to provide a low-salt diet. (N.D. 5, 7)

Include student in educating fellow students as to side effects of steroids and chemotherapy, including cushingoid features, alopecia, muscle atrophy, increased facial hair, special dietary needs, and altered activities. (N.D. 8-10)

Instruct student in medication actions, potential side effects, dangers of abrupt discontinuation, and benefits (N.D. 8-10)

Provide student and family with referrals to area support groups, especially teen-directed ones. (N.D. 8-10)

Provide disease and medication educational materials to staff and student. (N.D. 8-10)

Refer to school guidance counselor. (N.D. 8-10)

Explain to student, staff, and fellow students physiological reasons for fatigue—systemic inflammation, muscle weakness, disease activity, and chemotherapy. (N.D. 8-10)

Request to the principal that the school guidance counselor meet with student on a regularly scheduled basis. (N.D. 8, 9)

Stress to student that weight and appearance changes related to steroid and chemotherapy use are temporary and will resolve over time. (N.D. 8-0)

## Expected Student Outcomes

The student will:

- Use at least two rest periods in her schedule throughout the day to minimize fatigue and conserve energy. (N.D. 1, 7)
- Identify three main causative factors of fatigue. (N.D. 1, 10)
- Choose appropriate activities, diet, and rest schedule during school day. (N.D. 1, 2, 9)
- Successfully perform all scheduled activities throughout the day without experiencing fatigue and/or increase in pain. (N.D. 1, 2)
- Demonstrate proper joint-protection techniques while in school setting. (N.D. 2)
- Make proper choices in regard to activities that are nonstressful to joints during gym class. (N.D. 1, 2)
- Identify at least three activities that can be performed during joint flare. (N.D. 1, 2, 10)
- Participate with staff in developing and following section 504 service agreement and emergency evacuation plan as determined on _____. (N.D. 1, 2)
- Apply sunscreen and wear sun-barrier clothing during the school day when leaving the building. (N.D. 3, 8)
- Be able to identify halogen and fluorescent lighting in school building and apply appropriate protection. (N.D. 3, 10)
- Identify lupus rashes and report them to school health personnel. (N.D. 3, 10)
- Navigate through building without injury by being dismissed 5 minutes earlier and using elevator if needed. (N.D. 1, 2, 4)
- Identify signs of low platelet count. (N.D. 4, 10)
- Maintain dietary diary, recording fluid, sodium intakes for the day. (N.D. 4, 5, 7, 10)
- Maintain a nutritionally sound diet developed by family and school personnel. (N.D. 7, 10)
- Maintain good hydration. (N.D. 7, 10)
- Take extra precautions when notified there is an increased incidence of flu and/or strep throat in the school environment. (N.D. 4, 6)
- Successfully identify and report signs of infection other than fever. (N.D. 4, 6, 10)
- Practice good hygiene. (N.D. 6, 10)
- Wear medical alert bracelet at all times. (N.D. 4, 6, 10)
- Identify symptoms relating to specific body systems that are involved with lupus. (N.D. 10)
- Communicate with her teachers, friends about lupus and her symptoms. (N.D. 8-10)
- Maintain peer contacts and participate in at least one extracurricular activity while at school. (N.D. 8, 9)
- Be able to recite medication schedule, correct doses, potential side effects, and importance of compliance (N.D. 9, 10)
- Be able to list at least two outside resources available to provide information and support. (N.D. 9, 10)
- Meet with guidance counselor (as scheduled). (N.D. 8, 9)

# Case Study

Margie is a 15-year-old student in the 9th grade. She was diagnosed with systemic lupus erythematosus at the age of 13, approximately 8 months after beginning menstruation. She presented to her physician with a 3-week history of persistent fever, profound fatigue, fine malar rash over her face and neck, persistent mouth ulcers, pain and stiffness, and mild swelling of her elbows, knees, and hands.

At the time of her visit to the pediatrician, Margie had a temperature of 100.4°F and a fine malar rash over her cheeks, neck, and arms. She had inflammation of her wrists and metacarpal phalangeal joints bilaterally and warm, swollen knees. There were oral ulcers on the mucous membranes of her mouth, palpable cervical nodes in her neck, and bruising on her arms and legs.

Laboratory values were positive for an elevated sedimentation rate, mild anemia, decreased white blood cell count and platelet count, positive antinuclear antibody, positive anti-DNA antibody, and decreased serum C3 and C4 complement levels. Her urinalysis was positive for +4 proteinuria and + cellular casts.

Based on her history, physical, and laboratory findings, a diagnosis was made of systemic lupus erythematosus, with probable involvement of the skin, joints, blood, and kidneys. A kidney biopsy at a later date showed diffuse inflammation of the kidneys, and Margie was started on a regimen of high-dose steroids, a nonsteroidal anti-inflammatory drug, and intravenous Cytoxan at monthly intervals.

When she returned to school, a 504 service agreement was initiated, focusing on the following issues:

1. Mobility. Because of the inflammatory joint pain, profound fatigue, and the proximal muscle weakness resulting from the high-dose steroid use, Margie will need extra time to negotiate between classes, a buddy to assist her with her back pack, and use of the school elevator. An emergency evacuation plan was also developed.

2. Skin involvement. Because of her persistent malar rash and history of feeling sick after sun exposure, it was presumed that Margie was photosensitive. She is to use a sunscreen with 15 SPF when going outside during the school day and light coverings and hats during direct sun hours. She is to sit away from the windows in class. Because of mouth ulcers, she is to avoid hot, spicy foods and will be offered alternative meals on days when tacos, etc., are served.

3. Fatigue. Because of fatigue associated with the disease process, the effects of chemotherapy, the altered sleep patterns from the high-dose steroids, and the joint pain, Margie will be allowed to rest in the health office during study halls, after lunch, and as needed.

4. Susceptibility to infection. Because of depressed white blood cell count relating to the disease process and chemotherapy effects, we are to notify her mom if there is an increased incidence of cases of strep or flu resulting in greater than 5% of the school population to be out sick.

**Lupus**

| Assessment Data | Nursing Diagnosis | Goals | Nursing Interventions | Expected Outcomes |
|---|---|---|---|---|
| Profound fatigue associated with disease activity, poor nutritional intake, and side effects of chemotherapy. | Fatigue related to: disease activity, depressed body defenses, proximal muscle weakness, poor nutritional intake, depression. | The student will participate in an energy-conservation plan for completing school activities. | Collaborate with the student parents, and other school staff to develop a 504 plan. Allow Margie to rest in the health room during her study hall, nonacademic classes. Meet with guidance counselcr, teacher to arrange class schedule that will provide Margie wth adequate rest periods in the daytime. Provide a hall pass to enable Margie to leave classes 5 minutes early, allowing adequate time to change classes. Provide Margie with an elevator pass, allowing access to the school elevator if needed. Prepare an emergency evacuation plan to be instituted for evacuation. | Margie will use at least 2 rest periods in her schedule throughout the day to minimize fatigue and preserve energy. Margie will identify 3 main factors that cause fatigue. |
| Joint pain, stiffness, and swelling of her wrists, hands, and knees related to arthritis associated with lupus. | Chronic pain related to joint inflammation. | Margie will participate in an exercise program developed in conjunction with school personnel to protect joints, maintain range of motion, and reduce pain and stiffness. Margie will be able to perform activities without excessive fatigue or pain. | Meet with physical education instructor(s) and principal to suggest adaptations in gym curriculum, providing alternative activities when contact or high-endurance units are being taught. | Margie will be able to successfully perform all scheduled activities without experiencing pain or fatigue. Margie will make proper choices in regard to activities that are nonstressful to joints during gym class. |

**Systemic Lupus Erythematosus**

| Assessment Data | Nursing Diagnosis | Goals | Nursing Interventions | Expected Outcomes |
|---|---|---|---|---|
| | | | Collaborate with school physical and occupational therapists for in-school therapy to maintain muscle tone, improve activities of daily living, and instruct staff and student on energy conservation and joint protection.<br><br>Instruct staff to identify and observe for signs of internal/external bleeding:<br>• pain, swelling at pain site<br>• abdominal rigidity<br>• signs of shock<br>• gum, nasal bleeding<br>• petechiae of skin<br>• increased bruising | Margie will be able to identify at least 3 activities that can be performed during periods of joint flare.<br><br>Margie will be able to demonstrate proper joint protection techniques while in the school setting. |
| Photosensitive skin rash of the face and sun-exposed areas, mouth ulcers, and impairment of wound healing. | Impaired skin integrity related to skin manifestations of lupus and side effects of medications. | Margie will be protected against impaired skin integrity. | Facilitate student applying sunscreen with SPF 15 or higher to sun-exposed areas when in direct sunlight or near fluorescent or halogen lighting. Inform principal and scheduling counselors that classrooms with fluorescent and halogen lighting should be avoided when possible.<br><br>Encourage student to wear long-sleeved shirts and wide-brimmed hats when out in the sun. | Margie will not leave the building without application of sunscreen and sun-barrier clothing during the school day. She applies sunscreen daily in health office.<br><br>She reduces time in classrooms with high degree of florescent and/or halogen lighting.<br><br>Margie identifies signs of potentially low platelet counts, potentially infected wounds, and new rashes. |

| Assessment Data | Nursing Diagnosis | Goals | Nursing Interventions | Expected Outcomes |
|---|---|---|---|---|
| Has low white blood cell count from disease and immunosuppressive therapy. | Risk for infection related to disease process and use of immunosuppressive therapy. | Margie will practice good hygiene (hand washing) before eating and after toileting. | Reinforce student's ability to recognize the signs and symptoms of infection. | Margie will identify halogen and fluorescent lighting in school building and apply appropriate protection. |
| Steroids can mask signs of infection. | | Margie will recognize signs and symptoms of infection. | Reinforce hand-washing technique. | Margie will identify lupus rashes and report them to school health personnel |
| Skin integrity is compromised. | | | Monitor school environment for communicable/infectious diseases. | Margie will wash hands after toileting and before meals. |
| | | | Margie's family will be notified immediately if she has a fever. | Margie will be aware of any increased incidence of communicable disease activity, such as flu or strep, in the school. |
| | | | Margie and her family will be notified if there is increased incidence of communicable diseases such as flu and strep or if the absenteeism rate is greater than 5% of the student population. | Margie will successfully identify and report signs of infection other than fever. |
| | | | | Margie will identify and report any symptoms related to possible infection, either systemic or localized. |
| Mouth ulcers painful, especially with spicy foods. | Imbalanced nutrition: less than body requirements related to disease process and medication therapy. | Margie will maintain adequate and proper dietary intake. | Facilitate collaboration with cafeteria staff and teachers to allow Margie to eat frequent, nutritional snacks during day, following the guidelines of a low-salt diet. | Margie will maintain a nutritionally sound diet developed by family and school personnel, maintaining a stable weight. |
| Cytoxan causes extreme nausea. | | Margie will understand and participate in food management plan as developed by the school. | Margie will be allowed to keep a water bottle at her desk during the day. | Margie will maintain hydration. |
| Experiencing anorexia related to physical symptoms (bleeding gums, dry mouth, oral ulcers) and medication (steroids, Cytoxan). | | | Margie will be instructed and assisted in keeping a food diary with fluid and food intake | Margie will maintain a dietary diary during the school day. |

| Assessment Data | Nursing Diagnosis | Goals | Nursing Interventions | Expected Outcomes |
|---|---|---|---|---|
| Does not understand severity of disease and need for aggressive treatment.

Unable to explain disease to fellow students. | Deficit in knowledge related to lack of understanding of disease process and treatment. | Margie will have an increased understanding of lupus and treatment regimens.

Margie will establish a support network within the school setting. | Instruct Margie in medication actions, potential side effects, and danger of abrupt discontinuation and benefits.

Provide Margie with disease and medication educational materials, as well as staff.

Include Margie in educating fellow students as to the side effects of medications, special dietary needs, and altered activities.

Provide an opportunity for Margie to meet with the school guidance counselor on a regularly scheduled basis. | Margie will be able to identify symptoms relating to specific body systems that are involved with lupus.

Margie will be able to correctly recite medication schecule, doses, potential side effects, and importance of compliance.

Margie will communicate with her teachers and friends about lupus and her symptoms.

Margie will be aware of at least 2 outside sources available to provide information and support. |

# Emergency Evacuation Plan
# Lupus

**Student:** Margie Brooks
**Disability:** Systemic lupus erythematosus
**Medical Diagnosis:**

**Building:** North Middle School
**Grade:** 9
**Teacher:**

**Affected personnel:** Teachers, Administrators, Counselors, School Nurses, Parents, Student

**Background:** Margie is a 15-year old student in 9th grade at North Middle School who was diagnosed with systemic lupus erythematosus at the age of 13. She currently has chronic joint pain and inflammation, skin rashes associated with exposure to the sun and disease flaring, inflammation involving her kidneys, and depressed blood cell counts relating to the use of chemotherapy and disease process. Her activity level is directly dependent on the degree of joint inflammation and fatigue on any given day. Therefore, an emergency evacuation plan needs to be in place should she need assistance.

## Evacuation plan:
- Margie's schedule is to be posted in the elevator and in the health office.
- If evacuation is occurring when Margie is on the first floor, she will be met at her class by the school nurse or designated personnel and will be escorted out of the building via wheelchair.
- If evacuation is occurring when Margie is on the second or third floor and elevator is not be used, she will be escorted down the stairwell closest to her class by her teacher and met at the bottom of the stairwell on the first floor by the school nurse or designated personnel and escorted out via wheelchair.
- Margie will have a container of sunscreen with her at all times and will take it with her during evacuation. There will be a backup container in the school's emergency box, along with an umbrella, in case the evacuation warrants a lengthy period of time outside. Margie will be moved to a shaded area. The school nurse will carry a backup container.

## Signatures:

Student: _____ Date _____

Parent Nurse: _____ Date _____

Counselor: _____ Date _____

Principal Homeroom teacher: _____ Date _____

# Section 504 Service Agreement

**Student name:** Margie Brooks      **Birth date:** 8/26/89

**School:** North Middle School      **Grade:** 9

**Parent(s) name**_____      **Phone Number:**_____

**Initial agreement date:** 8/24/03      **Review date:**_____

**Modified date:**_____      **Service end date:**_____

1. **Describe the nature of the disability:** Margie is a 15-year-old student in the 9th grade with systemic lupus erythematosus. Margie is having difficulty caring for herself because her disease affects a variety of systems, is constantly changing, and requires close monitoring.

2. **Describe the basis for determining the disability:** Margie was diagnosed with systemic lupus erythematosus in 2001 at Children's Hospital. A copy of the diagnosis and plan of treatment is on file in the school health office.

3. **Describe how the disability limits access to school program(s), learning, or extracurricular activities:** Margie's chief complaint is profound fatigue related to both disease activity and treatment. Systems involved include the musculoskeletal system, which presents with joint pain and stiffness; the skin, which presents with photosensitivity, oral ulcers, and alopecia; and the renal system, which has the potential for fluid retention. Margie may have difficulty following the daily schedule and activities. Her rest, activity, and meal times must be monitored and adjusted, if needed.

4. **In response to a request for services under Chapter 15 and after consideration of evaluations (supporting document attached), the team recommends these reasonable accommodations:**
- Margie's schedule will be adapted to provide at least one study hall in the morning and one nonacademic classroom in the afternoon.
- Margie will be allowed to leave class 5 minutes early in order to avoid injury in the crowded hallway.
- Margie will use elevator to access different floors. She will be accompanied by another student. Her schedule will be posted in the elevator.
- An emergency evacuation plan (see attached) will be followed.
- Margie will have a student buddy assigned to her to assist with book carrying and to ride the elevator with her.
- Alternative nonstressful full gym activities will be provided when gym curriculum involves high-endurance or joint-stressing activities.
- Physical and occupational therapy will be consulted to instruct Margie and staff on energy-conservation, joint-protection, and isometric and isotonic exercises.
- Margie or the school nurse will apply sunscreen for any outside activities or when in classrooms with high florescent or halogen lighting.
- Cafeteria will provide Margie and her family with a list of alternative foods that are low in protein and salt.
- Margie may keep water bottle with her at all times.
- Margie will be allowed to rest in the health room when she identifies periods of excessive fatigue.
- Parent will be notified if there is an increased incidence of flu or strep causing greater than 5% of the school population to be out, according to district procedure.

5. **The following procedures are to be followed in the event of a medical emergency (if applicable):** Parents are to be called if Margie experiences change in mental status, acute bleeding episode, fever or signs of infection, new onset of rash, changes in breath sounds, or persistent nausea and vomiting. In the event of an acute emergency as determined by the school nurse, and her parents cannot be notified, she will be transported via emergency medical services to Children's Hospital.

Name                                    Title

_____          _____

_____          _____

_____          _____


**Directions: Please check one of the options and sign this form.**

_____ I agree to my son's/daughter's identification as a protected handicapped student and give permission to proceed as recommended.

_____ I do not agree and do not give permission to proceed as recommended.

_____ I would like to exercise my right to an informal conference to discuss my concerns.


My reason for disapproval is _____


**Signatures:**

Parent: _____ Date _____

# References

Hochberg, M. C. (1997). Updating the American College of Rheumatology revised criteria for the classification of systemic lupus eythematosis. *Arthritis and Rheumatism, 40,* 1725.

Lupus Foundation of America, Inc. (2001a). *What is lupus?* (Brochure). Washington, DC: Author.

Lupus Foundation of America, Inc. (2001b). *Laboratory tests used in the diagnosis of lupus.* (Brochure). Washington, DC: Author. Retrieved April 24, 2004, from http://www.lupus.org/education/labtests.html

Lupus Foundation of America, Inc. (2001c). *Lupus fact sheet* (Brochure). Washington, DC: Author.

NANDA International. (2003). *Nursing diagnoses: Definitions & classification 2003–2004.* Philadelphia: Author.

National Institutes of Health, National Institute of Arthritis and Musculoskeletal and Skin Diseases (NIAMS). (2001). *Lupus: A patient care guide for nurses and other health professionals.* Bethesda, MD: Author. Retrieved April 29, 2004from http://www.niams.nih.gov/hi/topics/lupus/lupusguide/credits.htm

Sullivan, K. E. (1999). *The complex genetic basis of systemic lupus erythematosus.* Retrieved April 29, 2004, from http://www.lupus.org/education/articles/geneticbasis.html (Reprinted from *Lupus Foundation of America Lupus News, 19*(4), Fall 1999, and *20*(1), Winter 1999-2000.)

Tan, E. M., Cohen, A. S., Fries, J. F., Masi, A. T., McShane, D. J., Rothfield, N. F., et al. (1982). The 1982 revised criteria for the classification of systemic lupus erythematosus. *Arthritis and Rheumatism, 25,* 1271–1277.

# Bibliography

Aladjem, H. (1985). *Understanding lupus.* New York: Macmillan. This book was written by a woman with lupus who is the head of the National Lupus Foundation. It is a first-hand account of living with lupus.

Katz, R. S. (2001). *Immune suppressants and related drugs used for lupus* [Brochure]. Washington, DC: Lupus Foundation of America, Inc. Retrieved April 24, 2004, from http://www.lupus.org/education/brochures/immune.html

Klippel, J. H. (Ed). (1997). Systemic lupus erythematosus. In *Primer on rheumatic diseases* (11th ed., pp. 96–110). Atlanta, GA: Arthritis Foundation.

Lehman, T. J. (2001). *Childhood lupus* [Brochure]. Washington, DC: Lupus Foundation of America, Inc. Retrieved April 26, 2004, from http://www.lupus.org/education/brochures/child06.html

Millard, T. P., & Hawk, J. L. (2003, September 9). *Photosensitivity and lupus* [Brochure]. Washington, DC: Lupus Foundation of America, Inc. Retrieved April/May 26, 2004, from http://www.lupus.org/education/brochures/photosensitivity.html

Phillips, R. H. (2001). *Coping with lupus.* Garden City Park, NY: Avery.

Phillips, R. H. (Ed.). (2002, Fall). Lupus: Its impact on young people. *Lupus News 22*(3). Retrieved February 16, 2005, from http://www.lupus.org/education/articles/impact.html

Schur, P. H. (Ed.). (1996). *The clinical management of systemic lupus erythematosus* (2nd ed.). Philadelphia: Lippincott Williams & Wilkins.

# Resources

American College of Rheumatology
Association of Rheumatology Health Professionals
1800 Century Place
Suite 250
Atlanta, GA 30345
404-633-3777
www.rheumatology.org

Arthritis Foundation
1330 West Peachtree Street
Atlanta, GA 30309
1-800-283-7800
www.arthritis.org

Lupus Foundation of America, Inc.
2000 L Street, NW
Suite 710
Washington, DC 20036

800) 558-0121
www.lupus.org
(Many states have a state foundation)

National Institute of Arthritis and Musculoskeletal
and Skin Diseases (NIAMS)/National Institutes
of Health
1 AMS Circle
Bethesda, MD 20892-3675
318-495-44844
www.nih.gov/niams

SLE Foundation
149 Madison Avenue
Suite 205
New York, NY 10016
215-685-4118
www.lupusny.org

## Chapter Seventy-three

# Tourette Syndrome

Lorali Gray

## Introduction

Gilles de la Tourette syndrome, more commonly known as Tourette syndrome (TS), is a neurologic spectrum disorder characterized by multiple involuntary vocal and motor tics. It is the most severe of the tic disorders and is usually first observed in infancy or childhood but may also manifest itself in early adolescence. The average age at onset is 7 years, and some children have periods of remission (American Psychiatric Association, 2000). TS is always diagnosed before age 18, and symptoms are generally present for life; however, improvement may occur in late adolescence and in adulthood (American Academy of Child & Adolescent Psychiatry, 2001). As represented in **Table 1**, there can be multiple types of motor and vocal tics associated with TS.

Some children may exhibit motor tics that are self-injurious or that may be harmful to others. These may present as scratching, head slapping, or jerking of an extremity. Safer physical alternatives may need to be learned, such as hitting a soft object or a safer place on the body. For example, the student could clap or hit his or her thigh (Prestia, 2003).

## Pathophysiology

The etiology of TS is unknown; however, there is mounting evidence that it is a genetic disorder. Through the use of genetic studies, it has been found to be inherited as an autosomal dominant gene (National Alliance of the Mentally Ill, 2004). The severity of TS may be influenced by factors such as prenatal or perinatal hypoxic injuries (Wong, Hockenberry, Wilson, Winkelstein & Kline, 2003). TS occurs in four to five of every 10,000 people, and the ratio of male to female is 4:1 (American Psychiatric Association, 2000).

For those diagnosed with TS, there has been found to be associated genetic abnormalities that affect the metabolism of the brain neurotransmitters dopamine, serotonin, and norepinephrine, such as an overproduction of dopamine or an increased sensitivity to neurotransmitters that impact inhibited urges or tics (DeStefano & Bear, 2002). Family members, however, do not always exhibit the same symptoms. A parent with TS has a 50% chance of passing the gene on to his or her children. The gene may be expressed as a milder tic disorder, obsessive-compulsive disorder (OCD), or no tic disorder at all (Tourette Syndrome Association, Inc., 2004).

**Table 1. Types of Tics**

| Simple motor | Eye blinking, grimacing, neck jerking, shoulder jerking, tongue and mouth movements |
|---|---|
| Complex motor | Jumping, squatting, stamping the foot, thrusting out an arm, hitting or biting self, ritualistic movements (smelling an object, touching own or another's body, obsessive or compulsive patterns of behavior), grooming behaviors |
| Simple vocal | Throat clearing, sniffing, grunting, coughing, snorting, lip noises |
| Complex vocal | Echolalia (repeating last-heard sound, word, or phrase of another, palilalia (repeating own sounds or words), coprolalia (use of socially unacceptable sounds or words, often obscene), shouting words out of context |

Reprinted and adapted from *Wong's Nursing Care of Infants and Children* (7th ed.), by D. L. Wong, M. J. Hockenberry, D. Wilson, M. L. Winkelstein, and N. E. Kline, 2003, St. Louis, MO: Mosby with permission from Elsevier.

In addition, there is an emerging theory that identifies a possible relationship between TS and a strep infection. Current recommendations suggest an evaluation for infection if a child has a sudden onset of tics or OCD behaviors (Vleck, 1998).

Furthermore, comorbid conditions may exist, and often teens who are diagnosed with TS will have accompanying symptoms of depression, anxiety, obsessive-compulsive behaviors, mood disorders, distractibility, impulsiveness, and learning disorders (DeStefano & Bear, 2002). According to the Tourette Syndrome Association, Inc. (2004), the following are associated comorbid conditions:

*Obsessive-compulsive disorder.* This disorder involves behaviors that are repeated over and over. Children with both TS and OCD have a modestly elevated rate of anger control problems, coprolalia, and a moderately elevated rate of social skills problems. Of children with TS, 50% to 60% will also have OCD; 10% will have severe symptoms (Vleck, 1998).

*Attention deficit hyperactivity disorder (ADHD).* Children with both TS and ADHD have a higher rate of anger-control problems, social skills, school difficulties, and sleep disorders (Vleck, 1998). Approximately 50% of clients with TS meet the criteria for ADHD (National Alliance of the Mentally Ill, 2004).

*Learning disabilities.* These may include dyslexia, perceptual disorders, impaired sensory processing, and difficulty with math and writing. It is reported that 40% of individuals with TS will have accompanying learning difficulties (Lingui Systems, Inc., 1999).

*General behavior disturbances.* Concerns with behavior may result from poor school performance, poor self-esteem, and an inability to suppress tics. Additionally, short tempers, argumentativeness, conduct disorder, and depression contribute to behavior problems (Vleck, 1998). There also appear to be some exhibitionism and sexual acting-out associated with TS.

*Sleep disorders.* Sleep disorders appear to be fairly common among people with TS. Frequent awakenings and talking and walking in one's sleep occur (Tourette Syndrome Association, Inc., 2004).

A diagnosis of TS is made by clinical observations of symptoms and a thorough history taking about the tics and abnormal behavior from the family and individual. Evaluating the history of the onset of symptoms is also important. In addition, the child's neurologic and mental status is assessed through tests such as an electroencephalogram, computed tomographic scan, and blood work, all of which are used to rule out other conditions that may be confused with TS. (Alsaraf & Robertson, 2003). Many children with TS are misdiagnosed and are often thought to have a behavioral or psychological disorder (Tourette Syndrome Association, Inc., 2004). Furthermore, it may take years from the onset of the symptoms to the time of an accurate diagnosis. However, early diagnosis is critical to the child's normal growth and development, self-esteem, and mental and emotional well-being. **Table 2** shows the diagnostic criteria for TS.

**Table 2. Diagnostic Criteria for Tourette Syndrome**

| |
|---|
| A. Both multiple motor and one or more vocal tics have been present at some time during the illness, although not necessarily concurrently. (A tic is a sudden, rapid, recurrent, nonrhythmic, stereotyped motor movement or vocalization.) |
| B. The tics occur many times a day (usually in bouts) nearly every day or intermittently throughout a period of more than 1 year, and during this period there was never a tic-free period of more than 3 consecutive months. |
| C. The disturbance causes marked distress or significant impairment in social, occupational, or other important areas of functioning. |
| D. The onset is before 18 years of age. |
| E. The disturbance is not due to the direct physiologic effects of a substance (e.g., stimulants) or a general medical condition (e.g., Huntington's disease or postviral encephalitis). |

Reprinted with permission from the *Diagnostic and Statistical Manual of Mental Disorders,* Copyright 2000. American Psychiatric Association.

## Management

According to the Tourette Syndrome Association, Inc., (2004), the majority of people with TS are not severely impacted or disabled by their tics or associated behaviors. However, children and adolescents with TS can present with many complex characteristics that can significantly impact social, behavioral and academic interactions (Prestia, 2003). Therefore, therapeutic management can consist of multiple modalities involving support by both the family and school staff. School nurses are an important part of the management of TS for the school-aged child because monitoring and management of symptoms and efficacy of medication at school are critical to effective treatment. In addition, the fostering of positive self-esteem is needed by all involved, especially the child's parents (Wong et al., 2003).

Nonmedication treatment consists primarily of counseling, cognitive behavioral therapy, and psychotherapy. Relaxation techniques and support to the family and child through education regarding the condition and expectations are also important. Children whose symptoms are severe and not relieved by supportive methods, as well as those whose symptoms are disabling or interfere with their ability to function, may benefit from medication. Medications are usually used as a last resort and are chosen on the basis of the child's symptoms and the potential side effects. Target symptoms are identified in an effort to prescribe appropriate medication. As seen in **Table 3**, many therapeutic agents are available for the treatment of TS.

**Table 3. Medications Used in the Treatment of Tourette Syndrome**

| Drug Classification | Generic Name | Brand Name | Therapeutic Effects | Side Effects |
|---|---|---|---|---|
| "Typical" neuroleptic<br><br>Antipsychotic | Haloperidol | Haldol<br><br>Mainstay treatment since the 1960s | Tic suppression | Fatigue, weight gain, muscle rigidity, cognitive blunting, personality change, tardive dyskinesia, photosensitivity, depression |
| "Typical" neuroleptic | Pimozide | Orap<br><br>Approved in 1984 for TS | Tic suppression | Same as haloperidol, electrocardiographic changes (prolongation of Q-T interval) |
| Antihypertensive<br><br>Alpha-adrenergic agonist | Clonidine | Catapres<br><br>Has been used since 1979 with some benefits | Broad spectrum of TS symptoms and tics | Fatigue, dry mouth, sedation, irritability, dizziness, headache, insomnia, skin rash |
| Anticonvulsant<br><br>High-potency benzodiazepine | Clonazepam | Klonopin | Decrease in emotional excitement | Fatigue, irritability, dizziness, disinhibition, sedation. Risk of habituation with prolonged use. |
| Antipsychotic neuroleptic | Fluphenazine | Prolixin | | Orthostatic hypotension, mild photosensitivity, dry mouth, constipation, urine retention, tardive dyskinesia |
| Antipsychotic neuroleptic | Thiothixene | Navane | Tic supression<br><br>Anger suppression | Dry mouth, nausea, vomiting, orthostatic hypotension, respiratory depression, seizures, neuroleptic malignant syndrome |
| "Atypical" neuroleptic<br><br>Antipsychotic | Risperidone | Risperdal<br><br>Introduced in 1994 | Emotional instability | Nausea, dystonia, insomnia, headache, tardive dyskinesia, agitation, and weight gain |

Adapted with permission from *Clinical Guidelines for School Nurses* (5th ed., revised), 2002, Nashville, TN: School Health Alert; and *Medications Primarily for Treatment of Tics*, 2004, Denver, CO: Tourette Syndrome Association, Inc., Rocky Mountain Region Chapter.

# Individualized Healthcare Plan

## Assessment
### History
- Child's medical and developmental history
- Known allergies
- Medication history
- Family history of mental health disorders
- Age at onset of symptoms or observation of tics
- Motor or vocal tics observed
- Duration of multiple motor and vocal tics
- Does the condition cause distress or impairment in social and academic functioning?
- Are there any other significant medical conditions or comorbidities?
- What medical interventions or treatments have been instituted?
- What other treatment modalities are being used?
- Does treatment include medication?
- Review of medical and educational assessments

### Current Status and Management
- Child's relationship with healthcare providers and mental health specialists
- What is the current management and treatment plan?
- Are there any medications being taken? Are side effects being experienced?
- Is there impairment of social or academic functioning?
- Is the child able to participate in activities of daily living?
- What is the child's current level of cognitive and social/emotional functioning?

### Self-care
- Child and family's knowledge/understanding of TS and its impact on self-care and school activities
- Knowledge of possible stressors
- Self-management and/or participation in treatment regimen
- Ability to self-administer medication
- Knowledge of side effects of medication and who to report to
- Ability and motivation to participate fully in personal care
- Ability to self-regulate activity when fatigued
- Current coping strategies: child and family

### Psychosocial Status
- How is the child responding to his/her diagnosis?
- Social stigma
- Feelings of peer rejection
- Embarrassment and shame
- Self-consciousness
- Social isolation
- Possible strained family relationships
- Anxiety and/or depression
- Peer acceptance and friendships

### Academic Issues
- Child's academic history
- Inability to complete work
- Lack of organizational skills
- Handwriting difficulty leading to poor quality of written work
- Inattentiveness and difficulty maintaining attention
- Possible side effects of medication
- Difficulty in testing
- Associated learning disabilities
- Fatigue
- Compulsive behaviors

- Short temper; argumentative
- Behavioral and discipline issues
- Poor self-esteem
- Possible associated comorbid conditions i.e. ADHD, OCD, and depression
- Disruptive vocal and motor tics
- Impulsivity
- Sensory processing difficulties
- School staff need to be aware of educational implications
- Current assessment of academic needs to determine if a 504 accommodation plan or an individualized education plan (IEP) is needed.

## Nursing Diagnoses (N.D.) (NANDA, 2003)

**N.D. 1** Deficient knowledge (NANDA 00126) related to:
- recent diagnosis of TS
- developmental understanding of TS and his/her management and treatment plan

**N.D. 2** Anxiety (NANDA 00146) related to:
- uncertainty of condition
- fear of tics occurring in school and during social interactions
- possible comorbid conditions

**N.D. 3** Risk for powerlessness (NANDA 00152) related to:
- inability to control symptoms
- dependence on family and school staff in managing treatment modalities

**N.D. 4** Chronic low self-esteem (NANDA 00119) related to:
- academic difficulties
- perceived isolation from peers
- embarrassment and shame
- chronic social and behavioral problems
- presence of chronic tics

**N.D. 5** Fatigue (NANDA 00093) related to:
- attempts to suppress tics and impulsive behaviors
- repetitive large muscle tics
- depression
- side effects of medication
- chronic stress
- difficulty sustaining handwriting
- associated sleep disorders

**N.D. 6** Ineffective coping (NANDA 00069) related to:
- stress regarding possible social and academic failure
- lack of coping strategies
- developmental level/skills
- inability to identify and express feelings
- stressors that exacerbate symptoms

**N.D. 7** Compromised family coping (NANDA 00074) related to:
- family adjustments to TS diagnosis
- strained family relationships
- fear
- challenges of the management and treatment program
- parental feelings of guilt
- difficulty understanding that behaviors and vocal tics are involuntary

**N.D. 8** Impaired social interaction (NANDA 00052) related to:
- behavior patterns
- social stigma associated with motor and vocal tics
- possible comorbid conditions
- anxiety
- presence of tics
- ridicule and rejection by peers

**N.D. 9** Ineffective health maintenance (NANDA 00099) related to:
- poor self-esteem
- frustration and anger
- depression or anxiety
- fatigue
- lack of knowledge of TS and its implications
- inability to provide self-care due to interference of tics

**N.D. 10** Risk for injury (NANDA 00035) related to:
- severe complex tic release
- impaired sensory processing
- impaired motor planning
- impaired visual perception
- presence of self-injurious tics

## Goals

The student will increase his/her understanding of TS and its management. (N.D.1)

The student will share information regarding TS with school staff to increase understanding of his/her behaviors. (N.D. 1)

The student will assist in the development of an individualized healthcare plan (IHP). (N.D. 1, 4, 6)

The student will maintain positive socialization with peers. (N.D. 4, 8)

The student will maintain an adjusted schedule to accommodate fatigue. (N.D. 5)

The student will work with the school physical education teacher to meet his/her physical needs. (N.D. 5)

The student will participate in self-care activities at home and school. (N.D. 9)

The student will verbalize his/her feelings to identified school staff in appropriate ways. (N.D. 6)

The student will maintain a positive self-image. (N.D. 4)

The student will identify signs and symptoms of concern (tics, anxiety, etc.). (N.D.1, 6)

The student will identify and reduce stressors that exacerbate symptoms. (N.D. 1, 6)

The student will develop acceptance of his/her disorder. (N.D. 6)

The student will communicate his/her fears. (N.D. 2, 6)

The student will remain involved in school activities as tolerated. (N.D. 7, 8)

The student will increase his/her ability to cope with symptoms and associated stressors. (N.D. 6)

The student will identify signs of anxiety and depression. (N.D. 2, 6)

The student will maintain healthy sleep patterns. (N.D. 5)

The student will prevent injury. (N.D. 10)

The student will become more independent in the management of his/her treatment plan. (N.D. 3)

The student will, along with his/her family, become knowledgeable about local community TS resources. (N.D. 6, 7)

The student will work with his/her family to become knowledgeable about strategies to increase family coping skills. (N.D. 6, 7)

## Nursing Interventions

Assist the student in learning about TS, his/her individual treatment regimen, and the implications for school social and academic interactions. (N.D 1)

Provide education to teachers, school staff, and student's peers about TS. (N.D. 1)

Develop and implement a school IHP. (N.D. 1)

Praise positive behaviors, encourage independence, promote self-esteem and self-confidence. (N.D. 3, 4)

Promote understanding of those with TS by educating the student's peers as well as school staff. (N.D. 1, 4)

Promote acceptance of those with differences. (N.D. 4, 8)

Educate staff and other classmates if appropriate regarding student's inability to control actions. (N.D. 1, 8)

Facilitate as needed a family referral to local social services, support groups, and community resources for individuals and families with TS. (N.D. 7)

Encourage the family to enlist support services at school for the student. Facilitate any needed academic assessments and secondary accommodations through a 504 plan or IEP. (N.D. 7)

Initiate a referral to an occupational therapist if needed for interventions that support self-care, prevent injury, and facilitate independence. (N.D.10)

Collaborate with the student's physical education teacher for possible accommodations related to fatigue. (N.D. 5)

Teach the student and his/her teacher about signs and symptoms of related depression and anxiety. (N.D. 6)

Teach coping strategies and assist student in identifying and using his/her current coping strategies. (N.D. 6)

Be a liaison between the family, physician, therapists, and school in the management of the school care plan. (N.D. 7)

Implement and monitor a medication program at school, if needed, and teach staff about possible side effects and therapeutic benefits of the prescribed medication. (N.D. 1)

Teach the student to identify and report medication side effects. (N.D. 1)

Teach the student about the need for removing himself a situation or taking a "time out". (N.D. 2, 6)

Assist teaching staff in providing a predictable structured routine for all daily school activities. (N.D. 6)

Provide regular "check-ins' with student to monitor compliance with treatment plan. (N.D. 1)

Provide one-on-one contact with the student to allow for teaching, and to assist in exploration of feelings and development of a healthy sense of self. (N.D. 1, 4, 8)

Assist in developing a plan that allows the student to become independent in activities of daily living. (N.D. 3, 9)

Discuss with the student the risk of injury associated with severe and self-injurious tics and possible prevention strategies to decrease that risk. (N.D. 10)

Discuss classroom strategies with the student's teachers that reduce stress for children with TS; for example, provision for alternate methods of task completion, untimed tests, using multisensory approaches, modified assignments, and opportunities for breaks. (N.D. 4, 6) (National Alliance for the Mentally Ill, 2004)

## Expected Student Outcomes

The student will:

- Demonstrate an increase in knowledge about TS and his/her treatment and management plan. (N.D. 1)
- Maintain regular daily positive social interactions with his/her peers. (N.D. 8)
- Assist with the implementation of the IHP. (N.D. 1)
- Demonstrate a healthy sense of self as evidenced by a positive self-image, positive attitude, and involvement with peers. (N.D. 4)
- Describe feelings of shame and embarrassment, fear, frustration, and anger to identified school staff in appropriate ways. (N.D. 4, 8)
- Describe difficulty with school work to appropriate school staff. (N.D. 4, 8)
- Identify three age-appropriate ways to interact with peers. (N.D. 4, 8)
- Experience less anxiety as evidenced by participation in school activities. (N.D. 2, 6)
- Along with his/her family, identify two local community TS resources available for students and families. (N.D. 6, 7)
- Along with his/her family, identify two effective family coping strategies for dealing with TS. (N.D. 6, 7)
- Describe how he/she feels when experiencing tics. ( N.D. 6)
- Demonstrate what to do and identify who to talk to when anger or frustration occurs. (N.D. 6)
- Identify three coping strategies to reduce stress and anxiety. (N.D. 6)
- Identify three contributing stressors that exacerbate symptoms. (N.D. 6)
- Follow recommended interventions that support self-care, independence, and prevent injury. (N.D. 9, 10)
- Work with his/her physical education teacher to meet physical needs related to fatigue and identify appropriate accommodations. (N.D. 5)
- Identify and implement two physical alternatives to self-injurious tics. (N.D. 10)
- List three signs of anxiety and three signs of depression. (N.D. 2)
- Demonstrate increased independence in the management of his/her treatment plan as evidenced by an increased responsibility, ownership. and control of said treatment plan. (N.D. 1, 3)
- Develop healthy sleep patterns as evidenced by a restful state and decreased lethargy. (N.D. 5)

# Case Study

Peter is a 13-year-old junior high student who was recently diagnosed with Tourette syndrome (TS).

Peter lives with his parents and two younger siblings. His mother reports that he was always a healthy, compliant, easygoing child, who got along well with all family members. He had numerous friends and did well in school.

At age 7, Peter started to blink his eyes rapidly, unable to stop for more than 10 or 20 minutes. When his parents would ask him what was wrong, he would always answer that something was in his eye. Between the second and sixth grades he began a long history of social problems: talking in class, disturbing others, and making very strange comments and noises. His parents mentioned these concerns to their family physician more than once over the years; however, they were usually advised to continue to observe his symptoms and return at some future time if they were still concerned. It was during this time that Peter also began to experience the first of many tics, such as repeating words six or seven times, blurting out random phrases, and pushing and touching other students. Despite these behavioral and social problems, Peter continued to be an outstanding student; however, he began having difficulty with his handwriting and was given additional writing support. Students started to tease him and laugh when his behavior was out of control. His friendships became compromised, and he began to have outbursts of anger. It became clear that Peter did not have effective coping strategies and was unable to express his feelings or needs.

As Peter entered adolescence, school staff were often unable to differentiate voluntary versus involuntary behaviors. Because of the school's perception that disciplinary measures were needed, they began to notify his parents repeatedly regarding his behaviors. The family once again sought a medical evaluation. Because of previous failed attempts to get help from the medical community, Peter's parents took him to a psychologist, who concluded that he had no social or psychological abnormalities. The frustration continued as his symptoms became worse; belching out loud, snorting, grunting, repeated facial tics, and letting out high-pitched noises. The interference of his tics was causing some difficulty in physical education activities as well as his ability to manage his lunch tray. In addition, he was now in trouble in the classroom and on the bus because of this behavior. He became argumentative, scared, and ashamed. As hard as he tried, he could not control his actions; some now included self-injurious motor tics, such as scratching and extreme jerking of his arms. These tics had the potential to harm not only himself but those around him as well.

Peter was finally referred by the school counselor to a pediatric neurologist, who was able to correctly diagnose him with TS.

Peter and his family experienced tremendous relief to know what it was that had caused years of uncontrollable actions and behaviors; however, they also realized it was just the beginning of a lifelong adjustment to the many behavioral, social, academic, and medical issues that accompany the disorder.

# Tourette Syndrome

| Assessment Data | Nursing Diagnosis | Goals | Nursing Interventions | Expected Outcomes |
|---|---|---|---|---|
| Recent diagnosis of TS.<br><br>Long history of undiagnosed symptoms. | Deficient knowledge related to:<br><br>Recent diagnosis of TS.<br><br>Developmental understanding about the management and treatment regimen. | The student will demonstrate an increased knowledge of TS and the management of his/her individual treatment regimen.<br><br>The student will be able to identify signs and symptoms of concern. | Assist the student in learning about TS, his/her individual treatment regimen, and the implications for school social and academic interactions.<br><br>Develop an IHP for school staff to follow. | The student will describe TS and his/her individual treatment plan.<br><br>The student will describe 3 symptoms of concern.<br><br>The student will assist with the implementation of the IHP. |
| Teasing by peers and classmates.<br><br>Feelings of shame, embarrassment, anger, and fright.<br><br>History of ongoing behavioral and social concerns. | Chronic low self-esteem related to:<br><br>Academic difficulties.<br><br>Perceived isolation from peers.<br><br>Chronic social and behavioral problems.<br><br>Presence of chronic tics. | The student will maintain a positive self-image.<br><br>The student will maintain positive socialization with peers. | Praise positive behaviors; encourage independence; promote self-esteem and self-confidence.<br><br>Promote understanding of those with TS by educating school staff and students f family and student agree.<br><br>Promote acceptance of those with differences. | The student will demonstrate a healthy sense of self as evidenced by a positive self-image, positive attitude, and involvement with peers.<br><br>The student will describe feelings of shame and embarrassment.<br><br>The student will participate in social and school activities as tolerated. |
| Student's poor peer relationships.<br><br>Vocal and motor tics.<br><br>Pushing and touching other students.<br><br>Compromised friendships. | Impaired social interaction related to:<br><br>Behavior patterns.<br><br>Social stigma of motor and vocal tics.<br><br>Possible comorbid conditions.<br><br>Anxiety.<br><br>Presence of tics. | The student will remain involved in school activities.<br><br>The student will identify 2 support systems within the school. | Educate staff and other classmates if appropriate regarding student's inability to control actions. | The student will maintain positive socializations and relationships with peers on a daily basis.<br><br>The student will identify 3 age-appropriate ways to interact with peers.<br><br>The student will experience less anxiety as evidenced by participation in school activities. |

| Assessment Data | Nursing Diagnosis | Goals | Nursing Interventions | Expected Outcomes |
|---|---|---|---|---|
| Lifelong adjustment to the many behavioral, social, academic, and medical issues that accompany TS.<br><br>Difficulty receiving help from the medical community.<br><br>Many years before a diagnosis was made. | Compromised family coping related to:<br><br>Family adjustments to TS diagnosis.<br><br>Possible strained family relationship.<br><br>Fear.<br><br>Challenges of the management and treatment program.<br><br>Parental feelings of guilt as they are overwhelmed with their child's odd behaviors. | Family will utilize positive coping strategies to adjust to a family member diagnosed with TS.<br><br>Family will understand that behaviors and vocal tics are involuntary. | Provide the family with local educational and support resources for TS.<br><br>Encourage the family to enlist support services at school for the student; for example, a 504 accommodation plan or possible IEP. | The student and family will identify 2 local community TS resources available for families.<br><br>The student and family will be actively involved in the planning of a 504 accommodation plan or an IEP.<br><br>The student and family will identify 2 effective family coping strategies for dealing with TS. |
| Anger, lack of effective coping skills, and an inability to express his/her feelings or needs.<br><br>Chronic social stress. | Ineffective coping related to:<br><br>Stress regarding possible school failure.<br><br>Developmental level.<br><br>Stressors that exacerbate symptoms.<br><br>Anxiety. | The student will communicate fears.<br><br>The student will increase ability to cope with symptom-associated stressors by identifying effective coping strategies.<br><br>The student will verbalize anger, frustration, and difficulty with schoolwork to appropriate school staff. | Teach coping strategies and assist the student in identifying his/her current effective coping strategies.<br><br>Teach the student about the possible need to remove himself from the situation or take a timeout.<br><br>Provide for a private area to express or release tics.<br><br>Teach the student and school staff about classroom strategies that reduce stress. | The student will describe how he/she feels when he/she experiences tics.<br><br>The student will identify 2 ways to express his/her needs.<br><br>The student will demonstrate what to do and identify who to talk to when anger or frustration occurs.<br><br>The student will identify 3 strategies that reduce stress.<br><br>The student will identify 3 contributing stressors that exacerbate symptoms. |

| Assessment Data | Nursing Diagnosis | Goals | Nursing Interventions | Expected Outcomes |
|---|---|---|---|---|
| Occasional difficulty managing lunch tray and participating in some physical education activities.<br><br>Self-injurious behaviors, such as scratching. | Risk for injury related to:<br><br>Severe complex tic release.<br><br>Impaired sensory processing.<br><br>Impaired motor planning.<br><br>Tics that are self-injurious. | The student will identify nonacademic tasks that are difficult due to the interference of complex tics.<br><br>The student will learn physical alternatives to self-injurious tics (Prestia, 2003). | Referral to an occupational therapist for interventions that support self-care, prevent injury, and facilitate independence.<br><br>Collaborate with the school physical education teacher for accommodations as needed. | The student will follow interventions that support self-care and independence and prevent injury.<br><br>The student will work with his/her physical education teacher to identify appropriate accommodations to physical education activities as needed.<br><br>The student will identify and implement 2 physical alternatives to self-injurious tics. |

# References

Alsaraf, S., & Robertson, M. (2003). They just can't help it. *Student British Medical Journal, 11,* 12–14.

American Academy of Child & Adolescent Psychiatry. (2001). *Glossary of symptoms and mental illnesses affecting teenagers: Tourette's syndrome.* Retrieved January 16, 2004, from http://www.aacap.org./about/glossary/tourette.htm

American Psychiatric Association. (2000). *Desk reference to the diagnostic criteria from DSM–IV–TR.* Washington, DC: Author.

American Psychiatric Association. (2000). *Diagnostic and statistical manual of mental health disorders* (4th ed., text revision) (DSM-IV TR). Washington, DC: Author.

*Clinical Guidelines for School Nurses* (5th ed., revised). (2002). Nashville, TN: School Health Alert.

DeStefano, Lewis, K., & Bear, B. (2002). *Manual of school health* (2nd ed.). St. Louis, MO: Saunders.

LinguiSystems, Inc. (1999). *The source for syndromes.* East Moline, IL: Author.

NANDA International. (2003). *Nursing diagnoses: Definitions & classifications 2003-2004.* Philadelphia: Author.

National Alliance of the Mentally Ill. (2004). *NAMI facts: Facts on Tourette's.* Arlington, VA. Retrieved February 20, 2004, from www.nami.org

Prestia, K. (2003). Tourette's syndrome: Characteristics and interventions. *Intervention in School & Clinic, 39*(2), 67–71.

Tourette Syndrome Association, Inc. (2004). *What is Tourette syndrome?* Retrieved February 20, 2004, from www.tsa-usa.org

Tourette Syndrome Association, Inc., Rocky Mountain Region. (2004). *Medications primarily for treatment of tics.* Retrieved February, 2004, from www.sensiblenet.com/tsa/home.htm

Vleck, B. (1998). *Tourette's syndrome update. Child and Adolescent Neuropsychiatry: Critical Issues and Psychopharmacologic Update II.* Seattle, WA: Children's Hospital & Regional Medical Center.

Wong, D. L., Hockenberry, M. J., Wilson, D., Winkelstein, M. L., & Kline, N. E. (2003). *Wong's nursing care of infants and children* (7th ed.). St. Louis, MO: Mosby.

# Bibliography

Allen, P. J., & Vessey, J. A. (2004). In *Primary care of the child with a chronic condition* (4th ed.). St. Louis, MO: Mosby.

Biotech Week via NewsRx.com. (2003). *Antipsychotic drug risperidone reduces tics in children and adults.* Retrieved February 11, 2004, from EBSCOhost database.

Carter, A. S., O'Donnell, D. A., Schultz, R. T., Scahill, L., Leckman, J. F., & Pauls, D. L. (2000). Social and emotional adjustment in children affected with Gilles de la Tourette's syndrome: Associations with ADHD and family functioning. *Journal of Child Psychology and Psychiatry, 41,* 215–223.

Clark, M., Bray, M., Kehle, T., & Truscott, S. (2001). A school based intervention designed to reduce the frequency of tics in children with Tourette's syndrome. *School Psychology Review, 30*(1), 11–23. Retrieved February 11, 2004, from EBSCOhost database.

Hornsey, H., Banerjee, S., Zeitlin, H., & Robertson, M. (2001). The prevalence of Tourette syndrome in 13-14 year olds in mainstream schools. *Journal of Child Psychology and Psychiatry, 4,* 1035–1039.

Ludder Jackson, P., & Vessey, J. A. (2000). *Primary care of the child with a chronic condition* (3rd ed.). St. Louis, MO: Mosby.

Ottinger, B. (2003). *Tictionary: A reference guide to the world of Tourette syndrome, Asperger syndrome, attention deficit hyperactivity disorder and obsessive compulsive disorder for parents and professionals.* Shawnee Mission, KS: Autism Asperger.

Piacentini, J., & Chung, S. (2001). Behavioral treatments of Tourette's syndrome and tic disorders: State of the art. *Advanced Neurology, 85,* 319–331.

Sallee, F. R., Kurlan, R., & Goetz, C. G. (2000). Ziprasidone treatment of children and adolescents with Tourette's syndrome: A pilot study. *Journal of American Academy of Child and Adolescent Psychiatry, 39,* 292–299.

*TIC disorders and tourette syndrome: School care plan.* (1999). Olympia, WA: Washington State Office of the Superintendent of Public Instruction.

Wong, D. L., Hockenberry, M. J., Wilson, D., Winkelstein, M. L., & Kline, N. E. (2003). *Wong's nursing care of infants and children* (7th ed.). St. Louis, MO: Mosby.

# Resources

## Organizations, Agencies

American Academy of Child and Adolescent
    Psychiatry
3615 Wisconsin Ave NW
Washington, DC 20016
www.aacap.org

American Psychiatric Association
1000 Wilson Boulevard
Suite 1825
Arlington, VA 22209-3901
703-907-7300
www.psych.org

American Psychological Association (APA)
750 First Street, NE
Washington, DC, 20002-4242
202-336-5500
www.apa.org

National Alliance for the Mentally Ill (NAMI)
Colonial Place Three
2107 Wilson Blvd, Suite 300
Arlington, VA 22201-3042
www.nami.org

National Institute of Mental Health
Office of Communications and Public Liaison
6001 Executive Boulevard
Room 8184, MSC 9663
Bethesda, MD 20892-9663
1-88-88-ANXIETY
www.nimh.nih.gov

National Mental Health Association
2001 North Beauregard Street
12th Floor
Alexandria, VA 22311
703-684-7722
www.nmha.org

Obsessive Compulsive (OC) Foundation
676 State Street
New Haven, CT 06511
302-401-2070
www.ocfoundation.org

Tourette Syndrome Association, Inc.
42-40 Bell Boulevard
Bayside, NY 11361
718-224-2999
1-800-237-0717
www.tsa-usa.org

## Videos

*A Regular Kid, That's Me: Tourette Syndrome*
Target: Teachers (44 minutes)
Tourette Syndrome Association, Inc.

*Be My Friend: Tourette Syndrome*
Target: Children and classmates ages 8 to 15, health-
    care providers, teachers and parents (8 minutes)
Minnesota Tourette Syndrome Association

*I'm a Person Too: Tourette Syndrome*
Target: Parents & Young Adults (21 minutes)
Tourette Syndrome Association, Inc.

*Stop it! I Can't: Tourette Syndrome*
Target: Elementary grade classmates (13 minutes)
Tourette Syndrome Association, Inc.

*Tourette Syndrome: Handling It Like a Pro*
Target: Children and classmates over age 9 (36 min-
    utes)
Kansas City Tourette Syndrome Association

# Chapter Seventy-four

# Tuberculosis

Margarita Fernan Granthom

## Introduction

Tuberculosis (TB) has been described as the most important chronic infectious disease in the world (Starke, 1999). Tuberculosis is still a leading killer of young adults worldwide. Each year, 8 million people worldwide develop active TB and 3 million die. Several forces, often interrelated, behind TB's resurgence in the United states include the connection between human immunodeficiency virus (HIV) infection and TB, increased number of foreign-born nationals from countries where many cases of TB occur, increased poverty, injection drug use and homelessness, failure of patients to take prescribed antibiotics against TB as directed, increased number of residents in long-term care facilities, and diminished effectiveness of public health care in many areas of the United States. (Gravatt, 1999)

Children with TB infection or disease can attend school and daycare if they are receiving chemotherapy, clinical symptoms have disappeared, and an acceptable plan for completing the course of chemotherapy has been developed and begun. Most children recover from the primary infection (Wong, Hockenberry, Wilson, Winkelstein, & Kline, 2003).

Screening high-risk populations for TB and treating those with infection have been shown to be a cost-beneficial component of a comprehensive TB elimination strategy. Routine source case investigations for young children with TB disease are an effective way of identifying individuals with active TB and others requiring treatment (American Thoracic Society [ATS] & Centers for Disease Control and Prevention [CDC], 2002).

## Pathophysiology

Tuberculosis (TB) is an airborne communicable disease caused by *Mycobacterium tuberculosis*, or the tubercle bacillus. A primary infection usually goes unnoticed clinically, but sensitivity to tuberculin protein (skin tests) usually appears within 2 to 10 weeks following primary infection. Infection begins with the multiplication of tubercle bacilli in alveolar macrophages, some of which spread through the bloodstream; however, the immune system response usually prevents the development of disease. Persons who are infected but who do not have TB disease are asymptomatic and not infectious. Most people who are infected have a positive reaction to the tuberculin test within 2 to 10 weeks after infection (Chin, 2000).

Tuberculosis is spread person to person by airborne particles, called droplet nuclei, that contain *M tuberculosis*. Droplet nuclei may be expelled when a person with infectious TB coughs, sneezes, speaks, or sings. Persons at the highest risk of becoming infected with *M tuberculosis* are close contacts, those persons who often spend time with someone who has infectious TB, such as family members, roommates, friends, coworkers, or others. The source of infection in children is, in most situations, an infected adult or a teenager, usually a member of the household) (Wong et al., 2003)

The probability that TB will be transmitted depends on three factors:

- the infectiousness of the person with TB,
- the environment in which exposure occurred, and
- the duration of exposure (Chin, 2000).

The incubation period, the time between infection and demonstration of a primary lesion or significant tuberculin reaction, is 2 to 12 weeks (Chin, 2000). Communicability persists as long as living tubercle bacilli are being discharged, usually by coughing. Appropriate chemotherapy can reduce communicability within several weeks. Children younger than 12 years of age with primary pulmonary TB usually are not contagious because their lesions are small, cough is minimal or nonexistent, and there is little or no expulsion of the bacilli (American Academy of Pediatrics [AAP], 2000; Chin, 2000). Extrapulmonary TB is rarely contagious.

The lung is the usual portal of entry in human beings; the organism enters less often by ingestion. In the lungs, a proliferation of epithelial cells surround and encapsulate the multiplying bacilli in an attempt to wall off the invading organisms, thus forming the typical tubercle. After primary infection, lesions may become inactive or progress to active pulmonary TB. Extension of the primary lesion at the original site causes progressive tissue destruction as it spreads within the lung, discharges material from foci to other areas of the lungs, or produces pneumonia. Erosion of blood vessels by the primary lesion can cause widespread dissemination of the tubercle bacillus to near and distant sites (Wong et al., 2003).

Infection can progress to disease very quickly or many years after infection. In the United States, in approximately 5% of persons who have been recently infected with *M tuberculosis*, TB disease will develop in the first year or two after infection. In another 5%, disease will develop later in their lives. The remaining 90% will stay infected, but free of disease, for the rest of their lives. The risk of developing disease is highest in children under the age of 3 years old. It is lowest in late childhood and high again in adolescence (Chin, 2000). Infection with HIV is an important risk factor for TB infection progressing to active disease (ATS, CDC, & IDSA, 2003).

People are susceptible to both the human (*M tuberculosis*) and the bovine (*Mycobacterium bovis*) organisms. The *M bovis* bacilli are transmitted by ingestion of infected milk or milk products. In those locations where TB in cattle is not controlled or pasteurization of milk is not practiced, the bovine type can be a source of infection. (Chin, 2000).

Pulmonary TB is the most common type of disease worldwide. However, it can affect any organ or tissue in the body, including pleura, central nervous system, lymphatic system, kidneys, genitourinary system, bones and joints, larynx, skin, intestines, peritoneum, middle ears, and eyes (Chin 2000).

Symptoms of pulmonary TB include cough, chest pain, and hemoptysis. Systemic symptoms of TB include fever, chills, night sweats, easy fatigability, loss of appetite, and weight loss. Symptoms of extrapulmonary TB depend on the site of the disease. (e.g., TB of the spine may cause pain in the back; TB of the kidney may cause blood in the urine).

Tuberculin skin test (TST) is the single most important test to determine whether a person has been infected with the tubercle bacillus. Two types used for skin tests are old tuberculin and purified protein derivative (PPD) of tuberculin). The PPD is most widely used, and standard dose is 5 TU in 0.1 ml solution, injected intracutaneously (ATS & CDC, 2000).

Techniques for injection are as follows:

1. Mantoux tuberculin test (standard and preferred method)

Intradermal injection of .01 ml of PPD tuberculin containing 5 TU into either the volar or dorsal surface of the forearm. Injection should be made with a disposable tuberculin syringe, just beneath the surface of the skin, with the needle bevel facing upward. This should produce a discrete pale elevation of the skin (a wheal) 6 to 10 mm in diameter. Reaction should be read by a trained healthcare worker 48 to 72 hours after injection.

2. Multiple-puncture tests: tine, Heaf, Sclavo, Sterneedle, or MonoVac. A positive reaction indi-

**Table 1. Classification of persons exposed to and/or infected with *Mycobacterium Tuberculosis***

| Class | Type | Description |
|---|---|---|
| 0 | No TB exposure<br>Not infected | No history of exposure<br>Negative tuberculin test |
| 1 | TB exposure<br>No evidence of infection | History of exposure<br>Negative tuberculin test |
| 2 | TB infection<br>No disease | Positive tuberculin test<br>Negative bacteriologic studies<br>No clinical or radiographic evidence of active TB disease |
| 3 | TB disease, clinically active | Clinical, bacteriologic, and/or radiographic evidence of current TB, further defined by location of the disease<br>Positive tuberculin test |
| 4 | TB disease, not clinically active | History of previous episode of TB<br>No clinical, bacteriologic, or radiographic evidence of current disease<br>Positive tuberculin test |
| 5 | TB suspected (diagnosis pending) | Diagnosis of TB is being considered<br>Persons should not remain in this class for more than 3 months; when diagnostic procedures are completed, the person should be placed in class "1, 2, 3, or 4" |

Adapted from "Diagnostic Standards and Classification of Tuberculosis in Adults and Children," by American Thoracic Society and Centers for Disease Control and Prevention, 2000, *American Journal of Respiratory and Critical Care Medicine, 161,* pp. 1391-1392

cates that the individual has been infected and has developed sensitivity to the protein of the tubercle bacillus, but it does not confirm the presence of the actual disease.

The TST should be read by a trained healthcare worker 48 to 72 hours after injection. This is the time when induration would be maximum. The basic reading is the presence or absence of induration by inspection and palpation of the injection site. The diameter of induration is measured and recorded in millimeters. For each tuberculin skin test, documentation should be made of the technique of administration (Mantoux or multipuncture), kind and dose of tuberculin, and size of reaction (in millimeters of induration) (ATS & CDC, 2000).

Diagnosis of TB disease requires other procedures, such as a chest x-ray. Lesions may appear anywhere in the lungs and may differ in size, shape, density, and cavitation. Abnormalities often occur in the apical and posterior segments of the upper lobe or in the superior segments of the lower lobe. In some instances, other views or additional studies (e.g., computed tomographic scans) may be necessary. Diagnosis is confirmed by isolation of the tubercle bacilli by culture from sputum, gastric washings, and/or pleural fluid (ATS & CDC, 2000) (**Table 1**).

## Management

Management is most effective when both medical and significant social issues are addressed (ATS, CDC & IDSA, 2003). In children, management usually consists of chemotherapy, adequate rest, a healthy diet, avoidance of unnecessary exposure to other infections, and supportive measures. The regular immunization schedule should be followed. Children with TB infection can attend school and daycare if they are asymptomatic, effective medication therapy has been instituted, and adherence to the therapy has been documented (AAP, 2000). Only children with serious forms of the disease are hospitalized (Wong et al., 2003).

Chemotherapy is the most important therapeutic modality. Appropriate completion of preventative chemotherapy can reduce the lifetime risk of clinical TB (TB disease) by 95% and is effective in persons with HIV infection (Chin, 2000). The goal of chemotherapy is to achieve sterilization of the TB lesion in the shortest time possible (AAP, 2000). The most commonly used combination of drugs include

- isoniazid (INH),
- rifampin,
- pyrazinamide, and
- ethambutol (EMB) or streptomycin (SM) (ATS, CDC, & IDSA, 2003).

For most children, the recommended length of medication therapy is 9 months. New, shorter regimens of preventive therapy (e.g., rifampin and pyrazinamide for 2 months and rifampin alone for 4 months) are currently being evaluated (AAP, 2000). The initial regimen for treating TB disease should include four drugs and can be adjusted when results of drug susceptibility become available.

In children and adolescents, a specific treatment and monitoring plan should be developed in collaboration with the child's physician and local health department and should include a description of the treatment regimen, methods of assessing and ensuring adherence, and methods of monitoring for adverse reactions. A major determinant of the successful outcome of treatment is compliance with consistent and complete medication treatment. When student compliance with the medication treatment plan is poor, direct observation therapy at school may be an appropriate public health treatment strategy (Hootman, Schwab, Gelfman, Gregory, & Pohlman, 2001).

Teachers should also be educated about TB to ensure that they have the ability to identify TB symptoms in their students.

Limited immunity to TB can be produced by administration of the only successful vaccine to date, BCG (bacille Calmette-Guérin). It contains a live weakened bacteria, the bovine bacilli, which prevents *M tuberculosis* from speading within the body and therefore preventing TB disease from developing. The vaccine can cause a false-positive reaction to the tuberculin test. The vaccine is not used extensively in the United States; however, in parts of the world where TB is common, the World Health Organization recommends that infants receive BCG

The American Academy of Pediatrics (2000) continues to encourage focusing tuberculin skin testing on children who are at increased risk of acquiring TB. Therefore, children without risk factors who reside in low-prevalence regions do not need to have routine tuberculin skin testing.

If schools require screening for TB:

- The goals of any screening should be clearly defined and mechanisms must be in place to ensure that students receive any follow-up (e.g., chest radiographs, medical evaluation, preventive therapy) that is needed.
- Widespread screening of the general student population should not be done. Instead, students at high risk for infection (for example, international or foreign-born students from countries with high rates of TB, students working in healthcare settings, and immunocompromised students) should be targeted for screening.
- Only the Mantoux method for skin testing should be used.
- Students vaccinated with BCG should not be excluded from screening.
- Results of screening (all skin test results and demographic, clinical, and follow-up information) must be collected and periodically analyzed to evaluate the usefulness of screening and ensure that the goals of screening are met.
  - The modification and/or continuation of any screening program should be based on these analyses (Hennessey et al., 1998).

All screening activities should be accompanied by a plan for follow-up care for persons with infection or diseases and should always be carried out in consultation with the health department.

# Individualized Healthcare Plan

## Assessment

### History

- Tuberculosis infection diagnosed, disease diagnosed (dates)
- Previous TB testing (including x-rays): dates and results
- Healthcare provider's involvement in management of the student's TB
- Illness symptoms: fatigue/weakness, anorexia, weight loss, night sweats
- Fever, hemoptysis, aching, tight chest
- Known exposure to TB: lived in TB-endemic community/country, person with TB
- Involvement of support persons/systems
- Experience with self-medication at home
- Tuberculosis management plan: medications, child and family education, counseling
- Compliance with medical management plan
- Previous medical treatment for TB, including prophylaxis
- History of immunocompromised status
- Prognosis

### Current Status and Management

- Current immunization status—needs
- Cultural issues regarding infection and treatment
- Family ability to follow treatment plan—barriers (financial, housing, access to care, transportation)
- Knowledge about TB (student, parents/guardians, teachers)
- Current symptoms: cough, fever, thick/bloody sputum
- Current treatment plan, including medication and follow-up
- Student's health, school, family, and activities of daily living

### Self-care

- Self-care skills
- Decision-making skills
- Ability to self-administer medication
- Motivation for self-care, self-medication
- Barriers to self-care, self-medication
- Parent perception of student's ability for self-care

### Psychosocial Status

- Student's locus of control
- Student's perception of his/her health and TB
- Parent's perception of the student's health and TB
- Impact of diagnosis and health condition on student's normal daily activities
- Impact of diagnosis/health status on: peer relationships
- Ability to participate in activities with peers

### Academic Issues

- Student's attendance pattern, past and current
- Student's cognitive abilities and academic performance
- Accommodations/modifications needed
- Health needs at school—medications
- Individualized education program (IEP)
- Section 504 services and accommodations
- Activity tolerance in the school setting

## Nursing Diagnoses (N.D.) (NANDA, 2003)

**N.D. 1** Risk for infection (NANDA 00004) related to:
- exposure to infectious person
- immunocompromised health status

**N.D. 2** Deficient knowledge (NANDA 00126) related to:
- cultural beliefs
- cognitive limitations
- lack of interest/motivation in learning
- lack of information

**N.D. 3.** Deficient knowledge (NANDA 00126) concerning:
- spread of this infectious disease
- hand washing
- prevention and treatment measures

**N.D. 4** Ineffective health maintenance (NANDA 00099) related to:
- denial of chronic disease (infections)
- lack of medical health assessment/healthcare
- noncompliance with medical treatment plan
- cultural beliefs

**N.D. 5** Risk for situational low self-esteem (NANDA 00153) related to:
- chronic infectious disease

**N.D. 6** Ineffective therapeutic regimen management (NANDA 00078) with prescribed medications related to:
- knowledge deficit
- denial of need for medications
- inability to access medication

**N.D. 7** Fatigue (NANDA 00093) related to:
- infection
- energy expenditure
- malnutrition
- poor physical condition

## Goals

The student will participate in identifying possible exposure to TB. (N.D. 1)

The student will increase knowledge about TB. (N.D. 2, 3)

The student will comply with prescribed TB management plan. (N.D. 4, 6, 7)

The student will develop TB self-care skills. (N.D. 3, 4, 6)

The student will participate in school/class activities, including physical education class with modifications made as necessary. (N.D. 4, 5, 7)

The student will demonstrate good school attendance pattern and classroom participation. (N.D. 2, 4, 5)

The student will maintain a good nutritional intake pattern. (N.D. 4, 7)

The student will maintain a good sleep pattern. (N.D. 7)

## Nursing Interventions

Review assessments, observations, and recommendations with student and parent. (N.D. 4, 7)

Exclude student suspected of having TB for medical assessment
(N.D. 1–3) referral to:
- Healthcare provider
- Community resources

Provide educational opportunities for the student and family to learn about TB. (N.D. 2, 3, 6)

Encourage parents/guardians to maintain health maintenance care: immunizations, good sleep pattern, good nutritional pattern, good hygienic practices. (N.D. 4)

For student diagnosed with TB: (N.D. 1–4, 7)
- Advise school staff that student may return to school when the healthcare provider determines that the student is not contagious and is able to participate in school activities.
- Reinforce healthy practices of covering nose and mouth when coughing or sneezing.
- Assist staff to obtain answers to questions they have.

Provide an accepting environment in school that allows the student to ask questions and express feeling and concerns. (N.D. 5)

Provide educational opportunities for student and family to learn about TB: (N.D. 2, 3, 6)
- Infection
- Disease
- Cause
- Signs/symptoms
- Treatment measures and medications

Medication administration in schools: (N.D. 1–3)
- Obtain medication orders and authorization for medications needed at school.
- Ensure compliance with the drug regimen by instructing student/parents and staff regarding the importance of giving the medication as often and for as long as it is ordered.
- Monitor student's medication compliance. (N.D. 6)

Provide in-service training for school staff, (N.D. 1–7) including:
- Signs and symptoms of TB
- Infection versus disease
- Causes
- Preventive measures
- Treatments
- Preventive therapy
- Demonstration of appropriate technique to prevent droplet spread
- Hand washing—the most critical infection control practice

Assist physical education teachers to modify physical education activities and requirement, if needed. (N.D. 7)

Assist student to self-manage his/her activities at school with rest periods as needed to prevent fatigue during the school day. (N.D. 7)

Assist the student (and his/her parent) to access adequate nutritional resources, as needed:
- School breakfast and lunch program
- Community social services/community food bank

Encourage parents/guardians to establish and maintain health maintenance care.(N.D.4)
- Immunizations
- Good sleep pattern
- Good nutritional pattern
- Good hygiene practices

In collaboration with local public health agency: (N.D.1)
- Assist in identification of possible contacts.
- Assist in notification of students/parents as recommended by health officer regarding possible exposure to TB.
- Assist in medical management programs.
- Assist in the provision of TB screening in consultation with health department's TB control program.

## Expected Student Outcomes

The student will:
- Comply in answering questions asked and testing to determine possible exposure or infection with TB. (N.D. 1)
- Participate in regular classroom activities, with modifications made when necessary. (N.D. 1–7)
- Actively participate in school activities with peers. (N.D. 5)
- Define what TB is. (N.D. 1–7)
- Describe the benefits of taking medications as prescribed. (N.D. 5, 6)
- Describe the consequences of not taking medications as prescribed. (N.D. 6)
- Demonstrate a good school attendance pattern. (N.D.4, 7)
- Demonstrate compliance with medication management plan. (N.D. 6)
- Demonstrate compliance with medical management plan for TB; follow-up appointments with health care provider are made and completed. (N.D. 1–6)

- Demonstrate age-appropriate sleep pattern. (N.D. 3, 4, 7)
- Demonstrate good nutritional intake pattern. (N.D. 3, 4, 7)
- Demonstrate good hygiene pattern and appear clean and neat at school. (N.D. 3, 4)
- Demonstrate use of disease prevention measures by covering mouth and nose when coughing or sneezing. (N.D. 3)

## Case Study

You are a school nurse in a school district of 5,000 students. You are responsible for five school buildings—four elementary schools and a combination elementary/middle school. It is the first week of January and you get a call from the principal asking you to make a phone call to the parents of a ninth grader. The principal says that Cici, 15 years old, has been diagnosed with TB. The principal wants you to figure out what the school needs to do and expresses safety as well as health education concerns for other students and teachers in the school building.

Cici is a 15-year-old student at White Mountain Junior High. She has just been diagnosed with TB. She lives with her mother and father and is an only child. The family had a relative visit their home who has had a history of TB. Cici's mother took her to the community health nursing office due to frequent coughing, night sweats, and fever with thick, bloody sputum. The family does not have any medical insurance, and Cici's father had just gotten laid off from work. A local physician diagnosed Cici as having TB, and chemotherapy has been initiated and continued for over 2 weeks. Cici appears to be pale, tired, and malnourished.

Cici tells her school counselor that she is embarrassed to let her friends know that she has been diagnosed with TB. She says she is afraid they will not want to be with her or do things with her. She does not understand a lot of things about TB and would like to know more about it.

What can you do to help Cici and her family? Who else needs to be involved? What is your priority? What kinds of nursing care will Cici need for the rest of the school year? What additional data do you need? What outcomes do you want to achieve? What should Cici's IHP look like? How can the school nurse collaborate with the community health nurse?

It is important to develop the IHP with input from the parents and the student. For an older student, being a partner in the planning process and participating in her own care are important for her self-esteem. The school nurse writes up a draft of the plan and gives Cici a copy to go over with her parents and physician. The school nurse will identify and assist in dealing with cultural and communication/language barriers. Signing the IHP may indicate their agreement and willingness to participate. The IHP will be shared with appropriate school staff as needed. Using the nursing process, confidentiality will be maintained in line with the standards of practice and school policies

# Tuberculosis

| Assessment Data | Nursing Diagnosis | Goals | Nursing Interventions | Expected Outcomes |
|---|---|---|---|---|
| Cici states she has frequent coughing, night sweats, fever, thick bloody sputum. Diagnosed with TB and under care of local physician Chemotherapy has been initiated and continued over 2 weeks.<br><br>Cici appears pale, fatigued, and malnourished. | Fatigue related to chronic infection and symptoms and knowledge deficit. | Cici will maintain an adequate nutritional pattern.<br><br>Cici will maintain an adequate rest/sleep pattern.<br><br>Cici will maintain good hygiene practices.<br><br>Cici will participate in school/classroom activities, with modifications made as necessary. | Provide educational opportunities for Cici and her family to learn about TB: infection, disease, cause, signs and symptoms, treatment measures, and medications.<br><br>Emphasize that good nutrition, hygiene, and sleep patterns are a very critical part of the treatment plan.<br><br>Assist Cici to eat breakfast at home or school every day and lunch every day at school.<br><br>Assist Cici to self-manage her activities at school, with rest periods as needed to prevent fatigue during the school day.<br><br>Assist Cici and her teachers to modify her activities and schedule, as needed. | Cici demonstrates a good nutritional intake pattern, eating breakfast and lunch every day.<br><br>Cici demonstrates a good sleep pattern, as reported by her and her parents.<br><br>Cici demonstrates good hygiene pattern by appearing clean and neat at school every day.<br><br>Cici utillizes rest periods in school as needed and prevents fatigue and appearing tired during the school day. |
| Cici has no medical insurance coverage and no financial resources.<br><br>Family uses community health nursing office as a health resource. | Ineffective therapeutic regimen management related to economic difficulties and family patterns of healthcare. | Cici will continue to utilize community health resources to meet her health/medical needs.<br><br>Cici will develop TB management self-care skills. | Collaborate with Cici, her parents, the community health nursing services, and the physician to maintain adequate medical care for Cici: keeping reevaluation appointments, medication compliance, education for Cici and her parents, monitoring health status, etc. | Cici is compliant with medical treatment plan.<br><br>Cici goes to all follow-up appointments with physician and community nursing services.<br><br>Cici describes the benefits of taking her medication as prescribed. |

| Assessment Data | Nursing Diagnosis | Goals | Nursing Interventions | Expected Outcomes |
|---|---|---|---|---|
| Cici is embarrassed and afraid to let her friends know she has TB infection because she thinks they will not want to be with or do things with her. | Risk for situational low self-esteem related to having a chronic infectious disease. | Cici will maintain a good school attendance pattern.<br><br>Cici will participate in school activities with her peers. | Provide an accepting environment, allowing Cici and her friends to ask questions and express feelings and concerns.<br><br>Provide in-service training for school staff regarding TB infection and disease, causes, preventive measures, treatments, and general infection control practices. | Cici demonstrates a good school attendance pattern.<br><br>Cici actively participates in school activities with her friends. |
| Cici does not always cover her mouth and nose when coughing or sneezing. | Deficient knowledge regarding the spread of TB infection and prevention measures. | Cici will increase her knowledge about tuberculosis.<br><br>Cici will increase her use of disease prevention strategies. | Provide educational opportunities for Cici regarding disease, cause, prevention measures including hand washing and covering mouth and nose with cough or sneeze. | Cici defines what TB is, both infection and disease.<br><br>Cici consistently demonstrates covering her nose and mouth with coughing and sneezing. |

## References

American Academy of Pediatrics (AAP). (2000). *Red book 2000: Report of the committee on infectious diseases* (25th ed.). Elk Grove Village, IL: Author.

American Thoracic Society (ATS) & Centers for Disease Control and Prevention (CDC). (2000). Diagnostic standards and classification of tuberculosis in adults and children. *American Journal of Respiratory and Critical Care Medicine, 161,* 1376–1395.

American Thoracic Society (ATS), Centers for Disease Control and Prevention (CDC), & Infectious Disease Society of America (IDSA). (2003). Treatment of tuberculosis and tuberculosis infection in adults and children. *American Journal of Respiratory and Critical Care Medicine, 167,* 603–662.

Chin, J. (2000). *Control of Communicable Disease Manual* (17th ed.). Washington, DC: American Public Health Association.

Gravatt, B. (1999). Current concepts in the pharmacologic treatment and management of tuberculosis. *Journal of School Nursing, 13*(4), 28–38.

Hennessey, K., Schulte, J., Cook, L., Collins, M., Onorato, I., & Valway, S. (1998). Tuberculin skin test screening practices among US colleges and universities. *Journal of the American Medical Association, 280*(23), 2008–2012.

Hootman, J., Schwab, N. C., Gelfman, M. H. B., Gregory, E. K., & Pohlman, K. J. (2001). Chapter 6. School nursing practice: Clinical performance issues. In *Legal issures in school health services: A resource for school administrators, school attorneys, school nurses.* North Branch, MN: Sunrise River Press.

NANDA International. (2003). *Nursing diagnoses: Definitions & classification 2003-2004.* Philadelphia: Author.

Starke, J., R. Jacobs, and J. Jerreb. (1992). Resurgence of tuberculosis in children. J. Pediatrics. 120:839-855

Wong D. L. , Hockenberry, M. J., Wilson, D., Winkelstein, M. L. & Kline, N. L. (2003). *Wong's nursing care of infants and children* (7th ed.). St. Louis, MO: Mosby.

## Bibliography

American Academy of Pediatrics. (1996). Tuberculosis/AAP guidelines. *Pediatrics, 97*(2).

Besser, R., Pakiz, B., Haverkamp, J., Schulte, J., Moser, K., & Onorato, I. (1998). *Source case investigations of children with tuberculosis disease in San Diego.* Atlanta, GA: Centers for Disease Control and Prevention.

Boyles, S. (1995). Primary school teacher in Amsterdam infects 19 students. *Infectious Disease Weekly.* 17–19.

Hootman, J. (1996). *Quality nursing interventions in the school setting: Procedures, models, and guidelines.* Scarborough, ME: National Association of School Nurses.

Huang, M. (1998). Fighting tuberculosis. *Journal of the American Medical Association, 280*(19), 1724.

Marx, E., Wooley, S., & Northrop, D., eds. (1998). *Health is academic: A guide to coordinated school health programs.* New York: Teachers College Press.

Mohle-Boetani, J. C., Miller, B., Halpern, M. (1995). School-based screening for tuberculous infection. *Journal of the American Medical Association, 274,* 613–619.

National Institute of Health (March 2002) United States Department of Health, Human Services Data

Pong, A., Anders, B., Moser, K., Starkey, M., Gassmann, A., & Besser, R. (1998). Tuberculosis screening at two San Diego high schools with high-risk populations. *Archives of Pediatrics and Adolescent Medicine, 152,* 646–650.

# Resources

American Academy of Family Physicians
11400 Tomahawk Creek Parkway
Leavenworth, KS 66211-2672
1-800-274-2237
http://www.aafp.org/afp/2000050/2667/html

American Academy of Pediatrics
141 Northwest Park Boulevard
Elk Grove Village, IL 60007-1098
847-434-4000
http://www.bol.ucla.edu/-
    ofattal/tuberculosisAAPguidelines.htm

American Lung Association
61 Broadway
Sixth Floor
New York, NY 10006
212-315-8700
http://www.lungusa.org/diseases/pedtbfac.html

Centers for Disease Control and Prevention
1600 Clifton Road
Atlanta, GA 30333
404-639-3311
http://www.cdc.npin.org/scripts/tb/guide/special_op
    o.asp

Centre for Public Services
One Sidney Street
Sheffield S14RG, United Kingdom
44 (0) 114 272 6683
http://www.centre.public.org.uk

Columbia University
622 West 168th Street
New York, NY 10032
212-305-5780
http://www.cpmc.columbia.edu/resources/tbcpp/

Fairbanks NorthStar Borough School District
520 Fifth Avenue
Fairbanks, AK 99701
907-452-2000
http://www.northstar.k12.ak.us/schools/ndl/faculty/s
    mith/chronic.html

Francis J. Curry National Tuberculosis Center
3180 18th Street
Suite 101
San Francisco, CA 94110-2028
415-502-4600
tbcenter@nationalTbcenter.edu
http://www.nationaltbcenter.edu

Hawaii Department of Health
1250 Punchbowl Street
Honolulu, HI 96813
808-586-4400
http://www.state.hi.us/doh/aboutpress/p9_tb.htm

National Institute of Allergy and Infectious Diseases
Building 31, Room 7A-50
31 Center Drive MSC 2520
Bethesda, MD 20892-2520
http://www.niaid.nih.gov/factsheets/tb.htm

University of Alabama in Huntsville
Office of Environmental Health and Safety
Huntsville, AL 35899
256-824-2352
http://www.uah.edu/pedinfo/index.html/SubSpec_Ot
    her2.html#School

## Chapter Seventy-five

# Vision Problems and Eye Disorders

### Maureen C. Maguire and Anne M. Biddle

## Introduction

Undetected or inadequately treated vision problems or eye disorders have a profound effect on a child's ability to benefit from educational opportunities. Vision is a complex neurologic process in which stimuli come through the eye and are transmitted to the brain for interpretation (Lewis & Bear, 2002; Miller, Menacker, & Batshaw, 2002). Our sense of sight is dependent upon many systems, muscles, and parts. When our eye focuses on an object, the process of seeing begins.

Light rays reflected from an object enter the eye through the cornea, which is smooth, clear, and curved. Next, light passes through a watery liquid, the aqueous humor, in the front chamber of the eye. The refractive properties of these structures allow the light rays to converge as they pass through the pupil, hit the lens, and the muscles in the iris expand and contract so the correct amount of light is available. The lens further focuses the rays so they will form clear images where they strike the retina. When the image doesn't focus on the fovea of the retina, the object appears blurry. Receptors in the retina convert light rays into nerve impulses by a photochemical reaction, and they are then transmitted along the optic nerve to the visual cortex of the brain. In the emmetropic eye, the light rays are brought to focus on the fovea without the use of corrective lenses or accommodation. When any of these structures are disturbed, focusing of images on the retina could be in jeopardy (Holbrook, 1996; Kirk, Gallagher, & Anastasiow, 2000; Miller et al., 2002; Lewis & Bear, 2002; Kline & Bloom, 2003).

Approximately one child in 10 enters school with some visual impairment. Most can be corrected with glasses. For about one child in a thousand, visual impairments are not correctable (Kirk et al,. 2000). Children with vision problems are at risk for academic and social problems. A child in school needs to be able to see near and far, to focus and move the eyes in unison, and to have peripheral vision. If there are problems in any of these areas of visual function, it will, to some extent, impair the child's ability to learn. "The nurse's role is one of assessment, prevention, referral, and sometimes rehabilitation" (Kline & Bloom, 2003, p. 1000). School vision screening programs are discussed in the "Vision Screening" section of this

chapter. In the school setting, impairments are classified as moderate, severe, and profound, and are based not on tests of visual acuity but on the special adaptations required to help these children to learn (Kirk et al.).

This chapter addresses problems of vision, screening for vision deficits, and eye disorders. The eye problems and disorders addressed are not comprehensive but are those most likely encountered by a school nurse. Samples of individual health plans are provided at the end of the discussions.

### Vision Problems
### Pathophysiology

Blindness is the inability to see. *Legal blindness,* a legal term and not a medical diagnosis, in the United States is defined as a visual acuity of 20/200 or less and a visual field of 20 degrees or less in the better eye. It is estimated there are 20 to 40 million blind people worldwide (Thomas, 1997; Kline & Bloom, 2003).

Visual acuity that cannot be corrected medically, surgically, or with glasses to better than 20/70 is termed *low vision* or *partially sighted.* Children with low vision can usually attend regular schools with some assistance. They will need to be oriented to the school environment. Often they will require assistive devices, such as tape recorders, talking books, or adaptive computer technology (Lewis & Bear, 2002; Kline & Bloom, 2003).

*Visual impairment* is commonly caused by trauma, refractive error, strabismus, cortical visual impairments, congenital/hereditary problems, infections, ocular pathologies/functional losses, and field defects.

1. Trauma results in structural damage to one or more parts of the eye essential to vision. Various aspects of trauma are discussed in the "Eye Disorders" section of this chapter.

2. In refractive error, the eye is unable to correctly focus images on the back of the retina. The most common refractive errors among school-aged children are:

   a. Myopia (nearsightedness)—cannot see distant objects clearly, appear blurred; parallel light rays from a distant object focuses in front of the retina.

   b. Hyperopia (farsightedness)—difficulty seeing near objects clearly, appear blurred; parallel light rays from a near object focuses behind the retina

    c. Astigmatism—uneven curvature of cornea; light rays are bent in different directions; images appear blurred. May be associated with either myopia or hyperopia.

    d. Anisometropia—each eye has different refractive strength, acuity usually differs by 2 or more lines. Eyes are unable to function as one unit (Lewis & Bear, 2002; Kline & Bloom, 2003; Miller et al., 2002).

3. Strabismus is a condition in which the muscles of the two eyes are not coordinated. The eyes do not focus on the same point at the same time, which results in two different images being transmitted to the brain simultaneously. One type of strabismus, often referred to as cross-eyed, is esotropia, in which the eyes turn in. The other common type, "wall eyed," is exotropia, in which the eyes turn out. Some children exhibit this only when tired, or intermittently, whereas in others, it is apparent all the time (Miller et al., 2002). Persistence of this double image during the critical period of vision development (birth to 9 years of age) will result in suppression of the vision from the deviating eye at the visual cortex of the brain; this is called amblyopia, sometimes referred to as "lazy eye." Treatment of strabismus before the age of 2 years is most successful in preventing amblyopia. If untreated before the age of 8 or 9 years, vision loss in the deviating eye is probably irreversible. The underlying cause for strabismus may be congenital, neurologic, mechanical, or poor vision (Miller et al.; Kline & Bloom, 2004).

4. Cortical visual impairments are due to damage to the part of the brain that interprets visual information. Impairment may result from infants who sustain hypoxic-ischemic encephalopathy. Although testing in infancy may show extremely poor vision, vision does seem to improve in some children with cortical visual impairment. "It is hypothesized that either alternate neuronal pathways or cortical areas take over some visual function" (Miller et al., 2002, p. 177).

5. Congenital/hereditary or other acquired problems include congenital blindness, rubella syndrome, diabetes mellitus, glaucoma, cataracts, nystagmus, albinism, Down syndrome, retinitis pigmentosa, retinopathy of prematurity. Children with these conditions will have a range of visual impairment from total blindness to only minor deficiency. With conditions such as these, the child may also have other developmental problems related to physical, cognitive, and psychosocial development (Lewis & Bear, 2002; Miller et al., 2002; Kline & Bloom, 2004).

6. Infections may include histoplasmosis, toxoplasmosis, congenital infections, and inborn metabolism errors (e.g., Tay-Sachs disease) resulting in eye damage, especially damage of the retina. Retinal damage may also occur with shaken baby syndrome due to retinal hemorrhage, detachment, or

scarring. Retinoblastoma and other tumors can also lead to blindness (Miller et al., 2002).

7. Ocular pathologies/functional losses include photophobia (varying degrees of intolerance to light, slow recovery from glare, difficult adjustment to light) or color distortions. Photophobia may occur from eye disease, injury, or infection, or from systemic reaction to drugs, or may exist without any underlying cause. Color vision is a function of the cones in the eye. An individual with color deficiencies is unable to distinguish between the colors of red, green, and blue. The degree of this color confusion can vary from minor to severe. This condition may be hereditary, which primarily affects males, or it may be acquired through injury or disease. Whereas congenital color blindness does not decrease visual acuity, the onset of acquired loss of color vision may be an optic nerve disorder (Lewis & Bear, 2002; Vision–light sensitive, 2003 ).

8. Field defects include no peripheral vision and hemianopsia (half of field missing right, left, top, or bottom). These defects are usually associated with one or more of the other visual impairment etiologies list in the above discussion.

## Management

Management depends on the cause of the vision loss or distortion. A student who lost vision as a child has a different perspective of the world than the child who has congenital visual impairment or blindness. A sudden adjustment to vision loss requires more psychological support than if it were from birth, but visual memory can be very helpful in learning. As a single issue, vision impairment related to diminished acuity may be managed with corrective lens, or it may involve other devices and accommodations. Additionally, the visual impairment may be only one of several health and developmental issues that need to be addressed for the child in the school setting. The age at which vision became impaired is important in addressing one's emotional and educational needs.

There are many technological aids for reading books and computers, with frequent advances all the time. Children with low vision should be encouraged to develop keen listening skills and use residual vision as communication tools. Often, optical aids such as magnifiers, telescopes, and glasses are used. Large print is helpful to many students, too. Assistive devices provided on a loan basis with follow-up sessions allow the students to practice in their individual environments. Many new technological aids are available, including devices that convert print to readable vibrating form, print scanners for computers, and tools that read text with a speed-adjustable synthetic voice. Assistive help for computers includes devices to magnify images or systems using speech recognition to tell the computer what to do. Braille is also used for blindness and other severe impairment (Miller et al., 2002).

All visually impaired students should receive instruction in special orientation (one's position relative to the environment is established through the remaining senses) and navigational/mobility skills (moving efficiently and safely from one point to another) (Kline & Bloom, 2003). Helpful classroom modifications include tilt-top desks, increased illumination, off-white paper with dull finish, and chairs with wheels to view the board better. Colored paper, for example, is more difficult to read and should be avoided as a background for text in classroom presentations or projects. A dark pen may be used to go over text on copied papers, making them easier to read. These minor adjustments can provide an important educational benefit to the visually impaired student along with other assistive devices that may be prescribed. Biomedical research may provide a form of artificial sight sometime in the future.

New advances are constantly being made in the area of technological and computer aids as well (Heward, 2000).

Management in school should be carefully coordinated with community and state services for the visually impaired. School nurses serve a vital role in assisting parents, teachers, and students to find assistive devices. The nurse can be instrumental in connecting parents with a state or local agency serving visually impaired who may, for example, provide a hand-held magnifier to empower a student with diabetes independence when drawing up insulin. Awareness in assessing and providing appropriate interventions for all of the student's health-related conditions requires the nurse to have keen observations, education, and ongoing communication skills.

## Individualized Healthcare Plan

### Child With Low Vision
### Assessment
*History*
- Age of child when vision deficit was identified
- Probable cause of the deficit/confirmed diagnosis
- Complications related to the deficit
- Health conditions associated with the deficit
- Healthcare providers involved in assessment and treatment of the student's vision deficit
- Past ophthalmologic findings
- Past and current use of assistive devices and effectiveness
- Student's academic progress
- Past and current school experiences—academic and social—type of setting
- Specialized vision education/training, e.g., Braille
- Support systems at home and school
- Involvement with organizations for children with vision deficits

*Current Status and Management*
- Parents' knowledge and understanding of the deficit
- Teachers' knowledge and understanding of the deficit and of teaching strategies for vision-impaired students
- Current medical management
- Parents' perception of child's deficit
- Current visual acuity and ophthalmologic status—with and without assistive devices
- Appearance of eyes, any unusual markings on face
- Student's need for orientation to school environment
- Use of cane or guide dog

*Self-care*
- Proper use and care of assistive devices
- Decision-making skills
- Level of independence
- Social skills
- Student's knowledge and understanding of the deficit
- Student's ability to communicate and function in classroom setting
- Barriers present to participating in self-care
- Need for any assistance when moving from place to place
- Ability to care for guide dog
- Skill in moving about independently with/without cane

*Psychosocial Status*
- Student's involvement with peers, family, school, and community activities
- Relationship with family members
- Participation in extracurricular activities
- Support system

*Academic Issues*
- Seating in classroom, obstacles to view of board, teacher, etc.
- Spare glasses kept in school
- Current and past academic achievement
- Past schools
- School health services needed
- Use of large print, books on tape, Braille, telescopic device, field enhancer, etc.
- School environment accommodations needed with regard to obstacles in the classroom, access to assistive devices, proximity to nurse, door, and restroom
- Classroom/school modifications needed with regard to assistive devices, assistance to and from class, common areas, locker, and bus
- Curriculum adjustments—workload, special books, resource materials
- Special education status—current and past
- 504 plan—current or past
- Emergency evacuation plan from building
- Transportation needs, e.g., assistance to and from bus, help on the bus

## Nursing Diagnoses (N.D.) (NANDA, 2003)

**N.D. 1** Disturbed sensory perception, vision (NANDA 00122) related to (cause of the vision deficit)

**N.D. 2** Impaired verbal communication (NANDA 00051) related to vision deficit

**N.D. 3** Risk for injury (NANDA 00035) related to visual impairment

**N.D. 4** (Risk for) ineffective role performance of educational attainment, learning (NANDA 00055) related to limitations of vision deficit

**N.D. 5** Deficient knowledge (NANDA 00126) about use and care of assistive devices related to:
- vision deficit
- lack of information
- lack of interest or motivation to learn
- developmental unreadiness

**N.D. 6** (Risk for) impaired social interactions (NANDA 00052) related to:
- communication barriers
- self-concept disturbance
- noncommunicative behaviors

**N.D. 7** Chronic low self-esteem (NANDA 00119) related to perception of differences due to physical characteristics

**N.D. 8** (Risk for) powerlessness (NANDA 00125) related to:
- physical impairment
- dependence on others for activities of daily living at home and school

## Goals

The student will not sustain injury/additional injury. (N.D. 2, 3, 5, 8)

The student will eliminate any contributory factors to vision deficit. (N.D. 1, 2, 5, 8)

The student will improve communication ability and skills. (N.D. 2, 5, 6, 7, 8)

The student will participate in plans to maximize and maintain his/her ability to learn. (N.D. 2, 4, 5, 8)

The student will enhance effective social interaction in school, home, and community. (N.D. 2, 4, 5, 6, 8)

The student will achieve/maintain positive self-esteem. (N.D. 2, 5, 7)

The student will experience a sense of adequacy in activities of daily living (N.D. 2, 5, 7, 8)

The student will limit additional injury to eyes from sun exposure by using protective items. (N.D. 2)

The student will achieve/maintain maximum potential for vision. (N.D. 1)

The student will increase knowledge and skills and use vision amplifiers. (N.D. 2, 4, 5, 8)

## Nursing Interventions

Orient student to school building. (N.D. 1–8)

Determine if rooms or other areas are inaccessible. (N.D. 1, 3, 4)

Implement modifications needed to make facility accessible for the student. (N.D. 1, 3).

With the student, determine the time needed to move through the daily schedule (from one class to another, to lunch, and to bus home, etc). (N.D. 1–6)

Arrange for modifications in release of times from classes to allow for the student's safe and efficient movement during the day. (N.D. 1, 2, 3, 8)

With the student, verify that all classrooms will accommodate student's needs (e.g., outlet, space for assistive devices, etc.). (N.D. 1, 2, 4, 5).

Collaborate with vision specialists to educate teachers about mechanics of assistive measures needed in classroom. (N.D. 1, 2, 4).

Collaborate with other adults who work with the student in the school setting to develop emergency evacuation plan that clearly indicates how student will be evacuated from the building during emergency situations. (N.D. 1, 2, 3, 4, 8)

Discuss with parents, healthcare providers, teachers, and special education teachers the type, cause, and severity of vision deficit, and ways to maximize vision, how the deficit does or may impact student's ability to learn. (N.D.1, 2, 4)

Discuss with student factors that increase risk of injury. (N.D. 2, 3, 5)

Inform teachers/staff of potential risks to student. (N.D. 2)

Provide a place for the student to keep items needed to protect skin and eyes—sunglasses, wide-brimmed hat, and sunscreen. (N.D. 2)

Evaluate student's knowledge about use of amplifiers. (N.D. 5)

Teach student care and skills in use of amplifiers. (N.D. 4, 5)

Utilize measures to decrease or eliminate causative or contributory factors to vision deficit. (N.D. 1, 2)

Provide in-service training for teachers and staff who work with student on ways to enhance student's ability to learn and communicate by: (N.D. 1–7)
- Arranging for preferential seating
- Describing use of multi-modality approach
- Suggesting use of both visual and verbal cues to assist her to understand the information.
- Demonstrating how to check equipment batteries, how to replace batteries, and how to adjust equipment.

Keep extra batteries or other supplies in cool, dry, safe place known to student and all applicable staff. (N.D. 1, 4, 8)

Encourage student to inform teacher if devices not working properly. (N.D. 1, 2, 4, 5, 7, 8)

Monitor function and proper use of assistive devices by student daily. (N.D. 1, 3, 4, 5)

Provide positive reinforcement to student for demonstrating new knowledge and skills in use and care of assistive devices. (N.D. 2, 4, 5, 8)

Emphasize student's strengths and abilities. (N.D. 6, 7, 8)

Assist student to maintain good communication with teachers and parents. (N.D. 2, 6, 7, 8)

Provide ample opportunity to make decisions regarding health management, assistive care, and school and peer activities. (N.D. 2, 7, 8)

Maintain communication with the other school personnel working with the student. (N.D. 7)

Discuss positive support for student with teachers/staff. (N.D. 7)

Provide opportunities for the student to interact and communicate with other students. (N.D. 6)

Provide opportunity for self-responsibilities and control of identified factors of student's life, (relaying information to teachers/parents, getting homework done and turned in on time, getting missed assignments if student is absent, and being to class on time). (N.D. 4, 5, 8)

Collaborate with parents, student, and school personnel to: (N.D. 1, 3, 4)
- Explore need for 504 plan
- Develop 504 plan
- Implement 504 plan

## Expected Student Outcomes

The student will:

- Eliminate factors that contribute to vision deficit. (N.D. 1–8 )
- Describe how the vision deficit can affect ability to learn. (N.D. 1–8 )
- Achieve independent mobility in school setting, or increase in independence if currently dependent on others for assistance. (N.D. 1, 8)
- Utilize adaptive devices to increase mobility. (N.D. 3, 5, 8)
- Participate in the development and implementation of emergency evacuation plan (EEP). (N.D. 1, 2, 3, 8)
- Demonstrate effective communication skills when interacting with teachers and peers. (N.D. 2, 4, 6,7)
- List ways to decrease vision-related barriers in the classroom (glare, illegible writing/too small, contrast, etc.). (N.D. 1, 4, 8)
- Describe correct use and care of assistive devices. (N.D. 5)
- Wear glasses at school as prescribed. (N.D. 1, 3, 4, 6)
- Demonstrate correct care of aids, how to replace batteries, and how to adjust the settings. (N.D. 5)
- Tell parents/teachers if assistive devices not working properly. (N.D. 1, 2)
- Demonstrate use of good social skills in classroom and social time at school—lunch, recess, before and after school. (N.D. 6)
- Be involved with at least one social activity—club, sport, organization, etc. (N.D. 6)
- Demonstrate consistent use of protective items. (N.D. 2, 3)
- Communicate effectively with peers and teachers. (N.D. 2, 7)
- Describe personal strengths and special abilities. (N.D. 7)

## Case Study

### Student With Low Vision

Lauren is an 11-year-old girl in the fifth grade with a diagnosis of ocular albinism since birth. This is a congenital lack of pigment in the iris, retina, hair, and skin that can result in reduced visual acuity with photophobia. Her hyperopic astigmatism causes her to need prescriptive lenses on account of farsightedness and an irregularly shaped cornea that does not focus light rays into the eye properly. Her corrective lenses achieve a vision of 20/100 in both eyes.

She has annual evaluations with her ophthalmologist and monthly visits from the itinerant teacher consultant for the visually impaired. To enhance her learning, she uses a 3X illuminated stand magnifier, a 4X telescope, and closed-circuit TV in school. Lauren appears to lack knowledge about care and use of these devices. She attends a regular education school and cites problems occasionally with seeing the board, maps, and overheads, and small print or small pictures and maps. Regular print materials cause her enough visual fatigue to negatively impact her reading efficiency, so she uses 18-point large print as much as possible. Sometimes glare is a problem; sitting close to the front with her back to the window will defuse glare. Oversized chalk is used on the board, as well as black ink on dry erase boards and overhead transparencies to increase contrast. When going outdoors, Lauren must wear sunglasses and a brimmed hat to shield her eyes from the sun.

Lauren is doing well academically. Her parents' chief concern is her current and future independence, e.g., driving a car, safely crossing streets. Socially, Lauren's concern is "blending in" with her peers. She fears looking different or "sticking out." Her younger sister has the same diagnosis (a recessive gene was identified), which comforts her and helps greatly. Her mother reports this to be beneficial also: "At least they have each other." Teachers and school personnel report her to be very noncommunicative and are concerned about her needs being met. She is often encouraged to speak up and communicate more with teachers and classmates.

# Child with Low Vision

| Assessment Data | Nursing Diagnosis | Goals | Nursing Interventions | Expected Outcomes |
|---|---|---|---|---|
| Best vision with glasses is 20/50 in both eyes. | Disturbed sensory perception–vision related to ocular albinism. | Student will achieve/maintain maximum potential for vision. | The nurse will:<br>• Orient student to school building<br>• In collaboration with the student, verify that classrooms will accommodate student's needs<br>• Educate teachers/staff about mechanics of assistive devices needed in the classroom | The student will:<br>• Achieve independent mobility in school<br>• Wear glasses at school as prescribed<br>• List ways to decrease vision-related barriers in the classroom |
| Because of photophobia, Lauren needs to wear sunglasses and a brimmed hat when going outside to be protected from the sun. | Risk for injury related to visual deficit. | The student will limit additional injury to eye from exposure to sun. | Discuss with the student factors that increase risk of injury. Provide opportunity for student to make decisions about health management. Inform teachers/staff of potential risk to student.<br><br>Provide space for student to keep protective items—brimmed hat and sunglasses. | Lauren will demonstrate consistent use of protective items when in the sun. |
| Requires assistive devices to improve vision; appears to lack knowledge about care and use of the devices. | Knowledge deficit related to lack of information. | Student will increase knowledge and skills in use of vision amplifiers. | Evaluate student's knowledge about use of amplifiers.<br><br>Teach student care and skills in use of amplifiers.<br><br>Provide positive reinforcement to student for demonstrating new knowledge and skills in use and care of assistive devices. | Name the assistive devices she needs.<br><br>Demonstrate correct use and care of assistive devices. |

| Assessment Data | Nursing Diagnosis | Goals | Nursing Interventions | Expected Outcomes |
|---|---|---|---|---|
| Teachers and school personnel report Lauren is very noncommunicative. | Impaired social interactions related to noncommunicative behavior. | Student will enhance effective social interactions in school. | Provide opportunities for the student to interact and communicate with other students. Emphasize Lauren's strengths and abilities. | Demonstrate use of good social skills in classroom and social time at school. |
| Lauren fears "sticking out" and not blending in with peers. | (Risk for) chronic low self-esteem related to perception of differences due to physical characteristics. | Student will achieve/maintain positive self-esteem. | Emphasize student's strengths and abilities. Discuss positive support for student with teachers/staff. Maintain communication with other school personnel working with Lauren–school counselor. | Demonstrate effective communication skills when interacting with teachers and peers. Describe personal strengths and special abilities. Describe positive feelings about personal accomplishments. |

# Emergency Evacuation Plan
## for Students With Disabilities

**Student:** Lauren

**Disability Area:** 6

**Concerned personnel:**
    Teachers
    Counselors
    Administrators
    Parents
    Student
    Social worker
    Paraprofessional working with student

**School:** Newark Charter School

**Grade:** 7

**Concern:** Lauren is physically impaired—partially sighted—and may have difficulty evacuating the building in the event of an emergency. The elevator may not be used in an emergency.

**Plan for emergency evacuation from first floor:** Lauren will be accompanied by paraprofessional from Learning Resource Room and will exit with her class.

From second floor, she will be assisted by paraprofessional from Learning Resource Room and will exit with her class.

## Vision Screening

The visual system isn't fully developed until 7 to 9 years of age and permanent vision loss can result from undetected problems (Kline & Bloom, 2003; Lewis & Bear, 2002). School nurses, typically the first-line screeners in schools, conduct vision screening programs to detect vision problems in children. There are a number of tools that can be used in a vision-screening program (Hockenberry, 2004). Whatever methods are used, the screening program should include screening to determine who does and does not meet the screening criteria, referral for an evaluation by an eye care professional, and follow-up to determine if financial resources are available for the evaluation and glasses, if needed, and to learn the results of the examination. Final phase of the screening program is determining if the child is using the corrective lens or other devices that may have been prescribed as a result of the referral.

Each state and/or local school district may determine appropriate screening tools, population to be screened, and referral criteria. For example, Delaware's *School Nurses Technical Assistance Manual* (2001) recommends that students' vision be evaluated for the following: near (8 to 10 inches), intermediate (16 to 40 inches), and far (10 feet) acuity and refractive errors, eye muscle coordination, accommodation, color vision, and general health of the eye. During school years, children should be screened once in preschool, twice in elementary school, and once during the middle and high school years. The American Optometric Association (1994) recommends that children who wear corrective lenses should be checked annually. The association also stresses that vision screening is not a substitute for a thorough professional eye examination. However, many children would not get that examination unless they were first identified through a school screening program.

Teachers are often the ones who recognize that a child is having difficulty seeing clearly. Clinical signs that a child is having vision problems and should be screened include excessive eye rubbing, tilting the head or closing one eye to visualize objects, putting the head close to the table to write, squinting, and complaints of dizziness or headache after doing school work (Kline & Bloom, 2004).

Students with significant visual impairments are followed with regular evaluations by their eye care professional and don't typically participate in school vision screening programs.

# Eye Disorders

## Pathophysiology and Management

### Foreign Body in the Eye

Small particles that enter the eye with low velocity can usually be removed with careful technique. To look for a foreign body in the lower conjunctival sac, have the child look upward while pulling the lower lid downward. To examine under the upper lid, it is usually helpful to evert the upper lid. While the child looks downward, a cotton-tipped applicator or similar tool is placed at the upper border of the tarsal plate and the lid is pulled out and up over the applicator. A loose particle may be removed with a cotton swab or flushed out with saline. It is important that the child does not rub the eye (Kline & Bloom, 2003; Eisenbaum, 1999).

### Corneal Abrasion

When a foreign body injures the cornea, an abrasion results. An abrasion may be superficial, meaning that it does not penetrate Bowman's membrane. Because the cornea has great self-healing capabilities, a superficial abrasion is usually gone in 24 to 48 hours and does not leave a scar. A deep abrasion that does penetrate Bowman's membrane will take longer to heal and will usually leave a corneal scar. The symptoms of a corneal abrasion include acute pain in the eye, excessive tearing, and the sensation of a particle in the eye. The child may be very reluctant to open the eye because of the discomfort and photophobia. It is impossible to determine how serious the abrasion is by gross examination, so the child should be transported to an ophthalmologist or emergency care provider. Putting a pressure bandage on the eye is no longer common treatment but may be used, if necessary, to increase comfort until the child gets to the doctor. Ophthalmologists may put a soft contact lens "bandage" directly onto the cornea to improve healing and take away the pain (American Academy of Pediatrics [AAP], 2002; Sowka, Gurwood, & Kabat, 2001d).

### Hordeolum (Stye)

A stye is a localized infection along the margin of the eyelid. It may involve the hair follicles of the eyelashes (external type) or the meibomian glands (internal). It is a red, painful, pointed lesion that will produce purulent discharge. The entire lid may be swollen. The organism most commonly involved (90% to 95% of the time) is *Staphylococcus aureus*. Most styes are self-limiting and are treated with warm compresses four times per day. Antibiotics may be used if the inflammation spreads beyond the stye itself. On rare occasions, an abscess may form, which would require drainage by an ophthalmologist (Kline & Bloom, 2003; Bessette, 2001).

### Chalazion

A chalazion is a painless nodule caused by inflammation and blockage of one or more of the meibomian glands of the eyelids. Although it may result from an accumulation of cells following an eyelid infection such as a stye, it is not infectious. About one fourth of chalazia go away without treatment. The first-line treatment for those that do not is application of warm compresses to the area for about 15 minutes, four times a day, followed by gentle massage to break up the nodule. If the chalazion persists, the child should be referred to an ophthalmologist for antibiotic drops or injection with triamcinolone acetonide (Kline & Bloom, 2003; Sowka, Gurwood, & Kabat, 2001c; Children's Hospital, 2003).

### Blepharitis

This is an inflammation of the eyelids and is most often caused by seborrhea. Yellow crusts are apparent at the base of the eyelashes, and there may be tiny flakes of dandruff on the lashes. The condition responds to cleaning the lids with baby shampoo and warm compresses once or twice a day (Ball & Bindler, 2003; AAP, 2002).

### Conjunctivitis

*Acute bacterial conjunctivitis:* Although the eye has defense mechanisms to ward off bacteria, sometimes they are overcome and bacteria infect the conjunctiva. This is commonly called pinkeye. It is contagious from person to person. The bacteria act like antigens and trigger an antigen-antibody reaction and inflammation. The most common organisms involved are *Staphylococcus aureus*, *Hemophilus influenzae*, and *Streptococcus pneumoniae*. The conjunctiva is red, and there is a mucopurulent discharge that often sticks the eyelashes together during sleep. A healthy eye can eventually rid itself of the bacteria, but usually antibiotic eye drops are used to hasten the process. Antibiotics eradicate the bacteria but do not cure the inflammation, so the eye usually continues to be red even after the infection is gone (Gunn & Nechyba, 2002; Sowka, Gurwood, & Kabat, 2001a; Eisenbaum, 1999). Parents of children with infectious conjunctivitis should be informed of the high degree of communicability of the condition and instructed about thorough hand washing and keeping anything that might touch the infected eye, such as a washcloth, away from other family members. Also, parents may need to be taught how to remove exudates from the eye and how to instill eye drops or ointment (Kline & Bloom, 2003; Ball & Bindler, 2003). Children with bacterial conjunctivitis should be excluded from school until all symptoms are resolved or after 24 hours of treatment with antibiotic eye drops (Ball & Bindler; Albanese, 1998).

*Viral conjunctivitis:* Viral conjunctivitis is prevalent in school-aged children (D'Alessandro & Huth, 2004). Several types of adenovirus are the most common causes of viral conjunctivitis. The eye symptoms occur with or after an upper respiratory infection. The conjunctiva becomes red and there is a serous, not purulent, discharge (Kline & Bloom, 2003). The eyelid usually becomes swollen, and pinpoint subconjunctival hemorrhages appear. Commonly there is enlargement of the preauricular lymph node. The condition is self-limiting and usually resolves in 8 to 10 days. However, it is highly contagious, and the child should be excluded from school until there is no discharge (Kline & Bloom; Eisenbaum, 1999).

*Allergic conjunctivitis:* Individuals with seasonal allergies often experience ocular symptoms also. When an allergic individual comes in contact with an antigen to which he or she is hypersensitive, mast cells release chemical mediators such as histamine that cause the characteristic signs and symptoms of red, itchy, watery eyes (Kline & Bloom, 2003). Eyelids become swollen, and the papillae of the conjunctiva take on a "cobblestone" appearance. Avoidance of the allergens is the best management strategy but often not possible. Treatment is geared to reducing symptoms such as with cool compresses, artificial tears, and prescription eye drops that work as antihistamines and mast cell stabilizers. These children are not infectious and do not need to be excluded from school (Sowka, Gurwood, & Kabat, 2001b). However, parents do need to know the signs and symptoms of infectious conjunctivitis so that it is not overlooked in a child with a history of allergic conjunctivitis (Ball & Bindler, 2003).

### Eye Emergencies

*Chemical splash in the eye:* When any kind of chemical enters the eye, immediate flushing with copious amounts of water for about 20 minutes is essential (Kline & Bloom, 2003). It is important to keep the eye open during the irrigation. If no eye wash station equipment is available, other methods can be effective. A water fountain is a very good way to wash out the eye. Cupping hands under running water and putting the affected side of the face into the hands will also work. After the eye is thoroughly rinsed, the student should be transported to an emergency department. Appropriate referral is important to prevent complications, so the nurse should determine that an ophthalmologist will be present at the emergency department (Lewis & Bear, 2002; Twanmoh, 2005.).

*Penetrating injury of the globe:* Any kind of projectile at high velocity can penetrate the globe of the eye. No pressure should be put on the eye, nor should any attempt be made to remove the object. The nurse should wear sterile gloves when examining the eye and observe for hyphema, abnormal shape of the pupil or iris, and leakage of aqueous or vitreous humor leaking from the site of the penetration. A Fox shield should be applied if available but not a regular eye patch (Kline & Bloom, 2003). If the nurse does not have the appropriate shield, a paper-drinking cup (with the bottom partially cut out if necessary) can be secured over the injured eye with a triangle bandage or something comparable. The other eye should be patched to prevent consensual movement. The child should be transported immediately to an ophthalmologist (Kline & Bloom).

*Trauma to the eye:* A strong blow to the eye can cause an orbital fracture, intraocular bleeding, or a detached retina. There are many eye injuries associated with sports; the highest incidence is seen with basketball. It is estimated that protective eyewear could prevent 90% of sports-related eye injuries (Rodriquez & Lavina, 2003; Hoffman, 1997). School nurses should monitor the use of protective gear by student athletes. When a student has been hit in the eye, the nurse should use a light to carefully examine for blood in the anterior chamber (Kline & Bloom, 2003). With blunt force trauma, the eye can be lightly covered by a cool compress, but no pressure should be applied. The child should immediately be transported to an ophthalmologist or emergency care provider (Rodriquez & Lavina; Hoffman).

# Individualized Healthcare Plan

## Acute Eye Disorders or Injury

*Assessment*

Regardless of the origin of an eye disorder, whether traumatic or infectious, the nurse must take a careful history of the circumstances leading up to the problem and thoroughly examine all the visible structures of the eye.

*History*
- Description of event/circumstances leading up to the problem
- Symptoms
  - Pain—severity rated on 1 to 10 scale or Wong-Baker FACES pain scale (Hockenberry, 2003, p. 1905)
  - Tearing or discharge
  - Reduced or blurred vision
  - Photophobia
- Location
  - One eye or both
  - Any specific area of eye involved
- Onset/duration
  - When problem began; continuous or intermittent
  - Previous experience with problem, any treatment, outcome
- Any action/treatment tried to help the problem
  - Now or in the past
- Student's use of corrective lenses—glasses or contacts
- Use of protective eyewear at the time problem occurred
- Student/parent's concerns

*Current Status*
- Physical assessment findings (Hockenberry, 2004; Ball & Bindler, 2003)
  - Intactness of globe
  - Eyelids—color, any swelling, condition and direction of eyelashes, any crusting
  - Sclera—any color present other than white or ivory
  - Pupils—shape, clarity, equal, react to light and accommodation
  - Cornea—clarity, intactness
  - Conjunctiva—color, any irregularity of surface, e.g., cobblestone appearance
  - Discharge/tearing—amount, color, consistency
  - Ability to move eye in all positions of gaze
  - Presence of foreign body in eye
- Visual acuity

*Self-care*
- Knows to use protective eyewear when using chemicals, tools, machinery, some sports
- Knows to wash hands frequently
- Knows not to rub eyes
- Properly cares for contact lenses if worn
- Able to instill eye drops as prescribed by a doctor or nurse practitioner
- Able to change any eye dressing properly

*Psychosocial Status*
- Family's financial ability to delay seeking medical attention for eye disorders
- Family's financial ability to purchase protective eyewear

*Academic Issues*
- Accommodations needed in order for the student to return/participate in classes and activities
- Absence from school can lead to missing important information and have a negative effect on academic performance
  - Students with infectious disorders of the eye will be excluded from school
  - Students with traumatic injuries of the eye may miss considerable time from school

**Nursing Diagnoses (N.D.)** (NANDA, 2003)

**N.D. 1** Impaired tissue integrity (NANDA 00044) related to:
- inflammation
- trauma

**N.D. 2** Acute pain (NANDA 00132) related to:
- inflammation
- trauma.

**N.D. 3** Risk for infection (NANDA 00004) transmission related to communicability of eye infections

**N.D. 4** (Risk for) ineffective therapeutic regimen management (NANDA 00078) related to possible multiple medications and instillation into eye.

**N.D. 5** (Risk for) disturbed sensory perception, vision (NANDA 00122) related to:
- pain
- inflammation
- trauma
- photophobia

## Goals

The student will incur no further damage to eye structures. (N.D. 1)

The student will not experience anything in school to lengthen healing time. (N.D. 1)

The student will receive pain reduction treatment. (N.D. 2)

The student will report pain level is decreased. (N.D. 2)

The student will avoid transmitting the infection to others. (N.D. 3)

The student will follow directions correctly to manage eye condition. (N.D. 4)

The student will have environmental modifications made in the classroom to compensate for vision problem. (N.D. 5)

## Nursing Interventions

*Wound Care*

Remove any foreign body or chemical substance from eye using appropriate methods. (N.D.1)

Document appearance of eye condition. (N.D. 1)

Instruct student and family on management of eye condition. (N.D. 1)

Instruct student/family about signs and symptoms that condition is getting worse. (N.D. 1)

*Medication Administration: Eye*

Determine student's/family's knowledge of medication and administration. (N.D. 1)

Reinforce teaching of self-administration of medication. (N.D. 1)

Administer prescribed medication according to school district medication policy. (N.D. 1)

*Pain Management*

Use developmentally appropriate tool to measure student's perception of pain. (N.D. 2)

Use nonpharmacologic and pharmacologic (where permitted) methods to relieve pain. (N.D. 2)

Teach student/family nonpharmacologic methods to control pain. (N.D. 2)

Reinforce teaching about pharmacologic pain management. (N.D. 2)

*Infection Control*

Teach student/family to wash hands frequently. (N.D. 3)

Teach process of infection transmission. (N.D. 3)

Reinforce teaching of aseptic administration of eye medication. (N.D. 3)

Teach how to dispose of any contaminated dressings in the school setting. (N.D. 3)

*Teaching: Psychomotor Skill*

Evaluate student's ability to properly carry out any procedures, such as instilling eye drops. (N.D. 4)

Communicate with student's family regarding ability to carry out procedures in school. (N.D. 4)

*Environmental Management: Safety*
Identify safety hazards in school environment, including school bus if used. (N.D. 5)
Remove hazards in school setting if possible. (N.D. 5)
Modify school environment to decrease risk. (N.D. 5)
Educate student about hazards in school environment. (N.D. 5)
Inform teachers/staff about student's risk for injury. (N.D. 5)

## Expected Student Outcomes

The student will:
- Not have damage to the cornea or other eye structures. (N.D. 1)
- Have return of structural intactness and physiologic function that is not impeded by anything in school. (N.D. 1)
- Have pain controlled. (N.D. 2)
- Report perception of improved physical well-being. (N.D. 2)
- Describe mode of infection transmission. (N.D. 3)
- Follow procedures to prevent transmission. (N.D. 3)
- Not return to school until no longer capable of transmitting infection. (N.D. 3)
- Describe purpose of procedures to manage eye condition that need to be carried out in school. (N.D. 4)
- Do procedures correctly. (N.D. 4)
- Be placed in an advantageous position in the classroom to maximize visual ability if vision is compromised or eye is patched. (N.D. 5)
- Be provided with adequate lighting to do school work while vision is compromised or eye is patched. (N.D. 5)

# Case Study

## Student With Foreign Body in Eye

Juan, a 9-year-old fourth grader, comes to the school nurse in an agitated state with his hand covering his left eye. He says that the point of his pencil broke off when he was writing and flew into his eye. He rates his pain as 8 out of 10. He reluctantly removes his hand and opens his eye partially. The conjunctiva is red, and there is considerable tearing of clear fluid. On examination, a very small piece of pencil point tip can be seen in the lower conjunctival sac.

# Child with Foreign Body in Eye

| Assessment Data | Nursing Diagnosis | Goals | Nursing Interventions | Expected Outcomes |
|---|---|---|---|---|
| There is tearing of the left eye. The conjunctiva is red. Foreign body is visible in eye. | Impaired tissue integrity of conjunctiva related to trauma as evidenced by redness and tearing. | Student will:<br>• Incur no further damage to eye structures.<br>• Experience nothing in school to lengthen healing time. | The nurse will:<br>• Document the appearance of the eye.<br>• Use aseptic technique<br>• Remove foreign body by holding open the eye, having the child look upward, and using a moistened cotton-tipped applicator to lift out the foreign body.<br>• Rinse out the eye with saline to be sure there are no other particles.<br>• Carefully examine eye under both upper and lower lids.<br>• Document the appearance of the eye. | The student will:<br>• Not have damage to cornea or other eye structures. |
| Pain rated at 8/10. | Acute pain related to presence of foreign body in eye and trauma to conjunctiva as evidence by report. | Student will report that pain level is decreased. | The nurse will:<br>• Use nonpharmacologic methods to relieve pain: apply a cool compress to eyelid after FB is removed.<br>• Use developmentally appropriate tool to measure student's perception of pain: use 1 to 10 scale. | The student will:<br>• Have pain controlled.<br>• Report perception of improved well being. |

# References

Albanese, B. (1998). *Communicable disease summary—guide for schools and child care settings.* Baltimore: Maryland Department of Health and Mental Hygiene, Community and Public Health Administration, Epidemiology and Disease Control Program.

American Academy of Pediatrics (AAP). (2002). *Common vision and eye problems.* Retrieved April 18, 2004, from http://www.belredcenter.com/Pediatric_eye_problems.htm

American Optometric Association. (1994a). *A school nurse's guide to vision screening and ocular emergencies.* St. Louis, MO: American Foundation for Vision Awareness.

American Optometric Association. (1994b). *Optometric clinical practice guideline: Pediatric eye and vision care.* St. Louis, MO: Author.

Ball, J., & Bindler, R. (2003). *Pediatric nursing: Caring for children* (3rd ed.). Upper Saddle River, NJ: Prentice Hall.

Bessette, M. (2001). *Hordeolum and stye.* eMedicine. Retrieved January 28, 2004, from http://www.emedicine.com/emerg/topic755.htm

Children's Hospital of The King's Daughters Health System. (2003). *Chalazion.* Retrieved January 28, 2004, from http://www.chkd.org/Ophthalmology/chalazio.asp

Cooper, J. (2004). *All about strabismus. Development of vision (critical periods).* Optometrists Network. Retrieved March 8, 2004, from http://www.strabismus.org/critical_period_Hubel.html

D'Alessandro, D., & Huth, L. (2004). *Pink eye.* Virtual Children's Hospital. Retrieved March 8, 2004, from http://www.vh.org/pediatric/patient/pediatrics/cqqa/pinkeye.html

Eisenbaum, A. M. (1999). Eye. In W. W. Hay, A. R. Hayward, M. J. Levin, & J. M. Sondheimer (Eds.), *Current pediatric diagnosis & treatment* (14th ed., pp. 360–383). Stamford, CT: Appleton & Lange.

Gunn, V. L., & Nechyba, C. (2002). *The Harriet Lane Handbook* (16th ed.). Philadelphia: Mosby.

Heward, W.L.(2000). *Exceptional children: An introduction to special education* (6th ed.). Upper Saddle River: Printice Hall, Inc.

Hockenberry, M. (2003). *Wong's nursing care of infants and children* (7th ed.). St. Louis, MO: Mosby.

Hockenberry, M. (2004). *Wong's clinical manual of pediatric nursing* (6th ed.). St. Louis, MO: Mosby.

Hoffman, R. (1997). Evaluating and treating eye injuries. *Contemporary Pediatrics, 14*(4), 74–98.

Holbrook, M. C. (1996). *Children with visual impairments: A parent's guide.* Bethesda, MD: Woodbine House.

Kirk, S. A., Gallagher, J. J., & Anastasiow, N. J. (2000). *Educating exceptional children* (9th ed.). Boston: Houghton Mifflin.

Kline, N., & Bloom, D. (2003). In M. J. Hockenberry, D. Wilson, M. L. Winkelstein, & N. E. Kline (Eds.) *Wong's nursing care of infants and children* (7th ed., chap. 24). St Louis, MO: Mosby

Lewis, K. D., & Bear, B. J. (2002). *Manual of school health* (2nd ed.). St. Louis, MO: Elsevier Science.

Miller, M., Menacker, S.J., & Batshaw, M.L. (2002). In M.L. Batshaw (Ed.), *Children with disabilities* (5th ed.). Washington D.C.: Paul H. Brooks.

NANDA. (2003). *Nursing diagnoses: Definitions & classifications* 2003–2004. Philadelphia: Author.

Rodriquez, D. O., & Lavina, A. M. (2003). Prevention and treatment of common eye injuries in sports. *American Family Physician, 67*:1481-8,1494-6.

Sowka, J. W., Gurwood, A. S., & Kabat, A. G. (2001a). Acute bacterial conjunctivitis; In *Handbook of ocular disease and management.* Retrieved March 8, 2004, from http://www.revoptom.com/handbook/oct02_sec2_4.htm
Sowka, J. W., Gurwood, A. S., & Kabat, A. G. (2001b). Allergic conjunctivitis. In *Handbook of ocular disease management.* Retrieved March 8, 2004, from http://www.revoptom.com/handbook/oct02_sec2_2.htm

Sowka, J. W., Gurwood, A. S., & Kabat, A. G. (2001c). Chalazion. In *Handbook of ocular disease management.* Retrieved January 28, 2004, from http://www.revoptom.com/handbook/sect1d.htm

Sowka, J. W., Gurwood, A. S., & Kabat, A. G. (2001d). Corneal abrasion and recurrent corneal erosion. *Handbook of ocular disease and management.* Retrieved March 8, 2004, from http://www.revoptom.com/handbook/SECT3F.HTM

Sowka, J. W., Gurwood, A. S., & Kabat, A. G. (2001e). *Viral conjunctivitis.* Handbook of ocular disease management. Retrieved March 8, 2004, from http://www.revoptom.com/handbook/SECT2B.HTM

Thomas, C. L. (Ed.). (1997) *Taber's cyclopedic medical dictionary* (18th ed.). Philadelphia: Davis.

Twanmoh, J. R. (2005, January 10). *Eye injuries.* eMedicine. Retrieved February 10, 2005, from http://www.emedicine.com/aaem/topic187.htm

Vision - light sensitivity. (2003) *Medical Encyclopedia.* Retrieval February 10, 2005 from www.nlm.nih.gov/medlineplus/print/ency/article/003041

## Bibliography

Carpenito, L. J. (1993). *Nursing diagnosis, application to clinical practice* (5th ed.). Philadelphia: Lippincott.

Dochterman, J. M., & Bulechek, G. M. (Eds.). (2004). *Nursing interventions classification (NIC)* (4th ed.). Philadelphia: Mosby.

National Association of School Nurses. (2001). *Issue Brief: Screening for vision impairment.* Scarborough, ME: Author.

Moorhead, S., Johnson, M., & Maas, M. (Eds.). (2004). *Nursing outcomes classification (NOC)* (3rd ed.). Philadelphia: Mosby.

Proctor, S. (2005). *Assessing visual status in schools* [Manual]. Scarborough, ME: National Association of School Nurses.

Strawhacker, M. T., Gustafson, J. K., Kinne, M. J., & Little, D. (2003). Vision screening practices in central Iowa: A follow-up evaluation. *Journal of School Nursing, 19*(2), 111–118.

## Resources

American Academy of Ophthalmology
    655 Beach Street
    Box 7424
    San Francisco, CA 94120
    415-561-8500
www.aao.org
    Medical Library, including *Eye Injuries,* is available online.

Medem, Network
649 Mission Street
Second Floor
San Francisco, CA 94105
Medical Library, including eye health, children's eye health, is available at:
http://www.medem.com/medlb/articleslb.cfm?sub_cat=117

U.S. National Library of Medicine
National Institutes of Health
8600 Rockville Pike
Bethesda, MD 20894
Eye emergencies

# Index

# Software for Individualized Healthcare Plans for the School Nurse

Automatically creates comprehensive healthcare plans that include:

1) nursing diagnoses
2) goals
3) interventions

4) outcomes
5) a column to add individualized assessment data

## *Makes creating healthcare plans <u>simple</u>!*

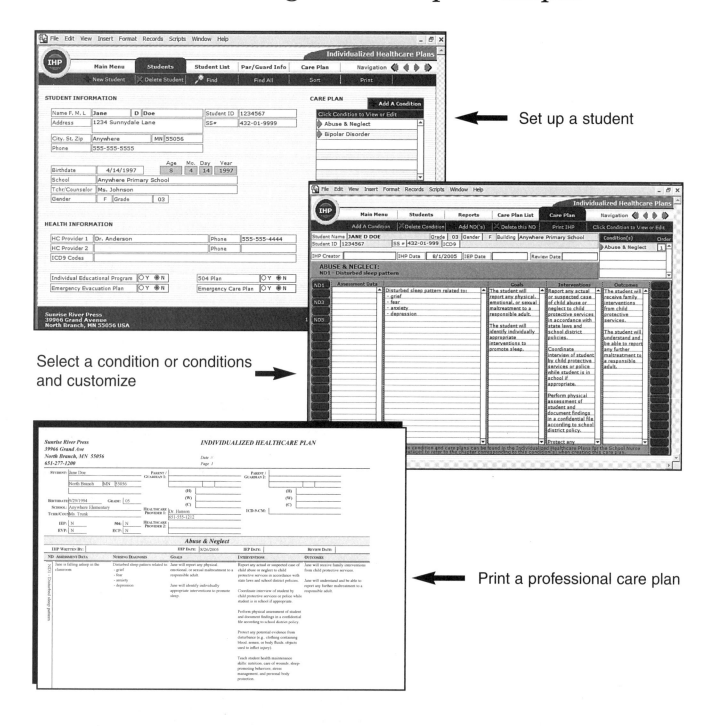

Set up a student

Select a condition or conditions and customize

Print a professional care plan